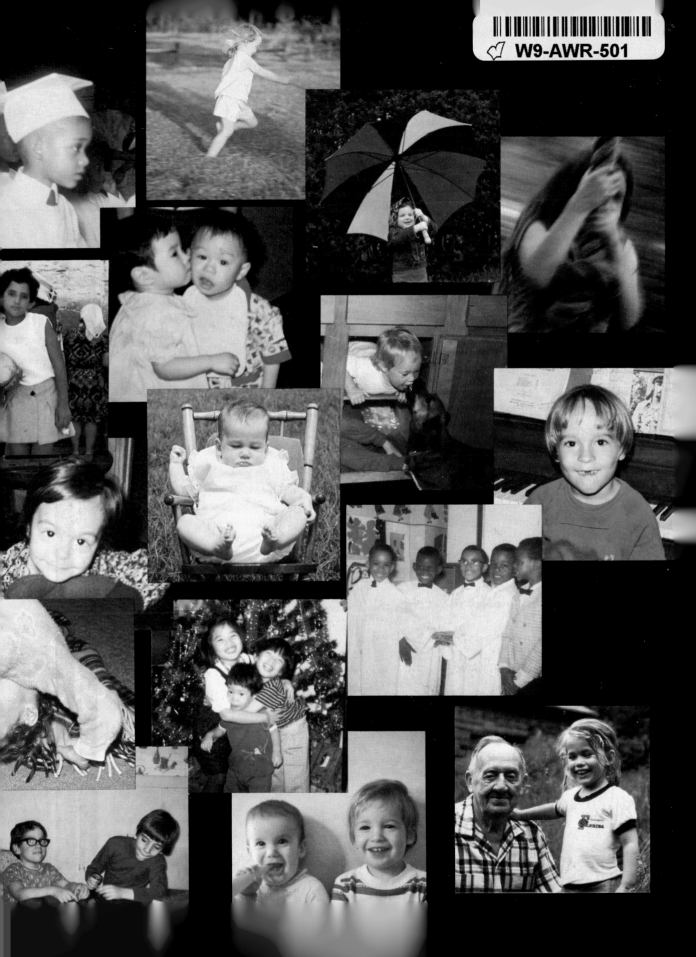

COMPREHENSIVE PEDIATRIC NURSING

COMPREHENSIVE PEDIATRIC NURSING

GLADYS M. SCIPIEN, R.N., B.S., M.S.
Assistant Professor
Boston University School of Nursing

MARTHA UNDERWOOD BARNARD, R.N., B.S.N., M.N.
Assistant Professor and Nurse Clinician
Department of Human Ecology and
Department of Nursing Education
University of Kansas Medical Center

MARILYN A. CHARD, R.N., B.S., Ed.M., M.S.
Associate Professor
Graduate Program in Maternal and Child Health Nursing
Boston University School of Nursing

JEANNE HOWE, R.N., Ph.D.
Associate Professor
University of Florida College of Nursing

PATRICIA J. PHILLIPS, R.N., B.S., M.S.
Assistant Professor, Practitioner/Teacher
Rush University
College of Nursing and Allied Health Sciences
Chicago

McGRAW-HILL BOOK COMPANY
A Blakiston Publication
New York   St. Louis   San Francisco   Auckland   Düsseldorf   Johannesburg
Kuala Lumpur   London   Mexico   Montreal   New Delhi
Panama   Paris   São Paulo   Singapore   Sydney   Tokyo   Toronto

COMPREHENSIVE PEDIATRIC NURSING

Copyright © 1975 by McGraw-Hill, Inc.
All rights reserved.
Printed in the United States of America.
No part of this publication may be reproduced,
stored in a retrieval system, or transmitted,
in any form or by any means,
electronic, mechanical, photocopying, recording, or
otherwise, without the prior written permission of the
publisher.

1 2 3 4 5 6 7 8 9 DODO 7 9 8 7 6 5

This book was set in Sans Serif by Monotype Composition Company, Inc.
The editors were Cathy Dilworth, Sally Barhydt Mobley, and Ida Abrams Wolfson;
the designer was Nicholas Krenitsky;
the production supervisor was Thomas J. LoPinto.
The drawings were done by Dorothy Merkel Alexander and J & R Services, Inc.
R. R. Donnelley & Sons Company was printer and binder.

Library of Congress Cataloging in Publication Data
Main entry under title:

Comprehensive pediatric nursing.

 "A Blakiston publication."
 1. Pediatric nursing. I. Scipien, Gladys M., ed.
[DNLM: 1. Pediatric nursing. WY159 C737]
RJ245.C63   610.73'62   74-11273
ISBN 0-07-055787-X

TO THOSE WHO HAVE HELPED

CONTENTS

LIST OF CONTRIBUTORS

Maud Adams, B.A., R.N., M.N., M.A.
Professor of Nursing
Department of Nursing Education and Department of
   Human Ecology
University of Kansas Medical Center
Kansas City, Kansas

Gaylene Bouska Altman, R.N., B.S.N., M.N.
Assistant Professor
Coordinator of Cardiovascular Nursing, Masters' Program
The Catholic University of America
Washington, D.C.

Anne Altshuler, R.N., M.S.
Assistant Clinical Professor
School of Nursing
University of Wisconsin—Madison;
Clinical Nurse Specialist School Age
   and Adolescent Unit
University of Wisconsin Hospitals
Madison, Wisconsin

Amanda Sirmon Baker, R.N., M.N.
Doctoral Student, Curriculum and Instruction
University of Florida College of Education
Gainesville, Florida

Pauline Hinton Barton, R.N., Ed.D.
Professor
University of Florida College of Nursing
Gainesville, Florida

Jeanne Quint Benoliel, R.N., B.S.N.E., M.S., D.N.Sc.
Professor and Chairman
Comparative Nursing Care Systems Department
University of Washington School of Nursing
Seattle, Washington

Jerry J. Bigner, Ph.D.
Assistant Professor
Department of Home Economics
Indiana University
Bloomington, Indiana

Luther Christman, R.N., B.S., Ed.M., Ph.D.
Dean and Professor of Nursing
College of Nursing and Allied Health Sciences
Professor of Sociology
Rush University College of Medicine
Chicago, Illinois

Barbara J. Clancy, R.N., M.S.N.
Assistant Professor
Department of Nursing Education
University of Kansas Medical Center
Kansas City, Kansas

Stephanie Clatworthy, R.N., B.S., M.S.
Assistant Professor
Boston University School of Nursing
Boston, Massachusetts

Laura Marie Bloomquist Cooper, R.N., B.S.N., M.S.N.
Pediatric Nurse Associate
Panama City, Florida

Deborah B. Dean, R.N., B.S.N., M.S.N.
Formerly Instructor, Human Development
Vanderbilt University School of Nursing
Nashville, Tennessee

Mary Jean Denyes, R.N., M.S.
Clinical Nurse Specialist
Assistant Clinical Professor
University of Wisconsin School of Nursing
Madison, Wisconsin

Jane Cooper Evans, R.N., M.S.
Nursing Service Administrator
St. John's Hospital
San Angelo, Texas

Mildred Fenske, R.N., B.S.N., M.S.
Assistant Professor and Clinical Specialist,
    Medical-Surgical Nursing
Vanderbilt University
Nashville, Tennesse

Edith L. Getchell, R.D., M.S.
Nutrition Coordinator for Staff and
    Student Education
Department of Dietetics
Children's Hospital Medical Center
Boston, Massachusetts

Christina M. Graf, R.N., B.S., M.S.
Associate Director
Nursing Service
Methodist Hospital of Dallas
Dallas, Texas

Patricia Ellis Greene, R.N., B.S.N., M.S.N.
Robbie Simpson Childhood Cancer Nursing Fellowship
St. Jude Children's Research Hospital
Memphis, Tennessee;
Pediatric Nurse Practitioner
Grady Memorial Hospital
Atlanta, Georgia

Jo-Eileen Gyulay, R.N., M.S.
Pediatric Nurse Clinician, Hematology-Oncology Team
Instructor in Pediatrics
University of Kansas Medical Center
Kansas City, Kansas

Dorothy Hall, R.N., M.N.
Associate
Department of Pediatrics
University of Mississippi
Jackson, Mississippi

Rosanne B. Howard, R.D., M.P.H.
Nutritionist, Developmental Evaluation Clinic
Children's Hospital Medical Center
Boston, Massachusetts
Lecturer in Nutrition
University of Massachusetts
Amherst, Massachusetts

Holly F. Hunt, R.N., M.S.
Head Nurse, Psychiatry
Veterans Administration Hospital
Gainesville, Florida

Judith M. Johnson, R.N., B.S., M.S.
Instructor of Nursing
Texas Women's University
Dallas, Texas

Virginia McDowell McClellen, R.N.
Nursing Consultant
University Affiliated Facilities
University of Kansas Medical Center
Kansas City, Kansas

Rosemary J. McKeighen
Associate Professor, Mental Health and Psychiatric Nurse
    Clinician
Department of Nursing Education
University of Kansas Medical Center
Kansas City, Kansas

Janet A. Marvin, R.N., B.S., M.N.
Instructor of Surgical Nursing, Health Science Center
University of Texas Southwestern Medical School
Dallas, Texas

Margaret Shandor Miles, R.N., M.N., M.A.
Pediatric Clinician
University of Missouri–Kansas City
Kansas City, Missouri

Judy L. Moore, R.N., M.N.
Assistant Professor
University of Florida College of Nursing
Gainesville, Florida

Alice H. Murphree, M.A.
Associate in Medicine
Department of Community Health and Family Medicine
University of Florida College of Medicine
Gainesville, Florida

Eileen Gallagher Nahigian, R.N., B.S.N.E., M.N.
Formerly Pediatric Clinical Nurse Specialist
Charleston Area Medical Center
Memorial Division; and Instructor
Mossis Harvey College
Charleston, West Virginia

Barbara L. Newcomer
Child Development and Mental Retardation Center
Assistant Professor
University of Washington School of Nursing
Seattle, Washington

Joyce M. Olson, R.N., M.S.
Pediatric Clinician
Department of Nursing Services;
Assistant Professor of Nursing
Department of Nursing Education
University of Kansas Medical Center
Kansas City, Kansas

Sherrilyn Passo, R.N., B.S., M.S.
Pediatric Clinical Specialist
James Whitcomb Riley Hospital for Children
Indianapolis, Indiana

Sarah Pasternack, R.N., B.A., M.A.
Instructor, School of Nursing
Boston University
Boston, Massachusetts

Dorris Brooks Payne, R.N., Ph.D.
Assistant Professor
Graduate Coordinator
University of Florida College of Nursing
Gainesville, Florida

Florence Bright Roberts, R.N., M.N.
Pediatric Nursing Consultant
Sumner County Guidance Center
Gallatin, Tennessee

Julia R. St. Petery, M.D.
Instructor
Department of Community Health and Family Medicine
Instructor
Department of Pediatrics
University of Florida College of Medicine
Gainesville, Florida

Mary C. Scahill, R.N., B.S., M.S.
Chief Nursing Consultant
Eunice Kennedy Shriver Center
Walter E. Fernald State School for the Retarded
Waverley, Massachusetts

Jeanne Schott, R.N., M.S.N.
Assistant Professor
Department of Nursing Education
Kansas University Medical Center
Kansas City, Kansas

Billie Marie Severtsen, R.N., M.A.
Assistant Professor
Idaho State University
Pocatello, Idaho

Rose Mary Shannon, R.N., B.S.N., M.N.
Nursing Care Coordinator
Children's Hospital of Pittsburgh
Pittsburgh, Pennsylvania

Rebecca Sisson, R.N., A.D., B.S., M.S.
Assistant Professor
School of Nursing
Medical College of Georgia
Augusta, Georgia

Inez L. King Teefy, R.N., B.S., M.N.Ed.
Assistant Professor of Nursing
Maternal and Child Health Coordinator
Texas Women's University
Dallas, Texas

Isobel H. Thorp, R.N., M.A.
Associate Professor
Director, Pediatric Nurse Practitioner Program
University of Alabama in Birmingham
Birmingham, Alabama

June Triplett, R.N., Ed.D.
Professor
University of Iowa College of Nursing
Iowa City, Iowa

Judith A. Trufant, R.N., M.N.
Pediatric Clinical Nurse Specialist
Charleston Area Medical Center
Memorial Division
Charleston, West Virginia

David D. Williams, R.N., M.N.
Doctoral Student, Curriculum and Instruction
University of Florida College of Education
Gainesville, Florida

Lorraine H. Wolf, R.N., M.A.
Associate Professor
Department of Nursing Education
University of Kansas Medical Center
Kansas City, Kansas

Patricia S. Yaros, R.N., M.N.
Instructor
University of Florida College of Nursing
Gainesville, Florida

Joyce Zadroga, R.N., B.S., M.S.
Assistant Professor
School of Nursing
Memorial University
St. John's, Newfoundland, Canada

PREFACE

Dramatic changes occurring in pediatrics and nursing have created demands for current and comprehensive pediatric nursing literature. Although existing pediatric nursing textbooks deal with growth and development, diseases, and nursing care, none takes a comprehensive approach. The editors of this text believe comprehensive pediatric nursing must be derived from an understanding of child and family development; a knowledge of normal and pathologic embryology, anatomy, and physiology; and the application of the nursing process in the care of children. In the belief that a single text was necessary to integrate, discuss, and apply these content areas, the editors developed this volume for use by students, practitioners, and educators. A multi-authored approach was chosen so that specialists could contribute knowledge from their various areas of expertise, geographical bias would be avoided, and the content—both experiential and theoretical—would be as current and as useful as possible.

The book is divided into five parts. Part 1 discusses the nursing process. It includes physical assessment as well as all other steps of the process which are essential to pediatric nursing practice. Part 2 examines principles and theories of human development in relation to children and their families. Health maintenance, preventive measures, and external influences on growth and development are included. The special problems and needs of mentally retarded children, emotionally disturbed children, and high-risk infants and their families are also discussed as deviations from the norm. Part 3 focuses on illness and hospitalization as they affect children of different ages and their families. In Part 4 normal embryology, anatomy, and physiology of the body systems are related to the pathophysiology of these systems at each developmental level. The nursing process is applied in the content on nursing care. Part 5 challenges the reader to explore the future of nursing education and practice and the evolving role of the pediatric nurse in episodic and distributive health care.

The editors hope that this text reflects their commitment to high-level pediatric nursing practice. This project could not have been realized without the contributions of the many authors who shared their expertise in an effort to better the quality of nursing care received by children and their families. The editorial board believes that this objective has been attained with the publication of this text.

ACKNOWLEDGMENTS

We wish to acknowledge the following persons for

their encouragement and support in this endeavor: Helen Adamson, Dorothy Alexander, Edward DeFoe, Burton Dudding, Patricia Grunder, Debra Hymovich, George Lazar, Helen Lillich, Katharine McCarty, Mary Murray, Patricia O'Brien, Lew Ann Packman, Penelope Peirce, and our families, friends, and colleagues. Special thanks go to McGraw-Hill editors Sally Mobley and Ida Wolfson for their editorial assistance and to Joseph Brehm and Cathy Dilworth for their patience, guidance, and endurance throughout this project.

Gladys M. Scipien
Martha Underwood Barnard
Marilyn A. Chard
Jeanne Howe
Patricia J. Phillips

1

**THE
NURSING
PROCESS
IN PEDIATRICS**

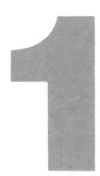

OBSERVATION AND INTERVIEWING

BILLIE MARIE SEVERTSEN

How can nurses best help their patients? It is in full and specific use of the nursing process that nurses most effectively play their role. To use the nursing process well, it must be understood. In this way help offered to the patient will be specific and useful, not merely a generalized, hit-or-miss set of activities and statements that often help no one.

The nursing process is built on four equally important and interdependent parts or foundations. Observation and interviewing are two of these parts. They help nurses assess where a patient is and where he wants to go. Then and only then specific help can be offered—help which will probably be accepted because it is perceived as useful by the patient and his family. For example, when a mother brings her child to a well-child clinic and reports that he constantly seems to contract colds and ear infections, she is doing something more than relating an interesting piece of the child's history. Observation and interviewing will reveal more specific information about this particular mother and child. The nurse may clearly see that her specific help should include teaching the mother to prevent and also predict the start of upper respiratory infections. Used in this way, the nursing process can raise the wellness level of the child.

OBSERVATION

What is observation and how does it feed into assessment? The dictionary defines observation as[1] "an act or the faculty of observing: an act of recognizing and noting a fact or occurrence often involving measurement with instruments: a judgment on or inference from what one has observed." Several concepts are presupposed in this definition. An attempt at summarization of these concepts is made below.

1 Observation is a process. *Process* means a two-way street or a reciprocal give and take between nurse and patient (and/or family). Process also tends to focus on *how*. Of course, some concern is, and should be, shown to the beginning and end of an episode, but the crux of process is *how* the beginning moved, *what* transpired, and *how* the episode drew to a close. A useful mental picture that can aid one who is considering process and its ramifications is that of imagining someone chewing gum. This is process in its purest form. Process is not static but is constantly changing. It includes both nurse (who observes the patient) and patient (who observes the nurse). As the process of observation begins, both nurse and patient tend to stereotype

3

each other. Joyce Travelbee has called this the "phase of the original encounter."[2] At this stage, observations (made by both parties to the process) are filtered through the prejudices which each person has about the stereotype of the other person.

For example, a nurse might consider a pediatric patient in the light of such stereotypes as "poorly developed," "undernourished," or "dirty." These stereotypes are, of course, based on what the nurse considers "normal" in children. The nurse often then goes on to draw conclusions about his stereotypes such as "parents who don't care or who are below average intelligence" or "a disadvantaged environment." While it is conceivable that these stereotypes are completely accurate, more often the impressions which the nurse initially received become tempered as he continues observing and interacting with the patient and family.

In addition, the nurse is constantly being seen and stereotyped by the child and his parents. A nurse may be seen as "friendly" or "mean," "helping" or "hindering," "accepting" or "judgmental." The way in which the patient and family stereotype the nurse influences in a major way the information they allow the nurse to possess. Very few children will not become frightened if they feel as though their examiner is "mean." If a parent receives an overall gestalt of a judgmental nurse who feels that she (the mother) is only marginally effective in mothering, she and her child will probably not waste their time on return visits to well-child clinic. A nurse who is concerned only about doing a physical examination on a child and who does not bother to explain what is being done or to spend time easing a frightened child is more apt than not to receive false, valueless information, from both mother and child, from the time the child is undressed until it is carried out the clinic door.

This seemingly vicious circle is broken in two ways. First, the nurse must be aware of the fact that stereotyping is occurring whenever an observational process begins. Awareness that this phenomenon is occurring should, it is hoped, enable the nurse to temper judgmental observations with a wait-and-see attitude. Secondly, as the process continues, the "original encounter" defined by Travelbee gives way to the "phase of emerging identities."[3] In this phase, stereotyping is superseded by increased perception of the patient and the nurse as individuals rather than extensions of the stereotyped "nurse" and "patient." As the nurse-patient relation progresses to this stage, it follows that the observational process has continued and has become more accurate in delineating both patient and nurse as individuals.

2 Observation is a method of data collection that implies use of all available and appropriate senses. In turn, several steps can be identified as components in this process. Initially, a message must be transmitted from the sender (in this case the patient or his family) to the receiver (the nurse). The message is usually visual or auditory, although it could conceivably affect any of the five senses as well as other senses (such as extrasensory perception) which are currently being investigated.[4] The first step is the sending of the message. Second comes the reception of the message. Involved here is the use of sensory organs plus sufficient stimulation of the reticular activating system to arouse the entire body, including the brain.[5] The third step in the process is perception of the message by the receiver.

It is imperative that the nurse maintain himself as an appropriate channel through which the message from the patient can flow relatively unobstructed. Implied in this statement are several things an observer can do to become and remain a valuable channel for observational messages.

First, when nurses observe, their sensory equipment must be ready to receive and interpret messages. This means that any event or substance which decreases sensory acuity should be avoided. It has been repeatedly demonstrated that a substance such as ingested ethyl alcohol or certain other drugs decreases considerably the accuracy with which one can receive and translate observational messages. It is not yet as well documented, but would seem to follow, that excessive monotony of job, job dissatisfaction, or preoccupation with routine tasks would tend to render an observer less sensitive as a channel for the receipt of messages.

Second, when an observer makes a premature judgment about something which has been observed, subsequent unbiased observation becomes difficult if not impossible. Naturally, there comes a time when judgments must be made about information which one has observed. The essential element is the timing of that judgment. Once the nurse decides what value or motivation prompted the behavior that was observed, a judgment has been made which may preclude further careful observation. The old adage about the foolishness of "leaping to conclusions" is applicable here. Nurses, as observers, must maintain open minds as long as possible. This is not to say that nurses should not focus particular attention on what they consider problem areas, giving these areas priority over seemingly less important material. Any observer, however, would be well advised to hold any judgment in abeyance until as much of the assessment data as possible has been collected.

Third, perception of what observation means is largely dependent upon the past experience and behavior of the observer. Inherent within the observational process is the task of perceiving what values and feelings lie behind the behavior which has been observed. Nurses deal with experiential knowledge, and it is essential that they validate with others (including the patient, if possible) their perceptions of what is happening. Validation of data which the nurse has collected is vital before goals for optimum health care are considered.

Consider this illustration: the prospect of surgery carries with it different value perceptions for different people. For one, surgery may connote speedy cure or at least great improvement from a disease process. For another person, an operation conjures up images of strange, frightening, brutally efficient people associated with the pain and suffering that he will certainly undergo. For a third individual surgery may suggest a threat no less than death. It is necessary for the nurse to initially consider his own perceptions of surgery and accept these perceptions as valid for him. Consideration must then be given to the thoughts a patient or patient's family may have about surgery. The perceptions of surgery from the patient's point of view may be similar to, or radically different from, the nurse's feelings. These perceptions, even if they differ substantially from the perceptions of the nurse are valid for the patient and should be considered as valid by the entire health team. One of the greatest mistakes which can be made by a health professional is to assume that the feelings of a patient or of his family about any aspect of the illness-wellness continuum are or should be the same as the feelings of the professional.

It has been pointed out earlier that an important task of the nurse is to validate with others the perceptions he has gained while observing the patient. The total health team can aid the data-collecting process immeasurably by the increased number of perceptions experienced and shared by a number of people as well as the heightened objectivity seen when perceptions are validated and shared.

Factors which help or hinder the nurse in observing the patient need to be considered next. It is always good to have a general plan to follow before one embarks on the actual task of observing someone or something. Various excellent tools have been devised as aids in the assessment of the patient. Usually these tools include observation as well as physical examination, testing, and interviewing. If no tool is available to the nurse, it is his responsibility in conjunction with other health team members to devise means of data collection that are reliable and comprehensive. Part of the means should be specifically oriented to observing behavior. The actual observation of the patient, however, often takes place within the confines of other means of data collection. For example, during the course of the physical examination does the patient wince, complain of pain, or seem embarrassed? Is the behavior of the patient during an interview apathetic and uncaring? Are the muscular movements of a patient smooth or jerky? Is the patient well groomed or poorly groomed?

Once general observations have been made, the nurse should go into more depth in observing so-called problem areas. For example, if a patient appears apathetic to the nurse and to others of the health team, what is the reason behind that presentation of self? A patient may appear apathetic for a number of reasons. He may feel, for instance, that his disease is fatal and be resigned to that perception. He may be convinced of his vulnerability in the face of hospitals, powerful doctors, awesome procedures, and expensive care. He may, for many reasons, seek to present himself to others as a perpetual "loser." Whatever his reason, it is the function of the nurse to make an observation of his behavior, validate with him and others that what was observed was indeed correct, attach a motivational value to the observation (using an informed judgment), and then employ this observational data to help the patient make choices and decisions based in reality.

When a patient is being observed, it is of major importance that the process of observation be of priority to the nurse. Far too often observation is thought of as a "nice but not necessary" nursing activity and because of this categorization is placed behind other activities, such as giving physical care or passing medications, in importance. Naturally there can be no quarrel that passing medications or giving physical care is of only minimal value: the point to be made is simply that if observation is accepted as a central tool in assessment, time and energy must be allowed for the nurse to observe.

Another factor which can help or hinder nurses in observing is their amount of knowledge or expertise in the particular problem area. This means that the nurse must be familiar with the disease process affecting the patient as well as with related theories of wellness-illness. Theories such as Dunn's health grid, Selye's general adaptation syndrome, Engel's stages of grieving, Maslow's hierarchy of needs, and

Erikson's stages of development are particularly valuable in assessment of a patient. These theories provide the observer with added insight into the various stress-producing situations affecting patients. For more detailed discussion, the reader is referred to the texts by these authors listed in the Bibliography at the end of the chapter. Observation of behavior becomes much more significant if (for instance) anger is seen and validated as part of the denial stage of adaptation to chronic illness. It cannot be stressed too emphatically that the nurse is the health professional best equipped by education and experience to apply these theories selectively to specific patients. This can be called *therapeutic* in the truest sense of the word. The nurse is now using her complemental role to work with the individual patient rather than with the disease process. Little has been said up to this point about observing things or individuals other than the patient. There are times when events or people external to the patient deserve the scrutiny of the observer even more than the patient. Accuracy of observation is largely dependent on the observer's ability to focus attention and energy on the crucial thing or person at the crucial time.

One example of a crucial thing at a crucial time would be the environment of the patient. To what extent and degree does the environment affect the patient's behavior? To answer this question, comparative observations need to be made on the patient both in his customary environment and away from it. The classic example of a comparative observation on a patient in the hospital and later in the home environment is that of a primipara patient and her baby. The observer can often see major changes in the infant in the home environment as compared with the hospital nursery setting. Such variables as temperature in the home, noise level, adequate or inadequate space, and activity and fatigue levels of the mother all contribute to the infant's adaptive response to the environment. Observing a cold, crowded, noisy apartment in combination with a harried, exhausted mother will, in many cases, produce the picture of an infant unable to tolerate the same formula which he tolerated easily in the hospital. A similar observation tool might be used in a classroom setting when a child experiences difficulty in school. Observing the child in the home and then at school will often yield valuable clues as to what the problem may be.

Closely related, of course, to environment per se are the people (most specifically the family) in close relationship or association with the patient. This is especially evident in pediatric patients.[6] It can be predicted with almost cause-and-effect accuracy that parental anxiety over a hospitalized or ill child will snowball and cause the child to behave with an increase in his own anxiety. This, in turn, tends to reduce the amount of available energy that the child has, perhaps causing a definite lag in his progression from illness to wellness. Perhaps as dramatic a change is not seen in the adult patient, but numerous well-documented studies and case histories[7] show the clear interrelation between environment, family, and patient.

Hence it follows that if the observer of the patient is to note what is crucial, he must be well attuned to the need for observing both environment and family, in addition to the patient. This may mean observing in the home—perhaps one time in the absence of the patient and another time with him present. For a patient who attends school, a visit to the school might be a necessity just as a visit to another patient's place of employment might be invaluable prior to obtaining reliable base line observational data about that patient.

It cannot be emphasized too strongly that in order to assess a patient, a nurse must strive to gain as complete a picture of the patient as possible. Observation is one of the tools used to gain that picture. The observational tool is neither valid nor reliable if great gaps exist in the nurse's observational knowledge of the patient. Nurses, therefore, are bound to observe completely, to observe accurately, to observe adjacent people or environmental factors as well as the individual patient, to observe at crucial times, and to focus their attention on specific "trouble" spots. Next, nurses must interpret and validate with others their interpretations of the motivations and values behind the behavior of the patient. The tool of observation, when used in this way, becomes (along with interviewing, testing, and physical examination) the foundation upon which specific and helpful nursing intervention can be planned, implemented, and evaluated.

INTERVIEWING

Interviewing is the second method of patient assessment which will be examined in order to understand its use in the building of a sound data base. Interviewing can properly be called a part of observation; however, it stands apart as a specific and crucial part of the larger observational tool. A dictionary definition is perhaps the best way to isolate and examine *interviewing*. It is defined as[8] "A formal consultation usually to evaluate qualifications: a meeting at which information is obtained." Consultation (the act of consulting) is further defined as "providing professional or expert advice."

As with the analysis of observation, it would be wise to examine concepts relating to the tool of interviewing. In this way parallels can be drawn between interviewing and observation.

Interviewing is a process just as observation is. Process, as has already been seen, is a two-way street, a give and take between patient (and/or family) and nurse. Process in interviewing is also concerned with the breaking down of stereotypes which one person has about another person. The definition of interviewing alludes to a mutual sight or view. The nurse must consider that the major task which he or she wishes to accomplish is the receipt of valid and reliable data from the patient. If the data collected are neither reliable nor valid, it follows that the information which the nurse interprets to the patient as reality may not be real to him at all. From this, it follows that goals which the nurse helps the patient formulate may be of only minimal value to him. Such a situation (of inaccurate information feeding into marginally valued goals) is not likely to motivate the patient. The final result of this process is very often nursing intervention which serves no useful purpose other than to alienate a patient, frustrate a nurse, and waste valuable time.

How is one to obtain valid and reliable data from a patient or family via the technic of interviewing? Here, as in observing, senses are involved in a process of reception, perception, and interpretation. The nurse must also be aware that two separate kinds of information are being received and processed by both interviewer and interviewee. It is worth our effort to examine these two types of information:

1 Verbal information: that which is obtained via oral or written communication.
2 Nonverbal information: that which is received in ways other than verbal, including attitudes, feelings, and thoughts conveyed intentionally or unintentionally by posture, gesture, vocal tone, and facial expression.

The nurse must use care in sorting out the kind of information received from either patient or parent. For example, a mother may state that she is happy that her child is going to undergo a tonsillectomy because "maybe now we won't be bothered with such terrible sore throats." This seems perfectly normal and logical. However, if the health worker notices that it is a dejected, slumped over, apathetic-appearing mother who relates how happy she is, a message with a distinct double meaning is being sent. Or a parent may receive instructions on what to do with her baby who is suffering from an upper respiratory infection. The parent may say she understands and is capable of following the instructions in regard to medication, treatment, and general care. However, if she appears ill at ease, rather than comfortable, it would be well for the nurse to inquire further into the situation. The mother's self-confidence may need a great deal more reinforcing before she will feel relaxed in caring for her sick baby.

As with observation, the next task of the nurse after receiving the message or messages is to perceive and validate the information. Again, it must be pointed out that the motivation or the value behind the overt work or act is the crucial element. This can be stated more simply as *Why* is the patient or his family saying what they are saying and *why* are they acting in this or that manner? An important corollary to remember here is that the patient and/or his parents may perceive that his importance is being measured in terms of the seriousness or unusualness of his problem. He also may know that in many health care facilities he is exempt from treatment if certain facts pertaining to him become known (for instance, if he is a drug addict). Very often, then, it is to the patient's advantage to modify in some way the information he gives to the nurse. A parent, for instance, may know that he has physically abused or neglected his child but may fear recriminations of many kinds if this information becomes known. The implication for the health professional in interviewing situations is to be alert to either gaps in the story related by the patient (or parent) or to a dichotomy between verbal and nonverbal communication.

Another important motivational force behind the giving of valid or nonvalid information to the nurse by the patient is the manner in which the nurse presents himself to the patient. A nurse with a very businesslike, efficient manner may be perceived by a patient as condescending; such a nurse is not likely to be given information about a patient's embarrassment over an anticipated pelvic examination, for example, or a mother's concern over her inability to successfully breast feed her baby. When interviewing a patient or family, the nurse must be constantly aware of the way in which he presents himself to the patient and how the patient responds to that presentation. If the patient and/or his family are not motivated to cooperate with the nurse, that nurse will not receive accurate information, and the entire vicious circle of inappropriate goals, based on inaccurate data, is repeated.

Just as with the tool of observation, the nurse is bound to validate with others, including the patient and his family, the information received via the interview. Naturally, some items require more clarification than others. If doubt exists with regard to what a patient meant or why he said what he said, clarification of that particular item should be made. It should also be remembered that because each human being is a product of experiences which have bombarded him since before birth, such intangibles as culture, language, religious values, socioeconomic status, and educational background must be considered before a patient can be understood. To understand these various factors is the task of the nurse. Translated into practical action, does a nurse continue to relate to a child's parents who have indicated that they are not married with an open mind—presenting the interviewer as nonhostile, noncondescending, and nonrecriminating—or does the nurse immediately make and transmit to the parents negative judgments of them as parents?

Another parallel of interviewing to observation is the advisability in both cases of an overall plan prior to beginning the data collection. Things which should be considered as important to the general plan of an interview would certainly include the clinical history (past and present), chief complaint and present illness, and social and family history.

A certain part of the information gained from an interview provides little feeling to the nurse. Included in this category would be questions about age, marital status, and number of children, which traditionally evoke a one-word or one-sentence answer. However, questions such as "How do you feel now?" or "What seems to bother you the most?" can often yield valuable data. A particularly valuable question for gaining insight into the emotional components of the situation for the patient and/or family is "Tell me what happened when you first got sick?" Nurses must keep in mind that with a question of this sort they are asking patients to reveal things which are an intimate part of themselves. It is crucial that the nurse listen carefully and specifically to what the patient says, noting along with his words, his posture and attitudes. When a patient reveals himself in this way to the nurse (provided the patient perceives the nurse as a warm and open human being), the situation can evolve into a kind of "peak experience" as described by Maslow.[9] During such an experience both interviewer and interviewee feel more "totally integrated"[10] with subsequent heightened perception of what the other is feeling and saying. Travelbee[11] has called this phenomenon the "stage of empathy" and has defined it as "the ability to instantaneously and accurately predict the patient's behavior because of knowledge about what the patient is thinking."

It cannot be overemphasized that a prerequisite to the peak experience just described is the ability and facility with which the nurse listens to the patient and his family. Listening means, in a literal sense, trying to somehow get into the other person's mind in order to find out what is going on. It follows that there are certain requirements for good listening.

THE ENVIRONMENT

One requirement of good listening (as well as of good interviewing) has to do with one's environment. It is certainly logical to assume that a patient or his parents will be apt to speak much more freely and honestly if they are relaxed and somewhat casual than if they feel pressured to give factual medical data with rapid hairline precision. Allowing for a relaxed environment often means sitting down beside the mother or child rather than pontificating behind a desk; it generally means questions asked not in rapid-fire succession but more slowly (perhaps during a physical exam or a child development test). Nurses continually must use their sensitivity to gauge the amount of tension the parents and/or the child exhibit and must subsequently seek to reduce tension by every method at their disposal. This certainly involves bending or changing a rigid, preset, interviewing sheet whenever necessary.

Another requirement of good listening is specificity. This refers to the act of "tuning in" on the specific information being shared by the patient. An aid to specific "tuning in" is asking the patient a very specific question of clarification occasionally. For example, if a mother relates that her baby is irritable, the interviewer might question what exactly the mother means by "irritable." Is the baby screaming constantly, whimpering, or restless? Is he irritable at certain times of the day or night or whenever certain people or elements are present in the environment? By questions such as these the interviewer has not only gained a great deal of in-depth information but has demonstrated to the mother that he is attentive to that mother's specific situation. Another useful, more general, question to ask the mother might be, "What is your baby's name?" This question also demonstrates a personal sort of interest—the mother to whom it is directed is not likely to feel that she is being stereotyped with all other mothers who have irritable babies.

Another requirement of good listening is the ability of the listener to withhold judgment as long as possible in the observational situation. In interviewing, however, when a judgment has been made, a verbal indication of that judgment is often forthcoming. For instance, the interviewer may say, "You seem to be angry about your condition." Once that statement (or a similar one) is made to the patient, he may feel that defense of his statement or even denial of the feeling (of being angry) will only strengthen the point of the interviewer, i.e., that he indeed *is* angry. Productive communication often stops at this point, the patient feeling that he has been cut off, while the interviewer feels that all worthwhile data have been collected. Nurses should remember that while they must always attempt to validate what is perceived as feeling or reaction, this does not give license to cut off the patient by indicating in any way that further discussion or clarification is not necessary or appropriate.

A corollary to the point just discussed is the caution the interviewer must use in offering advice. It is well to remember that very few, if any, people fundamentally change their behavior because of the desire of another person; people change rather because they themselves wish to change. The nurse who seeks to change a patient's life by offering "good advice" is apt to find that the "good advice" is "good" only as it applies to his own life and values. The patient and his family are products of a different genetic heritage, a different environment, and most likely a different life-style. It is clearly illogical to suppose that a decision which strikes the nurse as quite reasonable will apply equally well to the patient.

It must be pointed out that the offering of advice and the offering of realistic alternatives are two different things. The nurse must use caution in giving advice; however, when he points out realistic alternatives to the patient and/or family, a truly valuable nursing intervention is being rendered. Careful assessment is always a necessary forerunner of this specific nursing intervention (as it is with other nursing actions). Care must be taken to make sure that through assessment the nurse is equipping the patient to make an informed choice rather than trying to live his life for him. The nurse must keep in mind that a patient or his parents may not yet be at the point in their acceptance of a disease process to clearly delineate "good" from "bad." The choice of life goals always belongs to the patient and his family in the last analysis. Nursing responsibility consists both of assessing whether the patient is ready to decide upon goals which he perceives as "good" or "the best for me" and of offering various realistic ways to go about meeting his goals.

This principle can perhaps be more clearly illustrated by means of an example. If a nurse, while interviewing the mother of a baby, is informed by the mother, "My baby's not eating too well," the nurse must then assess the situation further. Let us assume that upon further assessment the nurse ascertains that the infant tolerates his commercially prepared formula only moderately well. The nurse may observe the baby hungrily gulping down formula, only to regurgitate a large portion of it. Further observation may show that the mother bubbles or burps the baby only twice during an 8-oz feeding. The mother may, in addition, appear very anxious when holding the baby and may jiggle and bounce him about constantly. The nurse is also aware (on the basis of a preliminary medical assessment) that the pediatrician feels nothing organically is wrong with the baby. In light of this evidence logical nursing intervention would be to teach the mother to bubble the baby more frequently during its feeding; to feed the baby frequently enough so that it does not become ravenously hungry by the time of the next feeding; to hold the baby in a quieter, calmer way. How the nurse goes about this task is crucial. The nurse may say to the mother, "You are too nervous when you hold the baby; try not to jiggle him around." Or he may say, "You should try to feed him more frequently; he's probably too hungry and eats too fast." Or again, "Three or four burps every feeding will probably prevent the spitting up. Burp or bubble him after every 2 oz of formula." Clearly it is a nurse's responsibility to give advice, and the advice is a sound, logical suggested modification of behavior. The problem in this example is rather with the procedure used by the nurse, who assessed the patient by both observation and interviewing. On the basis of that assessment, the nurse postulated what helpful behavior modifications the mother could make that might relieve the problem. The error in nursing intervention was in the manner in which the behavior modification was presented to the mother. The nurse assumed without question (1) that the mother will realize that the hungry gulping of formula is a contributing factor to subsequent regurgitation; (2) that the mother understands that flexibility in a feeding schedule will not adversely affect the baby's health or disposition or the mother's own time schedule; and (3) that the mother will be able to modify "nervous" movements to "calm" ones simply by willing herself to do this. The nurse perceived the advice as "good," and it would be "good" indeed if the nurse were the mother. However, one cannot say that the mother has the same values, motivations, or understandings as the nurse. The "good advice" to the mother may not be good at all. In contrast, how could the nurse point out reality to the mother in order for her to make her own "informed choice?'' The nurse might indicate to the mother the following: ''Many babies who are very hungry wolf down their food so fast that it causes them to spit up. If your baby were fed more often, maybe every 3 hours for a week or so, he might not be so hungry and drink his bottle so fast.'' In this intervention an attitude of ''try it and see'' coupled with understanding—''this is the reason it might work''—has been established. The mother retains both the prerogative to ask a question, such as, ''You mean that it's not good for a baby to be so hungry?'' as well as the option for changing her behavior because *she* wants to change it.

In the whole scheme of changing or modifying behavior, it is well for the nurse to remember that a patient or the family of a patient is using energy to constantly change and modify their respective self-concepts. The adaptation they must make to maintain an accurate and acceptable self-image becomes harder to accomplish in the face of other stresses such as illness. It is important for nurses to realize that at least three components can be identified as playing a part in the alteration of self-concept. These components (isolated by Putney and Putney[12]) are (1) self-thought or thinking about oneself in the new and different way, (2) action or practicing the new way of behaving, and (3) indirect self-acceptance or receiving feedback from significant other people that the new way of acting and behaving is appropriate. Since most people who suffer from illness must modify the way they view themselves, i.e., change their self-concept, the nurse is in an enviable position to facilitate the process of modification. This is accomplished in several ways. First, time must be allowed for the patient to think about himself in a new way (e.g., a formerly pregnant woman needs to consider herself a mother rather than pregnant). The nurse must also allow for action on the part of the patient in order for the patient to practice acting in his new role; e.g., the new mother needs to practice doing the things that new mothers do (as opposed to the things that pregnant women do). Lastly, the nurse must indicate approval of the appropriate new way in which the patient is thinking and acting. The new mother, for example, will feel that she can more easily accept her new, modified self-image if the nurse (as an expert on diseases and patients) indicates that he feels the new mother is acting the way a new mother should act.

Table 1-1 ILLUSTRATION OF AN ASSESSMENT RECORD: PATIENT PROFILE

Presenting-problem illness

Natal history—Prematurity: Ponderal index

Past medical history (immunizations, childhood diseases, dental care)

Family/Social history, including ordinal rank, age, height, weight, health history, education, occupation
  Mother
  Father
  MGM
  MGF
  PGM
  PGF
  Siblings

Summary of family and social history

Health care record

Review of systems
  Eating patterns
  Elimination patterns
  Sleep patterns
  Discipline patterns
  Enrichment
  Growth
    Height
    Weight
    Dentition
  Development
    Gross motor
    Fine motor
    Socialization
    Language

Physical assessment
  General appearance
  Head
  Eyes
  Ears
  Nose
  Mouth
  Throat
  Neck
  Chest
  Heart
  Abdomen
  Genitals
  Rectal
  Hips
  Extremities
  Torso
  Skin
  Central nervous system

Problems

Courtesy: Martha Barnard, University of Kansas Medical Center.

RECORDING

Little has been said about the methodology of recording data which are gathered by observation or interviewing. The importance of accurate, complete recording cannot be overemphasized since it is on the basis of recording that subsequent goals for care are formulated. Several characteristics of useful recording need to be mentioned:

1 Recording should reflect as nearly as possible the episode exactly as it occurred. This refers to the need for accuracy: precisely what happened is more accurate than a nurse's judgment of what happened in terms of usefulness of recording. Descriptive terms are valuable because they give authenticity and specificity to the episode. Consider these two examples: "Patient complains of dyspnea" and "10-year-old child with history of asthmatic attacks complains of dyspnea associated with sternal retraction. Appears very apprehensive, stating 'I've never had it this bad.' " These examples illustrate one very specific and one very general observation. It is easy to see that the specific account is a better one in terms of planning nursing intervention.

2 Recording should be done as soon as possible after the observation or the interview has taken place. Obviously, this is intended to minimize lapses of memory on the part of the nurse, who is very likely to forget points over a time span. These "forgotten details" may later prove to be critical ones underlying the patient's needs. It should be emphasized also that the continuity of an interview may be disrupted if the nurse constantly stops to write down observations or comments. Discretion must be used as to the appropriate time to record, but generally speaking the sooner the material is written down, the better for the patient.

3 Recording should list problems which the patient exhibits based on the data gathered by the nurse. With a problem orientation to recording, observations relevant to each problem will be listed at the time the problem is listed. Subsequent information which is obtained about the patient will be appropriately filed under the problem to which it pertains. The logic behind recording in this manner is to view the patient in an orderly, problem-oriented way, rather than a haphazard one. Ideally all health professionals, doctors, nurses, ancillary workers, dietitians, social workers, etc., should familiarize themselves with this manner of recording. Perhaps then we can move toward truly comprehensive care based on comprehensive analysis of the patient.

A specific patient assessment sheet is illustrated here. This kind of assessment tool is invaluable in ascertaining whether gaps in continuity of observation exist. It should serve as a check to comprehensiveness in the observational process as well as a guide to physical assessment.

REFERENCES

1 *Webster's New Collegiate Dictionary*, 8th ed., G. & C. Merriam Company, Springfield, Mass., 1973.
2 Joyce Travelbee, *Interpersonal Aspects of Nursing*, 2d ed., F. A. Davis Company, Philadelphia, 1967, p. 130.
3 Ibid., p. 133.
4 For a fascinating analysis of higher sense perception the reader is referred to Sheila Ostrander and Lynn Schroeder, *Psychic Discoveries behind the Iron Curtain*, Prentice-Hall, Inc., Englewood Cliffs, N.J., 1970.
5 Judith Chodil and Barbara Williams, "The Concept of Sensory Deprivation," *The Nursing Clinics of North America*, 5(3): 455, September 1970.
6 Florence Bright, "The Pediatric Nurse and Parental Anxiety," *Nursing Forum*, 4(2): 30–46, 1965.
7 For an informative account of this interrelationship the reader is referred to L. Schwartz and Jane Linker Schwartz, *The Psychodynamics of Patient Care*, Prentice-Hall, Inc., Englewood Cliffs, N.J., 1970.
8 *Webster's New Collegiate Dictionary*, op. cit.
9 A. Maslow, *Toward a Psychology of Being*, 2d ed., Van Nostrand Reinhold Company, New York, 1968, p. 71.
10 Ibid., p. 77.
11 Travelbee, op. cit., p. 135.
12 S. Putney and Gail J. Putney, *The Adjusted American: Normal Neurosis in the Individual and Society*, Harper & Row, Publishers, Inc., New York, 1966, pp. 23–36.

BIBLIOGRAPHY

Dunn, H.: *High-Level Wellness*, R. W. Beatty, Ltd., Arlington, Va., 1967.
Engel, G.: "Grief and Grieving," *American Journal of Nursing*, 64(9), September 1964.
Erikson, E. H.: *Childhood and Society*, 2d ed., W. W. Norton & Company, Inc., New York, 1963.
Selye, H.: *The Stress of Life*, McGraw-Hill Book Company, New York, 1956.

2
TESTING

LORRAINE H. WOLF

The traditional definition of testing as a diagnostic procedure to determine the nature and/or progress of a disease process, or identifying a change in the function or character of an organ or system, has limited this valuable process primarily to the physician member of the health care team. A broader definition of testing that includes the collection and comparison of data to determine the health status of an individual, or to identify the health problems of an individual, as well as aid in the diagnosis of dysfunction, is postulated by this author as relevant for nursing practice. Testing (assessing) in this context is the use of standardized procedures for measuring objectively the biochemical, physical, psychologic, and/or developmental status of an individual relevant to providing the basis for a nursing diagnosis upon which nursing intervention will be determined. This definition indicates that the goal, or objective, of the testing is to identify patient problems relevant to nursing practice. This broader definition thus enables the nurse practitioner to participate in the assessment of the patient.

This chapter presents two major areas of testing that are critical in the nursing assessment of the health status of infants, children, and adolescents, i.e., developmental and biochemical testing. Each of the two sections includes, where appropriate, test selections, goals, conditions, and protocol according to five age categories (birth to 1 year, 1 year to 3½ years, 3½ to 6½ years, 6½ to 12 years, and 12 to 18 years).

DEVELOPMENTAL TESTING

The growth and development of the human being is a dynamic and complex process that proceeds, within limitations, in a sequential pattern. Accordingly, developmental testing provides a means of ascertaining whether the infant, child, or adolescent is meeting the developmental milestones appropriate for his age.

Test Recommendations

Developmental milestones are listed in textbooks of nursing, pediatrics, psychology, psychiatry, neurology, special education, and others. Since these fixed timetables for the acquisition of skills that represent man's movement up the phylogenetic scale are more and more accepted, it is necessary to point out the wide variation in developmental patterns. While accepted developmental stages or milestones are widely used, they in no way represent a fixed or inflexible scale. Rather, developmental

Table 2-1 ASSESSMENT OF DEVELOPMENTAL PATTERNS

Skill	Assessment Instrument
Motor (fine and gross)	Birth–6 months: Physical assessment. 6 months–6 years: Physical assessment augmented by direct developmental testing (e.g., Denver Developmental Screening Test) or indirect testing (e.g., Preschool Attainment Record). School-age to adult: Physical assessment augmented by direct developmental testing (e.g., Valett Psychoeducational Test) or indirect testing (e.g., Vineland Social Maturity Scale). Children with physical handicaps evaluated by observation and use of reinforcers to obtain maximum effort. Suspected perceptual motor difficulties may be screened by the Ayers Test (Southern California Test Battery) for ages 4–11.
Language	Same instruments as for fine and gross motor skills. Additionally, the Vocabulary Language Test helps pinpoint deficits in language development. After 8 years, articulation errors may be assessed with the Templin Darley Screening Test. Suspected childhood aphasia may be evaluated with the Eisenson Examining for Aphasia Test.
Social and emotional	Same instruments as for motor and language development. Presenting emotional problems may further be screened with the Devereaux Child Behavior Rating Scale. The nurse who holds clinical membership in transactional analysis may find script analysis useful with the adolescent.
Cognitive	Assessment of cognitive or intellectual development is seldom a screening procedure. When there is a question about the potential of the child of 3 to 18 years, the Peabody Picture Vocabulary is an excellent tool. The Wide Range Achievement Test will also give an indication of the level at which the child or adolescent is functioning academically.

patterns are viewed as a guideline and include the most appropriate test currently available to nurses practicing with infants, children, and adolescents.

Test Selection

Most developmental tests (screening and diagnostic) are based on samples of social behavior, gross and fine motor skills, and communication skills. It is extremely important that the nurse select those tests that (1) are standardized on a large population, (2) have a high reliability (measure what they claim to measure), and (3) are valid (perform well related to outside nontest criteria). Nurses should be familiar with sources that report information about the standardization of the tests they select and that discuss the level of competency necessary to administer and evaluate the test, e.g., Buros' *Mental Measurements Yearbook* and Anastasi's *Psychological Testing* (see the Bibliography at the end of the chapter).

Assessment by testing may be done routinely, i.e., developmental testing on all well babies (after 6 months), toddlers, and preschoolers, or selectively when a deviation is suspected (e.g., language development testing, emotional development testing). In order for the nurse to exercise judgment regarding the selection of tests, it is necessary to distinguish the various purposes tests serve. For example, tests may perform the following functions:

1 Provide base line data for ongoing nursing action
2 Obtain data not otherwise readily available by observation, examination, or history
3 Distinguish between the individual's present and potential functioning
4 Determine the area and level of dysfunction
5 Assist in determining intervention by nurses or other members of the health care team
6 Provide information on which the nurse may wish to make a referral

Another consideration in test selection is whether it is more advantageous to do an indirect evaluation of the child or a direct assessment of the child's behavior.

In an indirect approach, for example, the examiner asks specific questions of the parent (or responsible adolescent) about the child's behavior. Typical items are: (1) "Is your child able to (or at what age did your child . . .) climb about? (skip? jump? unwrap covers? fasten shoes?)'' (2) ''Is your child able to (or at what age did your child . . .) help with simple tasks? (play competetively? sing harmoniously?)'' (3) ''Does your child (or at what age did your child . . .) imitate or echo your sounds and words? (talk in phrases? describe and share events?)'' and (4) ''Does your child (or at what age did your child . . .) mind? (get a drink? toilet self?).'' The Preschool Attainment Record (PAR) is an example of this approach to assessment and is extensively used by developmental specialists when it may not be expedient to observe the child directly because of illness of the child, absent at time of interview, or other reasons. Data from this approach are not obtained by observing the child directly.

The other major approach to developmental testing is for the examiner to directly observe the child's behavior wherein he is asked or induced to perform specific and predetermined acts. The child may be asked to perform the following kinds of behaviors, for example: (1) Place the infant on its stomach and observe if it lifts its head and chest (age 2 to 4 months). (2) Tell the child to walk backwards and observe if it can take two or more steps retaining balance (age 12 to 22 months). (3) Ask the child to hop on one foot and observe if it can do this two or more times (age 3 to 5 years). (4) A block is placed in each hand and the child encouraged to bang the blocks together (age 7 to 12 months). (5) Ask the child to show its eyes, ears, nose to the examiner (age 13 to 21 months). (6) Place colored blocks on the table and ask the child to identify the red block, blue block, etc. (age 2½ to 4½ years). (7) Give the child a toy and try gently to pull it away observing if the child resists having the toy taken away (age 4 to 10 months).

The Denver Developmental Screening Test (DDST) is an example of this approach to testing. The direct-observation approach enables the examiner to observe the child's behavior pattern in relation to parents and examiner, thus providing additional clinical information.

Both the direct and indirect approaches to developmental assessment are well-accepted procedures, and the choice depends on the time available for testing, cost, convenience, and the examiner's preference (See Table 2-1).

Test Considerations

Testing may be done in the eco-setting (home), clinic, or inpatient hospital unit. The nurse should be aware of several considerations before proceeding with testing. Four major considerations are as follows:

1 Age of child
   a Short testing periods are needed for infants as they tire easily.
   b A frequent change of activity for preschool children is useful because of their short attention span.
2 Eating and sleeping patterns
   a Infants may regurgitate if tested in the areas of mobility immediately after eating.
   b Preschool and school-age children should be tested 1 to 2 hours postprandial in order to elicit maximum effort at the time of high energy levels.
   c School-age children need to be tested during early school day. Fatigue and need for creative play are high after school hours.
3 Facilities
   a Inasmuch as possible, the environment should be regulated for light, temperature, and noise. Distractions may alter test results at all age levels.
   b Adequate space should be available before testing developmental levels requiring movement or the placement of objects at specified distances.
4 Health of child
   a Physical well-being is necessary to maximize the child's ability to perform the requested tasks. Defer testing when child is ill.
   b Stress in the testing situation is a normal response, but testing should be deferred if the child has suffered shock or trauma in the week preceding the examination.

Attending to these considerations increases the validity and reliability of the test results and provides the most satisfactory milieu for the nurse to focus on the child and his parent(s).

BIOCHEMICAL TESTING

In addition to the data secured from the history, physical assessment, and developmental tests, the employment of selected laboratory screening tests will yield pertinent information regarding the internal physiologic status of the infant, child, or adolescent. Early indications of potentially serious health problems may be identified and prevented. In the case of a presenting health problem the information obtained by biotesting provides the basis for referral to the physician for differential diagnosis and medical therapeutics.

Screening laboratory procedures have been developed for immediate routine analysis of blood, urine, and stool specimens. These tests use sources that are remarkably consistent in their normal state, e.g., blood and urine. Special procedures, such as the Papanicolaou and pregnancy tests, are also available to the nurse working with adolescents.

The purpose or objective of biochemical testing needs to be clearly defined within the context of the nursing process. As with developmental testing, the information sought and elicited will be utilized by the nurse to:

1 Provide base line data for nursing intervention or referral
2 Obtain data not available by other means of nursing assessment
3 Set priorities and plan nursing intervention appropriate to the needs of the individual
4 Make an appropriate referral to the physician for diagnosis and treatment

Within these criteria, the tests selected will be standardized screening tests that are within the competency of the practicing nurse.

Tests Selected

For clarity and readily accessible reference, the test selection is discussed and presented in terms of the source of the specimen. Normal ranges for the age levels are presented when relevant, as well as the common problems encountered by the nurse.

Urine The composition and characteristics of urine are reasonably constant. Abnormal findings on a routine urinalysis will yield information about abnormal products of metabolism, as well as an indication of kidney function. A word of caution is expressed by Green and Richmond: "The fact that a random urinalysis is normal does not eliminate the possibility of renal disease."[1]

Urine is routinely examined for *physical properties* (color, appearance, specific gravity, and reaction), *chemical properties* (glucose, albumin, and occasionally acetone), and *microscopic analysis* of sediments. The following tables list the screening tests usually employed, normal values or presence, and selected comments on deviation (see Tables 2-2 to 2-4).

Urinary tract infections are very common in children. It is recommended that every child have a complete urinary tract evaluation after the first episode of infection. This would include urine culture, creatinine clearance, urine concentration, intravenous pyelogram (IVP), voiding urethrocystogram, a cystoscopy, and a cystometerogram. Tucker[2] lists the following signs and symptoms of urinary tract problems by age.

Age	Signs and symptoms	Cause and incidence
Birth–2 mo	Unexplained jaundice; no fever; failure to thrive	Pathogens (under 2 yr) Incidence: 2 boys to 1 girl
2–18 mo	Unexplained fever; febrile convulsions; gastrointestinal upset; failure to thrive	Obstructive uropathy Incidence: 2 boys to 1 girl
18 mo–3 yr	Unexplained fever; gastrointestinal upset; failure to thrive	Nonobstructive uropathy (over 2–3 yr) Incidence: 30 girls to 1 boy
Over 3 yr	Dysuria; abdominal pain; costovertebral angle (CVA) tenderness; hematuria; failure to thrive	

Table 2-2 URINALYSIS: PHYSICAL PROPERTIES

Properties	Test	Procedure	Normal findings	Comments
Color	Observation	Look at specimen with naked eye	Straw to amber color	Acid urine usually darker than alkaline urine. Red-brown if blood present. Yellow-brown or greenish if bile present.
Appearance	Observation	Look at specimen with naked eye	Clear	May become cloudy on standing. Abnormal cloudiness due to mucus, bacteria, urates, phosphates.
Specific gravity	Observation	Place urine sample in urinometer, spin float, and read	1.002–1.030	Early morning specimen usually has higher specific gravity. If quantity not sufficient, add equal parts distilled water and multiply last two figures of finding by 2.
Reaction	Nitrazene paper	Dip paper in specimen three times, wait 1 min, compare with color chart	6.0–6.5 neutral 6.0 acid 6.5 alkaline	May be fixed alkalinity after pneumonia crisis or in some anemias. Normal range 4.8–7.5.

Table 2-3 URINALYSIS: CHEMICAL PROPERTIES

Properties	Test	Procedure	Normal findings	Comments
Glucose	Clinistix Bili Labstix	Moisten with urine, compare with color chart in 10 sec	Negative	Patient receiving large amounts of ascorbic acid will negate test. Abnormal (positive) in diabetes.
Protein	Bili Labstix	Moisten with urine, compare with chart immediately	Negative	May have false results if urine stands too long. Usually indicates damage to kidneys if abnormal. Associated with acute and chronic glomerulonephritis, nephrosis, dehydration, diabetes mellitus, lead poisoning among others.
Ketone	Bili Labstix	Moisten with urine, compare with chart in 15 sec	Negative	May have a false positive in presence of phenylpyruvic acid (PKU). Associated with diabetic acidosis, persistent vomiting, starvation, lead poisoning, acute febrile disease among others.
Occult blood	Bili Labstix	Moisten with urine, compare with chart in 30 sec	Negative	May have a false positive from contaminants or presence of myoglobin. Associated with acute glomerulonephritis, acute pyelonephritis, or septicemia.
Bilirubin	Bili Labstix	Moisten with urine, compare with chart in 20 sec	Negative	May have atypical results if patient is on Pyridium, Thorazine, or phenothiazine metabolites. Associated with viral hepatitis, chemical injury to liver, biliary obstruction among others.

Table 2-4 URINALYSIS: MICROSCOPIC PROPERTIES

Properties	Procedure	Normal findings	Comments
	1 Shake and centrifuge specimen 2 Pour off supernatant fluid 3 Pour a few drops on a clean slide 4 Place cover slide over drops 5 Examine six fields for casts under low power 6 Examine six fields for cells and other structures under high power		

Cells
  Epithelial
    Squamous
		Normally present	Arise from superficial layers of the urethra.
			Large, flat, irregular cells with round or oval nucleus.

Small round		Not normally present	Arise from deeper layers of urinary tract. More than a few are abnormal. Round cells with nucleus.
Transitional		Not normally present	Arise from kidneys and ureters. More than a few abnormal. Pear-shaped, spindle-shaped, or round (May have tail-like process).

Table 2-4 URINALYSIS: MICROSCOPIC PROPERTIES (*Continued*)

Properties	Procedure	Normal findings	Comments
Cells (*Continued*)			
Leukocytes		A few present (0–3/HPF)	Usually indicates a suppurative process. Round or oval, granular, have an irregular periphery.
Erythrocytes		Normally (0–2/HPF)	Large number indicates bleeding. Tiny round or oval, slightly concave disks.
Casts			
Hyaline			
Granular		Normally not present	Usually present when albumin in urine.
Fatty			Indicates pathologic change in kidneys.
Waxy			
Mucous threads		Present in moderate amounts	
Bacteria		Normally free, but may be a few from urethral contamination	*Escherichia coli* in 80% of infections.
Crystals			
Acid urine			
Uric acid		Not present	If found in fresh specimen in presence of blood, may indicate kidney stones. Yellow or reddish-brown rosette-like clusters.
Calcium oxalate		Not present	Commonly found after ingestion of foods rich in oxalic acid. When presenting in clumps may be suggestive of kidney stones. Glistening crystals in small squares.
Amorphous urates		Not present	No significance.
Alkaline urine			
Triple phosphate			May at times also be found in neutral or acid urine. Colorless prism-shaped stars or rosettes.
Calcium phosphate			No significance. Large flat crystals with irregular or jagged edges.
Aluminum biurate			No significance. Opaque yellow spheres or needlelike clusters.
Others			
Trichomonas vaginalis			
Yeast			Usually contaminants.
Mold			

The vagueness of the symptoms associated with some urinary tract problems, and the inability of the infant and young child to communicate location and intensity of discomfort, make it mandatory for the nurse to assess this source of biophysical data carefully on each visit, or to take into account the need for this information in assessing the hospitalized infant or child.

The ability of the older child and adolescent to communicate, as well as the increase in specific body responses to illness and trauma related to the urinary tract, allow the nurse to be more selective in assessment procedures.

Blood (Hematology) The blood is a critical indicator of the internal physiologic status of the infant, child, and adolescent (also adult). Circulating blood comes in contact with every tissue in the body. The cell constituents are produced in various organs and structures (e.g., spleen, lymph nodes, and red bone marrow). As a result, any change in body tissues or organs and structures related to the formation of blood constituents will affect and change the circulatory blood. The ready accessibility of a sample of this tissue for screening increases the value of this assessment procedure. Most of the screening examination can be carried out on drops of blood obtained by pricking the heel or big toe in infants and young children, or the finger of the older child and adolescent. Normal blood values for specific age groups are found in Table 2-5.

Testing procedures Procedures for obtaining specimens and determining the specific blood values by any of several methods are available to the practitioner. Data may be used diagnostically; procedures are well within the skill and expertise of the nurse.

Special Tests All previous tests apply across the age continuum that is the focus of this book (infancy, childhood, and adolescence). There are a few tests that are age-specific for the adolescent, i.e., the individual who is at puberty or beyond. While two of the three tests described below are obtained from swabs or scraping of a mucous membrane, the third is performed on a urine sample.

Vaginal and cervical fluid It is important to collect this specimen before normal examination of the vagina and cervix. The speculum is lubricated *only* with water or saline.

Papanicolaou test (carcinoma determinant) Haynes, Meonegert, and Huffman (1965) state, "Annual cytologic studies on all women over 25 years of age will permit detection of precancerous lesions in time to avoid development of invasive cancer." With the number of sexually active adolescents on oral contraceptives, the age to begin periodic cytologic examination is 13 to 15 years.

The following is a procedure for performing the Papanicolaou test:

1 Using an Ayer spatula or wooden applicator, completely circle the cervical os.
2 Spread smear on slide no. 1, and treat immediately with a commercial fixative on a 50:50 solution of 95 percent alcohol and ether.
3 Repeat procedure securing smear from the posterior fornix (cul de sac) and add fixative.
4 Send specimens to pathologist for interpretation.

Table 2-5 NORMAL BLOOD VALUES

	Child	Adult
Erythrocytes	4 million	4.6–6.2 million/mm³ 4.2–5.4 million/mm³
Hemoglobin	12–14 Gm/100 cc	14–18 Gm/100 ml 12–16 Gm/100 ml
Hematocrit	3-month drop to 36 cc/100	40–54 cc/100 37–47 cc/100
Reticulocytes	1-week 0.5–1.5%	0.1–0.8%
Platelets		250,000–350,000 mm³
Leukocytes	8,000–11,000 mm³	5,000–10,000 mm³
Total	50%	50–70%
Lymphocytes	40%	20–20%
Monocytes	8%	3–9%
Eosinophils } Basophils	2%	1–2%
Bleeding time		1–3 min
Clotting time		2–6 min

Leukorrhea culture Secretion from the vaginal tract increases at puberty. Although many adolescent girls adjust to the increased secretion, a "discharge" is still a common presenting health problem.

Lewis[3] states

> When leukorrhea is brought up as a non-physiologic phenomenon, it is essential to search for clues that will identify the etiology.... In general, most of the patients in the reproductive group will have monilial or trichomonal infections whereas postmenopausal or prepubertal infections will be related to some form of bacterial infection.

The following is a procedure for obtaining a culture for leukorrhea.[4]

1 Using a fresh swab, secure a specimen of the vaginal discharge and add to test tube of normal saline.
2 Place a drop or two of this solution on a slide and check under the microscope for motile trichomonads.
3 The subsequent addition of 10 percent KOH to the slide will aid in the detection of *Candida* infection.
4 Using another fresh swab, secure a second specimen and swab it on Nickerson's medium for identification of *Monilia* infection.

Urine test for pregnancy This particular test is included in this category rather than under urinalysis because of the direct relation of the test to this specific age group. One of the most common screening tests available is the UCG test. This test requires approximately 2 hours to complete. The procedure for this test is included below, but it should be pointed out that several tests are available in clinics that do not require filtration or centrifuging and take approximately 2 minutes with high correlation to clinical findings, e.g., Pregnosis, Gravidex, and Pregnosticon.

The following is a procedure for performing the UCG test.

1 Patient usually advised not to eat or drink anything after 8:00 P.M.
2 Collect first early morning specimen.
3 Refrigerate specimen until ready for testing.
4 Dilute one volume of urine with two volumes of distilled water. Filter or centrifuge if turbid.*
5 Using two supplied test tubes, label one C for control and the other P for patient and place vertically on rack.*
6 Fill to line (on included dropper) from control solution (bottle no. 1) and place in control test tube.*

* Developed from information provided by Wampole Laboratories, 1971.

7 Repeat procedure using UCG—antiserum (bottle no. 2) and place in patient test tube.*
8 With dropper (clean) or pipette, place ¼ ml diluted urine in each tube.*
9 Shake "cell suspension" (bottle no. 3) well and place 1 drop in each tube.*
10 Holding each tube, one at a time, flick with finger to create a homogeneous mixture.*
11 Allow tubes to remain undisturbed for 2 hours and read according to included chart.

Gonorrhea The third test included in this special group is the test for gonorrhea. Additional smears may be taken for dark-field study to identify *Treponema pallidum*, but the test is carried out in a laboratory. The test for *Neisseria gonorrhoeae*, however, is frequently done by the nurse in the clinic setting.

The following are the procedures for performing the test for gonorrhea.

Female
1 Swab vaginal vault with charcoal-coated swabs.
2 Place immediately in transport media.
3 Use second swab for urethral orifice after examination of Skene's glands.
4 Interpret.

Male
1 Swab urethral orifice.
2 Place in transport media.
3 Interpret.

SUMMARY

Data collected from biochemical testing are added to the data elicited by history, physical assessment, and developmental testing to provide a health status base line on the initial (or early) contact of the nurse and infant, child, or adolescent. Subsequent assessments will include, when appropriate, one or more biochemical analyses to support clinical nursing observations and continuity of care, or to provide the necessary data for referral to the physician. In order to prevent fragmentation of nursing care, the collection and interpretation of the data must be systematic, and problems must be identified and recorded concisely.

REFERENCES

1 M. Green and J. B. Richmond, *Pediatric Diagnosis*, W. B. Saunders Company, Philadelphia, 1962.
2 V. Tucker, "Urinary Tract Infections in Children," lecture presented to undergraduate nursing students at the University of Kansas Medical Center, Kansas City, Kansas, 1970 and 1971.

3 G. C. Lewis, "Office Gynecology," *American Family Physician*, 5(3):130, March 1972.
4 F. J. Hofmeister, "Guide to the Complete Gynecologic Examination," *Hospital Medicine* 7(7), July 1971.
5 Wampole Laboratories, Directions and Technical Information UCG-Test, Stanford, Conn. 1971.

BIBLIOGRAPHY

Allport, G. W.: *Pattern and Growth in Personality,* Holt, Rinehart and Winston, Inc., New York, 1961.
Al-Rashid, R. A.: *Pediatric Hematology Case Studies*, Medical Examination Publishing Co., Inc., Flushing, N.Y., 1972.
Anastasi, A.: *Psychological Testing*, The Macmillan Company, New York, 1959.
Bauer, J. D., Ackerman, P. G., and Toro, G.: *Bray's Clinical Laboratory Methods*, The C. V. Mosby Company, St. Louis, 1968.
Buros, O. K.: *Mental Measurements Yearbook*, Rutgers University Press, New Brunswick, N.J., 1972.
Erikson, E. H.: *Identity—Youth and Crises*, W. W. Norton & Company, Inc., New York, 1968.
———: *Childhood and Society*, W. W. Norton & Company, Inc., New York, 1963.
Flanell, J. H.: *The Developmental Psychology of Jean Piaget*, Van Nostrand Reinhold Company, New York, 1963.
Frankels, S., Reitman S., and Sonnenwerth, S.: *Gradwahl's Clinical Laboratory Methods and Diagnosis*, The C. V. Mosby Company, St. Louis, 1970.
Haynes, D. M., Meonegert, N. F., and Huffman, J. W.: "Essentials of Gynecologic History and Examination," Smith, Kline and French Laboratories, Philadelphia, 1965.
Illingsworth, R. S.: *The Development of the Infant and Young Child: Normal and Abnormal*, E. and S. Livingstone, Ltd., Edinburgh, 1960.
Kunin, C. M.: *Detection, Prevention and Management of Urinary Infections*, Lea & Febiger, Philadelphia, 1972.
Nelson, W. E.: *Textbook of Pediatrics*, W. B. Saunders Company, Philadelphia, 1964.
Sutterby, D. C., and Donnely, G. F.: *Perspectives in Human Development*, J. B. Lippincott, Philadelphia, 1973.

PHYSICAL ASSESSMENT

MARTHA UNDERWOOD BARNARD

The skill of doing a physical assessment on a child is one of many tools that provides the nurse with an accumulation of data on the patient and his present health status. It is by no means the only tool that should be used in the nursing assessment, but should be used with other skills that lead to the problem list and eventually the nursing diagnosis. The purpose of this chapter is to present the application of the significant techniques used in the examination of the pediatric-aged child.

THE ART OF ASSESSMENT

Physical assessment is accomplished by observation, auscultation, palpation, and percussion. At no time can one technique be used alone to determine the normal from the abnormal. These four techniques, along with interviewing and observation used during history-taking and testing, can help determine the problem list and nursing diagnosis that will be discussed in later chapters.

Observation and interviewing have been defined earlier, in Chapter 1. Both are used either separately or together along with auscultation, percussion, and palpation while doing the physical assessment. At no time should these latter three be used without observing, instructing, and asking the patients questions at the same time.

Palpation is the technique of applying the hands to parts of the patient's body to determine any underlying deviations from the normal. Auscultation is the technique of listening, either with the naked ear or with a stethoscope, for sounds in specific areas of the patient's body in order to distinguish normal from abnormal sounds. Percussion, on the other hand, is "the technique of tapping an area of the body and noting the sounds produced and the resistance encountered."[1]

The sounds produced by percussion in health and disease are arbitrarily classified into four major categories, each recognized by its distinctive acoustic properties of pitch, intensity, quality, and duration.[2] They are (1) resonance; (2) dullness; (3) flatness; (4) tympany and variations; (5) impaired resonance (relative dullness intermediate between resonance and dullness); and (6) hyperresonance (lower pitch than resonance) (see Fig. 3-1).

INSTRUMENTS

The instruments used for the physical assessment are ophthalmoscope, otoscope, flashlight, stethoscope, sphygmomanometer, percussion hammer, and tuning fork. In addition, toys for the child from

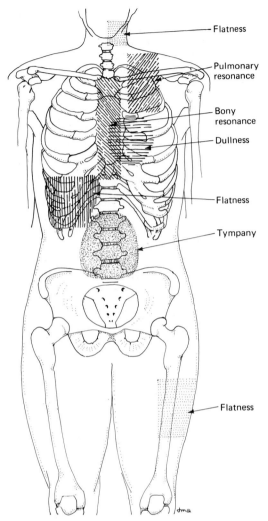

Flatness

Pulmonary resonance

Bony resonance

Dullness

Flatness

Tympany

Flatness

Figure 3-1 Areas where some sounds can be elicited during percussion.

1 to 6 or the Denver Developmental Screening Test (DDST) kit should be used to evaluate development, special senses, and the central nervous system. Special instruction should be given to all nurses concerning the use of these instruments and techniques for physical assessment.

GENERAL CONSIDERATIONS

Physical examination in the child is a very unique skill. Much of it can be carried out while the mother, with the child, is being interviewed by just observing the child and his actions and reactions to his environment and the individuals in the environment. When the actual examination starts, the age of the child and his previous experience with an examination must be taken into consideration when determining what part of the body is inspected first and whether the child is to be held on his mother's lap (Table 3-1). If developmental milestones are taken into consideration, one should be able to eliminate the anxiety that many children go through when the privacy of their body is intruded. The majority of the time the nurse should not assume that the child will not be embarrassed or frightened by having a physical examination performed on his body.

The significant difference between the examination of an adult and the examination of a child is that the basis of the entire physical examination is growth and development. The nurse should know the changes the child goes through at different stages of development and their significance to identifying normal and abnormal characteristics during the examination.

Realizing that any approach toward the child may set him off into a crying spell, the examiner must keep in mind that while the child is calm and not threatened should be the time to elicit as much information as possible. For example, while the child is sitting in the secure position of his mother's lap, the examiner might want to count respirations, watch for color changes, and observe for some developmental tasks. On the other hand, the examination of the newborn may start with auscultation of the chest and heart in order that an accurate examination can be done before the neonate is awakened and starts crying. The examination on the young child begins with the least threatening part of his body, for example, the extremities, and proceeds to the most threatening. The examination of the older school-age child or adolescent could be performed in a systematic manner very similar to the approach taken with the adult. In all approaches to the pediatric-age child the examiner should bear in mind that the age of the child and/or the developmental level determines the approach taken.

PHYSICAL ASSESSMENT
Linear Measurements

The first section of the physical assessment to be considered is the vital signs and linear measurements. It comprises height, weight, blood pressure, and pulse and respiration rates.

Height and Weight Height and weight should be measured at each physical assessment and should be done at least five times during the first year of life. After vital signs of the newborn infant have been

Table 3-1 APPROACH TO PHYSICAL EXAMINATION

Age	Physical examination	Approach
0–4 months	1 Observe color and respirations first.	Approach while asleep or quiet.
	2 Auscultate heart and chest. Count pulse and respirations.	
	3 Palpate anterior and posterior fontanels.	Place infant in mother's arms.
	4 Measure head circumference.	
	5 Palpate the abdomen.	Give infant bottle.
	6 Examine genitalia and rectum.	
	7 Examine eyes, ears, nose, and throat.	Place infant in mother's arms.
	8 Test central nervous system development.	Observe and examine infant on table.
4–12 months	1 Observe color and respirations first.	Place infant in mother's lap.
	2 Auscultate heart and chest.	Distract infant with bottle or rattle.
	3 Palpate anterior and posterior fontanels and measure head circumference.	
	4 Examine abdomen, genitalia, and rectum.	Upright position first in mother's lap and lying down after this.
	5 Examine eyes, ears, nose, and throat.	In mother's lap.
	6 Test central nervous system development.	
1–3 years	1 Observe for general appearance and growth and development.	Child should be allowed to play with familiar tools, e.g., tongue blade, flashlight, stethoscope.
	2 Examine extremities and central nervous system.	
	3 Examine neck.	
	4 Examine chest and heart.	In mother's lap or walking in examining room.
	5 Examine abdomen.	
	6 Examine genitalia.	Allow child to have a security object.
	7 Examine rectum; head; eyes, ears, nose, and throat; mouth.	
3–6 years	1 Examine head; neck; chest; heart; abdomen; extremities.	Talk to the child. Use flattery.
	2 Evaluate central nervous system development.	Allow to sit in mother's lap if he so desires.
	3 Examine eyes; ears; mouth; throat; genitourinary system.	Use familiar instruments, e.g., telephone, stethoscope. Allow child to play with instruments.
6–9 years	Perform physical in orderly fashion with genitourinary last.	Mother present in room. Use flattery. Ask child questions. Familiarize patient with instruments. Encourage cooperation. Give patient choice if parents should remain in room for examination.
9–12 years	Perform physical in orderly fashion with genitourinary last.*	Obtain history from adolescent. Provide privacy for examination. Offer anticipatory instruction.

* Development is assessed throughout entire history and physical.

maintained and the body temperature stabilized, the initial assessment for height and weight should be performed. The average length for the newborn infant is 18 to 20 inches; the male infant is on the average longer than the female. The weight of the newborn infant should range from 7 to 7½ lb. Again, the male infant is usually heavier than the female. At no time can the 6-lb newborn be regarded as small for his age or the 8-lb newborn heavy. Consideration must be given to the ratio of the weight to the length, and only then can the full-term newborn be regarded as normal, heavy, thin, or malnourished. This ratio can be calculated according to Rohrer's ponderal index, which is stated as follows:

$$\frac{100 \times \text{weight in grams}}{\text{length in centimeters}^3} = \text{ponderal index.}[3]$$

The ponderal index describes how heavy the baby is for his length and age; the larger numbers indicate a heavy baby for his length, and the smaller numbers describe an infant who is thin for his length (see Table 3-2).

Table 3-2   ROHRER'S PONDERAL INDEX RANGE

Range:
    3.00 = Heavy for length
    2.54 = Average
    2.21 = Light for length

Growth grids (standard anthropometric charts) should be used for recording the height and weight. These records will show the growth profile of a patient and whether the child maintains his own base line on the growth grid. Any child who is plotted on the chart and is found to be in the third percentile or lower or in the ninety-seventh percentile or greater deserves a careful evaluation; the height and weight of the parents and grandparents should also be evaluated. In addition, a careful examination should be made for possible nourishment, heart, endocrine, renal, and metabolic problems. It should be remembered that there is a wide range of normal growth and that individual children tend to have growth spurts at different times of their lives. A child that has been maintaining the 3 percent for all his life may be found to be perfectly normal, but the child that has been in the 50 percent group and suddenly drops below the 10 percent has to be considered for thorough evaluation. The most common causes for growth deviations of a child from the norm on a standard chart are nourishment causes and the genetic influences of both parents and grandparents.

In addition the crown to rump length should be calculated to determine if the child has child or adult body proportions (see Fig. 3-2). This is calculated by sitting the child and measuring from the vertex of the head to the point at which the child's buttocks touch the table. Crown to rump length represents 70 percent of the total height at birth, decreases to 60 percent at 2 years of age, and finally becomes about 52 percent at 10 years of age. The child is thought to have infantile stature if the sitting height is greater than one-half the standing height. However, if the sitting height is one-half or a little greater than the standing height, the child is said to have adult stature. If the child has an adult stature before 10 years of age, problems such as dwarfism and sexual precocity should be suspected. On the other hand, if the child is late in developing the adult stature, hypothyroidism or other serious pathologic problems should be suspected and thoroughly checked out.

Children that are found to be very high on the growth grids are rare but should be thoroughly evaluated for nutritional status. Obesity may be due to psychologic factors. On the other hand, the most common cause for the failure to gain weight is malnourishment. Pathologic problems must be kept in mind as possible causes for any of these deviations. A table has been developed to guide the practitioner in anticipating the amount of weight gain that can be expected of children at different ages.

The next measurement that should routinely be taken and plotted on the standardized chart is the head circumference. This in comparison with the chest circumference should help the nurse indicate if the circumference is progressing normally or if it is indicating any presence of pathology. At birth the average size of the head circumference is 37 cm and the average size of the chest is 35 cm. The tape is placed around the greatest circumference of the head (over the occiput and over the supraorbital ridges) for measurement. The chest circumference is measured midway between inspiration and expiration; the tape should be placed right across the nipple line. Measurements should be taken immediately after birth and then three to four days later to determine the head circumference after the edema and molding processes have resolved. A formula that can be used to evaluate head size is 0.5 of length in cm + 10 = normal head circumference in centimeters. Head circumference should be taken routinely on patients of all ages.

Vital Signs

Temperature   The normal temperature for the child is 99.6°F rectally, 98.6°F orally, and +97.4°F (36.3°C) axillary. These can vary greatly in the child with the least little disturbance of the metabolic rate. The temperature should be taken rectally in children up to 5 years of age and then orally. Axillary temperature can also be used if the need arises. The temperature should be taken before the newborn, or child, has been disturbed. The length of time for taking a temperature depends on the method initiated and can range from a few seconds with the electronic thermometer to 3 minutes which should be allowed for taking the rectal temperature.

Table 3-3   ANTICIPATED WEIGHT GAIN

Newborn (NB)	7 lb
NB–5 months	second 7-lb gained
12 months	third 7-lb gained
24 months	fourth 7-lb gained

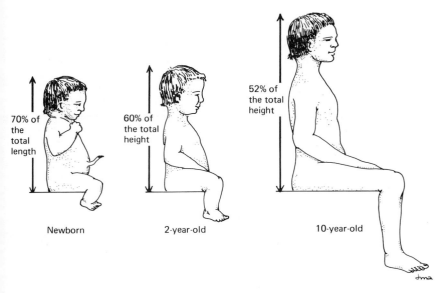

70% of the total length

Newborn

60% of the total height

2-year-old

52% of the total height

10-year-old

Figure 3-2 Average crown-to-rump length for a newborn, a 2-year-old, and a 10-year-old.

After the birth, the newborn's temperature drops and varies with the temperature of his environment. Usually the temperature does not stabilize before the first week of life. Hypothermia in the newborn may indicate infection as hyperthermia does in children.

If fever exists, the nurses should make every attempt to identify the cause. Low-grade fevers are of great significance and should be followed up with a medical evaluation. It may be of some importance for the nurse to have a mother keep a record of the child's temperature for several days. This may give important diagnostic information.

It should also be kept in mind that children tend to have convulsions after their temperature has reached 104°F (40°C). Every attempt should be made to identify a history of these febrile convulsions and to prevent them.

Heart and Respiration Rate   The pulse rate is also of some significance. It is usually obtained in children either apically or radially. Taking the temporal, carotid, pedal, popliteal, and femoral pulses is also important to evaluate circulatory status. In the young child the pulse should be counted for a full minute since there are some irregularities. If the older child is being evaluated for cardiac status, his pulse should be taken for 1 minute. In addition to rate and rhythm, the location should be noted.

Respirations are the next measurement. Rate, rhythm, and any retractions should be noted at this time. Again, it is preferable to take these for a full minute, especially in the infant or the ill child. These, like the pulse, should be compared with the norms for the age of a particular child (see Table 3-4).

Blood Pressure   The blood pressure is the final vital sign to be measured. Again, this should be measured after all others and before the child has the chance to become excited. Blood pressures can be measured several ways, such as by auscultation, palpation, or the flush method. The blood pressure cuff should be measured in all these methods and should never be less than one-half or more than two-thirds of the part of the extremity used. A narrow pressure cuff will give an abnormally high reading, and a wide cuff will give an abnormally low reading (see Fig. 3-3). Usually the arms are used for measuring the blood pressure; however, in the case of cardiac patients or suspected cardiac patients, the

Table 3-4   NORMAL PULSE AND RESPIRATORY RATES FOR SPECIFIC AGES

Age	Pulse	Respirations
Newborn	110–160	30–40
2 years	100–140	28–32
4 years	90–96	24–28
6 years	80–90	24–26
8 years	80–84	22–24
10 years	80–84	22–24
12 years	78–80	18–20

Note: These are averages only and vary with the sex of the child.

blood pressure should be taken in all four extremities for the purpose of comparison and also for the purpose of identifying the patient with coarctation of the aorta.

The flush method is most frequently used to obtain blood pressure in infants. The cuff is applied to an extremity. Then the extremity is elevated and an elastic bandage is placed on the lower or exposed part of the extremity (see Fig. 3-4). This will milk or occlude the blood from the exposed part of the inflated cuff. The cuff has been inflated above the expected blood pressure for this patient. The bandage is removed and the nurse starts to deflate the cuff while another nurse watches the pale extremity. At this point the pressure in the cuff is slowly reduced, and the observer states when the first flushing is noted in the extremity. It is at the point of the first flushing that the average between the systolic and diastolic pressures can be attained.

In addition, the pulse pressure should be noted. This usually varies from 20 to 50 mm of pressure. A widening pulse pressure may be a sign of increased intracranial pressure, and narrowing pulse pressure may indicate such things as aortic stenosis.

General Appearance

The general appearance should be included next in the physical examination. This can be evaluated by

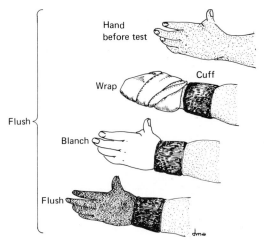

Figure 3-4 Flush blood pressure.

simply looking at the child during the history-taking and while the physical examination is being performed. The nurse should observe the child for acute distress, cleanliness, alertness, mood, color, size, and proportions.

Head

The physical examination will continue to the head. The measurements of the head have already been discussed above. In addition, the fontanels should also be measured. It should be stressed that the examination and measurement of the head should be done while the child is calm and in an upright position.

The anterior fontanel is the first one to be measured. Measurements vary with children, averaging about 1½ or 2 cm. The anterior fontanel, a diamond-shaped opening, can increase during the first 6 months of life and then start to diminish in size. It can also be as large as 4 or 5 cm and still be normal, but if it is this large, it should be referred to a physician for an evaluation. The anterior fontanel usually will be closed between 12 and 18 months, but can close as early as 9 months and still be normal. The posterior fontanel, a triangular-shaped opening, can be found in the midline of the occiput and usually is about the size of the end of an average-sized index finger. This can be expected to close from 2 to 3 months and as late as 4 months.

Bulging, tense, full, or sunken fontanels should be identified. A bulging fontanel can note serious problems such as hydrocephalus, hemorrhage, or any other cause of increased intracranial pressure. On the other hand, the sunken fontanel may indicate

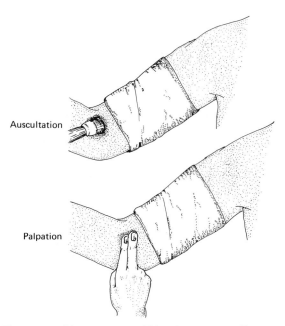

Figure 3-3 Measurement of blood pressure cuff.

dehydration or malnutrition. If the head is abnormally small in comparison with the size of the chest, length, or weight, microcephaly should be considered. In addition, if the size of the head and chest are disproportionate, increased intracranial pressure as well as microcephaly should be considered, depending on whether the head is large or small in comparison with the chest. It must be stressed that fontanels must be checked when the child is not crying. If a fontanel is bulging when the child is crying, the examiner must be sure that it returns to normal tensity when the crying has stopped.

In addition to the fontanels being examined, the suture lines must also be closely palpated and observed. Suture lines may overlap shortly after birth. However, this overlap disappears in a few days and can be palpated as small ridges until about six months of life. Abnormal sutures that are extremely wide should make the examiner suspect hydrocephalus or other causes of increased intracranial pressure.

In the examination of the rest of the head the examiner should palpate and observe for any abnormal ridges, caput succedaneum, cephalohematomas, craniotabes, asymmetry, growth, bruises, scratches, or flattening. These findings may indicate other types of pathologic conditions. For example, flattening of the occiput may be due to (1) lying in one position; (2) the intrauterine position; (3) premature suture closure or torticollis; or (4) abnormal intracranial growth.

Percussion of the head can determine the possibility of a subdural hematoma. This is done in the same manner that the heart is percussed. The percussion should take place over the saggital suture. Dullness would indicate one positive sign for diagnosing the subdural hematoma.

The skull can also be auscultated with the bell of the stethoscope for bruits. Continuous or systolic bruits can be heard in children up to 4 years of age and still be normal. These bruits can be heard over the orbital areas and considered normal. Any time the bruit is heard after that age, pathology must be suspected.

Additionally the need for transillumination of the skull may arise at any time there is a question about head circumference, size of the fontanel, or shape of the head. This is done by fitting sponge rubber around the head of the flashlight so that there is a tight fit when the flashlight is placed against the skull. The procedure is carried out in a dark room with the child in his mother's lap (see Fig. 3-6). The flashlight is then turned on and placed at different points on the head. If there is an increased luminosity, it may be indicative of a subdural hematoma or other causes of increased intracranial pressure.

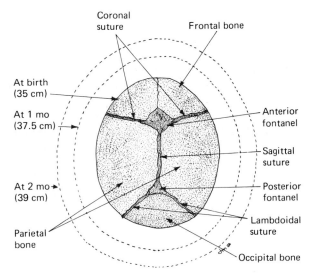

Figure 3-5 Head circumference and anatomical points.

During all the previous steps of the head examination the scalp should be checked for cradle cap, nits, ticks, scabies, and tinea capitus. Hair should also be checked for dryness, oiliness, and distribution.

Face

The face is then observed for symmetry and any evidence of paralysis. For example, when the newborn cries, the nurse should observe for any symptoms of one eye not closing, which may indicate a case of Bell's palsy. The older child should be able to smile and wrinkle his forehead so that the examiner can determine if any paralysis is present. Any twitching or ticks should also be observed for at this time. The examiner should follow this with attempts to elicit Chvostek's sign.

Color is evaluated next. Any cyanosis, jaundice, or pallor should be identified. Dark circles under the patient's eyes may signify allergies or fatigue. These dark circles should be differentiated from bruising.

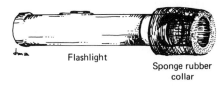

Figure 3-6 Flashlight used for transillumination of head.

Local edema around the eyes and over the parotid area should be observed for and palpated. The procedure for examination of the parotid area is done by having the child sit upright and look at the ceiling while the examiner runs his finger downward from the zygomatic arch to palpate for any swelling. Then the patient should be asked to lie down. If swelling is present, the parotid then falls back and moves the pinna of the ear forward. The sublingual glands and submaxillary glands should also be palpated for any enlargement. Any identified enlargement should be seen by the physician since it may indicate local infection, cystic fibrosis, or many other pathologic conditions.

Eyes

Examination of the eye should include the observation of the eyelids, eyelashes, conjunctiva, sclera, iris, and pupils. In addition, the examiner should palpate the eyes for turgor. A flashlight should be used to check the pupil reactions and their equality, and the ophthalmoscope should be used to check the opacity of the lens as well as the fundus. The examination should conclude with vision screening.

The eyes should be examined for any puffiness that might indicate edema. Questions should be aimed at identifying specific times of the day that the edema appears. If edema is present, the patient should be referred for further medical evaluation, especially in relation to renal problems. At this time the eyelid can be palpated to identify poor tensity as well as any tenderness or pain. The eyelashes should be checked to determine if the child has been either losing them or pulling them out. Observation for styes, foreign objects, infection, and scabies should also be included.

The nurse should note any excessive tearing or drainage. Drainage should be cultured if there is any question as to whether it is purulent. The cause of tearing, such as a foreign body, should be identified. Education should then be carried out in relation to the lacrimal ducts.

The conjunctiva should be examined for color and any type of abnormal growths. Following this, the sclera should be checked for any hemorrhage, discoloration, moles, or jaundice. The newborn's sclera may have a blue tint and be normal. However, a deep blue sclera may indicate a much more serious problem, such as osteogenesis imperfecta. Sclera may also have an occasional conjunctival hemorrhage during the first 2 to 3 weeks of life. Injected sclera may be indicative of an allergy, conjunctivitis, beginning glaucoma, eyestrain, or a foreign body, and should be followed up by a physician.

Pupil size, reaction, and accommodation should be checked. It should be noted if pupil reaction is present or absent. If present, the speed with which they react is observed. After reaction or before reaction the examiner should compare each pupil for size. Unequal pupils indicate a serious neurologic problem and should be referred immediately. The nurse should make sure that the light source used to determine pupillary response is equal to both eyes.

Muscle balance should be examined by checking the movements of the eyes as well as the corneal light reflex. Up to a few weeks after birth the newborn's eyes may wander individually. After the first 3 months of life vision should begin to fuse and become binocular. Some examiners may think that a child has strabismus but really have been mislead because there is a wide bridge to the nose of the child or there are prominent epicanthal folds. To rule this out, an examination by obtaining the corneal light reflex and a cover test will be in order.

The examiner now proceeds to rule out exophthalmos or endophthalmos. The two, if they occur, should be referred to the physician. The endophthalmos should not be mistaken for ptosis, which may be an important neurologic symptom. Exophthalmos is indicated when the eyeball appears to protrude, and endophthalmos when the eyeball appears to be sunken. The position of the eyes also should be noted. If the eyes appear to be below the lower lid, the child may have the setting-sun phenomenon. This could be normal if found in a premature or in some normal full-term newborns. However, it may be a sign of impending hydrocephalus.

Squinting or strabismus should be examined for early in life using the corneal light reflex and the cover test. The examiner performs the cover test by sitting directly in front of the patient and holding a light 2 to 3 ft in front of the patient's eyes. The patient is asked to focus on the light. The examiner then covers one of the patient's eyes and observes the opposite eye for motion. The test is repeated with the other eye. If the examiner observes motion in the uncovered eye, it suggests strabismus, esotropia, or exotropia. No movement of the uncovered eye means there are no abnormal deviations. Any deviation should always be referred to an ophthalmologist for evaluation if the child is past the age of 5 months.

Examination for nystagmus, an involuntary movement of the eyeball, should follow. The direction of the movements and whether they were in-

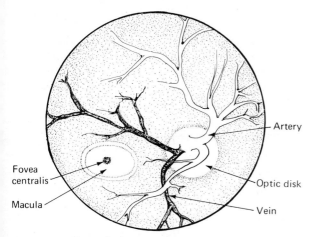

Fovea centralis

Macula

Artery

Optic disk

Vein

Figure 3-7   Normal eye ground.

duced should be noted. Their presence should alert the observer to some type of pathologic state.

Finally, the examination of the fundus should take place. It is preferable to do this in a darkened room. Many children need to be sent to the ophthalmologist so that their eyes can be dilated for accurate and thorough examination of the retina.

The child is placed directly in front of the examiner; a very young or frightened child should be placed in his mother's lap. The child is asked to look directly across the room. The examiner proceeds with the evaluation by sitting in front of the child and using his right eye to examine the patient's right eye and his left eye to examine the patient's left eye. The examiner should first select a +8 to a +2 lens for examination of the cornea, iris, and lens. Reassuring the child that he will see a bright light but that it will not be painful, the individual begins by shining the light in the pupil and moving closely. The examiner should immediately see the red-light reflex unless the lens is not clear. If the examiner is examining a non-Caucasian child, he will note that the red reflex is paler. If this red reflex is absent, cataracts or other pathologic conditions should be suspected. As the examiner moves closer, he will change the lens to a 0 to −2, making the landmarks of the retina much clearer. Abnormalities are then observed for in the retina such as a pale retina, blurred disk edges, papilledema, or a spot of blood that might indicate a retinal hemorrhage. The size of the veins and the arteries should be noted. They may be about equal in size, or the veins may be slightly larger. The vessels should then be noted for abnormal dilatation or abnormal pulsation. It should then be noted if they cup or dip down into the disk.

These conditions may indicate pathology and should be followed up by a referral to a physician.

Finally vision screening is carried out. Vision can be tested from very early in life and should be continued with routine examinations. The vision of the very young child can be tested by watching him track moving objects, bright lights, and bright colors. The child's pupil should also be observed to note accommodation. Vision is estimated to start in the first month and become much clearer by the sixth month. Any developmental retardation or the lack of interest of the child in his environment should make the examiner carry out a very thorough screening. Vision in the older child may be screened by the Snellen or the Titmus test. Any question about the vision should be followed with referrals.

Ears

The examination of the ear includes the position, the area immediately surrounding the ear, the outer auricle, the external canal, and the tympanic membrane. The presence of any tenderness or pain should be noted.

To begin with, the examiner should observe the position of the ears on all children. Low-set ears in newborns should lead the examiner to suspect the possibility of internal renal anomalies or the possibility of a trisomy. The top of the auricle should be equal with the level of the eyes. In addition, the nurse should note if the auricle of the ears stands out, which might indicate an outer ear infection, mumps, cellulitis, mastoiditis, or the possibility of congenital anomalies.

The area around the ears should then be examined for preauricular cysts and any type of fistulas. They can also be picked up with palpation of this area. If present, they should be referred for removal so that future infections can be avoided. The triangular fossa and other important landmarks are then observed for any abnormalities in shape.

The observer then will look for any evidence in the outer auricle of dried drainage. If found, the examiner should look for an otitis media. It is important while taking the history to see how long the drainage has been present and to eliminate the chance of the drainage being dried tears or dried milk.

At this point the otoscope examination should be initiated. The first and most important thing is to have an excellent light source. The ear can be manipulated by the examiner, and when doing so he should note if there is any pain. The speculum is fit so that the largest size is used and the tympanic membrane can still be visualized. This will avoid puncturing the membrane with the speculum. The otoscope is held firmly in one hand and that same hand rests on the head of the child in order to prevent the speculum from going through the membrane when the child moves suddenly. In the child under 3 years of age the auricle is pulled down in order for the examiner to view the eardrum. In the older child the membrane is pulled up and back for better visualization of the membrane. These manipulations are done because of the different ways the canal is positioned in children at different ages. The speculum is then placed very gently in the outer portion of the external canal to enable the examiner to visualize the outer canal. Any pain during manipulation or while the speculum is being placed into position may indicate the presence of a furuncle or otitis externa. At this time the examiner observes for any erythema of the canal which may indicate the presence of an infection or disease. However, if the child has been crying, this may cause the external canal to be injected, and therefore the examination should be delayed until the child has calmed down. If the membrane can not be visualized because cerumen is present, it may be viewed if a larger speculum is used to look over it. Additionally, if this does not work, the examiner should use a wire loop to remove the cerumen or irrigate the ear with tepid water or saline. Irrigation should never be done if there is any question that the eardrum might be perforated or if

any foreign body is present. Dizziness and/or vomiting may follow the irrigation.

The examination should be continued so that the tympanic membrane is viewed. The landmarks of the eardrum should be identified. First the eardrum is a pearl-colored membrane, translucent or opalescent. The light reflex, umbo, handle of malleus, and the short process of the malleus should be identified. The membrane may be injected either from infection, from crying, or from the process of manipulation. The light reflex starts at the umbo and goes anteroinferiorly. In any ear that is infected, the light reflex will be either dulled or absent. In addition, the translucency of the drum will be dull or gone. It may be bulging (from fluid) or there will be some injection of the membrane and the handle of the malleus will not be as clear. On the other hand, the membrane might be retracted. Any of these signs of pathology indicate a referral for treatment. Mobility of the eardrum can be tested, usually by the physician or a specially trained nurse. A tight-fitting speculum is needed. A rubber tube is connected to the outside of the otoscope, and air is gently blown into the canal. The examiner watches to see if the membrane is moved or if the light reflex moves. Absence of motion indicates disease, such as serous otitis.

The nodes are now felt about the ear. The tip of the mastoid is tapped, and the child is observed for any pain. Pain or tenderness might indicate a mastoiditis.

Hearing tests are performed as the final part of examination. Part of the developmental history may indicate a hearing loss. Examination can be done by using a watch to determine if the child can hear it ticking. Making statements to the child when he is not watching the examiner or when his back is turned may also help identify a hearing loss. Tuning forks can be used to identify either conduction or neurosensory losses. The vibrating fork's tip is placed over the tip of the mastoid and then placed over the examiner's. If the number of the seconds that the child can hear it is less than the examiner, there may be bone conduction loss, indicative of a neurosensory loss. If the child hears it longer, this indicates a conductive loss. Next the examiner places the tuning fork on the mastoid process, and then with the same number of vibrations places it about one inch from the ear. The child should hear the air-conducted vibrations longer than the bone-conducted ones. Last, the vibrating fork is placed in the middle of the forehead of the child. Normally the sound of the vibrations should be equal. However, if it is heard better in one ear than the other, it again indicates a neurosensory loss or a conductive loss.

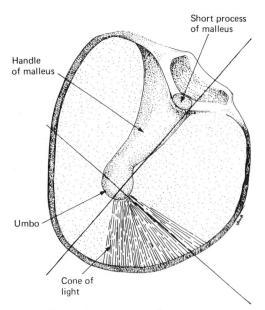

Short process
of malleus

Handle
of malleus

Umbo

Cone of
light

Figure 3-8 Normal tympanic eardrum.

In unilateral conduction hearing loss, the hearing is better in the good ear. If neurosensory deafness is present, the hearing is better in the affected ear.

Finally, the vestibular function test might be performed to rule out any brainstem or vestibular pathology. This is done by injecting cold water (65°F, 18.33°C) into the ear and turning the child around three or four times. Normally nystagmus should occur and if absent should be looked at as a definite sign of disease.

Any positive findings on these hearing tests behooves the examiner to send the child to an audiologist or physician for further evaluation.

Nose

A much-neglected area of the physical examination is the nose. It should be checked with the same care as any other part of the body.

To begin, observation should determine if the patient is breathing through his nose or his mouth. A newborn should have a stethoscope placed on both sides of its nares to determine their patency. This is done by blocking one side while listening to the other side. Any newborn with potential blockage of one or both sides of the nose must be considered a potential respiratory distress patient. A child who constantly breathes through his mouth may prove to have enlarged adenoids, allergies, polyps, or a deviated septum. These conditions are indicative of further follow-up evaluation.

The shape of the nose is then taken into account. One with a flat or saddle-shaped bridge may indicate a trisomy, congenital syphillis, cleft palate, or other conditions.

The alae should then be observed for flaring. Flaring indicates respiratory distress, and immediate follow-up should take place for respiratory assistance and to identify the cause.

The mucosa is then observed either by a speculum or by gently pushing the tip of the nose up. The color of the mucosa should be pink. Any paleness or extremely red or gray mucosa indicates pathology. Children with allergies have pale mucosa, whereas red mucosa indicates an infection. Gray mucosa should make the examiner aware of chronic rhinitis.

The characteristic of the secretions should be observed. Whether they are thin, watery, purulent, or bloody should be noted. Cultures should be carried out in the case of purulent discharge. Epistaxis should be noted. The point of bleeding is usually found in the lower anterior tip of the septum. Causes may be trauma, allergy, or a blood dyscrasia.

Finally, palpation and percussion should be performed over maxillary and ethmoid sinuses. Any tenderness may indicate sinusitis and may need medical follow-up.

Mouth/Throat

A careful examination of the mouth is frequently overlooked. To check the mouth and throat, the child should be in a sitting position, facing the examiner. The young child should preferably be in his mother's lap. In the case of an uncooperative child, the hands and feet should be restrained. In some instances it may be necessary to restrain the child in a supine position.

The examiner should ask the child to open his mouth. Sometimes some gentle stroking of the submandible helps the child relax and follow directions. As the examination proceeds, the lips and the area around the mouth should be examined for pallor, cyanosis, dryness, fissures, edema, and sores. The lips are more thoroughly examined for any asymmetry. This asymmetry should also be noted while the infant or child is crying. Then inspection should be carried out for the identification of cleft lips.

As the examination proceeds to the mouth, the examiner should ask the child to lift, move, depress, and stick out his tongue as much as possible without the assistance of the tongue blade. Asking the child to breathe through his mouth may help this procedure. If a tongue blade is a necessity, the examiner should give the child one to play with and examine first. The nurse might also have the child look in his or her mouth so that he knows what is being seen in his own mouth.

Any peculiar odors of the child's breath should be noted as they may indicate the presence of pathology such as caries, diabetes, diphtheria, mouth breathing, or poor oral hygiene.

The buccal mucosa is now inspected for moistness, distended veins, lesions, thrush, Koplik's spots, sores, cysts, or tumors. The gums and gingiva are then inspected for tenderness, inflammation, bleeding, edema, or any hypertrophy. Raised or receding areas of the gums should be noted. In addition, a black line at the margin of the gums may indicate some type of metal poisoning such as lead poisoning.

The teeth are now inspected for number, caries, fractures, abnormal formation, color, position, and hygiene. Teeth with flattened edges may be found in children that grind their teeth.

Salivation is next inspected. The consistency, amount, color, and odor of the saliva should be noted. Excessive drooling or the absence of salivation are significant symptoms.

The tongue should next be carefully inspected. The dorsal and inferior aspects are inspected for unusual color, tumors, sores, birthmarks, and moisture. The size is carefully inspected, and the position in which it is positioned in the mouth is carefully noted. The patient should be asked to protrude the tongue in order to note any deviation or tremors. The frenulum should then be examined to make sure that it is of appropriate length.

The geography of the tongue is then studied for any abnormal dryness, deep furrows, or scars. Scars may be an indication of a past history of convulsions.

Finally, the hard and soft palates are inspected for clefts, Epstein's pearls, abnormal areas of hypertrophy, and an abnormally high arch. All clefts, no matter what the size, must be referred to a physician. Any high palates or hypertrophy of the palates deserve close observation to make sure there are no impediments.

The throat is then examined. Placing the tongue blade back over the posterior aspect of the tongue, the examiner will most likely elicit the gag response. At this time a quick but thorough inspection should take place. The epiglottis should be observed during the gag for edema and erythema. If present, medical follow-up is indicated. The posterior aspect of the pharynx should be observed for drainage, erythema, edema, or abnormal growths or vesicles. The tonsils are also observed for edema, erythema, and the presence of exudate or a pseudomembrane. Red tonsils with an exudate may indicate a *Streptococcus* infection, and redness without an exudate is most likely a viral infection. A culture should follow most examinations where erythema is present.

The uvula is then inspected for mobility and length. When the patient says aaah, both the uvula and soft palate should move. Lack of motion may be an early sign of diphtheria or poliomyelitis. It may also be an early neurologic sign.

Finally, the examination is concluded when the patient is asked to speak. Abnormal hoarseness should have a follow-up, and for the older child who has difficulty pronouncing certain letters, a speech evaluation should follow.

Neck

The neck should now be carefully observed for any tilting, stiffness, or a painful motion. Both sternocleidomastoid muscles should be observed for any atrophy or signs of a tumor.

Children normally have palpable lymph nodes up to about 12 years of age. They may become quite enlarged with any infections of the throat or scalp. Any enlarged nodes should be palpated for tenderness, measured, and their location noted. Any that are tender and larger than a nickel should be seen by a physician.

Stiffness and nuchal rigidity should always have further medical examination.

The trachea should be palpated and inspected to note any deviation. This can be done by placing the thumbs to each side of the trachea above the suprasternal notches and carefully palpating up the side of the trachea.

The thyroid is also inspected and palpated. The examiner should stand behind the patient with the patient's neck hyperextended. Placing the fingers over the thyroid's lateral borders, the examiner asks the patient to swallow. Any enlargement or nodules can be felt.

Chest

The beginning of the examination of the chest is done through means of observation. The nurse should observe both the anterior and posterior aspects of the thorax. First the shape of the chest should be noted. A funnel chest, pectus excavatum, pigeon chest, barrel chest, or any other abnormalities are due careful consideration.

Any retractions should be noted and identified as to types and degree. At the same time any other signs of respiratory distress should be identified. Any grunting, rales, rhonchi, or wheezing should be listened for without the aid of the stethoscope.

Next, the chest should be palpated to rule out any cysts, tumors, or other abnormal growths. The clavicles should be palpated to determine the possibility of a fracture. The ribs are next to be palpated to determine if there is absence of any ribs as well as any tenderness over any part of the chest. Any lymph node enlargement should be examined for in the axillary and clavicle areas at this time.

Next place the hands at subsequent times over the lower chest, both anterior and posterior, with the thumbs adjacent to each other. Ask the patient to inhale, thus noting any asymmetry of the onset and the depth of the inspiratory movement. This procedure should also be carried out over the lateral aspects of the chest and over the shoulders below the clavicles as the patient is approached from behind.

The final technique of palpation should be to note the quality of vocal and tactile fremitus. This is done using the ulnar surface of the palm or the flat surface of the hand. Symmetrical palpation thus

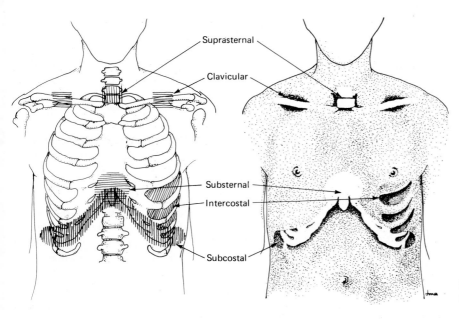

Suprasternal

Clavicular

Substernal

Intercostal

Subcostal

Figure 3-9 Areas of respiratory retractions.

follows when the examiner asks the patient to repeat the words *one, two, three,* and *ninety-nine*. The vibrations from the larynx should be transmitted to the thorax. The frequency of the voice should match the frequency *felt* in the thorax; this is known to be *tactile fremitus*. Also the frequency of the voice should match the frequency *heard* in the thorax, which is the *vocal fremitus*. The match is poor in adolescent females but there are good matches in males, newborns, and children. Any modification of the vocal fremitus indicates that either obstruction or consolidation of the respiratory tract may be present and should be considered a significant pathologic sign.

Percussion should now follow to identify any abnormalities of the percussion note. Abnormalities indicate the possibility of some pathology such as pneumonia, pleural effusion, enlargement of the heart, atelectasis, neoplasms, or birth defects.

Auscultation is the final part of the chest examination and most likely the most threatening. It again is done in a symmetrical manner over the anterior, posterior, and lateral aspects of the thorax. The auscultation of the thorax may be preceded by listening with the bell of the stethoscope in front of the nose or mouth; thus evaluation of breath sounds can begin to take place before disturbing the sleeping infant or child.

Following this, auscultation is done to note the breath sounds. The child is asked to breathe through his mouth and to breathe deeply. The younger child may be asked to blow on an object to accomplish

this. Children's breath sounds are almost always bronchovesicular or bronchial in nature. Decreased breath sounds may indicate pneumothorax, atelectasis, pneumonia, pleural effusion, or empyema. Increased breath sounds may be a good sign that a child is recovering from a bout with pneumonia. Any breath sounds heard over the sternum or vertebral column may signify the presence of a foreign body, mass, or some type of consolidation.

Abnormal sounds such as rales, rhonchi, pleural rub, wheezing, and grunting are listened for next. These abnormal sounds should be identified as being either inspiratory or expiratory in nature. Rales that disappear after coughing can be thought of as not being very significant.

Rhonchi must be distinguished from sounds that arise in larynx or trachea. Any sounds that are equal in intensity over the entire chest most likely originate from the larynx or trachea.

Throughout this examination the nurse should note any absence of voice sounds.

Heart

The examination of the heart follows the auscultation of the chest. The examiner should now auscultate the heart. The patient should be examined in the upright, supine, and left-lateral positions. Examination should also take place when the patient is leaning forward. The environment should be extremely quiet during the auscultation process. The newborn

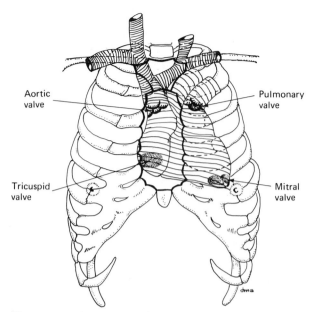

Figure 3-10 Areas of heart sounds.

and the infant should have their hearts auscultated while sleeping if at all possible.

The rate, rhythm, and any abnormal sounds are noted over the aortic, pulmonic, tricuspid, and mitral regions. If there is a slight speeding of rhythm during inspiration and decrease during expiration, this is known as a normal sinus arrythmia. Any tachycardia or bradycardia suggests pathology.

The heart sounds are evaluated next. First the location of heart sounds must be determined to rule out any heart displacement. The first heart sound is systolic in nature, and the second heart sound is diastolic in nature. The third heart sound is heard in many children. If three heart sounds are heard, they must be distinguished from the gallop rhythm, which is indicative of impending congestive heart failure. This might be done by palpating the chest. The gallop rhythm can be palpated, but the third heart sound can never be palpated. Also, the gallop rhythm would be present only if other signs of heart disease are present.

In some cases there is a turbulence of the flow of blood in the heart which is identified as a murmur. The examiner should identify the location, what heart sound they occur after, point of maximum intensity, pitch, and if it occurs regularly. He should also note if it disappears or increases after the child cries, exercises, or sits up. Any loud, continuous murmur diastolic in nature suggests medical follow-up.

After auscultation the nurse should determine if there is excess precordial activity. Then the point of maximal impulse (PMI), where the tip of the heart hits the chest wall, should be identified. This PMI is usually found inside the nipple line at the fourth to fifth intercostal space. In the younger infant it may be found outside the nipple line. If the PMI cannot be felt, this may signify the presence of fluid or increased air between the heart and the chest wall. Thrills may also be found during this palpation procedure.

Percussion should be initiated next and should be used to outline the cardiac margins. It might give the examiner some idea of the size of the heart; however, it does have limited value. Additionally any dullness should be listened for over the pericardial area during percussion; it may be suggestive of pericarditis.

Examination of carotid, radial, femoral, popliteal, and pedal pulses should identify presence, regularity, and intensity. Absence of any of these suggests pathology. For example, the femoral pulse is absent many times with coarctation of the aorta. In addition to examination of the pulses of the extremities, the temperature should also be noted. Cold, cyanotic, or pale extremities suggest the possibility of cardiac disease. In the older child, clubbing of the fingers should be identified.

The child should also be observed during or after exercise and feeding for color changes and exceptional fatigue.

Breasts

Breasts are examined in both male and female children. Engorgement is commonly found in newborns of both sexes. "Witches milk," equivalent to colostrum, can also be expressed from newborns' nipples.

No matter what age the patient is, the breasts should be examined for infection, abnormal growths, and tissue amount. Any child whose breasts develop before the usual, or normal, time should be observed for other signs of precocious puberty.

Abdomen

The examination of the abdomen requires a quiet child. The examiner cannot ascertain accurate data on a frightened and tense child. A bottle or nipple can be given a newborn or infant to relax the abdominal muscles. The older child is asked to breathe through his mouth and flex his knees to help him to relax his abdominal muscles. Any conversation that the examiner can conduct to distract the individual from the examination is most important. However, all these techniques will be of no avail if the examiner's hands are cold.

The examination begins by observing the newborn for a convex or concave abdomen. The concave abdomen suggests a diaphragmatic hernia, and the convex abdomen some type of obstruction. The neonate's umbilical cord should be observed for one vein and two arteries and for any signs of bleeding or infection. The older child's abdomen should also be examined for size and contour.

Peristaltic waves should be observed for in infants; they may indicate an obstruction. Also any distended veins should signify possible congestive heart failure.

Palpation begins with the lower chest or the inguinal areas. The beginning point should be determined by the point least likely to be the cause of difficulty. Using the hand lightly, the examiner should palpate for the liver below the midcostal margin. It should be palpable 1 to 2 cm below the right costal margin from the newborn period through infancy. More than 2 cm may suggest pathology. A small tip of the liver may remain palpable throughout childhood. The examiner should measure how far below the costal margin it is located and the consistency.

Next the spleen is palpated for lightly. Normally the spleen should not be felt. If it is palpable, pathology is suggested.

The hungry infant should be given a pacifier or a bottle when palpated for a pyloric tumor. The tumor can be found below the right costal margin just to the right of the midline of the abdomen. Other superficial masses are then palpated for over the entire abdomen.

Kidneys and deep abdominal masses are best felt on deep palpation when the child is inspiring or expiring deeply. Bimanual palpation by ballottement is useful for feeling retroperitoneal masses. This is done by placing one hand above the area being examined and one below the area. The ballotting hand should quickly thrust into the area being examined. Rebound tenderness may be elicited and masses felt.

Diastasis of the rectal muscles should be watched for. The protrusion's width should be measured and examined on subsequent visits.

The umbilical hernia is found commonly in infants. The defect of the abdominal wall should be periodically measured. Normally these disappear after the first 2 years of life or up to the time when the child begins to walk. They may be present up to the first 7 years of life in Negro children. The bladder is also palpated for distention and tenderness.

Inguinal areas are noted for any lymph node enlargement or any masses that might be present. Any mass of the inguinal area is always abnormal. Masses may be tumors, hernias, or undescended testicles and should always be followed up by a physician.

Percussion is carried out next over the abdomen. This is usually a tympanic sound. A dull percussive sound over the liver helps outline its borders; dullness over the other parts of the abdomen suggests abnormal growths or fecal masses.

Auscultation is finally carried out to determine the presence or absence of peristalsis. Hypoactive peristalsis suggests peritoneal irritation. Bowel sounds may increase with the condition of peritonitis. Absence indicates some obstruction. It is normally found in immediate postabdominal surgery patients.

Genitalia

The genitalia are carefully inspected for any abnormalities. Female patients are examined for synechia vulva, enlarged clitoris, masses in the labia majora, and imperforated hymens. Presence of pubic hair should be at the time of pubertal changes. Any vaginal or urethral discharge may indicate the presence of foreign bodies or some type of infection.

Male patients should be examined for the size of the penis. The position of the urethral meatus is noted in order to rule out epispadias or hypospadias. A urethral discharge should also be watched for in the examination. If uncircumcised, the penis should be inspected for phimosis or any type of infection.

The scrotum should be examined for the absence, presence, and size of each testis. The examiner should note any pain upon palpation. If the scrotal sac is enlarged, transillumination should be used to determine whether the enlargement is a hydrocele, a hernia, or a mass. An irreducible, transilluminated mass usually indicates a hydrocele. The mass that cannot be transilluminated may indicate a hernia. Any acute swelling of the scrotum should be seen by a physician since it may be due to torsion of the spermatic cord.

Finally, the cremasteric reflex is tested by stroking the inner aspects of the thighs. If the testis does not rise within the scrotum, it may be a positive neurologic sign or it may be normal.

Examination of the perineal area should follow to note any signs of abnormal growths or signs of

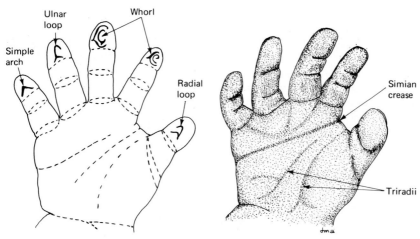

Figure 3-11 Palms, geographic creases.

any scratching. Scratching may indicate the presence of pinworms.

After this the anal region should be observed for any abnormal masses, rectal prolapse, or mucosal tabs. A well-lubricated finger is then used to perform the rectal examination. Any tear found in the mucosa indicates an anal fissure. Bleeding may follow this examination. Upon further examination the tone of the anal sphincter should be noted. A tight sphincter may be indicative of an anal stenosis and may result in constipation and pain upon defecation.

A shelf-like mass several centimeters above the anus may indicate aganglionic megacolon. It is also possible to palpate a retrorectal mass and the uterus during a rectal examination. The presence or absence of feces in the rectum should be felt for along with amount and consistency. Absence of feces in an ill child may indicate obstruction. Large amounts of feces may indicate anal stenosis, psychologic problems, or constipation.

Extremities and Spine

The extremities are examined by observing the child and his play activities. Any limited motion should be noted. Next observe the child while he is walking in order to identify any abnormal gaits or asymmetry and to rule out torsion of the legs or clubbing of the feet.

Next the extremities should be observed for any abnormal masses, sores, deviations, or extra digits. The temperature should be felt for as well as all the pulses mentioned under the examination of the heart. The hands and soles of the feet should then be checked for normal geographic creases or the presence of simian creases. Any signs of edema should be noted.

Following this the hips should be abducted passively to 180° to rule out hip dislocation. Each hip can only be rotated to a 45° angle if dislocation is present.

The spine is then examined for any abnormal curvature which might be present. The child may sit or stand in front of the examiner, and is then asked to bend over. In this way a curvature of the spine may be elicited. Lordosis can be identified from the lateral view.

The sacrococcygeal area is the last part of the examination. Any type of postanal dimple should have neurologic and cord defects ruled out. Any other mass, open areas, drainage, or signs of inflammation should be examined by a physician (see Chap. 40).

Neurologic Examination

The basis for the neurologic examination of the newborn through preschool-age child is development. A very thorough developmental evaluation should be performed, including the areas of gross motor, fine motor, language, and socialization development. This has been discussed more thoroughly under the section on testing. If at any time there are abnormal deviations in any area of development, a more thorough neurologic examination should be performed.

In addition to a developmental neurologic examination, the *mood* of the child should be observed, and a thorough interview conducted to elicit any information concerning his emotional health.

Any history related to gait deviations, dizziness, febrile convulsions, ataxia, muscle weakness, loss of muscle control, twitching, loss of any special sense, and meningeal irritation should be reason for a more thorough neurologic examination.

Meningeal irritation should be suspected if the patient complains of a stiff neck and resists flexing it. This resistance to bending the neck may not always be present in children with meningeal irritation. The examiner should also attempt to elicit the Kernig and Brudzinski signs. If either of these is elicited, the examiner should suspect meningitis.

The newborn should be examined for the presence of the primary reflexes. These should start to diminish around 3 months of age and be completely gone at 4 to 6 months. Any residual primary reflexes should be looked upon as a positive neurologic sign.

The primary reflexes that should be present are suck, grasp, Moro, tonic neck, sole plantar reflex, dance reflex, magnetic reflex, and spinal curvature reflex. In addition, the normal newborn should be in a flexed position, have good muscle tone, and should show no signs of muscle paralysis. Parts of this examination can be carried out while watching a newborn in his parent's arms. The reflexes should be tested systematically.

The older child's neurologic examination includes developmental history and evaluation, and evaluation of cranial nerves, cerebellum, special senses, motor development, and emotions (see Chap. 32). An adult can be normal and still have very strong deep tendon reflexes. However, when they occur in a child, it behooves the nurse to see that a neurologist follows up with a more thorough examination (see Chap. 32).

Skin

The last evaluation performed is that of the skin. Actually the examiner should have been performing this the entire time he was examining the rest of the body.

All areas should carefully be examined for color, abrasions, cuts, burns, and bruises at different stages of healing. This may alert the examiner to possible neurologic problems or the possibility of child abuse.

The head, forehead, ears, and skin creases of the newborn and infant should be examined for the presence of seborrheic dermatitis (cradle cap). In addition, the newborn's skin should be examined for milia, lanugo, vernix caseosa, petechiae, moles, and any birthmarks. Newborns may have erythema toxicum, but this can be considered normal. Moles and birthmarks should be evaluated medically.

Color is carefully appraised next. Any cyanosis, pallor, and flushing should be noted, and their relation to the child's activity considered (see Chap. 34). If jaundice is present, the examiner should note how many days since birth it began to occur and what parts of the body have it. The milligrams percent of the bilirubin can be predicted according to the area of the body that is involved. The only true bilirubin percentage can be determined by laboratory tests. If jaundice occurs within the first 24 hours after birth, it is considered a medical emergency.

Skin texture should be carefully evaluated for dehydration, malnourishment, edema, dryness, and scaliness. Signs of dehydration can best be checked over the sternal area and the medial malleolus. Edema found in dependent areas and around eyes should have further medical evaluation.

Skin rashes are common in children and may indicate allergic reactions, infectious disease, or heat rashes. These should be differentiated from petechiae which may be indicative of a blood dyscrasia. Rashes should be identified as to location and

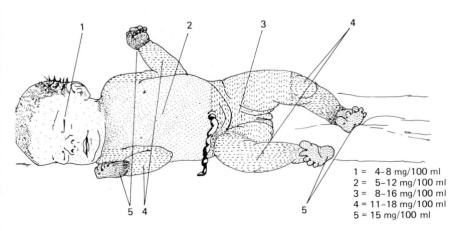

1 = 4–8 mg/100 ml
2 = 5–12 mg/100 ml
3 = 8–16 mg/100 ml
4 = 11–18 mg/100 ml
5 = 15 mg/100 ml

Figure 3-12 Estimating the degree of jaundice in the newborn. *(From Lloyd D. Kramer, "Advancement of Dermal Icterus in the Jaundice Newborn," American Journal of Diseases of Children, vol. 118, September 1969.)*

their characteristics (Chap. 41). The history should elicit any new allergens the patient has been exposed to or any exposure to individuals with communicable disease.

Diaper rash should be examined carefully to make sure that it is not caused by a monilial infection. If there is any question, a culture should be done.

Lesions, commonly found on the upper lip, but which are found in other areas of the body that are pustulovesicular in nature, may be impetigo. Again, any questions should be followed with a skin culture.

Herpes simplex is commonly found around the mouth and should also be referred for follow-up medical care.

The skin should also be carefully examined for tinea which is commonly found in the scalp and on the feet.

Pityriasis is another disease commonly found in children. The puritic papulosquamous eruption commonly found in skin creases may last 2 to 8 weeks. Again this dermatologic disorder should have medical follow-up.

Acne should also be examined for in the adolescent. History may elicit information that shows what aggravates this condition.

The hair and nails are also included under the examination of the integumentary system. Hair over the entire body should be examined for amount, distribution, and texture. Any signs of alopecia or dry or oily hair may be indicative of other systemic pathology. Early puberty hair (before 9½ years of age) should be followed up with a thorough medical examination to identify any others signs of precocious sexuality.

Finally, the nails should be examined for nail-biting, color, concavity, pitting, fissures, leukonychia, consistency, and inflammation. The presence of these deserve further evaluation.

In summary, the child's physical examination should be done in a systematic manner determined by the age of the child. This tool, along with history taking, developmental testing, and laboratory tests, should lead to the problem list that will determine what health professionals need to further evaluate and intervene with the individual patient and his family.

REFERENCES

1 E. Hochstein and A. Rubin, *Physical Diagnosis*, McGraw-Hill Book Company, New York, 1964, p. 140.
2 Ibid., p. 142.
3 L. O. Lubchenco, C. Hansman, and E. Boyd, "Intrauterine Growth in Length and Head Circumference as Estimated from Live Births at Gestational Ages From 26 to 42 Weeks," *Pediatrics*, 37:403–408, 1966.

BIBLIOGRAPHY

Alexander, Mary, and Brown, Marie: *Pediatric Physical Assessment,* McGraw-Hill Book Company, New York, 1974.
Barness, L. A.: *Manual of Pediatric Physical Diagnosis,* Year Book Medical Publishers, Inc., Chicago, 1972.
Green, M., and Richmond, J. B.: *Pediatric Diagnosis,* W. B. Saunders Company, Philadelphia, 1962.
Nelson, W. E., Vaughan, V. C., and McKay, R. J.: *Textbook of Pediatrics,* W. B. Saunders Company, Philadelphia, 1969.

THE NURSING DIAGNOSIS

BARBARA L. NEWCOMER and
VIRGINIA McDOWELL McCLELLEN

NURSING HISTORY AND ASSESSMENT
The Nursing Process—Diagnosis

A responsibility the professional nurse must assume is to design a system by which to make judgments regarding an individual nursing plan. The framework for this system must be based upon the collection of data through a nursing history and developmental and physical assessment. Data are gathered upon which to identify nursing problems, to formulate nursing objectives (goals), to determine plans for nursing care intervention based on scientific rationale, and finally to evaluate the nursing intervention. It is essential that the nursing objectives be well designed and carefully planned. The initial nursing plan must be retained as the basic framework, but must provide necessary flexibility as required for modifications and revisions.

To identify, understand, and meet the specific nursing needs of the patient, consideration must be given to specific steps of the nursing process. The first step in the nursing process is the initial assessment of the child's and/or family's need for nursing care intervention. This involves the collection of data regarding significant past history including developmental milestones, current patterns of daily living, present medical history, and current developmental level (see Table 4-1 for form and main items and "Case History" in Chapter 5 for a more comprehensive assessment). This step necessarily includes the analysis of objective and subjective data. It is imperative that objective data, exhibited actual facts not characterized by feelings and opinions of the nurse, be included in the data collection. Subjective data and introspective and reflective thoughts are also important sources of data, although it is important to keep such personal opinion at a minimum. The second step of the nursing process is a declaration of a problem list or nursing diagnosis. The third step is the formation of nursing care objectives. The development of nursing objectives forms the basis for the fourth step, which is the planning of the nursing care intervention. The planning of intervention must meet the objectives in relation to the nursing diagnosis. The fifth step is the actual initiation of the planned nursing care intervention. The sixth, and final, step is the evaluation of the planned and initiated nursing care intervention. Completion of the six steps forms a feedback system for continued reevaluation and modifications of the initial assessment, nursing diagnosis, and intervention.

When systematically assessing the child and family to obtain base line data, the pediatric nurse must begin by collecting information about the physiologic, psychologic, and social behavior of the child

Table 4-1 PEDIATRIC NURSING ASSESSMENT*

Child's name:	Informant:
Sex:	Date:
Birthdate:	Referred by:
Address:	Reason for referral:
Telephone:	Nurse:
Hospital number:	
Father's name:	Mother's name:
Occupation:	Occupation:
Age:	Age:

I	General observations
II	Parental view of presenting problem and/or medical diagnosis
III	Significant past history
IV	Early development milestones
V	Eating and drinking patterns
VI	Elimination patterns
VII	Sleeping patterns
VIII	Independence/dependence patterns
IX	Temperament
X	Play
XI	Discipline
XII	School
XIII	Present medical history
XIV	Current development level

* Expanded outline and completed form including answers, observations, and impressions are in Chapter 5, under "Case Study."

and the family. The nurse must also include as resources the family, other members of the health team, and all previous records. These resources will assist in clarifying and substantiating the initial data collected from the child. The primary techniques utilized in the collection of objective and subjective data are those of observation, interview, palpation, percussion, and auscultation. The nurse will find observation and interviewing techniques utilized in every nurse-patient interaction, but will find them directly valuable in the process of data collection.

In order to form a nursing diagnosis, the nursing history and assessment process to identify the child's strengths and problems must clearly be recognized as the function of a professional pediatric nurse. The unique function of the *professional* nurse may be conceived to be

"... (1) the identification or diagnosis of the nursing problem and the recognition of its interrelated aspects; (2) the deciding upon a course of nursing actions to be followed for the solution of the problem, in the light of immediate and long-

term objectives of nursing, with regard to prevention of illness, direct care, rehabilitation, and promotion of highest standards of health care possible for the individual."[1]

This statement necessarily implies the need for clinical thinking in addition to the clinical practice of professional nursing. Clinical nursing practice includes analytical thinking and direct observation of the patient for the assessment, planning, and implementation of nursing. The professional nurse collects data for evidence relative to nursing problems, evaluates the data, and arrives at clinical judgments.

The clinical judgments that the professional nurse makes on the basis of the nursing history and assessment process are the determinants of a nursing diagnosis. A diagnosis is

"the art or act of identifying a disease (or problem) from its signs and symptoms; investigation or analysis of the cause or nature of a condition, situation, or problem; a statement or conclusion concerning the nature or cause of some phenomenon."[2]

Even more specifically, McCain describes the nursing diagnosis as "... the identification of the patient's functional disabilities, or symptoms, as well as identification of his most important functional abilities."[3]

Problem identification is a result of nursing judgments which are based upon nursing skills. Therefore, a diagnosis is made intuitively when nursing problems are identified. An understanding and statement of the diagnosis are essential to the planning and implementation of nursing care intervention. It is not possible to effectively practice nursing skills without a clear-cut delineation of the nursing diagnosis in relation to nursing problems. In conclusion, the definition of the nursing diagnosis may be stated to be the identification of the patient's total problems as well as his assets.

In the process of collecting data to arrive at a nursing diagnosis, consideration of Faye Abdellah's 21 nursing problems is imperative. Abdellah presents in a logical, orderly method the problems that nurses must consider in the history and assessment process when forming a data base. Abdellah's list of nursing problems encompasses the total range of physiologic and psychologic aspects of human function, especially in relation to the promotion and maintenance of these functions. The 21 nursing problems are identified in Table 4-2.[4]

OBSERVATION AND COMMUNICATION

The skills of observation and communication are of primary importance in assessment, not only during the pediatric nursing assessment, but in any nurse-patient interaction. It is essential that the professional nurse become a highly skilled observer and communicator and continually work to develop and refine these skills.

Good observation requires several characteristics. Good observation is intentional; it has a purpose; it is outlined and planned in advance; and it is objective and truthful. Often the nurse may observe the child for both general and specific reasons, but observation is always purposeful. General observation is somewhat nonstructured and often is not focused on any one aspect of the child's behavior. An example of general observation would be the observation of a group of children playing together to determine parallel or group play performance. However, in specific observation the nurse is focusing attention upon a certain aspect of the child's behavior for a very specific reason. An example of specific observation would be the observation of the child for side affects after administration of a new drug.

Good observation is outlined and planned in advance. The nurse plans specific situations he wishes to observe and arranges to be present at the most opportune times to observe those situations. For instance, if the pediatric nurse wishes to observe the child's interaction with his mother, he arranges to be present during some part of the day when the mother is with the child. The nurse also makes general plans for the number and frequency of his observations in order to gain the most realistic sampling of observational data possible.

Objectivity and truthfulness are characteristics of good observation. It is sometimes helpful to compare and discuss observations with other members of the health care team in order to become aware of the similarities or differences in the data that others have observed. Professionals of other disciplines, such as psychology, nutrition, and physical therapy, observe children within a framework of criteria specific to their discipline. Comparison of findings from all disciplines increases the objectivity and truthfulness of the observations.

Recording of Observation

Once the nurse has become proficient in observation, the observation itself must be recorded accurately and perceptively in order to be effectively communicated to other members of the health care team. The events or behaviors observed should be recorded in the chart as soon as possible after they occur to ensure accuracy in recording the sequence and details. It is important to record exactly what the child did or said in descriptive terms. Personal opinion and interpretation should not be included.

Table 4-2 TWENTY-ONE NURSING PROBLEMS

1 To maintain good hygiene and physical comfort.
2 To promote optimal activity; exercise, rest, and sleep.
3 To promote safety through prevention of accident, injury, or other trauma and through the prevention of the spread of infection.
4 To maintain good body mechanics and prevent and correct deformities.
5 To facilitate the maintenance of a supply of oxygen to all body cells.
6 To facilitate the maintenance of nutrition of all body cells.
7 To facilitate the maintenance of elimination.
8 To facilitate the maintenance of fluid and electrolyte balance.
9 To recognize the physiological responses of the body to disease conditions—pathological, physiological, and compensatory.
10 To facilitate the maintenance of regulatory mechanisms and functions.
11 To facilitate the maintenance of sensory function.
12 To identify and accept positive and negative expressions, feelings, and reactions.
13 To identify and accept the interrelatedness of emotions and organic illness.
14 To facilitate the maintenance of effective verbal and nonverbal communication.
15 To promote the development of productive interpersonal relationships.
16 To facilitate progress toward achievement of personal spiritual goals.
17 To create and/or maintain a therapeutic environment.
18 To facilitate awareness of self as an individual with varying physical, emotional, and developmental needs.
19 To accept the optimum possible goals in the light of limitations.
20 To use community resources as an aid in resolving problems arising from illness.
21 To understand the role of social problems as influencing factors in the cause of illness.

Note: A logical, orderly method for identifying nursing problems resulted from two studies carried out by the Division of Nursing Resources, U.S. Public Health Service in 1953–1955. These problems are presented and described in *Patient-Centered Approaches to Nursing* by Abdellah and others and are reprinted here by permission of The Macmillan Company.

If the recording is accurate and descriptive, the person reading the record will decide for himself whether certain behaviors and interactions are appropriate or deviant.

Communication

Stressing the importance of communicating to other members of the health care team cannot be overemphasized. Opportunity for sharing facts, ideas, and feelings is provided through charting, shift-change reports, and clinical patient-care conferences.

The primary advantage of charting is that the material is written and remains permanent as a record. A disadvantage of charting is that frequently the written material is not objective or clearly stated. Too often, charted material is not read since reading it is felt to be time-consuming.

Communication shared during shift-change report provides staff members with knowledge of the immediate status of the patient's condition. The primary disadvantage is that shift-change report usually includes only members of the nursing staff for two 8-hour periods; therefore, information is not always communicated to the following shifts.

Patient-care conferences are advantageous, since members of more than one discipline attend. This provides the opportunity for sharing facts, ideas, and feelings of all health team members involved with the patient's care. There are two distinct disadvantages in communicating through patient-care conferences. First, such conferences are usually held only during day shifts, and so other staff members who would benefit are not present. Second, the entire staff cannot be included because of ongoing patient care responsibilities of the unit.

It is through communication that ideas and feelings are shared and exchanged by both verbal and nonverbal methods. Verbal communication uses words to convey these ideas and thoughts, and is expressed through written or oral channels. Clarity in expression enhances the probability of the idea or thought being accurately comprehended by others. Nonverbal communication includes posture, facial expression, voice inflection, and gesture to convey ideas and feelings. Often the use of nonverbal communication is unintentional, the communicator being unaware that either positive or negative influences are being conveyed to others. Nonverbal communication is inevitable whenever two or more persons interact. "It may well be that the science of communication is more pertinent to nursing than the science of disease or pathology."[5]

PROBLEM-ORIENTED RECORD SYSTEM

It is proposed that nursing accept the format of the problem-oriented record system[6] utilizing the techniques of observation and communication (interview) in the process of data collection. This system is effective, since it provides for long-term continuous feedback. Feedback is provided by the statement of all problems and a definite plan based upon scientific rationale for each identified problem. The progress notes are the evaluation of the problem and the evaluation of the intervention. Such a note serves as follow-up feedback. Continual feedback allows for correcting the statement of the problem whenever it is in error or for making a more precise, specific classification of identified problems. The problem-oriented record system is applicable to nursing in all environmental situations in that it can be utilized in both episodic and distributive areas of concentration in nursing practice. This form of problem identification is pertinent when considering the curative and restorative aspects of nursing as well as the prevention of disease and maintenance of the health aspects of nursing practice.

Initial Data Base

The initial data base forms the basic framework for identifying or diagnosing the nursing problem; for planning a specific course of nursing actions based upon scientific rationale; for evaluating the problem utilizing the progress notes; and finally, for evaluating the nursing care intervention. The data base is a guideline for further data collection when the period of study extends over a period of time,

Table 4-3 FORMAT FOR PROBLEM-ORIENTED RECORD SYSTEM

Problems:
1
2
3
Plan:
1:01
1:02
1:03
2:01
3:01
3:02
Progress note:
Plan no. 1
S: (Subjective)
O: (Objective)
A: (Assessment)
P: (Plan)

and it serves to determine validly designed objectives for care in the form of identified problems. The amount of time required to collect the data base, utilizing the pediatric nursing assessment format, varies from child to child and depends upon the nature and number of identified problems. The collection of pertinent information about the child serves as an initial data base and, in addition, as a basis for the collection of interval information during the period of study. The data base consists of information appropriate to the age of the child in the categories of environmental data, significant past medical history, early developmental milestones, present medical status, levels of impaired function due to illness, and current developmental level.

Problem List

When the format of the problem-oriented record system is utilized,[6] the problem list of identified nursing problems is apparent and readily available once it has been constructed. The format illustrates all problems at various stages of resolution and provides continuity with the identification of unsolved major problems. Critical factors relating to the child's nursing care plan and intervention are evident at a glance as the problem list is the first and most valuable part of each record. Each problem on the list must be numbered, titled, and dated, containing complete information in a precise manner. New problems may be added in a sequential manner whenever they occur. For example:

Problem list
10/13/71
1　Inadequate care of ileoconduit, appliance, and stoma.

Nursing Plans

The plans for all nursing care intervention must be keyed to the problem list. The list of nursing objectives and the plan must provide methods for further collection of data, for specific treatment, and for the education of the child and his family in relation to the identified nursing problems. Nursing objectives and plans must be based on the rationale of the biological and social sciences and the skills based upon them. For example:

Problem list
10/13/71
1:00　Inadequate care of ileoconduit, appliance, and stoma.

1:01　The social worker will record number of leakage episodes and time occurred for 1 week at home.
1:02　The teacher will record number of leakage episodes and the time of day occurred for 1 week in school.

PROGRESS NOTES

Progress notes are the evaluation of the nursing problems and intervention, and provide for considerable organization of factual data. The progress notes should include objective and subjective information. Results from physical examination or laboratory study, as they relate to specific problems, are a part of the objective findings. Statements by the child or family, clearly recorded as they relate to an identified problem, may be included as subjective information. The analysis of the objective and subjective data is utilized in further assessment for the gathering of interval data. In the process of evaluating the nursing problem and intervention, the nurse must include in the progress note specifically what the child and family are told in relation to problems and intervention. Stating specifically what the child and family are told will foster continuity of care and will indicate an orderly progression toward reaching nursing objectives. It is also necessary to include all counseling that is given to the child and family about episodic (curative and restorative aspects) versus distributive (prevention and maintenance aspects) areas of care in nursing practice. In addition to these two factors, in the final progress note at the end of the period of study the nurse must include exactly what medications are prescribed and their dosages, and where the child and family are referred for follow-up health care. Such information is vital for future health care and is readily available when included in the final discharge summary. An example of a progress note is:

Progress note
Problem 1
10/21/71
S:　Not applicable.
O:　Records were kept by the nurse for 1 week with the following results:
　　Thurs. 5:00 P.M.; 7:15 P.M.
　　Fri. 7:00 A.M.
　　Sat 9:30 A.M.; 12:30 P.M.; 4:15 P.M.
　　Sun. 8:10 A.M.; 9:45 A.M.
　　Mon. none
　　Tues. 7:30 A.M.; 12:15 P.M.; 7:30 P.M.
　　Wed. none

A: Data as to frequency and hour of day that urinary leakage occurred served as base line data.
P: Continue for 1 additional week.

The format utilized in problem-oriented charting is shown in Table 4-3.[6] Procedures for filling it out follow in Chap. 5.

INTERPRETATION

It is important that consideration be given to the analysis of the process of nurse-patient interaction. Interpretation, or analysis of interaction of the child's behavior, is the process of clarification, explanation, and elaboration. Interpretation is important since two individuals may view an episode of behavior within very different frames of reference. For example, two individuals observing the same child may view different behaviors as the primary problem. Also, two individuals observing the same portion of a child's behavior might give very different interpretations of it. Behavior is interpreted in relation to the observer's knowledge and experience as a frame of reference.

Once the data are gathered, they must be organized to show patterns of behavior. First, the data must be examined carefully and organized according to the systematic form provided by the pediatric nursing assessment (Table 4-1). Second, data must be analyzed, and generalizations or hypotheses must be derived. Third, the reliability and validity of the generalizations or hypotheses made about the data must be checked.

The pediatric nursing assessment of the child is the primary source for data collection. Personal observations of the child and of the socioenvironmental context of his behavior are vital components of the total nursing history and assessment. This necessarily includes observation of the child's family unit in regard to the dynamics and the interpersonal relations. Other data available for interpretation are the results of previously performed physical examinations and laboratory tests. It is also extremely important to analyze and interpret the reports from other health team members. Professionals of other disciplines, such as psychology, nutrition, and physical therapy, interpret the child's behavior within a framework of criteria specific to their discipline. Findings from all disciplines are important to consider in continuity of care. Conferences in regard to the child's nursing care plan and intervention are a source of additional data which must be included in the total analysis and interpretation process.

In addition to the above resources of available data, information about the community in which the child and family live, the home in which the child lives, and the level of development which the child has attained will be important in interpreting the collected data. Generalizations or hypotheses regarding the analysis and interpretation of the child's behavior may be affected by lack of sufficient knowledge about the data.

The procedure of data analysis is actually the objective assessment of collected data and the determination of the reliability and validity of the data. This includes the comparison of developmental milestones to the accepted norms, the determination of normalcy of the child's relations and interactions with others, and the evaluation of adaptation to the environmental setting. Determining trends in the child's behavior necessitates analyzing and interpreting all the available data collected from various sources.

The reliability of the generalizations or hypotheses may be determined by two general methods. One method is to ask an expert to analyze the data and then to compare the outcome or differences in interpretations. Another possible method is to reason through the data from generalizations (hypotheses) to specific facts and then from specific facts to generalizations.

In summary, the professional nurse has a responsibility to make a systematic assessment of a patient and his family. Once this assessment has been done and recorded, the nurse will identify the problems from the data base, make judgments on those problems, and plan a nursing intervention.

REFERENCES

1 Dorothy Smith, "A Clinical Nursing Tool," *American Journal of Nursing*, 68:2384–2388, November 1968.
2 *Webster's New Collegiate Dictionary*, 7th ed., G. & C. Merriam Company, Springfield, Mass., 1965.
3 Faye McCain, "Nursing by Assessment Not Intuition," *American Journal of Nursing*, 65:82–84, April 1965.
4 Faye G. Abdellah, *Patient Centered Approaches to Nursing*, The Macmillan Company, New York, 1960.
5 Dorothy Smith, "Myth and Method in Nursing Practice," *American Journal of Nursing*, 64:68–72, February 1964.
6 J. C. Bjorn and H. D. Cross, *Problem Oriented Practice*, Modern Hospital Press, McGraw-Hill Publications Co., New York, 1970.

BIBLIOGRAPHY

Abdellah, Faye G.: "Overview of Nursing Research 1955–1968," *Nursing Research*, 19:6–17, January-February 1970.
———, and Levine, E.: *Better Patient Care Through Nursing Research*, The Macmillan Company, New York, 1965.

"American Nurses Association's First Position on Education for Nursing," *American Journal of Nursing*, 65:106–111, December 1965.

"ANA/AAP To Draw Guidelines on Preparation of Pediatric Nurse Practitioners," *American Journal of Nursing*, 70:1833, September 1970.

Brown, Esther L.: *Nursing Reconsidered: A Study of Change*, J. B. Lippincott Company, Philadelphia, 1970.

Brown, Martha M., and Fowler, Grace R.: *Psychodynamic Nursing: A Biosocial Orientation*, 3d ed., W. B. Saunders Company, Philadelphia, 1966.

Campbell, Emily: "Not Education, Not Service, But Nursing: The Process of Change," *American Journal of Nursing*, 67:990–994, May 1967.

Cheitham, Evonna, Bautch, Judy, and Roberts, Sara: "Not Education, Not Service, But Nursing: Effecting Change," *American Journal of Nursing*, 67:995–997, May 1967.

Chioni, R. M., and Panicucci, C.: "Tomorrow's Nurse Practitioners," *Nursing Outlook*, 18:32–35, February 1970.

———, and Schoen, E.: "Preparing Tomorrow's Nurse Practitioners," *Nursing Outlook*, 18:50–53, October 1970.

Christman, Norma J.: "Clinical Performance of Baccalaureate Graduates," *Nursing Outlook*, 19:54–56, January 1971.

Committee on Nursing: "Medicine and Nursing in the 1970's: A Position Statement," *Journal of the American Medical Association*, 213:1881–1883, September 14, 1970.

Conant, Lucy H.: "Closing the Practice-Theory Gap," *Nursing Outlook*, 15:37–39, November 1967.

Corona, Dorothy F.: "A Continuous Progress Curriculum in Nursing," *Nursing Outlook*, 18:46–48, January 1970.

Dickoff, J., James, Patricia, and Wiedenbach, Ernestine: "Theory in a Practice Discipline," pt. I, Practice Oriented Theory, *Nursing Research*, 17:415–435, September-October 1968.

———, ———, and ———: "Theory in a Practice Discipline," pt. II, Practice Oriented Research, *Nursing Research*, 17:545–554, November-December 1968.

Dineen, Mary A.: "Current Trends in Collegiate Nursing Education," *Nursing Outlook*, 17:22–26, August 1969.

Elliott, Jo: "A Conversation on Nursing Service, Nursing Education and Economic and General Welfare," *American Journal of Nursing*, 68:792–799, April 1968.

Erikson, E. H.: *Insight and Responsibility*, W. W. Norton & Company, Inc., New York, 1964.

Etzioni, Amitai (ed.): *The Semi-Professions and Their Organization*, The Free Press, New York, 1969.

Goerke, L. S.: "Changes in Preventive Medicine," *Journal of School Health*, 38:1–8, January 1968.

Greenough, Katharine: "Determining Standards for Nursing Care," *American Journal of Nursing*, 68:2153–2157, October 1968.

Hurst, J. W., and Walker, H. K. (eds.): *The Problem-Oriented System*, Medcom Medical Update Series, New York, 1972.

Jacox, Ada K.: "Who Defines and Controls Nursing Practice?," *American Journal of Nursing*, 69:977–982, May 1969.

Johnson, Dorothy: "Consequences for Patients and Personnel," *American Journal of Nursing*, 62:96–100, May 1962.

———: "Professional Practice and Specialization in Nursing," *Image Sigma Theta Tau National Honor Society of Nursing*, 2:2–7, November 1968.

———: "The Significance of Nursing Care," *American Journal of Nursing*, 61:63–66, November 1961.

Kibrick, Anne: "Why Collegiate Programs for Nurses," *The New England Journal of Medicine*, 278:765–771, April 1968.

King, Imogene M.: *Toward A Theory for Nursing—General Concepts of Human Behavior*, John Wiley & Sons, Inc., New York, 1971.

Lambertsen, Eleanor: "Changes in Practice Require Changes in Education," *American Journal of Nursing*, 66:1784–1786, August 1966.

———: "The Emerging Health Occupations," *Nursing Forum*, 7:87–97, Winter 1968.

Leonard, R. C.: "Developing Research in a Practice-Oriented Discipline," *American Journal of Nursing*, 67:1472–1475, July 1967.

Levine, E.: "Nurse Manpower: Yesterday, Today, and Tomorrow," *American Journal of Nursing*, 69:290–296, February 1969.

Lifson, S. S.: "Our Changing Society—The Years Ahead: The Outlook for Health Education Practice," *American Journal of Public Health*, 58:678–683, April 1968.

Mauksch, Ingeborg G., and David, Miriam L.: "Prescription for Survival," *American Journal of Nursing*, 72:2189–2193, December 1972.

Murphy, Juanita F. (ed.): *Theoretical Issues in Professional Nursing*, Appleton Century Crofts, New York, 1971.

"Nursing in the Decade Ahead," *American Journal of Nursing*, 70:2116–2125, October 1970.

Orem, Dorothea E.: *Nursing: Concepts of Practice*, McGraw-Hill Book Company, New York, 1971.

Rogers, Martha E.: *The Theoretical Basis of Nursing*, F. A. Davis Company, Philadelphia, 1970.

Schell, Pamela L., and Campbell, Alla T.: "POMR—Not Just Another Way To Chart," *Nursing Outlook*, 20:510–514, August 1972.

Seward, Joan: "Professional Practice in a Bureaucratic Structure," *Nursing Outlook*, 17:58–61, December 1969.

Sheldon, A., et al.: "The Developing Role for the Nurse in a Community Mental Health Program," *Perspectives in Psychiatric Care*, 5:272–279, November, December 1967.

Silver, H. K.: "Pediatric Nurse—Practitioners Perform Expanded Care Role," *Hospital Topics*, 46:71–74, October 1968.

Smirnoff, V.: *The Scope of Child Analysis*, International Universities Press, Inc., New York, 1971.

Smith, Dorothy: "A Discussion of the 'Into, Out Of, Overall' Syndrome in Nursing," *International Journal of Nursing Studies*, 5:33–39, 1968.

———: "From Student to Nurse," *Nursing Outlook*, 11:735–736, October 1973.

———: "Writing Objectives as a Nursing Practice and Skill," *American Journal of Nursing*, 71:319–320, February 1971.

Thompson, Alice M. C. (ed.): "Focus on the Future," *International Nursing Review*, 16:195–196, 1969.

Weed, L. L.: *Medical Records, Medical Education, and Patient Care*, The Press of Case Western Reserve University, Cleveland, 1969.

PLANNING
AND
IMPLEMENTATION

BARBARA L. NEWCOMER and
VIRGINIA McDOWELL McCLELLEN

Before considering particular nursing functions of the extended role of the professional nurse, the nurse must survey the scope of nursing practice in this dynamic role. Pediatric nursing practice involves the provision of direct nursing services to children and their families as well as consideration of the total family unit. Regardless of whether episodic or distributive health care is involved, the interpersonal relation between the child, his family, and the nurse can be of short or long duration. Within the framework of episodic and distributive areas of concentration in health care, nursing practice functions must include primary care, acute care, and long-term care. An extended role for professional nurses performing nursing practice functions will increase the potential for availability and effectiveness of health care.

According to a report to the Secretary of Health, Education, and Welfare, prepared by the Secretary's Committee to Study Extended Roles for Nurses, in the current system of health care an important opportunity for change involves altering and expanding the practice of nurses so that they may assume considerably greater responsibility for delivering health care services. In addition, the Secretary's Committee has stated that as health care becomes increasingly valued in our society, nurses will be expected to take more responsibility for the delivery of nursing care, for coordinating preventive services, for initiating and participating in diagnostic screening, and for referring patients who require differential medical diagnoses and medical therapies.[1] The professional nurse functions as a member of the health care team by collaborating with professional colleagues in the planning and implementing of health services. In addition to functioning as an interdependent practitioner on the health care team, the nurse must also function as an independent practitioner when the needs of the patient (child and family) and standards and principles of nursing practice so warrant. As an interdependent practitioner on the health care team, the nurse functions in a mutually dependent manner with other health professionals involved with the child's care. The nurse as an independent practitioner exercises authority to think and to act in a self-governing manner.

Professional nurses are expected to function as independent and interdependent members of the health care team. In relation to nursing functions, the Secretary's Committee has drawn up lists (see below) of primary care, acute care, and long-term care functions for which nurses are now generally prepared and responsible and for which other nurses could be prepared.[2] The Committee's report states that certain of these functions should be the shared responsibility of both nurses and physicians. However, it is mandatory that professional nurses include these functions within the scope of extended nursing practice.

PRIMARY, ACUTE, AND LONG-TERM FUNCTIONS
Primary Care Functions

Primary care consists of assisting the individual in attaining and maintaining health. The major emphasis in primary care is on promotion of health and prevention of disease. Primary care functions for which nurses are now generally responsible are the following:

Case finding and medical referral.
Case finding and community resource assessment and referral.
Health surveillance of well babies and children.
Identification of the need for, and assisting in, the planning and implementation of needed changes in living arrangements affecting the health of individuals.
Evaluation of deviations from normal.
Assessment of the responses of patients to illness and prescribed treatment.
Prescription of modifications needed by patients coping with illness or maintaining health.

Primary care functions for which many nurses are now prepared and others could be prepared are

Routine assessment of the health status of individuals and families.
Institution and supervision of health care of normal children.
Management of care for selected patients within protocols mutually agreed upon by nursing and medical personnel.
Screening patients having problems requiring differential medical diagnosis and medical therapy.
Eliciting and recording a health history.
Making physical and psychosocial assessments, recognizing the range of normal and the manifestations of common abnormalities.
Making diagnoses, choosing, initiating, and modifying selected therapies.
Providing appropriate information to the patient and his family about a diagnosis or plan of therapy.

Acute Care Functions

Acute care consists of services that treat the acute phase of illness or disability and has as its purpose the assistance of the individual in activities contributing to health or recovery that will help him gain independence as rapidly as possible. Acute care functions for which nurses are now generally responsible are the following:

Recognizing syndromes and making clinical inferences.
Providing appropriate emergency treatment.
Providing appropriate information to the patient and his family about diagnosis or plan of therapy following physician-nurse appraisal.
Carrying out selected diagnostic and therapeutic procedures.
Translating research findings into practice.

Acute care functions for which many nurses are now prepared and others could be prepared are

Securing and recording a health and developmental history and making a critical evaluation of such records as an adjunct to planning and carrying out a health care regimen in collaboration with medical and other health professionals.
Performing physical and psychosocial assessments and translating the findings into appropriate nursing actions.
Discriminating between normal and abnormal findings in physical and psychosocial assessments.
Initiating actions within a protocol developed by medical and nursing personnel.

Long-term Care Functions

Long-term care consists of services designed to provide symptomatic treatment, maintenance, and rehabilitative services for patients of all ages. Long-term care functions for which nurses are now generally responsible are the following:

Teaching patients and family members to carry out the medical and nursing plans, taking into consideration cultural background, personal preferences, and financial status.
Observing and evaluating patients' physical and emotional conditions and reactions to therapeutic intervention.
Reporting new signs or symptoms and arranging for or initiating intervention when the patients' condition warrants it.
Assisting the patient and family to identify resources which will be helpful in maintaining him in the best possible state of health.
Making necessary changes in a treatment plan in regard to changes in the patient's physical or emotional tolerance.
Giving families correct information and emotional support and encouragement which may help them to adopt attitudes and practices which promote health and reduce anxiety, tension, and fatigue.
Making appropriate referral for continuity of care.

Long-term care functions for which many nurses are now prepared and others could be prepared are

Thoroughly assessing physical status of patients.
Securing and maintaining a health history.
Within protocols mutually agreed upon by medical and nursing staff, making adjustments in medications; initiating requests for certain laboratory tests and

interpreting them; making judgments about the use of accepted pharmaceutical agents as standard treatments in diagnosed conditions; assuming primary responsibility for determining possible alternative care settings and for initiating referrals.

Conducting nurse clinics for continuing care of selected patients.

Conducting community clinics for case finding and screening for health problems.

Assessing community needs in long-term care and participating in the development of resources to meet them.

Assuming continuing responsibility for acquainting selected patients and families with implications of health status, treatment, and prognosis.

Assuming responsibility for the environment of the care setting as it affects quality and effectiveness of care.

It is clear, then, within the framework of these episodic and distributive areas of concentration in health care that one of the most important opportunities for change in the current system of health care involves altering and expanding the practice of nurses so that they assume considerably greater responsibility for delivering all health care services.

When considering the primary, acute, and long-term care functions for which nurses are now generally prepared, it remains the responsibility of the professional nurse to plan and implement nursing care. The identification or diagnosis of nursing problems, the recognition of the interrelated aspects of the problem, and the decision about a course of nursing actions to resolve the problems in relation to immediate and long-term objectives may be conceived to be the unique functions of the professional nurse.[2, 3]

PLANNING AND IMPLEMENTATION OF NURSING INTERVENTION
Nursing Objectives

Following the identification or diagnosis of nursing problems, the professional nurse, utilizing the format for problem-oriented charting illustrated in Table 4-3, formulates immediate and long-term nursing objectives to resolve the identified problems, thereby making a decision regarding a course of nursing actions. An objective (goal) is something toward which effort is directed: an aim or end of action.[4] Behavior is any activity displayed by a patient that is observed by the nurse in the nurse-patient relation. Terminal behavior refers to the expected demonstrated behavior of the patient as a result of the nursing plans (orders) instituted to meet the nursing care objectives and to resolve the identified problems. Therefore, a nursing care objective may be stated in terms of the terminal behavior which

the individual will be assisted by nursing plans to demonstrate satisfactorily.[5]

It is essential that the nursing objectives be well-designed and carefully planned in order to assist the individual to demonstrate satisfactorily the behaviors expected.[5] The data recorded during the nursing history and assessment process form the primary source upon which nursing care objectives are based. The professional nurse's knowledge of the biological and social sciences, as well as of the skills based upon these sciences, is also a source which is utilized in the formation of nursing objectives. Data recorded by other members of the health team in the patient's chart, as well as the physician's plan of care, must be given consideration when formulating nursing objectives. In addition to being well-designed and carefully planned, behavioral objectives for patient care must reflect realistic judgments of what results can be expected.

The principal characteristics for writing objectives as guidelines for nursing care intervention must be considered by the nurse. The first principal characteristic is that the objective must be stated in terms of a subject responsible for demonstration of the behavior. For example, a subject responsible for demonstration of the behavior may be "the child," "the family," or "the nurse." The specific, precise, observable behavior that the person is expected to demonstrate is a principal characteristic guideline for writing a good objective. Examples of overtly observable behavior might include "will weigh," "will draw," and "will label." The circumstances, situations, or settings in which the behavior will be expected to occur are an additional principal characteristic for writing objectives. "Given 10 minutes" is an example of a situation in which behavior may occur. The level of performance or proficiency is another principal characteristic that must be included in a well-written objective. Examples of minimum levels of performance might include "a glass," "30 cc (ml)," and "10 ft." A completed objective might read: "The child will drink 60 cc of juice every 2 hours (8 A.M., 10 A.M., . . .).[5–7]

The purpose of planning and implementing nursing objectives is to provide a means of communicating to the patient, the family, the nursing staff, and the other members of the health care team the terminal behavior state. Terminal behavior refers to the expected demonstrated behavior of the subject. The nurse uses the terminal behavior as a measurement when evaluating whether the identified problems have been resolved. These will be resolved and the terminal behavior will be met when the nursing plans have met the nursing care objectives. The nursing objectives also provide criteria by which the patient's progress can be determined. The nursing staff should use the nursing objectives to help them focus on the specific nursing care that needs to be given. The objective guides the professional nurse in the decision-making process as to what nursing methods or techniques need to be planned.

The principal characteristics for writing objectives as guidelines for nursing care intervention have been described. The following questions must be asked when the wording of nursing care objectives is evaluated:

1   Is the objective stated in terms of a subject responsible for demonstration of the behavior?
2   Is the behavior that the person is expected to demonstrate written in specific, precise, observable terms? Could another competent nurse observe the subject and agree that the subject does or does not attain the objective?
3   Does the objective include the circumstances, situations, or settings under which the subject must perform the specified behavior?
4   Does the objective include the level of performance or proficiency that the subject must attain?[5-7]

Nursing Plans

An important reason for developing a nursing intervention plan is that it is the primary means of communicating the methods or techniques by which the nursing care objectives are to be met. Meeting these objectives serves as the only assurance that the scientific plan of care can be delivered. Because nursing plans are written, they afford some consistency in the kind of nursing intervention performed. Methods, practices, and techniques of nursing intervention are included in the nursing plan. The time, or times, when the specific action or nursing intervention is to occur is another reason for developing plans for nursing intervention. Nursing plans are also a method of letting the patient, his family, and other health team members know what intervention will be included to achieve the nursing objectives. Another purpose of a written nursing plan is to guide the activities of the nursing staff for health care intervention.

The characteristics for writing plans as guidelines for nursing care intervention have been described. The following questions must be asked when evaluating the written nursing plan:

1   Is the nursing plan developed from the information recorded in the nursing history and assessment? Is the nursing plan developed according to the nurse's scientific knowledge base of biological and social sciences?
2   Is the nursing plan developed in accordance with the data recorded in the patient's chart by other members of the health care team? Is the plan developed in accordance with the physician's plan of care?
3   Does the nursing plan include the specific person who is to receive the nursing intervention, the specific action, the content area, and a notation of the time, or times, the specific action is to occur?[8]

Progress Note

A summary of the patient's progress is a valuable method by which the attainment of nursing objectives may be evaluated. In addition, the effectiveness of the nursing intervention plan may be evaluated in a continuous manner in the progress notes. Communication to other health team members is provided via the progress notes in a concise manner at periodic intervals throughout the time of contact with the patient. A summary of current information concerning the patient's health status is provided in a continuous, ongoing manner in progressive form.

The requirements of a good written progress note must be considered by the professional nurse. An indication of the patient's response to the nursing intervention plan must be included. Another requirement of a good progress note is that it include any additional data collected as well as the new objectives and plans based on the additional data collected. It must include a notation of the future plans for nursing intervention.

The primary source of information to be included in the progress note is the observation of the child by the professional nurse. Reports of other members of the health care team must be included in the progress note, and also the reports of the patient and the family regarding the nursing intervention received.

The requirements for writing a good progress note have been described. The following questions must be considered when evaluating the written progress note:

1   Does the progress note include an indication of the patient's response to the nursing intervention plan?
2   Does the progress note include any additional data collected as well as the new objectives and plans based on the additional data collected?
3   Does the progress note include a notation of the future plans for nursing intervention?

The final progress note written at the termination of patient contact includes the same requirements as the interval progress note. In addition, the final one must include a résumé of the patient's total nursing intervention.

CASE STUDY

The process of planning and implementing nursing intervention described above will be illustrated with reference to the following case study.

October 9, 1971

   Timmy is an 8-year-old Caucasian male referred to the outpatient pediatric clinic for nursing care follow-up. The presenting problem is that he is "not being cooperative in the public school classroom" and "not taking care of his ileoconduit, i.e., not keeping his bag clean, not wearing the proper equipment, and occasionally wetting or soiling his clothes." Timmy is referred because he lives in a Children's Home as a ward of the state and has complex physical and emotional problems.

October 13, 1971

   A home visit was made to the Children's Home for the purpose of gathering developmental and environtal data to complete the Pediatric Nursing Assessment.

PEDIATRIC NURSING ASSESSMENT

Child's name: T. W.
Sex: Male
Birthdate: 10-23-62
Address: 9201 Fourth Street
Telephone: 823-9062
Hospital number: 0479022

Informant: Social worker at Children's Home
Date: October 13, 1971
Referred by: Social worker at Children's Home

Reason for referral:
(1) not cooperating in the public school classroom.
(2) not taking care of his ileoconduit.
Nurse: J. Smith, R.N.
Mother's name: Mrs. S. W.
Occupation: Housewife
Age: 37
Father's name: Mr. J. W.
Occupation: None
Age: 38
I   General observations
   A   *Home environment and living quarters*
       The Children's Home is located on a large acreage at the edge of the city. The home is a large stone building built in 1928. The rooms are large and drafty with wooden floors. Furnishings consist of light iron cots and one dresser per room. The walls have no pictures and the windows have no curtains. It is apparent that the accommodations are overcrowded and understaffed, providing minimal adult supervision.
   B   *Appearance and behavior*
       T. appeared thin, pale, and small for his age. His clothing was much too small and inappropriate for the coldness of the weather, i.e., he wore no socks and wore a sleeveless cotton shirt. Initially he was quiet, appeared very dejected, and showed no eye contact. Verbalizations were limited to single-word responses offered in a low, monotonous tone to specific questions directed toward him.
   C   *Parent-child interaction*
       There was no physical interaction between T. and his social worker and his verbal responses to her were as indicated above.
   D   *Siblings*
       T. is the ninth child in a family of nine children ranging in age from 8 to 16. T. is the only sibling who has not been placed in foster care during the past 6 months. At the present time T. has no contact with any of his siblings. (At this point in the interview, T. left the room to go outside to play.)
II   Parental view of presenting problem and/or medical diagnosis
   A   *Direct quote of problem*
       Social Worker, "T. doesn't take care of himself like he should and he's having problems in school, too."
   B   *Description of duration and specific details*
       Social Worker: "T. came to the Children's Home about 8 months ago when the nine children were removed from the natural parents' custody and made wards of the state. T. did not finish the last school year, and the public school teacher reports that he will not cooperate in following directions in his current classroom situation. The teacher also has reported that he appears shy and withdrawn and spends most of the day crying. Apparently T. does not assume responsibility for his ileoconduit, as the other children have complained that he frequently 'smells bad.' It has also been noted that he has had occasions of fecal incontinence during the school day."
III   Significant past medical history
   A   *Family history*
       1   Chronic illnesses and diseases
           Unknown and unobtainable.

2 Relationship to child
Unknown and unobtainable

B *Prenatal*
1 Maternal age
Unknown and unobtainable.
2 Obstetrical and gynecological history
Unknown and unobtainable.
3 Complications relating to pregnancy
Unknown and unobtainable.
4 Parental views of pregnancy
Unknown and unobtainable.

C *Birth history*
5 lb, 9 oz: Born with congenital imperforate anus which was surgically repaired by a pull-through procedure at one day of age. Continual fecal soiling due to lack of bowel control or sensation.

D *Medical history*
1 Illnesses
Unknown and unobtainable.
2 Hospitalizations
  a January 1970 (7 years): Sacral anaplasty with relocation of rectum through a levator sling. Observed to have urinary retention due to lack of motor innervation to the bladder.
  b February 1970 (7 years): Suprapubic cystostomy, rectal dilations, and rectal fistual abscess.
  c March 1970 (7 years): Incision and drainage of scrotal abscess.
  d April 1970 (7 years): Large hypotonic bladder which was not emptying. Noted on IVP to have reflux of both ureters. Ileoconduit performed.
  e December 1970 (8 years): Large amount of feces noted in colon via x-rays at clinic appointment. Continual fecal incontinence, therefore hospitalized to regulate bowel function on daily enema regime.
3 Separations from parents
It was the impression of the social worker that, prior to the children's removal from the natural parents, the children were left alone for extended periods of time. No more specific details are available.

IV Early developmental milestones
A *Age, in months, when child:*
1 Smiled
2 Followed objects with eyes
3 Held head up when prone
4 Turned self from prone to supine

5 Cut tooth
6 Sat with support
7 Sat without support
8 Crawled
9 Walked alone
10 Fed self with spoon
11 Said first words
12 Spoke sentences
13 Bowel and bladder trained during day
14 Bowel and bladder trained during night
All unknown and unobtainable.

B *Early behavior patterns as viewed by parents*
Unknown and unobtainable.

V Eating and drinking patterns
A *Meal patterns and appetite*
Eats his meals family style with the other 64 children and members of the staff. Breakfast is served at 6:30 A.M. and usually consists of bacon, eggs, toast, juice, and milk. Lunch is eaten in the school cafeteria at noontime. Dinner consists of a meat, vegetable, bread, and milk and is usually served at 5:00 P.M.

B *Food likes and dislikes*
T. prefers most meats and seems to dislike vegetables and eggs.

C *Medications or dietary supplements taken*
T. receives 30 ml of mild liquid laxative every night and a more potent liquid laxative is administered by the staff p.r.n.

D *Allergies to food or medication*
None known.

E *Problems related to nutrition*
T. seems to have a poor appetite in that he eats only a few bites of each food served. He is a slow eater and spends most of the mealtime playing with the food on his plate.

VI Eliminating patterns
A *Usual patterns*
T. has an ileoconduit and wears an appliance over the stoma. He empties the bag on demand during the day, and at night it is attached to a continuous dependent drainage system. T. is on an enema regime to control fecal incontinence which occurs almost every day, primarily at school.

B *Difficulties with elimination*
T. is receiving a 500 ml tap water enema after dinner every evening at 6:00 P.M.

VII Sleeping patterns
A *Usual patterns*
T. usually retires about 9:30 P.M. along with

the other children in the home. He apparently sleeps well and arises at 5:30 A.M.

B *Sleeping arrangements*
T. sleeps on an iron cot in a room with seven other boys approximately his age. The room is drafty, and each bed is covered with two sheets and a pillow.

C *Special rituals*
None.

D *Problems with sleeping*
T. appears to sleep well. Occasionally he is restless and awakens in the night with apparent nightmares on an average of once a week.

VIII Independence-dependence patterns

A *Level of independence-dependence*
T. functions relatively independently in all activities of daily living with the exception of his daily enema program. The staff requests that T. be completely responsible for this function. Most of the time T. begins the regime when reminded by staff; however, much of the time he does not follow through the entire process.

B *Patterns of self-care*
T. is not able to independently care for his ileoconduit, and he does not perform the enema regime independently. Medications are administered by staff.

C *Occurrence of dependent behavior*
T. tends to be most dependent when it is time to take his enema. He apparently needs consistent staff supervision which is not available.

D *Reaction to stress, illness, or hospitalization*
T. appears quiet and withdrawn, has no eye contact, and minimal verbal expression. He maintains a slumping posture with a hanging head.

IX Temperament

A *Description of temperament*
T. usually appears with a flat affect when talking with adults, and his face shows no expression. He appears happy and has been observed to laugh and smile while interacting with peers.

B *Means of response when:*
1 Angry
He cries and denies anger. T. will go to his room and lie face down on the bed.
2 Sad
T. goes to his bed or sits on a chair in an empty room.

3 Happy
Observed to smile and laugh only when with peers and no adults.
4 Frightened
He appears quiet, withdrawn, with no eye contact and no verbal expression.

X Play

A *Appropriateness of available toys*
There are few toys apparently available—several bats, balls, and mitts. There is a large swing set in backyard. Toys appear appropriate and safe for age level of children.

B *Availability and safety of play areas*
Large fenced-in yard surrounds the home. The children are required to play outside or to sit in chairs to watch TV while inside. There appears to be adequate adult supervision in the play areas.

C *Favorite toys and activities*
T. likes to play baseball with other children and occasionally with the staff.

D *Child's initiative and amount of creative play*
There are no apparent resources for creative play. T. will sometimes play tag and other interactive games with peers.

E *Preferred play*
1 Solitary
He spends considerable time inside sitting alone in a room watching TV. He prefers to play by himself for long periods of time.
2 Parallel
There has been minimal parallel play observed.
3 Cooperative
T. plays cooperative interactive outdoor games with his peers, but must be encouraged by staff to do so.

F *Peer interaction*
T. appears to "get along well" with peers, but he must constantly be encouraged by staff to interact with peer group.

XI Discipline

A *Responsibility for discipline*
Discipline is enforced by staff members.

B *Methods utilized*
He is required to sit in chair in corner of an empty room for specified time limits.

C *Effectiveness of methods*
It is apparently effective since T. will not repeat behavior after he is punished for it.

D *Child's reaction*
T. reacts by crying the entire time he is in the isolated situation.

XII School
A *History*
1968–69 Kindergarten
1969–70 Kindergarten
1970–71 First grade
1971–Present: Ungraded special education classroom; he functions at a preprimer and primer level in all subjects.

B *Child's reaction*
T. does not want to go to school each morning. He likes to play with peers at school. He seems to find schoolwork very frustrating.

C *Problems as viewed by parents or teacher*
Teacher reports that T. is subject to perplexity and confusion when required to do schoolwork. His attention span is short and difficult to maintain. His visual motor coordination is poor. He relates aggressively when confronted with frustration and will pull up his shirt and tear off the ileoconduit appliance when angry at teacher. This occurs approximately six to eight times per school day.

XIII Present medical history
A *Review of systems*
1 Skin
Intact. Appears dirty. Nailbeds unclean. No rashes, abrasions, or ecchymotic areas noted.
2 EENT
a Eyes: 20/20 vision without correction.
b Ears: Audiological testing reveals hearing is within normal limits. Ears are symmetrical and in line with eye level.
c Nose: Negative.
d Throat: Negative. Six-year molars are present. Both front upper incisors are absent. Several dental caries in need of repair are noted.
3 Respiratory
Rate 24 per minute while sitting. No congestion, cough, or dyspnea noted.
4 Cardiovascular
Pulse rate 88 per minute while sitting. No murmur noted. Does not fatigue easily. No cyanosis.
5 Central nervous system

Alert and responsive in single words to questions. Oriented to person and place. Does not tell time or know days or months. Cranial nerves I to XII are intact. Uses right and left hand equally well.
6 Gastrointestinal
Congenital imperforate anus with relocation of rectum through a levator sling. Fecal incontinence occurring nearly every day—primarily at school.
7 Genitourinary
Permanent urinary diversion—ileoconduit. Undescended left testis. Repaired hypospadias.
8 Skeletal
Height 50 inches and below the third percentile. Weight 49 lb on the tenth percentile. Face pulled to left reportedly due to scoliosis. Asymmetry of left shoulder lower than right. Minimal postural kyphosis.

B *Immunizations*
DPT #1 2/4/64
DPT #2 3/4/64
DPT #3 4/8/64
Booster 8/16/66, 8/19/71
Polio-Salk 8/8/67
OPV Series 1968
　　　Booster 7/25/69
Smallpox 4/22/66
Rubeola 1/22/66
Rubella 1/15/71
TB skin test 8/16/66 Negative
　　　　　8/8/67 Negative
　　　　　12/29/69 Negative
　　　　　1/1/70 Negative

XIV Current developmental level
A *Gross motor skills*
Runs, jumps, and skips. Appears coordinated. Is not able to backward heel-toe walk.
B *Fine motor—adaptive skills*
Fine-motor coordination is poor. Drawing and writing are inappropriate to age. Prints letters of words many varied sizes.
C *Language skills*
Primarily responds with single words, but will use five- to eight-word sentences appropriately if encouraged.
D *Personal—social skills*
Performs all activities of daily living. Reluctant most of the time to socialize with

peers. Appears withdrawn and dejected when with adults.

After the data are collected the professional nurse must proceed to analyze them and make the nursing diagnosis. In relation to the available data collected, four problems were identified as the nursing diagnosis. These problems are recorded in the format of the problem-oriented record system (see Table 4-3).[9]

In order to plan and implement nursing intervention, consideration must be given to the problem list. For this case it includes the following:

10/13/71

1 Inadequate knowledge and understanding of body systems and functions.
2 Inadequate care of ileoconduit, appliance, and stoma.
3 Inadequate maintenance of enema regime.
4 Poor self-concept.

Utilizing the format of problem-oriented charting (Table 4-3),[10] the professional nurse must proceed to plan the nursing objectives in relation to the identified problems before the implementation of nursing intervention. Table 5-1 includes only the initial planning and implementation process based upon the nurse's initial history and assessment of the child. Modifications, additions, and deletions of nursing intervention will necessarily follow in subsequent contacts with the child. For illustration purposes of this chapter, the process of planning and implementation is developed for problems (1) and (2). Also, it will be noted that the objectives and rationale are included for each problem. In addition to the identification of nursing problems, the formation of nursing plans ultimately involves the formulation of objectives on the basis of a scientific rationale. Although these categories are not included in the nurse's written communication (charting), they are included in this chapter to assist the reader in identifying the basis for the proposed nursing problems and plans.

The effectiveness of nursing plans is evaluated in the written progress note. Following the nurse's second visit to the Children's Home, the initial planning and implementation were evaluated and recorded.

Progress note
10/20/71
3:30 P.M.

Problem 1
S: T. needed much encouragement to draw and label the genitourinary system. T. was reluctant to verbalize regarding one function of the genitourinary system.
O: T. was able to correctly draw and label the diagram. At this time T. was not able to identify one function of the genitourinary system.
A: Not satisfactory.
P: Repeat session in 1 week. T. needs much encouragement and reinforcement.

Problem 2
S: T. appeared quiet, withdrawn, had no eye contact and no verbal expression.
O: Records were kept by the social worker for 1 week with the following results:
Thurs. 5:00 P.M.; 7:15 P.M.
Fri. 7:00 A.M.
Sat. 9:30 A.M.; 12:30 P.M.; 4:15 P.M.
Sun. 8:10 A.M.; 9:45 A.M.
Mon. none
Tues. 7:30 A.M.; 12:15 P.M., 7:30 P.M.
Wed. none
Records were not kept by the teacher because she was absent from the classroom.
T. was able to complete categories (b) and (d) perfectly for the entire week. T. was reinforced with a total of 14 pennies for the week.
No symptoms of decreased urinary output were noted. Output was difficult to accurately assess due to frequent leakage.
A: Data were incomplete from school reports. Pennies as a form of positive reinforcement appear to be an effective reward for T. at the present time. Urinary output was difficult to assess accurately because of frequent leakage.
P: Records to be kept by the teacher for 1 week. Social worker will continue daily charting with T. Social worker continues to reinforce T. with a penny for each star on the chart. Social worker and nurse will continue observation for decreased urinary output. Output will be measured with a graduated cylinder as accurately as possible in spite of frequent urinary leakage.

The process of planning and implementing nursing intervention as illustrated is a function of the professional nurse. The case study serves to illustrate the process of planning and implementing nursing intervention which must be developed by the professional nurse.

Table 5-1 PLANNING AND IMPLEMENTATION PROCESS

Problem 1   Inadequate knowledge and understanding of body systems and functions.

Objective	Rationale	Plan
I T. will correctly identify parts of the genitourinary system.	1a Correct identification of body parts is preliminary to knowledge of body functions. b Presentation of one system per session will enhance integration of material.	1:01 Using a torso model, the nurse will identify parts of the body by a systems approach. a Genitourinary b Eyes, ears, nose, throat c Respiratory d Cardiovascular e Central nervous system f Gastrointestinal g Skeletal h Skin
	2a Correct placement of body parts on the diagram indicates a knowledge of the physical body. b Correct placement of body parts on the diagram will show the relation of one system to another.	1:02 On a previously drawn torso diagram, T. will correctly draw and label the genitourinary system in appropriate locations.
II T. will correctly identify one function of the genitourinary system.	1a Correct identification of one function of each system is preliminary to a knowledge of interrelations of the systems. b Presentation of one system per session will enhance integration of material. 2a Verbal discussion of each system will enhance the clarification of functions for T.	1:03 Using a torso model, the nurse will identify at least one function of the genitourinary system per session. 1:04 T. will verbally discuss one function of the genitourinary system with the nurse.

Problem 2   Inadequate care of ileoconduit, appliance, and stoma.

Objective	Rationale	Plan
I To collect base line data concerning frequency and the hour of day that urinary leakage occurs as evidenced by a plotted graph recorded by the social worker over 1 week's time.	1a Data as to frequency and the hour of day that urinary leakage occurs will serve as base line data.	2:01 The social worker will record number of leakage episodes and time occurred for 1 week at home.
	2a Data as to frequency and the hour of day that urinary leakage occurs will serve as base line data.	2:02 The teacher will record number of leakage episodes and time occurred for 1 week in school.
II To increase self-care of ileoconduit, appliance, and stoma, T. will complete a weekly chart.	1a Being rewarded with a star on the chart for each category will act to reinforce self-care.	2:03 The nurse will develop a chart to be completed daily by T. and his social worker. The chart will include: a Proper application of glue. b Wear appliance belt. c Keep appliance clean and alternate bags daily. d Attach bag to dependent drainage system at night.
	2a A penny will serve as a form of positive reinforcement.	2:04 The social worker will positively reinforce T. with one penny for each star on the chart.
III The social worker and nurse will observe T. for decreased urinary output.	1a Early detection of decreased urinary output will demonstrate the need for medical intervention.	2:05 The social worker and nurse will observe T. for decreased urinary output. Signs of decreased urinary output in a child with an ileoconduit include absence of urinary output, discomfort in pelvic area, or restlessness. 2:06 Measure urinary output in a graduated cylinder.

REFERENCES

1 "Extending the Scope of Nursing Practice," *Nursing Outlook*, 20:46–52, January 1972.
2 Virginia Henderson, "The Nature of Nursing," *American Journal of Nursing*, 64:62–68, August 1964.
3 Dorothy Smith, "A Clinical Nursing Tool," *American Journal of Nursing*, 68:2384–2388, November 1968.
4 *Webster's New Collegiate Dictionary*, 7th ed., G. & C. Merriam Company, Springfield, Mass., 1965.
5 R. F. Mager, *Preparing Instructional Objectives*, Fearon Publishers, Inc., Palo Alto, Calif., 1962.
6 R. M. Gagne, *The Conditions of Learning,* Holt, Rinehart and Winston, Inc., New York, 1970.
7 N. E. Gronlund, *Stating Behavioral Objectives for Classroom Instruction*, Collier-Macmillan Canada, Ltd., Toronto, 1970.
8 R. F. Mager and P. Pipe, *Performance Problems*, Fearon Publishers, Inc., Palo Alto, Calif., 1970.
9 J. C. Bjorn and H. D. Cross, *Problem Oriented Practice*, Modernal Hospital Press, McGraw-Hill Publications Co., New York, 1970.

BIBLIOGRAPHY

"ANA/AAP to Draw Guidelines on Preparation of Pediatric Nurse Practitioners," *American Journal of Nursing*, 70:1833, September 1970.
Aradine, Carolyn R., and Hansen, M. F.: "Nursing in a Primary Health Care Setting, *Nursing Outlook*, 8:45–46, April 1970.
Christman, Norma J.: "Clinical Performance of Baccalaureate Graduates," *Nursing Outlook*, 19:54–56, January 1971.
"Comprehensive Planning of Health Facilities and Services," *Journal of the American Medical Association*, 204:808–810, May 1968.
Dickoff, J., James, Patricia, and Wiedenbach, Ernestine: "Theory in a Practice Discipline," pt. I, Practice Oriented Theory, *Nursing Research*, 17:415–435, September-October 1968.
——, ——, and ——: "Theory in a Practice Discipline," pt. II, Practice Oriented Research, *Nursing Research*, 17:545–554, November-December 1968.
Elliott, Jo: "A Conversation on Nursing Services, Nursing Education and Economic and General Welfare," *American Journal of Nursing*, 68:792–799, April 1968.
Etzioni, Amitai (ed.): *The Semi-Professions and Their Organization*, The Free Press, New York, 1969.
Goerke, L. S.: "Changes in Preventive Medicine," *Journal of School Health*, 38:1–8, January 1968.
Greenough, Katharine: "Determining Standards of Nursing Care," *American Journal of Nursing*, 68:2153–2157, October 1968.
"Health Occupations Supportive to Nursing," *American Journal of Nursing*, 68:559–563, March 1966.
Hurst, J. W., and Walker, H. K. (eds.): *The Problem-Oriented System*, Medcom Medical Update Series, New York, 1972.
Jacox, Ada: "Who Defines and Controls Nursing Practice?," *American Journal of Nursing*, 69:977–982, May 1969.
James, G.: "Competition in Providing Community Health Services," *Nursing Outlook*, 18:42–45, February 1970.
Johnson, Dorothy: "The Significance of Nursing Care,"
American Journal of Nursing, 61:63–66, November 1961.
——: "Consequences for Patients and Personnel," *American Journal of Nursing*, 62:96–100, May 1962.
——: "Today's Action Will Determine Tomorrow's Nursing," *Nursing Outlook*, 13:38–41, September 1964.
——: "Professional Practice and Specialization in Nursing," *Image Sigma Theta Tau National Honor Society of Nursing*, 2:2–7, November 1968.
Lambertsen, Eleanor: "Changes in Practice Require Changes in Education," *American Journal of Nursing*, 66:1784–1786, August 1966.
——: "The Emerging Health Occupations," *Nursing Forum*, 7:87–97, Winter 1968.
Leonard, R. C.: "Developing Research in a Practice-Oriented Discipline," *American Journal of Nursing*, 67:1472–1475, July 1967.
Levine, E.: "Nurse Manpower: Yesterday, Today, and Tomorrow," *American Journal of Nursing*, 69:290–296, February 1969.
Lifson, S. S.: "Our Changing Society—The Years Ahead: The Outlook for Health Education Practice," *American Journal of Public Health*, 58:678–683, April 1968.
Lysaught, J. P.: "Continuing Education: Necessity and Opportunity," *Journal of Continuing Education in Nursing*, 1:5–10, September 1970.
Mauksch, Ingeborg G., and David, Miriam L.: "Prescription for Survival," *American Journal of Nursing*, 72:2189–2193, December 1972.
"National Commission for the Study of Nursing and Nursing Education," *American Journal of Nursing*, 70:279–296, February 1970.
Nordmark, Madelyn, and Rohweder, Anne W.: *Scientific Foundations of Nursing*, 2d ed., J. B. Lippincott Company, Philadelphia, 1967.
Orem, Dorothea E.: *Nursing: Concepts of Practice*, McGraw-Hill Book Company, New York, 1971.
Paulsen, F. R.: "Nursing Goals beyond Commitment," *Nursing Outlook*, 14:57–59, December 1966.
Schell, Pamela L., and Campbell, Alla T.: "POMR—Not Just Another Way To Chart," *Nursing Outlook*, 20:510–514, August 1972.
Seward, Joan: "Professional Practice in a Bureaucratic Structure," *Nursing Outlook*, 17:58–61, December 1969.
Sheldon, A., et al.: "The Developing Role for the Nurse in a Community Mental Health Program," *Perspectives in Psychiatric Care*, 5:272–279, November-December 1967.
Silver, H. K.: "Pediatric Nurse—Practitioners Perform Expanded Care Role," *Hospital Topics*, 46:71–74, October 1968.
Smith, Dorothy: "From Student to Nurse," *Nursing Outlook*, 11:735–736, October 1963.
——: "A Discussion of the 'Into, Out of, Overall' Syndrome in Nursing," *International Journal of Nursing Studies*, 5:33–39, 1968.
——: "Writing Objectives as a Nursing Practice and Skill," *American Journal of Nursing*, 71:319–320, February 1971.
Thompson, Alice M. C. (ed.): "Focus on the Future," *International Nursing Review*, 16:195–196, 1969.
"Toward Real Continuity in Patient Care," *Nursing Forum*, 2:21–25, 1964.
Weed, L. L.: *Medical Records, Medical Education, and Patient Care*, The Press of Case Western Reserve University, Cleveland, 1969.
Wolford, Helen G.: "Complemental Nursing Care and Practice," *Nursing Forum*, 3:8–20, 1964.

EVALUATION

ROSEMARY J. McKEIGHEN

The history of nursing practice reflects the evolvement of many changes. In most instances, historical and/or social factors effected these changes, yet, in each instance, evaluation was also in operation. Whenever change occurs or is being considered, evaluation becomes a necessary ingredient as it is responsible for justifying the change or demanding its occurrence. As John F. Kennedy said,

> All this will not be finished in the first one hundred days. Nor will it be finished in the first one thousand days . . . nor even perhaps in our lifetime on this planet. But let us begin.

Evaluation is not a new concept for nurses. Nurses have always based their actions upon changes they have observed. The new thought is that skill in evaluation procedure and competency of nursing practice are related. Thus to improve their practice, nurses must improve their evaluative skills.

To acquire effectiveness in evaluative skills, two things are requisite: (1) An understanding of evaluation as process, and (2) a precise and orderly method for moving through the evaluative process.

This chapter provides information relevant to these two categories by discussing evaluation as process. It also addresses itself to the nurse's role and responsibility for operationalization in each step of the process.

EVALUATION AS PROCESS

A price tag represents the terminal point of evaluation. The method used to determine the price of something may range from simple to complex, dependent upon the number and types of variables involved. The first step of this process is measurement against a standardized criterion, guaranteeing its utility at a prescribed level and under specified conditions. Measurement is inherent in the process, yet evaluation goes beyond this by considering facts that are enmeshed with a wider scope of variables: value standards, particular circumstances, and goal attainment. It embodies both a quantitative and qualitative dimension. For example, if one wished to know the value of an old ring, he would simply take it to a jewelry appraiser and allow him to examine it. Depending upon the materials the ring was fashioned from, the quality of workmanship, how much wear was manifest, and market conditions, the jeweler could assign a price. This would be an evaluation. However, if the ring had been given to Marie Antoinette by Louis XVI, this would indeed require a different value appraisal as other variables —antiquity and ownership by a prominent historical personality—were added. If Marie Antoinette was of his lineage, still another dimension, personal heritage, needs to be considered. If this ring happened to be one his fiancée found while sharing a pleasant experience with him, and if she voiced the desire to have it as an engagement ring, the evaluation becomes even more complex.

Evaluation, then, is a process whose end product is a value label. It begins with measurement and moves to introduction of variables that carry the potential of change and dictate its rate of movement and quality of content. The sum total of the specific impact of every given proposal yields the terminal statement.

Attempting to evaluate the behavioral change of the patients in a specialized situation, who are receiving services from nurses with varying personalities, educational preparation, and skill competency, is not a simple task. Complexity comes from knowledge that the care being given rarely is a singular patient-nurse interaction, but instead, a network of multiple encounters with ministrations planned in a sequential pattern. The nature of the variables, the multicausation factor, the time span involved, and the lack of standard measures specific to nursing actions are some of the obvious difficulties. The fact that the care given has the potential of affecting the recipient's well-being while he is in the situation and after he leaves it necessitates its accomplishment.

This evaluation must reflect both qualitative and quantitative aspects and also include examination of predetermined goal achievement and measurement of behavioral change. The behavioral change must be assessed in four areas: attitudinal, functional, personal, and social.

The *attitudinal* area is concerned with the feelings the patient experiences that stem from the explicit meaning the label holds for that person. The implication that coughing behavior has for a patient who has associated it with death as a result of seeing a parent die of tuberculosis is quite different from that of a patient who has associated coughing with an environmental irritation.

The *functional* area speaks to the patient's ability to perform a specific task in maintaining or regulating his body needs, i.e., range of motion regarding a limb or changes in the excretion of waste materials.

The *personal* area embodies those aspects that carry the potential of affecting or distorting the patient's self-image; i.e., a cardiac-arrest patient has

difficulty maintaining his image of prowess on the tennis courts, being independent and self-sufficient if experiencing thoracic discomfort while breathing and being totally reliant upon others to meet basic needs.

The *social* area refers to interactions that are altered to accommodate this unique condition. This impingement begins with the patient's adjustments and radiates to each person within his life space and social sphere. The depth of penetration into his social realm and the severeness of accommodation of all involved needs to be taken into account.

It is apparent that the data for evaluation in the usual clinical experience differ from those of the nurse using the nursing process. In the former, a one-sided report of a two-person interaction becomes the substance of a nursing action. In the latter the nurse, to be effective, must or should include the patient's perspective as well. The two-person interaction, between patient and nurse, serves as raw data.

It should be clear that evaluation then becomes a process for determining how well the nursing care plan, as developed and organized, is producing the desired results. It will identify the strengths and weaknesses of the plan. This helps check the validity of the nursing diagnosis, upon which the nursing care plan has been formulated. It further serves to monitor the effectiveness of the nursing interventions, the nurse's impact, and other conditions that exert influence upon nursing care.

In each stage of the process evaluation activity is mobilized around formulation of answers to the specific questions generated by the content of that stage. It is this constantly increasing and changing fund of knowledge that the nurse uses to formulate a plan of action for meeting the patient's unique need requirement in the most effective and expedient manner. Evaluation determines the degrees of accomplishment.

EVALUATION OF NURSING PROCESS

When undertaking an evaluation, it is important to keep two points in mind: (1) Evaluation is a process that must be continuous to be effective, and (2) it takes place at various levels and to different degrees, dependent upon extraneous variables. For examination purposes it is possible to set down a logical cognitive schema to follow; however, individuals and circumstances are equally unpredictable, and yet they are the cardinal factors that dictate deviations in progression and determine rate of movement through the process.

When we speak of evaluation of the nursing process, we refer to examination of the behavior outcomes that are continually occurring within an intricate system. Simultaneous interactions between patient behaviors, nursing actions, and environmental constraints for the purpose of study make up the complex system. These interactions are components of each step of the process, data collection, nursing diagnosis, nursing orders, interventions, and evaluation.

The evaluation includes examination of each of these phases as well as the final step of the nursing process, evaluation. In this final step the material which is to be evaluated is the compilation of all the evaluations and modifications that have occurred in each of the preceding phases. In this instance, evaluation occurs on a primary and secondary level as well as sequentially and cumulatively.

Since nursing objectives are fundamental to produce specific changes in the behavior and functional ability of the patient, evaluation is the method for specifying the degree to which these changes are being realized.

This conception of evaluation has two important aspects. (1) It implies that evaluation must appraise the behavior of patients in order to note the desired change of behavior. (2) It also suggests that evaluation must involve more than a single assessment and that, by comparing these periodic assessments, one may identify the change as it occurs.

The behavioral outcomes of the patient can be viewed as the culmination of the nurse's effort at problem solving and decision making. It reflects the nurse's ability at analysis of patient data, formulation of a nursing problem list, arrival at a nursing diagnosis, prescription and implementation of nursing ministrations, and evaluation of the consequences of those specific actions.

When the nurse reaches the stage of stating a nursing diagnosis, he has begun some formulation of nursing care objectives. At this point in the process, evaluation becomes examination of patient behaviors for predicting possible outcomes as consequences of specific nursing action. Up until this stage, primary and secondary evaluation was taking place. *Primary* is synonymous with examination of all the data the patient presents upon admission. *Secondary* refers to examination of the consequences of interactions within the therapeutic system.

For greater clarity, each phase of the nursing process will be discussed as to the nursing action, type of evaluation applied, intellectual process operation, and the cumulative effect relevant to the next stage. All intellectual process operation discussions are adaptations from J. P. Guilford's collected works on the human intellect.[1]

DATA COLLECTION

In a sense, certain preliminary evaluation of the patient and his general situation has already been made prior to his coming to the attention of the nurse. This includes all manner of hard testing data such as laboratory tests, radiologic studies, psychologic measurements, screening device results, i.e. glaucoma, tuberculosis, eye, growth, development, and tissue biopsy.

Primary nursing evaluation begins with these measurements, derived by means of a number of valid and reliable instruments, and then goes beyond this comparison by examining the results of measurement in the light of the immediate goals of the patient. The immediate goals can be associated with limitations on usual activities or could even be analogous with the patient's reason for entry into the health care system, i.e., surgery, relief of pain, diagnosis, and so forth. This collection of facts is heavily skewed to reveal body steady states and functional ability, and produce a tentative medical label. The nurse's action at this point is to recall or gather information regarding the nature of the label and proper care and cure components unique to that label.

The cognitive operation of memory is heavily relied upon. The nurse must know or be able to recall specific nursing measures that are applicable to maintaining body steady states. Identification of disequilibrium is essential. In conditions which are produced by gross disruptions in a patient's physiologic state, i.e., temperature or fluid imbalance, the nurse routinely manipulates the structural support system in adjusting thermals or fluids. However, when a subtle distortion is operating and an internal or a metabolic change is required, the nurse must know where to seek direction to effect the desired results, i.e., obtain a medication order or obtain instruction for closed-system chest aspiration.

For evaluation to proceed, additions to patient data must be made to build a sufficient knowledge base from which a nursing problem list and diagnosis can evolve. Content representative of physical, psychologic, and social behavior is needed. The functional limitations significance to other phases of life must also be determined.

The nursing history, physical examination, and additional specific testing, if warranted, are the methods used to gather this information. Objective data are obtained from observation of the patient, and subjective facts by interview. The physical examination serves to substantiate subjective beliefs and augment objective and observational data. Findings of the routine areas assessed during gross physical examination include such data as blood pressure, eye examination, temperature, and a general assessment of the 12 cranial nerves.

Substance that speaks to secondary or long-term goals and to each level of Maslow's hierarchy of needs would satisfy the criteria used for this stage of appraisal. According to Maslow (1943) man's needs are the operational force that motivate his behavior. He postulates that these needs develop in a sequential manner from lower (physiologic) to higher (esteem) needs. He adds that at any time the person can reaffirm a need, even though there has been prior need fulfillment. Conceivably disruptions of health have the potential of creating a condition in which the person is vulnerable to responding in this manner.

Since patient behavior is one aspect that nursing practice is based upon, it is important for the nurse to determine if this has happened. In the hospital situation children anticipating surgery frequently express apprehensive crying and clinging behavior. An experienced nurse knows that tactile support is the intervention necessary to alleviate this regression to the safety need.

Secondary evaluations take place at this level. Suggestive hypotheses that were considered on the basis of information gained during the primary evaluation are compared, corroborated, or viewed from another vantage point. Elementary working knowledge is needed about those features of the environment that serve as stimuli for the patient and cause him to respond. Careful notation of his response reactions must be made. Activity levels and body language are both communicative realms that are individually determined yet extremely important for both placement on the dependence-independence continuum and interpretation of nonverbal messages.

When nurses observe the activity levels of patients, they are focusing upon objective conditions of attention. Such indices as *intensity* (i.e., speech, play, visitation), *size* (i.e., content discussed, treatment, amount eaten), *change* (i.e., verbal to nonverbal, passive to assertive), *suddenness of onset, movement*, and *repetition of behavior* are noted. The position the patient takes in the patient-nurse dyad and the ward structure are also revealing data. The stance of continually being administered to conveys quite a different message from a reciprocal "give and take" interchange.

It is important to learn whether the patient uses *isolation*. Does he remove himself from others or does he include himself in a group? Most behaviorists agree that seeking proximity, physical contact, help, attention, reassurance, and approval are dependent behaviors. This aggregate of factual data will reveal patterns of behavior that the nurse will need to rely upon when manipulating variables in the patient's immediate surroundings in order to assist him in meeting his needs.

Formulation of a pattern of behaving enables the nurse to identify the underlying feeling that is the instigator for the action. Any action constitutes a message to ourselves as well as to others, and effective nursing care embodies quite a different approach for a patient that is angry or hostile regarding his upcoming death from the patient who has accepted the inevitable.

It is at this juncture that the cyclic nature of the process becomes apparent, that is, a commitment to inquiry, compilation of assessments of data received, incorporation of facts into a system, imputation of a value, and validation of the judgment given. If any discrepancies are detected at any stage, the process must be repeated and the value refined. For example, if the objective is to teach a patient about diabetes and the nurse learns the patient's scoring of the menu cards is not compatible with that required for diabetic maintenance, the nurse needs to reactivate the cycle, redefine values, and revise the nursing care plan. At a later point in time if recreational therapy reports the patient's activity performance is such that frequent trauma is possible, the process is again repeated because introduction of new data also demands reactivation of the cycle.

Rate of movement through successive stages is predicated upon nurses familiarity with the steps of the process and the effectiveness with which they apply them. This is important because the process becomes more complex in the succeeding phases as additional steps are added and the frequency of new data is increased.

For an adequate evaluation to be made, observation and cognitive skill are vital and necessary. *Observation* is defined as the act or practice of noting facts and events. When approaching a patient, the nurse's most effective tool is observation. The facts the nurse should be most perceptive of are the aspects of symmetry, deviance, color, texture, gait, and the like. The events are achievement of goals as reflected against cultural norms and values, biologic capacity, personal experience, and accessibility.

Cognition is the process of knowing, discovering, and recognizing, including some reasoning. At the close of this phase, the nurse should have some basic information regarding how the patient will be helped in utilizing his strengths in order to meet his needs, maintain his body steady states, correct his deviation, and obtain relief of disturbing behavior. The success of the forthcoming phases is determined by identification of the patient's strengths and weaknesses in the four areas of evaluation—attitudinal, functional, personal, and social.

The evaluation process is an interesting one and continues to receive attention throughout the nursing process, either deliberately, using a planned scientific approach, or unconsciously in an "intuitive manner."

NURSING DIAGNOSIS AND NURSING PRESCRIPTION

Here the evaluation activity is focused upon the efficacy with which the nurse has executed the two cardinal tasks indigenous to this phase, that is, establishing a nursing diagnosis and formulating a plan of action.

Before a nursing diagnosis can be determined, a patient problem list must be assembled. This list contains the patient's unique requirements for need fulfillment such as maintenance of body steady states, correction of deviation, and relief of distressing behaviors. Divarications fall into two categories: deficiencies and overloads. Problem origin may be developmental, pathologic, situational, or combinations of any of these.

Evaluation implies determining that all new manner of viewing the data has been exhausted. After extracting relevant facts and concepts from each patient contact and information sources, extraneous applications or possible variations are discarded. The data are sorted and classified, and interrelations are established. The basic questions that the evaluation should answer are: Is the information relevant to the patient's situation? Do I have enough information? Are these all the facts that are needed to draw accurate conclusions? These results reveal a definitive and differential diagnosis of the patient's problem. From this one develops the nursing diagnosis.

Convergent thinking is the intellectual operation employed to determine a nursing diagnosis. It is explained as generalization of new information from known and remembered knowledge. This mental activity produces the "best conventional answers and solutions" to the problems. An effectual evaluation can occur when the patient's behavior is perceived as the problem rather than the problem itself. For example, following anesthesia, nausea and vomiting are frequently considered as the problem, when in fact, aspiration is the definitive problem. Anesthesia is the causal or differential problem, and nausea and vomiting are simply behavioral manifestations of the problem. Another instance of nonproductive evaluation exists when the nurse's goal supersedes or is in conflict with the patient's goal.

The nursing problem list complements the patient list by grappling with how each problem might be solved. A nursing problem is an exercise to ferret out the nursing measures that might enable the patient to solve or adapt to his problem. It is the nurse's responsibility to select, from all alternatives possible, the approach best suited to the patient's situation. This method of solution becomes the goal of the nursing orders, and changed patient behavior becomes the objective.

This exercise introduces other evaluative areas, the quality of decision and priorities. Reality supports the notion that a patient rarely has a single problem; instead, he has multiple problems, and an order of attention must be arranged for effective problem solution. Evaluation reveals the criteria by which the order of rank is determined and whether the decision made was the best for the patient's predicament.

Evaluation of written objectives substantiates the intent of their design. Well-written objectives contain the criteria by which the behavioral change will be evaluated. Three judgments are made for validation purposes. The desired outcome must be stated in behavioral terms. The required time span perspective must be elucidated and the method by which this is to be accomplished must be specified. Objectives under examination should also contain specificity and clarity. They need to state the sphere in which change is desired—either functional information, skill-related, or attitudinal. Objectives serve as guides for nursing care, while specifications are parameters for evaluation.

Divergent and discriminative thinking are the intellectual process operations employed. *Divergent thinking* is described as generation of new information from known and remembered information as well as production of numerous, diverse, and unconventional answers and solutions. It implies a branching off toward new ideas and methods. *Discriminative thinking* is the intellectual process of considering differences between intervals, divisions, or values, and recognizing differences. It is required to make judgments regarding relative importance and for distinction of strategies which are being considered for use.

The expansion of the cycle in this phase is involved with defining and stating a problem, determining the intended solution, and developing methods for achieving the solution. A rank ordering of ministrations, their calculated results, and a time parameter are stated along with the criterion for measuring the effectiveness of the methods used.

It is helpful to check the validity of the nursing diagnosis by demonstrating a relation between use of relevant theories from other disciplines or research studies and stated nursing theory. Together they generate the hypotheses that serve as the basis for the nursing orders.

NURSING ORDERS AND MANAGEMENT

The composite of all previous mental activity of the preceding stage is clinically tested and applied in this phase. Because the process of evaluation implies a series of evaluations, the nurse cannot rely upon observing patients only at the end of their hospital stay or therapeutic regimen. Instead he must use the feedback gained during validation of the nursing measures selected for accomplishment of the goals the patient has in mind. Actual patient responses are used as evaluative statements that give indication of success or failure of the nursing interventions.

The feasibility of every solution is judged according to the following four criteria: Are the actions designed to aid the patient in coping with his environment? Do they direct help to the patient for achieving a stable pattern of self-regulation? Do they serve the function of preventing additional pathology from developing, slowing the process of existing pathology, and increasing the rate and degree of recovery? Have they adapted the therapeutic regimen to the patient's unique rhythmic cycle?

Evaluation delimits four major distinctions of this period.

First the evaluation should reveal the unique sifting exercise this phase was portended to do. It should produce designation of the nursing orders that are efficacious, the ones that must be dis-

carded, and the interventions that, with some modification, are workable.

A list of variables influencing the patient's behavioral response and explanations of how they may affect the response is necessary. Expansion of these variables, of the relations between them, and of their combined potency upon patient behavior is also required.

Information that identifies the nursing actions including techniques and goals appropriate to any maintenal problems should be organized and communicated. These communications reflect the effects of single or combined variables. Nursing orders are explicit as to what needs to be done, when, and under what circumstances.

The second evaluative distinction can be made referent to the frequency with which data are acquired. This phase should differ from the earlier ones in that frequency rate and amount of data have vital significance. These measures are indicators of efficiency. For a cogent rating to be made, an exacerbation of both realms should be noticeable.

If the nursing order is adequate and correct, an expression is generated that signifies change. The circuitous action of nursing order exercise, incorporation of patient reaction, appraisal, and action should be self-evident.

Documentation of alterations in objectives should be made directly proportional to behavioral modification. This employs fluidity, and since activity increases the probability of change occurring, it follows that amount of data will show the same directionality.

A third distinction adding validity and enhancing evaluation is evidence confirming use of the multiformity of roles that nursing strategies embrace. Not only those focused upon curing pathologic situations are studied, but also such nursing measures as prevention, rehabilitation, counseling, and health teaching. These should be patently clear with the teaching component asserting prominence. The criteria are selections for use and demonstrations of variability of roles employed, instead of compatability or appropriateness of role selection. The efficiency with which the nurse employs the role is evaluated in the next section.

This fourth and final dimension to be reviewed derives its salience from its concentration with the time index. This is reflected in the standard for evaluation of this stage. It is expected that all short-term goals should have been met and some statement of the intended correction or solution and a schematic progression toward achieving long-term goals should have been stipulated.

The adequacy of planning for care is under careful consideration. Appropriateness and effectiveness of content were assessed earlier. Here they are reviewed in regard to a time dimension. Because learning theory and the process of planned change undergrid nursing practice to a Herculean degree, some evidence of sophistication with the process must be obvious for a nursing action to accomplish its goal. Specifically one must comprehend the employment of those time-related concepts such as motivation, reinforcement, and transfer of learning. The mode and manner of instigating change must be particularized with a model of mechanisms and a time for each of the three designated stages.

Related to some degree are time period considerations of provisions for diagnostic and therapeutic services. This responds to measuring the constancy with which the effectiveness of all the nursing interventions are monitored. Effectiveness is judged with regard to patient safety and degree of change attained.

Time allotments for planning and completing beneficial operations, which are focused on prevention, control, or alleviation of the maintenance problem through appropriate response to patient behaviors and manipulation of the major influencing variables, are noted. Also, the amount of time spent must be determined by varying nursing interventions in accordance with any single or combination of related variables and behavioral responses.

Evaluation is described here in the following terms of "reaching decision as to the goodness, correctness, suitability, or adequacy of what we know, what we remember, what we produce in productive thinking."[1] Its relevance to the next stage stems from the duality of its purpose. Its authority originates in responsibility to transmit knowledge that has been fruitful and to set the stage for a deeper insightful overall evaluation.

SYNTHESIS OF EVALUATION

This final stage reviews the extent that the fusion of the three components, patient behavior, nurse action, and situational constraints, has made toward achieving the collective, stated objectives for patient goal attainment. This stage stipulates what is needed from each constituent for speculation upon his specific imputation. For the sake of clarity, the discussion presents the patient's perspective first, then nursing input, and last, situational constraints. It must be kept in mind that this is an artificial separation and that in reality these factions interact simultaneously and are continually exerting influences each upon the other.

From the patient's perspective, it is important to have information about each kind of patient behavior specific to each of the major nursing care objectives; attitudinal, functional, personal, and social, available for examination. For example, if one of the objectives is for the patient to acquire knowledge about his disease process, then it is a requisite that "the evaluation" yield some evidence of the information the patient has gained. If another is to develop methods of analyzing his problems of living and assessing proposed solutions, then inspection requires demonstration of the patient's ability at problem analysis and judgment of possible resolutions. Evaluation should promote this two-dimensional analysis that functions as the basis for planning nursing experiences and for evaluation procedure. Again, examination is made to ascertain that the behavioral objectives have been clearly defined by the nurse. It should be explicit that objectives act as a concrete guide in the selection and planning of nursing experiences. Evaluation forces persons who have not previously clarified their objectives to do so. Unless there is some distinct conception of the type of behavior implied by the objectives, no one can know the precise action to look for in the patient to learn to what degree change has come about.

Evaluation has a powerful influence upon learning, and evaluation procedures have great importance in the individual guidance of patients. It can be used continuously as a basis for identifying particular points needing further attention.

Objectives operate as communicative forms that ensure involvement of all health team members with patient care and guarantee alertness to his condition. They provide a central point of view by stating each team member's impression of the situation, projected plan, and rate of accomplishment toward the patient's goal.

The next step of the process is concerned with deciding whether identification of situations that provide opportunity for the patient to express the desired behavior was afforded. Frequently nurses, in their enthusiasm to get on with care, give meager attention to this requirement, assuming the patient is able to grasp the concept and will operationalize it at a more convenient time. Data are perused for not only availability of situations to indicate the altered behavior, but also the number of times opportunity was given.

The care plan is scrutinized for disclosure of creative use of environment and nursing measures for patient need fulfillment and growth. If we are going to see how patients are developing personal-social adjustment, we must use situations which give patients a chance to react with other patients. It is only after the objectives have been identified and clearly defined, and conditions listed which give opportunity for the expression of the behavior desired, that it is possible to examine results.

Any appraisal of human behavior should be analytic rather than subjective. Three measures necessary for making an appraisal are objectivity, reliability, and validity. *Objectivity* is defined as having to do with a known or perceived object as distinguished from something existing only in the mind of the subject or person thinking, and *reliability* is applied to a person or thing that can be depended upon to do what is expected. Nurses are familiar with objectivity and reliability as concepts and can relate them to the patient without much difficulty. Most of the nursing-patient data represented in the care plans have "face-validity"; that is, they have *validity* because they directly sample the kind of behavior they desire to appraise, as when one directly observes the food which patients are selecting and then evaluates their food habits.

There is interest with confirming role performance as well. Indication of the extent of qualitative nursing actions that develop verification of direct and indirect care to patients, their families, and significant others is sought. Functions such as teaching, directing, and supervision of others engrossed in care, and collaboration with other health professionals, are inclined to reveal these indices. Visibility of use of a shared plan based on manipulation of the major influencing variables, employing a variety of techniques modified on the basis of evaluation of each aspect of intervention as well as evaluation of the total effectiveness of intervention, making creative modifications based on theoretical explanations, is the objective.

Every nursing care program entails several objectives, and some objectives will have many descriptive indices to summarize their products. Results obtained from evaluations will not be a single definitive measure, but rather a composite of calculations of many tangibles.

The patient's functional response comes closest to allowing a discrete interpretation. The appraisals of the nursing components accrue from elements utilized by the nurse in planning care. These reflect behavioral, intellectual, and technical attributes, based upon theories and principles of the physical and social sciences.

All aspects of the nursing role have basic importance to the care of patients and need to be evaluated. Intellectual skills are composed of modes of gathering information, examining data in innovative ways, creating new ideas, and generating unique methods of application for problem solution. These abilities can be appraised with the concepts of convergent, divergent, discriminative, and evaluative thinking, which were explored earlier.

The nurse's repertoire of technical knowledge must be comprehensive. The skill bank must contain a variety of techniques ranging from simple to complex, supportive to restorative, applicable to the present condition. The technical realm needs to be continually validated, and techniques must be exercised with skill and discrimination. Responsibility of the nurse extends beyond judicious use and expert application of the technique to teaching the art to others and supervising those who employ these practices.

Behavioral skills are the focal point of all nursing action. Communication, success in interpersonal relations, coordination and leadership ability, all depend upon a sound theoretical knowledge base, utilization of approaches dictated by patient readiness, and situational demands. Supportive responses to others indicate an understanding of people.

Watching different nurses at work can be very revealing. Each has his own personality, level of experience, educational orientation to nursing, and different skills in varying degrees of competence. Some act as nuturing parents, others as sources of wisdom, others as automatons; still others as jailors. The manner in which patient needs are met is one means of distinguishing these differences. Some nurses respond to the overt, conscious needs of their patients; others to what appears to them as more significant unconscious wants and drives; still others have no visible criterion upon which responses are patterned. However, all are different and perhaps each must fufill all these roles at specific times when dictated by patient problem and circumstance. The point is that for effective evaluation the nurse must be committed to self-examination in each patient-nurse interaction in order to learn the role he has utilized, effect it has produced, and determination as to whether this was the role required by the patient's situation.

This suggests looking at the nurse's role to identify and describe problems which may be encountered by those who undertake an evaluation of nursing process, and to demonstrate the basic premise that nurses are patent factors in the total interaction. Their influence must be considered in order to achieve cogent understanding of the evaluation of the nursing care process.

For nursing process to be effectual, a condition that allows for an integration of emotional and cognitive learning must exist. The nurse's task is primarily one of creating an atmosphere that is conducive to patient learning and adaptation to a changing situation.

Accurate assessment by the nurse of the amount and rate of learning that the patient is able to benefit from is critical: the success of the nursing care plan depends upon the nurse's ability to correctly evaluate the patient's potential. This view of the nursing role emphasizes the nurse's sensitivity in the selection of suitable goals as a factor of prime importance increasing the possibility of doing a competent job.

In their work, nurses cannot avoid involvement in the course of activity of patients. This allows them to pick up the cues that enable them to provide the kind of assistance that helps patients work out problems. Their capacity for discovering cues and ability to determine appropriate courses of action are extremely important. This type of involvement serves to indicate the nurses' involvement, knowledge level, attitude, and adequacy of communications skill. In all situations the nurses' roles are defined by how they act on their perceptions. A clinical frame of reference is used. Viewing nursing behavior in its psychodynamic aspects admits nurse personality as a fundamental variable in the process of the nurse-patient relation. It challenges the validity of the structural and functional properties of the patient that are studied apart from the nurse. Sensitivity to patient behavior, listening, and physical presence of the nurse are overt behaviors that have value.

Two hypotheses underlie the clinical point of view. First, the nurse is a constant source of motivational stimuli for the patient; second, the stimuli put forth by the nurse are a direct function of his total personality organization and philosophical orientation.

Assertion that the nurse is a constant source of motivational stimuli for the patient implies that the nurse is always a force for encouragement, facilitation, hindrance, or inhibition to the patient. By tracing the source of these motivational stimuli to the personality organization of the nurse, one is able to assess his behavior as a function of his needs, beliefs, values, and attitudes. Thus, the nursing role is the result of a constellation of such factors as the degree and kind of education nurses possess, their

imaginative capacity, direct responsiveness to the environment, outlook toward past, present and future, range of experiential data, and general pattern of technical skills.

It is desirable not only to analyze the results of an evaluation to indicate the various successes and failure, but it is also necessary to examine these data to suggest possible explanations or hypotheses about the reason for this particular pattern of strengths and weaknesses and to isolate unusual problems not generally experienced and not usually predictable with that particular set of circumstances.

Again the implements of evaluation are simple to reiterate: those tangibles germane and unique to the individual are observation, cognition, knowledge, and skill bank. The implements the person employs are theories of behavior from the social and applied sciences, tests, and written objectives. However, most crucial to all this are people with inquisitive minds.

The realm of the situational input to the evaluation are those features in the environment that engender strong emotional states, such as anxiety, alienation, or hopelessness, in either the patient or the nurse. Also factors in the immediate situation apart from the immediate dyad can influence or modify the learning processes. The type of material to be learned, the time parameter, features that can affect sensory perception, the social-cultural system position and organizational rules, all affect the process. Nursing care planning is a continuous process, and as materials and procedures are developed, they are tested, their results appraised, their inadequacies identified, and suggested improvements indicated. There is replanning, redevelopment, and then reappraisal. In this kind of cycle it is possible for nursing care to be continuously improved. Through these methods we hope to have a more effective nursing program, rather than depending on a hit-and-miss judgment for patient care.

It would be erroneous to believe it always occurs in such an orderly fashion. Depending on the situation, nurses' cognition, individuality, philosophy, and orientation to learning will dictate the manner in which they approach evaluation. These qualities determine whether evaluation occurs in a systematic orderly fashion, simultaneously, or in a sequential manner.

The hope here was to present a framework by which evaluation can be understood, its relevance to the nursing process grasped, and a dedication to its use engendered.

The study of nursing process has a circular aspect, in which everything is related to everything else. The thread that ties all these together is evaluation.

REFERENCES

1 Adapted from J. P. Guilford, "The Three Faces of Intellect," *American Psychologist*, 14:469–479, 1959.

BIBLIOGRAPHY

Bennis, W. G., Beene, K. D., and Chin, R.: *The Planning of Change: Readings in the Applied Behavioral Sciences*, Holt, Rinehart and Winston, Inc., New York, 1962.

Bigge, M. L.: *Learning Theories for Teachers*, Harper & Row, New York, 1964.

Brinling, Trudy: "Tearing Down a Wall," *American Journal of Nursing*, 71(7):1406–1409, 1971.

Cipolla, Josephine, and Collings, G. H., Jr.: "Nurse Clinicians in Industry," *American Journal of Nursing*, 71(8):1530–1534, 1971.

Cornell, Sadie H., and Brush, F.: "Systems Approach to Nursing Care Plans," *American Journal of Nursing*, 71(7):1376–1378, 1971.

Fast, J.: *Body Language*, J. B. Lippincott, New York, 1970.

Fox, Madeline J.: "Talking With Patients Who Can't Answer," *American Journal of Nursing*, 71(6):1146–1149, 1971.

Francis, Gloria M.: "This Thing Called Problem Solving," *Journal of Nursing Education*, 6:27–30, 1967.

Goldsborough, Judith D.: "On Becoming Non-Judgemental," *American Journal of Nursing*, 70(11):2340, 1970.

Gronlund, N. E., *Measurement and Evaluation in Teaching*, 2d ed., The Macmillan Company, New York, 1971.

Hardiman, Margaret A.: "Interviewing or Social Chit Chat," *American Journal of Nursing*, 71(7):1379–1381, 1971.

Hazzard, Mary Elizabeth: "An Overview of Systems Theory," *Nurse Clinicians of North America*, 6(3):385–393, 1971.

Guilford, J. P.: *Frontiers in Psychology*, Scott, Foresman and Company, Glenview, Ill., pp. 125–147, 1964.

——: *The Nature of Human Intelligence*, McGraw-Hill Book Company, New York, 1967.

Jourard, S. M.: *The Transparent Self*, 2d ed., D. Van Nostrand Company, Inc., Princeton, N.J., 1971.

Klapsbreen, S. C.: "Communications in the Treatment of Cancer," *American Journal of Nursing*, 71(5):944–948, 1971.

Little, Dolores, and Carnevali, Doris: "The Nursing Care Planning System," *Nursing Outlook*, 19(3), March 1971.

Maslow, Abraham H.: *Motivation and Personality*, Harper & Row, New York, 1954.

——: *Toward a Psychology of Being*, 2d ed., Van Nostrand Reinhold Company, New York, 1968.

Mayers, Marlene Glover: *A Systematic Approach to the Nursing Care Plan*, Appleton Century Crofts, New York, 1972.

Mouly, G. J.: *Psychology for Effective Teaching*, Holt, Rinehart and Winston, Inc., New York, 1962.

Paterson, Josephine G.: "From a Philosophy of Clinical Nursing to a Method of Nursology," *Nursing Research*, 20(2):143–146, March, April 1971.

Popham, W. J.: *Criterion Referenced Measurement, An Introduction,* Educational Technology Publications, Englewood Cliffs, N.J., 1972.

Redman, Barbara Kluz: *The Process of Patient Teaching in Nursing*, The C. V. Mosby, Company, St. Louis, 1968.

Roy, Sister Callista: "Adaptation, A Conceptual Framework for Nursing," *Nursing Outlook*, 18(3):42–45, March 1970.

Ruesch, J.: *Therapeutic Communications*, W. W. Norton & Company, Inc., New York, 1961.

——, and Bateson, G.: *Communication, The Social Matrix of Psychiatry*. W. W. Norton & Company, Inc., New York, 1968.

Schein, E. H.: *Professional Education, Some New Directions*, McGraw-Hill Book Company, New York, 1972.

Schweer, Mildred E., and Gardella, Frances: "Planning, Orienting and Preparing for a New Kind of Nurse Leadership," *Nursing Outlook,* 18(5):42–46, 1970.

Smith, Dorothy: "Writing Objectives as a Nursing Practice Skill," *American Journal of Nursing*, 71(2):319–320, 1971.

Straus, David, et al.: *Tools for Change*, 2d ed., Interaction Associates, Inc., San Francisco, 1971.

Zimmerman, Donna S., and Gohrke, Carol: "The Goal-Directed Approach: It Does Work," *American Journal of Nursing*, 70:306–310, 1970.

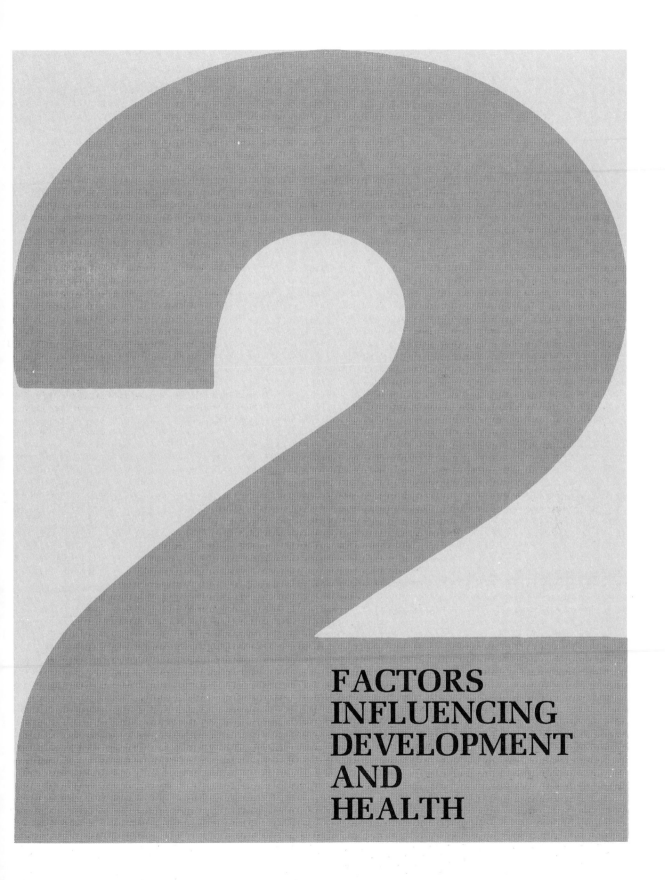

2

FACTORS
INFLUENCING
DEVELOPMENT
AND
HEALTH

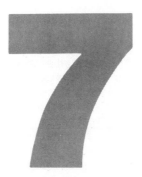

PRINCIPLES AND THEORIES OF CHILD DEVELOPMENT

JEANNE HOWE

Comprehensive health care aims at a much broader target than just the treatment, or even the prevention and treatment, of illness. One of the goals of pediatric health care is to assist and support the growing, changing child so that he may achieve his potential, whatever it may be in his individual case.

Children and the larger society at times needlessly fail to develop their capabilities to the fullest because of illness, handicap, emotional imbalance, or living conditions which produce these problems. Health professionals have unique opportunities and skills for safeguarding human potential. There is a very long tradition among the health disciplines, including nursing, of attempting to prevent or correct conditions which are known to threaten the quality of life. Despite the adoption of this goal, however, and in spite of scientific advances to make it increasingly attainable, the health care professions have by no means always made adequate provisions for the broad range of needs of children and families, nor do they consistently do so even today. There have been numerous reports of children who suffer temporary or long-term handicapping emotional disturbance following hospitalization or treatment which was otherwise successful in correcting some physical disorder. Parents' abilities to love and nurture and find satisfaction in their parenting have suffered in some families as a result of prolonged separation during a child's hospitalization or because of inadequate professional management of fear, guilt, resentment, or misinformation relating to a child's illness. It is obviously desirable to keep the emotional, social, and developmental "costs" of health care at an absolute minimum. Excellence is attained only when, in addition to adequate physical care, all appropriate and feasible efforts are made to safeguard the patient's progress toward achieving his overall potential.

Helping the child and family to reach their highest level of development requires understanding patterns of human change across time, familiarity with hazards which threaten successful progress during various periods of life, and the knowledge and resources necessary to avoid those hazards or to ameliorate their effects. This chapter presents principles and theories of human development in order to provide a basis for understanding children and the processes by which they progress toward maturity. Although it is somewhat artificial and awkward to present child development separately from overall family and other social considerations, the bulk of family and cultural material has been reserved for later chapters.

THE RELEVANCE OF CHILD DEVELOPMENT TO NURSING

Human development is one of the sciences which provide the knowledge base on which the practice of nursing is constructed. Perhaps because change is rapid and apparent in the childhood years, human development has become a more prominent part of pediatric nursing than it generally is in adult nursing.

Child Development and the Nursing Assessment

Assessment has been shown to be an early phase of the nursing process, and the effectiveness of the entire process depends upon the adequacy of the nursing assessment. One simply cannot evaluate any patient without knowing what is important to look for, what is usual, and what constitutes deviation beyond the range of normalcy. The statement that children are not small adults has been made so often that it has become trite. This concept, however—that children can be evaluated only if their special developmental characteristics are taken into consideration—is inescapably basic to the success of the pediatric nursing assessment. Strabismus (crossed eyes), low hemoglobin, tremors, specific fears, and unnumbered other phenomena are within normal limits during some periods of childhood but indicate pathologic conditions at other ages. Child development is the science of child growth and behavior which makes meaningful assessment possible.

Child Development and the Implementation of Nursing Care

An understanding of child development is essential, too, if the nursing actions that follow the assessment phase are to be effective and safe. There was a period in the earlier part of the twentieth century, for example, when infants in institutions such as foundling homes were rigorously protected from infections by keeping their social contacts at the minimum required for feeding and hygiene. The more nearly germ-free their environment, it was believed, the better the babies would fare. History documents that in fact those children had inordinately high rates of emotional disturbance, growth failure, speech maldevelopment, and the like, and that in some institutions many died. Child care experts now generally agree that infants cannot thrive without quantities of human contact and stimulation and that protective seclusion can easily be a greater threat than microorganisms.

Today such blatant, damaging offenses against the needs of pediatric patients are infrequent, but lesser misjudgments that lead to difficulties for children and families still occur and constitute a needless "cost" of health care. Even well-intended treatment, when based on insufficient understanding of the recipient, can place children and their families unnecessarily at risk. *The most effective pediatric nursing is that which, in addition to being otherwise highly skilled, is translated into the idiom of the patient's developmental characteristics.* For example, the explanation offered about procedures, the self-care responsibility given, the behavioral controls imposed, and the methods of communicating and teaching must be fitted to the child.

Child Development in Pediatric Health Maintenance

As nursing and the other health care fields become more concerned with the promotion and maintenance of health, as contrasted to the historically more prominent emphasis upon treatment of illness, anticipatory health guidance becomes an increasingly important facet of pediatric nursing. Some health maintenance needs of children are different not only from adults but also children of other ages.

Accident prevention provides a ready example. The incidence and types of accidents vary throughout childhood and differ from those of adults. In the pediatric age group accidents are the leading cause of death and the major reason for outpatient treatment or hospitalization. Accident prevention requires anticipating the growing child's increasing ability to reach dangerous places and to manipulate his environment in ways that may be hazardous to him and must take into account the child's inexperience and immature judgment about what is safe and what is not. All this needed information—about age-typical progressions in motor ability, patterns of exploration and manipulation of the environment, and cognition and risk-taking behavior—is obtained through a study of child development.

Child Development and the Nurse's Satisfaction

Finally, a knowledge of child development is valuable to nurses because in helping them to understand and succeed with pediatric patients, it expands the enjoyment they find in their work. Children, particularly when they are hurt, sick, or scared, can create distress, discouragement, frustration, and anger in adults who undertake their care. An inconsolably crying infant, an enraged 4-year-old, an adolescent who refuses needed medicines, or a patient who will not rest can play havoc with the self-concept and job satisfaction of a nurse who does not understand the child's actions or know how to respond appropriately. It is sometimes overlooked that nurses, as well as patients, need opportunities for maximum satisfaction and development in their work and life situations. Pediatric nurses appropriately place themselves in an advantaged position by learning to understand and contribute to the development of their patients so that their nursing will be enhancing to themselves as well as to the consumers of their services (Fig. 7-1).

USEFUL PRINCIPLES OF CHILD DEVELOPMENT

Effectively working with children—understanding them, providing for their requirements, helping them develop, and enjoying them (which is likely to follow) —can be learned. Skill in relating to children is not a mystique that some persons have and others do not. Children's growth and development follow orderly, predictable patterns. There are several summary statements or principles which can be extracted from the large body of child development literature to provide a framework for understanding children.

Children Are Competent

Children are well endowed with the qualities and abilities needed to ensure their survival and promote their development. Even the rather helpless-appearing newborn is physiologically equipped for ingestion, digestion, respiration, excretion, and tissue growth and repair.

The neonate has an alarm system to summon assistance when he is hungry or uncomfortable. He has many protective neuromuscular reflexes which, among other things, enable him to cough or sneeze foreign materials from his respiratory tract, withdraw his extremities from pain-producing objects, locate and operate a nearby food supply, react with a startle reflex that tends to place his extremities in a protective position over his face and abdomen, and cry for help. The infant is capable of actions which elicit and reward caretaking responses from adults so that, in a sense, he helps to ensure the availability of needed assistance. Newborns, for example, ordinarily stop crying when fed, thus effectively communicating to parents that their efforts have been successful. Older babies respond to other persons with eye contact, vocalizations, smiles, and generalized excitement which parents and others welcome and which not only strengthen the caretaking relationship but also increase the adult-infant interaction so that the infant has access to the stimula-

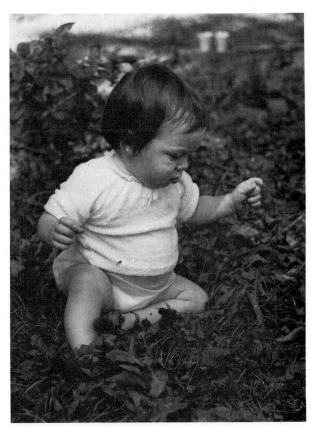

Figure 7-1 At each age the healthy child has specific capabilities for interacting with his environment in ways that can provide stimulation and learning to ensure his continuing development.

tion and experience he needs to promote his continuing development.

Throughout childhood the young human organism's fundamental capabilities to survive, grow, and develop are repeatedly demonstrated. Children are strong and competent and are "programmed" to adapt and thrive if given an environment that meets them halfway.

Children Resemble One Another

The physical and behavioral characteristics of each age and the changes that occur with increasing age are conspicuously similar from child to child. It is usual for children to have physical skills and measurements, physiologic characteristics, and behavioral qualities that closely approximate those of age mates but differ from children of other ages. This developmental principle has obvious implications for nursing assessment. Comparing a child to the norms for his age is a useful and simple preliminary screening technique.

A hemoglobin concentration of 18 Gm/100 ml, for example, is within normal limits for newborns but suggests a pathologic condition at any other age. Similarly, a hemoglobin value of 10 Gm/100 ml is not surprising in a child of 3 months but would be suspect at another age. The limited oxygen available during intrauterine life prompts the fetus to produce an abundance of hemoglobin to maximize oxygen transport. This high hemoglobin is still present at birth. Because the life-span of a red blood cell is about 3 months, and because the red blood cell production rate depends in part on the need to replace dead cells, it is usual for infants to have a progressive drop in hemoglobin that reaches its lowest point around 3 months of age.

Normative data by age and sometimes also by sex are available for many physical and physiologic features with which pediatric nurses are concerned, and for some of the behavioral characteristics as well. Detailed normative descriptions are presented in the chapters that follow and in the appendices.

Each Child Is Unique

Although comparing an individual child to the norms for his age group is a useful screening technique, those averages must not be accepted as absolute standards, and variations from the norms must not be considered defective ipso facto. An awareness of the process by which norms are derived is helpful in preventing their misuse.

The quality of interest—say, height at age 4—is measured on a large number of 4-year-olds. Statistical computations are then performed to find the height that is most representative of the group. The statistic most frequently used is the median (also called the 50th percentile), which is the midpoint of the group; 50 percent of the children are taller than that height, and 50 percent are shorter. The median height of any group of 4-year-olds in the United States is around 103 cm (40½ inches). The median of 103 cm does not mean that *any* of the children in the group were actually 103 cm tall, only that half the children were taller than that and half were shorter. More important, the median does not in any way indicate that a 4-year-old *must* be 103 cm tall, that it is more advantageous to be 103 cm than another height, or that a 4-year-old who *is* 103 cm tall is in good health.

Normative charts or tables are more useful if

they also show how much the members of the group varied from the average. A height table for 4-year-olds, for example, might include the information that only 10 percent of the children measured less than 99 cm (39 inches) and only 10 percent were taller than 109 cm (43 inches). The fact that 80 percent of the group were somewhere between 99 and 109 cm tells more about that group of children than the median value alone. The nurse or other person referring to the norms can now ascertain whether a particular child is like or different from an 80 percent majority of the reference group. However, he still cannot definitively say on the basis of how well the child conforms to the norms whether or not that child is well and growing properly.

Every child has his own unique qualities and consequently is likely to differ in several ways from the norms. Even newborns differ from one another and from a hypothetical "average" baby in length and weight, degree of physiologic stability, assertiveness, feeding behavior, and so forth. Especially as children grow older and varieties in their experience increase, they reflect their individual enrichments or deprivations in addition to their unique inborn traits, and considerable difference is to be expected from child to child.

It can be difficult to know how much deviation from the norm is compatible with well-being and at what point differences should arouse professional concern. No general rules are available to show infallibly "how much is too much." In the case of a child who differs from normative expectations in size, rate of growth, motor ability, language development, social relationships, or in some other manner, it is important to include all other relevant considerations in his assessment. Some other possibly explanatory points to consider are discussed next.

Family Patterns The family history may show that siblings or other relatives of the child in question have also been atypical in the same way. If so, this information can help the nurse decide whether intervention is required or whether the long-term outcome may be expected to be satisfactory.

Cultural, Ethnic, or Racial Influences A child's background may be substantively different from that of the group used for comparison, making assessment difficult; he may appear deviant in terms of the group when in fact he is not exceptional in his own group.

For example, Orientals and blacks are generally smaller at the same age than the Caucasians of Western

European and Nordic backgrounds that have predominated in the growth studies from which the norms were developed. And language patterns vary widely among subcultures and regionally, so that a child whose speech and language may seem aberrant to the nurse may be at the age level for his group. Similarly, umbilical hernia is common and usually self-correcting in black children even into the preschool years but has probable surgical significance in whites.

The Child's Past History   Since each child grows and develops according to his own pattern, his history can be used as a standard to which he is compared. Allowing for the occasional spurts and levelings that occur at some points during the maturation process, each child generally follows a consistent pattern with respect to early or late acquisition of new skills, early or late growth, large or small size, and so forth. For this reason, a loss of pace with his own usual pattern may be a more meaningful sign than conforming to or deviating from norms.

Expert Opinion   Collaboration with colleagues, including those in medicine, psychology, education, physical therapy, and other appropriate fields, can be of invaluable assistance in assessing deviant children and planning any indicated therapies.

Growth and Development Are Directional

The cephalocaudal and general-to-specific principles of development provide predictability that can be helpful to nurses. The law of *cephalocaudal* (from head toward tail) progression of development describes the observed fact that growth, motor skill, and perhaps sensory acuteness are more advanced in the newborn at and near the head and gradually progress downward to the neck, trunk, and extremities. Thus a child gains control of his neck muscles to steady his previously wobbly head before he has sufficient strength in his trunk muscles to allow him to sit. Similarly, hip control for sitting precedes leg control for walking. In the upper extremity, sufficient strength and coordination to move the shoulders and direct the arms to reach an attractive object antedate being able to coordinate the hands to pick it up. This directional progression from head toward buttocks and from proximal toward distal end of the extremities allows the nurse to anticipate, for example, that a child who is still at the stage of large, uncoordinated arm movements will not need to be restrained from picking at IVs, dressings, or sutures except as required to protect against random arm movements.

Development proceeds also *from the general to the specific*, from the global to the precise. An infant makes varied, random vocal sounds before he refines them into speech. Large muscle activities such as throwing precede the fine motor coordination required for fastening buttons or tying shoelaces. Perceptual phenomena and social relationships, as well as these speech and motor examples, seem to develop in accordance with this progression from the more general to the more specific.

Development Is Timely

The concept of *critical periods*, which has received more attention to date with respect to the lower animals than to humans, appears at least implicitly in most of the major child development theories. A critical period is a span of time maximally favorable for the accomplishment of a new developmental process. That same developmental change is said to be more difficult or impossible to master either before or after its critical period.

An often-cited example that seems to demonstrate the critical period phenomenon and that has applicability to nursing is the development of the special social bond between an infant and his mother or primary caretaker. Observations of inadequately parented babies, such as orphanage residents who lack a continuing relationship with a significant caretaking adult, have indicated that such a relationship is necessary during approximately the second half of the first year of life. The "classic" institution babies, fortunately now quite rare outside long-term hospitalization settings, developed normally for about the first 4 to 6 months following birth and then began to show signs of progressive developmental retardation, including distorted interpersonal relationships. Those who survived the increased mortality rates of infancy in institutions often demonstrated long-lasting inability to form trusting, loving relationships and exhibited enuresis, speech impediments, asocial or delinquent behavior, learning disabilities, and a complex of other developmental difficulties that seem to be sequelae of maternal deprivation during the critical second 6 months. Although research is not totally consistent about the limits of the critical period for the formation of the primary social bond between infant and principal caretaker, it is generally accepted that before about 3 to 6 months of age and after about the first birthday maternal deprivation does not have the same impact or produce quite the same kind or degree of developmental distortion.

In contrast, the infant reared within a sufficiently continuous relationship during that period typically demonstrates a progressive exclusiveness in his preference for the caretaking person. The baby learns to recognize the primary caretaker as distinct from other persons, shows special fondness for that person, and at about 7 to 9 months begins to react to strangers (sometimes to *all* others) with avoidance and apparent fear. This response to strangers is called "8-month anxiety." Many developmentalists believe it is the human equivalent of the fear phase that closes the critical period for *imprinting* (forming the primary social bond) in many infrahuman species and ensures that the young animal will recognize and stay with its mother until old enough to care for itself.

Critical periods in human beings have not yet been demonstrated with the same precision as those in lower animals, but the premise that they exist is expressed in the familiar concept of developmental task and in those theories of human development which are classified as stage theories.

A *developmental task* may be defined as a skill, a competency, or a learning which is necessary for a child to accomplish at a particular time in his life. Delay or failure in doing so is said to make his subsequent development more difficult.

For example, a developmental task of the newborn is to adapt physiologically to air breathing, body temperature maintenance, and the other changes required for survival and continued development in his extrauterine environment. A task of the school-age child is to become adept at using symbols—numbers and the written word—and at understanding the concepts symbols represent. Among the tasks of late adolescence is mastery of the diverse range of advanced self-care skills and judgments which can permit termination of reliance upon parents.

Stage theories of development are those which break the life-span into sequential periods, each characterized by some developmental quality which is more prominent at that period of life than before or after it. Freudian theory, with its oral, anal, and phallic stages, is a familiar example.

New Skills Tend to Predominate

Especially in the earlier years of childhood, while the child remains relatively simplistic and incapable of dealing with several things at one time, there is a strong tendency for the current developmental issue to become a preoccupation. The appearance of a new ability is accompanied by a strong drive to practice and perfect that ability.

For example, infants around 9 to 12 months old, which is the usual age to learn to pull from a sitting to a standing position, may be so eager to exercise their new ability that they insist on standing for meals. Even when quite ill, babies this age often appear driven to stand up in their hospital cribs rather than lie down. Similarly, the application of a plaster cast to one or both extremities of a child who has just learned to crawl or walk generally does little to impede his practice of his new mobility, as is evidenced by the worn-out knees or feet of the cast.

As a corollary to this tendency to attend fully to one aspect of development at a time, the situation in which a child must deal with more than one developmental feature can be very stressful and probably should not be imposed unnecessarily. It is said, for example, that a child who is adapting to a recent loss or addition of a family member should not be simultaneously subjected to the anxieties of hospitalization if it can feasibly be postponed. Similarly, the occasional request that hospital personnel "break" a child of having a bedtime bottle or impose other habit training during hospitalization, already a period of stress, probably should be declined (and this principle should be explained to the parents).

It seems reasonable to suppose, although it has not been substantiated, that the preeminence of one developing skill may actually delay the onset of subsequent skills. This writer has noticed, for example, that talking, which ordinarily follows walking, may appear several months early and be especially well developed in children in whom paralysis or some similar physical debility has prevented walking at the time it would ordinarily begin.

This principle of one developmental feature being more prominent than others at a given period of time is central to the stage theories and will be further described in the following section about theories. At this point it is sufficient to note that most developmentalists consider the chronologically earlier accomplishments, tasks, and stages to be prerequisites for success with later skills. That is, each developmental step is viewed as a necessary foundation for subsequent development.

The Many Aspects of Development Are Interrelated

It is artificial and therefore somewhat misleading to speak of subcategories such as physical, social, cognitive, emotional, or ethical aspects of behavior and development as if they were separate entities. Such categories, contrived as they are, nevertheless are commonplace because they seem to assist in understanding the complex human organism. Child development, being a cross-disciplinary field of study, helps describe the essential unity of the developmental process by showing how one category is related to another.

Emotional self-reliance, for example, cannot develop more rapidly than the *physical* strength and coordination plus the self-care *judgment* (a *cognitive* function which requires *experience* as well) which make it possible. And bone growth depends on *nutritional* adequacy, which has strong *physiologic* and *socioeconomic* determinants; on *gravitational* pull, which in turn is influenced by the *maturational* ability to assume various positions and to move about; on the amount of *force* applied by attached muscles, which is dependent on *neurologic* function and the *work load* applied; and by many other circularly interrelated factors. In summary, the so-called physical, cognitive, and other aspects of the developing child act upon and react to one another extensively and inseparably.

Health care directed at producing change in one realm of development without giving sufficient consideration to the prerequisites or consequences in the other areas has a limited chance of accomplishing the larger goal of supporting the total child in his progressive movement toward realizing his fullest potential.

THEORIES OF CHILD DEVELOPMENT

There are many ways to study children and to interpret the results. In simplest terms, a theory is essentially a detailed, organized, internally consistent framework for such study and interpretation.

There are probably more than a dozen different theories which could be called upon to help nurses understand children, although far fewer are widely used in nursing and only five will be included here. One point is worth noting about the number and variety of applicable theories, however; none of them is completely satisfactory for all purposes or to all who study children. One reason is that the several theories vary in the scope of phenomena they attempt to explain. For example, Darwin's biology-based theory of evolution or Malthus's bioeconomic theory might be useful for explaining and predicting the consequences for the human race of correcting birth defects so that genetically atypical children can survive to reproduce; a learning theory like Piaget's presumably would be irrelevant in that kind of research. Another factor limiting the widespread applicability of a single theory is that any theory may be unacceptable to some persons because its basic assumptions conflict with some of their values. Darwinian theory, for example, has historically been offensive to some who hold to fundamentalist Christianity; and the Freudian concepts of id, ego, and superego are rejected by some who believe behavioral science must be based only upon more directly observable and measurable phenomena.

The theories selected for inclusion in this chapter are those of Freud, Erikson, and Piaget; the stimulus-response theory; and a group of concepts from what might be termed social interaction theories. Freudian and Eriksonian theories were chosen because they have been emphasized in nursing for the past 20 or 30 years. There are unmistakable indications at the present that these approaches (especially Freud's) to explaining or modifying behavior are not as broadly accepted as they once were, but since they are still in sufficiently common use, pediatric nurses need to be familiar with them. Piaget's work appears at this time to have limited applicability to nursing but is touched upon because currently it is probably the most talked about theory in many of the other child study disciplines; and consequently, nurses who may look into the wider scope of child development literature or work with interdisciplinary teams will be handicapped if they do not understand at least its fundaments. Stimulus-response theory likewise has produced a rapidly expanding literature and, as the basis of behavior modification, is being widely and somewhat controversially used in the nursing of mentally retarded and emotionally disturbed children as well as in the education and training of normal children.

The sociologic theories and their concepts of role, interaction, group dynamics, and social systems are just beginning to become popular in the health disciplines. Medicine and nursing have in the past stayed mainly within the conceptual limits of theories which deal with individual persons rather than with groups or even with individuals in interaction. Individual psychotherapy and the case study method of research are familiar and undeniably productive ways in which physicians and nurses have used the one-to-one orientation to treatment and study which has resulted from the preeminence of psychologic theories in the health fields. An unfortunate narrowness has resulted, however. Individual patients have too often been approached as if their health and behavior depended only upon them as individuals, when in truth each person is continually influenced by his family, the staff in the clinical setting, other patients, his school or work group, and endless other small or large groups with whom he interacts socially. Patients, particularly pediatric patients, seldom if ever relate to a nurse in isolation from family members and others with whom the nurse must skillfully relate if the patient's health care program is to be effective. Without minimizing the importance of the individual or de-emphasizing the usefulness of individual growth, development, and behavior as bases of nursing practice, this book has been developed with a focus on nurses working with families, with teams of other health care workers, and with patients who interact among themselves as members of groups. For these reasons, sociologic constructs are included in the following material about theoretical underpinnings of development and behavior.

Freudian Theory

Probably the developmental theory that is most widely familiar to nurses and has the longest history of inclusion in nursing education is Freudian psychology. Sigmund Freud (1856–1939) was an Austrian physician whose ideas about behavior and development became popular in the United States in the 1930s. It would be difficult to name another person whose thought has been as pervasively integrated into the American way of life. A very extensive school of child study, child bearing, and behavioral interpretation has developed around the tenets of psychoanalysis. Among the concepts Freud is credited with originating or popularizing are the unconscious mind; the defense mechanisms; the oral, anal, phallic, latency, and adult sexuality stages of development; early childhood as the origin of emotional disorders; the id, ego, and superego; and the classic psychoanalytic "couch" technique of retracing past experiences to discover the historical causes of present maladjustments.

The *unconscious* is conceptualized as the portion of the mind which contains memories, motives, facts, fantasies, fears, etc., of which the person is unaware. The unconscious, although ordinarily inaccessible to recall or recognition, asserts a very active influence on behavior. The well-known premise that "all behavior is meaningful" is a reference to the Freudian belief that even the most seemingly trivial or illogical behavior makes sense if its unconscious motivations can be discovered. Thus dreams, irra-

tional fears, habits and mannerisms such as smoking and tics, and slips of the tongue (Freudian slips, technically known as parapraxes) are viewed within the Freudian tradition as evidences of the unconscious mind's pervasive influence on thought and behavior.

Freud conceived the mind as consisting of three structures: the *id*, the *ego*, and the *superego*. The id is the part of the psyche concerned with obtaining as much enjoyment as possible as soon as possible and by any means available. The newborn, for example, is said to be all id—he wants what he wants without consideration of others or of the consequences of his demands, and he protests any delay or compromise. The id is said to be the origin of lust, greed, aggression, and any other manifestation of unrestrained pleasure seeking.

The ego is a very complex part of the psyche whose functions include intelligence, memory, cognition, separating reality from fantasy, problem solving, compromising between the instinctual drives of the id and the pressures of reality, and incorporating experiences and learning into one's future behavior. The overall function of the ego is to enable the person to operate successfully within the realities of his social, psychologic, and physical environment. The ego presumably begins to develop during the first year of life, as the infant's accumulating experience begins to assert influence upon his earlier, purely id-motivated behavior. Ego development continues throughout childhood and to some degree throughout the life-span.

The third part of the psyche is the superego, which can simplistically be equated with the conscience. Development of the superego probably begins as early as infancy, then is seen more clearly in the toddler, and progressively becomes more apparent in the preschool and school-age child, as he learns socially acceptable behavior. As people in the child's experiential environment socialize him to the rules and regulations of his social setting, he gradually adopts behavioral, ethical, and moral standards and incorporates them as his expectations for his own behavior—his superego.

A major theoretical contribution of Freudian theory has been the description of defense mechanisms. These are essentially unconscious coping mechanisms contrived by the ego for distorting awareness in order to reduce stress. The stress may have arisen out of conflict among the three parts of the psyche or between the mind and external reality. Something too painful to be acknowledged, for example, may be "forgotten" (*repression*) and thereby rendered unavailable to the conscious mind.

As another example, a person who engenders intolerable amounts of hostility may become the object of excessive affection and kindness instead (*reaction formation*). Or a specific emotion may be transferred to a distantly related situation (*displacement*) as in the case of a person whose extreme fear of needles is actually a displacement of his unconscious fear of phallic intrusiveness. The major point to be understood about the defense mechanisms is that they operate unconsciously to distort the person's awareness to protect him from the discomfort he would feel if he were conscious of his feelings. There are numerous defense mechanisms. It is not feasible to deal with them here in detail. The interested reader is referred to the readings at the end of the chapter or to any basic psychology text.

Freud identified the underlying motivation for human behavior at all ages to be sexuality, which he termed libido. His concept of sex and sexuality was considerably broader than is implied in the ordinary usage of those words, which has caused misunderstanding and created resistance to psychoanalytic ideas. In psychoanalytic language, libido refers not only to sexuality in its genital manifestations but to pleasure seeking in general. The libidinous thoughts or activities of infants and young children are referred to as pregenital in order to make this distinction.

Psychoanalytic theory states that there are oral, anal, phallic, and latency stages of childhood development. The infant's libidinal pleasures are believed to center about the gratification he finds from using his mouth for sucking and for satisfying his hunger. The first year of life is said to be orally dominated, with pleasure, hostility, aggression, and any other feelings and acitivities being focused on and expressed by the mouth. Even the infant's use of eyes, hands, and interpersonal interactions is viewed as being used to symbolically carry out the oral behaviors of grasping and incorporating. The child's oral experiences are believed to be the foundation of his personality development, so that either too much or too little oral gratification in infancy can produce in an older person an "oral personality" characterized by passivity, dependence, eating problems, speech disorders, and so forth.

With the beginning of neuromuscular control over the anal sphincter, the child transfers his predominating focus and expression of libido from his mouth to his anal region. The erotic experiences, both frustrating and satisfying, which accompany control over withholding and expelling, containing and releasing, now become the hub of the child's mental life and take predominance in the development of his personality. Possessiveness, retentiveness, aggressiveness, pronounced messiness or tidiness, punctuality, and shame are among the personality characteristics psychoanalysts associate with the anal stage. Toilet training, which requires that the toddler compromise between his libidinal enjoyment of his bowel function and the controls imposed by social expectation, is seen as the crucial issue in the anal stage.

Around age 4 the child's interest, activity, and erotic pleasure focus around his genital region. Self-stimulation, self-comfort, curiosity, questioning, play, and social activities and relationships, according to Freudians, are best understood if viewed in the context of genital libidinous interests. Both sexes of preschoolers are said to place a great value on the penis, with boys treasuring their sex organ and fearing some injury to it or attack upon it by hostile others (*castration anxiety*) and girls wishing they had a penis (*penis envy*) and sometimes imagining that they previously had one which was taken away by a hostile, jealous mother. The general intrusiveness with which the 4-year-old attacks his environment is interpreted as symbolic of phallic assertiveness.

As genital sexuality becomes the primary mode of libidinous expression, the young child's relationship with his parents becomes infused with his sexual feelings and ambitions. The preschool boy, although his concepts of a sexual relationship may not include a realistic knowledge of sexual intercourse, is described by Freudians as wishing an intimate sexual possessiveness of his mother. His physical approaches to her and his other expressions of affection toward her—protectiveness, gift giving, stories about someday living alone with her and bringing up their children, etc.—are interpreted in terms of the *Oedipus complex*. The boy is thought to be jealous and competitive toward his father, as is indicated by his striving to appear bigger and stronger and to outdo his father both in general and in his appeals for his mother's exclusive attention and love. He fears that his father will take retribution on him, either in the form of a direct genital assault (castration) or in a more generalized punishing or annihilating way.

A similar sexuality and preference for the opposite-sex parent is believed to dominate the preschool period for girls. Sometimes called the *Electra complex* by laymen, this developmental phase is said to be characterized by sexual fantasies and strivings involving her father, coy or seductive behavior toward him, and jealousy, petulance, and fear toward her mother.

About the age of 6, the child is said to learn that a sexual relationship with a parent is not feasible. Because of the futility he sees in pursuing his incestuous wishes, and because of the anxieties produced by castration anxiety and fears of losing parental love, the school-age child turns his attention from sexuality. He becomes intent upon the tasks of socialization, including the things he learns at school and the refinement of his roles and role relationships. Freud termed the school-age years the *latency period* to signify the quiescence of sexuality between the oedipal period and adolescence. According to theory, as the child gives up his oedipal ambitions, he increasingly identifies with his same-sex parent and spends his latency period learning and practicing the skills and roles which will prepare him for adulthood and for winning a mate of his own.

Adolescence begins the stage of *adult sexuality*, although psychoanalytic psychology considers adolescence to have several distinguishing characteristics of its own rather than to be just a part of a homogeneous, final developmental phase. Freud considered adolescence a resumption of the preschool libidinous interests, now possible in an overt, nonincestuous heterosexual relationship. With the resurgence of sexual pressures and conflicts, the intrapsychic tranquility of latency is lost, and great turmoil ensues before defense mechanisms and life-style adaptations make mature adult adjustment possible. Adolescent ego functions (behavior and thought) are expected to be disturbed and bizarre, even to the extent that some psychoanalysts refer to adolescence as "the normal psychosis."

Freud believed that the essentials of personality formation are completed by the end of the phallic stage and that personality and adjustment in later life depend upon the development that took place in the oral, anal, and phallic phases. Consequently, mental illness is believed to have its roots in early childhood. Psychoanalytic therapy hence consists of reexploring the experiences of infancy and early childhood to uncover and resolve disturbances. The "couch" techniques—*free association* (unpremeditated verbal responses to thoughts, or the flow of ideas unrestrained by logic) and recall of early experiences in order to uncover material in the unconscious mind—are not considered appropriate or effective therapeutic techniques for children. Psychoanalytic therapy for children frequently is based on observations of the child's nondirected play as the means of discovering unconscious mental processes. Psychoanalysts believe that, since all behavior reflects unconscious feelings and thought associations, the play of even preverbal children reveals the content of the child's unconscious mind and hence makes that material accessible for therapeutic intervention.

Critique of Freudian Theory Psychoanalytic theory is virtually unlimited in the range of behavioral phenomena it attempts to explain. Everything, including the meaning of dreams, consumer responses to advertising, vocational and marital selection, international relations, habits, and art forms, falls within the scope of psychoanalytic interpretation. The theory is very fully developed, with an expansive literature dealing in detail with most of the structural aspects of the theory and its applications in behavior and therapy.

With the emergence of alternative theoretical basis for psychotherapy (reality therapy, behavior modification, transactional analysis, drug therapy, etc.), psychoanalysis with its lengthy, expensive, and questionably effective methods of treatment has been replaced to some extent as a therapeutic approach. A major limitation of psychoanalysis is that it deals rather exclusively with intrapsychic phenomena rather than with the person's current interpersonal setting which is, after all, the context within which thought and behavior take on meaning as either effective and acceptable or not. Also, as the behavioral sciences become better developed and take on more of the scientific rigor that has previously been more characteristic of the physical and biologic sciences, many persons have become dissatisfied with the "unscientific" imprecision of psychoanalytic theory and with the induction (as opposed to deduction, which is an earmark of scientific theory and the scientific method) required to make psychoanalytic interpretations. Psychoanalysis has been criticized as being a dogma, rather than a science, which can be understood and used only by the "priesthood" who have themselves undergone analysis and have thereby gained special insight not shared by persons trained in the sciences. The basic assumptions of psychoanalytic theory (the existence of the id, ego, superego, libidinal energy, the unconscious, etc.), the basic data of the psychoanalytic method (thoughts, memories, fantasies), and the basic methods of data collection (remembering, responding to suggestion) are perhaps all reliable and valid constructs, but the fact that they cannot be tested for reliability and validity by any scientific evaluative procedure leaves psychoanalysis vulnerable to criticism against which it has offered few substantive defenses. Since Freud constructed his theory on the basis of his work with neurotic adults, its validity with respect to the normal development of children is in question.

Eriksonian Theory

Erik Erikson (1902–) is a lay (not having a medical degree) psychoanalyst who, in contradistinction to Freud, has worked very extensively with children. Erikson's famous eight ages of man, presented at the 1950 White House Conference on Children and Youth, has been adopted by many disciplines, including nursing, as a useful theory of human development.

Erikson describes the life-span from birth through senescence as consisting of a sequence of eight stages. Each stage is dominated by a major developmental problem which takes an either-or configuration; that is, for each stage there is a central task or problem which will be resolved either favorably, so that the foundation is well laid for the subsequent stage, or unfavorably, which will make later development more difficult. In none of the stages is the problem resolved totally and forever; instead, it holds a zenith position during the stage it dominates and then remains less dominant but arises again from time to time to be further resolved. Also, no problem is expected to be mastered so that the favorable alternative is achieved to the complete exclusion of the unfavorable one; good adjustment consists of developing the desirable alternative so that it *predominates* over the undesirable one.

During infancy, according to Erikson, the central task is to establish a sense of *basic trust* in predominance to *mistrust*. The infant who finds that his needs for food and other kinds of comfort are consistently and effectively met learns that his world is a safe and predictable place and that he can trust others and his own organism.

A toddler phase constitutes the period in which the child must establish a sense of *autonomy* rather than *shame and doubt*. The toddler who has learned to trust is developmentally driven to assert his growing awareness that his behavior is under his own control. He can move about and do things, and his will and ability are effective in producing his desired outcomes. "I can do it myself, and that delights me" is the earmark of autonomy. Shame and doubt are the developmental hazards for the toddler, to which he is especially vulnerable if he has brought a substantial quantity of mistrust from his infancy or if he finds as a result of his autonomous assertiveness that his independent actions are unacceptable (shame) or ineffectual (doubt).

About the time he has become able to walk easily without having to attend the motor manipulations walking involves (Erikson says the child is confident that he can "stand on his own feet"), he moves into the third developmental stage, in which the central task is to develop a sense of *initiative* in preponderance to a sense of *guilt*. The preschooler is bent on exploring what he can attain and create and on seeing what he can do with the motor, language, interpersonal, and other skills of which he is almost daily becoming more capable. The vigorous, phallic preschooler throws himself full force into his expanding physical and social worlds. His behavior is characterized by intrusiveness, manifest in his endless thrusting of questions, noises, and physical and intellectual explorations. Guilt is the major developmental hazard for the preschooler because a good deal of what he plans or undertakes cannot be permitted or accomplished, and some of his schemes do not win the praise of the people he wishes to please. He is also vulnerable to guilt because the superego becomes prominent during the preschool years and the child often disapproves of his own actions (or fantasies, which he does not clearly distinguish from reality).

The child who successfully attains the ability to initiate acceptable goals and to persevere in his attempt to reach them is in good stead for entering the school-age period, in which the central task as identified by Erikson is to develop a sense of *industry* rather than a sense of *inferiority*. The school-age child uses the physical, cognitive, and social skills he has brought from the preschool phase and now turns his attention to learning what he must know in preparation for success in the adult world of facts and tools. Setting aside his former explorations of fantasy and preoccupation with his family, he now focuses upon reality and the larger social sphere. There is a lot to learn—mathematics, reading, writing, history, geography, science, the rudiments of religion and politics, social roles, and the social and physical skills required for dealing successfully with the realities of the almost-adult world in which he operates. The child who finds his abilities wanting becomes discouraged in his development of industriousness and may conceptualize himself as inadequate and inferior.

Erikson characterizes adolescence as centering around the task of developing a sense of *identity*, with the undesirable alternative being *role confusion*. In his quest to find out who he is and who he will be as an adult, the adolescent identifies with and "understudies" a gamut of persons which may include missionaries and mobsters, parents and rock heroes, politicians and artists, and almost anyone else observable. The adolescent's clannishness and intolerance of those who are different are interpreted as ways of helping to establish who he *is* by isolating and condemning that which he *is not.* Erikson describes the attainment of identity as the young person's coming to feel that his views of himself are internally consistent and consistent with others' views of him. The major hazard of adolescence, role confusion, arises from the rapid changes in experience of self and from the sometimes overwhelming number of ways to behave and roles to select. Some young people adopt delinquent or other disapproved, "negative" identities as a way of resolving their need for some identity rather than continuing confusion.

The young adult, having established his sense of identity, seeks next to share himself in *intimacy* with other persons. The hazard during the intimacy stage is *isolation*, or the inability to expose the self by sharing it with another in mature friendship and love.

Following the stage of intimacy versus isolation, the majority of the adult years are seen by Erikson as devoted to the developmental task of establishing a sense of *generativity*, which essentially means productivity and satisfaction with it. The well-developed adult is productive in his work, as a citizen, and in his establishment and management of a home and family. Producing and rearing children comprise a major part of generativity for most adults, although there are other expressions of the attainment of generativity, such as care and provision for other groups and causes besides one's own offspring. The developmental hazard of the generativity phase is *stagnation*, which is characterized by self-absorption, lack of productivity, and an uncharitable or competitive attitude toward one's children or others.

The final stage of adulthood requires developing what Erikson calls *ego integrity* rather than its opposing sense of *despair.* Ego integrity is a satisfaction that life has been what it had to be, that living has been good and meaningful, and that on the whole one has acted responsibly and has succeeded. Despair is characterized by a dread of dying, disgust with oneself and one's failures, and bitterness that it is too late to start over and do better.

Critique of Eriksonian Theory　Erikson has done a great deal to broaden Freudian theory and to make it more explicit and more useful to those who wish to understand children's development. He has enlarged Freud's fairly exclusive attention to the child's *inner, psychodynamic* influences and has emphasized also the *sociocultural* and *biophysical* factors

that affect development; that is, Erikson has presented human development as inseparably interrelated with culture and with physical growth as well as with the psychology of the growing person. For example, in Eriksonian theory the stages of development change in concert with the emergence of new physical attributes (such as the ability to control the whole motor apparatus as an initiator of autonomy, which is more directly observable and therefore conceptually more manageable than Freud's shift of libidinal investment from the mouth to the anus). As another example, Erikson's description of adolescence as a search for identity, with all its cultural and social influences, is far broader and again more observable than the Freudian position that the pubescent hormonal changes initiate a resurgence of preschool sexual strivings.

A problem with Eriksonian theory is the difficulty with which some of his basic postulates are operationalized; therefore, they cannot be confirmed or refuted using the scientific method. For example, what observable, measurable *behaviors* indicate that a baby has developed basic trust? If basic trust could be measured in terms of sleep patterns, feeding and bowel activity, crying, or other identified qualities, Eriksonian theory could be tested, which is a characteristic of a good theory, and would likely generate extensive research, another identifying mark of a good theory. Trust, mistrust, autonomy, shame and doubt, etc., have not been precisely enough delineated by Erikson to permit these kinds of tests of the theory.

Piagetian Theory

Jean Piaget (1896–), a Swiss zoologist, epistemologic philosopher, and psychologist, has worked during the majority of his lifetime to develop a theory of cognitive development. His very extensive writings and those of his Geneva colleagues and students report their thousands of ingeniously designed experiments and the theory derived from those studies of children's intellectual activity and its change as children get older. Without doubt, the Piagetian framework has produced the largest body of theoretical and observational literature about children's thinking now in existence.

There are a number of difficulties in understanding Piagetian theory. Piaget, as a biologist and philosopher, approaches his work with concepts and a specialized language that most behavioral scientists have not previously become familiar with. In addition, he writes in French, so that the necessity for translating not only his words but also some of their underlying concepts has contributed to difficulty in understanding his ideas. The following passages present a highly simplified, brief overview of the theory.

Piaget's work can be classified as a stage theory. It presents cognitive development as undergoing qualitative change across the ages of childhood. The earliest kind of thought, according to Piaget, is characteristic of the first 2 years of life. This time span he calls the *sensorimotor period*, which is broken into several chronologic substages. The main quality about the sensorimotor period is that thought derives from sensation and movement and so is inseparably linked to (and in fact limited to) the child's motor and sensory experiences. Without doing, there can be no cognition. The child's intellectual experience during the sensorimotor period consists of observing and adaptively manipulating himself and his environment. Beginning with the earliest sensorimotor input revolving around the feeding experience, for example, the infant gradually becomes able to organize information and to mentally coordinate the several related components of his experience, such as sucking, feeling, seeing, and tasting.

Piaget stresses the importance of the infant's learning that objects continue to exist even when they are out of sight. The understanding that an object covered by, for example, a blanket continues in existence and can be reclaimed by removing the blanket or reaching under it does not appear to be within a child's grasp until he is around 8 months of age, when he begins to search for an absent object rather than immediately turning his attention from it when it disappears. The concept of object permanence, which is a prerequisite for being able to think about things when they are not presently a part of the sensorimotor input, and which also precedes awareness that one can intentionally control some aspects of one's environment, is more than a matter of developing memory. It is related to the infant's progressing ability to deal with matters of time (continuing existence) and space (existence in other places besides the one presently experienced).

Goal-directed behavior begins to appear in the infant's behavioral repertoire and gradually includes alternative ways of achieving a goal. Thus by 12 months an infant is able not only to search for a toy that has rolled out of sight but also to go around a chair the toy has passed beyond in order to repossess it, rather than having to follow the same path the toy took under the chair. He begins to find a variety of ways of producing an outcome other than the process by which the event occurs. "Experimenting" and deliberate manipulation are taken up, although the discovery that, for example, an object will move if kicked comes from sensorimotor experience and cannot yet be foreseen or conceptualized in the abstract.

During the sensorimotor period the infant gains a primitive grasp of the connection between cause and effect and becomes active in making things happen in accordance with his intention. He can carry out a short series of related, goal-directed activities, combining behavioral elements into a sequence. Even by his second birthday, however, the child is severely limited in his ability to "think," as he is bound to the concrete aspects of his sensation and activity and cannot conceptualize or deal abstractly with things beyond the scope of his sensorimotor experience.

Piaget's second stage of cognitive development is sometimes presented as a single period extending from age 2 to age 11, and sometimes as two stages running from ages 2 to 7 and then from 7 to 11. The latter approach will be followed here. Like the sensorimotor period, these phases have been broken down into several sequential substages which are not discussed separately here.

From 2 to 7 years of age the child progresses through the period of *preoperational thought*. In comparison to the child of 2 and under, whose thinking is restricted to his sensorimotor experiences, the preoperational thinker deals at a much higher level with symbols. He uses language and memory and has a growing understanding of past, present, and future. The word preoperational, however, indicates that the child is not intellectually capable of understanding the fundamental *relationships* between or among phenomena. The preoperational thinker, for example, may deny that just because A is bigger than B, it follows that B is smaller than A. Additional examples characteristic of the 4- to 7-year-old child will make clearer the nature of preoperational thought. A child at this age, if given a marble and a penny, then a second marble and a second penny, and so forth one by one until he has an equal number of each, will report that he has more marbles than pennies because the marbles take up more space, or he may say that he has more pennies than marbles because the coins make a tall stack. He cannot understand that if one of two clay balls that he agrees are the same size is flattened into a new shape as he watches, the two masses still contain equal amounts of clay. Piaget attributes these errors in understanding to the child's not having yet developed the concept of *reversibility*, or the ability to conceptualize that a completed process can also be performed in reverse order so that the materials involved are returned to their initial condition. He does not grasp the basic relationship between objects or between events or understand the process of transition.

Preoperational thought is characterized by *egocentrism*. The preschooler is unable, and the early school-age child only poorly able, to take another person's point of view. Hence, especially at the younger age, he is annoyed because another does not know what he has dreamed, or he expects even a stranger to know a person or event he refers to in conversation. He believes that his experiences are universal and even that they revolve around him to the extent demonstrated by a preschool child who, when asked to explain the sun's daily movement across the sky, replied, "It follows me."

Another characteristic of preoperational thought is *centering*, which is the tendency to center attention on one feature of something and to be unable to see its other qualities. The child with the marbles and pennies attended to the size of his collection to the exclusion of its numerical features. A child who is aware of the pain-producing potential of a hypodermic needle has great difficulty conceiving of its therapeutic properties (although this is a somewhat adulterated example).

Thus, the preoperational period is characterized by symbolic, conceptual thinking, but at a level which does not permit simultaneous coordination of spatial, temporal, numerical, and certain other qualities of things and events. The child remains illogical by adult standards and commits cognitive errors which seem quite surprising to older children and adults.

Between the ages of 7 and 11, cognitive development proceeds through the stage of *concrete operations*. The child gradually overcomes his egocentrism and his propensity to center and masters the concepts of reversibility, mentioned above, and *conservation*. Conservation refers to the ability to understand that a thing is essentially the same even though its shape or arrangement is altered. The example of the clay masses previously presented is a problem in conservation of mass.

As an example of conservation of volume, a 2- to 7-year-old child who watched an invariant quantity of water poured from a short, wide bottle into a tall, thin bottle would say that the water was of greater volume in the taller container (or, perhaps, in the fatter container instead), whereas a child in the stage of concrete operations would recognize that the volume is not affected by the shape of the bottle.

Conservation of number is demonstrated by the Piagetian experiment in which a child watches as a fixed number of objects are clumped together or spread out over a surface; a preoperational child judges that the number of items is modified by their concentration in space, but a child in the stage of concrete operations does not make that mistake.

During the period of concrete operations, the child becomes skilled at classifying objects by any of their several characteristics. He can say, for example, that dogs, people, and horses have in common the property of being alive; that apples, nuts, and meat are all edibles but that among them only apples and nuts share the quality of being grown on plants; that all spaniels are dogs but not all dogs are spaniels; that parts are smaller than the whole they compose in combination; and so forth.

But the child does not attain a fully adult quality of thinking until the last stage of cognitive thinking, which Piaget calls the *formal operations* period. According to Piagetian theory, there is a qualitative change in thought between ages 11 and 15 which results in the child's becoming able to introspectively think about his own thoughts and to solve complicated, abstract problems as are found in formal logic and calculus. He can now formulate and test hypotheses which require imaginative departures from reality but which are still within the laws of the scientific method. The *content* of thought has become less important than the *form* of the abstract problem, so that the child in the stage of formal operations becomes able to deal with the *structure* of thought sequences without being limited to *empirical testing* or to his experiences with what seems true. By age 15, then, he is cognitively mature.

Critique of Piagetian Theory Piaget and his associates have unquestionably made massive contributions to the understanding of the development of thought processes. The usual criticisms of his work center about the lack of experimental controls that have been used in the studies and about the still incomplete state of the theory.

It does not seem appropriate here to present a complete critique when the treatment given the theory in this chapter has been so brief. What might more profitably be noted is the fact that Piagetian theory deals *only* with the development of *thought*. This statement is not in any way a criticism of the theory. The fact is, however, that it yet remains for nursing to derive for itself whatever applications of Piaget's work can be made to children's thought and behavior in health-related situations. Piaget's formulations suggest ways in which children's concepts about their bodies and about their health care experiences might be better understood. Likewise, nurses can draw implications for gearing their teaching methods to a child's learning and perceptual characteristics, both as related to overall developmental requirements and to more specific clinical situations. But it is not apparent at this time how or whether Piaget's contributions can be used to explain, predict, and modify the broad range of behavioral phenomena encompassed by the other theories discussed here.

Stimulus-Response Theory

The basic premise of stimulus-response theory (also sometimes called learning theory and behavior modification theory) is that behavior is *learned*. Behaviorists (persons who subscribe to this theory) believe that the child initially responds to his environment in random ways consistent with his developmental capability (motor, cognitive, etc.) and that the rewards and punishments that result from his action influence the child's subsequent behavior. Acts which bring pleasure are retained in the behavioral repertory and are repeated in similar situations, while behavior which results in punishment, disappointment, pain, or frustration tends to be discontinued. Behavior thus is a consequence of experience, of *learning*.

There are two types of learning situations, that is, two ways in which learning (called *conditioning*) takes place: *classical conditioning* and *instrumental conditioning*. The Russian physiologist Ivan Pavlov's early twentieth-century work with dogs is a widely known example of classical conditioning. Pavlov noted that if he consistently rang a bell just before feeding a dog, eventually the dog would begin to salivate at the sound of the bell before the food was presented. Thus, a reflex *response* (salivation) normally associated with the *stimulus* of feeding became linked to another stimulus (the sound of the bell) which has not produced the response before the dog learned to associate the bell with eating. Learning in which a response that is part of the organism's normal repertory of activities comes to be produced by an associated stimulus which previously would not have produced it is called *classical conditioning* or *pavlovian conditioning*.

In the other type of stimulus-response learning, called *instrumental conditioning* or *operant conditioning*, the animal or person learns to deliberately manipulate his environment in order to produce a desired response from it. For example, a pigeon in an experimental situation learns by trial and error that pecking a food-release disk while a light is on inside his cage will cause food to drop into the cage, whereas the same acitivity in the absence of the light will not. He learns to confine his pecking to the periods during which the light is on. Similarly, a young child will often cry over a slight injury if his mother is present and has comforted him on similar previous occasions, but will not cry if she is not nearby.

The distinction between classical and instrumental conditioning can be summarized as follows. In classical conditioning an already existing response to a stimulus comes to be produced by another stimulus which the organism has learned, because of temporal proximity (*contiguity*) of the two stimuli, to associate with the first stimulus. In instrumental conditioning a behavior that was not previously linked to any particular stimulus comes to be elicited by a stimulus when the organism has learned that performing that behavior in the presence of that stimulus produces a reward.

In stimulus-response theory the developmental process is not subdivided into stages as in Freudian, Eriksonian, and Piagetian theories. Behavior is viewed as the outcome of learning, and the learning process is considered to be the same at all ages. Learning takes place by *association*, which is the cognitive or perceptual linking of phenomena so that the presence of the stimulus tends to produce the response.

Stimulus-response theory stands in sharp contradistinction to the idea that behavior and development occur primarily under the influence of some internal psychologic pressure (such as libido). The basic data of stimulus-response theory are observed acts rather than such hypothetical inner constructs as feelings, ideas, and intention. Said another way, a person working within the stimulus-response theoretical framework is interested only in external behavior, not in unobservable and therefore speculative subjective phenomena such as thoughts and attitudes.

Behaviorists postulate that acitivity results from an organismic state of imbalance or need which they call *drive*. Examples of drive are hunger and fear. A hungry or frightened animal or person goes into action in order to relieve his hunger, remove himself from danger, or take some other goal-directed action aimed at reducing drive. Drive reduction is inherently rewarding, and behavior which effectively reduces drive becomes learned and is repeated in future similar states of heightened drive.

Generalization is the phenomenon by which learning is transferred from the learning situation to other, similar situations. A young child who develops fear of hospital personnel in white clothes may subsequently show the same fear response to barbers, grocers, or other persons dressed in white. Generalization is said to occur more readily among similar than less similar objects or situations. A child's actions in response to his mother tend to generalize to his nursery school teacher, for example, in proportion to the extent to which the teacher resembles the mother in appearance, mannerisms, approach to the child, and so forth.

Learned behavior can usually be "unlearned" (*extinguished*) if the situation can be modified so that the reward which previously was associated with the behavior no longer results from the behavior. For example, a child who has learned that he can get what he wants by having a tantrum theoretically will eventually give up his tantrum behavior if it ceases to bring him rewards. But certain kinds of learning are difficult to extinguish. Somewhat paradoxically, behavior which results in reward only part of the time is more likely to be continued in the absence of reward than behavior which previously was always rewarded. A gambler, for example, continues to play when he is losing because he is not accustomed to winning every time he plays. In contrast, a laboratory animal which has always received food for pressing a button rather quickly stops his button-pressing activity if he is not rewarded several times in succession.

Since stimulus-response adherents believe behavior is the product of experience with rewards and punishments, they believe behavior can be changed by a planned program of rewarding, punishing, or ignoring. Control over reward and punishment is, of course, the basis of animal training, and in behavior modification the same principles and similar procedures are applied to human behavior. Praise or material reward consistently given when a child performs some socially desirable act generally has the effect of leading him to repeat that act in order to gain additional reward. Ignoring or punishing an act tends to result in its discontinuation. Rather extreme forms of *reinforcement* (rewards or punishments) have sometimes been used to change intolerable behavior in children who for various reasons do not respond well to other forms of therapeutic intervention. Painful electric shocks, for example, have been used to deter mentally retarded or emotionally disturbed children from sticking their fingers into their eyes, banging their heads, or performing other self-mutilating habits which sometimes lead to blindness or other serious injury. Disturbed, retarded, or delinquent children frequently can be induced to work either for some immediate reward, such as candy, or for tokens which can be accumulated for repeated good behavior and eventually exchanged for some desired object or privilege, much as one would save money until he had enough to buy something he wanted.

Stimulus-response theorists have studied behavioral issues far broader than implied by the above discussion. The effects of *modeling* (watching another receive rewards or punishments for a specific behavior such as theft, aggression, or generosity) have been researched within a stimulus-response theoretical framework, for example, and have potentially great implications with respect to social policy regarding pornography, violence on television, and the like. Such basic issues in child development as dependency, sex-role behavior, and the development of conscience have been examined by *social learning theorists*, who have combined the tenets of psychoanalysis with those of stimulus-response psychology. Since space does not permit deeper exploration of these broader applications of the basic stimulus-response postulates, the reader is referred to the works of Robert Sears, Neil Miller, John Dollard, Albert Bandura, and Richard Walters (see Bibliography at the end of this chapter).

Critique of Stimulus-Response Theory As a theory of behavior, the stimulus-response framework has several strengths. There can be little doubt that classical and instrumental conditioning and behavior modification are everyday occurrences in human life. Learning by association and the effects of reward and punishment are major parts of child rearing and socialization. The research within the stimulus-response theoretical tradition has much to commend it in that it is characteristically of experimental design, as opposed to the more loosely structured observational studies of several other theories, which often lack controls or are poorly amenable to quantification. Behavior modification can be used as a therapeutic technique for persons with deviant behavior, a fact which gives stimulus-response psychology a pragmatic quality less easily developed from, for example, Eriksonian or Piagetian theory.

In criticism of stimulus-response research, however, it is often pointed out that the majority of research has been conducted with animals in artificial laboratory settings and therefore is not justifiably applicable to human beings in actual life situations.

In addition, many persons have expressed serious doubts about the wisdom and ethics of behavior modification programs because the children whose actions are affected do not choose the behaviors selected for reinforcement. Hence behavior modification imposes and perpetuates another's values. It is not known how being "paid" to perform will affect children's ethical and moral development, including their materialistic and humanitarian values. Finally, many developmentalists feel that stimulus-response theory deals too simplistically and atomistically with isolated aspects of behavior rather than with the "whole child."

Sociological Concepts Relating to Children and Families

Sociology and even the subspecialty of sociology of the family are extremely broad areas involving several theories and approaches. Although these theories cannot be included here, several sociological constructs are presented in this chapter because they provide helpful concepts for understanding children and, especially, families.

Sociological theories, far more than the psychologic theories previously discussed, focus upon the characteristics (including behavior) of *groups* instead of individuals. A basic premise of sociology is that groups—families, for example—are *social systems* which operate according to the principles of systems theory. Systems theory states that there is constant and reciprocal interaction among the several members within a system, that is, that all members continually influence and are influenced by all others. The interrelatedness of members of a system is illustrated by the familiar example of ecology, in which people affect and are reciprocally affected by the other organisms and elements in their environment. Another application of the systems concept is the physiologic phenomenon of homeostasis. In the family system, as in ecology and homeostasis, not only do the several parts of the system interact reciprocally with one another, but any change brought to bear on one member of the system inevitably affects in some way all other members of the system.

If a child becomes ill or injured and requires hospitalization, for example, he is by no means the only person in the family affected. The demands upon parental concern, time, and finances cause reallocation of those resources so that family members experience change in the availability of the resources and in those interactions. Parents cannot be home while they are with the hospitalized child; substitute caretakers may be brought into the home; siblings may miss the absent child, worry about him, feel responsible for his misfortune, and resent the heightened attention he receives. Individuals and the family as a unit may be affected by changes in their interactions with *other* systems such as the health care delivery institution, the parents' occupational systems, the children's school and play groups, and the extended family. The family system and its members undergo continual change as reestablishment of equilibrium is sought. No member of the family is unaffected, and none is only an actor or only a reactor.

Sociology differs from psychology with respect to its explanations of the origins of self and behavior. The self-concept is believed by sociologists to be derived in large part from the person's perceptions of other persons' attitudes toward him. His behavior is a product of not only his perception of himself but also his relationship to others. Behavior hence is not a result of some fixed internal psychic structure but is elicited by the social setting. Thus, a person presents himself quite differently to a parent than to a sibling, for example, and acts differently at a ball game than at a wedding.

The concept of *role* is integral to sociologic approaches to the understanding of behavior. A role is essentially a collection of consistent behaviors that a person "acts out" in his social relations. Family life includes many roles—mother, caretaker, wage earner, sex roles, age roles, and of course many others, sometimes including black sheep roles, scapegoat roles, and sick roles. There are normative expectations that go with every role to define how people in those roles are "supposed" to act. A family or other social system functions smoothly as long as all the roles necessary to keep the system operating have been assigned to persons in the group and as long as those to whom the various roles are assigned are competent and willing to perform them. Crisis may be expected if the members of the family are required to realign the role structures within the family, as may certainly happen in the event someone relinquishes his customary roles because of a change in health status or developmental status.

BIBLIOGRAPHY

Adler, A.: *Understanding Human Nature*, Premier Books, Fawcett World Library, New York, 1959.

Baldwin, A. L.: *Theories of Child Development*, John Wiley & Sons, Inc., New York, 1967.

Bandura, A.: *Principles of Behavior Modification*, Holt, Rinehart and Winston, Inc., New York, 1969.

———, and Walters, R. H.: *Social Learning and Per-*

sonality Development, Holt, Rinehart and Winston, Inc., New York, 1963.

Bossard, J. H. S., and Boll, E. S.: *The Sociology of Child Development*, Harper & Row, Publishers, Incorporated, New York, 1960.

Bowlby, J.: *Child Care and the Growth of Love*, Penguin Books, Inc., Baltimore, 1953.

Cooley, C. H.: *Human Nature and the Social Order*, The Free Press, New York, 1956.

Erikson, E. H.: *Childhood and Society*, 2d ed., W. W. Norton & Company, Inc., New York, 1963.

Freud, S.: *Three Essays on the Theory of Sexuality*, Avon Books Division, The Hearst Corporation, New York, 1962.

Gordon, I.: *Human Development: Readings in Research*, Scott, Foresman and Company, Glenview, Ill., 1965.

Gray, P. H.: "Theory and Evidence of Imprinting in Human Infants," *Journal of Psychology*, 46:155–166, 1958.

Hadley, B. J.: "Becoming Well: A Study of Role Change," Fourth Nursing Research Conference, American Nurses Association, New York, 1968.

Hall, C., and Lindzey, G.: *Theories of Personality*, John Wiley & Sons, Inc., New York, 1957.

Hebb, D. O.: *The Organization of Behavior*, John Wiley & Sons, Inc., New York, 1952.

Hunt, J. McV.: *Intelligence and Experience*, The Ronald Press Company, New York, 1961.

Irish, D. P.: "Sibling Interaction: A Neglected Aspect in Family Life Research," *Social Forces*, 42(3):279–288 1964.

Lorenz, K.: *Evolution and Modification of Behavior*, University of Chicago Press, Chicago, 1965.

Mabrey, J. H.: "Medicine and the Family," *Journal of Marriage and the Family*, 26:160–165, 1964.

Maier, H. W.: *Three Theories of Child Development*, Harper & Row, Publishers, Incorporated, New York, 1965.

Medinnus, G. R.: *Readings in the Psychology of Parent-Child Relations*, John Wiley & Sons, Inc., New York, 1967.

Miller, N. E., and Dollard, J.: *Social Learning and Imitation*, Yale University Press, New Haven, Conn., 1941.

Mowrer, O. H.: *Learning Theory and Behavior*, John Wiley & Sons, Inc., New York, 1960.

Munroe, R. L.: *Schools of Psychoanalytic Thought*, Holt, Rinehart and Winston, Inc., New York, 1955.

Mussen, P. H. (ed.): *Manual of Child Psychology*, 3d ed., John Wiley & Sons, Inc., New York, 1970.

———, Conger, J., and Kagan, J.: *Readings in Child Development and Personality*, Harper & Row, Publishers, Incorporated, New York, 1965.

Parsons, T.: *Social Structure and Personality*, The Free Press, New York, 1964.

———, and Bales, R. F.: *Family Socialization and Interaction Process*, The Free Press, New York, 1955.

Phillips, J. L.: *The Origins of Intellect: Piaget's Theory*, W. H. Freeman and Company, San Francisco, 1969.

Piaget, J.: *The Origin of Intelligence in Children*, International Universities Press, New York, 1952.

———: *Genetic Epistemology*, Columbia University Press, New York, 1970.

Scott, J. P.: "Critical Periods in Behavioral Development," *Science*, 138:949–958, 1962.

Sears, R. R., Maccoby, E., and Levin, H.: *Patterns of Child Rearing*, Row, Peterson and Company, Evanston, Ill., 1957.

Spitz, R.: "Hospitalism, an Inquiry into the Genesis of Psychiatric Conditions in Early Childhood," *Psychoanalytic Study of the Child*, 1:53–74, 1945.

Stolz, L. M.: *Influences on Parent Behavior*, Stanford University Press, Stanford, Calif., 1967.

Sullivan, H. S.: *The Interpersonal Theory of Psychiatry*, W. W. Norton & Company, Inc., New York, 1953.

Sutton-Smith, B., and Rosenberg, B. G.: *The Sibling*, Holt, Rinehart and Winston, New York, 1970.

Toman, W.: *Family Constellation: Theory and Practice of a Psychological Game*, Springer Publishing Co., Inc., New York, 1961.

PRENATAL DEVELOPMENT

JEANNE HOWE and HOLLY F. HUNT

The processes involved in conception and intra-uterine growth are among the most remarkable occurrences of human development. Furthermore, the events that precede birth, and even those that precede conception, profoundly influence the kind of individual that is born and the kind of person he can grow to become. In concordance with one of the premises of this book, that effective nursing is designed upon an understanding of the individualistic qualities of the particular child and family with whom the nurse interacts, this chapter describes the background and beginning of the new individual and traces his progress to the time of birth.

PRECONCEPTION FACTORS

With the merging of spermatozoon and ovum, the blueprint, or master plan, for the new person is unalterably completed. The many aspects of his human potential which are dependent upon his genetic makeup are determined at that moment, and he can by no process yet known to humankind be made to become anything beyond the possibilities that are established by that blending of his two parents' contributions to his heredity.

This is not to say that the infant born 9 months later will fulfill the promise presented in the blueprint 100 percent or that the mature human being, 20 or 80 years after conception, will have become all that his heredity would have made possible. Environmental influences, before as well as after his birth, will set limits upon the extent to which the capacities included in the blueprint will be realized. A person whose genetic inheritance calls for tallness will not reach his maximum potential height if, for example, growth hormone deficiency or starvation intervenes. A child conceived with the potential for normal intellectual functioning may become mentally retarded as a result of brain tissue damage inflicted by infectious organisms, chemicals, or trauma at any point in his prenatal or postnatal life.

Heredity

Both parents contribute equally to the heredity of their new child. The nucleus of the father's reproductive cell (the sperm cell, also called *spermatozoon*—plural, spermatozoa), like the nucleus of the mother's reproductive cell (*egg* or *ovum*—plural, ova), contains 23 chromosomes. Each *chromosome* is a tiny strand made up of the fundamental hereditary components called *genes* (Fig. 8-1). These basic hereditary units convey all the inherited character-

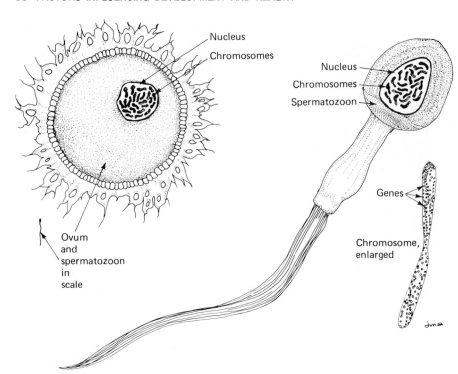

Figure 8-1 A schematic representation of ovum and spermatozoon, showing the relative locations of genes and chromosomes.

istics, the totality of the qualities which parents can pass on to their children.

Genes are made of the remarkable substance *deoxyribonucleic acid* (DNA). DNA has two characteristic properties which have earned it recognition as the basic substance of living matter. One is its capacity to copy itself. This quality makes it possible for the fertilized ovum to duplicate its chromosomes and divide into two cells exactly like itself which, in turn, will copy themselves again and again so that the single fertilized egg can become the multicellular embryo. The other fundamental property of DNA is that it carries the basic "instructions," a kind of blueprint in code, to determine inherited characteristics. Each gene has its own specialized function; that is, each conveys to the developing embryo the instructions for *one single characteristic* such as eye color, finger shape, or presence of a hereditary disorder such as hemophilia. There are perhaps several thousand genes on each chromosome.

Each of the chromosomes is unlike all the others. For each, however, there is one other which closely resembles it in size and shape. Hence the 46 chromosomes are considered to be 23 pairs. Geneticists have given each pair an identification number based on its size (Fig. 8-2).

Chromosomes are a part of the nucleus of every body cell, including the reproductive cells (*gametes*),

spermatozoa and ova. However, since 46 is the characteristic number of chromosomes in each cell of the human species and since a cell from each of *two* human beings combines to form the beginning of a new generation, it is immediately apparent that some special process is necessary to halve the number each parent contributes so that the fertilized ovum (*zygote*) will not contain twice the appropriate number. Reproductive cells are unique among the body's cells in that, as they mature and become available to participate in fertilization, a special kind of cell division (called *maturation division, reduction division,* or *meiosis*) takes place. The 46 chromosomes of the immature sex cells are, like the 46 chromosomes in all other human body cell nuclei, actually 23 pairs rather than 46 dissimilar, independent chromosomes. Each member of the pair separates from its partner during the maturation of the sex cells in such a way that from a cell of *23 pairs* of chromosomes, *two* cells are formed, each with *23 unpaired* chromosomes (Fig. 8-3). Thus, each mature spermatozoon and each mature ovum carries 23 single chromosomes, and they combine during fertilization to restore, within the single cell of the fertilized egg, the 23 pairs, the full human complement of 46 chromosomes.

The members of each chromosome pair share another similarity besides size and shape. The genes

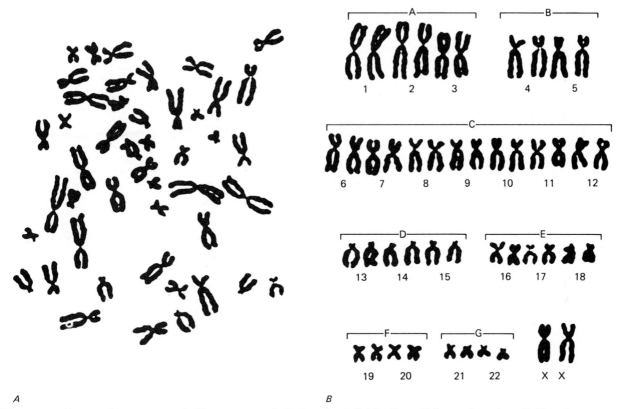

Figure 8-2 Human chromosomes. *A.* Chromosomes in their natural distribution within a cell nucleus. *B.* The chromosomes have been arranged in pairs and labeled in conformity with internationally standard nomenclature. The presence of two X chromosomes identifies the donor as female. The male configuration consists instead of one X and one Y, which is a very small, dissimilar-looking chromosome.

carried by the two have *the same function*; that is, they affect the same anatomic parts of the developing child. Each individual gene determines a specific, single hereditary characteristic. As far as is now known in the very young science of genetics, a gene for eye color is not the same as a gene for ear shape or hair color, has no influence on anything *but* eye color, and is the *only* hereditary determinant of eye color. The gene for any specific hereditary characteristic is invariably located on a particular chromosome and presumably has its own particular place among the thousands of genes on that chromosome. A second gene for the same characteristic is present in the corresponding location on the other member of the chromosome pair.

Dominance and Recessiveness Each gene has its partner on the other chromosome in the pair, as just described. The two genes work together to determine the heredity of the specific tissue they affect. The two genes may or may not be alike. One of the chromosomes in each pair, and consequently one of

the pair of genes for each unit characteristic, was inherited from the mother, the other from the father. For example, if a child has inherited a gene for blue eyes from each of his parents, both of his genes for eye color will be alike. He will be blue-eyed. If he inherits genes for brown eyes from both parents, again both of his genes will be alike. In this instance he will have brown eyes. But if he receives from one parent a gene that instructs the embryo to have blue eyes and from the other parent a gene that carries the instructions for brown eyes, he will in a sense have contradictory messages that require some resolution. In this instance the child will be brown-eyed, just as if the gene for blue eye color were not present. Such a child will be brown-eyed even though he carries the gene for blue eyes because *when the two genes for a single characteristic are not alike, one of them dominates the potential influence of the other.* The overshadowed gene is said to be *recessive*. Genes for brown eyes are dominant; those for blue eyes are recessive.

A recessive trait, such as blue eyes, appears

Immature reproductive cell

(Contains 23 pairs of chromosomes, 46 total)

Spermatzoon

Ovum

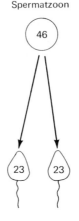

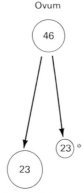

Mature reproductive cell

(Each of the original 23 pairs has split, and one member of each pair has gone into each mature sex cell.)

*Only one of the two mature ova is viable; the other rapidly degenerates and is never a candidate for fertilization.

Figure 8-3 A simplified representation of reduction division.

only in persons whose genes for that trait are *both* recessive. In a person with both a dominant and a recessive gene, the dominant quality will appear and the existence of the gene for the recessive trait will not be observable. The recessive gene, however, is unchanged by its association with its dominant partner. It continues to be duplicated with each cell division so that, with maturation division, it is passed on to half of the mature sex cells and thus retains its potential to appear in the subsequent generations of the family tree (Fig. 8-4).

Dominance and recessiveness take on great practical importance in pediatrics because numerous diseases are of genetic origin and hence can be passed on to one, several, or even all the children of spouses with certain genetic combinations. A couple who knows that inheritable disorders have appeared in their families can receive genetic counseling to advise them of the statistical odds that their children will be afflicted. Figure 8-5 shows how a dominant or recessive hereditary characteristic can appear among the offspring of various parental genetic combinations. It must be emphasized that the percentage of a couple's children shown in Figure 8-5 as inheriting each particular combination is only the long-range probability that would be statistically predicted if the couple were to produce a great number of children. It is easily possible for deviation from that probability to occur in any given family of four children, just as four tosses of a coin produces a number of results besides two heads and two tails. Of course, no dominant or recessive gene can appear in the spermatozoa or ova of a parent unless it was already present in his chromosomes as he inherited them from *his* parents, so in

the case of spouses whose genes are all dominant or all recessive it can be said with assurance that 100 percent of their offspring will receive the all-dominant or all-recessive genetic combination. (The rare exception to this certain predictability results from *mutation*, which is the spontaneous appearance of a new gene which has not been present in previous generations of the family.)

Several important hereditary diseases are carried by recessive genes and do not appear unless the child receives two recessive genes for the disease. Both parents must donate a recessive gene or none of their children will have the disease. If one parent is a carrier (Gg) (see Fig. 8-5) and the other is double dominant (GG), the full-blown disease (gg) cannot appear among their children; but on the average, one-fourth of their children will be carriers (Gg) capable of having children on their own who are carriers or who actually have the disease, depending upon the other half of their inheritance. If both parents are carriers (Gg), the odds that they will have a diseased child (gg) rise to one in four, while half their children are expected to be carriers (Gg) and only one-fourth are expected to be genetically free from the disease and the carrier state. If between the parents, only one type of gene exists (both parents are GG or gg), it is obvious that all the children will have the same type as their parents.

From the preceding discussion it should be apparent that the probabilities for producing a child with a double recessive inheritance are greater if both parents come from the same kinship group in which the recessive gene is present. Although the double recessive condition is not always undesirable, matings of close blood relatives are usually discouraged by law or by custom because of the increased probability that their offspring will receive and transmit recessive genes which *do* produce illness or deformity.

Boy or Girl? It was noted in Figure 8-2 that the 23d pair of chromosomes is alike (XX) in females but unmatched (XY) in males. The sex of the new person depends upon which of these two combinations he receives. Every child inherits the X chromosome from his mother, since at reduction division every ovum receives one member of her XX pair. But the immature sperm cell contains both an X and a Y, so that half of the mature sperm cells receive an X and the other half receive a Y. The sex of the child hence depends upon whether the spermatozoon that fertilizes the X-bearing ovum (Fig. 8-6) carries an X or Y chromosome. The maturation division of the spermatozoa produces equal numbers of X-bearing and Y-bearing mature sperm cells, so the odds for having a girl are numerically the same as for having a boy. In reality, however, the number of males conceived exceeds the number of females by nearly 10 percent, a fact that has not yet been satisfactorily explained.

X-linked (Sex-linked) Inheritance The X chromosome contains other genes besides those that determine sex. Genes producing color blindness, hemophilia, and baldness, for example, are among those carried on the X chromosome. Such genes and the traits they produce are called *sex-linked* or, more precisely, *X-linked*. X chromosomes are larger and carry *more* genes than Y chromosomes. Some genes on the X chromosome are recessive and therefore produce their effect only when there is no opposing, dominant gene present on the other chromosome in that pair. When the other 23d chromosome is an X, it may very well carry the dominant counterpart for the recessive gene. But when the other chromosome is a Y, the opposing gene for that trait is absent altogether and the X-carried recessive trait appears. Thus males, with their XY combination, more often demonstrate sex-linked disorders than females, who have a second X with (usually) a dominant gene to suppress the recessive gene. Because males transmit their sole X chromosome to all their daughters and to none of their sons, all the daughters of men who have an X-linked trait are carriers of the trait and all the sons of such men are normal unless they happen to have inherited the gene from their mother. X-linked traits are demonstrated by females only in

Both members of the chromosome pair have the dominant gene (*G*). This person demonstrates the dominant trait and all his reproductive cells carry a dominant gene.

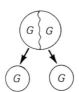

Immature sex cell (before reduction division)

Mature sex cells

Both members of the chromosome pair have the recessive gene (*g*). This person demonstrates the recessive trait and all his reproductive cells carry a recessive gene.

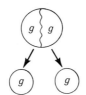

Immature sex cell (before reduction division)

Mature sex cells

One of the paired chromosomes has the dominant gene (*G*); the other has the recessive gene (*g*). This person demonstrates the dominant trait, but his reproductive cells can transmit either dominant or recessive genes.

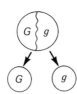

Immature sex cell (before reduction division)

Mature sex cells

Figure 8-4 The possibilities for distribution of dominant and recessive genes at reduction division. *G* represents a dominant gene for a particular trait; *g* represents a recessive gene for the same trait.

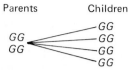

Both genes in each parent are dominant. Parents demonstrate the dominant trait and can give all their children only dominant genes. Hence all children appear dominant and can pass only dominant genes to their children.

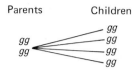

Both genes in each parent are recessive. Parents demonstrate the recessive trait and can give all their children only recessive genes. All children show the recessive trait and can transmit only recessive genes to their children.

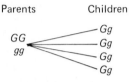

One parent has both dominant genes, the other both recessive. All offspring receive one dominant and one recessive gene, appear dominant, and can transmit either kind of gene to their children.

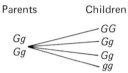

Each parent has a dominant and a recessive gene. One-fourth the children are pure dominant, one-half are mixed dominant and recessive, and one-fourth are pure recessive. The three-fourths at the top appear dominant. The three-fourths at the bottom can pass the recessive gene to their offspring.

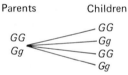

One parent has both genes dominant, the other has one dominant and one recessive. Half the children are pure dominant. The other half are mixed dominant and recessive; they appear dominant but can transmit either kind of gene to their children.

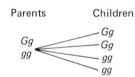

One parent is mixed dominant and recessive, the other is pure recessive. Half the children appear dominant, half display the recessive trait. All can transmit the recessive gene to their offspring.

Figure 8-5 Inheritance possibilities and probabilities for every combination of parents' dominant and recessive genes. *G* represents a dominant gene for a particular trait; *g* represents a recessive gene for the same trait. Each child receives one of each parent's two genes. The percentages of children receiving each combination are long-range statistical probabilities only and cannot be relied upon for any specific four children of a couple.

the rare instances in which both parents have donated an X chromosome which carries the recessive gene (see Fig. 8-7).

EVENTS FOLLOWING CONCEPTION
Intrauterine Growth Patterns

Following the combination of spermatozoon with ovum, the new person-to-be begins to emerge according to the instructions of his genetic blueprint. He is unique—a new blend of genetic traits randomly selected from both of his parents and their ancestry. But he has also inherited much that he shares in common with his relatives and with the whole human family. Among these commonalities are the basic patterns of his growth. He can be expected to

progress through an orderly sequence of intrauterine changes that will produce, from his tiny one-celled beginning, a 7-lb, 20-inch infant whose hundreds of millions of cells perform such specialized functions as manufacturing digestive juices, producing blood cells, moving food along the digestive tract, breathing, perceiving pain, and the myriad other abilities that give the newborn the competencies for sustaining life and continuing toward further development.

Within a few hours after fertilization the chromosomes of the *zygote* (fertilized ovum) duplicate themselves and separate into two new cells. Each of these in time repeats the process. By the end of the first week or 10 days the cell mass has multiplied to about 200 times its initial cell number, has secured itself

Immature reproductive cell containing, among its chromosomes, a *pair* of sex chromosomes (before reduction division)

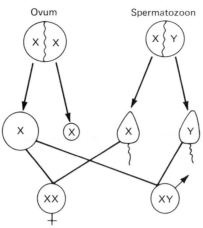

Mature reproductive cell containing only one member of the original pair of sex chromosomes

The possibilities for sex chromosome combination at fertilization

Figure 8-6 The X of the ovum is complemented at fertilization by either an X-carrying or a Y-carrying spermatozoon. The XX combination produces a female child, the XY a male.

in the protective and nurturing wall of the uterus, and has begun the development of the fetal membranes and placenta which, respectively, will constitute its housing and means of access to maternal supplies and services for the rest of its intrauterine stay.

    The 7- to 10-day-old embryo has also begun to specialize its cells into the three layers that will eventually form the nervous system and skin (*ectoderm*), the digestive system and adjoining structures

(*endoderm*), and the skeletal, cardiac, renal, and associated tissues (*mesoderm*). The process by which genetically and chromosomally identical cells can produce dissimilarly functioning, specialized cells which compose the diverse bone, muscle, nerve, glandular, and other tissues is not yet adequately understood.

    In the first month, the embryo develops rudimentary arms and legs, immature brain, eyes, ears, and mouth; some of its abdominal organs, a beating

Normal male mated with carrier female

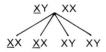

Of their daughters, half are expected to be normal and half to be carriers of the recessive gene. Of their sons, half are expected to be normal and half to demonstrate the trait.

The affected male may mate with any of three possible types of female (XX, XX, or XX). His potential offspring are predicted as shown, depending upon their mother's type.

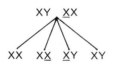

All daughters are carriers; all sons are normal.

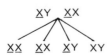

Half their daughters demonstrate the trait, half are carriers. Half their sons demonstrate the trait, half are normal.

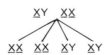

All children demonstrate the trait.

Figure 8-7 Inheritance probabilities for an X-linked gene. X represents an X chromosome with the recessive gene, which will produce the trait unless counteracted by a dominant gene for the same trait. The Y chromosome does not carry a gene for the trait and hence cannot suppress the gene on the X.

heart, and circulating blood.[1,2] By the end of the second month, although only about an inch long, the embryo has developed nearly all its specialized structures. Fingers and toes are well defined where previously there has been only limb buds; the nose, ears, and eyelids are present; and in fact the baby has almost finished forming all his component parts. The remainder of his intrauterine life will be spent in progressive growth, strengthening, and maturation of what is, after 8 gestational weeks, a fairly complete human body. Subsequently he is referred to as a fetus rather than an embryo.

The third intrauterine month sees further refinement of some of the baby's already present structures. The child moves about in his fluid chamber but is not yet large enough or vigorous enough to be felt by his mother. Respiratory and swallowing movements are present.[1] Because the first 3 months are the *vital* period of organ formation, they constitute the stage of greatest vulnerability to the major malformations. This is the time during which certain viruses infecting the mother and certain drugs she may use, among other fetal insults, are most dangerous to the unborn baby. Unfortunately, this is also the period in which the pregnancy may be yet undiscovered, so that precautions may not be taken against exposure to infectious diseases and x-rays, use of medicines, and other *teratogenic* (anomaly-producing) influences. The end of the first 3 months (*first trimester*) of pregnancy is regarded as a turning point in fetal development, beyond which the threat of birth defect is greatly reduced.

It is usually during the fourth month that the baby makes himself felt by his mother. He grows rapidly so that he is about 9 inches long and weighs ½ lb at the end of 4 months, 12 inches and 1 lb after 5 months, and 14 inches and 1¼ lb at the end of 6 gestational months.[1]

The last trimester of his intrauterine stay is one of tremendous growth, particularly the ninth month. As the last trimester proceeds, the fetus becomes progressively strong and mature and his chances of survival, if born prematurely, grow with the passing weeks. Important events occur during the last trimester that make it highly beneficial for the fetus to remain in utero for the full duration. He receives antibodies from his mother which will give him several months' protection against infectious diseases to which she has developed immunity. These commonly include diseases which could be serious for young infants, such as measles, scarlet fever, and chickenpox. Immature organ systems undergo maturational changes in the last weeks of pregnancy without which the infant cannot survive after he

leaves the uterus. The respiratory system is a notable example, with the infamous hyaline membrane disease (respiratory distress syndrome), which is a direct result of lung immaturity, taking a heavy toll of babies born before term. The advantages of a full 9 months in utero are made more fully apparent in Chapter 20 and in Part 4, where the risks of prematurity are discussed in detail.

Multiple Pregnancy

Two or more babies may be born from one pregnancy. There are two distinct types of multiple pregnancy progeny—identical (also called *monozygous, monovular,* or *duplicate*) siblings and fraternal (also called *dizygous, diovular,* or *dissimilar*) siblings.

Identical siblings are produced from only one ovum. Occasionally, in an early stage of the cell duplications that follow fertilization, the cellular conglomerate splits into separate cell masses and each of them becomes an individual embryo. It is apparent that each of these babies will have identical genes, since they receive their inheritance from a single egg fertilized by a single sperm cell. Hence, identical siblings always are of the same sex, have the same blood type and hereditary diseases, and bear a very strong resemblance to one another. Nevertheless they commonly differ in certain respects such as birth weight because of differences in the adequacy of their placental supplies, position or crowding inside the uterus, or other environmental differences. Some identical siblings are mirror images of each other: handedness, birthmark placement, location of hair whorl and direction of hair growth from it, and other right- and left-sided physical features are reversed in the children. Mirror imaging presumably results from the symmetric way the chromosomes split when the division of the young cell mass produces multiple embryos.

Nonidentical twins (or triplets or larger groups) occupy the uterus at the same time but develop from different ova. Occasionally more than one ovum are released at ovulation and subsequently fertilized, each of course by a different sperm cell. The embryo that develops from each zygote has its own unique inheritance and is genetically no more like his birthmate than like any other sibling born to the same parents.

Twins are born approximately once in 88 births. Three sets of fraternal twins are born for each set of identical twins. Triplets occur once in just fewer than 7,800 births; quadruplets are born once in around 680,000 pregnancies. Multiple births have become more common since the introduction of estrogenic birth control pills. These medications are effective contraceptive agents because they prevent ovulation; but when the pills are discontinued, several eggs which had been held back may be released in a single ovulatory period.

Multiple births tend to run in families, although the father's and mother's roles in transmitting this hereditary tendency remain unclear. Maternal age is also a factor, but only for nonidentical siblings. Older women are more likely to release more than one ovum at once.[2, 3]

It is not always easy to tell whether birthmates are identical or fraternal. Fraternal siblings, like singleton children in the same family, may look very much alike, and environmental factors may produce differences in identical siblings in spite of their common genetic inheritance. Examination, at delivery, of the placenta(s) and the membranes that have enclosed the babies may provide the answer in many cases, but the tearing of the membranes during birth and the growth patterns of the placentas often make the diagnosis difficult. It should be apparent from the preceding discussion that it is possible, in the case of three or more babies from the same pregnancy, for some of them to be identical and others to be fraternal.

Prenatal Diagnosis

Because of the advancement of knowledge and technology in recent years, it is possible to know quite a lot about a child before he is born. Radiologic studies confirm the number of fetuses present in cases of suspected multiple pregnancy or reveal skeletal or positional peculiarities of the unborn which can be expected to necessitate special delivery room management, such as cesarean delivery. Radioisotope placental scan makes it possible to determine if the placenta is implanted in the uterus in a way that will interfere with the normal passage of the baby during delivery. Sophisticated methods of electronically monitoring the fetal heartbeat, fetal electroencephalogram, and fetal motor activity now allow the collection of data about the baby's condition before and during labor. *Amniocentesis*, the aspiration of amniotic fluid through a needle inserted through the mother's abdomen, yields information about the chemicals and body cells released by the embryo or fetus into the fluid in which he lives. Amniocentesis makes it possible, for example, to diagnose blood type incompatibilities, certain intrauterine infections, fetal gestational age, and certain chromosomal and metabolic disorders. A positive prenatal diagnosis of these problems per-

mits preparation for treatment at birth or, in some cases, even before. The discovery of fetal aberrations is a useful adjunct to prenatal counseling of parents and is sometimes used as an indication for therapeutic abortion. Chromosomal material collected by amniocentesis also reveals the sex of the baby, but since amniocentesis is neither without risk nor widely available yet, it is not presently practicable solely for the purpose of diagnosing sex.

THE IMPROBABILITY AND UNIQUENESS OF EACH CONCEPTION

Fertilization cannot occur unless viable sperm cells are deposited in sufficient numbers into a healthy female genital tract within a day or so before or after a healthy ovum is released from its ovary to be brought into contact with the sperm cell. If, as believed, an egg is capable of being fertilized for about 12 to 24 hours and sperm cells remain capable of fertilization for about 30 to 48 hours,[1–3] then there is at most a 3-day span of time per ovulatory cycle during which intercourse can result in conception. A portion of the life-span of both sperm cell and egg is spent in traveling through the uterine tube, where they most commonly meet. The overall resultant likelihood that an ovum will be available for fertilization at any randomly chosen part of the menstrual cycle, and hence that conception will result from any single sexual encounter, is mathematically relatively low—actually about 1 chance in 10 or 15 for a 30-day cycle.

The tremendous number of sperm cells released at a single ejaculation (estimated to average around 200 million) increases the probability that one of them will contact the tiny ovum if in fact one is present and still young enough to be fertilized. If the sperm cells and egg do meet during the fertile part of their brief life-span, one sperm cell moves into the interior of the egg, and their nuclei fuse. With the successful entry of that sperm cell, the ovum becomes impermeable to all other sperm cells.

However, the unique combination of genetic qualities which occurs with the union of a *particular* ovum and a *particular* spermatozoon happens against almost infinite numerical odds. About 400 ova become available for fertilization during a woman's childbearing years. Theoretically, each of these ova is unlike all the others, so that the child produced by any one of them would have a different genetic makeup from the child produced by any other. This difference among ova results from the previously described separation of chromosome pairs to produce a mature sex cell containing only half the original 46 chromosomes. The yet un-counted thousands of genes contained in each chromosome are, at least in many cases, not identical with the genes on the other chromosome in the pair, so that when the pair members separate, each half takes to its sex cell a genetic component unlike that which the other member would have contributed. From the immense numbers of genes per chromosome and the 23 pairs of chromosomes, an estimated 17 million different genetic combinations are possible at the moment the chromosomes leave their pairs.[4] (This number does not include the additional combinations which result from the *crossover* phenomenon, in which a chromosome may sometimes exchange some of its genes with its pair partner before they separate, or from *nondisjunction*, in which the splitting of the pairs is occasionally imperfect, resulting in an unequal distribution of chromosomal material to the two sex cells.) *Which* 400 or so of these millions of possibilities actually materialize as ova available for fertilization is evidently a matter of chance.

A similar random allotment of genetic combinations occurs in the maturation divisions which produce the mature sperm cells. Untold billions of theoretically unidentical spermatozoa are produced in a reproductive lifetime, in contrast to the few hundred ova, and several hundred million compete to fertilize a single egg.

In summary, chance selections and combinations of inheritable qualities that occur in the formation and union of sex cells result, at conception, in the creation of a child who is literally one among billions of babies who might have been conceived in his place. These considerations perhaps serve to point up the uniqueness inherent in each person. It is immediately apparent that even persons with the same parents, unless they are identical twins, are genetically different from one another in a great many ways.

THE PREGNANT FAMILY

The pregnant woman and her family constitute a miniature social system. Pregnancy not only produces changes within the woman herself but also brings stress to bear upon the family system to which she belongs. Change in relation to others, as well as to self, begins from the moment a suspected pregnancy is confirmed. In accordance with the concept that *a change in any part of a system produces change throughout that system*, it seems inevitable that pregnancy has an impact upon not only the pregnant woman but all members of the family.

Even the most seemingly "normal" family faces a pregnancy with ambivalent and mixed feelings. The whole system must change its modus operandi. No longer will the family be able to operate within the framework of old, familiar patterns. New ways of functioning must be developed. The nature and extent of change varies from one family to another, of course. But in almost every family the role of "pregnant woman" is different from that of "woman." Similarly, the identity and role expectation of "father" introduce new implications for the man who is about to become one. Becoming a sibling or a grandparent, usually without being consulted ahead of time, likewise forces upon those family members new and perhaps not entirely welcome roles and ways of operating. The most pragmatic matters may require modification: older children's sleeping arrangements may be changed to accommodate the new baby; parental sexual practices may be altered by preference or by necessity; family travel plans may be postponed; economic stresses may arise, especially if the pregnancy interrupts the woman's employment; and new communications have to be established or resumed, including those with the health care system. Once the reality of the pregnancy is acknowledged, the new patterns of functioning begin to take form and substance. Pregnancy arouses old and new feelings of anxiety, joy, wonderment, anger, anticipation, frustration, resentment, and fulfillment. The family has established certain modes of relating to life situations which must undergo alteration. No longer can the family or any member of it refer to "we" or "I" and mean the same thing as before.

It is apparent that any adaptation which occurs during pregnancy will ultimately affect not only the existing family but also the unborn child. His development in utero is shot through with his emerging uniqueness, yet families infrequently regard the new person-to-be as an individual unto himself. Many babies are born with circumscribed obligations in the form of role expectations—to carry on the family name, to save a marriage, to compensate for a previous disappointment, to confirm a parent's role, to be the long-awaited girl in a family of boys, and so forth. These family expectations mitigate against the inherent individuality which characterizes the child even at conception, more so at birth, and certainly as he grows. The health professional who helps the family to expect and appreciate in the new member the characteristics which only he can offer performs a substantial service to the child, his family, and the larger society.

Early in the pregnancy the developing infant asserts an impact upon the family system first by creating change in one family member, his mother. Even the most miniscule awareness that she is pregnant causes the woman to alter her feelings and behavior, which in turn causes the beginning shifts of energy in the family system. She is the first to suspect that she has conceived. In time the flutter of the infant's movement impresses upon her a reality for which other family members as yet see little evidence. The family does not long escape awareness of the impact made upon them by the imminent new person. As changes in the woman's input into the family system are felt throughout the system, and as the other members begin to react to the pregnancy and to contemplate their changing roles, system-wide change becomes an irrefutable reality.

The first trimester is characterized by this rendezvous with wonderment (that a new person is, unseen, relentlessly moving toward membership in their family circle) and preliminary exploration with new roles (becoming a sibling, father, or mother for the first time or to one *more* child). This is the time for the nurse to assist family members individually and as a group in exploring their thoughts and feelings about their changing roles and methods of operating. Providing opportunities for the family to search for these meanings and answers can assist them in reaching their ultimate goal of realistic change. Change is inevitable but does not become as overwhelming to the family that has the support and assistance of a professional who explores with them the current and future changes they must all absorb as the family grows.

The second trimester, when the pregnant woman begins to physically display the developing infant, requires a new nursing approach to the family's changing configuration. The woman is different in appearance and feelings. The family struggles with its adaptation process. Shifts in the system energy have begun and now must be faced even more directly. Yes, the infant is a reality and will increasingly impinge upon the rest of the family. Because of the obviousness of the changes, the family becomes more accepting of the helping professional's interpretation of what is to come.

Confirmation and growing awareness of pregnancy creates a family crisis. *Crisis* in this sense is defined as any situation which the family faces without previously learned patterns of adaptation; that is, any change in the status quo which requires new responses constitutes a crisis. Although all families deal differently with the impact of pregnancy, usually there is at least a fleeting entertainment of the question, "Why now?" (Understandably, the family who has awaited and perhaps sought medical assistance in consummating the pregnancy may not experience this crisis reaction and its associated resentments to a great degree.)

The importance of the nurse's role in the second trimester lies in the ability to assist the family in capitalizing on their assets to attain growth and equilibrium. Even the most abnormal-appearing family has inherent strengths which can be utilized to face the crisis of expecting a new child. This is the time to focus on the feelings and required changes in the family system rather than being prematurely caught up in the narrow game, so often played by professionals, of preparing for the labor and delivery process. It is more appropriate to focus attention upon the prenatal needs and other realities of the developing infant and on his impact on the family. No matter how well-adjusted the family has felt itself to be, doubts will arise as they now question their ability to adapt. The second trimester is the time to allay the couple's fears of being incapable of parenthood because of moments or days of mixed feelings about the new member or themselves. Now is the time for helping them try on new ways of operating in preparation for the new arrival. The family can be helped to realize the commonalities they share with all prospective parents who, like themselves, must cope with perceived threats to established and comfortable habits of living. Providing opportunities for group discussion with other families about how they deal with the crisis is a feasible means of creating positive attitudes and change. The professional's interaction with second-trimester families needs to deal with role playing and with extracting and coping with the real portion of their fantasies, not with the selection of baby fixtures and furnishings.

Third trimester places even different stresses on the existing family system. The pregnant woman characteristically now questions her ability to deal successfully with the labor and delivery process. The potential addition to the family becomes even more real to her, and the woman herself seeks support from family members in ways she has not done before. What does it mean to seek protection, to question one's ability to carry out labor and delivery with any amount of dignity and self-acceptance, to wish that the realities of labor and delivery could be avoided? The family becomes more and more aware of the vigor of the baby and realizes that, ready or not, soon the new voice will sound itself and assert new demands upon them.

The family which has succeeded during the first two trimesters in dealing with their changing roles, at least at some beginning level, is now ready for explicit teaching about the birth process and about each family member's responsibilities and functions during the time of the child's birth. The time is ripe for providing the opportunity to bind anxiety by more concrete forms of instruction in preparations for receiving the infant into postnatal life. Labor and delivery are an experience of intimacy for the woman and her baby (and their attendants), but the greater the involvement of the baby's father and other family members, the more they will feel participation *as a family unit*. By focusing on the family as a unit, pointing out their group strengths, and detailing how they can all assist one another in final preparations the nurse helps them to be able to share their mutual experience and strengthen one another as well as the family as a system. Group decisions about readiness for going to the hospital, temporary care for any existing children, and coming home after delivery are real and concrete points to consider during the last trimester.

Along with the selection, now, of suitable furnishings and other household and family preparations, the nurse appropriately listens to the expression of continuing and new concerns. Parents usually raise the possibility that the mother will be endangered by labor and that the baby will not be normal or that it will disappoint them with its gender or some other characteristic. It is time to assist the family in gathering factual information and in preparing for these possibilities. "What if . . ." is a technique which parents utilize and is a useful tool for the nurse in helping them to get ready for feasible alternatives.

Nursing of the expectant family continues after the long-awaited infant joins them at home. The 40 weeks from conception to term constitute but a phase of the family's need for health maintenance and intervention. Continuing exploration of the various family members' roles in relationship to the care and enjoyment of the baby is very important, for realities of his impact upon the family system almost inevitably exceed expectations. Even if the parents have had prior successful experience with adapting to a new baby, the necessity for extending parental attention, time, and other family resources to include an additional person requires adjustments with which the nurse often can assist. The previously youngest child in the family will not have adapted to a new baby before, and he as well as other family members may require some special approaches which the nurse can guide the family in providing.

The professional may need to intervene as advocate of the new child's individuality. Although the family members almost invariably make early comparisons to the effect that the new arrival looks like or acts like some other kinsman, it may be appropriate for the nurse to help individual family members call upon skills they developed throughout the pregnancy to accept and respond to the baby as himself. Obviously this is especially helpful for those infants who, because of special health conditions, for example, do not conform to previously learned ways of behaving toward children within the family or among the family's culture group and other child-rearing role models.

The family system is stressed by the experiences of pregnancy and by the entry of its new member. If resources are adequate, stress leads to strength. The system is changed, as has been shown, and continues its alterations as the family with a new baby progresses through its developmental phases. Skilled support and intervention of the professional are major resources that can be strikingly beneficial throughout pregnancy, delivery, and subsequent development of the infant, his family members, and the family unit itself.

REFERENCES

1 Geraldine L. Flanagan, *The First Nine Months of Life*, Pocket Books, a division of Simon & Schuster, Inc., New York, 1965.
2 B. M. Patten, *Human Embryology,* 3d ed., McGraw-Hill Book Company, New York, 1968.
3 J. P. Greenhill, *The Miracle of Life*, Year Book Medical Publishers, Chicago, 1971.
4 Patten, op. cit., p. 31.

BIBLIOGRAPHY

Batstone, G. F., Blair, A. W., and Slater, J. M.: *A Handbook of Pre-natal Paediatrics*, J. B. Lippincott Company, Philadelphia, 1971.
Carter, C. O.: *An ABC of Medical Genetics*, Little, Brown and Company, Boston, 1969.
Coleman, A. D., and Coleman, Libby Lee: *Pregnancy: The Psychological Experience*, Herder and Herder, Inc., New York, 1971.
Enelow, A. J.: "The Psychological Impact of Pregnancy on the Family," in James Blake Thomas, *Introduction to Human Embryology*, Lea & Febiger, Philadelphia, 1968, pp. 35–43.
Gedda, L.: *Twins in History and Science*, Charles C Thomas, Publisher, Springfield, Ill., 1961.
Hamilton, W. J., and Mossman, H. W. (eds.): *Human Embryology: Prenatal Form and Function*, The Williams & Wilkins Company, Baltimore, 1972.

Handler, P. (ed.): *Biology and the Future of Man*, Oxford University Press, New York, 1970.

Hilton, B., Callahan, D., Harris, M., Condliffe, P., and Berkley, B. (eds.): *Ethical Issues in Human Genetics: Genetic Counseling and the Use of Genetic Knowledge*, Plenum Press, New York, 1973.

Hooker, D.: *The Prenatal Origin of Behavior*, University of Kansas Press, Lawrence, 1952.

Howells, J. G. (ed.): *Modern Perspectives in Psycho-obstretrics*, Brunner/Mazel, New York, 1972.

Joffe, J. M.: *Prenatal Determinants of Behavior*, Pergamon Press, New York, 1969.

McKusick, V. A.: *Human Genetics*, Prentice-Hall, Inc., Englewood Cliffs, N. J., 1964.

Montagu, M. F. A.: *Prenatal Influences*, Charles C Thomas, Publisher, Springfield, Ill., 1962.

Nilsson, L., Ingelman-Sundberg, A., and Wirsen, C.: *A Child Is Born*, Dell Publishing Co., Inc., New York, 1966.

Rugh, R., and Shettles, L. B.: *From Conception to Birth,* Harper & Row, Publishers, Incorporated, New York, 1971.

Scheinfeld, A.: *Heredity in Humans*, J. B. Lippincott Company, Philadelphia, 1972.

———: *Your Heredity and Environment*, J. B. Lippincott Company, Philadelphia, 1965.

Schimke, R. N.: "Heredity for Clinicians—Genetics and the Practicing Physician," *The Journal of the Kansas Medical Society*, 69:1–9, January 1968.

THE NEONATE— BIRTH TO 1 MONTH

DAVID D. WILLIAMS

The neonatal period, the first 28 days of extrauterine life, is characterized by adaptation and change. As the newborn exits from the uterus, he leaves an environment that existed solely to meet his needs. Once delivered, he must adapt to a new environment in order to maintain homeostasis, grow, and develop.

The newborn's surroundings are vastly different from the custom-made home of the uterus. The intrauterine environment consisted of a fluid medium exerting equal pressure on all parts of his body. The rhythmic sounds and motion of the mother's body were constant and familiar. Fluid requirements, food requirements, and oxygen exchange were provided by the mother through the placenta. Temperature was maintained within optimum range for the developing fetus. All his needs were met through the symbiotic relationship with his mother.

At birth the newborn enters a gaseous atmosphere and must begin gas exchange in the lungs to obtain oxygen and rid the bloodstream of carbon dioxide. Drastic changes in environmental temperatures and uneven pressures on various parts of the body require physiologic adjustments. Transition from a symbiotic relationship with the mother to an interdependence with the family, and later a larger society, requires sociologic changes.

The normal newborn has the innate, though limited, ability to adjust to changes in temperature, pressure, sight, sound, position, and a myriad of additional conditions or requirements for extrauterine existence. There are, however, many variations among newborns, and many health hazards require medical and nursing intervention during the first 4 weeks of life. The infant's ability to adjust to extrauterine life and to realize his potential to grow and develop depends upon many enhancing and inhibiting factors. Some of these factors are related to his physical state; others are peculiar to his environment and social climate. This chapter discusses the effects of both enhancing and inhibiting factors on the development of the newborn. Although the focus of this chapter is the normal newborn, potential threats to health and preventive nursing intervention will be included to emphasize the importance of the nursing process in maintaining health.

PSYCHOSOCIAL INFLUENCES

The newborn has the potential to interact with persons in his environment and to begin establishing interpersonal relationships with members of his family. How this potential is realized depends upon a host of variables such as the infant's physiologic condition, personality factors, and position in the family. The success of his interactions also depends upon the family's attitude toward infants, their experience with babies and child rearing, and their responsiveness to this particular new member of the family (Fig. 9-1). It is not possible to list all the influences on each family; however, the following discussion will serve to illustrate the interactive nature of several common variables.

Development of Parenting

Parenting is a dynamic behavioral process based on the parents' philosophy, knowledge, attitudes, and emotions about themselves and their children. Parenting must be developed. It is not a set of feelings or a pattern of behaving that is acquired when a baby is born. Parenting begins well before birth, during the parent's own childhood. It is based on the parent's views of himself and the roles with which he identifies in his relationships with others, especially his own parents and his spouse. Attitudes and feelings may be modified during the preconception period of planning for a baby and during the prenatal period as the parent prepares for the birth process. Parenting is always in a state of development. As the child grows and develops and as the parent matures, the parent and child must continue to adjust in their changing relationship with each other.

The old stereotypes of mother as the principal caretaker and father as the breadwinner no longer seem as true. With today's life-styles, many mothers work outside the home and contribute to the family income while fathers assume an equal responsibility for the care of their children. The parents' views of their roles will influence the amount and kind of interaction they have with the baby (Fig. 9-2).

Development of Trust

The newborn is egocentric. His perceptual and cognitive development is understandably at a minimum, and his experience is so limited that he has little or no awareness of anything beyond his own physical sensations. As far as he can tell, the world *is* his body. His sole purpose is to achieve and maintain a comfortable, pleasurable state of existence.

In his dependent, almost completely helpless developmental state, he cannot provide for his own needs or even communicate the source or nature of any discomfort. His cry and uncoordinated muscular activity are his only means of expressing distress and demanding action to return him to a state of comfort.

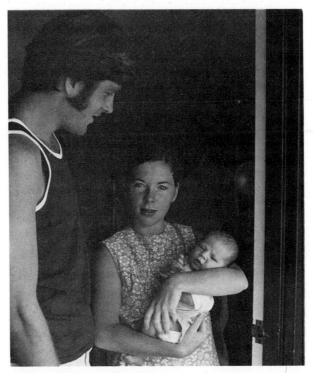

Figure 9-1 Parents and newborn, a family.

The manner in which his needs are met by others determines the newborn's view of his world and his response to it. Furthermore, the impressions he receives from his contact with caretakers are incorporated into his personality and begin even in the first month to contribute to his later attitudes and expectations. When his needs are met in a consistent and comforting manner, he begins to develop trust.[1] The world becomes a predictable and pleasant place to live. He learns that he can safely expect others to restore him to a state of comfort. If his caretakers are unresponsive, ineffectual, or inconsistent in their responses to him, or if his body is for some reason incapable of being comforted, the impressions integrated into his personality are much different. He does not develop confidence in those caring for him or in his own ability to attain a feeling of well-being. He learns to mistrust. This basic development of trust rather than mistrust extends into the second year of life at least, and has only its beginnings in the neonatal period.

Trust is a quality that not only develops within the infant as an outcome of his experiences with his body and with his caretakers but also is strengthened in the parents as they accrue success in the parenting of their new child. Thus, there develops a

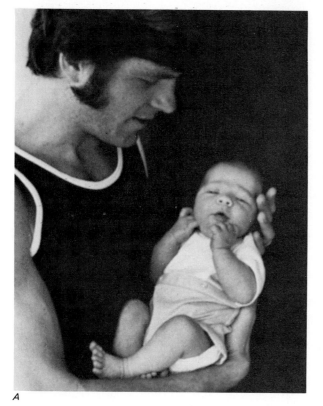

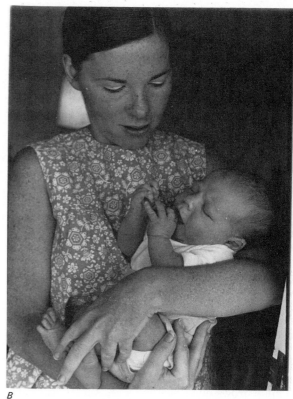

A

B

Figure 9-2 *A.* A father's touch, while gentle and secure, is typically less enfolding than a mother's (*B*).

mutuality of trust in self and in significant others, establishing a favorable base upon which both parents and child are launched toward their subsequent development as individuals and as a family unit.

Position in the Family

A child's position in the family constellation also has an influence on his beginning psychosocial development. If he is a first child, the attentiveness of his parents and the intimacy he shares with them are usually quite intense. For example, Sears and his associates[2] found that firstborn children were more likely to be breast-fed than those born later. The first child of inexperienced parents serves as a practice model. Parents who have had previous parenting experience are very likely to approach the care of subsequent babies with somewhat different expectations and methods. Even in the first month, experienced parents may be more confident, more relaxed, and more skilled in their approach to a non-firstborn infant.

The newborn who is one of several children enters a complex family system. The addition of the new infant to the previous family configuration may of course be an enrichment to all, but it also in a sense dilutes the intensity of interpersonal ties that existed before his arrival. Bossard and Boll[3] have shown that the *number* of relationships within a family increases geometrically with the addition of each new child according to the formula $x = \dfrac{y^2 - y}{2}$, in which x represents the number of relationships and y represents the number of persons in the group. Hence in a 2-parent family only 1 interpersonal relationship exists before a child is born. With the addition of the new baby, 3 relationships result. The second child enlarges this number to 6, the third brings it to 10, a 6-member family has 15, and so forth.

The non-firstborn child begins life with the involuntary role of replacement for the position of youngest. He becomes the baby of the family for his siblings as well as for his parents, which has inevitable implications for the older children as well as for himself. The extent to which older children are prepared for the birth of a new brother or sister affects the ease with which they are able to adapt. When older siblings are prepared for the baby's arrival and are able to view him as at least partially theirs, there is apt to be less competition and less jealousy, more shared pride and enjoyment, and a positive beginning for their lifelong association.

The non-firstborn child has the interest, expectations, and stimulation of siblings as well as parents. Because the several family members differ in their personal characteristics and in their role relationships to the new baby, he experiences considerable variety and intensity in his social interactions, even as a neonate. The potential is greater for inconsistency and conflict as well as for enriching variety.

Physiologic Factors Promoting Social Interaction

Certain of the characteristics of the newborn enhance social interaction, while others tend to limit the nature of social situations. He is unable to approach people in his environment. He cannot talk, which places another limitation on the nature of his associations with others. On the other hand, he is capable of physiologic responses which tend to enhance interpersonal relationships. For example, the normal newborn has a well-developed grasp reflex and automatically closes his fist around any object that touches the palm of his hand. The grasp reflex helps to elicit positive, adoring responses from persons in his environment. Adults who place their extended finger in the grasp of the baby's tiny hand often misinterpret this reflex behavior as a sign of acceptance or affection and thus prolong their contact with the baby.

Evidence of the reciprocal effect of the neonate's responses can be seen in the interaction between parent and child. The baby who is responsive, good-natured, and alert engenders a different set of feelings from parents than a baby who is lethargic and less sensitive to his environment and therefore less responsive to attention. Similarly, the infant who is fussy and frustrated because he is ill or has trouble sucking may create feelings of frustration and impatience in the parent trying to satisfy him.

Cognitive Development

An intact nervous system is necessary for the optimum development of the cognitive areas of personality. While all the nerve cells of the brain are present before birth, not all the cells and nerve centers are mature enough to function immediately after birth. Although research in this area is inconclusive, it is doubtful that cortical function is possible at birth. Fortunately, the simple reflexive actions of the newborn make it possible for him to function without cortical involvement for an indefinite period.

The newborn receives information about the world through his senses. Much of the cognitive development during the first month of life revolves around those processes that allow him to become more attentive to the outside world. In the next months he will develop the ability to actively seek stimuli, to make associations, and to take deliberate action based on his perceptions.

The tactile senses are well developed before birth and become a primary receptor of sensory input after birth. The newborn receives a great deal of tactile stimulation when held, cuddled, caressed, fed, bathed, rocked, or carried from one place to another. All these activities provide needed excitement to the central nervous system.

Frank[4] has observed that the fetus receives regular, rhythmic tactile stimulation from the mother's heartbeat. Heart sounds are transmitted as waves to all areas of the skin through the amniotic fluid. The baby carried by the mother in close skin contact continues to receive similar stimulation after birth. Frank also explains that tactile stimulation is the basis for deriving meaning from other stimuli. Sensory experiences of sound and sight are enhanced by association with touch.[4]

Recent investigations reveal a well-developed sense of hearing in very young babies. Bronstein and Petrova's research suggests that very young infants are able not only to respond to sound, but also to discriminate differences in sound.[5] These investigators recorded variations in sucking behavior in response to sound patterns. When a sound occurred the infant stopped sucking and when the sound was repeated in several trials, the baby gradually shortened the time in which sucking was discontinued. After enough repetition of the sound of one pitch, the infant continued to suck when it was played; however, when sound of a different pitch was introduced, the infant stopped sucking again. Simner and Reilly[6] have also produced research suggesting that newborns respond to the vocal qualities of the cry of other newborns.

The eyes are somewhat less developed at birth than other sensory receptors. Tear production is usually limited or absent the first 2 months. The newborn can fixate light momentarily, and the pupil constricts in response to bright light; but coordination, fixation, and focusing must be refined as the infant matures and gains experience in using his

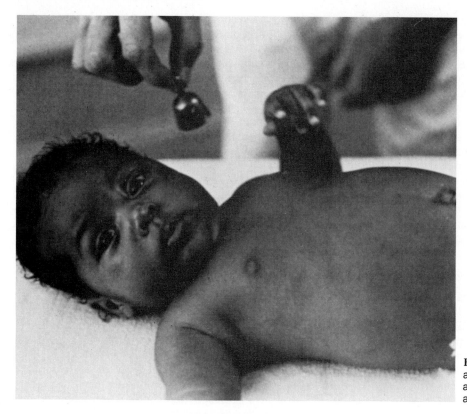

Figure 9-3 The neonate shows alert responsiveness to sound and fixes his eyes on persons about him.

eyes. Within a few days, most newborns are able to fixate a bright light for a short period of time, and by the end of the first month they are able to follow a moving light or bright object to the midline of vision.

Coordination of vision and hearing appears to be developed early in infancy. Although Wertheimer[7] reports a newborn responding with eye movements to a sound presented as early as 10 minutes after birth, and Leventhal[8] concludes that newborns can discriminate the location of sound source, it has been this writer's experience that most infants fail to look toward the sound of a bell within the first 2 months (Fig. 9-3).

Korner and Thomas,[9] studying 2- to 4-day-old healthy full-term newborns, found a surprising sensitivity to vestibular-proprioceptive (movement and position) stimulation. In their study, vestibular stimulation had a highly potent soothing effect on crying babies.

Babies seem to be able to perceive some kinds of pain stimuli more acutely than other kinds. A pinprick or intramuscular injection usually elicits a very brief crying episode, while gas in the gastrointestinal tract can produce a prolonged outburst of crying. The difference in response may be related to the length of exposure to the painful stimuli; however, surgical wounds which take days to heal do not appear to cause the neonate any degree of discomfort.

Lipsitt and Levy[10] studied crying and withdrawal responses to painful stimuli. Sensitivity to pain increased steadily during the first few days of life. It was also found that girls demonstrated greater sensitivity than boys. This result was attributed to the greater maturity of girls at birth.

HAZARDS TO HEALTH
Neonatal Mortality Rates

Even though the majority of newborns make a successful transition to extrauterine existence, the adjustment period is not without its hazards. The high death rate during the first 28 days of life emphasizes the importance of health care during the neonatal period. The neonatal mortality rate is an expression of the number of deaths in the first 28 days following birth as compared with the number of live births within a given year, and it is usually expressed as the number of deaths per thousand live births. In

1970 the United States experienced a total mortality rate during the neonatal period of 14.9. In other words, for every 1,000 live-born infants nearly 15 died during the first 28 days following birth.

Although the mortality rates for both white and nonwhite neonates have decreased over the past several decades, the rate for the nonwhite population remains higher than that for whites (see Table 9-1). Since the figures given for the nonwhite population include Negro, Indian, and Oriental births in the United States, socioeconomic rather than racial factors are thought to be the cause of their higher rate.

The establishment of prenatal programs, nutrition projects, free clinics, and neonatal intensive care units, together with increased emphasis on planned parenthood and prepared childbirth, has contributed to a lowering of the neonatal death rate. Nevertheless, the newborn sustains the greatest risk of death in the immediate period following birth, when the transition is made from intrauterine symbiotic existence to extrauterine independent life. Of all the deaths occurring before the age of 1 year, nearly one-half occur on the first day following birth and approximately three-fourths during the first 28 days.

Congenital malformations account for a fair number of neonatal deaths. However, a greater number of deaths result from asphyxia, atelectasis, birth injury, infection, and erythroblastosis combined than from congenital malformations. Prematurity and problems related to the establishment and maintenance of adequate respiration remain chief causes of early death.

PHYSICAL ASSESSMENT

By completing a physical assessment of the newborn, the nurse establishes a basis for his care. Data gathered by the nurse become the foundation

Table 9-1 MORTALITY RATES

	1950	1960	1968	1970
Infant	29.2	26.0	21.8	19.8
White	26.8	22.9	19.2	NA*
Nonwhite	44.5	43.2	34.5	NA
Neonate	20.5	18.7	16.1	14.9
White	19.4	17.2	14.7	NA
Nonwhite	27.5	26.9	23.0	NA

* Figures for white and nonwhite not available for 1970.
Source: Figures from *Statistical Abstract of the United States,* U.S. Bureau of the Census, 1972.

for planning both nursing and medical care and for evaluating subtle changes in the newborn's condition. An understanding of the normal characteristics of the newborn is essential in order for the nurse to be able to evaluate his physical findings. Normal characteristics and their variations, most of which require no therapy, are discussed below in considerable detail. A few abnormal or pathologic findings are included, but these will be presented in greater detail in the later chapters devoted to specific organ systems and their disorders.

Initial Assessment

Apgar Scoring System Assessment of the infant begins at birth. The healthy newborn has a heart rate of 120 to 160 beats per minute, a good strong cry, well-flexed extremities, irritable reflexes, and a healthy pink color at birth. The Apgar scoring chart is used in most delivery rooms to evaluate these five signs (see Table 9-2). A score of 0 to 2 is recorded for each sign, depending upon the degree to which it is present or absent. The total score reflects the infant's general condition 60 seconds after birth. The nurse computing an Apgar score should begin the evaluation 55 seconds after both the top of the head and the bottom of the feet are visible, taking no more than 5 seconds to observe the five signs. A score of 10 indicates an infant in the best possible condition. An infant with a score from 5 to 10 usually requires no treatment; however, a baby scoring 4 or below requires immediate medical attention. The first score should be decided at 60 seconds even though resuscitation is in progress. A second score may be computed 5 minutes later to measure how well the infant is adjusting to extrauterine life.

Gross malformations such as spina bifida, cleft lip, or omphalocele may be observed on preliminary examination at birth. A more thorough physical examination should be performed as soon as possible after a clear airway has been established and the infant has demonstrated that he is able to maintain respiratory function. When the infant has been delivered in the hospital, a physical assessment may be made by the nurse as soon as the infant arrives in the newborn nursery. If the infant has been delivered at home, the mother should be made comfortable and a physical examination of the infant performed immediately. Increasing numbers of hospitals offer rooming-in or family care facilities. If such facilities are available, the parents may be present for the initial examination of their baby. The nurse needs to be skillful in interpersonal communications and sensitive to the emotions expressed by the parents when

Table 9-2 APGAR SCORING CHART

Sign	0	1	2
Heart rate	Absent	Slow (less than 100)	Greater than 100
Respiratory effort	Absent	Weak cry, hypoventilation	Good, strong cry
Muscle tone	Limp	Some flexion of extremities	Well-flexed extremities
Reflex irritability (skin stimulation to feet)	No response	Some motion	Cry
Color	Blue, pale	Body pink, extremities blue	Body completely pink

they examine their baby for the first time. The nurse should accompany the examination with careful explanation of the physical characteristic of the newborn. Ideally, the parents should have been prepared during the prenatal period for the baby's immediate postnatal appearance. The nurse can contribute significantly to the comfort of new parents at this time.

Appearance at First Sight Because the appearance of the newborn changes rapidly in the first several days, few people are prepared for his unattractive appearance immediately after birth. At first the newborn may appear "pinched," with a long head, short neck, and flexed extremities. He usually assumes his position of comfort, which is similar to his position in utero. The head is flexed, back bent forward, arms held close to chest, hands held in fists, hips flexed, knees bent, and feet dorsiflexed. Often a fussy baby can be comforted by placing him in this position. The body is cylindric and appears small in relation to the head. Head circumference equals or slightly exceeds that of the chest. The average head circumference of the full-term infant is 33 to 35 cm (13 to 14 inches) at birth. The average chest circumference is 30 to 33 cm (12 to 13 inches). Due to the natural molding of the head during the birth process, causing an elongated appearance of the skull and face, head circumference may be slightly smaller than chest circumference for the first 24 hours. For most infants, the normal contour of the head will return in 2 to 3 days. If a discrepancy between the head and chest circumferences is suspected or the proportion between the two appears abnormal, the nurse may wish to repeat the measurements for several consecutive days. A careful record should be kept of each measurement. An abnormally small head may indicate microcephalus, while an abnormally large head may indicate hydrocephalus or intracranial bleeding.

Measurement of head and chest circumferences should be made with the infant lying in the supine position on a firm surface. A flexible tape measure is placed under the head and drawn firmly around the head from the occipital bone to the brow (Fig. 9-4). This represents the point of greatest circumference of the head. With the measuring tape still under the infant, the chest circumference is measured at the nipple line.

Length The head of the neonate comprises approximately one-quarter of his total length. The average newborn male is 50 cm (20 inches) long, the average female 49 cm (19½ inches). The normal range for both sexes is 47.5 to 53.75 cm (19 to 21½ inches).

Weight A large percentage of full-term infants weigh between 2,700 and 3,850 Gm (about 6 to 8 lb 8 oz) at birth. The average girl weighs approximately 3,180 Gm (7 lb), and the average boy weighs approximately 3,400 Gm (7 lb 8 oz).

Variations in weight and length of infants at birth may be attributed to a combination of maturity at time of delivery, genetic characteristics, and the nutritional and metabolic condition of the mother and fetus during pregnancy. Parents of small stature are likely to have a small infant. Babies of diabetic mothers tend to be larger than the average infant at birth. Negro, Indian, and Oriental infants are usually smaller than Caucasian infants of the same gestational age. Children born to the same parents are rarely the same weight and length at birth. The first-born infant is likely to be smaller than later siblings.

It is usual for the newborn to lose 5 to 10 percent of his birth weight during the first few days of life. This loss may total 170 to 280 Gm, or 6 to 10 oz. The passage of meconium and urine and the withholding of water and feedings account for the majority of this weight loss. Most infants regain their birth weight within 10 days. Infants who are heavy at birth may lose more weight following birth than slender babies and may show slower gain records during the neonatal period.

Normal weight gain for the neonate is 140 to 190 Gm (5 to 7 oz) per week. The breast-fed infant may show a slower gain than the infant receiving formula

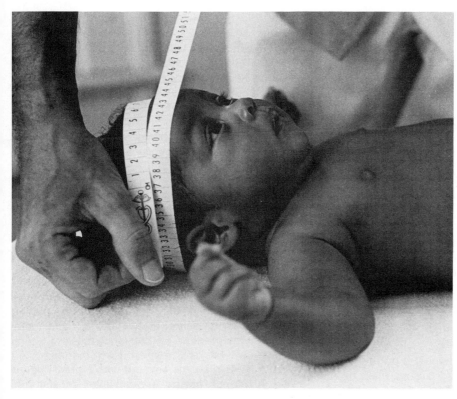

Figure 9-4 Measurement of head circumference.

feedings. Newborns are weighed routinely each day in the hospital. Although there are usually variations in weight from day to day, and some days there may be a loss rather than a gain, the progress of the infant is determined by the total deviation from the birth weight.

To ensure an accurate record of the infant's weight, care should be taken to weigh the infant at the same time each day, to see that the scales are properly balanced, and to be certain that the weight recorded does not include clothing or crib blankets. Precautions should be taken to provide for the baby's safety by placing him in the center of the scales and by posing a hand over him. Even a newborn can be active enough to roll off some infant scales.

Head The bony plates of the cranial vault are not joined to one another at birth. Following birth, ridges may be palpable in several places on the infant's head. These ridges are caused by an overlapping of the cranial bones as the head passed through the tight-fitting birth canal. By the second day following birth, minute openings called suture lines may be palpated where the ridges were earlier. The suture lines remain uncalcified for several months to allow the cranial vault to grow.

Fontanels are "soft spots" formed at the junction of the suture lines; They are spaces not yet filled in by bone. The anterior fontanel is at the junction of the sagittal and coronal sutures. (Refer to Chap. 3 for details about the anatomic landmarks of the fontanels.) This diamond-shaped fontanel may be as much as 5 cm (2 inches) at its widest part. Because of molding during the birth process, however, the anterior fontanel may be slightly smaller during the first 24 hours than afterward. The posterior fontanel is located at the junction of the sagittal suture and the lambdoid suture. This triangular opening averages 1 cm (0.4 inches) or less in size and may be difficult to locate on palpation.

The fontanels should be soft and flat; however, both the fontanels and sutures may initially be obscured by molding or by swelling of the scalp as a result of trauma to the head during birth. The anterior fontanel may be observed to pulsate with the heartbeat and to distend when the infant cries. Both of these findings are normal.

Caput succedaneum is a poorly defined area of edema of the presenting portion of the scalp. The edema is usually absorbed quickly so that the swelling disappears by the third day.

Birth trauma may cause a *cephalhematoma*, which is a collection of blood between the periosteum and a flat cranial bone. The mass is a soft gelatin-like enlargement which does not cross a suture line. It is irreducible, but due to the nature of the mass, it tends to fluctuate when external pressure is applied. Because the accumulation of blood lies between the periosteum and bone, crying does not increase the size of the mass. Since the sanguineous fluid is usually absorbed within a few weeks, it is seldom necessary to aspirate a cephalhematoma.

Eyes Although darkly pigmented babies have dark eyes at birth, the eyes of Caucasian babies are blue or slate gray. Permanent color may be detected by about 3 months; however, pigmentation of the iris may increase for as long as 1 year.

Small areas of subconjunctival hemorrhage, caused by impairment of venous return and rupture of capillaries in the sclerae during delivery, may be present for the first week or more. In addition to hemorrhage, there may be a moderate purulent discharge from the eyes for 2 to 3 days after birth. Although infection must be ruled out in every baby with eye drainage, this condition may be simply a chemical conjunctivitis caused by the instillation of silver nitrate eye drops shortly after birth. Neither chemical conjunctivitis nor subconjunctival hemorrhage is of any clinical significance.

Thorax The thorax should be examined for symmetry, size, and shape. Examination should reveal a thorax that is both symmetric and cylindric. Chest circumference should be measured as noted previously.

Normal newborns are abdominal breathers, producing very little movement of the thoracic cavity during ordinary respiratory activity. The characteristic respiratory pattern includes rapid, irregular respirations that fluctuate between 40 and 60 per minute. Frequent apneic periods, restlessness, flaring of the nostrils, noisy respirations, retractions, and cyanosis are signs of distress and require immediate attention.

For the first several weeks, a noticeable enlargement of the breasts may be present and a pale milky fluid called "witch's milk" may be secreted. This is a transient condition caused by the transfer of maternal hormones in the last weeks of pregnancy. As the baby gradually excretes residual hormones, the condition disappears. The breasts should not be pressed or squeezed.

The clamped umbilical cord should be examined when the baby arrives in the newborn nursery and periodically for the next several days. Traces of blood may indicate that the stump needs to be reclamped or tied. Purulent drainage is a sign of infection and calls for immediate culture and antibiotic therapy. The umbilical stump usually turns black and sloughs off between the sixth and tenth day.

Skin It is important for the nurse to examine the skin of an infant under adequate light which is free from surface reflections. Yellow, blue, or pink nursery walls tend to alter the infant's skin color, giving the false appearance of jaundice, cyanosis, or flushing. Sunlight or an overhead examination light in a white room is best for accurate observation. Racial variations occur in the color of newborns' skin, with Mediterranean, Latin, and black babies usually appearing darker than whites but considerably lighter than adults of their ancestry and lighter than they will become in subsequent months.

At birth the baby is covered with a greasy, gray-white substance having a cheeselike consistency. This substance, *vernix caseosa*, tends to make the newborn slippery to handle and gives him a "messy" appearance on first sight. Vernix caseosa is an accumulation of epithelial cells and secretions from the sebaceous glands. Most of the vernix is removed with the initial bath, or absorbs or is rubbed off on clothing within 12 to 24 hours. Occasionally it is necessary to remove accumulated secretions such as vernix caseosa from deep skin folds to prevent the development of intertrigo and to protect the child from cutaneous infection. After the first day, the skin may become dry and flaky.

Acrocyanosis is seen in most infants for the first several days. This condition is characterized by blueness of the hands and feet and is caused by venous stasis in the extremities. As circulation improves, acrocyanosis disappears.

The skin may show signs of a traumatic delivery. There may be *ecchymoses* (bruises) on the face and shoulders of a newborn delivered in the vertex position. Forceps marks may also be present if the delivery has been difficult. Extensive areas of ecchymoses may be found on the feet, buttocks, and sacrum of the newborn delivered from the breech position.

Pinpoint hemorrhagic areas (*petechiae*) on the upper trunk or face may result from increased intravascular pressure, producing ruptured capillaries during the birth process. Because ecchymoses and petechiae are collections of extravascular blood, they do not disappear when the skin is blanched. Red rashes from local engorgement of surface capillaries can be distinguished from petechiae by blanching. Rashes disappear when pressure is applied and blood is forced from the capillary bed.

Other characteristics are not associated with trauma. *Mongolian spots* appear as areas of blue pigmentation resembling bruises on the back, sacrum, or buttocks of Negro, Oriental, and Mediterranean infants. Parents may be assured that these darkened areas will disappear by the preschool years. There is no relationship between Mongolian spots and Down's syndrome.

Telangiectatic nevi, or "stork bites," may be present at the nape of the neck or, less commonly, on the head, face, or trunk. This condition is caused by a congenital widening of the surface capillaries and disappears momentarily with blanching of the skin. Because of their prominent position, stork bites can cause parental alarm. Although these marks ordinarily do not completely disappear, parents can be assured that they will gradually fade as the child grows older and the skin becomes thicker.

Milia appears as tiny white papules across the newborn's nose and face. The papules are accumulations of secretions caused by clogged sebaceous glands. Milia disappears spontaneously within a few weeks. No attempt should be made to wash, rub, or squeeze milia.

Between the 16th and 32d weeks of intrauterine development the fetus is covered with fine hair called *lanugo*. Although sloughing begins after the thirty-second week, many newborns retain a dense covering of hair on the shoulders, back, forehead, and cheeks. This downy covering continues to disappear during the first few weeks of life.

Erythema toxicum is a blotchy, transient rash which commonly appears in the first few days of life. Characterized by irregularly shaped, small reddened areas with pale centers, this eruption of unknown cause produces no symptoms and requires no treatment.

Normal physiologic *icterus* (jaundice) appears in over half of all healthy newborns. Jaundice is a yellow staining of the skin and sclerae resulting from high concentrations of the bile pigment *bilirubin* in the circulating blood. Bilirubin is one of the breakdown products of destroyed red blood cells; hence, serum bilirubin levels rise whenever red blood cells are broken down at a rapid rate. Because the high hemoglobin required for adequate oxygenation of the baby in utero is no longer needed after he becomes an air breather, red blood cell breakdown is part of his adaptation during the first days of extrauterine life.

Jaundice in the neonate may be a manifestation of this normal adjustment after birth, in which case it is called *physiologic jaundice*, or it may indicate a serious pathologic condition, such as sepsis or maternal-child blood type incompatibility. Hence, observation for the appearance and extent of icterus is a critical part of the nursing assessment of the newborn. The presence of jaundice at birth or within the first 48 hours is considered pathologic and may require phototherapy or exchange transfusion. Physiologic jaundice, on the other hand, ordinarily does not appear until after 48 hours of age and requires no special treatment. Time of appearance, however, cannot safely be relied upon for determining the significance of this clinical sign. The infant should be closely observed for any signs of illness or infection, and the blood level of bilirubin should be determined.

Darkly pigmented skin tends to mask the presence of icterus. Since the underlying pigment of dark-skinned persons normally appears yellow, the technique of blanching the skin is not a satisfactory method of examining the infant suspected of being jaundiced. Jaundice may be readily detected by examining the sclerae and the posterior portion of the hard palate.[11]

Reflexes Examination of the newborn should include an assessment of certain reflexes ordinarily present at birth. Since the central nervous system is immature in its function for some time after birth, the presence or absence of various reflexes and the time at which they appear or disappear are indicative of the infant's progress toward normal development.

Of those reflexes present at birth, several enhance the newborn's chances of survival. The coughing and sneezing reflexes help to rid the respiratory system of amniotic fluid and to protect the newborn from inhaling foreign substances from the environment. Yawning is a reflex which enables the newborn to draw in a supply of oxygen when his rate of respiratory exchange is insufficient to meet his needs.

Other reflexes that are protective or defensive include the ability to hiccup, to blink when exposed to bright light, to shiver when cold, to withdraw from pain, and to cry when uncomfortable.

Obtaining nourishment is primarily dependent upon a group of reflexes that are very active in the newborn. The *rooting reflex* functions to help the newborn search for food. This reflex may be elicited by touching the baby's cheek with a nipple or by stroking the cheek with a hand. The baby responds by opening his mouth and turning toward the source of stimulation.

The sucking reflex is so well developed at birth that many babies are born with the ability to suck their fist or thumb. Examination of the newborn's hands may reveal calluses or other marks indicative of prenatal sucking. So prominent is this reflex that sucking movements may be seen whenever the lips are stimulated by the touch of crib blankets, pacifier, nipple, or the infant's own hand. A weak or absent suck reflex is considered abnormal and may be evidence of immaturity, neuromuscular pathology, or depression. Infants without a suck reflex usually require intravenous therapy, gastrostomy, or nasogastric tube feedings.

The swallowing, gagging, and vomiting reflexes are also well developed in the normal newborn at the time of birth. The swallow reflex enables the baby to ingest food substances, while the gagging and vomiting reflexes provide for the rejection of irritating or toxic substances from the gastrointestinal tract.

The grasp reflex (Fig. 9-5) has been discussed previously in the section titled "Physiologic Factors Promoting Social Interactions." If the newborn is able to grasp an object securely enough to be pulled to a standing position, this action is referred to as the *Darwinian reflex*. Not all newborns are able to perform this movement, and it is not considered abnormal if the grasp is not this strong. Later the infant will gain control over this reflex and will be able to grasp or drop objects voluntarily.

When held in an upright position with the feet touching a solid surface, the newborn will respond with dancing movements of the legs. This reflex, called the *dance reflex*, is normally present at birth but soon disappears. The dance reflex may be absent at birth in babies who have sustained damage to either the central nervous system or the peripheral nerves to the lower extremity.

The *Moro reflex* also is present at birth in normal infants. When the baby is lying quietly, jerking the blanket beneath the baby or jarring the crib should elicit a startle response. Another common method of activating this reflex is to hold the infant quietly and suddenly remove support from beneath the head, allowing the head to drop slightly. The infant should respond by drawing up his legs and throwing his arms forward. If movements are absent or not symmetric, neurologic injury should be suspected.

Occasionally the Moro reflex is absent for the first 24 hours and appears on the second day. This delay may be due to the presence of cerebral edema shortly after birth. As the edema subsides, the reflex can be elicited. If the reflex is present at birth but disappears shortly after birth, increasing intracranial pressure should be suspected. The Moro reflex is usually present until the fourth or fifth month.

The *tonic neck reflex* is often referred to as the fencing position. As the infant lies on his back and his head is turned either to the left or to the right, he extends the arm and leg on the side to which he is facing, similar to the stance a fencer assumes when meeting an opponent. The arm and the leg on the opposite side are flexed. The tonic neck reflex is well developed at birth and gradually disappears over a span of several months. As the nervous system develops, the baby gradually gains control over his movements and assumes a symmetric position.

Anogenital Area Examination shows that the size of the penis and scrotum varies among newborn babies. In full-term infants the testes, which developed in the abdomen of the fetus, should have descended into the scrotum or be palpable in the inguinal canals. The *prepuce* (foreskin) may be long and may adhere tightly to the glans. Unless urination or hygiene are impeded, no treatment is required. In most hospitals circumcision is no longer considered a matter-of-course procedure to be performed on all newborn males. The urinary meatus should be visible near the end of the glans penis. Congenital malplacement of the meatus (*epispadias* if the urethra opens on the dorsal side of the penile shaft and *hypospadias* if it is located on the ventral side) usually requires surgical correction.

If the parents request circumcision, it is usually performed during the newborn period. Until the surgical wound has healed, the penis should be observed for signs of bleeding or infection and the incision should be covered with a sterile petroleum jelly dressing. It is thought that newborns experience little discomfort during circumcision, since many appear contented and suck on a pacifier during the surgical procedure.

In the female, the labia majora appear underdeveloped while the labia minora are swollen and enlarged. Maternal hormones transferred in utero are responsible for the enlarged labia minora and may also cause a blood-tinged mucus to be dis-

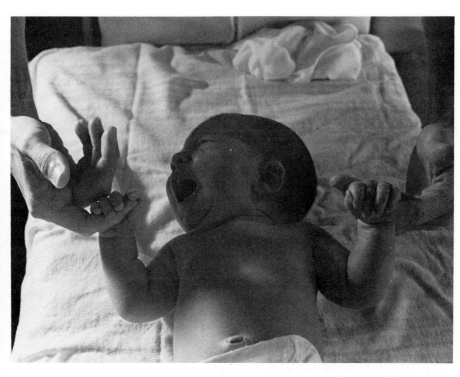

Figure 9-5 The neonate demonstrates a strong, bilateral grasp reflex.

charged from the vagina. This condition gradually disappears as the maternal hormones are excreted.

The kidneys begin to function well before birth, and urine is passed into the amniotic fluid. The nurse should be alert to the first voiding after birth. The time of the first voiding may be normally delayed for as long as 24 to 36 hours, since the kidneys are not very active until the infant begins regular feedings. Failure to void on the second day, an intermittent stream, or grimacing on voiding, however, may be signs of stricture and should be reported immediately. The kidneys are immature in the newborn and lack the ability to concentrate urine. Consequently, when the infant does void, the urine is dilute.

The anal area should be examined for patency and for fissures. A digital examination may be done to rule out imperforate anus and rectal atresia. The nurse should observe for the passing of the first stool (*meconium*). Meconium is a sticky, odorless material that appears greenish black. Failure to pass meconium within 24 hours of birth may indicate obstruction due to atresia of the gastrointestinal tract or to *meconium ileus*, a condition in which the meconium is too viscous to pass through the bowel and be excreted.

The character of the stools changes throughout the first week. The first meconium stools are followed by *transitional stools*, which appear dark greenish yellow and have a loose consistency. After the transitional phase, the characteristics of the stool depend upon the type of feedings. The stool pattern of the breast-fed baby tends to be more erratic than that of the baby fed cow's milk or commercial formula. Generally, however, the breast-fed baby has two to four yellow pasty stools daily, while the baby on cow's milk or formula produces one or two yellowish-brown stools a day.

Muscle Control The newborn lacks coordinated control of his motor activity. He moves his extremities in a random fashion and cannot direct his actions toward any purpose. In a prone position he is able to lift his head only slightly, although he may attempt crawling movements and some newborns push themselves across their cribs. Because his muscles lack strength, his head sags forward and his back bows, causing him to slump forward when held in a sitting position (Fig. 9-6). When picking up the newborn or holding him, it is necessary to support his head and back since he lacks the muscular strength to control his own posture. An evaluation of the newborn should include an assessment of muscle strength. The normal newborn has firm muscles and offers resistance to passive movement. This is most noticeable when the examiner attempts

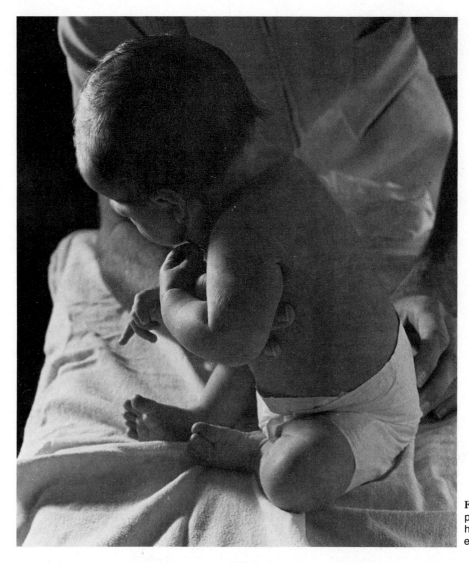

Figure 9-6 Neonatal sitting posture. The back curves, the head falls forward, and all extremities are flexed.

to extend the baby's flexed extremities. Flaccid muscles may indicate central or peripheral nervous system disorder or electrolyte imbalance.

SPECIAL CONSIDERATIONS FOR CARE

Immaturity is a major inhibiting factor in the newborn's adjustment to extrauterine life. If he is to survive and grow, special care will be required during his first weeks and months. In addition to assessment, the primary focus of nursing will be on planning, delivering, teaching, and evaluating care in many of the following areas to ensure the comfort and well-being of the newborn.

Nourishment

The newborn is not yet ready to assimilate a wide variety of foods. The digestive tract is efficient enough to break down the nutrients needed for growth; however, food offered to the infant must be prepared in a form that can be ingested and utilized. The absence of teeth and of coordinated chewing necessitates, initially, a liquid diet of milk or a milk substitute. Even when solids are eventually introduced into the diet they will be accepted more readily if diluted to a more liquid consistency. The newborn's stomach capacity is small, yet his rapid growth rate requires large amounts of food in proportion to his body size. Fortunately, food is not retained in the stomach but begins emptying into the duodenum almost immediately. Thus, frequent feedings are not only possible but required in the neonatal period.

Because the newborn has a well-developed suck reflex, he is well prepared to obtain nourishment from a nipple. He is capable of taking between 45 and 60 ml (1½ and 2 oz) at each feeding. The newborn who is satisfied at each feeding usually sleeps contentedly 3 to 4 hours before he experiences hunger pains and requires another feeding.

Unless contraindicated by some maternal or infant disease or disorder, the choice between breast-feeding or artificial feeding should be left up to the parents. If the parents are comfortable with breast-feeding, it can contribute to a warm mother-child relationship. On the other hand, artificial feeding provides an opportunity for the father to participate in feeding and thus an opportunity for him to establish a closer relationship with the infant. Some parents prefer to breast-feed and to offer a supplemental bottle once or twice a day.

Newborns have individual differences in their eating habits, and several trials are sometimes necessary to develop a successful feeding technique. Several research studies suggest that biologic and environmental factors influence individual eating habits. Nisbett and Gurwitz[12] discovered that heavy infants increased their intake more than lighter infants when given sweetened formula. They also observed that heavy infants were less willing than lighter infants to exert effort to obtain food when sucking was made difficult.

Elder[13] recorded sucking pressures as the environmental temperature was increased from 26.7 to 32.2°C (80 to 90°F). Sucking pressure was noted to decrease as environmental temperature increased to 32.2°C (90°F). Higher sucking pressures also were recorded in the morning feeding period than in the afternoon.

The infant with a weak suck or one who tires easily usually benefits from an enlarged nipple to enable him to obtain sufficient nourishment without overexertion. On the other hand, the infant with a strong, vigorous suck will need a nipple with a smaller hole. All babies swallow some amount of air in the process of nursing and require frequent bubbling. Some infants require bubbling more often than others, but it is good practice to bubble every newborn before placing him in bed. Air released from the stomach while the infant is in a recumbent position is often accompanied by gastric content, which can easily be aspirated. To prevent aspiration it is wise to place the infant in a prone position with his head turned to the side after feeding.

A few newborns tend to vomit a small amount routinely after each feeding, usually because of a poorly developed cardiac sphincter at the esophageal end of the stomach. Persistent vomiting, however, may be a sign of obstruction or illness and should never be taken lightly.

Feeding is the focus of an intimate relationship between parent and child. The manner in which the baby is fed can convey to him a feeling of security and warmth. He enjoys close physical contact when held and cuddled and soon comes to associate the parent's contact with pleasant experiences. Whenever possible, it is advisable to hold the newborn during feeding and until he falls asleep.

Additional information about the physiologic and psychosocial aspects of infant feeding is presented in Chapter 15.

Protection

At birth the infant is unable to produce antibodies in response to either naturally acquired infections or immunizations. Until he matures sufficiently to develop active immunity, precautions should be taken to protect him from infection. During the last months of pregnancy, certain antibodies the mother has developed are transferred, via the placenta, to the infant. This passive immunity offers temporary protection against a few infectious organisms. Other measures are needed to safeguard his well-being, including sterilization of formula, good physical hygiene and cleanliness, and isolation from persons with known infections.

Rest

The first month of life is characterized by a rapid rate of growth. The amount of sleep required decreases as the growth rate decreases and age increases. Sufficient opportunity should be provided for activity, for stretching new muscles, and for experiencing the world; however, for each hour of wakefulness the newborn requires approximately 2 hours of sleep.

Environmental sounds seem to have little disturbing effect on the newborn's sleep. In the nursery, he often sleeps while the infant next to him cries quite loudly. At first he sleeps day and night, waking for feedings and little else. Toward the end of the first month the intervals between awakenings during the night become longer, and a somewhat higher percentage of time is spent in sleep at night than during the daytime.

Awakening the infant for care usually presents no problem since he awakens easily and returns to sleep just as easily if he is comfortable. Part of the "settling in" process when the newborn is introduced into the household is his becoming accustomed to receiving routine care within reasonable intervals and coming to anticipate care by being awake in advance of those times. The newborn who does not sleep well between feedings and is fussy or cries for long periods may be hungry or uncomfortable, perhaps due to illness.

Bathing and Dressing

Immediately after birth the body temperature usually drops several degrees, often to as low as 35°C (95°F). A heated crib or incubator may be indicated until the baby's temperature has increased and stabilized within normal limits. In lieu of a heating device, he may be diapered and wrapped securely in soft lightweight blankets and placed in a warm room. It is often advisable to delay exposing large portions of the newborn's body for cleansing until his temperature has stabilized.

Although bathing becomes part of the daily routine for many babies, a sponge bath may be substituted from time to time in place of the regular bath. Because the newborn's body has a large surface area in proportion to his size, heat loss is rapid and precautions should be taken to prevent chilling during the bath. If the temperature of the room is between 23.9 and 26.7°C (75 and 80°F), bath time provides an opportunity for him to be free from the encumbrance and restraint of clothing and permits him to stretch and exercise underdeveloped muscles. Care should be taken to cleanse the deep creases and skin folds of the neck and groin with mild soap and water. Care should also be taken to dry these areas and then expose them to air as much as possible to prevent the development of intertrigo. A complete tub bath can be given as soon as the umbilicus has healed. There is suggestive evidence that hexachlorophene soap may cause brain damage in newborns, and its routine use is no longer advisable.

If the room temperature is comfortably warm, very little clothing is needed. Because newborns have poor circulation to their extremities, their hands and feet will often feel cool to the touch. However, adding clothing seldom remedies this situation. Feeling the nape of the neck with the back of the hand is a better method of judging the infant's relative warmth. Clothing should be selected that will permit the infant freedom of movement and that will be easy to put on and take off.

REFERENCES

1 E. Erikson, *Childhood and Society*, W. W. Norton & Company, Inc., New York, 1950.
2 R. R. Sears, E. E. Maccoby, and H. Levin, *Patterns of Child Rearing*, Row, Peterson & Company, Evanston, Ill., 1957.
3 J. H. S. Bossard, and E. S. Boll, *The Large Family System: An Original Study in the Sociology of Family Behavior*, University of Pennsylvania Press, Philadelphia, 1956, p. 77.
4 L. K. Frank, "Tactile Communication," *Genetic Psychological Monograph*, 56:209–225, 1957.
5 A. I. Bronstein and E. P. Petrova, "The Auditory Analyzer in Young Infants," in Y. Brackbill and G. G. Thompson (eds.), *Behavior in Infancy and Early Childhood*, The Free Press, New York, 1967, pp. 163–172.
6 M. L. Simner and B. Reilly, "Response of the Newborn Infant to the Cry of Another Infant," paper presented at the Meeting of the Society for Research in Child Development, March 28, 1969.
7 M. Wertheimer, "Psychomotor Coordination of Auditory and Visual Perception at Birth," *Science*, 134:1962, 1961.
8 A. S. Leventhal and L. P. Lipsitt, "Adaptation, Pitch Discrimination, and Sound Localization in the Neonate," *Child Development*, 35:759–767, 1964.
9 Anneliese Korner and Evelyn Thomas, "The Relative Efficacy of Contact and Vestibular-Proprioceptive Stimulation in Soothing Neonates," *Child Development*, 43:443–453, 1972.
10 L. P. Lipsitt and N. Levy, "Electrotactual Threshold in the Neonate," *Child Development*, 30:547–554, 1959.
11 L. B. Roach, "Skin Changes in Dark Skin," *Nursing '72*, 2:22, 1972.
12 R. Nisbett and S. Gurwitz, "Weight, Sex, and the Eating Behavior of Human Newborns," *Journal of Comparative and Physiological Psychology*, 73:245–253, 1970.
13 M. Elder, "The Effects of Temperature and Position on the Sucking Pressure of Newborn Infants," *Child Development*, 41:95–102, 1970.

10

THE INFANT— 1 TO 12 MONTHS

BARBARA J. CLANCY and JEANNE SCHOTT

PARENTING

The transition to parenthood is, at least for many persons in our society, more difficult than the adjustment to marriage or an occupation. Many adults have attended classes preparing them for marriage, and no one is expected to perform a work role without training. However, the majority have no formal education for parenting. The parent role, furthermore, requires continual modification as the child's development proceeds, so that parenting behaviors inevitably become obsolete rather quickly. Even the most successful parenting skills must eventually be relinquished as the child changes. Because of the rapid developmental progressions that characterize the infant's first year of life, parents are called upon to learn quickly and then discard a variety of parenting behaviors during the 11-month period discussed in this chapter.

It has been said that it takes 3 months for a new mother to establish a feeling of commitment to her infant.[1] A woman's need to mother is relative to the several other aspects of her life patterns, while an infant's need to be mothered cannot be compromised if he is to develop successfully. Mothering depends on significant past interpersonal experiences as well as on personal values concerning child rearing (see Chap. 8). The mother's development of narcissism during pregnancy and the early postpartum period increases her ability to be nurturant.[2] The early tasks of motherhood, according to Rubin[2] and Spaulding,[3] consist of identifying the new child as her own, defining her relationship to the child, altering her style of living, reconstructing the family constellation, assuming responsibility for the baby's care, learning to anticipate the infant's needs, and learning to regulate the infant's demands.

It may be difficult for a woman to express motherliness until her mate has adjusted to fatherhood.[4] Fathers need to be aware of the infant's developmental changes and the consequent changes that can be expected in family living. It may be difficult for a father to establish a relationship to the infant and hence to exhibit fatherliness until the child freely responds to stimulation, such as, for example, smiling and lifting his arms to be picked up by the father. Rubin[1] says feelings of fatherliness are usually established by the time the baby is 6 months old. Because of the changing roles of parents, fathering tasks currently include feeding, diapering, and cuddling. The father's involvement in these caretaking activities for infants younger than 6 months can enhance his feeling of commitment earlier than this time. In the past it may have been considered unmasculine for a father to participate in child care; however, presently both parents are encouraged to regard pregnancy and child-rearing experiences as mutual responsibilities. It is true that the infant is socially rather passive for several months, but a mature parent does not need continual gratification and reinforcement from the child. Satisfaction is received by meeting the needs of this dependent human being.

Although parenthood is considered a normal developmental phase, the required adjustments can still create a crisis. The transition to parenthood may be painful because of the reorganization of a two-person pattern of interaction into a three-person system. No longer are the father and mother always able to sit and have a quiet conversation. The pressure experienced by the new father may be increased because of added financial responsibility and his wife's additional need for him to help with household tasks. Eating and sleeping patterns may be altered along with the other changes in life-style. The father and mother may find little time for their own personal growth while adjusting to a new baby. But the media have romanticized the role of parenthood. It is easy to see why new parents wonder whether something is wrong when the arrival of a newborn causes a crisis in the family. Anticipatory guidance regarding family adjustments to the new baby is part of the nurse's role during pregnancy and throughout the first several months after the birth. The crisis of parenting can be lessened if the parents are made aware of changes that will be required and how they may react.

Adjustment to a new baby in the family is almost always somewhat difficult for siblings. No matter what their age or prior preparation, the other children will have their patterns of living disrupted by the baby. The adjustments required of siblings, like those parents must make, change at intervals throughout the baby's first year, so that the birth of a new child creates a recurrent crisis for them. Parents frequently find that the jealousies and regressions of their older children add to the stresses of caring for the new baby. On the other hand, siblings also commonly respond to the new baby with interest, protectiveness, and affection (see Fig. 10-1). Nursing guidance in helping parents incorporate children in the preparations for the infant and in the provision of his care can be extremely helpful to all the family.

New mothers sometimes complain of chronic tiredness and the loss of social contacts because of confinement to the house during the first year of the infant's life. They may have an idea of a perfect mother and feel guilty because they do not meet these expectations. New mothers are torn between a need for dependence on the one hand and a desire for independence and responsibility on the other. Mothers may also feel frustration because they think they are neglecting other members of the family. Mothers with professional education or experience may suffer more extensive or severe crisis in adjustment to motherhood than women who have not had a career that was important to them. There is no doubt that giving up a significant career and assuming the role of a mother can be traumatic. Again, guilt feelings may come to the surface.

The crisis of parenthood may alter previous sexual adjustment. The husband may feel that his wife is a less enthusiastic sexual partner because she is fatigued or distracted by the baby's requirements. Libido in either or both persons may be decreased because of fear of another pregnancy. Marital discord may arise if the husband, feeling tied down by his new family, seeks recreation outside the home while the wife feels unable or unwilling to go and yet is resentful about being left at home. All these factors can cause disenchantment with the sexual relationship.

Even in families which are well prepared for the birth of a baby, stress and ambivalence are to be expected as the family system adapts and continually readjusts to the infant's presence. The grief work associated with giving up a previous role is necessary and becomes a catalyst for taking on new roles.[5, 6] Parents need to know that feeling ambivalent about the parental role is common and natural.

SECOND AND THIRD MONTHS

The young infant is completely dependent upon his environment, with crying almost his only means of communication. He is awake more than during the neonatal period and shows increased interest in a variety of sights and sounds. As babies begin to exhibit increased awareness, they need and seek stimulation. They enjoy having people around and fuss if left alone. The type and amount of stimulation must be carefully considered. Infants need routine and continuity in their lives. Sudden changes or extensive alterations in daily activities can exert a damaging effect on the infant's development. Development of the child comes about by living. The child is always becoming and never "is" in the finished sense of the word. Habits are formed by repetitive use of reflexes combined with neurologic and physical maturation. Infants are more content when a

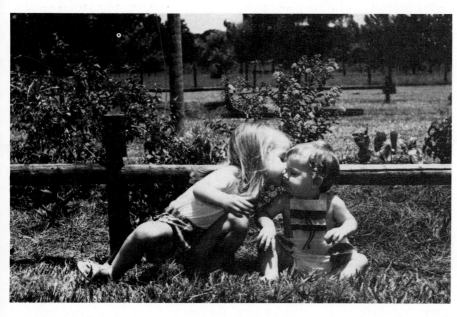

Figure 10-1 Having a sibling within a few years of his own age is a profoundly stimulating, developmentally enriching experience for each member of the relationship.

pattern is established early. Whereas the first stage of cognitive development is based solely on the use of reflexes, during the second and third months the reflexive behavior slowly begins to be replaced by voluntary movements. Neurologic maturity must reach a certain stage before an infant can comprehend his own sensations.[7]

Young infants have a great need to be touched. Touch is perhaps as important to the young infant as food. Infants who have not experienced adequate tactile stimulation frequently do not thrive. Bathing, diapering, and feeding times are opportunities for this needed body contact. Propping the bottle and leaving the small infant alone is unsafe because it predisposes to aspiration, but it is also developmentally hazardous because it deprives him of the experience, including but not limited to tactile stimulation, which he would receive if held for feedings. In addition, the practice of bottle propping prolongs the child's attachment to his bottle, since it has been his sole source of gratification.

By the second month, the baby begins to show that he anticipates being fed when he is placed in his customary feeding position. He eats at approximately 4-hour intervals and may still require one or two night feedings. Some physicians advocate starting cereals or fruit, or both, in the second month in order to eliminate the night feeding. The infant enjoys sucking and frequently places his whole hand in his mouth indicating hunger or sheer enjoyment. Finger sucking is common among infants and does not indicate a lack of mothering. Infants vary in their need to suck, and some breast-fed babies nurse long after the breast is empty. Bottle-fed babies who have an increased need for sucking may have a fluid intake that exceeds their nutritional requirements. These infants may legitimately need a pacifier to satisfy their desire for sucking.

By the third month, motor coordination is developed to the extent that the baby can purposefully get his hand to his mouth. At this time the infant can satisfy his own sucking needs and a pacifier is no longer needed. If foods besides milk have not been introduced earlier, they are usually started at this time. Solid foods should be introduced one at a time at intervals of at least a week (see Chap. 15 for details about infant feeding). This schedule helps the child acquire a taste for new foods and allows identification of foods which may produce allergies, since many allergic reactions take several days to develop. Infants who become allergic to foods usually do so by 6 months of age. If an infant balks at new foods, it is probably because of the difference in texture rather than the taste. The infant knows how to swallow liquid; solid texture, however, presents a new challenge. While he is learning how to swallow solids, it may appear that he is spitting the food out of his mouth (the extrusion reflex). In reality he is learning how to manipulate his tongue in the act of swallowing. Spitting up after feeding may occur until the child is able to sustain an upright position. Spitting up an ounce or so is normal, but if the regurgitation is projectile, a physician should be notified.

Between 2 and 3 months of age the infant becomes able to hold his head erect. He can focus his eyes on a bright object and follow a moving person or an object with his eyes. If he loses sight of an object he does not look for it; he does not have the concept of object permanence[8, 9] (see discussion of Piagetian theory in Chap. 7). Each time the mother comes into the infant's room, she is a new mother. The blinking reflex is present: the baby closes his eyes when an object approaches them rapidly. Accommodation of the lens of the eye is essentially mature by the age of 3 months, allowing eye convergence as an object approaches the infant's face.[10]

In the second month the infant who is active may roll over. By 3 months, the baby indicates a preference for the prone or supine position. If he lies prone, he will make crawling movements with his legs and arch his back, holding his head high (Fig. 10-2).

Because the infant engages in clutching and scratching movements, cutting his fingernails is a necessity. Some parents may wish to cover the hands with mittens; however, this practice diminishes the child's tactile exploration.

The baby seems to enjoy being held or propped in a sitting position for a few minutes. Until the child is about 3 months old, his neck muscles are not sufficiently controlled to prevent his head from falling backward when lifted from a lying position or to keep the head from wobbling while he is upright.

Early in the third month, the infant begins to reach out to the sides of his body. This activity is necessary before reaching forward is accomplished. He is unable to open his fingers to grasp an object but will strike an object in an attempt to do this. He watches his own hand as if it were an entertaining object.

Infants acquire a preference for a sleeping position as early as 2 months, and some may indicate a preference from birth. By 3 months, the infant has an established routine that precedes sleeping. This routine may include finding a comfortable position, sucking on fingers or a toy, listening to music, and crying.

The 2- and 3-month-old stops crying when someone enters the room or caresses him. The neonate's crying is usually tearless, but by the second month the tear-forming structures have matured enough to produce tears. By the third month, because of the infant's increased awareness of his environment and ability to interact with it, he has less need to cry. Crying still fulfills an important need for the infant, however. It enhances lung expansion and provides a means of exercise which increases the circulation. The mother must distinguish between crying that denotes pain, illness, or other distress requiring attention and crying that is necessary for physiologic well-being.

At 2 months the social smile begins. This is usually a delight to the family members. At this time the infant begins to pay more attention to stimuli that are different from those he usually encounters.[11] Infants who have been stimulated by hearing the human voice early in life may begin to vocalize in response. These early attempts at verbalization may be spontaneous as well as in response to siblings and adult members of the family. Infants with older siblings frequently begin vocalizing earlier than firstborn children. Around 2 months of age babies begin to squeal with delight when stimulated by touching, talking, singing, and roughhousing. Fathers are likely to interact more with the baby now that it is more responsive than previously.

Reaching can be encouraged by offering safe play objects. Rattles and mobiles provide auditory and visual stimulation. Research indicates that babies who are permitted to set a mobile in motion voluntarily persevere at that activity and that they learn at the early age of 2 months that they can make a change in their environment.[12] Repetitiveness is common during play activities and is necessary for learning. During their feeding infants enjoy playing and are usually good-tempered and receptive during this pleasurable time. Playfulness during feedings may be annoying to mothers but seems necessary for the development of social skills associated with eating.

FOURTH, FIFTH, AND SIXTH MONTHS

Uncoordinated movements of the hand and arm begin to progress to definite reaching and grasping. The infant spreads his fingers to grasp, but it will be several months before he will be able to coordinate his thumb for good hand control. Although the infant can pick up an object by around 4 months of age, he cannot intentionally release it until about the sixth month. The fourth month begins the age of exploration with eyes, fingers, hands, and mouth. Since everything the baby touches goes into his mouth, care should be taken to provide a safe environment. By 6 months he is reaching for everything in sight. He not only grasps but can hold and manipulate objects. His hands appear coordinated in the way he handles objects.

Intentional rolling over may appear earlier but is definitely to be expected during the fourth month. The baby now holds his head up (rather than letting

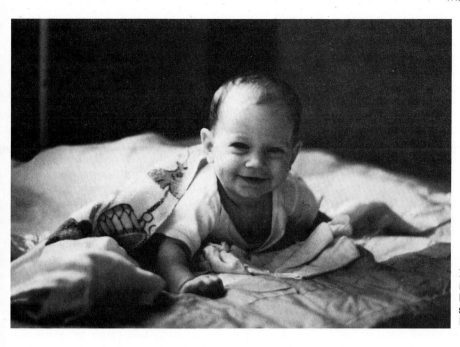

Figure 10-2 This child at 2 months actively interacts with her environment by raising up, smiling, vocalizing, and following people with her eyes.

his neck hyperextend) when he is pulled to a sitting position, and when held or propped in a sitting position he holds his head steady. Positioning the infant upright increases his perspective of the environment, since he is able to view his world in three dimensions. Although he can see more, the infant is believed to perceive and conceptualize his environment as simply a series of images appearing at random.[8, 9]

When being pulled to a sitting position at 4 months of age, the child may attempt to stand. This is a reflex response rather than an intentional movement. By the fifth month, the infant is able to sit for longer periods of time if well supported on pillows or in a baby seat. When his head rolls to the side and his body slumps, he needs to be placed in another position. At 6 months, the infant supports most of his weight on his hands rather than his forearms when lying in the prone position. He may begin creeping, or moving along with his abdomen on the floor. Creeping is a precursor to crawling, which requires the infant to support his weight on his hands and knees. The flexion motion of the legs is often stronger than the extension force at this time, which causes some infants to creep backward before attaining a forward motion. When rolling over, the baby may accidentally sit upright; however, intentional sitting does not occur until later. Toward the end of the sixth month, an infant may stand with little support.

Although the teeth usually erupt after the sixth month, the signs of teething may begin around the fourth or fifth month. Chewing on objects, especially cold things, may reduce the swelling of the gums. Rubbing the gums may also relieve discomfort.

A 4- to 6-month-old infant may go 4 or 5 hours between feedings. In the fifth month he may eat his meals with the family because he usually is able to tolerate being fed just three meals a day. His appetite may decrease due to his heightened interest in the environment and in practicing his developing motor activity. His weight gain, which has been rapid until this time (babies generally double their birth weight by 5 months), may decline. Eating less than previously and gaining less are normal during periods of preoccupation with new interests and developing skills. When a baby begins to hold his own bottle, it is a good time to initiate cup feeding. Cups that prevent spilling are recommended until the child is able to coordinate the cup in an upright position. At this stage he may be given a spoon or finger foods (but not a fork, since his hand and arm movements are still primitive and a fork presents a danger to the baby's eyes) to occupy his hands so he doesn't interfere with the feeding process. Later, he may imitate his mother's feeding gestures with his own utensils. The usual age for weaning is between 5 and 6 months. This may be a difficult time for both mother and infant. Weaning should be gradually accomplished over several weeks to allow for physiologic and emotional transition.

Around 4 months, the baby's sleep habits begin

to settle into a pattern which includes defined nap times during the day. Most infants of 4 or 5 months sleep through the night without awakening for feeding. Although they may awaken early in the morning, demanding attention, the early waking does not usually bother parents because they are happy to be able to sleep through the night. During waking periods the infant is content to stay alone for short intervals, permitting the mother to conduct her household tasks with few interruptions and to have additional time to enjoy the infant. The baby shows increased awareness of himself by the sixth month. He enjoys looking at himself in the mirror. This visual stimulation promotes his beginning awareness that he is an individual and distinct from the total environment. According to Piaget, the child's efforts are geared toward making events last or creating a sense of permanency. This is the child's first real acknowledgment of environmental objects and events.[7]

Around the fourth month, the baby's breathing and mouth activity begin to be coordinated in relation to his vocal cords. Breathing and sucking movements are used in beginning word formation.[13] Later, the infant vocalizes to anyone who will listen to him. He observes and imitates the facial expressions and sounds of people interacting with him. He may accidentally respond with "mama" and "dada," to the delight of the parents, and elicit positive reinforcement. He learns that repetition will continue to produce a positive response. At this time he is unable to associate the sounds he is making with their meaning. At 6 months, however, it is usual for motor activity to take precedent over vocalization, but the infant does begin to associate meaning with sounds used for mama and dada.

By 4 months of age, an infant begins to use his hands to explore the world around him. Transference of toys from one hand to the other is to be expected at 5 months. The 4- to 6-month-old loves his bath and uses this time to play with floating objects. He may laugh out loud for the first time, which pleases the family. Noisy toys are enjoyed by infants of this age. An infant's attachment for a special toy or object signifies awareness of something other than himself. These treasured objects are the earliest substitute for his previous exclusive attachment to parents and assist the infant with the realities and frustrations of his separations from parents. By 5 months of age, attention span has increased, making it possible for him to play alone for 1 to 2 hours. At 6 months perceptual and cognitive maturity are sufficiently advanced so that the baby responds with attentiveness to novel stimuli; for example, if one of two identical toys is replaced by a nonidentical one, the infant looks more intensely at the new, different toy.[11] Toys need to be within reach so he can touch, examine, and mouth each one.

SEVENTH, EIGHTH, AND NINTH MONTHS

Around the seventh month sufficient strength and coordination of the infant's trunk, arms, and hands are developed to allow him to move purposefully about by creeping. Some infants bounce on their bottoms ("hitch") rather than creep on their elbows and abdomens. They can pull up to a standing position and side-step while holding on to furniture, and later within this age period they can teeter from one leg to another. But they lack the coordination to sit down and must fall backward to sit. By the ninth month, a child is able to stand without holding onto furniture, an accomplishment which he seems to enjoy a great deal. Although this stage of increased mobility can be taxing for parents, it is a necessary stage of development and should not be curtailed by routinely using playpens, bounce chairs, harnesses, and small fenced areas.

The infant now uses both hands with equal importance. He loves to touch things as well as to put objects into his mouth. This latter accomplishment requires vigilance to protect the infant from electric outlets and appliances, sharp objects, and small items that could be aspirated. Safety must be achieved in a manner that does not impinge upon the normal developmental needs of the infant. Safety precautions relevant to infancy are discussed in Chapter 16.

The first teeth that erupt are usually the two lower incisors, followed by the two upper incisors. Babies are usually bothered by the first eruptions and the molars. They may display discomfort by rubbing and pulling on their ears, drooling, being irritable, running a low-grade fever, and showing a decrease in appetite.

Because of the infant's increased coordination and curiosity, he shows an interest in feeding himself. He is able to pick up small pieces of food with finger motions rather than using his entire hand, and finally around 8 months the infant can approximate his thumb and first finger in a pincer grasp. He uses several of his senses—not just taste—while eating. In the process of feeding himself, he smears and throws food on the table or floor or on himself, which can be exasperating for the family. It may seem more practical to feed the infant; however, he usually insists on doing at least part of his own feeding. He may show his determination by turning his head to one side, closing his mouth tightly, and grabbing for the dish and spoon or pushing others away. Every effort should be made to create a congenial atmosphere during mealtime. Force-feeding an infant or preventing him from helping to feed himself may well lay the groundwork for feeding problems in later years.

As an infant is learning about vertical space by getting up and down, he is becoming more aware of the world that surrounds him. This increased awareness may cause fear and insecurity. The baby begins to recognize at this age that his mother is different from others, and he seems to need her presence. He may actually cling to the mother when he is upset or fearful. His exclusive preference for her and his clinging to her can create separation problems for the infant and mother that had not been previously encountered. Later, the child learns to anticipate his mother's return after separation, making short separations endurable. It is wise to warn other persons of a change from the infant's earlier friendly behavior and encourage strangers to approach slowly. Toys and soft objects can also be the recipients of this clinging behavior.

The infant at 7 months smiles and laughs aloud often, responding to stimulation from familiar children and adults (Fig. 10-3). He makes talking sounds in response to others talking to him. He learns much from siblings by trying to imitate their speech and activities. Social behavior should be enhanced by smiling at the baby and engaging in eye-to-eye contact while talking to him. He should not be left alone for long periods of time while awake. Auditory, visual, and tactile stimulation are needed for the development of socialization skills. An infant around 8 or 9 months loves to play social games such as peek-a-boo, patty cake, and give-and-take. These activities apparently never become boring to the infant.

When the child begins to understand the meaning of "no," the parents may effectively begin to discipline him as needed. It is important to be serious and consistent about setting limits. The disciplinary role may be difficult, but parents must learn to feel comfortable in taking a stand even though the infant protests and appears disappointed.

When sitting and bending from the waist is accomplished with ease, the child may become quite interested in his genitals. He can now see as well as feel his genital region. This natural curiosity should be explained to parents.

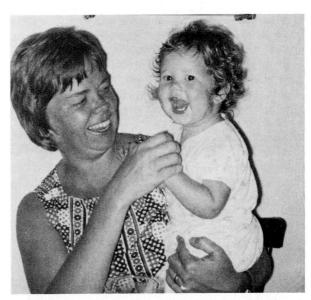

Figure 10-3 Vocalization, and speech and language development which follow it, like most other aspects of infant development, are dependent upon interpersonal interactions.

TENTH, ELEVENTH, AND TWELFTH MONTHS

The infant in the last quarter of his first year is able to side-step while holding on to furniture, or "cruise," fairly rapidly and easily. He learns to stand alone even with much distracting activity around him. He is able to take a few steps while holding on to an adult's hand. The child may begin to toddle by himself toward the end of the first year; however, to get where he needs to go he generally crawls on all fours, since he can accomplish this with speed and ease. As one author aptly stated, "Walking is for pleasure but crawling is the business approach to the world."[14] During initial attempts at walking the child needs to grip the floor with his toes, necessitating soft flexible shoes or bare feet. He experiences a period of increased dependency when he is accomplishing the momentous task of walking. With support and understanding from parents he is able to become more independent.

Hand dominance becomes evident at the end of the first year. There is an increasing use of the dominant hand to explore while the other hand is used to carry objects. This action is seen during feeding and playing.

Now the child may wish to use a spoon while feeding himself, although most of the time he prefers to use his fingers. The spoon is difficult for him to manipulate and often reaches his mouth upside down. Appetite and weight gain are small at this age, frequently causing parents to become concerned; however, this phenomenon is entirely normal, and the child should not be force-fed.[14] He is in perpetual motion and is often too busy to eat. As a rule of thumb, birth weight may be expected to triple by the first birthday.

Some parents may wish to begin toilet training around 10 to 12 months because infants begin to show a regular pattern of bladder and bowel elimination. This active age does not lend itself to the discipline of toilet training. There are more appropriate times during the second year when motor skills are more refined.

As the meaning of "no" becomes more clear, the infant realizes that he can also say "no" and elicit quite a response from his parents. This behavior, an important part of his ego development, can be difficult for parents to deal with. Negativism, including tantrums, may occur. Discipline is ineffective during a tantrum. The child needs patience until he is calm, and someone is there to comfort him. Parents are often afraid to set limits for fear of initiating a display of temper, but adult responsibility, of course, includes putting restrictions on behavior that conflicts with the standards of safety or socialization. An infant needs guidelines and pressure to conform to the family's life-style, including commands and consistent limit setting. For example, practically every older infant resists going to bed; however, for his own physical and emotional well-being plus that of his parents, he must establish a reasonable bedtime.

Toward the end of the first year the infant is able to say a few intelligible words, but generally his vocabulary is not easily understood. Parents should not become concerned about the child's speech pattern at this time; talking is a task to be accomplished during the second year of life and later.

By the time he is 1 year old, the child begins to adopt a sex identification as a result of the reinforcement of the family. A coy tilt of the head may be considered cute for a baby girl, for example, but may not earn the same reward for a boy.

A child experiences his environment through play (Fig. 10-4). He learns to navigate stairways, crawl under tables, and climb on chairs. Through these activities he is improving both motor and learning skills. He enjoys listening to music and trying to sing. Infants usually perform better on tasks they set for themselves. Play in general should be self-directed rather than parent-directed.

According to Piaget, by the end of the first year the infant applies previously learned sensorimotor activities to new situations. The capacity for intelligent reasoning has begun to emerge when the child displays searching behavior for an object that has disappeared.[7] At 12 months of age the infant's attention span is fairly long, suggesting the emergence of a new cognitive process called a *hypothesis*. The child begins to be able to conceptualize an unfamiliar event in terms of its resemblance to a familiar one.[11] Scientists are unsure whether changes in behavior affect a child's later intelligence. Most intelligence tests for children under 2 years of age are really assessments of motor ability, which has not proved to be predictive of later intelligence. One behavior, that of habituation, which is defined as the waning of response to a repeated stimulus, has been shown to predict later intelligence.[15]

SUPPORT SYSTEMS FOR THE FAMILY

Parenthood is becoming an increasingly complex task; however, it remains the greatest domain of the amateur. A parental and child health program offered through official and voluntary health agencies can guide the parents through the child's infancy, fostering healthful relationships and preparing parents for the physical and emotional hazards commonly experienced during the first year. Programs in the past have dealt mainly with the mother and the child rather than the entire family. Recently, some emphasis has been placed on including the entire family in preparation for childbirth and child rearing.

Professional persons in family health education can make significant contributions to improve the ability of adults to adjust to the parenting role. Groups of expectant parents continue to discuss pregnancy, labor, delivery, and the neonatal period. Other types of parent groups need to be formed that are concerned with infant development and parenting roles after the first month of life. Parents tend to discuss infant development informally in their neighborhoods, but recreation centers, for example, could offer organized information and support. Various family development programs can be offered in colleges and through continuing education. Nurses can be instrumental in sponsoring and presenting such programs.

Federal, state, and private monies must be obtained to improve and enlarge day care centers. Presently more mothers are working than in the past.

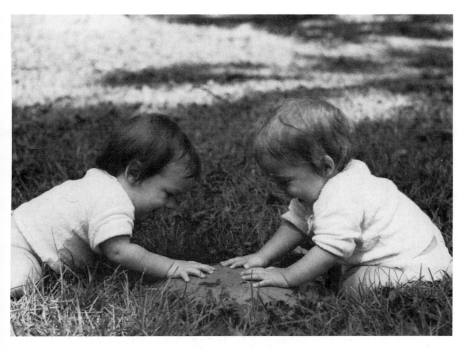

Figure 10-4 Exploratory involvement with the physical and social environments and with one's own self in relationship to them is well under way before the end of infancy.

Care for these women's infants must be more than custodial, and emphasis should be given to behavioral as well as physical needs.

In order to meet the needs of our society, patterns of health care delivery and child care will be changing. Collaborative planning by multidisciplinary providers of the care and by the lay consumers of services will be required. Nurses have a major role to play in the planning and provision of comprehensive services for young families. The role of family health care workers, such as the family nurse practitioner and clinician, will be mainly the maintenance and promotion of health rather than health teaching related to illness alone.

REFERENCES

1 R. Rubin, "Maternal Touch," *Nursing Outlook*, 11:828–831, 1963.
2 R. Rubin, "Cognitive Style in Pregnancy," *American Journal of Nursing*, 70:502–505, 1970.
3 M. R. Spaulding, "The Effectiveness of Tape Recordings with Primiparas of the Lower Socioeconomic Group in Coping with Mothering Tasks," in M. V. Batey (ed.), *Communicating Nursing Research*, Western Interstate Commission for Higher Education, Boulder, Colo., 1968, pp. 107–118.
4 P. Robischon and D. Scott, "Role Theory and Its Application in Family Nursing," *Nursing Outlook*, 17:52–57, 1969.
5 R. Rubin, "Attainment of the Maternal Role: Part I," *Nursing Research*, 16:237–245, 1967.
6 R. Rubin, "Attainment of the Maternal Role: Part II," *Nursing Research*, 16:342–346, 1967.
7 H. W. Maier, *Three Theories of Child Development*, Harper & Row, Publishers, Incorporated, New York, 1965.
8 H. Ginsburg and S. Opper, *Piaget's Theory of Intellectual Development: An Introduction*, Prentice-Hall, Inc., Englewood Cliffs, N.J., 1969.
9 J. Piaget, *The Construction of Reality in the Child* (trans. by M. Cook), Basic Books, Inc., New York, 1954.
10 L. J. Stone and J. Church, *Childhood and Adolescence*, Random House, Inc., New York, 1968.
11 J. Kagan, "Do Infants Think?" *Scientific American*, 226:74–82, March 1972.
12 J. Kagan and H. Moss, *Birth to Maturity: A Study in Psychological Development*, John Wiley & Sons, Inc., 1962.
13 M. Ribble, *The Rights of Infants*, Columbia University Press, New York, 1965.
14 T. B. Brazelton, *Infants and Mothers: Differences in Development*, Delacorte Press, Dell Publishing Co., Inc., New York, 1972.
15 W. H. Bridger, "Sensory Habituation and Discrimination in the Human Neonate," *American Journal of Psychiatry*, 117:991–996, 1961.

11

THE TODDLER— 1 TO 3 YEARS

ISOBEL H. THORP

The word *toddler* evokes various responses from different people. The parent who is currently attempting to rear one might describe a toddler as unpredictable, hectic, terrible, negative, or even angelic at times. The toddler's philosophy of life seems to be that holes need to be filled up; everything needs to be touched, tasted, and manipulated; no one except his mother is to be trusted; nothing should be agreed to; and displeasure should be shown often and loudly. These descriptions draw a composite picture of the toddler.

Descriptive and familiar as this picture may be, however, it is superficial and leaves the toddler more a puzzle than an understandable, developmentally rational little being. The nurse who understands the development of the young child not only finds his behavior predictable but also has a base from which to relate effectively to the child and his parents.

During the approximately 2 years ascribed to this age group, the young child has a number of developmental tasks to attempt and master. Built upon the successful attainment of earlier developmental tasks, the new ones reflect his widening environment, physical maturing, more complex quality of thinking, and growing ability to communicate verbally and nonverbally. The examination and analysis in this chapter of multiple factors contributing to the attainment of the age-typical developmental tasks should lead to a better understanding of the toddler.

DEVELOPMENTAL TASKS

Major developmental tasks for the child in the second and third years of life are:

1 To differentiate himself from other people and things
2 To tolerate separation from his mother
3 To control socially unacceptable emotional impulses
4 To learn the sex-role distinctions prescribed by his family's culture group
5 To reach a more mature, stable physiologic state
6 To become enculturated

A discussion of each of these tasks follows. It should be understood that, as is usually true of developmental tasks, most or all of these six actually arise before and are continued beyond this age period.

Self-Differentiation

Since the toddler is walking, his environment is increasingly accessible to him, and he is developmentally driven to explore it and involve himself with it (Fig. 11-1). Is it any wonder that the toddler is per-

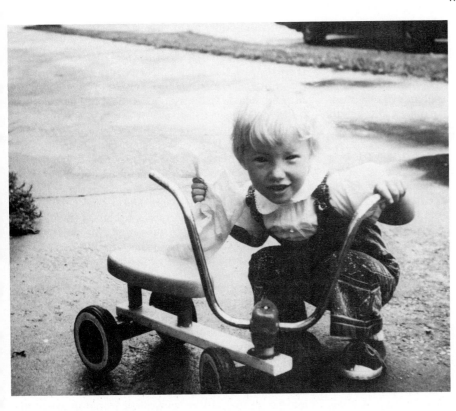

Figure 11-1 The toddler's natural curiosity and assertiveness, combined with his growing physical abilities, lead him to interact expansively with his environment.

petually in trouble as he investigates this new world about which he is so curious but understands so little? In order to differentiate himself from other people and things, he must develop his perception of objects and must test things from all angles for shape, size, weight, texture, color, function, spatial relationship, and interaction with self. Having discovered an object and identified its shape, weight, texture, and other qualities, he must *reexamine* it often within a short period in order to remember it and establish his relationship to it. Depending upon whether it is a "no" object or a "yes" object, he goes back frequently to reexplore it, or he weighs the "no" within the communication system he has established with his mother. If it is a prohibited item, he may observe it, check to see whether his mother is watching, and then touch it. Only when he can categorize many similar objects with similar relationships to himself is he free from his need to test and retest at every opportunity.

An example of this process is the ever-present electric wall outlet. Shortly after becoming mobile, the young child discovers the electric outlet in the main activity room. He looks, touches, traces the shape, and puts his finger to the holes. His mother sees his exploration, it is hoped, emphatically says, "No, no," and slaps his hand. This has been her past action for prohibiting an activity, and he expects and comprehends it. Perhaps his mother does not observe his activity, and he gets an electric shock. The pain may act as a prohibiting agent for that one electric outlet, but it also may not. One contact, whether pleasurable or painful, does not establish a memory pattern concerning size, shape, and relation to self. So he must try again. Perhaps he will test to see whether his mother really means no. After several reenactments he looks at the socket, looks at his mother, and says "no" himself. She reinforces his response and rewards him for having learned.

Now the toddler finds himself in another room with electric outlets differing very little in all qualities from the first. There is neither memory of these new sockets nor recognition of their similarity to the one he has experienced. He must go through the same process of testing both object and response. Having already learned about the other room's electric outlet, he will learn the same things about the new one in a shorter period of testing, if responses are consistent. He builds upon the developing memory scheme. Now he identifies the two outlets as having similarities to one another and a consistent relationship to him.

Many more may have to be tested before the child finally categorizes electric outlets easily and before he can overcome the spatial requirement of being able to recognize them only in one location. This categorization can occur as early as 18 months or maybe as late as 3½ years, depending upon consistency of response, number of chances to encounter the object, and length of encounters. The process is repeated for all objects.

The foregoing examination of the toddler's learning about his environment suggests some guidelines that adults can use to enhance his learning. Playing with a small number of objects over an extended period enables the child to retest his knowledge and perceptions. Providing objects with similarities and differences helps him learn discrimination and categorization which will assist his subsequent interactions with other items. Large objects with moving parts that he can successfully manipulate even with his immature motor and perceptual skills offer him maximal learning opportunities with minimal frustration.

Associated with the task of differentiating self from not-self, the young child attempts to develop a matrix of behavioral cues to assist him in viewing himself in relation to others. Since his family is the proving ground for most of this learning, it is usually his mother and father who must confront and modify the interpersonal manipulation the child exhibits.

Laura, 2½ years old, has well-established cues from her parents which indicate their approval or disapproval of her behavior. Her mother smiles, verbally encourages, and fondly touches when giving approval; her father echoes the same cues and frequently enhances them with an embrace. Disapproval is shown first with a negative word and shaking the index finger and head, increases with a slap on the hand, and eventuates in the ultimate punishment of a spanking given by her mother.

Laura has found that her mother responds with great approval when Laura puts her face up, opens her arms, and says, "Kiss, Mommy!" Her father responds to a beguiling smile and, as an extreme measure, offering him his slippers. Laura has been encouraged to become part of the family interaction and has just recently been permitted to climb onto a chair by the sink in order to help with the washing of dishes.

The stage is set. Her father has been cleaning his shoes with liquid shoe polish and has left the bottle on the sink. Laura, having had approval previously, moves her chair to the sink, removes the bottle, and proceeds to polish the kitchen floor, her clothing,

shoes, and body a lovely black. Her mother discovers the activity at this time.

The loud shout, accompanied by the mother's rush toward the scene, clearly tells Laura this is a disapproved situation. She begins to cry before the now-expected spanking. After sobbing for a short period, she turns to her mother, who is attempting to repair the damage, opens her arms, smiles, and says, "Kiss, Mommy!" Her mother, still angry, ignores the request. Laura then goes to her father and smiles through her tears but still gets no encouragement. Sobbing sporadically, she next appears at her father's side with slippers in hand, smile on face, and one plaintive sob. Her father gives up all efforts at sternness and gathers her into his arms. She settles down on his lap and commands his attention while her mother reminds him of his role in disciplining Laura.

Parents of toddlers relate unending tales of their children testing and manipulating them to the point of exhaustion. The toddler is exploring the cues exhibited by his parents in order to obtain guidelines for subsequent action. Since a parent's tolerance is affected by many variables not evident to the young child, the retesting must continue until the child can establish a parent-cue frame of reference. In his interpersonal setting, as well as in his physical environment, only by *doing* will the child ultimately learn successful behavior.

Separation from Mother

Becoming able to tolerate physical distance from his mother is a direct outgrowth of the toddler's seeing himself as separate from others. The very core of his life experience has been the physical presence of his most significant person (Fig. 11-2). His sense of control (an important aspect of autonomy) depends upon that person's response to his symbolic language in a way which is predictable for both partners of the interaction. He first tolerates separation by allowing his mother to be out of sight, but initially he wants to feel that he can recall her with his signal. As he gains the age-typical need to explore and strike out on his own, he voluntarily leaves his mother for short periods but runs to find her at intervals. It is interesting to note that he evidently feels it's all right for him to leave her at will, but he protests with screams of anguish when he does not find his mother in her expected place.

As he becomes adjusted to not seeing and interacting with the significant person for progressively longer intervals, a gradual transition occurs. The

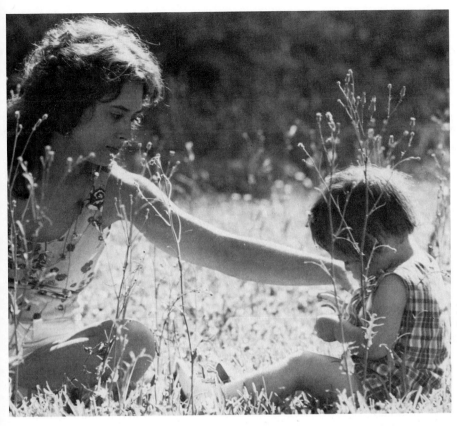

Figure 11-2 The toddler wants and benefits from a continuing relationship with his mother, but he becomes able to do without her for periods of time and to extend that relationship to include other adults in her place. *(Photo courtesy of George Lazar.)*

toddler's need for his mother's actual presence diminishes, and he gains reassurance instead from *symbols* of her and of her love. The symbols are usually those that have been important in the mother-child relationship. Now they become acceptable forms of reinforcement when offered to him by other people. The symbols may consist of a smile, affectionate body contact, and verbal endearments, although they vary between cultures and individual families. "Good boy" or "big girl" from one mother may have the same meaning as a fond "you're a mess" or "you're so bad" from another.

Nurses and others working with toddlers can help a child tolerate his mother's absence if they ascertain from the mother the particular symbolic language which has developed between the two. The child fears loss of love as much as loss of the love object. Another person utilizing the individual child's symbolic language can communicate love, thus reducing the anxiety of love-object loss.

The toddler responds to new love symbols if they are introduced gradually over extended periods, are repeated on several occasions, and *are observed by him to have his mother's approval.* Progress has

been made toward tolerating separation from his mother when the child can be consoled by a symbolic representation of her (for example, her purse, keys, or a piece of jewelry) which indicates that she will return.

Because the degree of separation tolerance depends upon several variables, a wide range of responses is observed in children of all ages. The variables, not necessarily in order of importance, are (1) the degree of intense and satisfying interaction with the mother which has provided a basis for trust, (2) the number and type of separations successfully achieved previously, and (3) the other stresses the child must handle at that time.

Bobby, age 18 months, demonstrates a growing tolerance to separation which is diminished when other stress is increased. Bobby has progressed to permitting his mother to be out of sight and hearing range for periods of 1 or 2 hours while he plays in other parts of the house or in the yard. He has stayed with baby-sitters for several hours without signs of stress.

However, since Bobby's world has grown, he has

recently become afraid of some objects he did not fear previously. His daytime activity extends into his sleep, occasionally producing night terrors, or fearful dreams. He awakens screaming, obviously frightened. He is unable to cope with his fearful dreams while in the dark with no way to get to his mother. His mother or father comes to him, pats him, and soothingly speaks to him. He returns to sleep.

As this reassuring sequence of parental behavior is repeated on several occasions, Bobby eventually needs only to hear his parent call to him from another room to know that mother or father is indeed readily available.

Children develop a variety of behaviors to reassure themselves of their mother's availability. One child may just need to hear her, another may need to see her, and still another may require touch. Under stress a child may need all three forms of contact.

When mother-child separation is anticipated, whether for hospitalization, the mother's employment, or entrance to preschool, there are numerous ways to help the child prepare. Usually by his first birthday the child can participate in peek-a-boo games and other forms of hide-and-seek, always being able to find and thus reclaim the lost object. These games are believed to symbolize the predictable return of the mother. The mother should be encouraged to begin transferring the dependency relationship to another person gradually and for short periods. This transfer is greatly facilitated if the mother spends time together with the substitute when the child is present, both to show the youngster her approval of the new person and to orient the substitute to the symbolic language known to her child. As the toddler accepts the substitute without excessive emotional response, additional persons can be introduced in the substitute role. Mothers must be cautioned not to sneak away while the child is not looking. Leaving without saying good-bye only heightens the child's suspicion that his mother can disappear and increases his need to keep in closer contact at all times for fear of losing her without warning.

Although dependency upon the mother as original love object lasts in some degree for many years and sometimes even into adulthood, developmental readiness to adapt to separation occurs during the toddler stage. When a toddler or older child is observed to have extreme separation anxiety, the causes must be explored. Are other stresses so great that they can be borne only if the mother is present? Has the child had opportunities to identify others as dependable? Has the mother given approval or op-portunity for other relationships to develop? Do the mother's own needs include a dependent young child?

Mastering Emotional Impulses

Gaining control over instinctual emotional responses is a very difficult and complex task for the toddler. Self-control takes years of conscious awareness of self and often is not fully achieved until adulthood. To begin developing self-control, the toddler must first identify his response to a situation as a deliberate behavior of his own making. Second, he must be motivated to emulate the behavior of an acceptable role model. The final stage is a result of the previous two: the child makes conscious efforts to control his own behavior. Success at self-control leads him to incorporate approving adults' positive responses to his behavior into his growing self-concept. Since the toddler period is characterized by a love of doing and a resistance to being done to, the beginning ability to set his own limits and abide by them satisfies his drive toward autonomy and, at the same time, builds self-esteem.

Many variables determine the child's success in mastering impulsive behavior. As he gains mobility but finds that his motor skills limit his ability to successfully manipulate things, almost everything he contacts can produce intense frustration and anger. When he was an infant, his indignant screams usually produced his mother, ready to perform in conformity with his wishes. Now that he is older not all wishes can be granted because of safety considerations or training in socially acceptable behavior. The toddler's immaturity prevents him from using reason or sharing his parents' understanding of the need for restraint. He has limited language skills with which to negotiate or articulate his position. What he *can* do is scream, kick, and shout his protests. When his desires are thwarted, his goal-seeking activity increases. In response, his mother shows disapproval and continues to impose the frustrating restriction. As continued and heightened activity only increase the mother's disapproval, the child experiences conflict between wanting to please his mother and wanting to please himself. Gradually he becomes aware that he perhaps has some control over his own behavior. As this awareness increases, he reverts to the previously developed practice of imitation in order to gain parental approval.

The child observes other family members' behavior which he knows has won approval. His imitation may be rather obvious, hilarious, or inappropriate as he attempts to incorporate action with intense feeling in differing situations. As approval or reward is received for his efforts, he incorporates more and more acceptable behavior into his reaction to his world. The desire and the ability to make his behavior conform to parental expectation are becoming evident, although they are far from being established. Continual testing and the reexperiencing of outcomes are required before the long-awaited socially acceptable behavior becomes reliable.

If the toddler is reinforced for his tantrum behavior in the first stage of identifying his behavior as deliberate and subject to his control, he will continue it, developing an awareness that he can control his family through his behavior. Since his ability to control others is compatible with his developmental drive for assertiveness, he receives pleasure from his successful manipulation through tantrums. This mode of control will be repeated until he finds that it produces an unrewarding response from others.

Concurrent to his tantrum behavior and his learning to distinguish differences within his environment, the toddler may learn that different people or different settings yield different responses to his tantrums. Even though a tantrum at home may get little reaction, he may find that the same stormy behavior is quite effective in controlling people at the store or when there are guests. It does not take him long to learn the value of temper tantrums in selected settings and to use that behavior only where he knows he will receive reinforcement.

The second stage of developing self-control, that of finding a role model for acceptable behavior, centers upon the behavior of other members of the family. Some of the problems associated with role-model selection are due to differing standards of behavior for male and female children, younger and older children, healthy and handicapped children, and so forth. The expectations for toddlers very often exceed their understanding of what is expected as well as their ability to make acceptable modifications in the behavior they observe and try to imitate. Awareness of role distinctions is just beginning for the toddler, and he makes progress by trial and error.

An angry, frustrated toddler in the midst of a tantrum cannot be effectively dealt with by reasoning or threats. Neither is it appropriate to try to terminate a tantrum by promising or providing the desired object or activity (which in any case often does not calm him). Probably the wisest approach is to ignore the behavior, reduce external stimulation, remove any objects which might prove injurious, and supportively reinforce control as it begins to be regained. A toddler in a rage may find his lack of

control and the disapproval it brings him quite a cause for insecurity. He benefits from judicious help to avoid extremely frustrating situations whenever possible, from rewards for visible attempts at self-control, and from the security of knowing that benevolent adults will help him to control his unacceptable behavior and support his efforts toward proper behavior after his temper episode has passed. Acceptable substitute methods of expressing his anger can be helpful—for example, toys for pounding, throwing, and attacking. In the later part of the toddler period the child utilizes dolls and toy animals to imaginatively enact his feelings of frustration and anger. It is helpful to adults to recall that the toddler must encounter frustration innumerable times in order to develop a frame of reference for socialized behavior and that as he becomes more mature and finds better ways of coping, he will be able to build on what he has learned from the experiences of this age period.

Sex-Role Distinctions

During the toddler period the child begins to identify sex roles by observing and emulating the behavior of his two main role models, his mother and father. The little boy is told to act like his father, and the little girl copies her mother in her daily activities. Since there is yet little oedipal competition, this developmental task usually produces few problems for the toddler.

Even very young children perceive sex-role distinctions, and observation of the activity of older toddlers usually discloses characteristic behavior which is identifiable as male or female. The culture of the parents determines their concept of the gender roles, and the young toddler is subjected to the same cultural roles as his parents. Mothers and fathers subtly and overtly introduce their concepts of the differing roles. The family acts differently toward boys than toward girls in preparing them for their social sex roles.

The toddler's recognition of the behavior peculiar to one sex or the other extends beyond task-oriented behavior and includes walking, talking, posturing, and temper control. In the later part of the toddler period, when play involves fantasy and acting-out behavior, it becomes obvious that the young child has assimilated much more about both sex roles than has been intentionally taught. It is not unusual to find children playing out both roles interchangeably with embellishments and accuracy.

An important factor in the toddler's learning his designated sex role is the agreement of both parents upon the role behavior. A child who must play one sex role with his mother and a different role with his father has a more complex and difficult task than if both parents agreed. When the parents' expectations of the child's behavior are contradictory, the toddler's confusion can be very burdensome indeed.

Somewhat different problems are encountered when one parent is absent and the toddler has no opportunity to observe differentiation of sex roles. Even in intact families, boys frequently have some degree of difficulty because they are in greater contact with the female role model than with older males and therefore have fewer opportunities to observe and replicate whatever constitutes "masculine" behavior in their culture. Animosity between parents, even when both are living in the home, sometimes prompts derogation of behavior which exemplifies the opposite sex. The young boy then sees himself as bad because he is like his father, and the young girl foresees no pleasure in being like her mother.

As counselors working with parents of toddlers, nurses must be aware of the wide variations among families of acceptable gender behavior. Some parents need help to see that their toddler has become a proving ground for their own gender-identity crisis.

This discussion has emphasized behavior identified with gender difference, which is not the same as sexual urges or sex organ identification, to be discussed later.

Physiologic Stability

As the toddler develops more physiologic stability, he gains increasing ability to control his own body functions. His development of a positive self-concept depends upon his feeling that he is in charge of himself for most of his activity.

The self-regulated activities which are important at the toddler level are toilet training, eating, sleeping, self-stimulation, and physical manipulative skills (as well as behavior related to intense emotion, which was discussed previously).

Toilet Training Toilet training usually begins between 18 and 24 months, with wide variance among individual children. Examining the mechanism required for effective bowel and bladder control shows that the process of toilet training is complex. First the child must be aware of discomfort after incontinent bowel and bladder emptying. Next, elimination must be identified as the cause of the discomfort. The child must also develop awareness of the characteristic sensations that precede excretion.

Finally he must want to do something about the physical discomfort and (if he has experienced it) the social discomfort of being untrained.

Methods of accomplishing toilet training vary directly with the number of authorities writing about child rearing and the number of mothers whose children have successfully accomplished the task. Most agree on the fundamentals necessary to attempt this training: (1) one or two significant people who are willing and able to devote time and effort to establishing patterns of toileting; (2) a mutual communication system between the child and the significant person; (3) reinforcement for success; and (4) no harsh punishment for failure.

Some difficulties related to toilet training seem to be associated with the child's desire to accomplish the task. It is not that he doesn't want to please his significant person or even prove his ability to control his own functions, but his other interests tend to keep him from reaching the toileting facilities until it is too late. More severe problems exist when the toddler manipulates the mother through over-controlling his body functions, either retaining over prolonged periods or expelling in forbidden places.

As the toddler progresses toward his second birthday, bowel movements become more regular and are preceded by specific, recognizable behavior. The alert mother can predict when her child is about to have a bowel movement and begin the learning sequence by placing him on a potty chair or similar furniture at those times. She becomes trained to pick up her child's cues. Only then can awareness on the child's part follow and develop into the ability to inform his mother of his need to eliminate.

Neuromuscular maturation must be reached prior to accomplishing successful training. Daytime bowel and bladder control usually can be attained by 30 months. Nighttime control is harder to master and can be a problem through the preschool years. Suggestions for reducing bed-wetting include reducing fluid intake after the last meal of the day, extending the quiet period before bedtime, and awakening the child for toileting during the night.

A typical picture is **Alan**, a 2½-year-old who was ready for training at 20 months. His 4-year-old brother has provided an example as well as motivation for Alan to imitate his behavior. Daytime control and training were accomplished easily. However, a typical accident occurred. He was playing in the yard with his brother and a neighbor. In the midst of very verbal and motor activity, Alan grabbed his pants and ran to the back door. The door was closed, and as he frantically manipulated the door knob with one hand, while holding his pants with the other hand, a large stream ran down his leg and formed a puddle. Mother came to the door to let him in and saw the problem. Alan began to cry, but his mother provided assurance, since she realized that he was trying to reach the bathroom when his accident occurred. A quiet change of pants without punishment or recrimination enforced his belief in his own ability to become aware when urgency threatens and enhanced his desire to please and do better next time. At the same time his mother was made aware of his involvement in other important activities and mentally promised to remind him every 2 or 3 hours.

Alan's mother also reports that nighttime control is established about 80 percent of the time. She can predict loss of night control when he eats watermelon before bedtime and when he has had a very exciting or unusual day. At no time is Alan made to wear diapers, even when his mother can predict he will wet his bed.

We can assume that with continued reinforcement Alan will achieve complete control without difficulty or emotional problems within a short period.

Because of the interest and motivation toward bowel and bladder control the toddler demonstrates a curiosity toward his and others' genital organs. Observing and feeling the urinary stream, touching and feeling feces, and touching and manipulating his own genitalia are common in this period. If viewed in relation to his curiosity about all other things, these activities can be placed in perspective as a desire to identify himself in relation to all things and do not seem "dirty" or "nasty." Parents can help a toddler satisfy his tactile and perceptual curiosity by providing simple explanations. They can also offer diversional play activities which involve water, clay, and containment and release themes, thus allowing him to gain understanding of the functions and materials he is interested in without emphasizing any negative connotations.

The nurse responsible for the toddler in the hospital should be aware of the level of training to which the toddler has progressed in order to reinforce his beginning control. The child's vocabulary and timetable can be easily ascertained from the mother in order to continue this ego-strengthening control of body function. The nurse working with well children should be prepared to discuss with parents a variety of methods of toilet training as well as to help the parent understand the toddler's behavior related to beginning and maintaining a training regimen.

Feeding During late infancy and the early toddler years, the child should be encouraged to practice feeding himself with utensils, with additional food being fed simultaneously by the parent. As the child gains proficiency in coordinating pronation of the forearm with wrist and hand movement, he demands to assume an increased responsibility for feeding himself. He begins to reject any offer of assistance and refuses to swallow anything fed to him. His insistence upon independence can cause each mealtime to become a battleground. The mother is sure her child will starve, and the child is equally sure that he will feed himself. A fact which is often reassuring to parents is that toddlers require relatively less food than they did as infants. The infant, as can be pointed out to parents, grows at such a rate that he usually at least triples his weight in the first year of life. The toddler's decreased rate of growth requires that he eat less, in proportion to his size, than the parent may have become accustomed to during infancy. If parents are concerned, however, suggestions for increasing the toddler's food intake include freedom for self-feeding and the provision of sandwiches and other "finger foods" which can be eaten "on the run," which is the toddler's usual activity state. Unless a physical or emotional disorder exists, the toddler will eat when hungry and when he can feed himself. Chapter 15 deals in greater detail with the nutritional requirements and eating patterns of toddlers.

Sleep During the toddler period, sleep and rest patterns change. Sleep requirements diminish to 10 to 14 hours daily. The need for a midmorning nap decreases, although an afternoon nap continues to be necessary for a majority of young children. Nap and sleep patterns more nearly coincide with family living patterns.

Since going to sleep requires a certain amount of acquiescence by the child, bedtime frequently becomes a setting for proving autonomy. The toddler cries and screams in rejection of being put to bed. He seems to say, "There is not enough time, there is too much to do, and I want to stay here where the fun is." Parents complain that toddlers fight sleep, become irritable, cranky, and horrible to live with, and still will not go to sleep.

Putting a toddler to bed does not guarantee that he will fall asleep. During the toddler period it is also easier to put him in bed than to keep him there. As the toddler gains proficiency in climbing and falls out of bed a few times, parents usually find some method of permitting the child to get in and out of bed with less danger of falling. This maneuver results in fewer falls but precipitates other problems. The toddler has a seemingly endless capacity to get into dangerous or destructive activities when unsupervised. His propensity to awaken early and get out of bed while the rest of the family is still asleep is a major safety hazard and annoyance.

Several things may combine to produce the "no sleep" syndrome. Although the child has set patterns, he is not always sleepy when relegated to bed. There may be excessive stimulation at bedtime which requires the child to spend additional time exploring or interacting or quieting down from these activities. Refusing to go to sleep may be the child's method of demonstrating his desire to control himself through his body's activities.

When a parent requests guidance from a nurse to help develop workable sleeping patterns for a toddler, the nurse must first find out what sleep and activity schedules are currently being used. Perhaps the awakening hour is unrealistically early or late, and perhaps household activity interferes with the child's bedtime. The entire activity schedule should be evaluated before any plans are made to work with the child's sleeping patterns. Overall suggestions for encouraging sleep include reducing stimulation prior to the desired nap time, providing quiet toys for bedtime use, and above all *not* using bed as a punishment. The toddler's age-typical love of ritual can be utilized to everyone's advantage by establishing a bedtime routine through which he becomes accustomed to a predictable chain of events ending in his going to bed. After-dinner bathing, selecting and dressing himself in pajamas, saying good-night to family members, choosing a bed toy, hearing a prespecified number of stories in bed, turning on his own night light, and being left to play with his toy is an example of bedtime ritual which can be adapted to the needs and preferences of any individual family. Such an established procedure—*and firm adherence to it*—can do much to ensure that the toddler gets the rest he needs without the insecurity he feels when allowed to exasperate his parents.

Some mothers, wearied by the child's early waking and day-long vigor, can enjoy a nap or other restful activity if they plan to fit it into their toddler's afternoon nap time.

Self-Stimulation or Self-Comfort Self-stimulation is an outgrowth of the child's interest in learning about his own body. In touching and manipulating parts of his body he experiences feelings of pleasure and thus returns to the pleasure-giving body areas for repeated effect. Probably the most common form of self-stimulation or self-consolation is thumb or finger sucking, which is especially frequent when the toddler is distressed or tired and ready for sleep.

Another form of stimulation observed in this period is masturbation. Tight diapers and inadvertent touching of the penis lead to the young boy's discovering his penis and the pleasure that accompanies manipulation of it. This is not exclusively male behavior as little girls also discover similar pleasure in clitoral stimulation, but sexual arousal is more obvious in boys because of visible erections. The only harm in genital self-stimulation is that it upsets parents and others and hence subjects the child to punishment or ridicule which he poorly understands and which may subsequently interfere with his self-concept.

These hazards to development are sufficient reason to appropriately discourage masturbation. In the young toddler, self-stimulation is usually easily interrupted by diversionary activity which requires use of the hands. The older toddler responds to a negative command. Self-stimulation is a normal activity for the toddler, although many parents become concerned when the child begins genital stimulation. When the toddler becomes preoccupied with masturbation to the exclusion of other interaction with his environment, a thorough assessment and referral may be necessary.

Physical Manipulative Skills A great part of the toddler's day is spent practicing his many physical skills through play. Early in the ambulatory phase, he enjoys items such as pull toys which help him practice walking and enhance the pleasures of being upright, mobile, and in control. Walking progresses to running, jumping, climbing stairs, and riding a tricycle. The toddler's hand and arm movements progress from gross hand-to-mouth movements to finer hand grasp and finger control, permitting turning of pages, scribbling, and holding items when walking. Throwing becomes purposeful. When this task is being mastered, the young toddler's favorite game is "I throw, you pick up," which can last until the retriever becomes exhausted. The toddler is able to copy a circle after mastering a straight vertical line. All these tasks require repeated practice. When he begins a new task and becomes discouraged, the toddler frequently returns to previously mastered tasks to regain self-esteem. Play and appropriate toys help the child work through and accomplish his developmental tasks.

Socially Acceptable Behavior

Since the family is the primary motivating force for the toddler and also the primary agent for transmitting cultural values, each child's behavior reflects the acceptable limits of his parents' cultural values. The family draws the perimeters of acceptable tolerance of tensions or frustrations, the amount and type of unique communication, the level of mother-child interdependency, the projected gender role, and the roles the child occupies within his social setting.

The diversifications of national origin, racial, religious, and economic factors preclude making absolute statements regarding the definition of acceptable behavior in all groups. The health worker must ascertain the patterns of behavior and cultural values in each family with which he works. Health care counseling for rearing the toddler must reflect the values of the family and the social setting in which the family lives.

The seeming apathy characteristic of the poverty culture is in itself a socially acceptable behavior for that family in that community. The nonintervention of the parents, the lack of child stimulation, and the differing expectations and practices regarding health provide the framework in which the toddler learns to function. With poverty families the nurse often must first work toward meeting the parents' identified needs and supporting their self-esteem before the parents can see the need for developmentally stimulating parent-child interactions. A more thorough exploration of culture and the family is presented in Chapter 18. Additional readings are included in the bibliography.

PHYSICAL CHARACTERISTICS

Body Dimensions The toddler shows a slowing in height and weight gains after the rapid increase that took place in infancy. By measuring and graphing the child's height, weight, and head circumference on a normative percentile chart, the nurse can determine whether the child is within normal limits for a range suitable to his morphologic structure. Serial charting at spaced intervals should reveal a toddler who remains within his own percentile range as he grows. For example, a child measuring within the 60th percentile would not be expected to drop to the 20th percentile in 6 months. Head circumference continues to be an important measurement until all fontanels are closed, usually after 15 months of age.

The toddler's body goes through *proportional* changes. Ossification and growth in the epiphyseal centers of the long bones provide the toddler with more rapidly lengthening legs and arms, while his trunk and head grow at a much slower rate. With the muscular strength resulting from increased ambulation and gross motor activity, the protruding abdomen diminishes and the lumbar lordosis disappears. The legs frequently show a bowing (tibial torsion) early in the ambulatory phase, along with flat feet, which usually correct themselves without assistance by the time the child reaches preschool age. The nurse's intermittent assessment of gait and posture can provide assurance to parents or can initiate a referral for orthopedic evaluation.

Vision Vision during the toddler phase continues to be hyperopic in decreasing degrees, so that he requires large objects for clear identification. Binocular vision does not usually provide fusion of images until the beginning of the toddler period, so stumbling and bumping into things during the early toddler stage are common occurrences. Despite hyperopia, distance fixation is very poor and requires the young toddler to be within a 6-foot range for clear vision. The several muscles of the eyes should be equally strong so that strabismus is absent or infrequent. When strabismus is consistently evident in the toddler, a referral should be recommended to the parents.

It is very important to provide the toddler with visual experiences which contribute to his overall intellectual and psychologic development. Large pictures of familiar scenes, people, and animals encourage development of image association. As language increases, the images acquire names and form the basis for effective communication of ideas.

Hearing Hearing, already mature at the onset of the toddler period, must be serially evaluated because of the toddler's susceptibility to otitis media and resultant hearing loss. Because language development and often the personality of the child are closely related to his ability to hear, interpret sounds, and incorporate their meaning, loss of hearing can disturb his development. Auditory screening must be part of every health appraisal.

Teeth Although the eruption of deciduous teeth begins in infancy, the first and second molars and cuspids erupt during the toddler years. Ossification and formation of permanent teeth, begun at birth, continue throughout the toddler period in preparation for later eruption. Care of the teeth and gums begins when the first few teeth appear. Mothers should be encouraged to gently wipe the teeth with a soft cloth at least weekly. As the young child begins finer hand and arm movement, he can be instructed in teeth cleaning. However, dental authorities recommend that the parent should gently but thoroughly brush and floss the child's teeth daily and continue close supervision of his self-care through the preschool period.

The toddler's early practice in teeth cleaning usually includes brushing everything within reach. The faucets, sink, bed, dolls, toys, and even the toilet bowl are fair game for practicing the scrubbing action. Some persons find that the teeth of the family dog suddenly become brighter during this practice period! Despite the revulsion adults feel upon viewing the range of the toothbrush in a toddler's hands, it seems necessary for the young child to practice brushing things he can see before he can master the complicated movement required for effective cleaning of his own teeth, which he cannot see.

Dental caries continues to be the most common disease in all age groups. Caries appears earlier in those toddlers who suck a bottle of milk while going to sleep. The steady supply of milk in the mouth over several hours provides an ideal glucose medium for early decay.

DEVELOPMENTAL ASSESSMENT THROUGH MOTOR SKILLS

Motor development patterns have been studied and documented and are used to assess the developmental level of the young child. Before the establishment of effective verbal communication, motor ability is the most reliable indication of developmental attainment. The extent of a child's progress in the activities which have been identified as normative landmarks can readily be evaluated.

As he gains practice in walking steadily without support, the toddler attains balance and is willing to attempt stairs with assistance. He soon manages climbing up stairs by himself but still needs assistance coming down them. He runs and can jump in place. By the age of 3 years he should be able to ride a tricycle and ambulate without concentrating.

The toddler's hand and finger movements become progressively refined. Self-feeding begins with gross movement of hand to mouth, the spoon frequently turning before his food gets to his mouth. Coordination becomes smoother, and he soon is able to insert the spoon into his mouth without spilling. Small objects are successfully manipulated with a high degree of finger, thumb, and hand precision. The toddler demonstrates a typical scribble when given a writing implement and can copy a vertical line by the time he is 3. He rolls or tosses a ball in the general direction of a ball game partici-

pant and progresses to a purposeful directed throw by 3 years.[1]

Motor maturation develops from gross, uncontrolled movements to fine, coordinated action during the toddler period. However, progress is made only with practice and encompasses many spills, many falls, and frequently broken equipment. Guiding parents in providing the opportunity for practice of motor activities is an often overlooked function of the nurse.

COGNITIVE DEVELOPMENT

The toddler period marks the transition of intellectual development from categorization of sensorimotor operations to a rudimentary system of concrete operations. The processes required to accomplish this transition are as follows: (1) The child can distinguish objects from the related scheme of activity; (2) he can distinguish end products from their means; and (3) he can discover new means for producing the same end products. Each of these cognitive steps is discussed next.

Since he has a beginning memory of numerous experiences, the toddler merely needs a beginning stimulus to be able to complete an experience as he remembers it. With increased activity and ambulation a rapid accumulation of complete experiences occurs, requiring him to generalize them into classes of experiences. One trial of a new experience is not sufficient for him to be able to categorize it, so his experiments must be tried and tried again. This cognitive process is the basis of the toddler's characteristic repetitious behavior, which has been pointed out throughout this chapter.

The next step is to experiment with alternative methods of getting the same results. This is the very beginning of concrete and logical intellectual operations. The toddler can create different ways of getting to his desired outcome.

Bobby, having spent time filling an assortment of empty boxes and jars with sand from a sand box, sees a dog dish complete with food. He proceeds to pack sand into that dish, along with his shoes, his mother's compact, and his father's tool box. A short time later his mother discovers the sand-packed articles and shows displeasure. Bobby becomes confused for a few seconds and then runs to his mother and embraces her legs, a display which has previously won him a positive response.

In his curiosity he has been experimenting with sand in its relationship to containers—filling, pouring, and refilling. The containers are immaterial; the sand behaves in a way which he must study additionally. In his attempt to discover all about sand, he must test it with everything within reach, including his mouth. When his mother offers a negative response, he must choose a behavior sequence which will recall the approval response (this explains the complete change in his focus of interest from his sand play to his embrace of his mother).

If given the opportunity to repeat the sand play several times with varying results, he will become able to conclude that sand is for boxes and bottles, not for the dog's dish, compact, shoes, or tool box. Similar experimentation with other objects produces comparable learning. Milk goes in a cup, a bottle, or the milk carton; milk does not go in shoes, the dog's ear, or the tool box. Shoes go on feet; shoes do not go in the bathtub.

The child begins experimenting in this manner usually by 18 months and continues unabated until verbal ability permits him to communicate his questions and logically think through alternative ways of reaching conclusions without having to enact everything in order to understand it (Fig. 11-3).

Language development closely follows alongside the cognitive development of the child. Shortly after attaining the ability to say "mama" and "dada" when they appear, the infant or toddler is able to imitate one- or two-syllable words when they are said to him. Soon he can recall and pronounce the word when provided with a picture or image stimulus: *dog, baby, bed, milk*. Nouns and single words characterize the beginning of verbal communication. Single verbs then appear attached to the noun: *baby cry, daddy go, dog bark*. Most 3-year-olds can combine a one-word subject, a verb, and a one-word object: *daddy go store, mommy go work, Dickie go bed*. Adjectives such as *small* and *big* are used with nouns but do not denote accurate awareness of the concept of size. Numbers and colors are learned as nouns without the usual cognitively mature meanings. A child who has learned that a particular picture is a brown cow will at first give the same name to another picture of a pink horse. New things are initially identified as things they resemble with which he is already familiar.

The toddler can comprehend much more than he can speak. In fact, some children seem reluctant to attempt additional vocabulary beyond that required to receive absolute necessities. These children, however, develop an adequate communication by pointing, grunting, and other language behavior. As long as such a child gets his request, he will continue not to verbalize.

Developmental norms for language usage have been established; some examples of these tests are the Denver Developmental Screening Test, Washington Guide,[1] and Vineland Social Maturity Scale. Frequently, however, the toddler's developmental testing shows him to be below average in language skills only.

Children learn language skills through hearing the spoken word, by imitating sounds, and by trials of using words appropriately. Encouraging mothers and fathers to talk to their toddlers strengthens the background for the child's verbal development. Even if all the words are not understood, the child begins trying to use them. Children who consistently test low in verbal development are usually those who receive little verbal interaction. Socially and economically deprived children typically test lower in language development than middle-class children, no doubt because of their lesser language experience.

When language skills are below average for age the nurse should attempt to ascertain the reason. Does the toddler lack verbal stimulation? Does he have little need to talk because he gets what he needs without verbalizing? Does a history of otitis media or familial hearing defect suggest that the child may have a hearing loss? Does he have enlarged tonsils and adenoids that interfere with his hearing?

Picture books and story reading assist the young toddler in developing memory skills, visual discrimination skills, and language. After having a story book read to him several times the child becomes able to tell the whole story by viewing the pictures or can fill in gaps when the reader hesitates.

All mental development requires the chance to practice new skills. The toddler who is not permitted to explore in order to find sameness and difference will have little ability to categorize; the toddler who is not spoken to has no chance to attach meaning to words.

PSYCHOSOCIAL DEVELOPMENT

The toddler's psychosocial development is dominated by his need to adapt to an increasingly large and complex environment. Adaptation, which requires compromise between opposing forces, must continue to build the self-esteem of the child. The toddler's need to explore his own muscular and physical strength opposes his reluctance to experiment with his capacity because of fear of hurt or reprimand. The need to gratify his impulses opposes a wish to remain safe in a previous state. The desire to do what he wants opposes the fear of being

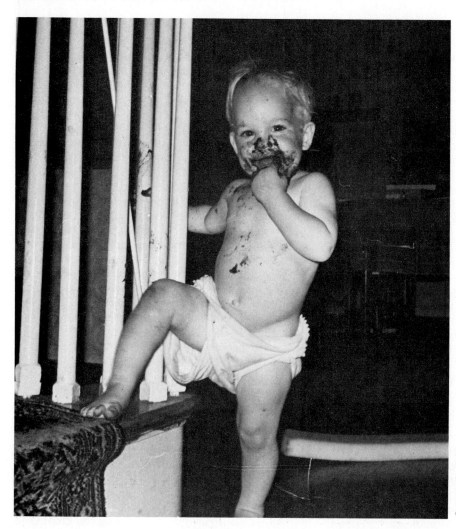

Figure 11-3 The toddler, in learning about his environment, characteristically uses materials (in this case, chocolate pudding) in ways adults do not expect or appreciate.

caught. The wish for self-regulation opposes and accompanies the desire to control others.

Practice of both fine and gross motor activity is essential to psychosocial development because the reinforcement of successfully attaining the goal provides positive self-esteem. A child learning to undress sees the activity as an accomplishment, whereas parents may see it as an undesired behavior requiring punishment. The child then must choose between practicing this new task, which can result in a reprimand, or giving up the activity and maintaining dependence on his mother for being undressed.

The power attained through growing independence permits the child to view himself as capable of self-control. The extreme negativism typical of many toddlers is their way of showing their control over other people and events. The de-

sire to control frequently overcomes the toddler's desire for what would happen if he did not try to prevent it. "No" is his spontaneous answer to most questions, even though the opposite—"yes"—would be expected to yield an attractive outcome. Offering a toddler a dish of ice cream provokes an instantaneous "no" followed shortly by dipping his spoon into the dish.

The great desire to act on his own terms is the prevailing theme in the toddler's age-typical assertion of his autonomy. Yet in order to become a social being he must learn a give-and-take relationship with others. The ensuing conflict causes blackmail behavior, tantrums, and returns to infantile acts. Early in toddlerhood the desire for self-regulation enlarges to include wanting to regulate others, since others interfere with his wishes. He attempts to manipulate others in order to enhance his self-regulation. His terms become unbearable to parents who find being with a tyrant, especially a 2-year-old tyrant, a threat to their own identity. Their refusal to bow to the toddler's manipulative behavior leads him to respond with frustration and tantrums. After repeated attempts fail to produce the desired outcome, the child develops other means of getting parents to do his bidding. Through trial and error he learns how to lead others to do things for him. He finds out that he must give in different ways to reach his desired objective, in this way conforming to socially acceptable methods of manipulating people. He learns that this conforming does not reduce his self-esteem but actually increases it, since he is able to control himself in his giving and receiving.

Erikson describes the toddler as characterized by conflicting wishes for "holding on" and "letting go," within the broad range of toddler activities. The need to hold on to self-regulation on his own terms progresses to giving up sufficient portions of his control to permit him to act within mutual regulations established with the parents.

Toilet training can be viewed in this framework. The final step which characterizes the knowledgeable act of releasing into a parent-specified repository in order to be acceptable conflicts with his desire to determine where and when he will release that which is his. Similarly, the temper tantrums discussed previously are examples of the blackmail behavior he utilizes in an effort to show his power. In essence he is saying, "I will be in charge or I will behave in a manner which you do not like."

Adapting to social restraints while at the same time building self-esteem is a very complicated process which must be refined throughout life. For the sake of future adjustment, the beginning adaptation must be accomplished during the toddler stage in order to permit him as a growing person to view frustration as a part of life and not a threat to life. Play is a critical factor in the child's learning to experiment with social expectations and to work out his own boundaries of self-restraint and self-assertiveness. In independent play he creates roles, makes restrictions, and controls the action of his imaginary characters within the boundaries. He can try many actions and manipulate objects, even destroying them and bringing them back to life again. Until he can accomplish the beginning steps of giving in order to receive, he is incapable of playing with a partner. Although the toddler enjoys the interaction of play with his mother or father, he must also have the opportunity to interact with toys and objects without adult intervention.

Parents of a child in this adaptive phase can be helped by guidance in setting and maintaining reasonable limits on the child's behavior, granting him freedom to exercise some control within the set limits, and supplying reinforcement when the child demonstrates beginning control. Awareness that negativism is an automatic response may help the parents learn to approach the child with questions that cannot be answered with a "no" but which still leave a choice for the child. Instead of asking whether the toddler wants lunch, the parent can ask which food he wishes to eat first. The toddler must be given the opportunity to make choices, or he will be unable to develop independent function, but the range of possible choices can be circumscribed by the parent. Encouragement to choose among alternatives which are all acceptable will build his belief in his ability to make decisions.

The toddler is motivated by his extreme desire to be independent, but since his development has not progressed to enable him to deal with all the variables which threaten his safety and adjustment, he must have limits of acceptable behavior established for him. Another prime motivating force is his need to be loved and approved. Being well informed about the behavioral manifestations of these two motivating forces provides guidelines for appreciating and working effectively with the toddler.

During the toddler period the foundation for adaptation to the world of reality is begun. From this foundation is developed the mentally and physically healthy child who can interact successfully with objects and people in a way which builds a positive view of himself.

The nurse functioning in primary health care has an excellent opportunity to assist parents in understanding and guiding the toddler. The nurse in the acute care setting can adapt nursing care to the needs of the toddler.

REFERENCES

1 Kathryn Barnard and Marcene Powell, *Teaching the Mentally Retarded Child: A Family Care Approach*, The C. V. Mosby Company, St. Louis, 1972.

BIBLIOGRAPHY

Almy, Millie: *Young Children's Thinking*, Teachers College Press, Columbia University, New York, 1967.
Anthony, E. J., and Koupernik C. (eds.): *The Child in His Family*, John Wiley & Sons, Inc., New York, 1970.
Bakwin, H., and Bakwin, R. M.: *Behavior Disorders in Children*, 4th ed., W. B. Saunders Company, Philadelphia, 1972.

Erikson, E.: *Childhood and Society,* W. W. Norton & Company, Inc., New York, 1950.

Furth, H.: *Piaget and Knowledge,* Prentice-Hall, Inc., Englewood Cliffs, N.J., 1969.

Gouin DeCarie, Theresa: *Intelligence and Affectivity in Early Childhood,* International Universities Press, Inc., New York, 1966.

Hughes, J. G.: *Synopsis of Pediatrics*, 3d ed., The C. V. Mosby Company, St. Louis, 1971.

Joint Commission on Mental Health of Children: *Mental Health: From Infancy through Adolescence*, Harper & Row, Publishers, Incorporated, New York, 1973.

Kagan, J.: *Changes and Continuity in Infancy*, John Wiley & Sons, Inc., New York, 1971.

Maier, H. W.: *Three Theories of Child Development*, Harper & Row, Publishers, Incorporated, New York, 1965.

Piers, Marie W. (ed.): *Play and Development*, W. W. Norton & Company, Inc., New York, 1972.

Senn, J. J., and Solnit, A. J.: *Problems in Child Behavior and Development*, Lea & Febiger, Philadelphia, 1968.

Silver, H. K., et al.: *Handbook of Pediatrics*, 9th ed., Lange Medical Publications, Los Altos, Calif., 1971.

Watson, E. H., and Lowrey, G. H.: *Growth and Development of Children*, 5th ed., Year Book Medical Publishers, Inc., Chicago, 1969.

Wesley, F.: *Childrearing Psychology*, Behavioral Publications, New York, 1971.

Whipple, Dorothy V.: *Dynamics of Development: Euthenic Pediatrics*, McGraw-Hill Book Company, New York, 1965.

Zaporozhets, A. V., and Elkonin, D. B.: *The Psychology of Preschool Children*, Massachusetts Institute of Technology Press, Cambridge, Mass., 1971.

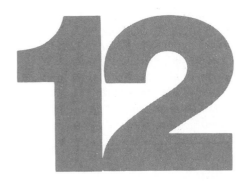

THE PRESCHOOLER— 3 TO 5 YEARS

EILEEN GALLAGHER NAHIGIAN

PHYSICAL DEVELOPMENT OF THE PRESCHOOLER
Overview

The child between 3 and 5 years of age is a conspicuously physical child. With the growth and development of his body comes the need to practice new skills. As new skills appear, earlier behavior is refined; a synchrony begins to develop as various aspects of growth interact to reveal the *preschooler*.

The preschooler loses his baby fat but retains an innocent and cherubic appearance which conceals the variety of behaviors of which he is now capable and his capacity to get into mischief. He has quiet and contemplative moods (Fig. 12-1), but more frequently he displays his activity and inquisitiveness, at once charming and disarming.

As in earlier stages, reliance on a timetable for the unfolding of specific skills is unwise; it is more helpful to evaluate the pattern and direction of development in terms of an appreciation for *ranges* and deviations from normal. Nevertheless, certain milestones are outlined in this chapter as a general guideline for observation.

Physical Milestones and Activities

Certain guidelines, such as those presented in Table 12-1, are necessary to the professional's clinical evaluation of a preschooler's physical development and health. These norms also assist the nurse in assuring worried parents that their child is indeed normal. Many investigations have arrived at generally accepted developmental scales; perhaps best known among these are the works of Arnold Gesell and his associates. The student is referred to the many publications of Gesell, as well as others, for elaboration of schedules included here and elsewhere in the text.

Pattern of Development in the Preschool Years

Observation provides fascination with, as well as information about, the preschooler's normally intrusive and inquisitive activity. During these years basic skills are being completed and refined; ease and economy of effort begin to replace earlier clumsiness. The days of gaining head control, upright posture, and basic manipulative abilities have long passed. Where concentration had been focused on the physical skill, the skill now becomes subservient to broader pleasures. For example, running formerly had been a goal in itself, but it now becomes the means to bigger and better ends. Previously iso-

139

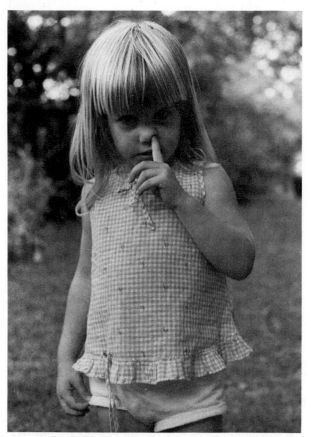

Figure 12-1 The preschooler's moods encompass a broad range and are reflected in a wide variety of behaviors. *(Photo courtesy of George Lazar.)*

lated activities are combined to form more obviously complex activities such as games of tag or ball.

The preschooler's level of physical achievement in part reflects his everyday opportunities and parental encouragement. The unfolding of any skill relies in one sense on his actual *practice* of it, but in a greater sense on daily activities which require coordinated use of limbs, vision, hearing, and other elemental motor and perceptual abilities. In fact, physical prowess is less a function of chronologic age than of sequential development through phases approaching proficiency.

Since no skill is an all-or-none proposition, and since the several aspects of development (language, hand coordination, social competency, and so forth) usually do not progress at the same rate, any one child may be accomplished in one skill while awkward in another. In addition, differences exist between the sexes. Girls are more efficient in some activities and boys excel in others, whether because of inborn sex differences or incidental sex-prescribed experiences. (It will be interesting in future years to note the continuance or discontinuance of this difference as a result of current efforts toward equality of opportunity for boys and girls.)

Adaptive behavior is also a part of physical growth and development but will be discussed in this chapter in the section regarding intellectual development, to which it more broadly applies. Elements of adaptation have already been presented in Table 12-1 in such activities as the use of hands and locomotion.

It must be understood that there are certain limitations to the preschooler's motor skills, chiefly his quickness of movement which compromises opportunities to judge distance, strength, and required sense of equilibrium. Thus, chairs *will* topple, and objects placed precariously on counters and tables will crash to the floor. Since he participates so fully in family life, it is imperative that the preschooler's parents recognize the normalcy of these accidents resulting from misjudgment (or inattentiveness—there are more important matters on the child's mind) so they can enjoy living with him without worrying over their "hyperactive" child. The nurse is given many opportunities to interpret behavior and to advise parents of means by which they might limit the inevitable accidents that mark preschool life. Provision of safe and sturdy toys and furniture, protection of valuable household objects, assignment of play areas, and the development of a parental art for diverting rambunctious children from dangerous activities are some suggestions the nurse can offer.

One Preschooler in Action

The overall body activity repertoire of a preschooler at any given moment is illustrated in the following 15-minute observation recorded by the author during a usual morning in nursery school. This record affords additional insights to the preschooler's cognitive and personality development.

Ted, 4 years old, strutted to his teacher, calling her by name and submitting his test result paper to her. He pivoted and started to return to his seat. He responded to the teacher's immediate signal to seat himself at another table. He half-bounced, half-walked, dragging each foot alternately till he arrived at the table. There he slung his right arm over the chair back, all the while trying to comprehend the activities of the teacher and boy to his left. His position changed almost continuously from slumping

Table 12-1 SCHEDULE OF PHYSICAL GROWTH AND MOTOR ACTIVITY OF THE PRESCHOOL CHILD

Measurement of development	Age 3 years	Age 4 years	Age 5 years
Physical growth			
Pulse	95/min	92/min	90/min
Respirations	25/min	25/min	24/min
Blood pressure	85–90/60	85–90/60	85–90/60
Height (mean)	96 cm (37½ in.)	103 cm (40½ in.)	108 cm (42 in.)
Weight (mean)	14½ kg (32 lb); slow, steady gain	16 kg (36 lb); five times birthweight	18 kg (40 lb)
Additional measurements of physical growth			Losing temporary teeth Stomachache a common complaint Handedness usually established
Motor activity			
Hands	Uses scissors with some success Strings large beads Good small muscle control evidenced by ability to copy circle or cross	Throws ball overhand Cuts out pictures Copies square Builds five-block gate from model	Hits nail on head with hammer
Position and locomotion	Pedals tricycle Walks backward Walks up and down stairs alone, alternating feet	High level of motor control Lighter, more graceful, more rhythmic movement Jumps and climbs well Manages stairs unaided Hops on one foot	Runs skillfully and plays simultaneously; runs on tiptoes Jumps rope Skips well Skates on one roller skate Rides tricycle with skill Good poise—maintains position longer than formerly

over the table to sitting straight back with his hands pressing against the chair seat for support, his legs waggling unceasingly.

The other boy, busy at the table, looked up and inquired, "You got somethin' you want?" Ted made no reply. "What's your name?"

"Ted." Then, after a pause: "I got new things." "I got new socks."

Ted muttered, pulling at his shirt, "I got a new shirt." He said no more, but his body continued to move. His mouth changed expressions under voluntary command as he grinned, bared his teeth, and wrinkled his lips.

(During this interval, a girl at the same table had been counting all the girls in the room. The other boy had commented that there were nine girls, but she ignored him.)

Ted defended the boy: "He said 'nine' too!" He emphasized the remark by pointing to the boy.

Ted reared back, stretched from head to toe, "wound-up," and displayed his muscles; then he began "boxing" with his new comrade who had just referred to himself as "superman." A short interval of playful fist-to-fist boxing ensued.

The teacher, seeming to ignore the boxing, soon interrupted pleasantly, "I have something for you to do."

Ted sat back, wiggling his legs. When his teacher handed him a paper and pencil, he noted merrily, "That's a bigger pencil!" [Bigger than what?]

After having received instructions to draw a line connecting similar shapes on the paper, Ted dawdled with his pencil. He encircled the pencil with four fingers, then experimented with alternate fingerings until he finally resumed the original grasp.

He drew one line with great flourish, held up his paper, and announced: "I did it, teacher, and I know the same things." To this there was no immediate response from the teacher; he sat down to wait. While idling, he attempted to secure the pencil behind his right ear, as his right elbow remained pressed against the table top.

The teacher arrived and he explained, "This the same, this the same." The teacher congratulated him and further instructed him to color the similar pictures the same color.

He found a purple crayon and proceeded with his assignment. The second boy interrupted, "I got a purple, too."

Ted observed, "That's not purple . . ." and for a moment surveyed the open box of crayons. As he looked at the crayons, he remained sitting and continued to color his paper; he jutted his chin and nose out over the box, with his eyes seeming to bulge downward in search of another purple crayon. A girl approached and located the purple crayon first.

With no comment, Ted settled back further in his chair and continued coloring. Regularly, his gaze was interrupted by activity elsewhere in the room. He busied himself with short, straight, back-and-forth scribbles.

Teacher returned and admonished him to follow the previous instruction. He returned to the task, being additionally reprimanded by the girl, "You know dat, you know dat!"

To this he responded only with a superficially gleeful, "Heh, heh, heh, heh, heh!" He continued to color, following the lines he had drawn earlier and coloring the circles. "I did one like that!" he observed to himself.

Just then, he glimpsed the teacher leading a 2-year-old "visitor" to the toilet room. "Teacher, I gonna go make water." This was said loudly, but was not shouted. No one seemed to heed him.

He examined his neighbor's drawing and admonished him, "That not how you do that, rubberhead. Rubberhead!" The repeated "rubberhead" carried a tone of "I like that so I'll say it again."

He and the other boy then traipsed off to the bathroom. Very shortly they returned, flying their arms as if imitating an airplane. Ted "flew" directly to the teacher and asked if "block corner" could be their next activity.

Such a word picture is more descriptive than a set of statistical averages showing when a child can manipulate a pencil, imitate an airplane, or initiate toileting. Whether in a daily living situation or during a relatively confined hospitalization, adults who remain unaware of the constancy of such normal activity may precipitate unfortunate misunderstandings and anxieties in themselves and in the child.

INTELLECTUAL DEVELOPMENT
Adaptation

Adaptive behavior, which implements motor, perceptual, and verbal-social abilities, is intimately related to physical, cognitive, and personal-social development. All these behaviors are based on early infantile activities which are further developed as intellectual development proceeds. From its simplest to its most complex aspects, adaptation is fundamental to the child's eventual mastery of his environment.

Early Adaptation Building structures from blocks is among the earliest of the child's adaptive skills. This skill is dependent upon the preschooler's prior establishment of basic relationships between eye, hand, and block. Progressively he employs these relationships as he learns to build towers, gates, bridges, and steps. Perceptual ability is summoned in an increasingly broad sense throughout the preschool years as perception of dimension, shape, or depth and memory of sequential maneuvers become essential to the child's adaptation.

Adaptation or intelligence can legitimately be evaluated according to these early building skills only if the evaluator takes into consideration extenuating circumstances such as experiential background, alertness, degree of health or illness, social ease with the observer, and integrity of the physical apparatus (visual acuity, for example). Fantasy also modifies the preschooler's performance; his constructions assume names and purposes and may easily be altered in process to suit his current fantasy.

Picture Drawing Adaptation extends to the child's ability to use pencil and paper to depict some aspects of his world. Much growth in this skill occurs as early as 3 years of age[1] when meaningless scribbles give way to purposeful attempts to copy and repeat specific forms. Eventually an intentional "creation" can be announced and subsequently drawn, showing ability to follow through on a specific idea.

Because of the characteristic subjectivity of drawing at this age, the primitive forms, especially, allow for creative adventures as they assume a variety of meanings to the child. For this reason adults are cautioned that to request identification of spontaneously drawn pictures may stifle the child's subjective explorations and thereby may hamper his future ability to reach mature levels of perception.[2]

The child also profits best from freedom to draw unguided, since he represents significant people (primarily) and objects according to his egocentric conceptualization of them. Simply providing appropriate materials will prompt expression of his inner feelings and conceptions in a way needed but not yet permitted by verbal language. If direction is given regarding what the child might draw, it should be offered more as a suggestion than as a mandate. Figures 12-2 and 12-3 are typical preschool drawings in response to an instruction to draw something about a story that had just been read. The story concerned a young female animal who felt rejected when a sibling was born. While only two children in the group depicted the story's theme, all the children accepted the opportunity to convey *some* thought. Although the observer could not establish the influence of the story on the other pictures, it is possible that it aroused either unexpected associations or an avoidance reaction in the children.

Drawing provides the preschooler an opportunity to experience a variety of tactile, visual, and kinesthetic sensations formerly foreign to him. These experiences will be broadened still more when the child is offered large sheets of paper and paints in lieu of pencil and paper. Because his representations also encourage progressive maturation, adults should avoid directing the child to draw specified objects except in testing or evaluation situations.

Gesell and his associates[3] have devised tests and norms for the evaluation of preschoolers' drawing ability. Analyses of drawings are made on the basis of the child's response to varying restrictions placed on his efforts: (1) to draw whatever he wishes to draw; (2) to draw a man; (3) to finish a drawing of a man; or (4) to imitate and copy geometric forms. Interpretation of the results is facilitated by careful recording of the manner in which the child draws as well as how he describes his drawing. Such additional data provide pertinent information regarding the child's ability in the larger spheres of perseverance, ingenuity, and independence.

Aside from actual evaluation situations, other valuable use of specific drawings may be advised. In clinical situations it is often desirable to request the child to draw a specific part of the body or a picture about some aspect of his treatment. In this way the nurse can achieve at least two goals: learning the child's concepts of an involved body part or a procedure; and finding a basis for discussing the child's illness or hospitalization with him (see Figs. 12-4 and 12-5).

Language   Children from 3 to 5 years old present delightful verbal insights for anyone who listens. Their use of language holds a fascination all its

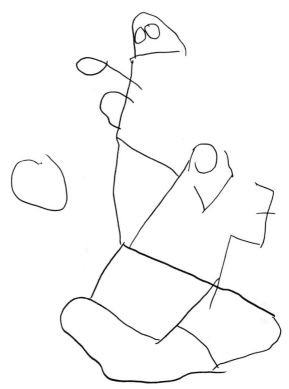

Figure 12-2   "Baby Frances, Frances' sister, Mother, and Daddy."

own. Preschool language may also prove a nemesis to parents who may inappropriately reward "cute" mispronunciations or unduly punish for the normal profanities.

The "cute" nature of preschool language is largely a holdover from earlier years and includes

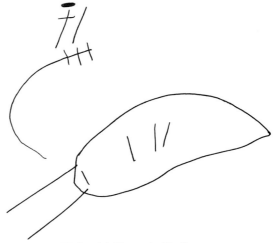

Figure 12-3   "Baby drinking a bottle."

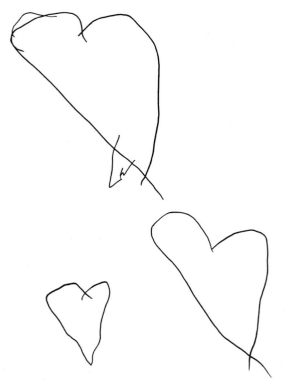

Figure 12-4 "My heart." This drawing was produced by a 4-year-old girl newly diagnosed to have rheumatic fever.

difficulties with personal pronouns (for example, "we" may be substituted for "you," "me" for "I"), words which sound alike, and placement of consonants in such words as "aminal" (animal) or "algerly" (allergy). At other times parents may be

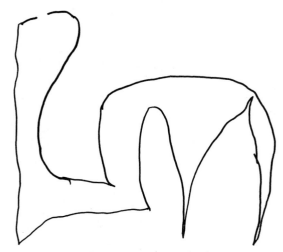

Figure 12-5 "Daddy's heart." This was drawn by the same child who drew Figure 12-4.

astounded by the preschooler's use of adult vocabulary, phraseology, and grammatic structure.

Like sounds may cause misunderstandings. A 4-year-old boy expressed horror that his aunt had spoken a naughty word when, after having exhausted herself playing with him, she announced, "I'm pooped!" "Poop" to him was a bathroom word. Hospitalized children are often plagued by strange vocabulary which proves frightening. For example, one physician had the habit of saying "shoot the dye" when he was about to inject dye. The child might confuse "die" and "dye," especially in conjunction with the term "shoot."

Many or most parents have occasion to overhear their preschooler repeat "bad" words; indeed, many have been innocently asked, "What does '*&#!' mean?" Most preschoolers experiment with words, including nonsense words and profanities. Language is for them another newly acquired skill which is sufficiently under control by age 4 or 5 to be manipulated for pleasure.

Language also is a learning mechanism for the preschooler. Whether egocentric or socialized forms of speech[4] are employed, the child continues to learn by naming objects, repeating words, experimenting with language forms, or seeking information. Although his speech is very often egocentric, the preschooler is equally prone to spontaneously conduct extensive conversations with adults on a variety of topics which may include birth, death, illness, the sky, and endless other things.

Although articulation improves by age 5, the younger preschooler continues to speak in an infantile manner. Although persons outside the family may understand these infantile pronunciations, the child should be encouraged to eradicate mispronunciations. Such encouragement becomes increasingly effective with age; in early preschool years the child can correctly pronounce ordinary conversation.

Language development is much more complex than can be discussed here and includes the eventual ability to read. The student is urged to read more about development of this phase of this stage of adaptation in other sources including those suggested here.[5, 6]

Perceptions of and Conceptions about the Environment

From age 3 onward, the child's view of the world changes significantly. Size and form, color discriminations, time, and space take on new meaning as the child relates one to the other, comparing and contrasting, for example, the apparent difference in size of an object viewed from nearby or far away. His demeanor and his vocalizations clue the observant adult to his increasing maturity, simultaneously revealing his confusion about appearances.

Some experience and development are required for the easy completion of tasks such as placing a square object into the correct opening when given a choice of round, square, oblong, diagonal, or other openings. Even as he approaches the correct opening the young child needs to experiment with positioning of the block in order to achieve success.

Concept formation requires increasing maturity and therefore remains primitive and confused for the preschooler. Nevertheless, he is active in determining subjectively suitable explanations for the origin of plants, of dreams, or of the heavens. Time concepts are primitive as he begins to separate afternoon from morning and weekends (maybe as "Daddy's no-work day") from weekdays. The cognitive material reported by Piaget (discussed in Chap. 7 and in the following pages) suggests some bases for the preschooler's perceptual and conceptual achievements and distortions.

Jean Piaget's Cognitive Theory

Cognition is discussed here for a specific purpose: to demonstrate the important fact that the preschool child thinks differently from anyone else. He is beyond the sensorimotor intelligence of the infant and toddler; but contrary to adults' expectation, the 3- to 5-year-old does not think like a grown-up.

Preoperational and Intuitive Periods Beginning in the symbolic, or preoperational, period of thought (1½ to 4 years), the characteristics of realism, irreversibility, concreteness, and animism appear. Definitions of these characteristics may help the reader see how the child's cognitive limitations influence his reaction to new experiences.

Realism and animism evolve from confusion between objective and subjective reality.[7] The young child is incapable of accurately differentiating inherent features of an object from those features he himself assigns the objective (realism). For a child under 6 years of age, activity and life are synonymous; therefore, anything that moves—no matter by what means—is alive (animism). (Consider how easy and how frightening it would be for the child to feel defenseless against active attack perpetrated by an unfamiliar object such as an elevator or electrocardiograph.)

Also limiting the young child is his relative in-flexibility or *concreteness* of thought. He lacks the adult ability to analyze and synthesize; thus, he readily misunderstands and may feel threatened and afraid when confronted with strange objects or experiences. Associated with this is his *irreversibility* of thought, which prevents realization that changes in the appearance of an object need not change the essence of the object. Consequently he is unable to anticipate reversal of a change despite his having observed the actual induction of change. (As an application, consider the familiar nurse changed into unfamiliar garb. How readily can the child be expected to accept him without question?)

Intuitive Period In addition to the characteristics just described, there are others which do not become apparent until the child is about 4 years of age. These attributes and limitations of preschool thought include egocentrism, centering, and focusing on states rather than on the process of transformation.

In this context, *egocentrism* is a neutral term with no derogatory connotations. The egocentric child has a private meaning within his symbols or language. He is also *unable* to see the viewpoint of another and *unable* to understand another's inability to appreciate his viewpoint. Adults who are unaware of this characteristic experience unnecessary consternation at what appears to be stubbornness and an extension of earlier negativism. The preschooler who disagrees with a parental judgment or statement frequently is operating under the delusions of egocentrism. He believes he is correct. When his private codes lead him to a conclusion differing from the parental conclusion, he may suffer undeserved defamation as "bold," "bad," or "obstinate." As time progresses and maturity emerges, the child may be helped to identify additional circumstances which alter his incorrect assumptions; for the present, however, it is helpful if adults understand the child's cognitive limitations.

Perhaps if a child could think about how a person or object moves from one state or position to another, anticipatory explanations of events would pose little challenge. Piaget's evidence, however, is to the contrary. Because the child is *less likely to concentrate on the transformations inherent in change than on the nature of the changed object itself*, he profits little from a discourse on the process of change. (The student is advised to recall this statement if ever tempted to elaborate on a clinical or surgical procedure when giving anticipatory explanations to preschoolers.)

Still another aspect of the preschooler's cognitive processes which both simplifies and complicates anticipatory explanations is *centering*, or focusing attention on a single detail of an object or situation and being unable to shift attention from one detail to another. Centering has been discussed in the Piagetian section of Chapter 7.

It is impossible to discuss thoroughly all the areas of intelligence which develop simultaneously throughout the preschool years. What has been presented in the foregoing section and in Table 12-2, it is hoped, will encourage further study. It is, furthermore, impossible to characterize the child and his responses to life on the basis of adaptive and cognitive behavior apart from his psychosocial development. The following section especially needs to be studied in association with the child's intellectual behavior if the preschooler is to be understood.

PERSONALITY AND SOCIALIZATION
Psychosocial Development

Preschoolers in a social environment are seldom unnoticed by the group. Although they actually have begun to control some areas of their behavior, they may seem to be always underfoot and uncontrollable, the 4-year-old being the most conspicuous offender. Evidence of budding self-control is recognizable in the 3-year-old's adherence to ritual in simple acts such as dressing or going to bed. Maturity, related to developing mental powers, eventually results in the child's being better able to cope with his environment by 6 years of age without reliance on rituals.

Much of the preschooler's total behavior is dependent upon his development in the personal-social realm. The present discussion, while presented from a predominantly psychoanalytic reference point, is broadened somewhat by the inclusion of selected concepts from other behavior theories. This expansion seems important for at least two reasons: psychoanalytic concepts and terminology have fallen into disfavor among some professionals; and the nurse's use of abstract psychoanalytic terms while counseling parents may only compound their confusion.

As the child's preschool personality develops, his ego—or his inner self—emerges more fully than at any previous time to assist him in his adaptation to the world. So strengthened, he is better equipped to decide whether, when, and how to seek satisfaction of his desires because he can test his judgments against reality. However, he remains too immature to cope directly with the newly developing and rigid superego, social conscience, or self-expectation for social conformity. To assist him in dealing with the gap between what he expects of himself and what he sees his actual performance to be, he evolves a repertoire of self-defensive mechanisms. These defenses (including sublimation, repression, reaction formation, isolation, and undoing) distort the child's perception, as if to eliminate real disturbances by psychologic gymnastics. Fantasy and daydreams are also frequently evidenced during these years, relieving the child temporarily from the demands of reality.

Probably the most burdensome feature of the preschooler's personality is his perfectionistic need to conform to social mores. The psychoanalytic position is that this perfectionistic self-expectation grows out of the oedipal situation and is an attempt to attain the unrealizable standards imposed by the parental conscience.[8]

Identification The preschooler's process of identification may be obvious at some times and very elusive at other times; for the observer it may be quite intriguing. Theoretically, it is related to the termination of the oedipal situation as described originally by Sigmund Freud. Simplified discussions of the process can be found in more recent and readable sources.[9, 10]

Essentially what occurs in the resolution of the oedipal situation is that girls identify with their mothers (femininity) and boys with their fathers (masculinity). Comfortable resolution entails satisfaction with and security within one's own sex role and develops from the child's growing ability to give as well as receive love. Before this can be achieved, the child must move, during the preschool years, from a period of primary, security-dependent, and asexual love for both parents to a preference for the love of the opposite-sex parent, as is described more fully in Chapter 7.

Parents, without choosing, participate vitally in the child's resolution of the oedipal situation and identification process. Parents' reality orientation provides the key for the resolution of the oedipal stage. Fraiberg[11] discusses this idea, indicating that the period is eased if the child has learned earlier that he cannot assert authority over his parents. Cautioning that the child ought not to be intimidated and that his feelings and frustrations ought to be acknowledged, Fraiberg believes that reality will inform the child that parents have a private life together which he cannot intrude upon or usurp.

The final outcome of the preschool phase of the

Table 12-2 NORMATIVE ACHIEVEMENTS OF THE PRESCHOOLER'S ADAPTIVE DEVELOPMENT

Area of development	Age 3 years	Age 4 years	Age 5 years
Motor achievements	Tries to draw a picture; may add an eye or leg when asked to draw a complete man Helps dry dishes Unbuttons front and side of clothes Undresses and helps dress self Uses toilet; stays dry at night Washes hands Feeds self May brush teeth	Makes drawings with form and meaning but rarely detailed Represents man by head and eyes Adds two parts to complete drawing of a man Buttons front and side of clothes Laces shoes Brushes teeth May bathe self with direction Takes partial responsibility for toileting May attempt to print letters	Makes drawing of man including body, arms, legs, feet Adds about seven parts to complete drawing of man Puts three or more details in drawings Prints first name and maybe other words; forms small letters well Dresses self except for tying shoes Washes self without wetting clothes
Verbal abilities	Has 900-word vocabulary Uses plurals Creates a phrase and repeats it Repeats six-syllable sentences Uses language more fluently and with confidence (whether or not anyone listens) Sings simple songs	Has 1,500-word vocabulary Uses mild profanities and name-calling Uses language aggressively Asks many questions Uses phrases and exclamations	Has 2,100-word vocabularly Talks constantly Uses adult speech forms Finds speech more important in peer relationships Participates in conversation without monopolizing it Asks for definitions Asks fewer but more relevant questions Laughs frequently during conversation
Perceptual and conceptual characteristics	Has beginning understanding of past and future—"tomorrow" and "yesterday" still confusing	Learning number concepts—counts to three, repeats four numbers, counts four coins Names one or more colors well Has poor space perception	Specifies what he will draw or paint Copies a triangle Constructs a rectangle from two right triangles Does not fully understand time gradations Knows weeks as units of time; names weekdays Knows four or more colors Knows his age and residence Determines the heavier of two objects Begining to understand kinship relations, such as uncle, grandmother, etc. Beginning to develop power of reasoning
Cognitive characteristics	Shifts frequently between intelligent adaptation and play or imitation In the symbolic or preconceptual period of cognition Shows persistence of realism, irreversibility, concreteness, and animism	In Piaget's period of intuitive thought—egocentrism and centering Focuses on present state of displayed objects rather than on process of change	Continues period of intuitive thought—egocentrism and centering

identification process, then, includes renunciation of parent as sex object and leads to security based in parental admiration of the child's appropriate femininity or masculinity.

Conscience, or Who's "OK"? The superego has been variously referred to as conscience, social conformity, and more recently as "parent."[12] "Parent" is part of the terminology of the psychologic theory known as transactional analysis, which points out that each person operates at any given moment from either a child, adult, or parent ego state. Transactional analysis and these three ego states are described in Chapter 22. For purposes of the present discussion, parent refers to the internalized judgmental attitudes and rules which a child adopts as his own in the process of learning to conform to social expectations. Hence, parent as used here is an approximate synonym for conscience.

If one considers the data incorporated from the parent to be the basis for many later judgments and admonitions, it is easy to accept Harris'[12] analogy of "tapes" being played and replayed throughout life. Accordingly, what a child incorporates into his conscience from his mother and father is recorded directly in his "parent" without benefit of elaboration from extenuating circumstances of which the youngster is not yet aware. Because details and justifications are often lacking, literal recordings indicating only that "big boys don't do that" or "it's a sin to eat the white part of the watermelon" or other equally ridiculous "principles" mingle with more rational, less judgmental teachings and standards to confuse and make inflexible the youngster's growing sense of right and wrong. The preschooler constantly records the dos and don'ts about black cats, clean hands, and idle minds. Recorded as *truth*, all such pronouncements can carry equal weight for the receiver who is unable to sift fact from fiction, reasonable rules from arbitrary ones.

Disharmony may exist among recordings and further confuse the developing conscience. Sometimes a parent instructs, "Don't cross the street in the middle of the block" but is observed to do so himself, or sometimes parents openly disagree about what constitutes right and wrong. Harris likens these instances to stereophonic recordings in which one track lacks harmony with the other; when played back, the dissonance is obvious and painful, and the messages are contradictory. The result is evidenced later in inconsistent persons who vacillate between right and wrong, strength and weakness. However, even though Erikson[13] also warns that one of life's deepest conflicts revolves around hating a parent found trying to transgress his own pronouncements while retaining the role of model, Harris is confident that people are capable of overcoming the maladjustments of childhood. This is a very important idea for adults who fear that child care is too heavy a responsibility.

Eriksonian Theory: Initiative and Intrusiveness
Conscience governs the child's struggle to develop a sense of initiative instead of a sense of guilt.[14] To develop initiative, on which his future ambitions are founded, a child requires opportunities to successfully resolve his own "crises." Fortunately the preschooler is endowed with an apparent excess of energy which permits him to attack problems anew as if ignoring any previous failures.

Intrusiveness, which Erikson[15] says also marks the preschool period, assists the growth of initiative by promoting increased goal-directed activity, including competition and conquest. Although his goals are desirable attainments, the intrusive child is also confronted by fantasy, which arouses a sense of guilt over the imagined commission of evil deeds.

The rigid conscience of the preschooler readily creates guilt feelings for real or imagined, secret or overt transgressions. Adults need to realize this in order to be prepared to intercept inflexible self-punishment and to deal with the inevitable dreams and nightmares growing out of the child's experiences with his conscience.

Body Image and Body Boundary Also integral to psychosocial development during the preschool period are the concepts of *body image* and *body boundary*. Body image is defined simply as a person's mental image of his own body.[16] Body boundary,[17] a closely related concept, is a person's perceived exterior body limit, the outer edge of his body image. As self-awareness develops in early childhood, and as the outside world of "not-me" becomes clearer in his mind, the child forms an increasingly accurate picture of his physical self and learns to differentiate his body from his environment. The body image is a changing, developing mental picture which adjusts in response to life experiences. From the physical sphere of experience, both sensation and mobility contribute to the formation of the body image. Interpersonal experiences likewise influence the body image, with the emphases the child observes others placing on their own body configurations and on his body helping to establish his image of himself. Finally, psychologic factors such as the person's attitudes toward his body and his interest in it strongly influence the body image.

The preschool child is renowned for his conspicuous concerns about his body and its intactness. The heightened interest in his genital apparatus, the vociferous protests and obvious anxiety with which he reacts to loss of body boundary intactness which occurs when he skins a knee or receives an injection, and the curiosity with which he regards people who have physical disfigurations are all earmarks of the intense body awareness characteristic of this developmental stage. Body image and body boundary concerns assume special importance in the case and understanding of the *ill* preschooler. Chapter 26 deals in detail with these considerations.

Socialization through Contacts Outside the Immediate Family

The preschooler becomes more and more a social being as his interests and environment expand. As the friendly but selfish 3-year-old, then as the noisy and somewhat less pleasant 4-year-old, and eventually as the sociable 5-year-old, the preschooler encounters a multitude of social experiences. Whether from the resolution of the oedipal situation, as some believe, or incidental to increasing physical mobility and verbal facility, he learns to meet and accept strangers of all ages.

Tentatively in the early days and with more confidence later, the preschooler learns to ease into social exchange and to accept brief separations from home and parents with a graciousness formerly unknown. Unexplained or misunderstood separation, however, may be interpreted as punishment for "bad" wishes or for earlier misconduct (now forgotten by the parent) and can consequently cause poor adjustment if undetected. Separation might also induce regression of varying degrees, normally temporary, even in the well-socialized youngster. Mahler's[18] studies of separation-individuation offer insights into this phenomenon. She relates that the most extreme separation reaction may be expected in children who have experienced too exclusive and too lengthy a symbiotic period with mothers who refused to acknowledge their growth toward independence.

Vocabulary and conversation skills play a big part in the preschooler's socialization. His well-known mild profanities and name-calling are an exercise of verbal aggression. He also talks incessantly and is a great mimic of overheard adult phrases and inflections. His questions become increasingly relevant, demanding reflective adult response. Especially in the earlier phase, the preschooler's conversation lacks clarity because he egocentrically expects the hearer to know and understand all the details lacking from his message.[19]

The child's imagination also assists in his interactions with others and in his learning about their reactions to him. The 4-year-old is particularly noted for his wildly imaginative tales which, often without total clarification even in his own mind, he presents as true. Through his dramatizations he holds the interest of others as he openly explores their responses to him and observes their opinions of what is likely to be factual and what is not.

Socialization through Fantasy and Play

To preschoolers, fantasy is as believable as reality. The child vacillates from fantasy to reality, with the two merging so that he separates them only with difficulty. This behavior produces both fortunate and unfortunate effects. Fantasy eases the hardships of everyday life, especially when the child may be exposed to experiences beyond his ability to cope. Unfortunately, fantasied misrepresentations and misinterpretations of the real world may be accompanied by terror. Preschool fantasy is not entirely fairy princesses and candy; in large measure it is evil monsters and punishment. The preschooler, after all, essentially *lives* in a fantasy because his egocentric and animistic view colors all that happens; this is one of the chief ways in which the two worlds of make-believe and reality become one for him. It also explains why reality-bound adults do not always respond with understanding to the child's other-world existence and his sometimes outlandish reports of it.

"All the world's a stage" for the preschooler more than for anyone else. Any object or being within his range may unknowingly become a prop for his current adventure. Blocks may become anything he desires; a cowboy hat sets an entire Western scene; Grandma's old clothes change several motley youngsters into the wedding party of the century (Fig. 12-6). Maturation from 3 to 6 years of age is reflected somewhat in more purposefully planned sequences of fantasy; the 5-year-old, for example, sets a stage and acquires realistic props for a fairly formalized production, but the 3-year-old more or less happens upon fantasy play.

Various kinds of diversions which interest preschoolers are included in Table 12-3. Each of the preschool years is characterized by the desire to experiment with new skills, whether riding a tricycle, dancing, matching pictures and forms, or completing simple number games. Dress-up and make-believe drama are favorite activities throughout the preschool period. Play and diversional activities can profitably be adapted to hospital situations to ease the preschooler's adjustment, which is readily threatened by disconcerting fantasies (see Chap. 26 for elaboration of this point).

COUNSELING PARENTS
Life and Its Origin

Discussing one of the most obvious aspects of human existence—life—somehow presents a stumbling block to adults who deal with young children. The preschooler is most curious about life, from

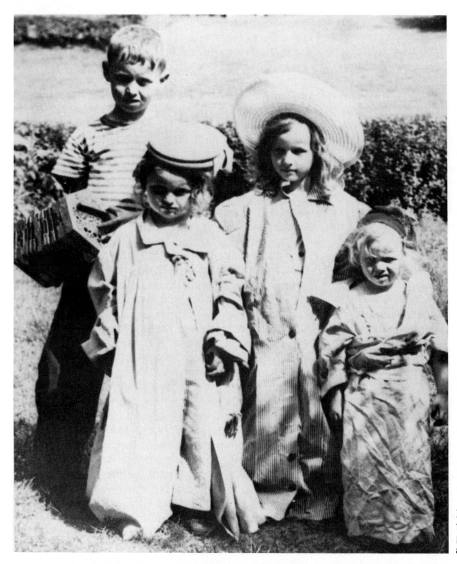

Figure 12-6 Dressing up is a favorite activity that helps the preschooler imagine himself in another world.

the tiniest form upward. Most of all, as his self-awareness grows, he becomes curious about himself and his genesis. His interest pervades numerous activities: he makes pets of ants, reaches to touch a caterpillar, pulls the cat's tail, peeks at his parents and siblings when they are dressing, and fondles his own genitalia. Searching for the mysteries of life, he inquires about the color of eyes, the role of ears, the need for a belly button, the quizzical thumping of his heart, and the strange experiences of elimination.

Eventually comes the inevitable question: "Where did I come from?" or "What was I before I was me?" or "How did I get borned?" Few adults relish the question because they cannot determine a "best" reply. Indeed, a reply is difficult, for the truth

may seem more unbelievable than fiction when heard from the preschooler's vantage! In answering his questions it is well to remember that the young child cannot retain all the details in one hearing and requires repetition. Hesitancy about the body, and about sex in particular, is easily communicated to a child even on a nonverbal level. Consequently, whether or not he has been given an accurate explanation of life and birth, he may deny and repress portions of his lesson and construct his own explanation to complete the gaps.

As part of the child's quest for life's mystery, he conducts personal research through physical exploration of self and playmates, usually to the distress of adults, who have forgotten or find little

Table 12-3 SOME FEATURES OF PRESCHOOL PERSONALITY, SOCIALIZATION, AND PLAY

Age	Psychosocial development	Diversion
3 years	Child in Erikson's stage of initiative vs. guilt (see description at age 4 years) Completes Mahler's subphase for object constancy; retains mental image of mother; more realistic about mother's good and bad qualities Develops concept of own identity and family Imitates others—boy exhibits penis as if to affirm body intactness Meets and accepts strangers Demonstrates much sexual curiosity; "masturbates"; knows his own sex Is jealous of sibling Is friendly, pleasing; alternates with periods of irritability, provocativeness	Participates in simple games Cooperates in play with others; takes turns; plays spontaneously with a group Enjoys reliving infancy through hearing stories Uses crayons and coloring book; plays "dress-up" Enjoys fire engine; rides tricycle; plays "house" Uses scissors and paper; likes materials he can practice "pouring"; enjoys books
4 years	Child in Erikson's initiative stage: adds to previously established autonomy the functions of undertaking, planning, and attacking tasks, very active and on the move Evidences intrusiveness by physical attack, aggressive talking, questioning, teasing Is exhibitionistic and bids for attention; noisy; less pleasant in a group Fabricates, exaggerates, boasts, and tattles; dramatizes experiences Has imaginary companion, often used to project blame for actions Is proud of accomplishments Volunteers to help group Is a keen observer Persists in sexual curiosity Has good sense of "mine" and "yours" Can perform simple errands Is more active with peers—success helps replenish depleted narcissism of former years	Stays with group activities longer Enjoys "dress-up" Participates in much dramatic play Enjoys drawing Likes to tell and hear stories Enjoys nail-pounding Engages in cooperative play with peers Takes opportunities to do things for self "Helps" adults Enjoys expressive materials for making things—clothespin dolls; pictures to sew; animals to stuff; paper chains Likes costumes Enjoys being read to Likes records; demonstrates rhythmic activity Participates well in organized, simple group play Shows creativity Likes scrapbooks
5 years	Child in Erikson's stage of initiative vs. guilt Has dreams and nightmares Is serious about self and abilities Is less rebellious Accepts responsibility for acts Glories in achievements Desires a companion Knows he is not serious when concocting tales; is generally truthful Is cooperative and sympathetic; generous with toys Evidences tension by nose-picking, nail-biting, whining, snuffling Is protective yet jealous of younger siblings and playmates Is relatively independent Regresses when first enters kindergarten, but adjustment is aided by this experience Asks searching questions Is interested in meaning of relatives	Plays with cars and trucks Plays war games Understands simple letter and number games Likes matching pictures and forms Demonstrates much gross motor activity Plays with mud, snow, leaves, rocks, stones, etc.

consolation in remembering their own curious childhood experiments. This type of learning can be used positively as a stepping-off point for explaining sex differences and for socializing the child to cultural and family standards of privacy. These may seem rather profound topics for discussion with one so young, but the preschool child is beginning to deal with fundamental truths and values which continue to be revised throughout the life-span.

It is important to remember that the preschooler

is not yet either moral or immoral. Morality develops later after the child has identified his self and established his social values. Cognizant of this fact, parents are advised to approach sex education on a rather neutral and forthright plane from the earliest days, perfecting their explanations as opportunities and the child's needs present themselves. One key may be to begin with a phenomenon familiar to the child and construct analogies; caution is prescribed, however, to de-emphasize pollination and other aspects of reproduction not duplicated in humans. All the while, it is imperative to realize the impact of attitudes and behavior observed by the child; words about respect for the beauty of life and its origins are empty if not confirmed in parental example.

Masturbation is a common preschool manifestation of developing self-awareness and is an often-used form of self-consolation for the hurts and distresses with which the young child has limited ways of coping. The difficulty associated with masturbation lies not in the child's curiosity or enjoyment, but in the moral implications of the adult's world and the associated adult guilt still unknown to the child. Guidance is necessary to protect the child and those about him from public embarrassment and discomfiture and to obviate arousal of the child's fantasies of guilt and self-mutilation.

Terminology for body parts offers one objective avenue to instruction related to the body and its functions. A parent never calls an arm, eye, or tongue by some "more neutral" term; the practice of devising an "acceptable" term for the genitals is unwise and tends to encourage attitudes of unacceptability toward genital and excretory matters.

Death

Another undeniable part of the human condition is mortality. Rather than attempting to explain death to preschoolers, many parents prefer to hide it. It is unnecessary and unfair to deny the child the experience of learning about death and the ways people react to it. This is not to say that death is simple to explain; it is in fact a difficult concept for young children to deal with cognitively and, because of its timing, is frequently fraught with emotion. Full human sharing requires sharing loss, and family life seems the appropriate place to learn this lesson. To deny one's own or a child's grief at the death of a favored person or pet is to imply that the loss causes no unhappiness and that the person or animal had no value. To so attempt to "protect" the child is to perform an injustice.

As with the beginnings of life, opportunities to help a child understand and deal with death present themselves subtly and often. Perhaps a crushed insect initiates his questioning. Flowers and trees also are observed to die, but since they return with each spring, they are not the best examples. In the child's magical mind it would be just as likely that a parent or pet could similarly return to life. (The preschooler equates death with separation, which he has learned is often temporary.)

A multitude of problems face parents who attempt to explain death to their child, not the least of which may be their own unresolved attitudes about dying and loss. Others include fear of arousing in the child anxiety about dying if ill, injured, or anorectic; reluctance to present God as an evil force that takes away that which the child desires; and fear that the child will protect himself from further loss by refusing to form close relationships.

Commonly the first test arises when a pet dies. Immediate parental response might be to substitute a similar animal before the child realizes his loss. This practice deceptively intimates that life is immortal and denies the child his opportunity for practice with the natural and inevitable experience of loss. Equally unwise is the immediate promise of, and acquisition of, a new pet to forestall the child's reaction. When this happens he is again denied a normal human need—to express a sense of loss. Later, when he has been helped to reconcile his loss, it is more appropriate to let the child participate in the decision of selecting a new pet.

Parents, siblings, grandparents, and friends die. When these realities occur they cannot and should not be concealed. Occasionally, in an attempt to comfort a child, an adult suggests that a new parent, sibling, etc., can be acquired to make up for the loss. This suggestion is obviously unwise. In addition to being unrealistic and disrespectful of both the child and the deceased, it may lead the child to infer that he too could be readily replaced in the affections of family and friends if he were to die.

Most families subscribe to some belief which conceives of life as continuing beyond its finite limits. For such families this belief provides a helpful basis for helping the child deal with death, especially when it promises eternal reward and offers hope of eventual reunion.

When a parent dies the explanation may be particularly difficult, but it must be given if only to preclude the child's fantasies about what might have happened. A preschool child may otherwise imagine that his own wishes or actions have caused the death or that the parent has voluntarily abandoned him. The following example illustrates how the death of a parent was explained to children in one hospital situation.

Two brothers, 4 and 5 years old, were hospitalized to recover from carbon monoxide intoxication. Their mother had been killed in the same accident; their father was suffering from mild toxicity compounded by his grief. Relatives milled around the children's beds, some rigid and some sobbing. When the grandmother learned that her daughter had died, she fainted at the doorway of the boy's hospital room. The boys watched silently and wide-eyed. The 5-year-old seemed especially desirous of an explanation but did not speak.

The father was aware that the boys must be informed, but he was too dazed to do it. A few days after admission, with the father and an aunt present (and with the father's permission), a nurse explained to the 5-year-old:

"We know you wonder where Mommy is and that you miss her. Daddy and Aunt Rosie miss her too. Well, Jimmy, when the gas made you and Toby sick, it also made Mommy so sick that she couldn't get better. Mommy can't come to see you and Toby because she was so sick—much sicker than you and Toby—and she died and went to heaven to be with God." The aunt was then able to participate in the explanation, emphasizing the family belief in heaven and eternal happiness. Later that day, the aunt was able to answer Toby's unasked questions, and Jimmy began to talk for the first time since admission—first about his games and then about his mother having been buried on the hill and being in heaven.

Discipline and Praise

Many uncertainties exist for the preschool child because of the increasing complexity of the demands placed on him by his expanding world and because of his developmental limitations in understanding and coping with those demands. His developmental propensity toward magical, prelogical thinking and his natural assertiveness and aggressiveness, combined with his mistaken ideas about why things happen, create a tendency to believe that wishing something can make it happen and that, furthermore, others' wishes (like his own) are sometimes hostile. As a consequence the preschool child can feel quite insecure. Good discipline does much to combat this insecurity.

The following guidelines are helpful to parents and other adults in relating to young children.

1 Discipline should be motivated by love and should have as its objective the child's long-range best interest.
2 Discipline should be consistent. Limits imposed upon the child's behavior must be consistent across time and among his disciplinarians. Discipline should also be consistent with the child's developmental level, so that disciplinary methods and expectations for his behavior are suited to his abilities and change as he matures. Without unnecessarily departing from the goal of consistency, it is appropriate to consider mitigating circumstances, such as unusual fatigue or periods of special stress.

The best discipline is that which is also consistent with the nature of the child's infraction. A child who abuses others' property may be forbidden to use it for a time, for example, or one who takes intolerable risks with a particular piece of playground equipment in spite of instruction may be restricted from using it.

Since the objective of discipline is to teach the child safe and socially acceptable ways of operating within his environment, discipline also needs to be consistent with the standards expected by his family and by the larger sociocultural setting in which he must operate successfully.
3 The child should know why he is being disciplined and should be helped to identify acceptable alternatives to his misbehavior. Unexplained or misperceived discipline misses its target and may engender hostility and retaliation.
4 Ineffective measures should be corrected. Repeating discipline which has been unsuccessful only frustrates both child and adult and can damage the self-concept of both as well as their appraisals of one another's competence.
5 The parent or other disciplinarian should understand his motivations in the disciplinary situation and try not to punish while angry.
6 Discipline should be limited to hazardous activities affecting the physical, emotional, or social well-being of the child.

Some people believe and others disagree that the undesirable *act, not* the child, should be disapproved and that the child should continue to be assured of his parent's unconditional love. To discipline a broken egg for having been smashed[20] is obviously not sensible, but neither is an uncontrolled verbal or physical attack against the child who broke it.[21] The child's self-worth must always be considered, but there is no more appropriate place to learn honest emotion and its expression—anger as well as love—than in the home. It may be meaningless and dishonest to discipline without admitting one's justified and controlled anger. On the other hand, discipline which permanently lowers self-esteem or causes a neurotic avoidance of pleasurable activities also severely limits the growing person. An aura of punitiveness or deprivation is *not* synonymous with discipline, but neither is the false pretense that nothing jeopardizes parental love.

The effectively disciplined child escapes not

only much insecurity but also unnecessary health hazards and social retribution. Good discipline fosters respect, not fear, of parents and of societal standards and safety regulations. In time, the well-disciplined child develops a functional level of *self*-control.

Good behavior deserves at least as much attention as misbehavior; its reinforcement is desirable and can be effected by favorable response directed toward the child's deeds. Preschoolers enjoy pleasing others, but their rigid self-expectations often cause them to distrust anyone who insists on praising their lesser attempts. It can also frustrate the preschooler to be repeatedly told he is "good" when he knows he has entertained "evil" wishes. As with discipline, then, praise is necessary to the growing child but ought to be offered thoughtfully and purposefully.

Health Needs

With the continual development of his body and his world, the preschooler is exposed repeatedly to numerous demands on his health and adjustment. Table 12-4 is presented to summarize some of the more evident health and developmental needs of the preschooler and to offer suggestions for care to maintain him in optimum condition.

REFERENCES

1 J. DiLeo, *Young Children and Their Drawings*, Brunner/Mazel, Inc., New York, 1970, pp. 28–50.
2 Ibid., p. 35.
3 A. Gesell et al., *The First Five Years of Life*, Harper & Row, Publishers, Incorporated, New York, 1940, pp. 138–169.
4 J. Piaget, *The Language and Thought of the Child*, Humanities Press, Inc., New York, 1926.
5 Gesell et al., op. cit., pp. 189–237.
6 R. I. Watson, *Psychology of the Child*, 2d ed., John Wiley & Sons, Inc., New York, 1965, pp. 321–333.
7 J. Piaget, *The Child's Conception of the World* (trans., by Joan and Andrew Tomlinson), Littlefield, Adams & Company, Totowa, N.J., 1969.
8 C. S. Hall and G. Lindzey, "The Relevance of Freudian Psychology and Related Viewpoints for the Social Sciences," in G. Lindzey and E. Aronson (eds.), *The Handbook of Social Psychology*, vol I, Addison-Wesley Publishing Co., Inc., Reading, Mass., 1968, pp. 245–319.
9 Irene Josselyn, *Psychosocial Development of Children*, Family Service Association of America, New York, 1969, pp. 64–74.
10 Selma H. Fraiberg, *The Magic Years*, Charles Scribner's Sons, New York, 1959, pp. 227–241.

Table 12-4 SUMMARY OF SOME MEASURES TO MEET THE PRESCHOOLER'S HEALTH AND DEVELOPMENTAL NEEDS

Age	Cues for adults	Health needs
3 years	Child responds better to suggestions than commands Handle fears at child's own pace (may fear animals, dark); explain at his level of understanding; encourage creativity; begin religious education Provide items he can "own" Understand pros and cons of thumbsucking Allow participation in self-care	Begin dental exams if not already begun Encourage a daily nap Have child tested for TB Provide good nutrition (child needs approximately 1,250 cal/day); include all food groups; give nutritious snacks, limit concentrated sweets; provide good example of nutritional habits
4 years	Base expectations within child's limitations Assist coping by providing limited frustrations from environment Maintain a calm, responsible attitude toward masturbation Provide opportunities for brief, nonthreatening separations from home and parents Prevent accidents (common causes: motor vehicles, drowning, fire, firearms, falling objects)	Provide professional health supervision every 6–12 mo Provide dental care—caries prevention and treatment Meet the total sleep need of about 12 hr, including nap Have child tested for TB Provide good nutrition (child needs approximately 1,400 cal/day) Serve regular meals; let child help plan meals
5 years	Provide reassurance and guidance in adjusting to group needs; allow self-care; may have toileting "accidents" because of other interests Prevent accidents as at age 4 Observe for prodromal symptoms of communicable diseases and seek medical advice Limit group contacts during epidemic period	Child should receive communicable disease immunization (DPT, OPV boosters); have child tested for TB Provide good nutrition (child needs approximately 1,600 cal/day)

11 Ibid., pp. 223–227.
12 T. A. Harris, *I'm OK, You're OK*, Harper & Row, Publishers, Incorporated, New York, 1969.
13 E. H. Erikson, *Childhood and Society*, 2d ed., W. W. Norton & Company, Inc., New York, 1963, p. 257.
14 E. H. Erikson, *Identity, Youth and Crisis*, W. W. Norton & Company, Inc., New York, 1968, p. 119.
15 Ibid., p. 116.
16 P. Schilder, *The Image and Appearance of the Human Body*, John Wiley & Sons, Inc., New York, 1950.
17 S. Fisher and S. E. Cleveland, *Body Image and Personality*, D. Van Nostrand Company, Inc., Princeton, N.J., 1958, p. 363.
18 Margaret S. Mahler in Collaboration with Manuel Furer, *Infantile Psychosis*, Vol. I, *Human Symbiosis and the Vicissitudes of Individuation*, International Universities Press, Inc., New York, 1968, p. 225.
19 J. Piaget, "Communication between Children" in Wayne Dennis (ed.), *Readings in Child Psychology*, Prentice-Hall, Inc., Englewood Cliffs, N.J., 1963, pp. 213–214.
20 Fraiberg, op. cit., p. 249.
21 H. G. Ginott, *Between Parent and Child*, Avon Book Division, The Hearst Corporation, New York, 1965, p. 112.

13

THE SCHOOL-AGE CHILD— 6 TO 12 YEARS

JERRY J. BIGNER

DEVELOPMENTAL TRENDS IN MIDDLE CHILDHOOD

Growth and development during the ages of 6 to 12 years reflect changes that are indicative of what has occurred previously during the preschool years and what will transpire in adolescence. The rapid physical growth rates of early childhood become slower and more even during the middle childhood years. Sex differences in almost every facet of development become much more obvious to the observer and to the child as well. The middle years are a time of psychologic tension between conflicting desires to attain adult status and to retain the prerogatives and privileges of childhood. During these years the culture of childhood is developed through games, contacts with peers, relationships with family members, and the environment of the school. It is a time for the child's active discovery of what the world is all about, while being positive that the world "is his oyster." Middle childhood is a period when making things and the process of making and building with friends are all-important. It is a time for testing limits and challenging established authority, both in the home and in the community, as a part of the process of self-discovery. The middle years serve the purpose of greater refinement, differentiation, and articulation of developmental trends that were evident during the early years, and they set the stage for further development in the years of adolescence.

AGE-SPECIFIC CHARACTERISTICS

Although professionals have reacted somewhat negatively in the past to describing the growth and development of children by particular age groups, it seems that much can be learned by becoming acquainted with the general expectations for growth and development that are evident in year-by-year normative descriptions. Individual differences between one child and another can be very noticeable, as critics of age profiles have suggested. However, the fact remains that norms are valuable in showing the organization and trends in development that are typical of the group as a whole.

Each of these descriptions is rather general and somewhat idealistic. It should be remembered that norms are only guides to the behavioral and developmental highlights that illustrate the cyclic nature of the age period from 6 to 12 years. These descriptions also aid the observer of child behavior in evaluating whether certain events are age-specific and appropriate or due to individual differences, or whether a physical or psychosocial pathologic condition is present. No particular child will fit the norms in all aspects.

It is helpful for the professional observer of child growth and development to remember that there can be no growth without conflict, as Elkind[1] has suggested. To illustrate this point, Gesell and Ilg[2] have shown that there is a high correlation between *periods of rapid growth* and *periods of disruption of established behavior patterns*. This correlation is presented graphically in Figure 13-1. The letters A through F pinpoint the ages of childhood investigated, and point A is repeated on the right side of the graph to reestablish the cycle of growth. Where the curve is straight and smooth, the growth of the child is proceeding at a relatively slow rate. Curves in the line illustrate periods of growth. More twists in the curves indicate that more rapid growth is taking place. This graphic illustration of growth rates should be referred to when studying the following age-specific characteristics of middle childhood.

The Six-Year-Old

The 6-year-old child can be described generally as having a high activity level. He enjoys a great deal of boisterous play and verbal aggression. He is constantly in motion, assertive, bossy, and opinionated. The 6-year-old still retains some of the characteristic behavior learned during his earlier years in that he continues to dawdle at many activities, particularly if those in authority are in a hurry. He is very capable of giving his authority figures a hard time by being argumentative, whiny, and a know-it-all. He is the center of his universe and has difficulty empathizing with the views and responsibilities of others. He wants to have his own way immediately and becomes disturbed with adults when his needs and wishes do not receive priority attention.

The 6-year-old is very involved in discovering both his self and his world. He is interested in playing simple games that have rules with other children or adults. Lottos and other matching games intrigue him. Making things from pliable and solid materials are high on his list of preferred activities. His large muscle coordination is far ahead of his fine muscle abilities, and he enjoys running, climbing, hopping, jumping, skipping, and other active pursuits. He has a positive attitude toward his world and those who populate it. He is proud of what accomplishments he can make both individually and within a group. While he is beginning to discover the value of friends, his frustration level and attention span have yet to be developed enough to allow him to continue alone at any particular activity for a long period of time. A major problem of the 6-year-old in relating to others through play activities is his inability to know when to stop before getting hurt, psychologically or physically. A child of this age will, on the other hand, leave a game or activity in which it is probable that he will lose. His contacts with friends are limited and erratic, although many children will have cultivated a "best" friend. While he plays well with children of the opposite sex, some evidence is beginning to show of the sex cleavage, or preference for his own sex as playmates.

Overall, the 6-year-old is characterized as egocentric, active, outgoing, charming, opinionated, and boisterous. His egocentrism is offset by his lack of vanity. To many, his halo is tarnished, yet he retains an innocence and naïveté that makes him a joy to behold.

The Seven-Year-Old

The 7-year-old differs considerably from the 6-year-old in his seriousness and in his approach to the world. Children at this age have been described as quiet and reflective. It is thought that the 7-year-old is concerned with accommodating the experiences he assimilated during his previous year.[1] The 6-year-

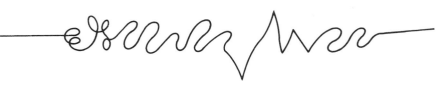

Figure 13-1 Wave of growth. *(Adapted from A. L. Gesell and F. L. Ilg, The Child from Five to Ten, Harper & Row, Publishers, Incorporated, New York, 1946.)*

	A	B	C		D	E	F		A
Age	2	2½	3		3½	4	4½		
	5	5½	6		7	8	9		
	10	11	12		13	14	15		

old was described actively investigating and discovering the world, while the 7-year-old is typically concerned with consolidating these experiences into a meaningful whole. Likewise, while the 6-year-old is physically vigorous and motor-oriented, the 7-year-old's activities become increasingly cognitive. Children of this age are growing in self-awareness and, in turn, are increasingly aware of others in their social environment. Accompanying this greater social awareness is a developing sensitivity of their actions toward others and of the reactions that others elicit from them.

The increased differentiation between self and others is evident in the concern that these children have about their bodies. The 7-year-old is characteristically shy or ashamed of his body and of the bodily changes that are occurring. Many children have entered into an "ugly duckling" stage at this time of their lives, with the absence or snaggled appearance of teeth as well as changes in hair texture and body proportion. For this reason, it is generally thought that the 7-year-old does not like to touch or be touched by others.

The enhanced sensitivity to others is manifested by a reluctance to expose himself to failure or to self-effacing situations. Criticism and teasing are tolerated very poorly by the 7-year-old child, and he frequently complains of being treated unfairly or unkindly by those he likes and admires. Very sensitive about the way he is treated by others, the child of this age is unusually polite and courteous toward adults and desires to please others in authority by cooperating with their wishes.

The 7-year-old has discovered the fun of school and of learning with others. His enhanced sensitivity to his social environment is manifested in an increased concern with what his teacher thinks of him, and he begins to see the teacher as a guide for intellectual activities. He is becoming more aware of being evaluated by those in authority, and his eagerness to please is shown in his more persistent work habits and the care that is taken in his productions. He shows a desire to play more cooperatively with his peers. Many children of this age come to regard books as friends and become interested in reading all types of stories, including the all-time favorite, comic books.

In summary, the 7-year-old is a more serious child than the 6-year-old. He is an insightful youngster who is attempting to accommodate experiences gained earlier in the world while becoming more cognizant of himself and others as social beings.

The Eight-Year-Old

The 8-year-old is an expansive, active, and gregarious child. Apparently, the time spent during the seventh year is only a reflective pause in the development trends of middle childhood, for during the eighth year the child approaches his world with vigor and a sense of well-being.

The 8-year-old may be termed a mature 4-year-old in his expansive attitude, mood, and approach toward life. However, an additional new characteristic is the pragmatic nature of the 8-year-old. He has an opinion on everything and advice for everyone. He is defensive and sometimes resentful of open evaluations of his character and behavior that are made by teachers, parents, and older siblings. Unlike the 6-year-old, the child of 8 is eager to learn the "why and wherefore" of the world about him, and he begins to be able to judge and appraise why things occur in the world in relation to himself.

The enormous curiosity of the 8-year-old is a characteristic that impresses most observers of this age period (Fig. 13-2). He is curious about everything and everyone with whom he comes into contact. This curiosity and his increasing ability to classify environmental objects and events are reflected in the phenomenon of collecting. His collections may include classifications of rocks, stamps, dolls, coins, or almost anything. In line with his phenomenal affinity for collecting objects is the development of the fine art of bartering for the purpose of increasing or refining his particular assets.

His curiosity about the world includes those who populate his social environment. He is anxiously attentive to adult conversations and can become extremely curious and eager to observe adult social activities. He is equally gregarious in his relations with others of his age. However, he now prefers the company of his own sex in play activities (Fig. 13-3). The relations between the sexes are of a "love-hate" nature that combines hostility with attraction. Boys thoroughly enjoy teasing girls, and while not eager to show their appreciation, girls do notice these activities.

During this period children begin to realize that parents are mere humans with shortcomings and lack the ability to be 100 percent right on every issue. The 8-year-old becomes somewhat self-righteous and dogmatic in insisting upon performing only those chores that he considers worthy of his time and effort. These jobs are the more mature, responsible tasks such as mowing the lawn, repairing items,

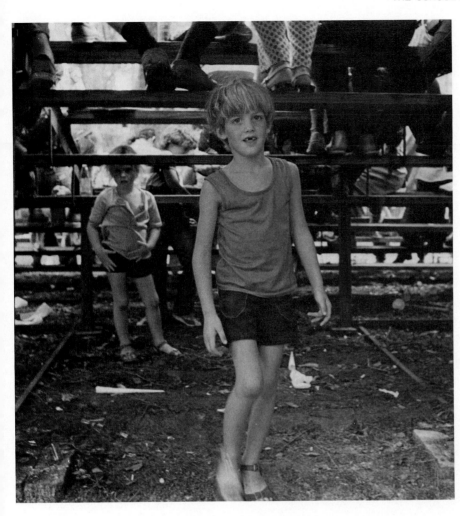

Figure 13-2 The school-age child's excitement over the world of people, things, relationships, and events, combined with his increasing freedom from parental supervision, leads him to new places and new experiences which are more likely to be shared with peers and siblings rather than with adults. *(Photo courtesy of George Lazar.)*

and cooking. When asking the 8-year-old to do something he considers beneath his dignity, parents quickly learn to expect grumbles and gripes from an otherwise cooperative child.

School is approached as a social activity now rather than an academic endeavor. It is a place where the child meets his friends, enjoys gossip about his playmates and teachers, thrills in passing notes in class, and dares to throw a spitball when the teacher does not seem to be looking. It is at this time, as well, that he learns about the teacher's innate ability to see these forbidden activities with the proverbial eyes in the back of her head.

To summarize, the 8-year-old is curious about the world, particularly the world of adults. He is ambivalent about growing up, and this attitude is reflected in his critical and dogmatic attitudes to-

ward adult authority and toward his position in the social order. His friends are now increasing in importance over the family as significant others to guide his behavior. He is a gregarious child who is eager to cooperate and learn, but only on his own conditions.

The Nine-Year-Old

Development during the ninth year shows greater refinement in behavior and conspicuous strides toward maturity. The self-confidence that emerged during the eighth year expands, perhaps because of increased involvement with peers and organizations that cater to the interests of children of this age. Parents come to the conclusion that they surely must be chauffeurs for their children in helping them meet what sometimes seem to be exhaustive social

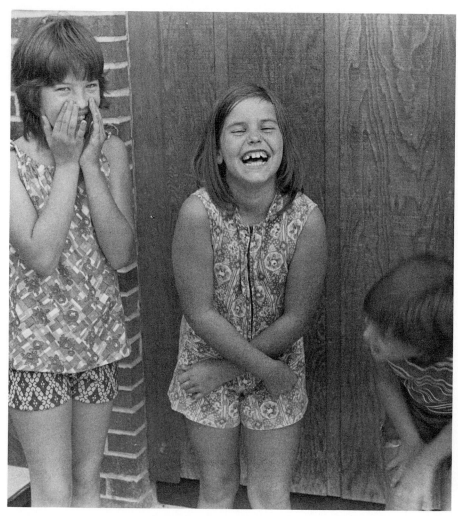

Figure 13-3 From the early school-age period through puberty, children in our culture electively segregate themselves into groups of the same sex. *(Photo courtesy of George Lazar.)*

schedules. Children of this age are particularly interested in group activities as well as those that develop individual abilities, including scouting and athletic groups and numberless lessons in music, art, dancing, judo, swimming, etc. Many children during this year eventually specialize in one main activity and become so inner-directed in perfecting or enjoying that activity that all sense of time is lost, meals are missed, and chores go undone.

The new self-confidence and maturity of the 9-year-old is seen in his ability to recognize his own faults and weaknesses as well as being able to accept blame for his actions. The tendency of the 9-year-old to make self-effacing remarks often disturbs parents and teachers. These remarks are in line with his new ability to differentiate himself from others and to accept responsibility for his own actions.

There is an increased awareness of sexuality and of appropriate sex-role behavior. Friendships are still determined on the basis of sex of the playmate, and close intimate bonds are often established between two or more children. Girls discover an interest in clothes, a fastidious appearance, and fashion, while boys are somewhat disdainful of cleanliness and of what they wear. The peer group lends its own special flavor of competitiveness to school as well as to play activities. Peers are useful for their evaluative purposes in determining how well a child stands in comparison with another. Good, not excellent, grades are the standard for achievement, and children who are exceptionally bright or slow can easily become social outcasts because of the group's inability to cope with them.

The 9-year-old, then, is a child who discovers a

new maturity, confidence, and independence from authority figures. He becomes more inner-directed and self-directed in his activities and is motivated more by his own interests than by obligations. He is a child who appears to have a solid base from which to grow in the next years.

The Ten-Year-Old

Growth and development through a decade of stormy conflicts and adaptations culminate in a plateau for the 10-year-old child. Elkind[1] has described this state in the tenth year as a *halcyon* period in human development, that is, a time when the child is at peace with himself and his world. It appears that the 10-year-old is in love with himself and the world, and this inner contentment results in a general feeling of well-being and satisfaction that generalizes to his relations with others. The 10-year-old is very peer-oriented, and this is an age when organized activities are especially preferred. It is a time when children discover the need to guard their secrets among friends their own age. "Secret" clubs are formed, with rigid rules of membership and conduct. Conformity to group principles and values is given great importance. Secret languages, codes, and gestures are formed for the exclusive use of the group members. Ostracism of those who fail to conform is standard procedure. Such activities are suggestive of the 10-year-old's desire to belong and to seek an identity of his own through association with his peers. His fascination with adventure is reflected by a strong interest in mystery and detective stories and television and movies.

Sex differences among 10-year-olds are prominent. Some girls begin the prepubertal growth spurt in this year. They show a rapid increase in height and weight, resulting in the "towering Amazon" appearance in comparison with boys of the same age. Girls who experience such rapid growth and accompanying secondary sexual development appear to become sensitive and concerned about their bodies, menstruation, and sexual matters in general.

The 10-year-old is generally characterized as a happy, cooperative, casual, and relaxed child who is congenial in his relations with others, affectionate in his relations with parents and family, and intense in his loyalty to peers. Because of his increasing ability to use logic and reasoning, many adults find that they relate best to children of this age. Perhaps it is because they realize that the tenth year is but the calm before the storm that will occur in the eleventh year.

The Eleven-Year-Old

Some adults say that they will go to great lengths to avoid working with a group of 11-year-olds. Such an attitude toward a particular age of childhood may appear to be extreme, but it is very understandable. The 11-year-old is typically critical of adults, especially of those in authority. He rebels at performing established routines, is moody, and resents being instructed to perform any particular task. Eleven-year-old children often strive for unreasonable independence from adult control. This desire is evident in "hero worship," cravings for being left alone, a strong urge to conform to peer group norms of behavior, and an intense interest in team or group efforts and activities.

Relations with peers become more intense during this year. Organized, competitive games become the vogue, and membership in clubs and community activities becomes crucial. Failure to be accepted by peers can be crushing for some children. Girls may "discover" boys at this age and become preoccupied with getting their attention. Boys begin to show an interest in girls as well and reciprocate the girls' interest by showing off, teasing, and going to great lengths to be daring.

Children of this age are generally interested in religion, earning money, and future vocational aspirations. Their highly moralistic approach to events and people is manifested in outright verbal attacks on what seem to them to be great injustices. Sometimes a rather fleeting paranoid attitude develops in an 11-year-old child, expressed by phrases that are commonly heard in adolescence: for example, "I can't ever do anything right! People are always picking on me!"

Much of the conflict and stormy behavior of 11-year-olds is thought to be due to pressures produced by the rapidly increasing growth rates during this year. Coupled with the rapid growth rates is the desire for independence and a renewed interest in self-identity and definition. The eleventh year heralds adolescence and perhaps indicates what parents and other adults should expect in the manner of wide swings in mood and temperament, questioning of established routines and rules, and the striving for autonomy and self-knowledge.

PHYSICAL MATURATION IN MIDDLE CHILDHOOD

The growth patterns of infancy and early childhood advanced far more rapidly than the growth that takes place between the ages of 6 and 12, which is less dramatic and slower than at any other time in the growth period. What *is* dramatic about growth during these years is the pattern of rapid spurts in height and weight which produce concomitant changes in the proportions of the body and in anatomic structures. During this period the pronounced rapid spurts and decrements in the rate of growth appear to follow a cyclic pattern.

The most pronounced growth spurt of middle childhood occurs toward the end of that period. The very rapid increases in weight and height during the tenth and eleventh years are closely related to approaching sexual maturity. In girls, sexual maturity is associated with the *menarche*, or first menstrual period, and the beginning appearance of the secondary sexual characteristics. In boys, this rapid period of growth closely parallels increases in penile and testicular size. Weight gains during this time are less regular than height gains. Boys continue to remain heavier than girls until the ninth or tenth year when girls catch up and overtake boys because of the growth spurt which precedes menarche. Girls begin attainment of sexual maturity roughly 2 to 3 years before boys. Physical development in preadolescence is described more fully in Chapter 14.

There appears to be little difference in body contour and proportion between boys and girls in the early years of middle childhood. Three types of body configuration, which are indicative of three stages of maturity, have been identified for the middle childhood period in attempting to provide some assessment of school readiness.[3] The characteristic "pot belly" of early childhood is lost during the middle years with a general slimming of the figure of both boys and girls. Toward adolescence, the appearance of secondary sexual characteristics in girls precedes that of boys and results in a more typically feminine, rounded figure. Maturity of the body configuration is thought to be associated with achievement in the first grade, and immaturity of the configuration with failure (see Fig. 13-4).

Physical maturity, however, isn't correlated or associated well with social maturity. The case of the early maturing child is an excellent example. It is somewhat paradoxic that an 8-year-old child who has the appearance of an 11-year-old *acts* like an 8-year-old. His size belies his age, but his behavior does not. There is a great deal of controversy surrounding the issue of the relation between body image, body build, and development of the self-concept. There is little question, however, that people react differently to others of different *somatotypes*. For example, it has been reported that boys as early as 8 years of age exhibit clear-cut, stereotyped

conceptions of behavior characteristics associated with particular body builds.[4] The *mesomorph*, or strongly muscular body build, is perceived and reacted to most favorably, in comparison to the *endomorph* (skinny body type) and *ectomorph* (heavily fatted body type). If these boys' reactions were indicative of attitudes held by others of their age and older, and if the reactions of one's peers have an effect on the development of the self-concept, then it follows that the body image and body build a child possesses will somehow influence how he feels about himself and how he will relate to others.

COGNITIVE DEVELOPMENT

The school-age child approaches the world in a manner that is characteristically different from that of a preschool child. The preschooler is inevitably bound to his rigid *egocentricity* in perceiving, assimilating, and accommodating to information gathering. The school-age child, by contrast, is characterized by his flexibility in thought and can delay in response until he has taken several alternatives into consideration. Continuity in cognitive development is present in middle childhood as it was in earlier years but differs in the school-age child's ability to be reflective, his greater storage of memories to rely upon, and a greater command of language. The school-age child's flexibility of thought is reflected in his increasing abilities to classify, group, deal with several parts of a whole, and understand that there are invariant elements of the physical and psychologic environments. However, his thinking is limited in a manner analogous to that of the preschool child in that he continues to respond to events and problems in concrete rather than abstract terms.

Piaget[5] refers to this stage of cognition during the middle years as the period of *concrete operations*. By the time a child reaches school age, he can understand and use certain principles of relationships between events, things, and objects. In using and comprehending these relationships, he operates with objects, symbols, and concepts. He now is able to internalize. He can add and subtract, classify and order, apply rules of logic to reach conclusions, and apply rules to his conduct. He becomes system-oriented in learning that certain operations result in addition, for example, while other operations result in subtraction. He is now able to use imagery to perform mentally certain actions that were performed physically in the past.

The application of operations is seen first in the

child's preoccupation with learning to group and to classify. The school-age child develops the ability to think about parts and the whole independently. For example, if a 4-year-old is given a box of wooden beads with more brown beads than white and asked, "Are there more brown beads or more wooden beads?" he responds that there are more brown beads. He is unable at this time in his development to deal simultaneously with two separate concepts, such as color and type of material. The child who is in the concrete operations period is able to comprehend that an object can be classified in two or more ways simultaneously, and the question would appear to be senseless to him.

The preoccupation with classification is evident in the collections that are loved and cherished by children during this period of their life. The collections that are begun by school-age children are numerous and varied and can range from the more common stamp, coin, and doll collections to pine cones, bubble gum wrappers, and bottle caps. At first, there is the collection and classification of anything and everything, but as a child grows older and has broader experiences with his environment, his collections begin to become more specialized. Specialization of interest is thought to be due to the child's ability to recognize more complex systems of classification. Refinement in object sorting is shown in the results of testing at various age levels from kindergarten to adulthood.[6]

Two other major cognitive events occurring during middle childhood are the attainment of understanding of *conservation* (of mass and volume, for example) and the awareness of *reversibility*. These cognitive phenomena are discussed in Chapter 7.

Cognitive Limitations

Like preschoolers, school-age children suffer from limitations in their cognitive approaches to the world. The preschooler is bound by his egocentric perceptions and point of view, while the school-age child is confined by his own hypotheses and assumptions about the world. After forming such hypotheses and assumptions, they then search for evidence to support their thoughts while disregarding evidence to the contrary. Such an approach results in what Elkind[7] has termed *cognitive conceit*. It will be remembered that during middle childhood children discover that parents are not entirely right all the time. This discovery leads to the conclusion that, therefore, the parent is wrong a good deal of the time, and his credibility is breached. Likewise, if a child learns that he is right on one matter, then it

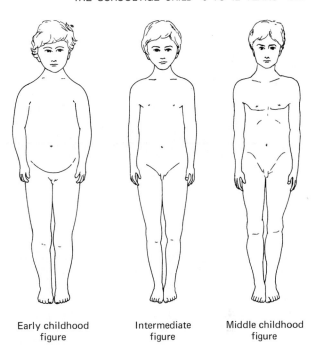

Early childhood figure Intermediate figure Middle childhood figure

Figure 13-4 Three types of body configuration observed in middle childhood. *(Reproduced with permission of Maria Simon and The Society for Research in Child Development; from Maria Simon, "Body Configuration and School Readiness," Child Development, 30:496, 1959.)*

only follows from his logic that he is right on all matters. It is possible that cognitive conceit may account for some of the negative feelings about growing up that 10- and 11-year-olds demonstrate.

PSYCHOSOCIAL DEVELOPMENT

As described in Chapter 7, Erikson's[8] presentation of the eight stages of man focused on the middle childhood years as a time when children are presented with the challenge to develop a *sense of industry vs. inferiority*. The major theme of this period of psychosocial development is the child's determination to master what he is doing. Great efforts are placed on producing, and there is the ever-present fear of not being able to do or produce enough. The child's fear of inferiority is founded on his knowledge that he is still a child and an incomplete person who lacks the abilities to compete successfully in the adult-oriented world. As a consequence of these feelings, there is an ambivalence about growing up. On the one hand, the child aspires to having the responsibilities and privileges of the adult world (Fig. 13-5), yet he wishes to retain the prerogatives of childhood.

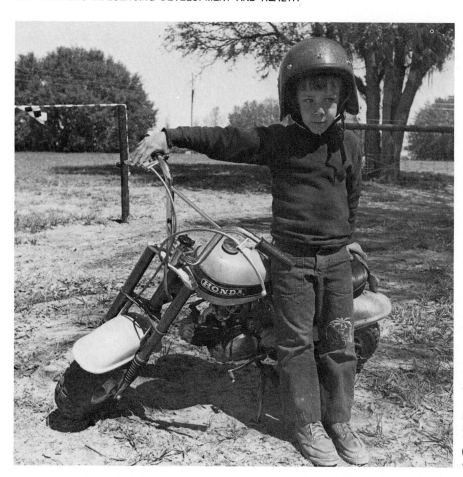

Figure 13-5 The wish to participate in "adult" activities is not new in the school-age period but becomes more possible to realize because of the child's developing abilities. *(Photo courtesy of George Lazar.)*

Peer Group Influences

The school-age child, then, finds himself to be a member of two worlds: that of adults and that of his peers. As he grows older through this period, he begins to invest a great deal of effort in his capacity to relate and communicate with the people who are most significant to him outside his family—his peers. He strives for accomplishment of something well done, of being the strongest, the best, or the wittiest among those of his own age and abilities.

While the family is the primary agent of socialization, the peer group aids the child in the socialization process by performing various functions that include (1) teaching the child how to get along with others, that is, how to persuade, cooperate, and compromise; (2) reinforcing appropriate sex-role behaviors; (3) assisting in the acquisition of values and attitudes such as fairness, sharing, taking turns, etc.; (4) teaching and encouraging fair play through com-

petitive efforts; and (5) aiding in the development of the child's self-concept and his attainment of autonomy.

Acceptance into the peer group is sometimes determined on a pass-fail basis. Children are judged by others of their age on the impression, skills, and abilities that they convey of themselves to the group. In the areas of skills and abilities, it appears that more intelligent and creative children are more readily accepted by their peers than slow learners and less adept children. Body size, muscular strength, and athletic ability appear to be criteria of acceptability among boys, whereas developmental maturity is associated with prestige among girls.

The social class of a child and his cultural heritage and traditions affect his relations with peers. Evidence suggests that substantially different patterns of peer relations exist among middle- and lower-class children.[9] Social class of the parents will affect peer relations accordingly, in that the family influences whom the child has contact with during this age period. Hollingshead[10] has shown that school-age children's group membership tends to be homogeneous within social classes. Furthermore, children appear to discriminate peer group membership on the basis of race and economic status of the family in which the child is a member.[11] As American social patterns change with time, these childhood friendship patterns probably are also changing.

One of the most important functions of the peer group is to help the child to form a picture of his own identity as a social person. Early in his group experiences, the child learns that his peers place him in a certain position on the social hierarchy and into particular roles. As he grows older, he becomes more proficient in interpreting his status in the eyes of other children. It has been found that high status in the group builds a positive self-concept in children, while lack of status and security results in unpopularity, dissatisfaction with self, and lack of self-esteem.[12] However, there is no conclusive evidence that peer acceptance is causally determined by the degree of a child's self-esteem.

Parental Influences

Relationships within the home environment have a profound influence on the development of children. Within the family are the primary forces that shape the personalities, values, norms of behavior, philosophy, and life goals of children.

As a child moves up the developmental ladder, changes in his needs and in his responses to these needs effect a corresponding shift in his parents' modes of response. Parents soon learn, for example, that they must change from being a physical helper of children to being a psychologic helper. This shift on the part of parents is prompted in numerous ways by their children. The striving for autonomy in the early years of childhood elicits entirely different patterns of parental caretaking than are called for in helping children to develop a sense of industry. Entrance into school often brings the realization for the child as well as the parents that the child is progressively growing up and taking on more adult responsibilities. It is with this event, then, that parental expectations for children become more sharply focused than ever. Parents now become greatly concerned with the child's achievement, moral development, and outlook on life, and with equipping him to cope with adult responsibilities. These adult standards of behavior as expressed by parents are acquired by *observation learning*, that is,

listening and watching the behavior and expressions of the parents, as well as by direct precept.

The influence of observation learning is well illustrated in the acquisition of sex-role identity. Freudian theory heavily emphasizes the school-age period as a *latency* stage in the psychosexual development of children. According to the theory, this is when children actively engage in pursuits that lead toward mastery of basic personality processes, such as sex-role identification. Identification with parents, and hence adoption of adult sex roles, has been explained in relation to the learning of behaviors, attitudes, and expectations involved in the *instrumental* and *expressive* roles played by the father and mother, respectively.[13] A child in an intact family (both mother and father present) has the opportunity to observe and imitate, consciously and unconsciously, these roles of the mother and father. In the typical family, the mother plays the expressive role primarily. Such a role involves sensitivity to others' feelings, being concerned with the welfare of others, being the peacemaker in resolving conflicts, and having the primary responsibility of emotional support and care of children. The father carries the responsibility of playing both expressive and instrumental roles. In addition to the behaviors and attitudes associated with expressiveness are those which involve the settling of disputes and conflicts, handling major disciplinary matters, and assuming the authority to make major decisions for the family as a whole.

It is the father, apparently, who plays an important part in ensuring that children acquire the behaviors and attitudes that society deems appropriate for their sex. The father represents the realities and expectations of the larger world to his children, and it is during the school-age period that the father assumes a greater impact on his children as they begin to loosen the close maternal ties that were established in earlier years. The father holds different expectations for his sons than for his daughters.[14] He tends to react expressively with his daughters in reinforcing and encouraging their feminine characteristics, while being more demanding with his sons and pressuring them to adopt characteristics which will conform with the expectations of what the world terms masculine behavior and attitudes.

While there is relatively little empirical information on the global effects of fathering, it appears that sex-role identification in boys is particularly facilitated by a warm, rewarding, nurturant father who openly expresses interest in his son's development of aggressiveness and other culturally pre-scribed masculine traits.[15, 16] The father's impor-tance to the sex-role development of daughters has been supported by similar findings.[17]

Since the father's importance in this aspect of his children's development has been found to be crucial, researchers have been interested in deter-mining the sex-role development of children in homes where the father is absent. It has been found that the absence of a father occurs more frequently among lower-class families and among Negro fam-ilies in all social classes.[18] Studies have shown that the father's absence produces a number of behav-ioral problems in the children and has deleterious effects on their intellectual and personality develop-ment as well. The relative feminization of males as a result of the absence of the father from the family setting has been one of the more prominent findings of studies conducted in recent years. This general finding has been cited by numerous authors who have presented data showing that both male and female children experience deleterious personality development due not only to the father's absence but also to the mother's shift to more authoritarian child-rearing procedures.[19–24] Although there is in-formation available on the development of boys when the father is absent from the home environ-ment, there is relatively little information on the effect of the lack of fathering on girls.[25]

Family configurations and sex-role behaviors are two of the fastest changing aspects of the cur-rent American social scene. It is likely that the in-creased appearance and acceptance of alternative family forms and the loosening of sex-role delinea-tions—which proceed at a faster rate than they are researched and reported—are making an impact upon children's family relations and their develop-ment. The student is referred to Chapter 17 and 18 for further discussion of variations in family and culture patterns and their effects upon children.

Sibling Influences

Children are influenced in their development by re-lationships with their siblings as well as those estab-lished with their parents. During the preschool years, siblings appear to serve a utilitarian function for each other that is expressed in terms of companion-ship, protection, etc.[26] As children grow through the school-age years, their attitudes toward their sib-lings change. Younger children appear to regard young siblings as playmates and older brothers and sisters in terms of caretaking and recreational ac-tivities.[27, 28] With increasing age, the older siblings

are viewed in more abstract terms, and the more positive social aspects of having a sibling are em-phasized. The value of siblings has not been exten-sively investigated. However, it appears that older siblings serve important functions for younger children in the areas of sex-role development, the discrimination of age roles and sex roles, and other related areas. For example, the older sibling is con-sistently viewed in terms of his higher social power over the younger sibling as well as his abilities to facilitate social interaction. Apparently, the younger sibling views himself as interfering or disruptive in interactions between himself and his older sibling, and as giving in to the wishes of the older sibling.[29] During the school-age years, children continue to perceive the older sibling in terms of the power present in his role, while the effectiveness of the older sibling in serving as a sex-role model ends between the ages of 9 and 13. Much of the data on sibling relationships has consistently indicated that siblings serve as *significant others* in the develop-ment of children and are useful to the developing child in defining roles and concepts of self.[30, 31] Un-til recently, the primary thrust of research on per-sonality development has been to show how parents produce differences in their children, as Sutton-Smith and Rosenberg[31] have pointed out. The cur-rent trend is to attempt to learn how siblings produce differences in each other in terms of personality development. It should be noted that the influence of one sibling on another is determined by numerous complex factors, such as age of the child, his sex, the sex of his sibling, and the age difference between the siblings.

REFERENCES

1 D. Elkind, *A Sympathetic Understanding of the Child Six to Sixteen*, Allyn and Bacon, Inc., Boston, 1971.
2 A. Gesell and F. Ilg, *The Child from Five to Ten*, Harper & Row, Publishers, Incorporated, New York, 1946.
3 M. Simon, "Body Configuration and School Readi-ness," *Child Development*, 30:493–512, 1959.
4 P. Johnson and J. Staffieri, "Stereotypic Affective Properties of Personal Names and Somatotypes in Children," *Developmental Psychology*, 5:176, 1971.
5 J. Piaget, *Six Psychological Studies*, Random House, Inc., New York, 1967.
6 A. Goldman and M. Levine, "A Developmental Study of Object Sorting," *Child Development*, 34:649–666, 1963.
7 D. Elkind, "Cognitive Structure in Latency Behavior," paper presented at the conference on "Origins of Indi-viduality," University of Wisconsin, Madison, 1969.
8 E. Erikson, *Childhood and Society*, W. W. Norton & Company, Inc., New York, 1950.
9 G. Psathas, "Ethnicity, Social Class, and Adolescent Independence from Parental Control," *American Sociological Review*, 22:415–423, 1957.

10 A. Hollingshead, *Elmtown's Youth*, John Wiley & Sons, Inc., New York, 1949.

11 M. MacDonald, C. McGuire, and R. Havighurst, "Leisure Activities and the Socioeconomic Status of Children," *American Journal of Sociology*, 54:505–519, 1949.

12 R. Lippitt and R. White, "An Experimental Study of Leadership and Group Life," in T. M. Newcomb and Ruth Hartley (eds.), *Readings in Social Psychology*, Holt, Rinehart and Winston, Inc., New York, 1947, pp. 315–330.

13 M. Johnson, "Sex-Role Learning in the Nuclear Family," *Child Development*, 34:319–333, 1963.

14 D. Aberle and K. Naegele, "Middle-class Fathers' Occupational Role and Attitudes toward Children," *American Journal of Orthopsychiatry*, 22:366–378, 1952.

15 P. Mussen and L. Distler, "Masculinity, Identification, and the Father-Son Relationship," *Journal of Abnormal and Social Psychology*, 59:350–352, 1959.

16 H. Biller, and L. Borstelmann, "Masculine Development: An Integrative Review," *Merrill-Palmer Quarterly*, 13:253–294, 1967.

17 P. Mussen and M. Rutherford, "Parent-Child Relationship and Parental Personality in Relation to Young Children's Sex Role Preferences," *Child Development*, 34:589–607, 1963.

18 M. Deutsch and B. Brown, "Social Influences in Negro-White Intelligence Differences," *Journal of Social Issues*, 18:24–35, 1964.

19 R. Sears, M. Pintler, and P. Sears, "Effects of Father Separation on Preschool Children's Doll Play Aggression," *Child Development*, 17:219–243, 1946.

20 P. Sears, "Doll-Play Aggression in Normal Young Children: Influences of Age, Sex, Sibling Status, and Father Absence," *Psychological Monographs*, Vol. 65, no. 323, 1951.

21 L. Stolz et al., *Father Relations of War-Born Children*, Stanford University Press, Stanford, Calif., 1954.

22 D. Lynn and W. Sawry, "The Effects of Father Absence on Norwegian Boys and Girls," *Journal of Abnormal and Social Psychology*, 59:258–262, 1959.

23 H. B. Biller, "A Note on Father Absence and Masculine Behavior in Lower Class Negro and White Boys," *Child Development*, 39:1003–1006, 1968.

24 H. B. Biller, "Father-Absence, Maternal Encouragement, and Sex-Role Development in Kindergarten Age Boys," *Child Development*, 40: 539–546, 1969.

25 H. B. Biller and S. D. Weiss, "The Father-Daughter Relationship and the Personality Development of the Female," *Journal of Genetic Psychology*, 116:79–94, 1970.

26 H. Koch, "Some Emotional Attitudes of the Young Child in Relation to Characteristics of His Sibling," *Child Development*, 27:393–426, 1956.

27 J. Bigner, "Children's Discrimination of Sibling Role Concepts," paper presented at the Biennial Meeting of the Society for Research in Child Development, 1973.

28 J. Bigner, "A Wernerian Developmental Analysis of Children's Descriptions of Siblings, *Child Development*, 1974 (in press).

29 J. Bigner, "Ontogenetic Changes in Children's Sibling Role Definitions," Final Report, Office of Research and Advanced Studies, Indiana University, 1973.

30 J. Bigner, "Sibling Position and Definition of Self, *Journal of Social Psychology*, 84:307–308, 1971.

31 B. Sutton-Smith and B. G. Rosenberg, *The Sibling*, Holt, Rinehart and Winston, Inc., New York, 1970.

14

THE ADOLESCENT

PATRICIA S. YAROS

ADOLESCENCE REFLECTS THE TIMES

For years people have looked at the adolescent as an "apprentice," a novice attempting to master the tasks of beginning adulthood. From the time of dependence until the prescribed time for independence, this apprentice practices what his role models teach. In the past this practice has fallen along lines of gender: the girl works alongside her mother in the kitchen, and the boy emulates his father's work role.

However, in our present complex society, adolescents are somewhat alienated from such an ascent into adult society. The high school youngster of today has a physical and intellectual maturity far more advanced than the youth of a century ago. Yet a century ago young people had a more concrete perception of their function in society than they do today. The contemporary adolescent hovers in a limbo-like world where he may seem physically and intellectually ready for adult tasks but lacks the necessary experiential or educational criteria demanded by the modern-day world. Young people are often kept at the edge of adult society, left with little to do but wait for the "golden age" of legal adulthood.

Young people of college age who can afford to go to school may bide their time fulfilling the requirements of a technologically oriented world in which they prepare for jobs that may not exist in 10 years. Longer and longer periods of education and training for more and more segmented and specialized areas of work leave adolescents feeling alienated and searching for deeper meanings in life. By prolonging dependency, modern civilization cultivates a perpetuated adolescence.

Adolescents cannot be understood unless viewed as products of a complex culture. While puberty can be seen as a transitional physiologic state with accompanying psychologic attributes, adolescence becomes the role the individual plays in response to the limbo in which he finds himself. The idiosyncrasies of modern American life become reflected in the behaviors of the adolescent generation. Unisex clothes, drugs, and pacifism are hallmarks of the current American scene, as were father-to-son businesses and extreme nationalism in another era. Since the passage into adulthood will always be unique to the society in which it occurs, it is understandable that the adolescent of today bears slight resemblance to the "apprentice" youth of the past.

THEORETICAL ISSUES IN ADOLESCENCE
Biogenetic Theories: Biology Determines Development and Behavior

Only since the turn of the century has passage into adulthood been observed and catalogued to any major degree. G. Stanley Hall[1] in 1904 published his monumental two-volume work and became the first to establish observational areas for adolescent developmental patterns, such as body growth, sexual development, emotional eccentricities, and delinquency. His ideals of adolescent development followed a Darwinian evolution theory of *recapitulation* so that each person was believed to pass through a predetermined set of stages from primitive behavior to civilized actions. Hall conceived these primitive-to-civilized stages as analogous to the evolution of the human race. He likened the turbulence of adolescence to the periods of storm and stress in the growth of modern culture.

In 1922 Hall was followed by Jones, a Freudian. Jones theorized that adolescence recapitulates and expands upon the individual's first 5 years of life, with sequential autoerotic, pregenital, genital-narcissistic, homosexual, and heterosexual stages.[2] Jones' and Hall's theories did not allow for environmental influences. Biology was considered the sole determinant of adolescent behavior.

Environmental Theories: Experience Influences Development and Behavior

The biogenetic theorists were soon challenged by the environmentalists, who reported cultural variability in patterns of adolescent growth and development. Margaret Mead in 1928 became world-renowned for her description of a startling cross-cultural difference in youth's rise to adulthood in *Coming of Age in Samoa*.[3] Samoan children accepted adult roles and responsibilities as early as 5 or 6 years of age and proceeded gradually to develop toward their full adult status. The idiosyncrasies of adolescence described by Hall and Jones were not to be found in Samoan youth. Mead and other sociocultural theorists tried to put to rest the simplistic biologic explanation of adolescent development. Despite the heavy influences of anthropologic theorizing and field work, current interpretations of adolescent developmental patterns still commonly follow the Hall tradition.

Contemporary theorists have attempted to explain the vast subculture that adolescents have formed in modern society. These theorists hope to understand the effect that the youth of America have had on the politics, dress, mores, and spirit of the society as a whole. Philippe Aries,[4] the French historian of the family, makes the intriguing assertion that the twentieth century is enthralled with adolescence. Today's youths have given the impression of "secretly possessing new values capable of reviving an aged and sclerosed society." Americans wish to come into adolescence earlier and live it as long as possible.[4]

Continuing Questions The long struggle by so many to explain or define adolescence has left a confusing diversity of opinions. Beyond the consensus that adolescence occurs somewhere between childhood and adulthood, theorists grossly disagree about when adolescence occurs, how it prepares people for adulthood, and what the "norms" of the period are. These differences of opinion revolve around the following major issues:

1 The age limits, if any, of the adolescent period
2 The relationship of puberty to adolescence
3 The conflict of the generations
4 The cross-cultural universality of adolescence
5 Disruption, delinquency, and stability in adolescence

This chapter explores these issues in order to introduce the student to the complexities of social, psychologic, and biologic processes at work in adolescent development.

ADOLESCENCE: PUBESCENCE, PUBERTY, AND BEYOND

It has been generally accepted that there are individual as well as cultural variations in the age of onset and termination of adolescence and in the length of time involved. This variability, however, has not kept writers from identifying some approximate age ranges. Holmes[5] cites ages 12 to 18 as the adolescent period. Somewhat arbitrarily Pearson[6] identifies 10½ years as the age of onset because it is in this year that the majority of physiologic changes begin to appear in Pearson's definition of pubescence. Others believe adolescence commences with prepubertal growth spurt. Adding confusion to the issue is the fact that many authors use physical landmarks for the onset of adolescence and psychologic processes as signs of its end.

Definitions: Pubescence, Puberty, and Adolescence

Clarification of terms is required if one is to understand both the physiologic and psychologic parameters of adolescence. *Pubescence* is the time span during which the young person's reproductive functions begin to mature. It may be equated with the term *early adolescence*.[7] Pubescence ends with the attainment of full reproductive capacity.[7] Erikson[8] states that pubescence is characterized by rapid body growth, full genital development, and an overwhelming sexual awareness.

Following the period of pubescence, the period in which the person reaches reproductive maturity is called *puberty*. This point has in the past been denoted in girls as the time of first menstruation.

However, studies have shown that most young females are not fertile for approximately 1 to 2 years after menarche. Their ability to conceive is therefore often delayed. The average age at menarche for American girls is 12½ to 13½ years.[9]

For boys, puberty approaches at or near the time of first ejaculations. This is not the most precise pubertal milestone because of the relative difficulty in obtaining an accurate history of its occurrence in young adolescent boys. As can be seen in Figure 14-1, first ejaculations generally occur at ages 13 through 16 in American boys.[10] True reproductive maturity is not attained until several years later, when viable sperm appear in the semen.[9]

Obviously, from what has just been mentioned, the terms *pubescence* and *puberty* deal most con-

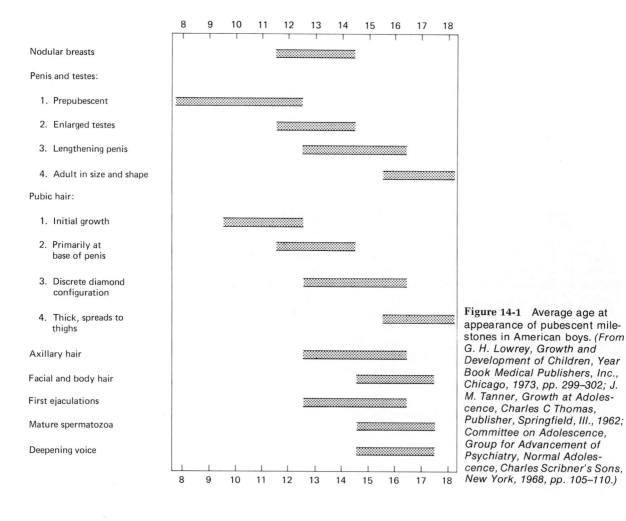

Figure 14-1 Average age at appearance of pubescent milestones in American boys. *(From G. H. Lowrey, Growth and Development of Children, Year Book Medical Publishers, Inc., Chicago, 1973, pp. 299–302; J. M. Tanner, Growth at Adolescence, Charles C Thomas, Publisher, Springfield, Ill., 1962; Committee on Adolescence, Group for Advancement of Psychiatry, Normal Adolescence, Charles Scribner's Sons, New York, 1968, pp. 105–110.)*

cretely with biology. The social and behavioral maturation that encompasses the period beginning with the onset of pubescence and extending beyond the time of reproductive maturity is called *adolescence* (Fig. 14-2).

The Growth Spurt

Until about 10 years of age, boys and girls grow at approximately the same rate. There is slight variance in children's height at the same chronologic age. However, a child whose biologic age (as measured by bone age) is more advanced than another's will attain sexual maturity sooner. Additionally, this means that the biologically older child has less growth potential. Girls start out in life with a more

advanced bone age, reach puberty earlier, and thus are shorter than male counterparts.[11]

The first body parts to increase in size during the growth spurt are the hands and feet. The calves and forearms then follow, with hips, chest, and shoulders next, in that order.[11] Because the trunk is the last to grow appreciably, the young adolescent almost invariably passes through a transitional phase when his hands and feet appear gigantic and awkward compared with the rest of his body. However, the trunk growth rate soon catches up and surpasses the rate of the lower extremities, causing the overall adolescent height increase to be due more to lengthening of the trunk rather than to growth of the legs.

For girls in the United States, the growth spurt

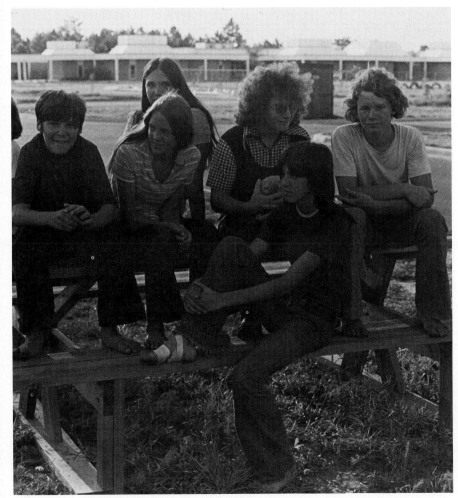

Figure 14-2 Wide variations in physical maturity are characteristic of early and middle adolescence, even at the same chronologic age. Similarities in clothing and hair style and aggregation in groups allow practice, sharing, and enjoyment of social experiences to help with the formation of self-identity without forcing premature intimacy. *(Photo courtesy of George Lazar.)*

begins at approximately 10½ years of age.[11] There may be a variability of about 3 years between two normal children. Until menarche, the young adolescent girl grows an average of 3 inches per year. At the onset of menstruation, growth slows but does not cease. Approximately 3 years later, at age 16, most young females have reached their adult height.[10]

The average adolescent male starts his growth spurt at age 13.[11] His later onset is compensated for by a longer duration and greater cumulative growth. For about 2½ years he grows at the phenomenal rate of 4 inches per year. (This gain is exceeded only in the toddler years.) Following this period of rapid growth, the adolescent continues to grow at a slightly slower rate into his late teens. Additionally, the average adolescent boy almost doubles in weight between 12 and 16 years of age. Much of this weight is new muscle. The muscles grow rapidly at this time and will continue to "fill out" the frame even after adult height is reached.[11]

Pubescent Development in Both Sexes

Along with the dramatic growth changes which occur at the onset of pubescence, there are equally dramatic alterations in the body shape because of the beginning sexual maturation. The angular preadolescent female form becomes smoother because of the deposition of fat in the thighs, hips, and breasts. The girl's pelvis broadens at this time, preparing her for childbearing. The young adolescent boy, meanwhile, becomes leaner than he will ever be again. His pelvic girth does not change appreciably, but his chest and shoulders broaden.

In girls, breast development is the first overt sign of beginning reproductive maturation. The increase in estrogen level from the maturing ovary promotes mammary tissue development, but most of the early breast enlargement is due to fatty deposits.[9] As shown in Figure 14-3, normal breast development has been categorized in four stages. Stage I denotes the prepubescent breast, in which there is only a slight elevation of the nipple. From approximately 9 to 11 years of age, the areola surrounding the nipple becomes protuberant. This stage II is characterized by the formation of a small mound, or "bud."[9, 12] Stage III begins as the nipple and areola further increase in size and pigmentation of the area becomes obvious. This breast change occurs about the same time as first menstruation.[9, 12] Two to 3 years later, the young adolescent girl should be the proud possessor of relatively mature breasts. This mature state is designated as stage IV

and is characterized by palpable gland and duct tissue in the breasts with the areola receded to the same level as the surrounding skin.[9, 12] Young adolescent males may experience a slight hypertrophy of their breasts at the beginning of the teen years. A nodular mound forms when the androgen and estrogen hormone balance becomes upset at this time.[9] Mammary enlargement (*gynecomastia*) is a condition which generally passes within a few months but which in the meantime can cause some embarrassment to a sensitive teen-age boy.

During early pubescence the girl also experiences endocrinologic imbalances. Estrogen production surges and then adjusts at a plateau after regular menstruation is firmly established.[9] Just before menarche, the hormones produce vaginal changes. The pubescent girl develops a milky vaginal secretion as the vaginal walls adjust to increasingly acidic conditions.[9] As can be seen in Figure 14-3, this vaginal change usually occurs before the age of 12.

Pubic hair growth follows quickly behind the initial pubescent phenomena in both the boy and girl (see Figs. 14-1 and 14-3). Stage I for both sexes is a preliminary sparse growth of downy hair barely evident around the genitals. In the girl, this growth precedes menarche by approximately 1 year. In the boy, it is concurrent with the beginning of the growth of the genitals. Stage II presents as a darkening of the initial hair with no spread to the thighs. The pubic hair growth in stage III becomes distinctly male or female in its distribution—a triangular configuration across the mons veneris for girls and, for boys, the characteristic diamond-shaped pattern spreading from the base of the penis upward. As this growth thickens and spreads to the thighs, it approximates the adult pattern for life. Stage IV of pubic hair development may not be fully completed for either sex until the early or mid twenties.[12]

The earliest secondary sex characteristic to appear in boys is an increase in the size of the testes and scrotum and later the penis. Since boys are usually 2 years behind girls in pubescent development, the gradual enlargement of the genitals does not commence until age 13 for most boys. Figure 14-1 shows that the development of male genitalia to adult size and shape takes 5 to 6 years.

For full reproductive maturity, the adolescent boy must produce viable sperm. As has been mentioned before, this level of maturity does not exist at the time of his first ejaculations. The early ejaculations usually happen while the boy is asleep and are termed *nocturnal seminal emissions*. These are physiologic reflex ejaculations and may occur with

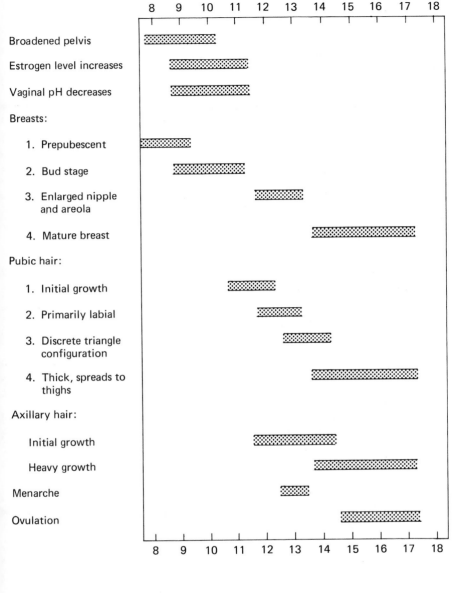

Figure 14-3   Average age at appearance of pubescent milestones in American girls. *(From G. H. Lowrey, Growth and Development of Children, Year Book Medical Publishers, Inc., Chicago, 1973, pp. 299–302; J. M. Tanner, Growth at Adolescence, Charles C Thomas, Publisher, Springfield, Ill., 1962; Committee on Adolescence, Group for Advancement of Psychiatry, Normal Adolescence, Charles Scribner's Sons, New York, 1968, pp. 105–110.)*

or without sexual stimulation. Mature sperm production is several years in developing, but most young men's reproductive maturity is reached by age 17.[9]

Regular menstruation and ovulation do not generally appear simultaneously in the pubescent girl. Irregular menstrual periods are the rule for this time in life. Production of mature ova in the female cannot be accurately measured in any one person but is generally thought to be firmly established approximately 2 years after the first menstruation.

Other changes during pubescence, which are probably not looked on so favorably as those previously mentioned, are the changes in skin secretions. During middle and late adolescence the sweat glands become hyperactive. *Hyperhidrosis*, abnormally increased secretion of perspiration, creates body odor which usually proves most embarrassing for young people. The appearance of skin blemishes at this time is not unusual and may be even more socially traumatic. Acne, which is caused by plugged sebaceous glands, is directly related to the hormonal changes of pubescence. Androgens evidently increase the secretion levels of the sebaceous glands, especially in persons predisposed to acne.

Psychologic Responses to Pubescent Changes

Girls' Reaction to Pubescence   The first concerns of the developing young woman are those dealing with her new body functions. This is not to say that menarche, rather than the altered physique, is more disquieting or satisfying for the girl. The young adolescent girl usually looks forward to menstruation as her badge of womanhood. However, this herald of approaching maturity can also have an adverse effect. Some girls believe they will "bleed to death." If the bleeding is accompanied by cramps, headache, backache, and nausea or vomiting, it is understandable that a girl might wonder whether she was seriously ill.

The attitude of the girl toward menstruation is in great part dependent upon her cultural background and the attitudes of those who give her information about it. Whether or not the girl is informed before the occurrence of first menstruation may be significant to her emotional response to the event. Most of all, if menstruation is explained to her as a normal function, she will be less inclined to fantasize about injury. When those around her believe menstruation is a "curse" or that it necessitates staying in bed, the girl will probably believe the same.[13]

After the menstrual cycle is established, the young adolescent girl is likely to resent menstruation, not so much because of the accompanying discomforts but because it may restrict her activities. Furthermore, her nonparticipation in certain sports, such as swimming, openly reveals her condition. None of this encourages her to welcome her new status.

The continual transformation of her body is also of great concern to the pubescent girl. She pays careful attention to the mirror at this time, often bemoaning every real or imagined disproportion she finds and wondering whether she will ever grow out of it. The normal transitions during the growth spurt may send her into a state of depression. It is difficult to convince such a youngster that her disproportions are temporary.

Unfamiliarity with a changing body often produces a very awkward adolescent girl. This awkwardness is mostly derived from lack of experience in coordinating the newly disproportionate body parts. The adaptability of the young person generally comes to her psychologic rescue if she makes a conscious effort at learning to use the unfamiliar body parts. Some girls find that dancing lessons, swimming, or modeling classes promote grace and coordination.

The appearance of secondary sex characteristics prompts the pubescent girl to compare herself constantly with her friends and classmates. The first girl in class to wear a brassiere is simultaneously held in awe and suspected: suspected of what, no one is really sure. Deviating from the norm is of great importance to young adolescent girls and boys, so when any one girl's maturation is markedly delayed or accelerated she may become a misfit in her peer group. This is a traumatic situation in the life of a pubescent girl and should never be taken lightly.

Since girls have a year or more head start on boys in pubescent maturation, they are interested in their attractiveness to the opposite sex much sooner than boys are. The girl tests her attractiveness on others to see how they regard her. She may agonize over the slightest uncomplimentary statement. When her father makes such a remark, it can be particularly significant to the girl and hurt her deeply. Similarly, any compliment by him can lift her spirits. As the young adolescent girl becomes more mature and attractive, her father may draw away from her because he feels it is inappropriate to be as close physically as before. This withdrawal can easily be misinterpreted by the daughter as rejection. A great deal of tact is necessary for a father to handle this dilemma.

Many girls are overwhelmed by the changes in the ways males relate to them. Male response to them is such an important part of their self-image that it often causes much embarrassment, discomfort, and pleasure. The young adolescent girl may scorn a brief flirtation with a young man, but if she were to observe the same scene between two others, she might feel envious and unattractive.

Intense attachments to certain adults may spring up in these early adolescent years. These "crushes" are transient but are often deeply felt by the young person. Girls' crushes are most often directed toward older males, including teachers, counselors, or friends of the family. In a few instances there may be an actual relationship, but in most cases it is more fantasy than fact. An attachment can form for someone of the same sex—a sort of hero worship—but this is more likely to occur in the preadolescent years. As the girl matures and becomes more certain about her own identity and more confident in interpersonal relationships, she typically finds less need to "try on" such relationships.

One important difference between pubescent boys and girls is their sexual awareness. Among girls there are, of course, many normal individual variations. Some girls experience rather diffuse sexual stirrings in their pubertal years, while others do not until later. For most young girls in their early teens, sensual pleasures are mixed with other intense internal responses to a stimulating environment. Usually, not until the late teens do girls experience the direct genital urge for sexual relations. However, external pressures may push a girl into early sexual encounters when social situations make sexual activity seem either obligatory or advantageous for some reason other than sensual pleasure.

Boys' Reactions to Pubescence The major stresses of maturation for the adolescent boy result directly from endocrinologic changes. Pubescent alterations in physique produce an almost entirely new body to which the boy must accustom himself. Especially striking are his rapidly increasing size and muscular strength. However, as the sexual aspects of his development become clear to him, the young adolescent boy usually sees his sexuality as the most important feature of his maturation and the greatest complication in dealing with his new and changing image.

Most boys are very conscious of genital sensations which appear in the early teen years. They become acutely interested in what is going on in their bodies with the onset of nocturnal emissions. In many instances, the boy knows about emissions before they occur, usually having been informed by friends. If a boy has not been properly prepared by his parents or a knowledgeable other person, he may fear that he has a serious moral or physical problem. Often, boys imagine that nocturnal emissions are a consequence of masturbation. If not educated to believe that nocturnal emissions are a normal phenomenon in his life, a boy can develop strong conflicts regarding the "good" and "bad," respectively, of his mind and body.

The acute sensations that arise from the penis demand action and relief. In our society, sexual urges in adolescence have no legitimate outlet. Traditional beliefs still hold masturbation to be an evil practice. Shame, embarrassment, and guilt feelings accompany masturbatory activities for most boys. In addition, many young people are led to believe that there are grave physical consequences such as acne, epilepsy, blindness, impotence, and insanity. Even though there is no evidence to support these assertions, such propaganda has caused a great deal of concern for many young people. The only real harm that can be attributed to masturbation is the worry and guilt boys *and girls* may experience because of it.

Another source of concern for the pubescent boy is the physical change in his sex organs. His penis and scrotum may seem so underdeveloped at the beginning of the pubescent years that he may fear they will never reach adult size and proportion. Then, at the time of the most growth, around the age of 15, the boy may think that his genitals are too obvious through his clothing. But some boys accentuate this development by wearing tight pants.

The late-developing adolescent may have great anxieties about undressing in front of his peers for fear that his diminutive organ will elicit ridicule. This is not an unfounded concern, because of the sense of competition and striving for a mature masculine image boys exhibit at this age.

As reproductive maturity nears, the pubescent male's sexual awareness affects his thoughts and behavior almost constantly. His sexual desires, which he usually would prefer to have satisfied by a female rather than masturbation, are complicated by many other feelings. Again, the universal adolescent feelings of embarrassment and uncertainty rear their ugly heads. The boy may be afraid that he will reveal his innermost sexual feelings by chance slip. He may be confused about how to act around girls at all. Not knowing what a girl might do when faced with his awkward advances, he feels safer not attempting them. Doubts about his own sexual adequacy may be prevalent and may also hamper his venturing into a male-female sexual encounter.

When a pubescent boy succeeds in overcoming his embarrassment at approaching a girl and she accepts his first advances, even in the most limited way, he may easily think that he is in love. This is an immature and romantic reaction but most appropriate for the middle teen years. This love is not like the love that he will feel later in his early adulthood. It is more a glow from being accepted and liked. It is also a reaffirmation that he will soon be a man. All this emotional response combines with the spark of sexual desire to make the young man feel he is in love.

The adolescent whose maturation has not kept pace with that of his contemporaries is in a predicament that seemingly takes forever to resolve itself. A slight build, short stature, or a soprano voice would make any 16-year-old boy feel left out and depressed. If he has no interest in girls or dating, he may well wonder whether he is normal, particularly since he is likely to want to imitate older boys in this as well as other behavior. The boy who matures may be in a somewhat more enviable position, but not necessarily. He looks older than his chronologic age and is expected to be emotionally and intellectually more mature. Of course, this is usually not so, and the boy may be branded "stupid" or a "dumbbell." It has been found that many boys who mature early lack the energy that their peers have and often fall behind in their schoolwork.[14] This decline tends to reinforce the "stupid" label given to the boy, making him quite unhappy.

Educating pubescent boys and girls about the wide variations in the norms for their growth and development is one way to help alleviate frustrations and uncertainties. It is important to emphasize that deviations such as early maturing in girls and late maturing in boys are temporary. For most pubescents, this knowledge can go a long way to forestall unhappiness concerning their changing appearance.

Late Adolescence

With the attainment of full sexual maturity and the development of effective coping patterns for dealing with the emotional onslaught it has brought on, the young person moves past the midpoint of this metamorphosis and into *late adolescence*. He must prepare himself for a place in the adult world. In middle-class American culture this means choosing a vocation, becoming independent of one's parents, and developing a commitment to responsible citizenship. As the older teen-ager is learning the feelings and behaviors of his new body, he must also progress to utilizing his body to share intimacy and love. The theme of the developmental transformations of late adolescence is the finding of one's self, or identity.

The term *identity*, which was popularized by Erik Erikson,[8, 15] refers to the older adolescent's coming to feel that he understands himself and that his image of himself is congruent with the way others view him. He learns to separate his ideas from the viewpoints of others. As all this comes about, the youth leaves behind his earlier intense preoccupation with himself and turns his energies toward discovering what ethics and values the outside world offers him.[15] He must fit these standards into a picture of himself.

The social and intellectual characteristics of late adolescence differ from those of early adolescence in that they are more complex and are more heavily influenced by society than earlier, when they were more exclusively affected by family and peer relationships. Decisions now are usually made after long discussions with those who have more experience with similar problems. As the adolescent matures, he attempts to deal with reality within the framework of his own value system and attitudes. In this way,

adolescents have a tendency to ignore specific rules or bend them to suit their goal (Fig. 14-4).

Morality in Late Adolescence In the early teen years, there was a rather strict internalization of the moral principles handed down from the adolescent's parents, teachers, church, or other external sources. However, with broadening social experiences, an increased number of conflicting situations arise. In other words, the young adolescent does not have a rule to guide him on every occasion. In order to resolve these situations to their own satisfaction, adolescents must develop their own concepts of right and wrong. In this process of selection, of course, they may discard moral precepts which parents and others have given them.

As his moral attitudes adapt to fit his life-style, the adolescent may become more tolerant of certain acts he would formerly have condemned. Students who turn to cheating in the classroom justify it on the grounds that society demands high grades in order to achieve success later and that cheating is therefore necessary to meet society's expectations. But just as there may be a growing tolerance for some things, there may be an increasing intolerance of others. For example, bribery and conceit are typically far more serious transgressions to the older adolescent than to the pubescent youngster.

Greater tolerance to formerly condemned sexual behavior is prevalent in the late adolescent years. Sexual sharing of oneself with another tends to occur as part of the developing capacity for intimate relationships.

Some adolescents formalize their sexually intimate relationships by marriage; others do not. Cohabitation is openly tolerated in some segments of adolescent society. Dependable contraception methods have allowed young people to explore their sexuality without the former risks of pregnancy and ensuing early marriage. The diminishing influence of the double standard has freed adolescent girls to engage in sexual experimentation without a serious commitment to the partner and, for many, with little or no guilt. However, there is still a stigma attached to outright promiscuity, so the definition of it has been modified. A girl may have successive affairs with several young men, and as long as they don't overlap appreciably she is not generally considered promiscuous by her peers or herself.

However, there are difficulties in the new adolescent sexual mores. Late adolescence is not yet a time of emotional stability, a fact which certainly influences intimate behavior. Relationships have a

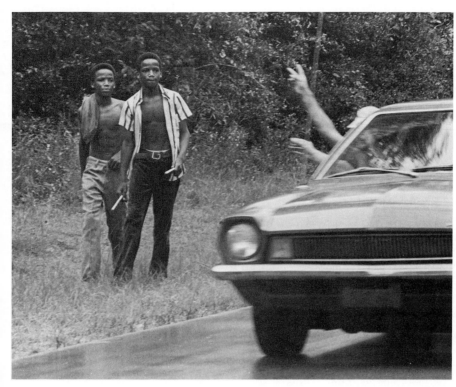

Figure 14-4 The adolescent subculture characteristically uses its own language and gestures to express attitudes regarding race relations, pacifism, and other concerns about which young people are forming values they will carry into adulthood. *(Photo courtesy of George Lazar.)*

tendency to be transitory, with both sexes reaching for new interpersonal experiences. Trouble arises when one person in the relationship invests more of himself than the other, who may still be treating the situation as a casual and passing encounter. This discrepancy between the two partners signals that one may have dependency needs that the other clearly does not recognize or, even more likely, is unable to cope with. Not until young adulthood are matters of lifelong commitment to one person likely to be seriously or effectively considered.

Vocational Interests in Late Adolescence As an inherent part of the quest for one's identity, the need to plan for a future occupation becomes an important concern of late adolescence. In the middle-class American household it is expected that the children will give some thought to the career they will follow. However, those from lower classes may not enjoy the luxury of having a choice. Financial pressures and a "present-oriented" outlook may force a lower-class adolescent into the first available job, whether or not schooling is finished.

Aside from the economic influence on the adolescent's vocational choice, identification with parents may profoundly affect the route the young

person takes. Many young men have been known to "follow in their fathers' footsteps." However, a young man may not have the same aptitudes that his father had, so he must seek a realistic appraisal of his abilities and interests. Some adolescents who do not do so become disappointed in themselves and feel that they have disappointed their parents as well.

Upward social mobility appeals to many young Americans today, and one consequence has been an overcrowding of colleges and universities. For many years, a college education was equated with future success. There is evidence now that this viewpoint is not held by as many young people and parents as it once was. Nevertheless, a college education is a consideration for older teens of either sex as they contemplate which road to take toward vocational fulfillment and financial security.

The main motivations that prompt young people to enter college stem from the cultural and educational traditions, ambitions, and hopes of the family.[16] If there is a tradition of college attendance in the family or if a college education is considered to be a way to improve one's lot, the young person may feel that college is necessary. Even without any support or encouragement from the family, some adolescents become desirous of higher education after seeing the frustrations of their parents' job circumstances or after being encouraged by teachers or others. The rejection of family educational traditions also occurs, but no definitive studies have been made to explain all the motivations of persons who seek less education than their parents had.

Whatever route the young person chooses, it may include an abundance of detours, as may be especially true of young women. Marriage and homemaking are seen by some adolescent girls as an occupation in themselves. Others plan for careers that will not be greatly interrupted by marriage and child rearing if they occur. Those girls who plan only for marriage may find themselves at a disadvantage if later life circumstances make it necessary or desirable for them to be employed. Young women planning for their future are benefited from the current social pattern which has done away with most of the stigma previously felt by working mothers and career women.

Intimacy and Love in Late Adolescence Group activities in childhood and early adolescence provide the training ground for dating behavior in the late teen period. School functions, parties, picnics, and dances bring together youthful members of the opposite sex for approved social interaction. Through these activities, the same-sex partnerships of the late childhood years begin yielding to the mounting heterosexual interests of the pubertal years. Pairing off begins to occur more and more frequently by the middle teens. Dating patterns become established as the appropriate opportunities for heterosexual association increase and parental restrictions are lessened.

Prestige is an important factor in dating in the high school and college age groups. The prestige hierarchy is denoted by symbols which identify attractive and unattractive dating partners. Many of these symbols change with the times. Additionally, they may differ from school to school and even for different cliques within a school, a fact which creates difficulty for adolescents who transfer to a new school or move into a new social setting. A "good" date may possess such status symbols as belonging to a fraternity or sorority, owning or having access to a certain type of automobile, having an athletic letter sweater, or wearing a certain brand or style of clothing. Lacking any or all of these symbols leaves a young person considerably lower in dating status. Many young people find themselves trying to conform to some ideal of dating potential. Romanticized and idealized versions of what one desires in a

partner and what is desired in oneself eventually give way to a more reality-based view as the young person succeeds in establishing his sense of identity.

As the adolescent becomes more secure, he can begin to cope successfully with intimacy. According to Erikson, intimacy involves being able to blend one's identity with that of another without fear of losing it.[5] Also, intimacy can be viewed as a state in which the happiness of another becomes as important if not more important than one's own happiness. The adolescent finds, perhaps without conscious awareness of it, that he can feel complete only when joined with and sharing with a member of the opposite sex. This emergence of the capacity for more mature love combines the affectional and the erotic and bears little resemblance to the crushes of the earlier adolescent years (Fig. 14-5).

The overwhelming need to gain acceptance from the opposite sex is accompanied by a great deal of anxiety on the part of any adolescent. Because of this some young people retreat into a more comfortable relationship with a member of the same sex. The range of intimacy that same-sex friendships may engender may be quite broad. In adolescent boys, the most frequent overtly sexual occurrence in this realm is group or mutual masturbation. Some young people who do not engage in explicit sexual relations find a "safe" relationship by associating with someone of the opposite sex who has avowed homosexual tendencies. There is no pressure for true heterosexual functioning in this kind of relationship, and the young person avoids the anxiety of fulfilling a heterosexual *or* homosexual role. It must be emphasized that any of the aforementioned behaviors are not to be conclusively labeled as precursors of later homosexuality or as explicit homosexuality as known in the adult. Some degree of affectional and/or frankly sexual interchange is very common in adolescence and, depending upon a number of influences not yet well understood, may or may not develop into a homosexual orientation to sexuality and love in adulthood.

The capacity for full sexual expression in the late adolescent years does not, of course, carry with it the guarantee that it will be utilized for the fulfillment of a mature sharing of onself. Transitory sexual relationships occur in which the goal is satisfaction of sexual needs and not much else. The balance must be attained by each young person when he is faced with making a stand for himself, either with or against the prevailing group mores. Going full force into a sexual relationship or declining to do so may be the norm in his group. Each young person decides at some point whether or not

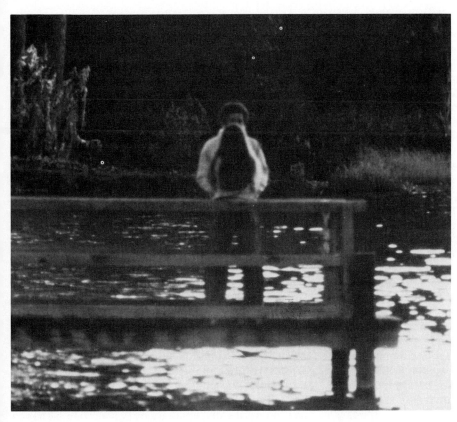

Figure 14-5   The successfully developing late adolescent or young adult is able to share himself in a mature love relationship.

to conform to his reference group. His decision becomes part of clarifying his identity.

Independence in Late Adolescence   A critical element in the establishment of a sense of identity is emancipation of the adolescent from his family and parental ties. This maneuver serves a necessary purpose in making it possible for the young person to someday fulfill an appropriate adult role. It is also a step that can be very painful and frustrating. Ambivalence on the part of both parent and teen is not at all unusual. Generally in the mid-teens the youth does not wish to do anything that suggests dependence on the family, but neither can he comfortably reject them or do without the functions they perform. The parents know that the adolescent must be pushed or allowed from the nest at some time but they may have difficulty admitting to themselves that they are no longer so necessary to the young person.

The task of establishing independence becomes doubly difficult for those who are financially dependent on their parents for their schooling at the same time they wish to break the magnetic emotional hold. This type of binding dependence may cause a youth to feel uncomfortable and somewhat ashamed that he is not managing without parental assistance, especially if he has reached the age of legal adulthood in his state. Most adolescents weather this bind by gradually loosening the ties in other ways. Physically moving away from the parents' household helps to give many adolescents the opportunity to see how they fare on their own.

It is understandable that many people believe that independent decision making on the part of immature and inexperienced young people can have serious consequences. However, withholding such opportunities from adolescents too long is a form of overprotection likely to hamper the achievement of independence for the youth. Some young people remain dependent upon their families and parents into adulthood or choose a parent substitute, perhaps as a spouse, and therefore never fully develop in a stable and mature manner.

CONFLICT IN THE HOME

Making the transition from childhood dependency and obedience to full responsibility for oneself is never easy. For most adolescents, the greatest problems arise in their own homes. There just is no smooth and conflict-free path that adolescents can follow when it comes to relationships within their family. Dealings between siblings are often fraught with rivalries of one kind or another. Relationships with parents are complicated by the fact that the world today is quite unlike that which existed when the parents were young. Consequently, the natural discrepancy in life-styles often sets off a powder keg of threatened values on both sides.

The harmony that the parent may have had with his youngster in childhood gradually disappears as the youth begins having strong stirrings to assert himself as a person in his own right. Values that the parent bestowed on his offspring are no longer accepted carte blanche. The ceaseless questioning and testing of values that were previously accepted on faith create parental anxiety and are perceived as a threat among adults. This natural and necessary—albeit conflict-producing—self-assertiveness in opposition to parental values is a sign of progress toward accomplishing a major developmental task of adolescence (and of parents of adolescents).

The idealistic attitudes of young people carry over into their criticism of the adults around them. They typically are highly critical of any adult who does not "practice what he preaches." It has been postulated that in the "saint with feet of clay" syndrome, an unexpected revelation may occur to the adolescent: adulthood is not the impossible dream of any distant attainment of perfection.[17]

Especially for the younger adolescent, a major disturbance in the equilibrium of the parent-adolescent relationship arises because of his testing of the limits set for him. Outrageous and unreasonable acts may be perpetrated by the youth in order to see whether he is still loved despite his behavior. These are not generally premeditated plots but are unconscious signals that the young teen is ambivalent about his approaching maturity. He wishes to receive again the attention and unconditional love that made him so secure in the past. His self-doubt and questioning about what others think of him may force him to act rashly in order to get an immediate resolution to his uncertainty and frustrations.

Quite a traumatic breech in family relations results as the adolescent acts to fulfill a natural inclination to break out from the family walls. This break exhibits itself in a variety of ways such as staying out later than the family's curfew time, keeping company with friends disapproved by parents, or running away from home. The independence-seeking youth runs afoul of parental authority when he is no longer unquestioningly obedient but be-

comes rebellious, assertive, and obstinate. A showdown between parent and child is likely to ensue.

Altercations in the household can be as severe as all-out screaming matches. These usually begin with small skirmishes of belittlement on both sides. The adolescent may burst into a rage and lash out in angry defiance at his parents, and the words shot out in anger may be fully meant at the time. Regrets about such behavior usually follow when both sides cool down. Of course, not all families act in this manner. Wars of silence may prevail in some households. Both of these behaviors take a toll on family relationships, some suffering irreparable damage.

When teens begin to view their parents as repressive or old-fashioned, communications between them and their parents may suffer. The adolescent may attempt to share experiences, thoughts, or feelings, but at the least misunderstanding he readily retreats behind the despairing and disparaging, "You will never understand me!"

Conflict and blocked communication in the home can be eased if parents and adolescents do more talking *with* each other rather than *at* each other. More favorable attitudes flourish where attempts to understand one anothers' point of view outnumber the attempts to dictate. The adolescent wishes to be taken seriously and not to be judged as if he were still a child. By not giving him a chance to express himself, parents may lose the opportunity to *help* a young person make up his mind about the values and beliefs he will keep.

THE CRITERIA OF ADULTHOOD ACROSS CULTURES

Becoming an adult and reaching maturity are two different states of being in many cultures, especially in Western society. Adult status may be a conferred privilege that has little to do with age or physical development. Being mature is actually a physical or psychologic characteristic. The difference in the two, generally in terms of time, is the cause of the "limbo" type of adolescence that presently predominates in the United States. However, in some cultures, maturity and adult status so approximate each other that there may be no identifiable adolescent period as we know it.

Simple *puberty rites* in many primitive societies, such as the Arapesh of New Guinea, give the young person full adult privileges including the right to marry and to own property.[18] The young people of such societies have the advantage of knowing when they will become adults. Their initiation period, which is timed to coincide with the onset of reproductive maturity, may last only a few days or weeks compared with Western society's 5 to 8 years. It is interesting to note, however, that there are still remnants of ancient puberty rites in our contemporary culture. The religious observances of Catholic confirmation and Jewish Bar Mitzvah, both held about the age of 13, originally ushered the young person into adult membership in the community.

In a culture such as the Manus society, the attainment of a prescribed amount of material wealth denotes adulthood for the male. The age for marriage is about 18. At this time, the young man loses his previous rights and independence; he must subjugate himself to others until, by any means possible, he has acquired the money and land necessary to have economic independence for his family and adult status for himself. This culture, then, has an expanded adolescence from the age of marriage at 18 until about 30 or 35 years old.[19]

Land ownership as the entitlement to adult status has carried over to Western culture for certain groups such as the Irish. Especially in the early and middle 1900s, the practice was that only the eldest son could inherit property. Since land was scarce, younger sons lost out unless some rare opportunity came along. The only other road to adulthood was to become a priest. Therefore, Ireland had many men who experienced a prolonged adolescence through waiting and perhaps never attaining what their older brothers did. One might comment that the moodiness and sometimes uncontrolled exuberance for which Irish men are noted is quite reminiscent of the way adolescence is usually described in the Western culture.[20]

Class and Cultural Distinctions in the United States

In the United States, lower-class adolescence is distinguished from middle-class adolescence by significant differences in life-style and life opportunity. The core concerns of the lower-class adolescent often center on survival, as he necessarily becomes preoccupied with the adversities he must suffer because of his socioeconomic status. He often develops a "toughness" to outmaneuver or "con" those whom he deems to have made a world only for themselves, the white middle class. In order to transcend their deprived circumstances, lower-class youth commonly spend a great deal of time in the pursuit of excitement. An antiauthoritarian and anti-intellectual attitude is often persistent among such young people, especially when they have feelings of powerlessness and resignation in regard to their destiny.[21]

Lack of achievement and of orientation toward success has consistently been found to typify lower-class young people. Since many of these adolescents are uninterested in educational or professional preparations, the length of their adolescence may be shorter in that respect when compared to middle-class youth. Their economic plight usually calls for a remedy of a more immediate nature, so they often drop out of the middle-class–oriented educational system to take a job at low income. Practical efforts to motivate these young people toward higher-paying skilled labor or finding financial support for higher education are only now becoming a national priority and beginning to succeed.

For the adolescent who comes from the lower class and is culturally different from the middle-class majority, the attainment of full adult status may be severely hindered. A case in point is the American Negro male. In the white society, the black male is made to feel powerless and impotent; his history of subservience to the white male haunts him. His reaction to this fact bears a likeness to normal adolescent behavior: frustration, rebelliousness, sexual adventuring, and transient self-defeating behavior. In the past, the attitudes toward the black male were implicit in the derogatory term "boy," which served to humiliate him. It is practically impossible, in such an environment, to achieve adult status.

The transitional development of the adolescent is not a uniform experience for every teen but is altered significantly by his socioeconomic class and racial and cultural background. There is much diversity in the adolescent experience, especially in the way he perceives himself and is viewed by others. These factors cannot be ignored by persons who wish to understand adolescence; neither can they reliably be used to "pigeonhole" any one adolescent. One does not achieve a perfect picture of adolescence by considering cultural manifestations, but they provide a sketch from which one can understand a great deal.

STABILITY, INSTABILITY, AND DELINQUENCY

The great inner turmoil of adolescence brings with it mood swings, rebelliousness, anxieties, frustrations, anger, and doubts. This emotional upheaval is so pronounced that some observers have called adolescence the period of the *normal psychosis*. Conflict and suffering seem inevitable. It is somewhat problematic, then, to assess whether an adolescent's behavior is a sign that he is getting into difficulty or whether he is following a stormy but normal path to adulthood.

There are many opinions as to when an adolescent is truly in trouble with himself. Since the adolescent is on a long road to achieving a workable sense of self, conflicts and problems along the way are natural. Assessing his progress is quite difficult while the young person is vacillating and struggling so. Signs of relinquishing the struggle should be taken as cues that the adolescent is in serious difficulty. If the youth is no longer (even awkwardly) seeking solutions to his conflicts and problems, if he becomes totally alienated and unable to make choices for himself, he is in danger of failing to accomplish the developmental tasks of his age period. A young person who begins to reject large parts of that which society has to offer and takes on an alien way of life is especially endangering himself.

The drug culture that has flourished in recent years has preyed upon young people wishing to "find" themselves through a mind-expanding experience. The illusion of direct access to the inner mind, of easy self-discovery, becomes a temptation for young persons suffering the pains of adolescence. Continuing drug abuse is a complex behavior that is indicative of the uncertainty and insecurity of those who indulge in it. The peer group pressures concerning drug use can be particularly strong and difficult to resist for an adolescent who is already under significant emotional strain. Among adolescents, the availability of many types of drugs, combined with exhortations from peers and teen idols, makes some drug experimentation almost inevitable. However, the danger of continuing into a life-style that is unproductive and antisocial makes drug use a hazardous complication in an already turbulent life.

The adolescent whose conflict with society has involved him in the legal process may be termed *delinquent*. It is virtually impossible to offer a definition for delinquency that would be applicable to all areas of the United States, because the level of tolerance for acts committed by adolescents is different in various communities. In a rural area, actions which would be labeled delinquent in an urban setting might be viewed as merely "high spirits" on the part of the youth. Also, different agencies that deal with youthful law offenders have their own guidelines of age, offense, and previous record of the offender to delineate a delinquent youth.

Since an adolescent in trouble with the law is no longer a child and not yet an adult, he may be victimized by vaguely worded legislation allowing wide discretion on the part of judiciary and law enforcement personnel. Additionally, the community biases and tolerance level may administer unfair or de-velopmentally inappropriate treatment for his "crimes."

Many theories have been suggested to help explain delinquent behavior. A prominent theory which has spawned many studies is the *differential association* theory[22] developed by the famed criminologist Edwin H. Sutherland. He presents his theory through nine axioms which interrelate delinquency and criminality as being caused by the types of social relationships a person forms. Sutherland stresses that social relationships constitute the means by which either criminal or law-abiding behavior is learned. In adolescence, with the intensity of peer influence at its height, the risk of delinquency is apparent when viewed from this theoretical framework.

The differential association theory is sharply opposite the thinking of psychoanalytic theorists who view criminal behavior as an outcome of flaws in the early development of the personality. Blos[23] has postulated that the inability to build basic trust and the overwhelming need to control his environment bring the child to behavior in adolescence which is antisocial and labeled delinquent. In a primitive attempt to control, delinquent acts are perpetrated against the environment when the adolescent feels that the normal stresses of his age are too great and the environment is the cause of the stressful situation.

Prevention of delinquency involves identifying and helping those who are vulnerable to a delinquent life-style. The strategies concern improving environmental and home conditions in an attempt to reduce the stimuli which would push a young person into delinquency. Legislation is constantly in progress to protect young persons' rights and to establish agencies which help rehabilitate youthful offenders into a more productive life pattern.

REFERENCES

1 G. S. Hall, *Adolescence: Its Psychology and Its Relations to Physiology, Anthropology, Sociology, Sex, Crime, Religion and Education*, vols. I and II, Appleton-Century-Crofts, New York, 1904.

2 E. Jones, "Some Problems of Adolescence," *British Journal of Psychology*, 13:41–47, 1922.

3 Margaret Mead, *Coming of Age in Samoa*, William Morrow & Company, New York, 1928.

4 P. Aries, *Centuries of Childhood*, Alfred A. Knopf, Inc., New York, 1962.

5 D. J. Holmes, *The Adolescent in Psychotherapy*, Little, Brown and Company, Boston, 1964, p. 26.

6 G. H. Pearson, *Adolescence and the Conflict of Generations*, W. W. Norton & Company, Inc., New York, 1958.

7 R. E. Muuss, *Theories of Adolescence*, Random House, Inc., New York, 1968, pp. 5–7.

8 E. H. Erikson, *Childhood and Society*, W. W. Norton & Company, Inc., New York, 1963, p. 261.

9 G. H. Lowery, *Growth and Development of Children*, Year Book Medical Publishers, Inc., Chicago, 1973, pp. 299–302.

10 J. M. Tanner, *Growth at Adolescence*, Charles C Thomas, Publisher, Springfield, Ill., 1962.

11 U.S. Department of Health, Education and Welfare, *How Children Grow*, U.S. Government Printing Office, Washington, D.C., 1972, pp. 47–48.

12 Committee on Adolescence, Group for the Advancement of Psychiatry, *Normal Adolescence*, Charles Scribner's Sons, New York, pp. 105–110.

13 A. Kinsey et al., *Sexual Behavior in the Human Female*, W. B. Saunders Company, Philadelphia, 1953.

14 Elizabeth B. Hurlock, *Developmental Psychology*, McGraw-Hill Book Company, New York, 1968, p. 377.

15 E. H. Erikson, *Identity: Youth and Crisis*, W. W. Norton & Company, Inc., New York, 1968.

16 G. E. Hill, "College Proneness, a Guidance Problem," *Personal Guidance Journal*, 33:70–73, 1954.

17 D. D. Williams, *Adolescent Needs Met by Reference Group*, unpublished manuscript.

18 Margaret Mead, *Growing Up in New Guinea*, New American Library, Inc., New York, 1935.

19 Ann Sieg, "Why Adolescence Occurs," *Adolescence*, 6:337–347, 1971.

20 C. Arensburg and S. T. Kimball, *Family and Community in Ireland*, Harvard University Press, Cambridge, Mass., 1940.

21 H. Sebald, *Adolescence: A Sociological Analysis*, Appleton-Century-Crofts, New York, 1968, pp. 320–347.

22 E. H. Sutherland, *Principles of Criminology*, J. B. Lippincott Company, Philadelphia, 1947.

23 P. Blos, "Delinquency" in L. Sandor and H. I. Schneer (eds.), *Adolescents: Psychoanalytic Approach to Problems and Therapy*, Paul B. Hoeber, Inc., New York, 1961, p. 132.

BIBLIOGRAPHY

Coleman, J. S.: *The Adolescent Society*, The Free Press, New York, 1961.

Sorensen, R. C.: *Adolescent Sexuality in Contemporary America*, World Publishing Company, New York, 1973.

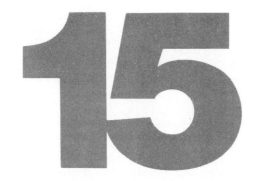

NUTRITION IN DEVELOPMENT

EDITH L. GETCHELL
and ROSANNE B. HOWARD*

The term "psychodietetics" has been coined[1] to describe relationships between the various sciences dealing with psychology and nutrition. Research in physiology, biochemistry, molecular biology, and nutrition has provided explanations concerning the functions of specific nutrients. The social and behavioral sciences have uncovered clues for understanding the various food habits observed around the world. Information has been pooled from these sources in an attempt to discover why the instincts tending to guide human beings in food selection become modified and, therefore, less reliable than those of animals. Food and feeding must be viewed in a wider context than the biochemical. Eating becomes a necessity dictated by needs beyond our physical survival; it is both complex and extremely personal. A publication of the National Dairy Council has beautifully described this human experience.[2]

> Food can bring to life my keen anticipation. . . . It can evoke my memory in all its pain and joy; it can pierce me with nostalgia. . . . Its preparation can be an act of relatedness, of creativity, of love; its eating can be participation and communion. Let us hope it also nourishes me physically, supplying me with the proteins, vitamins, carbohydrates and other nutrients I need to stay alive and healthy so that I can experience the fullness of human existence.

The nurse is in a position to enrich the eating experience. This chapter will attempt to convey the pervading influence of food on the total well-being of the developing child.

DEFINITION OF TERMS
Nutrition

Nutrition can be defined from the viewpoint of either the provider or the receiver. Nutrition can mean the act or process of nourishing as well as the act of being nourished. The interpersonal aspect is implicit. While in the past definitions were limited to the effect

* Supported in part through Project 928 Maternal and Child Health Services, Department of Health, Education, and Welfare.

The authors gratefully acknowledge the support of Allen Crocker, M.D., Project Director and Director of Pediatrics, Developmental Evaluation Clinic, Children's Hospital Medical Center; Maxine Gilson, former Director, Department of Dietetics, Children's Hospital Medical Center; and Ethel Trafton, Director, Children's Hospital School of Nursing. For editing assistance, they are indebted to Marie Cullinane, Director of Nursing, Developmental Evaluation Clinic, Children's Hospital Medical Center; Helene Marsh, Instructor of Pediatric Nursing, Children's Hospital School of Nursing; and Marguerite Queneau, R.D. (retired).

of food on individual organisms, current explanations reach beyond analyses or laboratory approaches and recognize that human nutrition, from infancy through senescence, embodies human relationships. Acceptance and availability of foods have direct bearing on what is given or received as nourishment. The acceptability of foods varies culturally, while the availability of foods is determined by geography, climate, and technology. Both are affected by politics and economics. Yudkin's definition of nutrition is both simple and inclusive: "Nutrition is the study of the relationship between man and his food."[3]

Nutritional Status

Nutritional status is concerned with the condition of the human body, which is the expression of that body's utilization of essential nutrients. Nutritional status may be good, fair, or poor, depending upon the availability of nutrients. Availability is affected by intake, individual body needs, and ability to use the nutrients provided, that is, efficiency of digestion and absorption. Evaluation of nutritional status requires the collection and interpretation of physical, biochemical, and clinical observations as well as a study of food intake.

Nutrient Needs

Nutrient needs (synonymous with minimum requirement) are highly variable. Each individual's need for a specific nutrient depends upon his height, weight, biologic age, sex, and state of health. Differentiation must be made between the commonly used terms minimum requirement and recommended allowance. The *minimum requirement* for any specific nutrient is defined as the least amount of that nutrient that will promote an optimum state of health. The term *recommended dietary allowance*, commonly referred to as RDA, applies to a table of values published periodically by the Food and Nutrition Board of the National Research Council at the National Academy of Sciences. The recommendations are intended to serve as goals for planning food supplies and for interpretation of food consumption data of groups of people. Except for calories, the allowances include margins of safety designed to allow for variations of need among the general population. This margin also provides a buffer for the increased needs of common stress and allows for full realization of growth and productive potential. RDAs do not represent minimum requirements but do suggest amounts that allow for the normal variations in individual

nutrient needs that would be found in the healthy United States population. Thus, the values recommended exceed many individual needs. However, the built-in safety factor should not be considered adequate to cover additional requirements of individuals depleted by disease, traumatic stress, or prolonged inadequate nutritional intake or utilization. The conclusion should never be made that individual food intakes short of recommendations constitute inadequacies.

Enrichment and Fortification

As both infant foods and staple foods may be enriched or fortified, clarification of these terms seems indicated. Commonly used foods can be enhanced in nutritive value by enrichment or fortification.[4, 5] *Enriched* foods (primarily those made from cereal grains) are those in which the thiamine, riboflavin, niacin, and iron that were removed in processing have been replaced. The basic four food selection guide of the National Dairy Council specifies the use of enriched or whole grain products in their bread and cereal food group. Any product labeled enriched must include all four of the above nutrients. Calcium and vitamin D additions are optional, but if made, it must be stated on the label. Minimum and maximum ranges are established by the Food and Drug Administration (FDA). Enrichment of food is not required by federal law, although many manufacturers voluntarily enrich their products.

Fortification applies to foods with certain added nutrients that may or may not have been present naturally in the food. Margarine may be fortified with vitamin A. Most fluid and evaporated milk is fortified with vitamin D. Some table salts have been fortified with iodine. Iron-fortified cereals provide iron at higher levels than enriched products. Levels of fortification are also defined by the FDA.

Nutrition Labeling

Because of increased public interest in nutrition and the need for accurate consumer information, the FDA published regulations in *The Federal Register* (Jan. 19, 1973) establishing criteria for nutrition labeling.[6] These criteria were designed to provide the consumer with information to enable him to assess the nutritional quality of the food he buys. Nutritional labeling is voluntary unless some nutritional claim is shown on the label. If a product makes any specific nutrient claim, or if the product is labeled "enriched" or "fortified," full nutrition labeling is required. Size of serving, servings per container, carbohydrate, protein, fat, and calorie content, as well as the percentage of the RDAs for protein and seven of the important vitamins and minerals must be stated on the label. Major nutrients present in amounts less than 2 percent of RDA must be identified.

Products designed and marketed for special dietary use ("dietetic" products such as those reduced in sodium and carbohydrate content) also have labeling requirements which identify ingredients and the amount of the altered nutrient still present in the product.

Members of the health team involved in nutrition education need to become proficient label readers. Some consumers may require assistance in order to make practical use of the information provided. For those with lowered or increased nutrient needs, skill in product analysis becomes imperative. Parents could find this information helpful in making wise marketing selections for their families.

THE IMPACT OF NUTRITION ON DEVELOPMENT
Nutritional Status at Conception

The influence of nutrition on growth has no point of beginning, and only death marks the end of its effect, for middle and later years are simply continuations of human development. The quality of the developing fetus is dependent upon maternal status at entry into pregnancy, which in turn reflects eating habits of the years preceding conception. Shank[7] reports that the two major reasons for low birth weight in babies are the youthfulness of the mother and her poor nutrition. It is no accident that these two factors emerge as being the most common, for poor nutrition is all too often characteristic of the adolescent. To existing risks of biologic immaturity and poor nutritional status, her poor food habits may add another—insufficient weight gain during pregnancy. The old practice of allowing a total weight gain of only 18 lb is no longer tenable. Improving dietary intake during pregnancy will help the unborn but cannot be expected to erase the deficits existing at the outset of gestation. Prenatal nutrition education must not confine itself to a brief 9 months, but must broaden its scope to include the preceding years.

Intrauterine Growth

The growth which takes place in the 9-month prenatal period is the most crucial and rapid of any period of human growth. Present evidence indicates that the influence of the uterine environment may equal that of genetic endowment.[8] The second through the tenth week of prenatal growth is the most vulnerable period because it is then that the cells for arms, legs, eyes, ears, and vital organs differentiate. If the concentration of nutrients traveling through the placenta is adequate, the birth weight of the infant is expected to be a minimum of 5½ lb (2,500 Gm).

Infant survival rate is inversely correlated with birth weight. The practice of classifying all infants below 5½ lb as premature has changed. Low-birth-weight infants are now more accurately grouped as either intrauterine growth retarded or premature. It is believed that intrauterine growth retardation accounts for one-third to one-half of all low-birth-weight newborns.

Although ounce for ounce the growth-retarded newborns (low weight for date) have better survival rates than premature infants, they do have a higher incidence of birth defects.[9] Poor nutritional status of the mother is associated with the occurrence of both prematurity and growth retardation. As mentioned earlier, nutritional status is the expression of long-standing preconceptional nutrition. Interestingly (though not to minimize the importance of nutrition during pregnancy), a mother arriving at pregnancy with normal nutritional stores has a good chance of producing a normal birth weight baby *even if* her intake during pregnancy is not adequate. The old wives' tale is true: the developing fetus has competitive advantage and will satisfy his nutritional needs at the expense of the mother.[10]

Much attention has been given to the relationship between nutritional deprivation and attainment of mental potential. Small-for-gestational-age infants carry an increased risk of mental retardation. Fetal undernutrition may seriously affect growth and development of the central nervous system. The deficits may not be completely reversed by good postnatal nutrition. It is important to realize that the inadequate nutritional supply to the fetus is more likely the result of inadequate placental function than secondary to maternal malnutrition. However, the deficiency in nutrient supply has far-reaching consequences, and postnatal nutrition of low-birth-weight babies requires scrupulous attention.[11]

Optimal Lifetime Development

An optimal state of health is contingent upon a properly balanced assortment of available essential nutrients. Choice of food influences every stage of growth and development. During times of accelerated growth such as infancy and adolescence, when nutrient needs are the greatest, the importance of the quality of intake is apparent. The periods of gradual growth, the mature years, and even advanced age are likewise affected by imbalances and shortages in supply. During growth and development (increase in size and complexity of function) each organ system has its critical time of development, so there is no time when interference with the supply line is without consequence. Prior to adolescence, although growth rate is slower, laying down nutrient stores will provide advantages for the growth spurts to follow. Mortality rates from all children's diseases are higher when malnutrition coexists. Less loss of growth potential results from infections in well-nourished populations. The onset of puberty can be delayed by malnutrition, and even though puberty will eventually be attained, maximum size will not. Malnourished children are smaller when they enter puberty in comparison with well-nourished peers and remain relatively smaller at the end of puberty.[12] Obesity, the opposite expression of malnutrition, is associated with a shortened life expectancy because of its correlation with such conditions as diabetes, atherosclerosis, and hypertension. Its occurrence can complicate respiratory difficulties and increase surgical risk.

THE INTERRELATIONSHIP OF NUTRITION WITH PHYSICAL AND PSYCHOSOCIAL DEVELOPMENT

Physical growth—an increase in the number and size of cells—is influenced by heredity, nutrition, hormones, and time. Throughout the world, children show very similar capacities for growth, although the attainment of potential may be dissimilar because of differences in environmental support. Even when all growth needs are met, development, although similar for all children, varies in rate, and each child proceeds to adulthood at his own pace. Before puberty, normal growth appears more dependent on environment than upon genetic makeup, hence the emphasis afforded to nutrition.

Personality development is influenced by the feeding experience. At the breast or bottle, the infant learns many things: what his mother looks like; how she sounds, feels, and smells; and what she tastes like. The infant's powers of perception begin developing very early. As his biologic needs of hunger and thirst are met, he experiences satisfaction (a full stomach) and comes to identify the one who provides that satisfaction. As needs are answered, trust develops. Unfortunately the feeding experience can also be the setting for the development of faulty interpersonal relationships in cases in which oppositional or passive-aggressive behavior takes place.[13]

Physical Development

Growth is often discussed in terms of two ages: the chronologic, timed from birth; and the biologic, which is a measurement of physical maturity. *Biologic age* is often determined by bone x-ray and is referred to as bone age. The extent of ossification (which progresses through puberty) and of epiphyseal closure increases with biologic age. *Chronologic age* can be gauged by the number of muscle cells and is related to a child's sex.

The old belief that growth after birth was due solely to increase in cell size has given way to the realization that specialized cells increase in *number* as well as size for many years after birth. Boys and girls are born with the same number of muscle cells, but by age 10, girls have a fivefold increase in cell number, after which there is little change in either cell size or cell number. In contrast, by the age of 18 years, boys have increased their birth muscle cell number 14-fold, and the size continues to enlarge for another 5 years. Once muscle cells stop growing, increase in size (as evidenced by muscle-building exercise) is due to an increase in the diameter of the fibrils within the muscle cell. Caloric needs for the sexes differ because basal metabolic needs are related to muscle mass; therefore, the female must consume fewer calories than her male peers if she is to avoid weight gain. From birth the female's fatty tissue exceeds that of the male. She enters the world more biologically mature and apparently less vulnerable to growth-retarding conditions.

Effects of Deprivation Marked deviation from the growth patterns exhibited by the normal population have been viewed with concern, especially when these apparent growth failures are seen in early life. The extremely rapid growth of the first year makes the infant especially vulnerable to shortages and imbalances in the nutrient supply. Genetic contributions to low heights and weights, while valid in some instances, are less common than originally believed, and current opinion leans toward environmental etiology. Many studies have been conducted and opinions expressed concerning long-term effects of malnutrition on growth and mental development.[11, 12, 14–17]

The most rapid brain growth takes place during the first year. Thereafter growth proceeds more slowly; yet by the third year a child's brain has reached 80 percent of its adult weight. The implications are most striking when this growth rate is compared to the rest of the body which, at this age, has only reached 20 percent of adult size. Undernutrition of sufficient magnitude to affect height and weight might be expected to place similar limitations on concurrent brain growth. Studies suggest that severe malnutrition in early infancy results in decreased brain size due to decreased cellularity. The earlier the infant develops malnutrition, the more marked the effect upon brain size.

Malnutrition has been associated with retardation of intellectual development, influencing learning, perceptual ability, and attention span. Agreement on interpretation of experimental data is lacking because of differences of opinion regarding validity of methods used to determine intelligence. In many studies, retardation is defined in terms of IQ scores which, admittedly, are most often designed for middle-class exposures. Poverty and malnutrition coexist, and the presence or absence of environmental stimuli conducive to learning has not always been examined. However, studies [18-20] aimed at controlling the many other variables—size of family, income, education of parents, home environment—seem to indicate that extreme malnutrition during the first year of life does indeed contribute to long-lasting intellectual limitations, which may not be reversed by suitable nutritional intervention.

Lowenberg's vicious circle[14] illustrates the cyclic nature of poverty engendering poverty. Lowered earning capacity spawns inability to procure an adequate food supply, which in turn results in educational lacks, poor housing, disease, and infections. All of these factors drain energies and capacites, and so the circle goes on.

At present, it is impossible to conclude that diet alone is responsible for stunting intellectual potential. Controlling the many variables, which in addition to malnutrition influence mental capacity, is exceedingly difficult. There is still more to be learned concerning the extent of the role of malnutrition and the permanence of its effect. We can conclude, however, that both social and nutritional deficiencies interact, and the correction of one deficiency without the correction of the other is inappropriate.

Concerns about Overfeeding

Patterning for Obesity Overnutrition can be viewed as a form of malnutrition. Among various school populations, 15 to 30 percent have been estimated to be obese. The chances are 4 out of 5 that overweight will persist into adolescence and adulthood. A high correlation exists between teen-age obesity and development in later years of heart disease, diabetes, hypertension, and respiratory problems. The question has been asked: "Is it possible that giving too much food too soon contributes to maturity obesity?"

Should we not consider the possibility that maximal rates of growth and maturation during infancy may be incompatible with vigorous maturity and the greatest life expectancy? Current infant feeding practices introduce solid foods long before biologic need requires it. Even reasonable dietary additions based on developmental and overall nutritional needs can exceed infant *caloric* requirements (see Table 15-10A and B). Perhaps an overzealous approach to early feeding does pattern for (predispose to) obesity. Hirsch,[21] using a method of cell sizing and counting, examined adipose tissue cellularity. He studied adults of normal weight, obese adults, and obese adults who had lost weight, as well as infants and children. He discovered that the obese had a 40 percent increase in fat-cell size and a 190 percent increase in fat cell *number*. Those with the earliest onset of obesity had the highest number of cells. The largest cell size was found in persons who were most obese and whose obesity had begun in adulthood. Cross-sectional examination of subjects who had successfully lost weight revealed that although their fat cell *size* decreased to values of the nonobese controls, their cell *number* remained high. Studies on 30 infants and children indicate that there is roughly a threefold increase in fat cell size from birth to age 6, with little change in size between the ages of 6 and 13. However, at 13 the fat cells still have not reached adult proportions. The *number* of cells, however, increases more rapidly, tripling during the first year of life and showing a more gradual increase throughout childhood. Adult numbers have not been reached at puberty. If overfeeding in infancy causes increase in adipose cellularity, current feeding practices may put many children at a disadvantage in terms of lifetime weight regulation. If most adipose tissue growth has taken place by adolescence, the need for caloric regulation before adolescence is apparent. The obese adolescent has a Herculean task cut out for him when he attempts to wage the battle of the bulge.

Excessive Sodium Intake The early ingestion of solid foods has been correlated with higher sodium intakes later in life.[22] Because mothers refuse foods judged unpalatable to their taste, salt is added to almost all baby and junior foods. The 4-month-old infant consuming cow's milk and a combination of commercially prepared infant foods ingests five times as much sodium as the breast-fed infant.[23] Although evidence associating salt intake with the development of hypertension is inconclusive, there are numbers of reports which do show a correlation between salt intake and frequency of hypertension in other cultures.[23, 24] Increasing salt intake has been shown to precipitate development of hypertension in the rat, but addition of salt to infant foods at levels currently used has not been proved either harmful or harmless. However, intakes of infants are substantially in excess of needs, and recommendations have been made that manufacturers reduce the level of salt used in infant foods.[25]

Type of Fat in Infant Diets Fatty streaking of arteries has been observed early in infancy. Fomon[26] suggests that manipulation of an infant's type of dietary fat (i.e., increasing polyunsaturates) even if proved effective, raises additional questions. Similarity of lipid concentrations in the serum of breast-fed infants with those of babies fed formula (cow's milk with butterfat) suggest that breast milk is equally hazardous. More practically, adjustments during infancy may be insignificant in relation to dietary intake throughout life.

Unnecessary Use of Vitamins Another form of overfeeding is the irresponsible addition of vitamins to the diet. Vitamin supplementation is common pediatric practice. However, as more infant staple foods are enriched or fortified, attention should be given to the total amount of each nutrient being consumed by infants and children. Adjustment in routine vitamin supplements may be indicated in terms of actual need and the greater availability in food. Although toxicity is an unlikely problem except for vitamins A and D, providing amounts of nutrients substantially in excess of needs is neither economically sound or medically indicated. At the present, opinions differ on iron fortification. Some authorities strongly advocate fortification because of the high incidence of iron-deficiency anemia,[27, 28] while others call for caution in view of our incomplete knowledge regarding iron absorption and because of the rare disposition some individuals have to excessive iron storage.[29]

Contributions to the Development of Motor Skills and Learning The part food and feeding play in the development of motor skills is often overlooked. Table 15-11 illustrates the many opportunities mealtime provides for developing coordination. Food can also be an early learning experience in discovering colors, shapes, and textures. A child's insatiable curiosity to explore and learn does not stop during mealtime. A new food offered may initially remain untasted, though fingers, eyes, and nose eagerly explore in attempts to become familiar with it. Tasting may await another time, and the wise parent does

not interpret his child's response as a refusal. The manual dexterity exhibited by an infant when holding his own bottle develops and becomes refined through progressive attempts at the cup, the spoon, and in later years, the fork and knife. The child whose parent interferes unnecessarily or offers too much help is deprived of many learning opportunities.

Psychosocial Development

Personality Development in the Feeding Situation The feeding situation provides a setting for many of life's most pleasant experiences. Unfortunately, the dinner table also becomes the arena for acting out conflicts between child and parent and among family members. Why do food and eating become so emotionally charged?

Unlike solitary experiences such as sleeping or defecating, eating from the very first exposure involves two people and throughout life continues to connote the interpersonal. We are so conditioned to the social aspect of food that few of us enjoy eating alone; when forced to do so, we dispense with the meal quickly. During feeding the infant is exposed to, and at the mercy of, the emotions and attitudes of the parent or parent substitute. Early feeding experiences can be either a foundation for the development of rich and fulfilling personal relationships or the beginnings of confusion, tension, withdrawal, and decreasing ability to communicate. Failure to thrive (of nonorganic cause), rumination, and anorexia nervosa are expressions of extreme distortion of family function and parent-child interaction. Well-meaning parents can unintentionally set up road blocks to a good feeding atmosphere. Overconcern for the child's nutritional health can lead to forcing or bullying. Failure to recognize developing individuality or faulty interpretation of the messages primitively communicated by a child can lead to inappropriate action on the part of the parent and confusion for the child. Bruch[30] has spent many years treating patients with appetite disorders and has observed consequences of faulty communications in early feeding experiences. Her clinical observation of the obese and anorexic indicate that a common denominator of these extremes in eating behavior is a distortion in the ability to recognize hunger. The experience of hunger contains elements of learning and develops out of reciprocal feedbacks between mother and child. If an infant expresses tension from discomfort or the desire for attention, and his expression is incorrectly interpreted as hunger and answered by the offer of food, the infant is confused and misled. Response to a verbal or conceptual communication should answer the child's *actual* need rather than the parent's opinion of the infant's need. Adults' powers of observation need to be developed so that communications from child to parent are accurately translated. With appropriate responses the child learns to recognize his bodily sensations. He recognizes hunger as a genuine need for food, and he does not confuse this sensation with other tensions. Eating then is not misused to serve complex emotional and interpersonal problems.

Mealtime provides the preschooler an opportunity for increased socialization. Parental behavior has tremendous impact at this time of increased imitation and sex identification. Attitudes about food and interactions between other family members are observed and accurately imitated. The feeding environment can be psychologically significant. Feeding problems are really a problem of development. The dinner table provides the child with a perfect opportunity to register dissatisfaction with what parents are giving or expecting. From infancy, nutritional needs and the approaches to satisfy them play an important role in personality and character development.

Symbolism in Food Hunger connotes need; appetite implies desire or preference which is based on previous experience. "Biological hunger becomes culturally patterned appetite."[31] Symbolic significance of food determines whether food is craved or refused. Human beings place the importance of symbolic aspects above the more practical consideration of nutrient contribution or need. Children learn from their families the meanings of food, patterns of meals, and what constitutes a proper food for a particular meal. Within any culture, food habits are the oldest and most deeply entrenched of behaviors. Milk, a staple of American culture, is rejected as an animal discharge by some societies. The Greeks center their meal around bread, and all else becomes secondary. The Moslem and Orthodox Jew shun pork, while the Seventh Day Adventist may be a vegetarian. Food becomes an expression of support or a means of sharing joy. At the death of a friend, concern is often expressed by preparing food for the bereaved family. Weddings, birthdays, christenings, bar mitzvahs, and graduations give food a place of prominence. For those involved in feeding children, it is wise to remember that a person accepts food best from those he considers a friend or an ally. The child who feels threatened by or antagonistic toward a nurse or dietitian will never eat well for him.

Of course the enormity of social influence on eating stems from the mother's original role. Moore describes eating as human and feeding as maternal.[32] A mother's image of herself as well as the image she projects to others is usually strongly colored by her role in the feeding situation. Her self-esteem is deeply involved. Nutritional suggestions and education should be directed at building upon good existing practices without overtly questioning maternal competence. The very young child may consider his mother the best cook in the world though her choices of food are poor and her skill in preparing them is minimal. Families from limited backgrounds or different cultures may have unshakable faith in their own customs, many of which are as valid as those of middle-class America.

Other meanings of food include the status afforded to such items as steak or caviar, and the "feminine" connotation of the cottage cheese and fruit salad as compared to the "masculine" ham and eggs. Some food items are assigned age categories; peanut butter is for children, olives for adults. The unspoken language of food is clearly understood and dictates the formation of long-lasting, difficult to alter food habits.

Inappropriate Use of Food At a very early age the child in a primitive society learns that eating is not a right but a necessity for survival. He discovers that food is essential but in no way satisfies needs, probably not even hunger. The status hierarchy probably dictates that men eat first, then women, and finally children, who are given the remains.

Wolff discusses the very different set of impressions given the American child.[33] Insecure parents establish hierarchies in which children place first, even to the detriment of others. The availability of food is casually accepted, with only a small segment of society being actually aware of real hunger.[62] Unfortunately, the child learns early that food is a reward or can be used as a pacifier. He is cajoled into performing certain tasks or curbing unacceptable behavior by the promise of a cookie or a piece of candy. His bruises and hurt feelings are soothed with a lollipop or ice cream cone. Certain foods may become so desirable that foods with necessary nutrients may be excluded from the diet.

Misuse of food may pave the road to obesity by dulling the perception of actual hunger, so that one eats even when the stomach is full. Food misuse can also deter the developing child from realistically approaching the challenges of life. This is not to suggest that pleasure should be removed from the eating situation. Impersonal aspects of modern life can be relieved by the family-centered mealtime when food becomes an expression of love, sharing, and genuine enjoyment. This exemplifies the proper use of food.

MEETING NUTRITIONAL AND PSYCHOSOCIAL NEEDS OF THE GROWING CHILD

Nurturing in the total sense of the word requires more than the provision of food. Education and physical and emotional support also promote development, and together with food they influence the expressions of human genetic potential. The requirements for total nutritional care, applicable to ill or handicapped as well as to normal and healthy children, include determining *individual* nutrient needs, recognizing levels of development, understanding expected behaviors which are characteristic of the development achieved, and recognizing and meeting psychosocial and emotional needs.

When all the above requirements are considered in the feeding situation, a sound nutritional approach is assured. Nutrient needs vary with age and maturation. Impaired health can place additional demands on nutrient supply. Physical limitations affecting ingestion, digestion, and absorption must be considered when determining individual nutrient needs.

To avoid unnecessary and harmful tension during feeding, expectations of ability and behavior must be realistic. Manual maturity of a child should dictate how much assistance or encouragement is given. Chronologic age is not always a reliable indicator of manipulative capability. With inaccurate observations of "readiness" signs, the feeder may expect too much and show impatience or may require too little and overprotect the child or thwart his natural desires to do things for himself. Certain behaviors are natural expressions of levels of maturity. Imposing standards of neatness on an infant still learning texture and shape by touch and handling will lead to frustration for everyone involved. Awareness of the growing child's changing emotional needs guides the student and parent in their approach. These important considerations are illustrated and discussed later in this chapter under "Establishing Sound Nutritional Practices."

Calorie-Yielding Food Components

Carbohydrate In the United States during the past 60 years there has been a marked decrease in the consumption of complex carbohydrate (starch from cereal grains and tuberous vegetables) and a sharp increase in the ingestion of simple sugars (sucrose). This change has been viewed with concern as various studies examine the role of sucrose in heart disease and the development of obesity. In pediatrics, concern centers on the contribution carbohydrate makes to the incidence of dental caries, as well as its influence on the development of tastes and preferences which may prove detrimental.

There is no specific recommendation for desirable carbohydrate intake. Diets known to be compatible with good health can vary widely in the proportions present. Eskimos, whose diets have a higher percentage of calories from fat than from carbohydrate, show no ill effects. Changes in total carbohydrate intake apparently elicit compensations by the body. Fomon[34] suggests that carbohydrate should comprise 29 to 58 percent of the calories in the infant's diet. Human milk furnishes 42 percent of calories as carbohydrate, and commercial formulas generally imitate this level. Laupus and Bennett[35] indicate that desirable carbohydrate levels can range from 25 to 55 percent of total calories. On the average, a well-balanced diet (for all ages) will provide approximately half the calories in the form of carbohydrate.

Storage capacity of carbohydrate is limited to 1 percent of the body weight. Glycogen deposits occur primarily in the liver where they act homeostatically to regulate blood glucose levels. Adult glycogen reserves supply sufficient energy for only 13 hours of very moderate activity.[36] The infant, whose liver is one-tenth the size of the adult, has much smaller glycogen reserves. Children with their proportionately higher caloric needs may quickly deplete this ready source of energy. Sufficient carbohydrate must be available (from stores or via absorption after eating) to prevent both excessive protein breakdown and development of ketosis. Development of ketosis demonstrates metabolic pathways of carbohydrate metabolism and the interrelationship with the oxidation of fat. Application of the principles involved can be made to various clinical situations—treatment of epilepsy, uncontrolled juvenile diabetes, and prolonged vomiting in the absence of eating, to name a few.

Ketosis is prevented by providing carbohydrate in sufficient quantities to insure complete metabolism of fat. For the adult, a daily 100-Gm carbohydrate intake is considered to be the lowest desirable level. This is roughly 20 percent of total calories. No minimal levels have been recommended for children. When carbohydrate levels fall below those necessary to support fat metabolism, acidosis develops. During the metabolism of the nutrients, oxaloacetate, produced by the oxidation of carbohydrate, combines with intermediary products of fat metabolism (ketones). This important combination reaction allows fat metabolites to enter the Kreb's (citric acid) cycle, resulting in the production of energy, carbon dioxide, and water. When carbohydrate metabolism is decreased, ketones accumulate, for they are produced at a faster rate than they can be oxidized. Since they are acidic, the body's acid-base balance is disturbed. Treatment is aimed at the cause of decreased carbohydrate metabolism. Therefore, the uncontrolled diabetic is given insulin to reverse his metabolic acidosis. Those unable to tolerate oral feedings or to consume a sufficient amount receive glucose intravenously. During fasting, the body mobilizes protein and adipose tissue for energy. However, the glucose provided by protein is insufficient to meet the demands of fat awaiting oxidation.

Dietary modifications designed for the treatment of epilepsy are based on the interrelationship of fat and carbohydrate metabolism just described. The diet purposely produces and maintains a state of acidosis by markedly decreasing carbohydrate and disproportionately increasing intake of fat. As early as 1921, accumulation of ketones was found to have a favorable effect on the irritability and restlessness of some epileptic children. Lasser[37] provided for a 3-year-old a diet containing only 4 percent of calories from carbohydrate (10 Gm) with 88 percent being derived from fat. Signore,[38] by using medium-chained triglycerides, which have a greater ketogenic effect because of their rapid absorption, did not restrict carbohydrate as drastically. Diets with carbohydrate providing as much as 19 percent of calories still produced the desired degree of ketosis; fat intake remained high at 70 percent of calories. Comparison of these levels with normal distribution (see Table 15-1) makes it apparent that ketogenic diets are difficult to design and follow. Without great care in planning they are very unpalatable.

It is interesting to note that several currently fashionable reduction diets restrict carbohydrate intakes far below recommendations. Some even state the establishment of ketosis as a goal. Weight loss is achieved as body fat is mobilized to meet energy needs and is incompletely metabolized in the absence of sufficient glucose. Because accumulating ketones must be excreted by the kidney, water intake should be increased. This approach to weight reduction (as all other "fad" diets) does not lend itself to improving faulty food habits. The effects of prolonged ketosis are not known. The extreme departure from customary food preferences required by the low-carbohydrate diets makes adherence difficult. The advisability of following such a regimen in the absence of compelling reasons (such as epilepsy) is highly questionable.

Malabsorption resulting from impaired carbohydrate digestion may be primary (due to disaccharidase deficiency) or secondary (resulting from epithelial cell damage, as in ulcerative colitis or gluten-induced enteropathy). Final carbohydrate digestion occurs at the microvilli extensions of the intestinal epithelial cell where disaccharidase enzymes (maltase, lactase, and sucrase) accomplish the final cleaving of double sugars. Glucose, fructose, and galactose are the end products. (See Table 15-1 for classifications of carbohydrate.) The intestinal cells limit entry to monosaccharides, as their carrier systems can only accommodate the molecular structure of these single 6-carbon molecules. Incompletely digested carbohydrate accumulates and is subject to degradation by intestinal microflora. The bacterial breakdown products and the accumulated unabsorbable carbohydrate act osmotically to produce distention of the bowel and troublesome diarrhea. When the specific missing enzyme is identified, the foods which must be eliminated become apparent. Lactase is the most common disaccharidase deficiency and requires omission of milk and milk products. Table 15-1 identifies major food sources of the various carbohydrate classifications.

Protein Protein is necessary to all biologic processes. Its major function is to provide nitrogen and amino acids for the synthesis of body proteins and other nitrogen-containing substances, such as nucleoproteins, creatinine, histamine, hormones, and hemoglobin. The characteristic properties of proteins depend upon their three-dimensional structure, hence, on the specific amino acids present and the *sequence* in which they occur. Synthesis is directed by the genetic material of the cell nucleus: DNA.

Protein synthesis is dependent upon a ready source of nitrogen and essential amino acids. Isoleucine, leucine, lysine, methionine, phenylalanine, threonine, tryptophan, and valine have been shown to be essential to the adult. Human beings cannot synthesize these individual amino acids but are able to manufacture the remaining amino acids found in cells. The essential amino acids, therefore, must be furnished by diet.

Amino acid requirements vary among different age groups and in certain disease conditions. Infants cannot synthesize arginine and histidine rapidly enough to accommodate growth needs, and so, for them, these two become essential. Tyrosine can be derived from phenylalanine and is not considered essential. However, in the metabolic disease phenylketonuria (PKU), diets limited in phenylalanine do not provide sufficient amounts to allow for conversion to tyrosine; consequently, tyrosine is essential to the child with PKU. Products commonly used in the treatment of this metabolic disorder are fortified with the amino acid tyrosine.

Protein synthesis requires that all essential amino acids be present in the diet simultaneously. The absence of only one amino acid will produce negative nitrogen balance. Requirements for amino acids are influenced by other nutrients. Recommended protein allowances assume sufficient calories from carbohydrate and fat, since caloric deficits will divert protein from synthesis and convert it to energy. Allowances must also consider food sources, for it is the amino acid balance that determines the total grams of protein that will be necessary. Animal proteins ensure a high concentration of essential amino acids and are referred to as *complete* proteins. Because vegetable protein has some essential amino acid deficiencies, vegetables represent *incomplete* protein sources. If protein is derived primarily from vegetables, the total intake must be higher to compensate for the lower concentration of essential amino acids. Choices can be made so that the resulting mixture is as effective as animal protein, but selection requires care and guidance. The recommended dietary allowances (RDA) shown in Table 15-1 were based on the following considerations:

1 The amount of protein necessary to replace nitrogen losses from urine, feces, sweat, and skin
2 Growth needs
3 Variability of need among different healthy people
4 Efficient utilization (65 to 70 percent)

The latter reflects our cultural use of a mixed diet—proteins from both plant and animal sources. Protein needs of the infant are based on the presumption that the amount in breast milk is adequate. Human milk provides 8 percent of calories as protein. Reference to Table 15-1 illustrates the high needs of early infancy, when the protein provided must be of optimum quality.

In the 1973 revision of the *Recommended Dietary Allowances*, protein recommendations are lower than previously presented. The adult allowance is 0.8 Gm/kg body weight (a 0.1 Gm/kg body weight decrease). Determination of children's allowances required estimation of growth needs, which was derived from limited data on body composition, applied to norms of height and weight of "Anglo" children at the different ages. The new allowances (see Table 15-1) are not significantly different for infants and children, but are 20 percent lower for adolescents.[39] Present protein allowances for all ages, however, are far lower than amounts voluntarily consumed—although preferred consumption should not be equated with requirement or advisable levels of intake.

The National Academy of Sciences has stressed that protein allowances are valid *only* if energy intakes are adequate to maintain weight in adults, or acceptable growth rates in children. Weight can be maintained over a range of caloric intake, however, nitrogen balance has been impaired by decreases in calories that have not caused noticeable loss of body weight.[40]

The protein standards have been established to meet the needs of healthy individuals in a population. Allowances were set at 2 standard deviations above the minimum requirement. This would exceed the needs of two-thirds of the population and meet the needs of almost all healthy individuals. Current recommendations will provide 7 to 9 percent of energy as protein. Common food practices can provide up to 20 percent of calories in this form.

The "all-or-nothing" aspect of protein synthesis requires that some complete protein food be offered at every meal to ensure the sumultaneous presence of all essential amino acids. When protein intake does not exceed actual protein needs, an adequate caloric intake is essential.

Vegetarianism, a long-established eating practice usually associated with religious or philosophic beliefs, is becoming more common among the adolescent and young adult population. Vegetarianism has presented a challenge to nutrition educators, who find it difficult to evaluate adequacy and make appropriate suggestions while using "traditional" tools of measure. Some vegetarian diets can be hazardous, while others generously meet nutritional requirements. Erhard[41] presents the various categories of vegetarianism and suggests educational tools which can be used in meeting needs of even the extreme adherents. Identifying the type of vegetarian diet is important. Lactovovegetarians include milk and eggs in their diet, while lactovegetarians use only milk. Pure vegetarians, or vegans, exclude all animal sources of protein. Fruitarians hazardously restrict their foods to raw or dried fruits, nuts, honey, and olive oil. Table 15-2 shows the amino acid composition of some foods and provides a guide for complementing low amino acid foods

Table 15-1   ENERGY-YIELDING NUTRIENTS

Nutrient	Functions	Energy yield per gram	Recommended allowances				
			Infancy	Ages 1–3 years	Ages 4–6 years	Ages 7–10 years	Ages 11–18 years
Carbohydrate	1 Energy source 2 Antiketogenic 3 Protein sparing 4 Source of bulk 5 Necessary for production of important body compounds: Ribose Deoxyribose Blood group materials Detoxifying agents Human milk	4 kcal (17kJ)	Minimum carbohydrate requirement unknown General recommendation: 40–50% of calories				
Protein	1 Provides nitrogen and amino acids for synthesis of body proteins and other nitrogen-containing substances 2 Energy source	4 kcal (17kJ)	8% of calories 0–6 mo 2.2 Gm/kg 6–12 mo 2.0 Gm/kg	10% of calories* 23 Gm daily	Usually increases to 20% of calories* 30 Gm daily	36 Gm	Boys: 11–14 years 44 Gm 15–18 years 54 Gm Girls: 11–14 years 44 Gm 15–18 years 48 Gm

* Reflects cultural preferences; exceeds recommended allowances.

Classifications	Examples	Major food sources	Pediatric concerns
Polysaccharides	Starch (composed of glucose units)	Cereals and cereal products and vegetables (corn, potatoes, legumes, winter squash)	Carbohydrate is restricted in the following metabolic disorders:
	Cellulose, hemicellulose	Skins, seeds, structural parts of plants	Diabetes Glycogen storage disease Galactosemia
	Pectin	Apples	Fructose intolerance
	Glycogen (storage form of glucose)	Muscle and liver of freshly slaughtered meat	Glucose intolerance Disaccharide deficiency
Disaccharides	Sucrose (glucose and fructose)	Cane sugar, candy, pastry, cake, pie, ice cream, condensed milk, fruits, jellies, vegetables	Excessive use of sucrose is associated with dental caries
	Maltose (2 glucose)	A product of starch hydrolysis	
	Lactose (glucose and galactose)	Milk, ice cream, yogurt, milk chocolate	
Monosaccharides	Glucose	Fruits (largest amounts in dates, dried figs, and prunes), sugar, corn syrup, honey, molasses	
	Fructose	Fruits (largest amounts in dates, dried figs, and prunes), honey, sugar, molasses	
	Galactose	Produced from milk sugar; minute amounts in peaches, beet sugar, casein, pears, apples, soybeans	
Complete protein	Proteins from animal sources which contain all the essential amino acids	Milk, eggs, meat, fish, poultry, cheese	Growth during first year of life requires high-quality protein. After first year, approximately half of the total protein intake should be derived from high-quality sources.
	Synthetic proteins	Protein analogues	Adolescents experimenting with vegetarianism need to learn vegetable protein combinations which assure balanced amino acid distribution.
Incomplete protein	Proteins from vegetable sources which lack one or more of the essential amino acids	Soybeans, peas, beans, cereals, nuts, lentils	Disorders in protein metabolism include aminoacidurias such as: Phenylketonuria Maple sugar urine disease (valine, leucine, and isoleucine) Histidinemia Glycinemia Protein-induced enteropathy (gluten)

(Continued)

Table 15-1 ENERGY-YIELDING NUTRIENTS (*Continued*)

Nutrient	Functions	Energy yield per gram	Recommended allowances				
			Infancy	Ages 1–3 years	Ages 4–6 years	Ages 7–10 years	Ages 11–18 years
Fat	1 Concentrated energy source	9 kcal (38 kJ)	30–35% of calories ————————————————→				
	2 Carrier of fat-soluble vitamins (A, D, E, and K)						
	3 Insulator						
	4 Cushion for vessels, nerves, and organs						
	5 Structural component of cell and nucleus membranes						
	6 Essential to growth (arachidonic acid or its precursor, linoleic acid)		3% of calories should be supplied by the essential fatty acid linoleic acid	After infancy, body stores of linoleate ensure against essential fatty acid deficiency, except in instances of extremely low fat intake.			
	7 Functions associated with fat-related compounds: phospholipids and cholesterol						
	8 Satiety value						

Source: Allowances taken from *Recommended Dietary Allowances*, Revised 1973, Food and Nutrition Board, National Academy of Sciences, National Research Council, *Journal American Dietetic Association*, 64:2, 1974, p. 150.

with others containing larger amounts. For example, corn, being low in lysine, threonine, and tryptophan, can be complemented by legumes, which improve the lysine and threonine shortage. Sesame seeds or sunflower seeds would provide additional tryptophan. Food combinations used in developing countries, where animal protein is in short supply, often result in good complementary mixtures of vegetable proteins.[42] Peanut proteins supplement wheat, corn, and rye. Soy and sesame have values comparable to milk. Legumes and leafy vegetables supplement cereals.

Textured vegetable protein products (analogues) are now available on the retail market. Purified protein fraction of soybean is fortified with or can be combined with foods providing nutrients commonly found in meat (such as iron or B vitamins). Although not inexpensive, they do simulate in form and in content the meat they are designed to replace.

Fat Adipose tissue normally comprises about 10 percent of body weight. A casual observation of any group of people demonstrates the wide variability in adiposity. During inanition (starvation), body fat may fall below 1 percent of body weight. In contrast, the fat depot in extreme obesity may exceed 50 percent of total weight.

Fat provides the most concentrated source of calories (9 kcal/Gm). The relationship of fats to coronary heart disease and atherosclerotic conditions has been widely debated. Epidemiology studies have shown an association between elevated serum lipids and an increased incidence of coronary disease. High intake of saturated fat is correlated with elevated serum lipids. Decreases in serum cholesterol and triglycerides can be accomplished by dietary manipulation, which lowers total fat, increases the ratio of polyunsaturated to saturated fat, and restricts total cholesterol intake. Reduction of body weight alone can contribute to decreasing serum lipids. The public has reacted to the emphasis given this issue. There has been a decrease in the use of lard and butter with a commensurate increase in the use of margarine, polyunsaturated shortenings, and vegetable oils. The Food and Drug Administration has responded to public and professional pressures by establishing guidelines for nutrition labeling relating to types of fat present in a product. To lessen

Classifications	Examples	Major food sources	Pediatric concerns
Saturated fat	Triglycerides primarily from animal sources; fatty acid composition is largely saturated Exception: coconut oil is the only saturated fat *not* an animal source Synthetic	Milk, butter, cream, fat surrounding or distributed throughout meat muscle Cream substitutes (except those labeled as polyunsaturated); some margarines MCT (medium-chain triglycerides) manufactured by hydrolysis of coconut oil or butter; 8 kcal/Gm	When fat content of the infant diet is less than 20% of calories, caloric needs must be met by increases in carbohydrate and protein. This may lead to excessive renal solute load and/or exceed disaccharidase activity ability. Use of skim milk in infancy is contraindicated. Varying levels of tolerance exhibited in:

Unsaturated
Monounsaturated
	Derived from vegetable sources
	Triglycerides composed primarily of monounsaturated fatty acids
		Olive oil, peanut oil, peanut butter	Biliary atresia
			  Obstructive jaundice
			  Cystic fibrosis

Polyunsaturated	Triglycerides composed primarily of polyunsaturated fatty acids	Vegetable oils from corn, safflower, cottonseed or soybean; margarines with one of above oils as major ingredient; walnuts	Short bowel syndrome
			  Obstruction of lymphatics
			  Inflammation of intestinal
			    mucosa

consumer confusion (not for the purposes of taking a position in scientific differences of opinion), the FDA will allow labels to show cholesterol content, in milligrams per 100 Gm of food, as well as amounts of polyunsaturated and saturated fats and other fatty acids present. The amount of fat in the product is to be expressed as percentage of total calories. Should the manufacturer use this form of labeling, he must also specify that the information provided is for those who are making modifications in their fat intake because of advice from their physician. As previously mentioned, questions concerning type of fat in infant diets and advisability of altering intake have not been resolved.

Minimal fat requirement is not known. During infancy, at least 20 percent of the calories must be provided as fat in order to meet caloric needs without taxing digestive and excretory capabilities. With lower fat intakes, carbohydrate and protein must be increased. Renal solute load may then become excessive, and the concentrations of disaccharides presented in the intestinal lumen may exceed existing disaccharidase activity. Fat in breast milk provides 50 percent of total calories. Most commercial formula mixtures provide 35 to 50 percent of calories as fat. During childhood and adolescence, fat intakes of 30 to 35 percent of the total calories probably represent desirable levels.

Arachidonic acid (or its precursor, linoleic acid) is an essential fatty acid needed for growth and dermal integrity in infants. To avoid deficiency (as evidenced by decreased growth and dermatitis) and to provide sufficient reserves, 3 percent of the calories should be derived from linoleic acid. Human milk contains 6 to 9 percent. After infancy, body stores of the essential fatty acid apparently protect against deficiency except in instances of severe fat deprivation.

Although the use of skim milk may be reasonable beyond infancy, Fomon believes it is unsatisfactory as a food for infants.[43] When infants 4 to 8 months of age are allowed to eat ad libitum, they consume approximately 100 kcal/kg of body weight/day. Since they appear "normal" (as opposed to overweight or underweight), it can be assumed that this intake reflects the infant's energy requirement. Energy necessary to support growth has been estimated to be around 100 kcal/kg of body weight/day. It can be

Table 15-2   AMINO ACID COMPOSITION OF SOME FOODS

Essential amino acids	Cheese, eggs, milk, meat	Corn	Cereal	Legumes	Whole grains (with germ)	Nuts, seed oils, soybeans	Sesame and sunflower seeds	Peanut protein	Green leafy vegetables, leaf protein	Gelatin*	Yeast
Cystine**			—	—			X				
Methionine			X	—	X	—	X	—	—	—	X
Isoleucine	X										
Leucine	X										
Lysine	X	—	—	X	X	X	—		—	—	
Phenylalanine											
Threonine	X	—	—	X	—	X		—			X
Tryptophan		—		—			X			—	
Valine	X										

* Gelatin is an incomplete protein and therefore is not a good source of all essential amino acids.
** Cystine is not an essential amino acid but has been included because it is hard to get in a vegetarian diet. Methionine and cystine can be compared as one.
Symbols:
   X High amount of amino acid present in that food
   — Low amount of amino acid present in that food
   Blank spaces indicate a generally good balance of amino acids present with respect to other amino acids in the food.
Source: D. Erhard, "Nutrition Education for the 'Now' Generation," *Journal of Nutrition Education*, Spring 1971, p. 137.

concluded, then, that intakes of less than 90 kcal/kg/day may interfere with growth. Observations of infants consuming skim milk have shown that they did indeed consume less than 90 kcal/kg/day, although their activity did not decrease. As these skim milk babies continued to grow, the energy deficits must have been supplied from body stores of fat. The depletion of these stores may be undesirable, as the infant must synthesize lipids for myelination of the nervous system.

When skim milk is used, the distribution of calories from carbohydrate, protein, and fat do not fall within desirable levels. It is likely that greater quantities of baby food will be consumed to compensate for the lower satiety value in a diet so low in fat. Patterning an infant to consume unusually large volumes of food may create the tendency to overeat. Attempts to control weight gain during infancy should never be drastic and should not reduce caloric intake below 90 kcal/kg of body weight/day. This minimum precludes the use of skim milk.

Several illnesses exhibit the clinical manifestations of malabsorption. In pediatrics the two most commonly encountered are gluten-induced enteropathy (celiac disease) and cystic fibrosis. The former is precipitated by intolerances to the protein fraction gluten, which is found in wheat, oats, barley, and rye. Treatment omits food products containing gluten. Although steatorrhea (passage of fatty stools) may be present, it is secondary to the inflammation caused by the primary offender, a protein derivative.

Clinical manifestations of cystic fibrosis, however, are the result of impaired *digestion* due to the decreased presence or total absence of pancreatic enzymes. Fat presents the largest problem to the child with cystic fibrosis, for unlike carbohydrate, which has been partially digested by salivary amylase, or protein, acted upon by gastric pepsin, fat arrives at the small intestine almost totally dependent upon pancreatic lipase. With insufficient lipase, fat is improperly prepared for the absorptive mechanisms available at the epithelial intestinal cell level. The pancreas also provides enzymes for carbohydrates and proteins (amylase and peptidases). Therefore, this decreased digestive capacity alters the nutritional needs of these patients. Requirements are increased for calories, protein, and vitamins, especially those which are fat-soluble (A, D, E, and K). The use of pancreatic replacement enzymes can normalize nutrient needs. Because cystic fibrosis patients lose substantial amounts of sodium through perspiration, sodium needs are likewise elevated.

Various commercial liquids, powders, and oils have been developed to meet a lowered ability to handle fat. The important ingredient in all these products is the medium-chain triglyceride (MCT). The ordinary diet contains a predominance of long-chain fatty acids (oleic, palmitic, and stearic acids). These are dependent upon bile salts and lipase for digestion and absorption. Only 5 percent of naturally occurring fat contains short- and medium-chain fatty acids, which are 6 to 12 carbons in length. These fats are much more easily digested and absorbed. MCT is commercially manufactured by the hydrolysis of coconut oil or butter. The free fatty acids thus released are then distilled. The short-chain fatty acids, being lighter, come off first and are collected and reconstituted with glycerol to form a synthetic triglyceride containing fatty acid chains no longer than 12 carbons. The caloric yield of this fat is 8 kcal/Gm.

A brief review of fats and their digestion and absorption should explain the rationale of MCT use as well as provide a background for many clinical observations. Dietary fat is composed of mixtures of triglycerides—3 fatty acids attached to a glycerol molecule. As fat arrives at the small intestine, it is initially emulsified by bile, which increases the surface area for enzyme action. Pancreatic lipase, in a stepwise fashion, breaks off 1 fatty acid at a time from the glycerol base. Each succeeding break is completed with increasing difficulty so that only about one-third of the dietary fat ever reaches complete breakdown, i.e., glycerol plus 3 fatty acids of varying chain lengths. Therefore, final products of fat digestion include glycerol, some free fatty acids, diglycerides, and monoglycerides. The villi of the small intestine handle these products in various ways. Glycerol, being water-soluble, is absorbed quickly and transported via the portal blood to the liver. The free fatty acids of *short* or *medium* length are likewise absorbed easily and directly via the portal system. However, the monoglycerides and diglycerides remaining, along with the free fatty acids with longer chains, are less soluble, and require bile salts to "ferry" them into the intestinal epithelial cell. Once these fatty acids are inside the cell, the bile is separated and returned to the liver for recirculation. Lipase, existing within the cell, then must complete the digestion of the diglycerides and monoglycerides ferried in. Final absorption (exit from the epithelial cell into circulation) still cannot be achieved until the fatty acids now available in the cell are resynthesized into new triglycerides. These newly formed triglycerides are made transportable by combining with protein to form a lipoprotein complex called chylomicron. Finally, in this form, they are transported out of the cell via the lymphatic system.

Knowledge of the body's complex handling of common sources of dietary fat explains difficulties encountered in malabsorption syndromes and provides a basis for understanding treatment. Clinical manifestations may originate from inadequate emulsification (such as occurs in biliary atresia), may arise during digestion (as with cystic fibrosis), or may be precipitated at the absorption level (as in short-bowel syndrome, Hodgkin's disease, regional enteritis, ulcerative colitis, and gluten-induced enteropathy).

Caloric Needs

Allowances   There is wide variation in the activity of infants and children. Therefore, even more than with adults, RDAs for calories are averages and approximations for groups. During the first 6 months of life, an allowance of 117 kcal/kg body weight/day is recommended.* Approximately 20 percent of these calories cover activity requirements. These needs, however, may vary widely from infant to infant.[44] To illustrate extremes in variation, a vigorously crying infant may temporarily increase his metabolism 100 percent. The phlegmatic infant may require only half the activity calories, while the unusually active may burn up four times that amount.[45] Therefore, assessment of appropriate calorie levels for individual infants requires observation of appetite, activity, and quality of growth.

During the first year, two caloric allowances are made (see Table 15-3). The infant grows at a rapid rate, but also at a decreasing one. The 117 kcal/kg/day recommended for the first 6 months decreases

---

* The kilocalorie (kcal) is the unit used to express the energy value of food. It is equivalent to 1000 small calories (cal), the unit used when minute amounts of heat are considered. Recommended allowances and food values are always given in kilocalories.

Table 15-3   CALORIC NEEDS OF CHILDREN

Age groups	Weight (kg)	Weight (lb)	kcal/kg	Total kcal	Total kJ*
Infants					
Birth to 6 mo	6	14	117	702	2948
6–12 mo	9	20	108	972	4082
Children					
1–3 years	13	28		1300	5460
4–6	20	44		1800	7560
Adolescents					
Males					
11–14 years	44	97		2800	11760
15–18	61	134		3000	12552
Females					
11–14 years	44	97		2400	10080
15–18	54	119		2100	8836

Pregnancy: +300 kcal, or 1260 kJ
Lactation: +500 kcal, or 2100 kJ
* Conversion factor: 1 kJ = 4.2 × kcal.
Source: Recommended Dietary Allowances, Revised 1973, Food and Nutrition Board, National Academy of Sciences, National Research Council, *Journal of the American Dietetic Association*, 64(2):150, 1974.

to 108 kcal/kg/day by the end of the first year. These allowances are three times that of the adult. The infant has proportionately more active tissue and more surface area and, therefore, greater energy needs and more heat loss.

Recommended requirements for calories per kilogram of body weight decrease progressively from infancy through adolescence, although *total* daily calories increase (see Table 15-3). After infancy, and up to age 10, daily caloric allowances for both sexes are approximately 80 kcal/kg body weight. Because of the difference in growth rates between boys and girls after age 10, separate allowances are made. Allowances are based on needs for resting metabolism, growth, maintenance of body temperature, activity, and excretory losses. Physical activity requirements average 15 to 25 kcal/kg/day. Peak activity may require as much as 50 to 80 kcal/kg for short periods of time, and the very active child may require caloric adjustment if his pattern of growth is not satisfactory. Childhood diseases may require temporary adjustments as there is a 10 percent increase in basal metabolism for every degree (centigrade) of fever.

The inherent variability in children renders tables and guides little more than rough indicators. Growth patterns and a child's sense of satiety and well-being are the only accurate indicators of whether caloric needs are being met.

The Calorie versus the Joule   The joule is the unit of energy in the metric system. In 1960, the joule was adopted as the unit of measure for electrical work, heat, mechanical work, and energy. The International Organization for Standardization (ISO) recommended the adoption of the joule as the preferred unit for energy, and the United States National Bureau of Standards adopted the ISO recommendation in 1964. Nine-tenths of the world is using or changing over to the metric system. The kilocalorie (the amount of heat required to raise 1 kg of water 1°C) is not derived from the basic International System of Units. The joule is coherent for energy measurements in all branches of science on which nutrition science ultimately depends.[46] The 1973 RDA includes the kilojoules conversion factor. During the next few years, energy values will be reported both ways, with the probable ultimate abandonment of the calorie in preference to the joule.

What is a joule (J)? The joule is based on Newton's law of motion and the meter-kilogram-second. It is a measure of force moving through a distance. A joule is defined as the energy expended by a current of 1 ampere flowing for 1 second through a resistance of 1 ohm. Though this definition has little meaning for those without a background in physics, persons familiar with measuring heat of combustion in calories can make the conversion using the following formula: 1 kcal equals 4.2 kilojoules (kJ).

Noncaloric Nutrient Needs

Table 15-4 summarizes some vitamin and mineral needs of infants and children. The table is not inclusive; many of the vitamins and minerals have been omitted. Omissions should not be interpreted as indicating nutrients of lesser importance but rather as an exercise in selectivity.

Fat-Soluble Vitamins   Vitamins A, D, E, and K, being fat-soluble, follow the same routes of digestion and absorption as dietary fats. Thus, any conditions interfering with the efficiency of fat utilization may increase intake needs and necessitate supplementation.

Fat-soluble vitamins are stored, and accumulated reserves can delay the clinical expression of their decreased consumption or dietary lack. Good vitamin A stores may require more than a year to deplete. Storage capability, however, also provides the opportunity for toxicity, and hypervitaminosis has been reported for both vitamins A and D.

Vitamin A   The recommended allowance for the infant is based on the amount found in human milk. For the first 6 months of life, 1,400 I.U. are suggested, which is equivalent to the amount found in 850 ml of breast milk. In the last 6 months of infancy, 2,000 I.U. are recommended. As the baby gets older and his need for the vitamin increases, so does the use of additional solid foods. Sources rich in vitamin A and carotene should be included. Recommended allowances for vitamin A are now given both as international units (I.U.) and as retinol equivalents (R.E.). As with the kilocalorie and the joule, the dual allowances represent transitional reporting. "Retinol equivalents" takes into consideration the varying activity levels of retinol (Vitamin A alcohol) and the provitamin A carotenoids. It is therefore preferred for general use, and probably will replace the I.U. by the next revision of allowances.[47] In a mixed dietary, about half of the vitamin activity is provided by the precursor carotene. Carotene becomes active only after conversion to vitamin A, which takes place during or subsequent to absorption through the intestinal wall. The conversion is not rapid enough to produce toxicity even when excessively large amounts are ingested. Hypercarotenosis produces a yellowing of the skin, which is particularly noticeable in the palms, ear lobes, and soles of the feet. When carotene sources are eliminated, yellowing disappears. Hypervitaminosis A (from preformed vitamin) is a more serious matter. Toxicity results from large doses (20 to 30 times the RDA) consumed or administered for long periods of time. Less extreme doses, although still greatly in excess, given daily for 1 to 3 months have been reported to be toxic for infants 3 to 6 months of age. Reports of acute hypervitaminosis in infants following a single massive dose have also been reported in the literature.[48] Symptoms include anorexia, hyperirritability, skin lesions, thickening of long bones, and increased intracranial pressure.

Deficiencies are most likely to be expressed as night blindness and irritating dryness of the eye (see Table 15-4, Functions). Extreme deficiencies, such as xerophthalmia, are found with severe malnutrition. Absorption of preformed vitamin A and its transport in the blood are impaired with protein deficiency.[49]

Vitamin A reserves can become depleted in patients with prolonged marginal intake, and vitamin A status needs to be watched in patients with celiac disease, cystic fibrosis, sprue, obstructive jaundice, cirrhosis, and biliary atresia.

When skim milk replaces whole milk, more attention must be given to other vitamin A and carotene sources. Every cup (240 ml) of whole milk contributes 350 I.U. of vitamin A, whereas skim milk contains only traces. For the toddler, milk may account for the majority of the day's vitamin A allowance. Even in adolescence, milk can contribute almost one-third of the RDA.

Vitamin D Few natural foods contain more than minute amounts of vitamin D; yet the vitamin is needed throughout the growth period, and a small need persists through adulthood. Fortunately, exposure to sunlight or the ultraviolet wavelengths of light converts 7-dehydrocholesterol in the skin to vitamin D, and the adult's requirement can be met entirely by skin irradiation. (Night workers might be wise to use milk fortified with vitamin D.) Amounts required in the diet fluctuate with exposure to sunlight; 400 I.U. daily is recommended during growth. This level has not been known to be toxic.

Intakes of 1,000 to 3,000 I.U. daily are known to be dangerous to children and adults and may lead to hypercalcemia. It becomes important, then, to consider the vitamin D content of all fortified foods and the amount of vitamin D being supplemented. Almost

all brands of commercial formula and evaporated milk have been fortified, as has most fluid milk. In North America, this undoubtedly accounts for the virtual disappearance, beyond infancy, of clinical rickets due to vitamin D deficiency. Human milk and unfortified cow's milk are minimal in vitamin D content. Rickets may occur in breast-fed infants or in those on unfortified formulas; therefore, supplementation is indicated. However, *total* vitamin D sources should dictate the amount of supplementation. Infant cereals are now being fortified, as are some milk flavorings.

Hypervitaminosis develops after large intakes have continued for 1 to 3 months. Vitamin D facilitates transport of calcium across the intestinal wall and probably is involved in incorporating calcium into the bone. Toxicity produces nausea, diarrhea, weight loss, polyuria, nocturia, and eventual calcification of soft tissues, including those of the heart, renal tubules, blood vessels, bronchi, and stomach. In Great Britain, increased incidence of idiopathic hypercalcemia of infancy was traced to the use of enriched cereals and dried milks in addition to the normal prophylactic supplementation. The nature and extent of hypercalcemia depend upon the time of exposure to excessive doses. Early severe damage can lead to permanent changes which remain after hypercalcemia is gone, including vascular changes, skeletal and facial changes, growth disturbances, and mental retardation.

Vitamin E The newborn is susceptible to vitamin E insufficiency. He is born with low stores because there is negligible placental transfer of this vitamin. Transfer is limited to immediate fetal needs. The amount transferred through mother's milk is much greater. Infants not receiving colostrum or breast milk require a longer time to attain normal serum vitamin E levels. Cow's milk may have as little as one-tenth the vitamin E present in human milk.

Normal resistance of red blood cells to hemolysis is reduced in vitamin E deficiency. Vitamin E preserves the integrity of the erythrocyte by inhibiting oxidation of the unsaturated lipid portion of the cell membrane (see Table 15-4, Functions). The recommended allowance for infants is 4 to 5 I.U. daily.

Allowances for vitamin E were made for the first time in 1968. For years the essentiality of the vitamin was not known, and even after determining that it was necessary to man, it was believed to be needed in such small amounts that a deficiency was impossible. Recent studies have added to our knowledge— and to our confusion as well. Association of vitamin E with reproduction in the female rat and sterility in

202

Table 15-4 NONCALORIC NUTRIENT NEEDS: VITAMINS

Nutrient	Functions	Recommended allowances						Sources	Pediatric concerns
		Infancy	1–3 years	4–6 years	7–10 years	11–18 years			
Fat-soluble vitamins									
Vitamin A (precursor, carotene)	1 Component of photosensitive pigment of the eye 　a Rods—rhodopsin (visual purple) 　b Cones—iodopsin 2 Maintains integrity of epithelial membranes 3 Essential to bone and tooth development	0–6 mo 1,400 I.U. 6–12 mo 2,000 I.U. 400 R.E.	2,000 I.U. 400 R.E.	2,500 I.U. 500 R.E.	3,300 I.U. 700 R.E.	Males: 5,000 I.U. 1,000 R.E. Females: 4,000 I.U. 800 R.E.		Liver, fish oils, whole milk, egg yolk, fortified margarine, butter Carotenes from dark green and yellow vegetables and fruits	Attention should be given vitamin A status in celiac disease, sprue, obstructive jaundice, cystic fibrosis, biliary atresia, and cirrhosis. Can be toxic when taken in excessive amounts. Supplementation should not be necessary with the use of whole milk formula or breast milk. After infancy, and often during adolescence, intake is marginal.
Vitamin D	Maintenance of calcium homeostasis and skeletal integrity: aids in absorption and utilization of calcium and phosphorus; regulates level of serum alkaline phosphatase	400 I.U.	Recommended for all ages from infancy to adolescence					Fish oils, yeast-fortified or irradiated milk, fortified oleomargarine, some milk flavorings, some infant cereals Exposure of skin to sun	With fortification of increasing numbers of infant foods, it is necessary to be aware of *all* vitamin D sources. Supplementation probably indicated only for breast-fed infants and those receiving unfortified milk or formula preparations. Hypervitaminosis may develop with intakes of 1,000–3,000 I.U. Excessive intake associated with idiopathic hypercalcemia of infancy. Absorption hindered in celiac disease, sprue, colitis, biliary disorders.
Vitamin E (tocopherol)	Antioxidant: stabilizes lipid portion of cell membrane, preventing oxidative deterioration and cellular damage; protects vitamin A, which is easily oxidized	0–6 mo 4 I.U. 6–12 mo 5 I.U.	7 I.U.	9 I.U.	10 I.U.	Males: 11–14 years 12 I.U. 15–18 years 15 I.U. Females: 11–14 years 10 I.U. 15–18 years 11 I.U.		Vegetable oils are a major source Some proprietary infant formulas Baby foods highest in content are peaches, apricots, sweet potato, spinach	Negligible placental transfer of this vitamin results in low reserves in the newborn. Supplementation indicated with malabsorption.
Vitamin K	Catalyzes synthesis of prothrombin in the liver (anticoagulants interfere with utilization)	1 mg at birth recommended Mandatory if breast	No allowances have been established					Synthesized by intestinal bacteria Widespread in food, green leafy vegetables, pork liver	Due to sterile intestinal tract of the newborn, vitamin K is lacking for prothrombin formation; deficiency is associated with hemorrhagic disease of the newborn. Absorption and utilization affected

Water-soluble vitamins	Functions						Food sources	Comments
Ascorbic acid (vitamin C)	1 Provides intercellular cementing substance necessary to formation and maintenance of bone matrix, cartilage, dentine, collagen, and connective tissue 2 Related to metabolism of phenylalanine, tyrosine, and tryptophan 3 Makes iron available for hemoglobin and maturation of red blood cells 4 Facilitates action of folic acid 5 Apparent role in resistance to bacterial infections and body's ability to cope with stress	35 mg	40 mg	⟶		45 mg	Citrus fruit, tomato, cabbage, potato, strawberries, melon	Breast milk has sufficient ascorbic acid if mother's intake is adequate. Supplementation is necessary with unfortified formula preparations. Citrus is not tolerated by many young infants. Gradual introduction should be made at 2 months, using diluted juice initially. When 2 oz of undiluted juice is tolerated, supplementation may be discontinued. Prolonged use of antibiotics interferes with intestinal synthesis.
Folic acid	Coenzyme in the formation of purines, thymine, and heme (iron-containing portion of hemoglobin)	50 µg	100 µg	200 µg	300 µg	400 µg	Glandular meats, yeast, green leafy vegetables, milk (except goat's milk)	Deficiency associated with megaloblastic anemia of infancy. Deficiency may result from celiac disease, chronic infectious enteritis, or enteroenteric fistulas; use of anticonvulsant drugs may lower serum folic acid levels. Increased need is associated with use of oral contraceptive drugs.
Cobalamin (vitamin B₁₂)	1 Involved in the synthesis of nucleic acid and vital cell proteins 2 Essential for maturation of red blood cells in bone marrow 3 Involved in the metabolism of nerve tissue	0.3 µg	1.0 µg	1.5 µg	2.0 µg	3.0 µg	Muscle and organ meats, fish, eggs, milk, and cheese	Vitamin B₁₂ will be deficient in vegetarian diets which exclude animal foods. Defect in absorption has been reported with surgical resection of terminal ileum, regional enteritis, and bacterial overgrowth of intestine

Source: Allowances taken from *Recommended Dietary Allowances,* Revised 1973, Food and Nutrition Board, National Academy of Sciences, National Research Council. *Journal of the American Dietetic Association.* 64:2. 1974. p. 150.

the male rat has triggered the popularity of large-dose self-medication. Interestingly, the new recommended allowances have not increased, but *decreased*.

The only known human function of vitamin E is that of an antioxidant. In this regard, the levels required are directly related to the amount of polyunsaturated fat in the diet. Because the general population was increasing their intake of this type of fat, and because figures available on vitamin E content of food suggested marginal intakes, concern seemed justified. However, we now know that 20 percent of the vitamin E activity in the American diet comes from gamma tocopherol. Although the latter is much less active than the alpha form (which was the form generally presented on food tables), the amount present in the diet has been increasing over the past 20 years. Vitamin E content of the United States diet has been underestimated. Nature seems to assist in this known association between vitamin E and polyunsaturated fats, for the best food sources of the vitamin are also those which contain high levels of polyunsaturated fatty acids.

This relationship also caused concern regarding the intake of vitamin E by infants on artifical formulas, when the butterfat of milk was replaced with vegetable oil. The type of oil used did not always satisfy the recognized desirable ratio of vitamin E to polyunsaturated fatty acids. There were reports of infants who did not thrive on these formulations. Adjusting the ingredients and adding vitamin E corrected the problem. Manufacturers are now aware of the importance of providing sufficient amounts of the vitamin.[50]

Vitamin E deficiency has been observed only in premature infants and in persons with impaired fat absorption. Supplementation is indicated in these instances. Although our knowledge of the function of vitamin E is still fragmentary, the absence of deficiency in the population does not support the fad of overdosing. While it is true that thus far no toxicities have been reported from the vitamin, suggesting mega-vitamin intake in the light of our present and incomplete knowledge is irresponsible.

Vitamin K This vitamin is needed in microgram amounts to maintain prothrombin and other clotting factors. It is present in a wide variety of foods, and usual intakes, in addition to the amounts synthesized by intestinal bacteria, insure adequacy. No minimal requirement has been established.

The newborn, with his sterile intestinal tract, lacks the vitamin K essential for prothrombin formation until the establishment of intestinal flora. The initial period of relative starvation in breast-fed infants plus the low vitamin K content of human milk may be involved in the hemorrhagic disease of the newborn. One milligram of natural vitamin K given parenterally at birth is adequate to prevent hemorrhagic disease. Infants born of mothers who have been receiving anticoagulants may have severe clotting defects and may required repeated doses of the vitamin.

Water-Soluble Vitamins

Ascorbic Acid (Vitamin C) Human beings are one of the few species unable to synthesize adequate amounts of ascorbic acid. Insufficient dietary intake results in scurvy. If a mother's intake was sufficient during pregnancy, her infant is born with adequate tissue levels of vitamin C. Breast milk of the well-nourished mother provides 4 to 7 mg/100 ml and is therefore an adequate source of the vitamin. Breast-fed infants can develop scurvy if their mother's intake of vitamin C is deficient. Supplement is often given to the infant being nursed (presumably as a safety factor). It should always be given the infant receiving formula if the preparation being used has *not* been fortified, as cow's milk is a poor source of ascorbic acid. Water-soluble vitamins are not stored beyond tissue saturation levels; therefore, any excess consumed is excreted and does not improve nutritional status. In the United States, scurvy, although uncommon, is no less prevalent in Florida than in states with less available citrus fruits. Fomon[51] concludes that the incidence of scurvy is associated with faulty nutritional education of the parent or failure of the physician to determine whether an infant's formula contains adequate amounts.

Many young infants do not tolerate citrus fruit in amounts large enough to supply their vitamin C need. It is safer, initially, to give supplementary vitamin C than to depend on citrus intake. Around the second month of life, diluted orange juice can be introduced. When the infant tolerates 2 oz, undiluted, of fresh, frozen, or canned orange juice, the ascorbic acid supplement can be discontinued.

Review of the functions of vitamin C (Table 15-4) underscores its importance to growth. There is a greater concentration in metabolically active tissues (adrenal gland, brain, kidney, liver, pancreas, thymus, and spleen) than in those less active. A child's multiplying tissue contains more ascorbic acid than adult tissue. Large concentrations of vitamin C in the adrenal glands indicate that the vitamin has a role in the body's reaction to stress (injury, illness, or shock). Infectious processes, especially bacterial, deplete tissue levels, as tissue saturation apparently aids resistance to infection. However, the use of megadoses of the vitamin to prevent the common cold has created controversy. Doses beyond those necessary to maintain tissue saturation, in light of current knowledge, are pointless because any excess amount is merely excreted. The importance of ascorbic acid during the hazardous growing years is apparent.

B Vitamins: Folic Acid and Cobalamin   Discussion of the B vitamins will be confined to folic acid and cobalamin (vitamin B_{12}) because of their role in anemias encountered during infancy and adolescence.

Folic acid deficiency (megaloblastic anemia of infancy) has a peak incidence between 4 and 7 months of age, a little earlier than the appearance of iron-deficiency anemia. The disease results from insufficient intake. The effect of this deficiency is intensified by rapid growth or infection, when folic acid needs are increased. Both human and cow's milk provide ample amounts, but goat's milk is deficient and, if used, should be supplemented. Deficiency of vitamin C impairs utilization of folic acid (see Table 15-4), functions of ascorbic acid).

Folic acid–deficient infants develop macrocytic anemia with a red blood cell count disproportionately lower than hematocrit. Megaloblastic nucleated red blood cells are often seen in the peripheral blood of such patients. Megaloblastic changes of the bone marrow are prominent. In addition to manifestations of anemia, the infant becomes irritable, fails to gain weight adequately, and develops diarrhea. Signs of scurvy may also be present.

Treatment includes folic acid supplementation. Doses as small as 50 μg have produced response. Because this amount does not effect primary vitamin B_{12} deficiency, these low doses can be used to differentiate between the two types of anemia.

In many patients, the use of anticonvulsant drugs has resulted in low serum folic acid levels, but symptoms of anemia do not usually develop. Should megaloblastic anemia become apparent, it is responsive to folic acid therapy.

The adolescent using orally administered contraceptives may need to consider folic acid status. Several types of contraceptive pills, both sequential and nonsequential, have been implicated in causing folate deficiency.[52] In such a situation, supplementation is indicated. However, this cause of folate deficiency is rare as compared to the usual causes, which are malnutrition, malabsorption, and pregnancy. Increased need for pyridoxine (vitamin B_6)

has also been suggested with use of oral contraceptives.[53]

Pernicious anemia results from the lack of intrinsic factor normally secreted by glands of the stomach. Only when dietary vitamin B_{12} forms a complex with this factor is vitamin B_{12} able to attach to the receptor sites along the ileum and subsequently be absorbed. Symptoms of pernicious anemia become apparent between 9 months and 4 years of age, when prenatal stores become exhausted. As the macrocytic anemia progresses, anorexia, listlessness, and irritability develop. The tongue becomes red, smooth, and painful. Neurologic complications include ataxia, paresthesias, hyporeflexia, Bakinski responses, clonus, and coma. Treatment involves parenteral administration of vitamin B_{12}, which bypasses the absorptive defect. Maintenance therapy must be continued through life.

Folic acid can cause blood cell regeneration in patients with pernicious anemia. However, its effect is not permanent, and it does not aid the degenerative neurologic problems. For this reason, nonprescription vitamin preparations should not contain more than 400 μg (0.4 mg) folic acid (the recommended allowance for age 10). The use of larger amounts can mask developing pernicious anemia and prevent its diagnosis.

The current increase in the popularity of vegetarian diets prompts a note of caution. The complete omission of animal food eliminates sources of vitamin B_{12}. The recommended allowance also may be compromised when animal sources are used, but too sparingly. Supplementation in these instances is indicated.

Minerals

Calcium   Of the body's calcium, 99 percent resides in bones and teeth. The remaining 1 percent, distributed in the plasma and other body fluids, remains remarkably constant, varying in total amount not more than 10 percent. This circulating calcium is involved with blood coagulation, muscle contraction, neuromuscular irritability, and myocardial function.

Not all dietary calcium is used by the body. Absorption requires the presence of vitamin D. Apparently with increased need there is increased efficiency of absorption, so that during periods of growth, intestinal uptake is greater. Average absorption is about 30 percent of intake, but efficiency is influenced by amount of dietary calcium available. As the amount of available calcium increases, the absorption rate decreases. For example, the breast-fed infant receives about 60 mg calcium per kilogram of body weight and retains roughly two-thirds, whereas the infant on cow's milk formula receiving 170 mg/kg only retains one-third to one-half.

Absorption can also be affected by the presence of oxalates. Calcium oxalate is insoluble and, therefore, unabsorbable. The effect of oxalate formation seems to be confined to calcium-containing foods, with the oxalate per se having little or no influence. To illustrate, the calcium found in spinach is present mostly as calcium oxalate, and as such is poorly absorbed. Chocolate has a substantial amount of oxalic acid, but not calcium, and therefore its oxalate has no effect on the absorption of calcium from other foods (as chocolate milk).[54]

The recommended daily calcium allowance for the infant is based on the amount available in breast milk. Between the ages of 1 and 10 years, skeletal growth requires retention of 75 to 150 mg calcium daily, which is adequately met by an intake of 800 mg. Because of the increased mineral needs during prepubertal and pubertal growth, the recommended allowances during these years increase to 1,200 mg.

The parathyroid hormone works synergistically with vitamin D to control serum calcium levels. Decrease in serum calcium stimulates osteoclastic activity, and calcium is mobilized from the bone and released into circulation to correct the imbalance. The intestinal mucosa is also signaled to increase absorption. The hormone regulates serum phosphorus as well, as these two minerals are normally maintained in a definite relationship—the serum calcium: phosphorus ratio (Ca:P). When serum phosphate levels increase, the hormone blocks renal tubular absorption of phosphorus, thereby increasing its excretion and returning the ratio to normal. The ratio is the solubility product of the two minerals, expressed in milligrams per 100 ml of serum. Normal serum calcium concentration is 10 mg/100 ml; that of phosphorus is 5 mg/100 ml (4 mg/100 ml for adults). Their solubility product, then, is 10×5, or 50. Any change in the serum concentration of one necessitates an adjustment in the concentration of the other.

Hypocalcemic tetany of the newborn illustrates the balance of this ratio. An excessive initial feeding of cow's milk presents the infant with an overload of phosphorus, for cow's milk has a greater concentration of minerals than breast milk. Temporary hypofunction of the parathyroid—that is, inadequate response to the need for calcium homeostasis—results in the kidneys' inability to clear the phosphate load. Phosphorus, accumulating in the serum, elicits a compensatory decrease in serum calcium in an attempt to maintain the Ca:P ratio. When serum calcium falls below 7 to 7.5 mg/100 ml, typical tetanic muscular spasms result.

Hypocalcemic tetany may also result from steatorrhea. The presence of excess fat in the intestinal tract leads to the formation of insoluble calcium soaps, which are then lost in the feces. If malabsorption is of sufficient magnitude to substantially reduce the total calcium absorbed, the serum calcium level may become low enough to precipitate claw-like cramps with the slightest stimulus.

Students may encounter the use of modified calcium diets in orthopedics. Prolonged immobilization causes resorption of calcium from bone stores into the blood. Since excess serum calcium must be excreted by the kidney, renal calculi may be avoided by not adding unnecessary amounts of dietary calcium for clearance. Adequate dietary calcium should be provided, but amounts should not exceed usual allowances. If renal stones have already formed, the diet should be further restricted.

Iron Iron-deficiency anemia is the most common hematalogic disease in infancy and childhood. It is rare before 4 months of age because of the iron stores laid down during the final weeks of gestation but is quite common between 9 and 24 months. Low-birth-weight and premature infants have increased iron needs as a result of early depletion of stores, and attention should be given to providing adequate sources of iron early.

Recommendations for intake are based on a 10 percent absorption of dietary iron. It is therefore necessary to ingest substantially more iron than the body needs. During the first year of life, relatively small quantities of iron-rich foods are given, and infants may be placed in a precarious situation, leading to iron deficiency. When iron-deficiency anemia has been diagnosed, supplementation is the treatment. The dose is determined by the elemental iron present in the supplement of choice. Ferrous sulfate contains approximately twice as much elemental iron by weight as ferrous gluconate. High bulk in the diet is believed to depress utilization of iron; on this basis, taking supplements before meals has been suggested. Ingestion of large amounts of milk may also decrease absorption, as phosphate binds iron, removing it from the body.

Nutrition education should emphasize iron-rich foods and reasonable (nonexcessive) use of milk. Although milk is an excellent source of many nutrients, it is a poor source of iron. In young children, drinking excessive amounts of milk may reduce their intake of solid foods which are important contributors of iron. Iron from animal sources is generally superior to vegetable sources. Phytates, found in outer hulls of many cereal grains, especially wheat, bind iron, rendering the mineral unavailable. Oxalate (as found in "iron-rich" spinach) also forms an insoluble complex. Mixed diets provide approximately 6 mg iron for every 1000 kcal consumed. As the caloric allowance for the year-old infant is approximately 1000 kcal, and his iron recommendation is 15 mg, it becomes apparent that choice of foods should be judicious. This problem persists through age 3 years and emerges again for adolescent girls whose 2100 to 2400-kcal intake will not provide the 18 mg iron needed unless especially rich iron sources are commonly used (see Table 15-5).

Iron intake also becomes important in the treatment of chronic lead poisoning, since a prominent finding is hypochromic microcytic anemia. Lead interferes with iron utilization and hemoglobin synthesis.

Unlike other minerals, iron does not have an efficient excretory mechanism. Regulatory mechanisms in the intestinal cells determine the amounts that are absorbed. Once iron has gained access to the body, there is no natural avenue for its elimination. Excess intravenous iron from repeated transfusions may cause iron accumulation beyond desired levels. A rare disease, hemochromatosis, occurring chiefly in males, results in abnormal iron storage which causes bronze discoloration, liver damage, and severe diabetes. A disturbance in the absorption mechanism apparently allows too much dietary iron to pass through intestinal cells, and capacity for storage is exceeded.

Because of iron's one-way route, accidental iron poisoning, resulting from ingestion of large amounts of medicinal iron, can be extremely serious. It is perhaps ironic that the nutrient which is the most difficult to obtain in the diet, the lack of which presents the most commonly encountered deficiency, can cause death in 50 percent of the cases of accidental iron poisoning. Ingestion of 2 to 4 Gm iron salts can result in a life-threatening series of events. Hemodynamic changes due to vasodepressor materials lead to shock and central nervous system depression. The excessive iron is irritating to the gastrointestinal tract and produces hemorrhagic necrosis of the mucosa, leading to vomiting and diarrhea, which is often bloody. Coma may develop 15 to 30 minutes after ingestion or may be delayed for several hours. In the absence of coma and shock, recovery is likely. Treatment involves the use of chelating agents to bind and remove excesses from the body.

Fluoride The incorporation of fluoride into mineral apatite crystals of the teeth appears to increase their resistance to dissolution and decay. When not present in the drinking water, fluoride supplementation is recommended from birth to 12 years. The protective role of fluoride is especially evident during infancy and early childhood. Beneficial effects are obtained with oral fluoride even after the teeth have erupted. Holding fluoride drops in the mouth for a minute or two, or using a chewable tablet, allows time for surface contact and enhances effectiveness. Supplements should not be used when drinking water supplies over 0.7 parts per million (ppm). Fluoride content in excess of 2.0 to 2.5 ppm produces a mottling of enamel. Water supplies providing fluoride in a concentration of 1 ppm have been shown to be safe and effective in reducing tooth decay (a 50 percent or greater reduction in incidence).

Too frequent between-meal, sucrose-containing snacks (candies and drinks) and poor oral hygiene influence susceptibility to caries. Fluoride alone cannot be expected to solve dental problems.

Water Although this nutrient is the last to be discussed, it is so vital to survival that it is second only to oxygen. The principal pediatric consideration is the infant's large body water content which makes him more vulnerable to dehydration and subsequent electrolyte imbalance. Compared to the adult, whose body water comprises two-thirds of his body weight, the infant is approximately three-fourths water. As a result, a baby must consume larger amounts of fluid per unit of body weight to maintain water balance.

Water turnover is more closely related to metabolic rate than body weight, and the metabolic rate per kilogram body weight in the infant is about three times that of the adult. As a result, the increased products of metabolism require more water for excretion. In addition, the infant has a greater proportion of his body fluid in the extracellular compartment. Daily water turnover in infants is normally one-half of the extracellular fluid volume. Therefore, in the infant, any interference with normal intake of water and electrolytes, or any condition which results in abnormal fluid losses, places the infant in precarious balance.

The requirement for water is determined by the amounts necessary for growth, amounts lost through skin and lungs, and quantities excreted in urine and feces. Rate of growth determines amount of fluid intake retained, which ranges from 0.5 to 3 percent. Losses from skin and lungs are substantial. At birth, an average of 175 ml per day are lost. The year-old

Table 15-5 IRON CONTENT OF SOME FOODS

Food sources	Quantity	Iron content (mg)
Breads and cereals		
Enriched or whole-grain	1 slice	0.5
Tortilla, yellow corn	1 cake, 6 in. diameter	0.9
Fortified cereals (read labels)		
Dry infant cereals	1 tbsp	2.0*
Farina, quick cooking	1 tbsp	1.0*
Ready-to-eat, dry cereals	1 oz	May contain up to 3 to 5*
Wheat germ	1 tbsp	0.4
Teething biscuit	1	0.2
Fruits *(Note:* For most, contribution is minimal, unless size of serving is generous)		
Dried fruits		
Apricots	1 large half	0.3
Prunes	1 large	0.4
Dates	1 medium	0.3
Figs	1 medium	0.6
Peaches	1 medium half	0.6
Raisins	1 tbsp	0.4
Prune juice	½ cup	5.0
Strained prunes (baby food, made with tapioca)	1 tbsp	0.2
Vegetables		
Beans	1 tbsp (cooked)	
Chick peas (garbanzos)		
Red kidney beans		0.4
Boston baked beans		
Baked beans with tomato sauce (white beans)		0.3
Lima beans		
Lentils		0.2
Greens		
Spinach and mustard greens	½ cup, cooked	2.0
(oxalate content may interfere with iron absorption)		
Strained baby spinach (creamed)	1 tbsp	0.1
Meats and fish		
Strained baby meat (beef, chicken, lamb, pork, turkey, veal)	1 tbsp	0.2
Most meat and poultry	1 oz cooked	1.0
Commonly used types of fish	1 oz cooked	0.3
The following represent rich iron sources, or those which can make substantial contribution to meeting total daily iron requirements:		
Organ meats	1 oz cooked	
Kidney		3.0
Heart		1.6
Liver		
Strained beef liver, baby food	1 tbsp	0.6
Calves', beef, or chicken liver		3.0
Lamb liver	1 oz cooked	4.5
Pork liver		6.0
Chitterlings (pork intestine)	1 oz raw	0.6
Liverwurst	1 oz (1 slice)	1.6
Sardines	2 medium (1 oz)	0.8
Mackerel (canned)	1 oz	0.6
Clams (canned with liquid)	1 tbsp (½ oz)	0.5
Eggs		
Yolk from medium egg	1 yolk	0.9
Strained yolk, baby food	1 tbsp	0.4
Additional sources		
Molasses		
Blackstrap	1 tbsp	2.3
Light	1 tbsp	0.9
Dark brown sugar	1 tbsp	0.4

* Iron in fortified cereals may be poorly absorbed.
Sources: Gerber Products Co., *Nutrient Values of Gerber Baby Foods,* Fremont, Mich., 1972; and Charles Church and Helen Church, *Bowes & Church's Food Values of Portions Commonly Used,* 11th ed., J. B. Lippincott Company, Philadelphia, 1970.

infant generally loses 500 ml per day. Fecal losses are small, and obligatory urine losses depend upon the renal solute load presented by body metabolism. Under ordinary circumstances, 1.5 ml/kcal will adequately take care of an infant's fluid requirement. The need decreases proportionately throughout life as the body becomes less hydrated and the metabolic rate per kilogram body weight decreases. For the adult, 1 ml/kcal is recommended. Table 15-6 includes allowances for various ages.

Special attention should be given to the fluid intake of infants and children given formula mixtures and diets which have a high protein content, thereby increasing renal solute load. Comatose patients and those unable to communicate thirst as well as those with fever, diarrhea, or polyuria require close observation of fluid intake and output.

Water is provided endogenously in the final oxidation of energy-producing nutrients. Every 100 kcal of carbohydrate, protein, and fat produce approximately 14 ml of water. Exogenous sources of water include oral fluids and the water content of foods. Baby foods are high in moisture content, and the diets normally given infants exceed their water requirements. Water balance becomes a primary concern in infant feeding when any of the following situations exist: (1) relatively low fluid intake (less than 100 ml/kg/day), (2) excessive extrarenal losses, (3) lowered renal concentrating ability, or (4) a diet with a high renal solute load.

Solutes that must be excreted by the kidney are referred to collectively as the renal solute load. Electrolytes and nitrogen are the principal solutes to be excreted, and therefore, protein is the primary contributor to renal solute load. Generous amounts of salt usually accompany the nitrogen that protein presents to the kidney. However, with a normally functioning kidney the infant's protein intake would have to exceed 20 percent of calories before renal solute load would become an important consideration. Although electrolyte balance is not included in this discussion, the sodium and potassium contents of some fluids commonly given to children are present in Table 15-7.

Altered Nutrient Needs of Low-Birth-Weight Infants

The incidence of low-birth-weight infants, whether the result of a shortened gestation period or retarded intrauterine growth, correlates with low socioeconomic status. Therefore, these infants' mothers show a high incidence of undernutrition, anemia, illness, inadequate prenatal care, and obstetric complications. At birth, these newborns have compro-

mised nutritional stores and are placed in further jeopardy by their growth needs, which are accelerated beyond those of the newborn whose weight is normal.

The premature infant may be limited in sucking ability and therefore may require a feeding approach which avoids fatigue. When sucking is limited, breast-feeding is least likely to be successful; when bottle feeding is necessary, small soft nipples with large holes are used to compensate for the limited ability to suck. Smaller, less vigorous infants may require gavage feeding initially, with a gradual change to bottle or breast as the infant develops strength. The premature infant's lack of body fat can result in substantial losses of body heat. These losses can be environmentally conserved by the use of external heat sources (incubators) to avoid creating excessive caloric need or expenditure.

When oral feedings are initiated, increasing amounts of 5 percent glucose solution are given, followed by dilute and, ultimately, full-strength formula mixtures. Amounts and concentrations are determined by the infant's condition and tolerance. If an infant is hungry or fails to gain weight, concentrations may be increased to 30 kcal/oz of formula (normal concentration is 20 kcal/oz). Small stomach capacities usually require that feedings be given often. After initiation of feeding, actual weight gain may not begin for a week or more.

Digestive enzymes are mature enough in premature and small-for-gestational-age newborns to allow the absorption of protein and carbohydrate. Fat is less well absorbed, with unsaturated fat and the fat of human milk being better absorbed than butterfat.

Small-for-gestational-age infants are more mature in their feeding capabilities than premature infants and may not require gavage feeding or such cautious introduction of oral feedings. However, like the premature infant, their nutrient needs are altered by their increased growth rate.

Calories Basal metabolic energy requirement may be higher in premature than in full term infants. However, because activity level is lower and heat losses are artificially conserved, the caloric level required to support growth and spare protein may not need to be increased beyond 125 kcal/kg body weight. (The recommended dietary allowance for full-term infants is 117 kcal/kg.) If an infant fails to gain weight, it may become necessary to increase calories to 130 to 150 kcal/kg.

Protein Because premature infants lack the ability to manufacture the amino acid cystine, dietary cys-

Table 15-6 NONCALORIC NUTRIENT NEEDS: WATER AND MINERALS

Nutrient	Functions	Recommended allowances — Infancy	1–3 years	4–6 years	7–10 years	11–18 years	Sources	Pediatric concerns
Water	1 Contributes to structure and form of body through tissue turgor 2 Provides aqueous environment necessary for cell metabolism 3 Solvent for transport of nutrients and metabolic waste products 4 Aids in maintaining body temperature	150 ml/kg	125 ml/kg	100 ml/kg	75 ml/kg	11–12 years 75 ml/kg 11–18 years 50 ml/kg	Oral fluids Water content of food Metabolic water of oxidation (14 ml for every 100/kcal of a mixed diet)	Infants are more prone to dehydration and subsequent electrolyte imbalances: infant's water content = 70–75% of body weight; adult's water content = 60–65% of body weight. Special attention to water needs required with coma, fever, diarrhea, high protein formula or diet, polyuria.
Minerals Calcium	1 Bone and teeth formation 2 Participates in blood coagulation 3 Initiates muscle contraction; vital to contraction and relaxation of cardiac muscle 4 Necessary to normal nerve transmission	0–6 mo 360 mg 6–12 mo 540 mg	800 mg →			1,200 mg	Milk, cheese, dairy products Secondary sources are green leafy vegetables, legumes, nuts, and whole grains	Hypocalcemic tetany may accompany the following: Newborn given too large an initial feeding Vitamin D deficiency Celiac disease Late stages of renal insufficiency Acute pancreatitis Prolonged immobilization leads to calcium resorption and increased serum calcium levels.
Iron	1 Constituent of hemoglobin and myoglobin; involved in O_2 and CO_2 transport 2 Component of cellular oxidative systems which release energy from the metabolic breakdown products of food	0–6 mo 10 mg 6–12 mo 15 mg	15 mg	10 mg	10 mg	18 mg	Liver, meat, egg yolk, green vegetables, whole or enriched grains, legumes, nuts Excellent baby food sources are dry infant cereals, quick cooking farina, Cream of Wheat, strained liver, strained beef with beef heart, and egg yolk	Iron-deficiency anemia is the most common hematologic disease of infancy and childhood; chronic iron deficiency anemia may result from lesions of the GI tract, Meckel's diverticulum, polyps, or hemangioma. Absorption is hindered by steatorrhea.
Fluoride	Structural component of bones and teeth	No specific allowances recommended; 1 ppm fluorine added to water supplies					Drinking water Plant and animal foods vary according to soil and water	Supplements should not be used where water supplies over 0.7 ppm; fluoride content in excess of 2.0–2.5 ppm produces a mottling of enamel.

Source: Allowances for water intake from W. E. Nelson, *Textbook of Pediatrics*, 9th ed., W. B. Saunders Company, Philadelphia, 1969, p. 129; other allowances from *Recommended*

tine is essential for them. The rapid growth rate of premature infants requires greater retention of nitrogen, and it is possible that the protein content of breast milk may be suboptimal. If birth weight exceeds 1,500 Gm, a protein intake of 2 Gm/kg body weight should be sufficient. Higher levels may be indicated for smaller babies. Since a high protein intake increases renal solute load, water balance must be carefully maintained.

Fat and Fat-Soluble Vitamins If fat absorption is significantly impaired, attention should be given to the fat-soluble vitamins. The premature infant's body stores of vitamin E are lower at birth than those of the full-term infant. In addition, absorption of the vitamin is also impaired, although it does attain a normal level as the infant approaches the equivalent of full-term gestational age. The vitamin is used in the treatment of hemolytic anemia because of its protective role in preserving cellular membrane integrity. The blood picture of the premature infant is complicated, for treating anemia with medicinal iron unfortunately has a two-sided effect. In addition to increasing the amounts of iron available to the body, the mineral also interferes with the already impaired absorption of vitamin E. Tocopheral supplement of 0.5 mg/kg body weight has been recommended.

Rapid growth can contribute to vitamin D de-

Table 15-7 SODIUM AND POTASSIUM CONTENT OF PEDIATRIC FLUIDS

Type (8 oz)	Sodium (mg)	Potassium (mg)
Pepsi-Cola	7	35
Ginger ale	18	1
Coca-Cola	2	88
Milk (whole)	122	342
Kool-Aid	0.7	0.12
Average fruit juices	4	20–585
Cranberry juice	2.5	20
Grape drink	2.5	88.5
Pear nectar	2.5	80
Grape juice		
Frozen concentrate, diluted	2.5	85
Bottled juice	5.0	290
Apple juice	2.5	240
Apricot nectar	1.28	372
Grapefruit juice (frozen, canned, fresh)	2.0	388
Orange juice (frozen, canned, fresh)	1.7	485
Prune juice	5.0	585

Source: Charles Church and Helen Church, *Bowes & Church's Food Values of Portions Commonly Used*, 11th ed., J. B. Lippincott Company, Philadelphia, 1970.

ficiency. Increase of intake to 1,000 I.U. has been suggested, beginning the second or third week of life. However, all food sources must be considered to avoid oversupplementation and toxicity.

Hemorrhagic conditions occurring in the premature infant as a result of hepatic immaturity are not ameliorated by vitamin K therapy. However, administration of vitamin K is prophylactic for postnatal decline of prothrombin factors which occur before intestinal flora become established.

Water-Soluble Vitamins In the low-birth-weight infant, the ascorbic acid requirement is increased because of its many growth-related functions. Intermediary metabolism of the essential amino acids phenylalanine and tyrosine (derived from phenylalanine) is incomplete without vitamin C. An intake of 50 mg is recommended.

Folic acid needs likewise increase with accelerated growth. Megaloblastic anemia has occurred in infants of low birth weight who were receiving cow's milk formula. Although the folic acid content of the formula was sufficient for full-size newborns, presumably, the low-birth-weight infant's needs exceed this amount. Some proprietary formulas provide folic acid at levels that are approximately twice the allowance recommended during early infancy.

Iron Early dietary sources of iron become very important, as low-birth-weight and premature infants have markedly reduced iron stores. Routine supplementation is 2 mg/kg body weight.

ESTABLISHING SOUND NUTRITIONAL PRACTICES
Infant

Growth and Psychosocial Characteristics A child's nutrient needs parallel his rate of growth. When considering infant feeding, one must begin by appreciating that during the first year of life, a healthy baby triples his birth weight and increases his length by 50 percent. This growth rate is second only to that of the intrauterine period and exceeds the rate of growth during adolescence. The infant's rapid growth makes him especially vulnerable to dietary inadequacies. Special attention should be given to both the *quality* and the *quantity* of foods in his diet. The manner in which the food is presented to the infant is also important. During the feeding process the infant and his parent establish their initial relationship. Food and love become synonymous as the infant is held in his parent's comforting arms. It is largely through this person-to-person interaction that the infant establishes basic trust in the world around him. He should be protected from unpleasant, tense feeding experiences which lead to the association of food and feeding with conflict and frustration and a consequent development of mistrust in human relationships. Parents need to understand that urging and cajoling are not necessary. When a baby's sucking comes to a full stop, it means that he is satisfied; he need not be urged to finish that last ounce. Parents in tune with their babies will be able to recognize the components of feeding behavior. O'Grady[55] describes infant feeding behavior in five distinct steps:

1 *Prefeeding behavior:* the level of arousal shown before feeding which indicates hunger
2 *Approach behavior:* the predominant physical mode of reaching out to food or showing readiness to eat
3 *Attachment behavior:* activities occurring between the time the nipple first touches the mouth and the time the infant is successful in nursing from it
4 *Consummatory behavior:* sucking and swallowing
5 *Satiety behavior:* the infant's acts which indicate that he has taken all the food that he wants

Since nutritional needs cannot be understood apart from overall maturation, it is helpful for parents and nurses to understand the natural characteristics of a child at various ages and stages. It is within this framework that food and feeding will be considered.

Food and Feeding

Formula   During the past 20 years feeding practices have changed. There is now a wide assortment of special food products manufactured for infant feeding. These changes reflect advances in technology and packaging. Pasturization and homogenization of milk and early supplementation of infant diets with vitamins A, D, and C have contributed to improved health and growth.

When more commercial formulas became available, the incidence of breast-feeding in the newborn period declined from 65 percent in 1940 to 26 percent in 1965.[56] Recently "the back to nature" movement and the publicity of the La Leche League (pronounced *lay lay' chay*) have influenced a resurgence in breast-feeding. Also, some pediatricians, in attempts to prevent overfeeding and obesity, are encouraging breast-feeding. They feel that the infant who is breast-fed relies on his own internal cues for satiety, whereas the bottle-fed baby may learn to rely on those external cues emanating from his mother, namely an empty bottle, thereby causing a functional deficit in proper hunger awareness.

The mother who finds breast-feeding comfortable and rewarding has made the choice that is best for her. Another mother may find bottle feeding more suitable. The mother and child are a feeding couple, and the needs of both should be considered in choosing the mode of feeding. Additional supplementary vitamins and minerals are necessary with formula and breast milk. The *type* and *amount* depend on the formula selected (see Table 15-8).

Most healthy infants want six to eight feedings a day by the end of the first week of life. The majority take enough at one feeding to satisfy themselves for approximately 4 hours, although intervals vary. Small, weak infants or those with an increased stomach emptying rate want milk about every 3 hours. Feeding schedules should be individualized.

The number of feedings per day decreases through the first year so that by 1 year of age most infants are satisfied with three meals daily.

Solid Foods   The age at which baby foods are introduced tends to be based more on contemporary trends than on nutritional requirements. At about 2½ months of age several significant changes take place. Birth stores of iron begin to diminish and caloric requirements exceed that which can be provided in 1 quart of formula. The extrusion reflex, which causes the younger infant to "spit out" solids rather than swallowing them, is diminishing. These changes seem to be natural indications for introducing solid foods. There is no firm evidence of harm in early feeding of solid foods, but there is *no* nutritional advantage. Some authorities are now associating early introduction of solid foods with obesity in later life.

Baby foods should be selected carefully because the feeding of solids which are nutritionally inferior to milk can lead to a poor nutritional state (see Table 15-9). At birth, an infant's stomach can hold only 2 tablespoons of food. By the end of the first year the stomach can comfortably accommodate about 1 cup of solids plus 8 oz of fluid, and the baby eats from one-third to one-half the amount of food an adult consumes. There is no room for foods that do not serve a real purpose.

Baby foods are concentrated in calories. Table 15-10 shows the amount of food needed for a male infant growing in the 50th percentile. A comparison between the calories recommended and *actual* food intake shows how easy it could be to overfeed a young child. Careful attention should be given to the *amount* and the *quality* of baby foods provided (in order to avoid foods high in calories and low in nutrients) so that optimum nutrition will be ensured and the patterning for childhood obesity avoided.

Frequent feeding of sucrose to infants has been recognized as a caries-producing practice. Discontinuing the use of sucrose solutions in infant comforters (small feeding bottles with sugar and water) or sweetened pacifiers (nipples with inserts of gauze dipped in sugar water) and deleting sucrose from vitamin mixtures, fruit, and fruit juices have been recommended.[57]

There are many possible sequences for introducing solids into infant diets. Practices vary according to the pediatrician and the parents' preference. The usual sequence is cereal first followed by fruits, vegetables, and meat, but a sequence of vegetables followed by meat, fruit, and cereal is just as acceptable and might lead the child to develop better food preferences.

Foods should be added one at a time in small amounts (1 teaspoon to 2 tablespoons) and placed well back on the tongue. Allergic reactions should be watched for. Foods that are common allergens (orange juice and egg white) should be introduced cautiously. Egg yolk can be added when beginning solid food. Whole egg is added toward the end of the first year. Orange juice, initially diluted with water, can be introduced around 2 months, and as the infant's tolerance increases, the water can then be eliminated (2 oz fresh, frozen, or canned orange juice provides the infant's daily vitamin C requirement).

A family history will help identify possible allergens. With older children, elimination diets are frequently used to determine the allergen. These diets need special attention to provide the necessary nutrients which may have also been eliminated. For example, a milk-free diet requires a milk substitute, which may not be readily accepted by the child because of the new taste. Another formula must be substituted or other milk-free sources of the missing protein, vitamins, and minerals must be found.

It has been shown that there are certain critical periods in the development of children when maturation brings them to a readiness for an activity.[58] For example, as the infant's extrusion reflex diminishes (around 2½ to 3 months), he becomes able to take solids well. When lateral motions of the jaw begin (around 6 to 7 months), he is ready to chew. Therefore, gradual increases in texture should begin toward the end of the fifth month to accustom the child to the new feel of food. Changes in texture can be accomplished by mashing table foods. There is no particular merit in junior foods other than convenience to the mother. Many mothers eliminate the cost of baby foods entirely by blenderizing all their own mixtures of baby food. Table 15-11 is a schedule

of acquiring new motor skills which influence readiness for new feeding behaviors.

As a child begins mouthing his hands and play objects, finger feeding can begin. Hard toast and teething biscuits can initiate the finger feeding experience. Thereafter as he sits alone, foods with bright colors, different shapes, and new smells will stimulate his food-learning experience. Finger foods should be selected according to their nutritional merit. Cooked vegetables, meat or cheese sticks, and enriched cereals are good choices. Stringy foods, nuts, and raisins can cause choking and therefore should be avoided.

Weaning Weaning is the transition from breast or bottle feedings to a more solid diet. Preparation for weaning begins in the second half of the first year. By the time a child is 5 months of age he can approximate his lips to the rim of a cup, and by the time he is 1 year old he can hold and drink from a cup with assistance. Developmentally, as he can take more fluids from the cup, he will need less from the bottle or breast.

Whole milk is generally introduced between 6 and 9 months of age. There is rising concern about the relationship between early whole milk ingestion and the occurrence of iron-deficiency anemia. The mechanism is not clearly understood. Investigators have identified malfunctions of the gastrointestinal tract with microscopic changes in the duodenal villi leading to impaired iron absorption.[59] These findings have prompted some pediatricians to delay the introduction of whole milk by giving a transition formula of evaporated milk and water or a commercial transition formula until the end of the first year.

Infant Feeding Problems *Infant feeding problems* have been defined as a difficulty exhibited by physically and physiologically healthy infants with respect to the ingestion of a diet designed to supply the necessary ingredients for optimal growth and health. This does not include obvious disease states such as malabsorption syndrome, alimentary tract abnormalities and anomalies, and early ulcerative colitis. Hughes and Falkner[60] have outlined a practical approach to infant feeding problems which begins after organic disease has been ruled out with five simple questions:

1 Is the intake of formula too large?
2 Is the intake of formula too small?
3 Is the technique of feeding incorrect?
4 Is the formula itself the wrong type?
5 Is there an emotional problem?

Table 15-8 INFANT FORMULA COMPARISON

Type	Description	Advantages and contraindications	Additional information
Breast milk	Water, solids, and fat content similar to cow's milk but has only about one-third of protein and ash content. In contrast, the amount of lactose approximately 1½ times that of cow's milk. *Colostrum*, yellowish secretion which appears 2–4 days after delivery, is not mature milk.	1 Human milk is a natural food for infants; however, the psychologic advantages are difficult to demonstrate. 2 Human milk is better tolerated; a small, flocculent curd is formed instead of a large casein. 3 Protein utilization is somewhat higher due to lactose content and amino acid pattern. 4 Lower renal solute load is due to lower levels of protein and minerals in human milk. 5 May prevent tendency to overfeed. 6 No sanitation or preparation problems. 7 Usually fewer and less serious feeding problems. 8 Constipation occurs less frequently. 9 Antibody immunization. This is questionable fact since antibodies do not survive ingestion. However, it is felt that maternal antibodies exert some production of local immunity in the gastrointestinal tract and cannot be expected to influence the frequency or severity of infections due to organisms that enter the body through other portals. 10 A substance present in human milk of some women appears to be responsible for persistent elevation of indirect reacting bilirubin. In such cases breast-feeding should be interrupted for 24–48 hours, which is generally sufficient to permit the concentration of bilirubin to fall below 10 mg/100 ml and subsequent resumption of breast-feeding with no associated increases in bilirubinemia. 11 Discontinue if mother supplies less than half the infant's needs. 12 Discontinue if mother has chronic illness (cardiac disease, tuberculosis, severe anemia, nephritis, chronic fevers). 13 Discontinue if mother returns to work. 14 Discontinue if infant is weak or unable to nurse because of anomalies of mouth. 15 Discontinue temporarily during acute infection of the mother. Milk should be pumped so that supply will not dwindle.	Milk is more mature at the end of the first month than earlier. Great variability in milk secreted by different women from one day to another, from one breast to another; however, volume averages out over a period of time. When a woman is poorly nourished, the volume of milk secreted will decrease but the percent of carbohydrate, protein, and fat will be little affected. However, *vitamin* content does reflect intake. Most drugs, including anesthesia used in dental treatment, taken by a nursing mother may inhibit milk production. Following is advised against: any drug or chemical in excessive amounts, diuretics, oral contraceptives, atropine, reserpine, steroids, radioactive preparations, morphine and its derivatives, hallucinogens, anticoagulants, bromides, antithyroid drugs, anthraquinones, dihydrotachysterol, and antimetabolites. Cigarette smoking also reduces the amount of milk produced.

	Description	Comments
Cow's milk, whole	Is lower in carbohydrate than breast milk but contains about twice as much protein and six times as much mineral matter. Therefore, for infant feeding it is diluted with water to reduce the vitamin and protein content and is mixed with a simple sugar to increase the carbohydrate content.	Negligible in iron content and ascorbic acid.
Cow's milk, skim	Alone is not suitable for infant formula's nutritional needs.	Alone is not suitable for infant formulas; 6 months of age is recommended for introduction of whole milk. Lacking linoleic acid and vitamin A.
Evaporated milk formula	Formula is a combination of evaporated milk, white corn syrup, and water. Average age evaporated milk formula 13 oz evaporated milk (1 can) 18 oz water 1 oz or 2 tbsp corn syrup	Caution mothers not to use sweetened condensed milk instead of evaporated milk. Avoid errors in formula preparation or sterilization. 1 Most economical of formulas 2 Supply of ingredients can be stored without refrigeration
Proprietary formula Similac 20 Similac with Iron SMA Enfamil	Artificial preparation designed to imitate the composition of breast milk in one or more of the following respects: 1 Lower protein content 2 Lower mineral content, particularly calcium 3 Substitution of vegetable fat mixture containing more unsaturated fat	Generally costs more than evaporated milk formula. Cost is related to ease of use (already prepared). Instruct mother to follow dilution directions: make clear differentiation between types. Combinations for mixing: powder—1 measure to 2 oz water liquid—1:1 ready feed—no dilution and no sterilization. 1 Convenient, easy preparation 2 A carbohydrate supplement has been added
Special formula preparations	Special preparations designed for the infant with allergy, digestive disturbances, or inborn errors of metabolism. These have been devised to approximate human milk but the offending agent is absent.	The use of special formulas allows the infant to grow and develop normally despite inability to handle regular formulas.
Prosobee Neomullsoy Cho-Free (undiluted) Lofenalac Lonalac Meat base Nutramigen Portagen		Milk-free Milk-free Carbohydrate-free and milk-free Low in phenylalanine Low in sodium Milk-free Hypoallergenic Lactose-free, contains medium-chain triglycerides
Pregestimil		Malabsorption disorders—carbohydrate as glucose, fat as medium-chain triglyceride, protein in a predigested, easily assimilated form

(Continued)

215

Table 15-8   INFANT FORMULA COMPARISON (Continued)

Type	Approximate composition									Vitamin and minerals considerations
	kcal/oz	Protein (Gm/100 ml)	Carbohydrate (Gm/10u ml)	Fat (Gm/100 ml)	Na (mEq/liter)	K (mEq/liter)	Ca (mEq/liter)	P (mEq/liter)	Fe (mg/liter)	
Breast milk	20	1.25	6.8	3.4	7	13	17	8	Trace	A supplement of vitamin D is needed, also ascorbic acid may need to be supplemented when the maternal intake is low. Fluoride must be provided when the water supply is not fluoridated. Breast milk does not supply iron.
Cow's milk, whole* †	20	3.5	5.0	4.1	25	35	63	62	1.0	Cow's milk does not supply iron, ascorbic acid, or fluoride.
Cow's milk, skim*	10	3.5	5.1	0.2	23	43	62	63	0.8	Skim milk does not supply iron, ascorbic acid, or fluoride. During processing, vitamins A and D are destroyed; therefore, skim milk is enriched with vitamin A and fortified with vitamin D.
Evaporated milk formula†	19	2.8	5.4	3.2	21	31	51	53	1.2	Same as for cow's milk.
Proprietary formula										Proprietary formulas are completely vitamin enriched. They may or may not provide iron. Labels should be read carefully. Fluoride must be provided when the water supply is not fluoridated.
Similac 20	20	1.8	7.7	3.4	12	22	35	32	Trace	
Similac with iron	20	1.8	7.0	3.6	13	25	35	32	12	
SMA	20	1.5	7.0	3.5	7	14	22	21	12	
Enfamil	20	1.5	7.0	3.7	11	18	32	32	1.4	
Special formula preparations										Same as for proprietary formulas.
Prosobee	20	2.5	6.8	3.4	24	28	47	42	8	
Neomullsoy	20	1.8	6.4	3.5	17	25	42	24	8	
Cho-Free (undiluted)	23	3.6	0	7.0	30	44	85	84	16	
Lofenalac	20	2.2	8.5	2.7	26	38	50	45	15	
Meat base	20	2.7	4.0	3.1	12	12	51	41	9.7	
Lonalac	20	3.4	4.8	3.5	1	27	58	68	2.1	
Nutramigen	20	2.2	8.5	2.6	17	26	50	45	9.5	
Portagen	20	2.7	7.7	3.2	17	33	49	52	11	
Pregestimil	20	2.2	8.8	2.8	17	23	45	45	12	

* Included in the table for purposes of composition comparison but not suitable for infant formula.
† Vitamin D supplement not necessary when milk is already fortified.

Sources: Charles Church and Helen Church, Bowes & Church's Food Values of Portions Commonly Used, 11th ed., J. B. Lippincott Company, Philadelphia, 1970; S. J. Fomon, Infant Nutrition, W. B. Saunders Company, Philadelphia, 1967; and Handbook of Infant Formulas, J. B. Roerig Div., Charles Pfizer & Co., New York, 1969.

Table 15-9 APPROXIMATE NUTRIENT CONTENT OF INFANT FOODS

Food item	Calories (kcal)	Protein (Gm)	Iron (mg)
Orange juice:			
Fresh or frozen (reconstituted and undiluted)	14/oz 56/4 oz	0.5/4 oz	0.1/oz 0.4/4 oz
Canned juice for babies	16/oz 65/4.2-oz can	0.5/4.2-oz can	0.1/oz 0.4/4.2-oz can
Ready-to-serve cereal			
Mixed dry cereal or high protein	9/tbsp	0.3/tbsp	2/tbsp
Wet-packed cereal	11/tbsp 101/4.7-oz jar	0.1/tbsp 1.3/4.7-oz jar	0.36/tbsp 3.40/4.7-oz jar
Strained fruit (average all kinds, including prunes)	12/tbsp 111/4.7-oz jar	0.5/4.7-oz jar	0.06/tbsp 0.06/4.7-oz jar
Strained dessert (average, all kinds)	13/tbsp 118/4.5-oz jar	0.1/tbsp 1.2/4.5-oz jar	0.38/tbsp 0.49/4.5-oz jar
Strained vegetables (average, all kinds)	6/tbsp 53/4.5-oz jar	0.2/tbsp 2.0/4.5-oz jar	0.2/tbsp 1.0/4.5-oz jar
Strained meat (average, all kinds, including liver)	16/tbsp 116/3.5-oz jar	2.0/tbsp 14.0/3.5-oz jar	0.3/tbsp 2.0/3.5-oz jar
Egg yolk	59/medium yolk	2.8/medium yolk	0.9/medium yolk
Egg yolk (baby)	28/tbsp 187/3.3-oz jar	1.4/tbsp 9.2/3.3-oz jar	0.4/tbsp 3.0/3.3-oz jar
Meat dinners (average, all kinds)	12/tbsp 84/3.5-oz jar	0.9/tbsp 6.6/3.5-oz jar	0.2/tbsp 1.0/3.5-oz jar
High meat dinner	12/tbsp 111/4.5-oz jar	0.9/tbsp 7.9/4.5-oz jar	0.1/tbsp 1.0/4.5-oz jar
Zweiback	31/average piece	0.9/average piece	

Comparison notes: Ready-to-serve cereal is higher in protein and iron than wet-packed cereal.
    Strained desserts create a "sweet tooth"; no need to introduce.
    Meat dinners and high meat dinners are poor sources of protein when compared to strained meat.
    One medium egg yolk equals 2 tbsp baby egg yolk.
Sources: Charles Church and Helen Church, *Bowes & Church's Food Values of Portions Commonly Used*, J. B. Lippincott Company, Philadelphia, 1970; Professional Communications Department— Gerber Products Company, *Nutrient Values of Gerber Baby Foods*, Fremont, Mich., 1972.

By following this approach the nurse can help in evaluating the type of problem or in determining whether a problem really exists (see Table 15-12).

Diarrhea and Constipation Diarrhea and constipation are commonly encountered problems often related to feeding and can be helped by adaptations of diet.

Common mild diarrhea and that caused by transient infections respond to reducing the food and formula intake, especially the carbohydrate and fat in the diet, and replacing it with water and clear liquids (diluted apple juice, liquid gelatin). If liquid gelatin is given in the bottle as a treatment for diarrhea, it is important to stress its discontinuance after the stool returns to normal. Gelatin is not a substitute for milk.

Constipation is practically unknown in breast-fed infants who receive adequate amounts of milk and is rare in artificially fed infants receiving an adequate diet. In artificially fed infants, constipation may be due to an insufficient amount of food or fluid. Simply increasing the amount of fluid or adding corn syrup to the formula may be corrective in the first few months of life. After this age, constipation may result from diets too high in protein or deficient in bulk. Improvement is achieved by increasing the intake of cereal, vegetables, and fruit while moderately reducing milk intake and increasing other fluids.

Iron-Deficiency Anemia Since iron-deficiency anemia is the most common hematologic symptom in infancy and childhood, special emphasis on iron intake is warranted. Often the following, singly or in combination, lead to an excessive milk intake (milk is a poor source of iron), crowding out other essential foods: prolonged bottle feeding, late weaning, nighttime bottle, and propping the bottle during feedings.

Table 15-10A FEEDING GUIDELINES FOR THE FIRST SIX MONTHS*

	0–2 weeks	2 weeks–2 months	2 months	3 months	4–5 months	5–6 months
Formula						
Ounces per feeding	2–3 oz	3–5 oz	4–6 oz	4–6 oz	5–7 oz	5–7 oz
Average total ounces	22 oz	28 oz	29 oz	30 oz	32 oz	30 oz
Number of feedings	6–8	5–6	4–5	4–5	4–5	4–5
Food texture	Liquids	Liquids	Liquids	Baby soft	Baby soft	Baby soft
Food additions						
Orange Juice		Give diluted juice; 1 oz juice and 1 oz water	2 oz, undiluted	3–4 oz	3–4 oz	3–4 oz
Baby cereal, enriched				1 tsp, B & S	2 tbsp, B & S	2 tbsp, B & S
Strained fruits				1 tsp, B & S	1 tbsp, B & S	1½ tbsp, B & S
Strained vegetables					1–2 tbsp, L	2 tbsp, L
Strained meats						1 tbsp, L
Egg yolk or baby egg yolk						½ med or 1 tbsp
Teething biscuit						½–1
Total calories	440	475	610	659–674	751–772	777–843
Recommended calories 117 cal/kg	410	410–608	608	667	725–784	784–878
Oral and neuromuscular development related to food intake	Rooting, sucking, swallowing ———→			Extrusion reflex diminishes; sucking becomes voluntary	Learning to reach hands to mouth; develops grasp	Chewing begins; can approximate lips to the rim of cup

* Calculations based on male growing at the 50th percentile for height and weight.

B = breakfast, L = lunch, S = supper

tsp = teaspoon

tbsp = tablespoon

Table 15-10B FEEDING GUIDELINES FOR INFANTS 6 TO 12 MONTHS*

	6–7 months	7–8 months	8–9 months	9–10 months	10–11 months	11–12 months
Whole milk						
Ounces per feeding	7–8 oz	8 oz	8 oz	8 oz	8 oz	8 oz
Average total ounces	28 oz	28 oz	24 oz	24 oz	24 oz	24 oz
Number of feedings	3–4	3–4	3	3	3	3
Food texture	Gradual increase →→		Mashed table →→			Cut fine
Food items						
Orange juice	4 oz	4 oz	4 oz	4 oz	4 oz	4 oz
Fortified cereal	⅓ cup, B	⅓ cup, B	½ cup, B	½ cup, B	½ cup, B	½ cup, B
Fruit, canned or fresh	4 tsp, B L, & S	4 tsp, B, L & S	2 tbsp, L & S	2 tbsp, L & S	3 tbsp, L & S	3 tbsp, L & S
Vegetables	1½ tbsp, L & S	2 tbsp, L & S	2 tbsp, L & S	2 tbsp, L & S	3 tbsp, L & S	3 tbsp, L & S
Meat, fish, poultry	1 tbsp, L & S	2 tbsp, L & S	2 tbsp, L & S	2 tbsp, L & S	2½ tbsp, L & S	2½ tbsp, L & S
Egg yolk or baby egg yolk	1 medium yolk, or 2 tbsp	1 medium yolk, or 2 tbsp	1 medium yolk, or 2 tbsp	1 whole egg	1 whole egg	1 whole egg
Teething biscuit or bread	1 biscuit	1 biscuit	½ slice bread	½ slice bread	½ slice bread	½ slice bread
Starch—potato, rice, macaroni				2 tbsp, S	2 tbsp, S	2 tbsp, S
Dessert—custard, pudding						
Butter		1 tsp	1 tsp	1 tsp	1 tsp	1 tsp
Total calories	859	876	937	974	1037	1069
Recommended calories 108 cal/kg	810–864	864–918	918–972	972–1015	1015–1048	1048–1083
Oral and neuromuscular development related to food intake	Begins using cup	Sits erect with support →→ Feeds self biscuit		Without support →→ Holds bottle	Picks up small food items & releases	Will hold and lick spoon after dipped into food; self feeding

* Calculations based on male growing at the 50th percentile for height and weight.

B = breakfast, L = lunch, S = supper

tsp = teaspoon

tbsp = tablespoon

Table 15-11 DEVELOPMENT OF FEEDING SKILLS

Age	Oral and neuromuscular development	Feeding behavior
Birth	Rooting reflex Sucking reflex Swallowing reflex Extrusion reflex	Turns mouth toward nipple or any object brushing cheek Initial swallowing involves the posterior of the tongue; By 9–12 weeks anterior portion is increasingly involved which facilitates ingestion of semisolid food Pushes food out when placed on tongue; strong the first 9 weeks By 6–10 weeks recognizes the position in which he is fed and begins mouthing and sucking when placed in this position
3–6 months	Beginning coordination between eyes and body movements Learning to reach mouth with hands at 4 months Extrusion reflex present until 4 months Able to grasp objects voluntarily at 5 months Sucking reflex becomes voluntary and lateral motions of the jaw begin	Explores world with eyes, fingers, hands, and mouth; starts reaching for objects at 4 months but overshoots; hands get in the way during feeding Finger sucking—by 6 months all objects go into the mouth May continue to push out food placed on tongue Grasps objects in mitten-like fashion Can approximate lips to the rim of cup by 5 months; chewing action begins; by 6 months begins drinking from cup
6–12 months	Eyes and hands working together Sits erect with support at 6 months Sits erect without support at 9 months Development of grasp (finger to thumb opposition) Relates objects at 10 months	Brings hand to mouth; at 7 months able to feed self biscuit Bangs cup and objects on table at 7 months Holds own bottle at 9–12 months Pincer approach to food Pokes at food with index finger at 10 months Reaches for food and utensils including those beyond reach; pushes plate around with spoon. Insists on holding spoon not to put in mouth but to return to plate or cup.
1–3 years	Development of manual dexterity	Increased desire to feed self *15 months*—begins to use spoon but turns it before reaching mouth; may hold cup, likely to tilt the cup rather than head, causing spilling *18 months*—eats with spoon, spills frequently, turns spoon in mouth; holds glass with both hands *2 years*—inserts spoon correctly, occasionally with one hand; holds glass; plays with food; distinguishes between food and inedible materials *2–3 years*—self-feeding complete with occasional spilling; uses fork; pours from pitcher; obtains drink of water from faucet

Excessive milk intake can be prevented by appropriate introduction of solids with special emphasis on foods high in iron (see Table 15-5). Iron-enriched formulas are now becoming popular as a preventive measure, especially in premature infants, infants of teen-age mothers, and infants of lower socioeconomic class. An iron supplement is necessary to replace iron stores (see discussions of iron under section on minerals).

Baby cereals and some table cereals are iron fortified; however, the amount of iron available to the child's body depends on the form of iron used. Cereals are commonly fortified with sodium iron pyrophosphate, which is poorly absorbed by the body. Therefore iron enriched cereals cannot be considered a reliable source of iron. Iron absorption can be enhanced by serving the cereals with orange juice.

Table 15-12   PRACTICAL APPROACHES TO INFANT FEEDING PROBLEMS

Problem	Signs and symptoms	Management
Intake of formula too large	Regurgitation Vomiting Diarrhea or frequent large stools Normal or excessive weight gain History of excessive intake for age	Reduce formula intake at feedings Explain the problem in detail to the parents and give reassurance
Intake of formula too small	Irritable Underweight Hungry Constipated History of inadequate intake for age	Increase the amount and frequency of formula and possibly the calorie content of the feedings
Improper technique of feeding	Any of the above signs and symptoms Following errors frequently encountered: 1 Hole in rubber nipple too small (providing too long feeding period) or too large (causing excessive swallowing of air, discomfort, and regurgitation)	A puncture with a needle will not increase the size of aperture; discard and use a new one
	2 Formula too hot	Moderately cold or room temperature formulas are well tolerated
	3 Improper placement of nipple in mouth	Place nipple far enough back in mouth
	4 Failure to bubble the infant	After feeding, hold the infant erect against shoulder to expel swallowed air
	5 Improper position of infant during feeding, such as horizontal or with propped pillow	The position should be inclined to at least a 45-degree angle
	6 Nursing from an empty bottle	Formula should fill the nipple throughout feeding, and ½ to 1 oz should be left in the bottle at termination of feeding
	7 Improper sterilization technique	Check sterilization technique Terminal sterilization technique consists of 1 Scrub bottles, nipples, equipment 2 Measure and mix formula 3 Pour mixture into bottles 4 Place bottle on rack in sterilizer and boil gently for 25 minutes 5 Store capped bottles in refrigerator
Improper composition of formula	*Carbohydrate*: Excessive amounts may produce diarrhea	Added carbohydrate in the form of corn syrup to evaporated milk formula need rarely exceed 1 oz or 2 tbsp per 24-hour volume
	Protein: Allergy to protein in cow's milk; allergic infants may have vomiting, irritability, diarrhea, with or without blood in the stool; onset 2–4 weeks after initiating of formula; history in other family members is significant	A few days' trial with a cow's milk substitute such as soybean milk, Nutramigen, or Cho-Free, with subsequent alleviation of symptoms, indicates milk allergy
	Fat: Improper fat digestion causes large bulky stools; digestion of cow's milk butterfat may be less complete than that of fat of breast milk	Substitute a formula free of butterfat, such as Similac, Enfamil, etc.
Emotional problems in the family	Irritability Colic Spitting up Vomiting Failure to gain weight	Explanation, education, patience, and understanding are needed along with constant reassurance and considerable tact

Source: Adapted from W. T. Hughes and F. Falkner, "Infant Feeding Problems: A Practical Approach," *Clinical Pediatrics*, 3:65, 1964.

Feeding Habits During the first year of life, the infant learns more mature ways of feeding as he makes the transition from relative passivity (sucking and swallowing) with a total milk diet to more active participation and a food with milk diet. Feeding and the enjoyment of foods are a learned experience which begins with the very first feeding. Good food habits are formed by a consistent approach with the expectation that he will eat, a reinforcement of positive behavior by good example, a pleasant relaxed atmosphere without pressure, and an offer of assistance only when needed. It is important to make a positive start, because the infant is forming his lifetime eating habits. At each age he will continue to build on these foundations.

Toddler

Growth and Psychosocial Characteristics At the end of the first year growth slows and weight gain is small. Approximately one-half of the weight gain during this period is due to muscle development. The plump infant begins to change gradually into a lean, muscular child. The overall skeletal growth is also slow. However, 50 percent of the adult height is attained by girls between 18 and 24 months of age and by boys between 24 and 30 months of age. The slower growth rate is reflected in decreased appetite.

During the second year, 8 more teeth erupt, making a total of 14 to 16, and by 3 years the child has most of his deciduous teeth, and he is able to handle adult foods well. The increased mobility of the toddler gives him a sense of independence which is reflected in his acceptance or refusal of food. His psychosocial development is characterized by an increasing sense of "I"—of being an individual. The increasing awareness of self is played out in the feeding situation; he wants to do more and more for himself, and refusals of food or of feeding assistance are common.

Food and Feeding The toddler's psychosocial development is pronounced, while physical growth proceeds at a slower rate. Knowledge of the child's decreased need for calories and his burgeoning sense of independence can help to avoid conflicts. Failure to recognize these features results in attempts to force-feed with subsequent rebellion and creation of feeding problems.

Adults who help toddlers with their eating should assume a calm, relaxed attitude. When an adult overreacts to food refusals by either forcing or replacing foods, negative behavior is being reinforced. A better response is to try to identify the real cause of the behavior. Sometimes appetite lag is due to such factors as overfatigue, overactivity, underactivity, or just too much attention. The older toddler can be expected to consume approximately one-half the amount of food that an adult consumes.

The toddler can bite and chew table foods and has the manipulative skills for self-feeding, although he may still require assistance and special attention to the size of the utensils. It is not appropriate to be concerned about his table manners while he is still learning these skills. Food should be presented with consideration of the taste preferences which arise as a part of the development of the individual child. A regular mealtime schedule is also important to the ritualistic toddler.

A variety of foods should be presented for tasting, touching, and eating, but the child will become confused if asked to decide what he wants to eat. Providing a variety of foods on his plate in appropriate size servings is a better approach. The diet should include a full range of foods: milk, meat, fruits, vegetables, breads, and cereals (Table 15-13) to provide optimum nutrition and cleansing action for the teeth. In order to prevent dental caries, concentrated sweets should be avoided, and their use as rewards for good behavior is inadvisable. Although the need for calories is lower than during the first year, protein requirements remain high as muscle mass expands. Accordingly, high-quality biologic proteins should be emphasized (see Table 15-1).

Appetite is sporadic during the toddler period, and food "jags" are common. Such situations should be treated in a matter-of-fact way: other foods should still be offered in small amounts along with those requested by the child. For example, if a child decides he does not like milk, he should not be forced. A small glass should be presented with each meal and then removed without comment if not taken. Milk can then be incorporated into the diet in other forms (see Table 15-13). Excessive milk intake is sometimes the source of the toddler's indifference to solid foods. As a result, he may be prone to develop a "milk anemia." During this period 16 to 24 oz of milk daily is sufficient for his needs. Iron-containing solids should be encouraged (see Table 15-5). Constipation can also be related to a high milk intake. Along with a moderate reduction in milk and an increase in other fluids, roughage foods or foods with natural laxative action should be promoted (raw fruits and vegetables; whole grain breads such as whole wheat or pumpernickel; raisin bread; whole grain cereals such as bran flakes, oatmeal, and oatmeal cookies; stewed fruit such as prunes and apricots; and prune juice).

Table 15-13 THE BASIC FOUR FOOD GROUPS THROUGHOUT THE GROWING YEARS

Food group	Servings per day	Average-size servings for age: Toddler	Preschool	School	Adolescent
Milk or equivalent	4	½–¾ cup	¾ cup	¾–1 cup	1 cup
½ cup milk equals 2 tbsp powdered milk 1 oz of cheese ¼ cup evaporated milk ½ cup cottage cheese 1 serving custard (4 servings from 1 pt milk) ½ cup milk pudding ½ cup yogurt					
Meat, fish, poultry or equivalent	2 or more	3 tbsp	4 tbsp	3–4 oz (6–8 tbsp)	4 oz or more
1 oz meat equals 1 egg, 1 frankfurter 1 oz cheese,* 1 cold cut 2 tbsp peanut butter, cut meat ¼ cup tuna fish or cottage cheese* ½ cup dried peas or beans					
Vegetables and fruits to include	4 or more				
Citrus fruit or equivalent	1 or more	4 oz	4 oz	4–6 oz	4–6 oz
1 citrus fruit serving equals ½ cup orange or grapefruit juice ½ grapefruit or cantaloupe ¾ cup strawberries 1 medium orange ½ citrus fruit serving equals ½ cup tomato juice or tomatoes, broccoli, chard, collards, greens, spinach, raw cabbage, brussels sprouts 1 medium tomato, 1 wedge honeydew					
Yellow or green vegetable or equivalent	1 or more	4 tbsp	4 tbsp	⅓ cup	½ cup
1 serving equals ½ cup broccoli, greens, spinach, carrots, squash, pumpkin 5 apricot halves ½ medium cantalope					
Other fruits and vegetables	2 or more				
Other vegetables including potatoes		2–3 tbsp	4 tbsp	⅓–½ cup	¾ cup
Other fruit including apples, banana, pears, peaches		½ med apple	½–1 med apple	1 med apple	1 med apple
Breads and cereals or whole grain or enriched equivalent	4 or more				
1 slice bread equals ¾ cup dry cereal ½ cup cooked cereal, rice, spaghetti, or macaroni 1 roll, muffin, or biscuit		½ slice ½ cup 2 tbsp	1 slice ¾ cup ¼–½ cup	1–2 slices 1 oz ½–1 cup	2 slices 1 oz 1 cup or more

* If cottage or cheddar cheese is used as a milk equivalent, it should not also be counted as a meat equivalent.
Source: Infant Feeding Guide, for use by professional staffs, Washington State Department of Social and Health Services, Health Services Division, Local Health Services, Nutrition Unit, 1972.

Pica Pica, the eating of dirt or any inedible material, is an aberration of eating and appetite which affects nutrition and is most commonly found in young children between the ages of 18 and 24 months and in pregnant women of the Negro race. Its cause is not understood. (Pica should not be confused with the normal oral examination of objects as the child learns to distinguish between food and inedible materials.) There has been little evidence associating pica with malnutrition.[61] Pica is felt to be a symptom of complex environmental, cultural, and psychologic factors seen more frequently in the urban ghetto. It is related to emotional deprivation rather than an effort to compensate for some dietary deficiency. However, investigators have found that milk, meat, and foods rich in vitamin C and iron are somewhat lacking in the diets of children who engage in pica.

Preschool Period

Growth and Psychosocial Characteristics During the third, fourth, and fifth years of life, gains in weight and height are relatively steady at approximately 4.5 lb and about 2½ to 3½ inches per year. This rate of growth, although far slower than that during infancy, continues to place heavy demands on the young body. An excessive energy outlay due to almost incessant activity during the waking hours, along with eager interest in his surroundings, frequently causes a diminished interest in food. However, the preschooler's fascination for color and shape can be applied to the feeding situation to stimulate his interest. This is a period of increasing imitation and sex identification; therefore, he identifies readily with parents at the table and will enjoy what they enjoy. A greater manual dexterity enables complete independence at mealtimes. The 5- or 6-year-old is even capable of cutting his own meat.

Food and Feeding According to the National Nutritional Survey, specific nutrients need emphasis during the preschool period.[62] Foods which contain protein, iron, thiamine, riboflavin, and vitamins C and A should be encouraged along with a continued use of iodized salt (see Tables 15-1, 15-4, and 15-5). Appetite tends to be sporadic, paralleling erratic weight gain. Failure to gain weight at a satisfactory rate creates parental concern. Parents are often so dismayed at the small quantity of foods the preschool child takes that they become willing to give him anything just to get him to eat. Emphasis should not be placed on the amount but rather on the *quality* of foods consumed. Snack times can be used to promote intake of nutritious foods; for example, crackers with peanut butter or cheese spread, fruit, cheese, yogurt or cottage cheese mixed with fruit, juices rather than soft drinks, dry cereals, oatmeal cookies, milk puddings, and custards. Some of the best childhood nutrition is received in the form of small, well-spaced snacks.

The preschool period is a time of frequent illnesses due to the child's increased exposure to communicable disease and his lack of immunity. These illnesses increase nutritional requirements and often leave a lingering impairment of appetite.

During preschool years, additional nutritional patterns and habits are shaped and become part of the child's lifetime practices.

School Years

From 6 to 12 years of age, the nutritional issues to be considered include the changing rate of growth, adaptation to the school experience, and childhood obesity.

Growth and Psychosocial Characteristics During the early years, growth proceeds at a moderate rate, culminating in a preadolescent growth spurt by about age 10 in girls and age 12 in boys (average gain in weight is 7 lb per year, and average growth in height is 2½ inches per year). Appetite parallels growth, and by 8 to 10 years of age the school child's appetite is usually good. His intake at this time is important, as he is laying down reserves for the demands of the adolescent period. His energy needs increase and approach the same as the adult.

As the child enters school he moves from dependence on parental standards to dependence on peers. He learns that only certain foods may be acceptable in his peer group and as a result may be unwilling to accept others. He wants the "in" foods in his bag lunch and when buying the school lunch will make choices in accordance with his peers. A good school lunch program may also serve to introduce new foods to the child since he is anxious to conform to the group.

School Adaptation Going to school can bring new problems. Classroom competition, school work, increasing participation in activities, and pressing schedules can bring about a decrease in appetite. Skipped or poor breakfasts and hurried lunches in the school cafeteria are common nutritional problems of this age group.

The school lunch program and the breakfast program (presently, the breakfast program is limited to schools with a large number of needy children) have been found to be a very important part of nourishment for many children, particularly in low income areas. The type A school lunch provides one-third of the recommended daily allowances for the 10- to 12-year-old child.

Childhood Obesity   During the school-age period, weight gain in anticipation of the adolescent growth spurt sometimes becomes excessive, leading to childhood obesity. (Obese children are those who exceed the mean weight for height and sex by 20 percent or more, provided that they are not edematous.) The "eyeball test" is usually a good determinant of body fat. However, it must be remembered that weight alone is not a good measure of body fat as weight also represents water and lean body mass. The use of skin fold calipers is considered useful to determine body fat, especially during the transition period from childhood to adolescence.

The cause of childhood obesity is hard to determine. It is often impossible to separate cause from effect. For example, is the child overweight because he is inactive, or inactive because he is overweight and therefore cannot easily keep up with his peers (which then causes him to become inactive, withdraw, and seek solace in food)?

The children of obese parents are at special risk. Heredity may play an important part. Also, obese parents are particularly prone to be concerned that their offspring are not eating enough, and therefore encourage them to eat more. The models, desirable and undesirable, which parents present in eating and exercise are transmitted to children.

Obesity during childhood can be *developmental* (that is, present over a period of time, beginning in infancy) or *reactive* to a particular stress period, such as that caused by death, divorce, separation, hospitalization, etc. Differentiation of these patterns gives clues for treatment.

Although diet is still the essential of treatment, psychologic factors and physical activity deserve equal attention. A *multidisciplinary* approach (doctor, nurse, nutritionist, social worker, child psychologist) is more successful in dealing with the many aspects of this problem. Appetite suppressants and the use of hormones are without merit in the treatment of obesity and can be harmful.

A weight reduction program should be tailored to the age needs of the total child. Psychologic support, heightened physical activity, and a realistic diet all need to be incorporated and moved forward simultaneously. Severe caloric restriction is not warranted and could interfere with growth; growth

represents an anabolic period, and diet implies catabolism. Therefore, a child may not be able to catabolize enough calories from his body fat for growth. A diet for age, height, and activity with a slight reduction in calories is recommended. Low-fat milk (comprising 1 to 2 percent calories from butterfat) is available and may be used.

Special consideration should be given to a child's food preferences and to his ethnic and economic background. Also, school lunches, birthday parties, and midafternoon and bedtime snacks should be considered in the diet plans. Special diet foods are not necessary and may only serve to separate the child further from his peers and perpetuate a notion that he can continue to eat volumes of food instead of learning to control the amount. Sweetening agents should be used in limited amounts if at all, for little is known about their long-term effects.

The child should not see his weight program as a diet per se, but rather, as a lifetime program. Parents should be helped to form an accepting and encouraging attitude in order to enable the child to develop a good self-concept and a positive body image despite weight fluctuations. Pressure only serves to reinforce a negative self-image and causes the child to become more passive and dependent.

It is estimated that 80 percent of fat children become fat adults. Obesity is a nutritionally related problem of significant public health concern in the United States today. Johnson, Burke, and Mayer classified 10 percent of a cross section of a Boston school as overweight.[63] Our affluence has led to important changes in our eating habits. For example, soft drinks have been substituted for water, and snacks such as potato chips and pretzels have become a must on every family's shopping list. Affluence has also affected exercise habits. The conveniences of modern life demand less energy expenditure. Children are bused to school and then come home to sit in front of television. Good attitudes toward exercise must be developed as part of the weight control program. Community facilities should be investigated to provide after-school activities. The thrust of weight control education should be *to encourage active minds and bodies instead of mouths*. The cure for obesity is prevention, which begins in childhood. The nurse is frequently responsible for keeping growth records and thereby holds the *key to prevention*, which is *awareness of the potential problem*.

Nutrition education integrated into the elementary and secondary school curricula gives the school-age child an opportunity to learn about the right foods for his body. Being informed enables him to select food wisely and prepares him for accepting more responsibility in the upcoming adolescent years.

Adolescence

Adolescence comprises nearly half the growing period in man. The implications for nutrition during this rapid growth period are great. Because growth spurts occur at different ages (10 to 14 years for girls and 12 to 15 years for boys) and because of other emerging growth differences, boys' and girls' nutritional requirements will be considered separately. However, there are some common problems that do not discriminate between the sexes, namely, the search for identity and the problems of acne and adolescent goiter.

Both sexes tend to assert their independence and as a demonstration of rebellion may reject the basic foods in favor of sweets, soft drinks, snack foods, or "natural foods." Family conflicts may have nutritional consequences as the teen-ager learns to avoid confrontation by eating away from home. A growing number of teen-agers, with diverse motivation, are adopting new eating patterns, some of which are extreme, faddish, eccentric, or grossly restricted. These diets (vegetarian, fruitarian, macrobiotic, etc.) tend to exacerbate parental and professional concern because they are different. Nutritional intervention can be viewed by young people as an attack on their cultural or value systems. A simple objective presentation of nutrition information can provide the teenager with an opportunity of choice, relevant to his life-style, whereas a nutrition lecture is almost certain to be ignored. The adolescent will listen if he can be shown how to incorporate nutrients into his diet rather than how to adopt a new life-style in order to incorporate his nutrients.

The problem of adolescent goiter, or simple goiter, is related to a lack of iodine in his diet. At the time of puberty, there is an increased demand for thyroid hormone, and in the presence of an iodine shortage the gland responds by simple hypertrophy. For this reason the use of iodized salt is encouraged.

Acne leads to physical and emotional burdens for both sexes during adolescence. It cannot be "cured" by any special diet; acne is a product of both changing hormones and stress. However, a well-balanced diet (meat, milk, fruits, vegetables, breads, and cereals) with avoidance of stimulants (coffee, tea, cola, and chocolate) may help to ameliorate the symptoms.

Adolescent Girls Many surveys show the adolescent girl to be particularly vulnerable to nutritional deficiencies. Girls more often than boys decrease their food intake to control their weight. Underweight is a commonly occurring problem. Skipping meals and reliance on vending machines for food further add to this deficiency picture. As a result, the adolescent girl may be malnourished at the very time her need for nutrients is the greatest.

Producing weight gain in undernourished girls can be a very delicate issue. An attempt should be made to understand the basis for food refusals and to work around the foods presently accepted. As tolerance improves, gradual increases in the amount can be made and better quality foods can be introduced. Supplementary foods such as frappes, eggnogs, and nourishing snacks (cheese or peanut butter with crackers, or milk puddings and custards) should be given in small amounts so as not to interfere with mealtime appetite. An extreme form of underweight, anorexia nervosa, is seen in adolescence, usually in girls. As the term implies, this is a psychologic disturbance and requires broader therapy than nutrition alone.

The use of oral contraceptives is now a consideration in planning for nutrient needs of adolescent girls. Vitamin supplementation is recommended for girls on the pill. Also, the use of intrauterine devices may cause increased menstrual loss, which increases the body's need for iron.

Early marriages and adolescent childbearing place additional demands on a young mother's body, with increased hazards to the developing fetus. In such cases, nutrition education becomes paramount, not only to alleviate the consequences of fetal malnutrition but also to provide optimum lifetime nutrition for the developing child.

Nutrition education programs directed towards the teenager's concern for her figure, complexion, and hair have more potential for success. Emphasis should be placed on foods which provide adequate protein, calories, calcium, vitamin A, iron, and thiamine. An iron supplement may be necessary when menses begin.

Due to physiologic sex differences associated with fat deposits and few opportunities for activity, teenage girls tend to gain weight easily. They often turn to fad diets to escape rejecting social attitudes, and these diets can be a potential health hazard. It is interesting to note that researchers find a high correlation between a female's weight and the socioeconomic position she achieves in life. The thin girls are found later in the top echelon, whereas the obese girls are in the lower strata of society.[64]

Adolescent obesity is not a condition particular to girls. It is a condition that erodes the physical health and emotional stability of one out of every ten teenagers in the United States.[65] Obese adolescents may come to feel that they deserve discrimination or may consider themselves ugly and loathe their body size, which can hinder the search for identity.

The principles of treatment outlined earlier in this chapter under "Childhood Obesity" apply also to the obese adolescent when combined with a realization of the adolescent's unique psychosocial development. He must be accepted for what he is and must be actively involved in the solution of his own problems. The prevention of obesity lies in early childhood intervention and education.

Adolescent Boys Where the adolescent girl tends to retain fat, the adolescent boy expands muscle mass. This rapid growth increases the body's need for protein, calcium, and iron. Increasing amounts of B vitamins are also needed to meet the extra demands of energy metabolism and muscle development.

Adolescent boys have large appetites which parallel their growth, and if provided with adequate amounts (2500 to 3000 kcal/day) of protective foods, they will have no trouble meeting their needs. The nutritional outlook for adolescent boys has been generally thought to be better than that for adolescent girls; however, the National Nutritional Survey showed that the male adolescent had more evidence of malnutrition than the female.[62]

Cigarette smoking decreases appetite and increases the body's basal metabolic rate and thereby can be a contributing factor to poor nutritional status in the adolescent population.

Boys are especially interested in physical fitness and competitive sports. Among athletes there often exists the belief that certain diets will lead to better performance. The most common fad is the high-protein diet. However, protein is not a special fuel for working muscle cells, whereas fats and carbohydrates are. During training, although the foods used to supply the calories (the athlete may need an additional 2000 to 4000 kcal/day) include more protein, the ratio of carbohydrate, protein, and fat should remain balanced. Just prior to an athletic event, an increase in the carbohydrate and fat in the diet can help replete glycogen and fat stores that will be called on during exercise.

Among the various age groups surveyed by the National Nutritional Survey, those between the ages of 10 and 16 years had the highest prevalence of unsatisfactory nutritional status.[62] The adolescent should therefore be the target for nutrition education programs. "Rap sessions" have been a useful tool to arouse interest and motivate adolescents to learn about their nutrition.

NUTRITIONAL FAILURE IN THE DEVELOPING CHILD

Now that we have taken a brief look at normal nutrition from birth to adolescence with its interrelationships to physical and psychosocial development, we will turn our attention to the nutritional evaluation of children who deviate from this pattern and will consider the causes of nutritional failure. The following section is not intended as a comprehensive review of diet therapy but rather as a conceptual basis for (1) examining the reasons for nutritional failure, (2) understanding the avenues available for compensation which will also provide for growth, (3) discussing the changes some adaptations bring to food-related learning experiences, and (4) illustrating the necessity for nutrition to be part of the interdisciplinary approach in health care. We will begin by determining the child's nutritional status.

Clinical Approaches to Evaluating a Child's Nutritional Status

Nutritional evaluation is not an easy task. Data on nutritional status have traditionally been derived from information obtained from a variety of sources.

1 *Clinical data*
    a Medical history: including birth weight, occurrence of serious illnesses, and the presence of disease or other disorders which could interfere with ingestion and utilization of nutrients
    b Clinical signs: general vitality; attention span; posture; condition of gums, teeth, skin, hair, and eyes; and development of muscles
    c Anthropometric measurements
       Weight and height: compared with the "average" weight and height for age (a series of measurements is more useful since it permits evaluation of growth over a period of time)
       Body measurements: head, chest, abdomen, calf, and pelvic circumferences; skin fold thickness
    d Radiographic examination: x-rays of hands and wrists to determine bone or biologic age, which is then compared to chronologic age
    e Dental examination: determination of the number of missing, decayed, or filled teeth; evaluate general condition of gums
2 *Laboratory data:* determination of hemoglobin, vitamin, and protein levels of the blood and examination of nutritional losses in the urine and feces can provide information on adequacy of intake or disturbances in absorption or utilization
3 *Dietary history* (see Table 15-14)

Table 15-14 DIETARY ASSESSMENT GUIDELINES

Methods of assessment
1 Daily recall: The interviewer makes a detailed listing of foods consumed during the previous 24 hours, obtaining estimates of the quantity of each food consumed during this period.
2 Food records: A record of everything consumed for a given period (3–7 days) is kept.
3 Dietary questionnaire: The following information is considered pertinent in determining actual food intake:
   a Social situation: family size, family economics, family feeding problems, family weight problems, ethnic background
   b Developmental stage: feeding age, texture of food, ability to chew, suck, and swallow
   c Growth: birth weight, height, weight gain, weight loss
   d Feeding behavior: food appetite, fluid consumption, favorite food, food dislikes, mealtime behavior problems, meals per day at home, meals out, school lunch, school hours, snacks per day, hungriest time of day
   e Food frequency per day: meat, fish, poultry _____ (including cold cuts, hot dogs, tuna fish), milk _____, eggs _____, cheese _____, peanut butter _____, bread _____, potato, macaroni, rice, noodles _____, crackers _____, fruit and fruit juices _____, vegetables _____, puddings, ice cream, custard _____, cookies _____, cake, pies _____, doughnuts, pastry _____, candy _____, potato chips, pretzels _____, tonic, Kool-Aid _____, vitamin supplementation _____

Analysis
1 Intake may be compared to food guide, such as basic four food groups.
2 Nutrient content may be calculated using tables of food composition.
3 Nutrient analysis made from a report of food actually consumed.

Evaluation
Nutrient intake is compared to some standard. In the United States the standard most frequently used is the Recommended Dietary Allowances of the National Research Council.

Limitation
1 Reliability of informant.
2 RDA standard cannot be applied to individuals. *Child's intake* applies only to groups of children.

Causes of Nutritional Failure

The term *malnutrition* means poor nutrition. It is usually thought to indicate a deficiency in one or more nutrients, but it can also mean an excess of certain nutrients. Obesity is an example of malnutrition in respect to excessive intake of food.

One may consider the causes of nutritional failure according to the following categories:

1 Defective food intake: qualitative and quantitative intake inadequate

2 Defective absorption: found in intrinsic disease states (regional enteritis, Hirschsprung's disease) or with exogenous stress (intestinal parasitosis, celiac disease, surgical removal of the small bowel)
3 Defective utilization: includes metabolic diseases (galactosemia), aminoacidopathies (phenylketonuria), and disturbed metabolic states (hepatic insufficiency and renal tubular acidosis, nephrogenic diabetes insipidus, adrenal cortical hyperplasia with salt loss)
4 Defects in function of major organ systems: severe congenital heart disease, severe chest disease (asthma, bronchiectasis), severe liver disease (cirrhosis), kidney disease (renal insufficiency), brain damage
5 Increased loss of food: vomiting and diarrhea of many causes and certain disease states in which there is increased movement of food through the gut
6 Increased metabolism: fever, infections, malignancy, hyperthyroidism
7 Excessive food or vitamin intake: in obesity caused by excessive food intake; vitamin intoxication caused by excessive intake of fat-soluble vitamins

The use of drugs in the treatment of a disease or condition can also contribute to the picture of nutritional failure. Drugs affect nutritional status by their influences on appetite, nutrient absorption, gastrointestinal flora, electrolyte balance, and metabolism. Antibiotics can affect nutritional status in a number of ways: neomycin produces a malabsorption syndrome which affects fat, glucose, carotene, and vitamin B_{12}; and isoniazid increases the requirement for pyridoxine (vitamin B_6). Corticosteriods have become a powerful therapeutic aid but may cause lowered glucose tolerance, loss of muscle protein, increase in liver fat, osteoporosis, and increased susceptibility to infection. There are numerous other examples. Folate deficiency is produced by anticonvulsant drugs used for epilepsy. Antibiotics are also known to inhibit the intestinal bacteria synthesis of vitamin K.[66]

Table 15-15 lists the above seven causes of nutritional failure and provides examples of available nutritional compensation which will also provide for continued growth.

Nutritional Status during Illness

The nutritional needs of the ill child differ from those of the healthy child. The sick child may spend his nutrient resources on body responses to illness. The body's reaction to moderate or severe trauma is a net loss of protein and other essential elements. Although increased secretion of glucocorticoid hormones increases catabolism of muscle protein, it also serves a useful purpose in the body's defense by stimulating synthesis of hepatic protein and enzymes. The increased nutrient losses resulting from bed rest and immobilization or the greater metabolic demands of fever are not sufficiently replaced when food intake is reduced, as is often the case during illness. The body's metabolic responses to surgery are determined by the extent of the surgery, the previous nutritional state, and the ability to digest and absorb nutrients after the surgery. Thus, illness alters nutrient demands. The amount of alteration will depend on the type, onset, severity, and duration of the disease. The basic nutritional needs of a particular growth period frequently need modification to meet the physiologic stress of disease or surgery.

In some instances special diets will be needed to accommodate a particular disease condition (see Table 15-15). Nutritional therapy is an integral part of the care of the sick child. To provide this therapy special consideration must be given to the *age group needs* along with the child's individual responses to illness and hospitalization.

The Hospitalized Child   The child's emotional reaction to illness is conditioned by his past experiences and by the usual growth and developmental patterns of childhood. Food often is the vehicle through which the child expresses his feelings. Since food is an essential component in the physical and emotional recovery from illness, mealtimes become therapeutic and should be made pleasant to ensure against possible rejections.

Pediatric nursing care includes thoughtful attention to the eating environment as well as the diet and the techniques of feeding. The nurse needs to apply knowledge of the total child: his ability to chew and swallow, his level of independence in self-feeding skills, his usual habits at home, nutritional requirements for his age, and the dietary management required by illness. Changes in eating patterns and regression in behavior are common while children are making emotional adjustments to hospitalization, but they can also occur when *the nursing approach encourages dependence and regression*.

The success of the plan for nutritional care depends upon the child's acceptance of the food. A number of factors may affect his appetite:

Physical factors
    General physical condition (too weak or too ill to eat)
    Position in which he is fed
    Cleanliness of the teeth and hands
    Comfort (need to void, dressed comfortably, room temperature), treatments (given before or after meals), environment (unpleasant objects in sight or clutter)
    Presentation of food (unattractive tray, inappropriately sized utensils, rushed meals with too little time to chew and swallow between mouthfuls)
    Medications (some cause drowsiness, nausea, altera-

tions of appetite, e.g., amphetamines cause decreased appetite, steroids increase appetite)
    Forced feedings
Emotional factors
    Anxiety
    Stress
    Loneliness

The nurse should analyze the factors underlying indifferent appetite and take the necessary measures to alleviate them.

A major responsibility for nursing care is observation and recording of food and fluid intake. The following will help the student in calculating amounts:

3 tsp	1 tbsp
2 tbsp	1 oz
4 tbsp	¼ cup
8 tbsp	½ cup
16 tbsp (dry)	1 cup
12 tbsp (liquid)	1 cup
2 cups	1 pt
4 cups	1 qt
5 Gm	1 tsp
15 Gm	1 tbsp
30 Gm	1 oz
120 Gm	½ cup
240 Gm	1 cup
1 kg	2.2 lb

Hospital mealtimes can be made pleasant if a warm, friendly atmosphere is created. Self-selection, group eating, proper sized portions and utensils, familiar foods, and parties help to build this atmosphere, but it is the nurse who "puts it all together."

When a child is unable to take food orally, tube feeding and parenteral nutrition become the means of providing his nutrients. These techniques represent marked departures from the normal methods of child feeding and therefore merit special attention.

Tube Feedings   When anorexia, nausea, or vomiting (not due to pyloric or intestinal obstruction) or facial paralysis is severe enough to limit caloric intake, tube feedings (by naso-esophageal tube, gastrostomy, or jejunostomy) are instituted. There are three varieties of feedings: blenderized food (meat, vegetables, fruit, and milk) with water, milk and egg base feedings (the use of fresh eggs is discouraged because of the possibility of *Salmonella* contamination), and commercial preparations. Whatever the choice, the mixture should fulfill the following criteria:

1   Diet should be nutritionally adequate, with a balance of carbohydrate, protein, and fat. There are certain guidelines to be observed regarding these proportions:

Table 15-15 CAUSES OF NUTRITIONAL FAILURE

Cause	Example	Disease or condition	Diet	Pediatric concerns
Defective food intake				
Quantitative	Maternal deprivation	Failure to thrive	High in protein, high in calories	Emotional and environmental support along with help to foster mother's capacity to nurture and protect her child
Qualitative	Judgmental errors			
	Low iron intake	Iron-deficiency anemia	High iron with initial supplementation to replete iron stores	Mothers may need support in the following areas: 1 To encourage the use of iron-containing foods the child may be rejecting 2 To wean the child in order to decrease milk consumption (large amounts of milk decrease iron absorption)
	High sugar intake	Dental caries	Low in concentrated carbohydrates (sugar, jams, jellies, honey, candy, cookies, cake)	Removal of sugar may cause conflict; mothers need positive reinforcement; frequency of sugar in the diet is as important as the total amount: if a sugar-containing food is allowed, it should be given once per day after a meal rather than throughout the day
Defective absorption	Gluten sensitivity	Gluten-induced enteropathy	Low gluten diet (avoidance of oats, wheat, rye, barley)	Offending grains are obvious in cereal forms, but are also used in many commercial products as thickeners or fillers; need for careful reading of product labels should be discussed
	Surgery	Surgical resection of small bowel (degree of malabsorption and general and specific nutrient deficiencies will depend on the amount and area of bowel resected)	Hyperalimentation, tube feedings, or high calorie, high carbohydrate (mostly simple sugar) diet with small frequent feedings	Compensations for lack of oral satisfaction and necessity to provide normal food-related experiences; when solids are restarted, food rejection and emotional problems are common
Defective utilization	Inborn error of metabolism	Galactosemia (absence of the enzyme galactose 1-phosphate uridyl transferase, one of three enzymes involved in the conversion of galactose to glucose)	Lactose-free diet (no milk or milk products)	A milk substitute must be used and careful attention must be paid to other food sources of lactose (drugs, breads, prepared mixes, etc.); careful reading of product labels should be discussed
Defective function of major organ system	Congenital anomalies	Cleft lip and palate	Adequate for normal nutritional requirements, but	Special attention to the feeding position and equipment (appro-

		Disease	Dietary management	Nursing considerations
			regarding the presence of the cleft; also should provide for nutritional stores in anticipation of surgery; acid and spicy foods may irritate the mouth and nose and may need to be eliminated	allay parents' fears that child may choke; explain to parents that patience is necessary, as feeding is apt to be a long, drawn-out process
		Cyanotic heart disease	High in calories, with small frequent feedings; need for sodium restriction depends on individual condition (normal diet for child contains 2–4 Gm Na++); adjustments in food texture may be necessary to prevent fatigue	Overdependence of child should be avoided; encourage normal age progression and independence in feeding
	Brain damage	Cerebral palsy with or without mental retardation	Adapted to the degree of handicap and level of independence; child's feeding position, food texture, and special equipment are specific considerations; muscular contractions (if present) increase caloric needs; immobile patients need supervision to prevent obesity	Same as that for cyanotic heart disease
Increased loss of food substances	Diarrhea	Ulcerative colitis	Nutritional management is primarily supportive, symptomatic, and nonspecific	Elimination diets are employed widely; despite occasional dramatic responses, there is no conclusive evidence that they are beneficial; when elimination diets are used, check to see that necessary nutrients have not also been eliminated
		Gastroenteritis (mild)	Reduction of food and formula (especially carbohydrate and fat) and restriction of liquids to water and clear fluids (broth, diluted apple juice, liquid gelatin)	A gradual return to a full diet should be stressed, and liquid gelatin in the bottle should be discontinued. Initially milk may be poorly tolerated, and should be added slowly
Increased metabolism	Malignancy	Leukemia	High in calories, high in protein (special frappes, eggnogs)	Child's appetite may be poor due to general condition and drug treatment; the diet should begin at the level of his appetite and work upward; avoid cajoling him and forced feedings
Excessive food intake	Overeating	Obesity	Appropriate for age, height, weight, and activity, with slight reduction in calories	Interdisciplinary approach: diet integrated with the psychologic factors and physical activity

  a *Calories:* intake should be sufficient to meet the child's needs, staying within the range of ⅔ to 1½ kcal/ml.
  b *Protein:* protein content should meet the child's requirement. Excess protein is unnecessary and will only be converted to energy or stored as fat, a process which obligates more water to be excreted by the kidney as urea.
  c *Carbohydrate:* sugar should not be used beyond the need for calories, as hypertonic solutions produce diarrhea.
  d *Fat:* only a sufficient amount to provide calories and essential fatty acids; excesses produce diarrhea.
  e *Water:* sufficient intake for proper fluid consistency and administration. Special attention is needed for the unconscious patient or the young child who cannot complain of thirst. (Patients given tube feedings who develop hypernatremia most frequently are found to have a water deficit rather than excessive electrolytes in feeding mixture.)
2 Foods are well tolerated by the patient.
3 Formula can be easily prepared.
4 Ingredients should be inexpensive.

Administration of tube feedings requires special regulation and close adherence to policy manuals for procedure techniques. The most common causes of diarrhea following tube feedings are bacterial contamination, improper administration (too cold or given too rapidly), and improper concentration (too much carbohydrate or too much fat).

Hyperalimentation   Hyperalimentation is the general term used for total parenteral nutrition. Its use is indicated *only* when oral or tube feedings are no longer sufficient for the patient's needs. With these indications, hyperalimentation may be lifesaving in a variety of clinical situations, including chronic intestinal obstruction, bowel fistula, inadequate intestinal length, extensive burns, birth weight less than 1 kg, and uremia, hyperkalemia of acute renal failure, and some cases of prolonged diarrhea.

Prior to initiating total parenteral nutrition, the child's nutritional requirements must be evaluated. In addition, his tolerance for fluid, nitrogen, glucose, and minerals (especially sodium and potassium) must be reviewed in the light of his cardiovascular, renal, gastrointestinal, and endocrine status.[69] From this evaluation, a basic unit solution is developed, providing a standard amount of calories and nutrients per unit volume. The number of units supplied will depend on the individual needs of the child. The insertion of a catheter into the superior vena cava and the use of a peristaltic pump to control the speed of delivery make it possible to administer hypertonic dextrose solutions which will ensure adequate caloric intake. In addition to protein hydrolysate, electrolytes, and vitamins, periodic infusions of whole blood or plasma will provide trace elements, essential fatty acids, and other unidentified factors. Control of infection and optimum treatment of trauma are necessary in reducing catabolic activity. Normal weight gain can be expected in children who are free of infection and who were not malnourished at the outset.

Reevaluation should be made on the basis of serial clinical and biochemical evaluations, which include accurate recordings of daily body weight, volume of urine output and other body fluid losses, and laboratory tests to determine the level of urinary sugar after each voiding, blood sugar concentration, and serum electrolytes and osmolarity. When the patient is stable, laboratory tests may be made less frequently.

Through the use of tube feedings and hyperalimentation, the child's nutritional state is maintained and improved. However, long-term maintenance can mean that the child totally misses those food-related experiences so important to his psychosocial development. It is necessary that compensations be made for the absence of oral satisfaction and that the child resume normal food-related experiences as soon as possible. Some of these same compensations must also be provided for the handicapped child.

The Handicapped Child   The handicapped child may have one or more deficient mechanisms which preclude normal feeding behavior. Therefore, he will need a special program to encourage the development of feeding skills in order to avoid overdependence on the part of caretakers. His diet should be adequate for his normal nutritional requirements and in addition must provide for his special needs in relation to *food texture, feeding position*, and *equipment*.

A Total Nutritional Care Plan[68]

A disease involving a special diet—namely, phenylketonuria—will be considered to show the interrelationships of diet and disease to the growing child and his internal, physical, and emotional environments.

The "Conceptual Visual Aid to Total Health" developed by Richmond and Lustman portrays some of the specific factors which interact significantly in the management of the nutritional needs for a child[69] (see Fig. 15-1). The outer circle has three subdivisions: (a) the internal environment of the child, (b) the physical environment of the child, and (c) his emotional environment. Each of the three "environ-

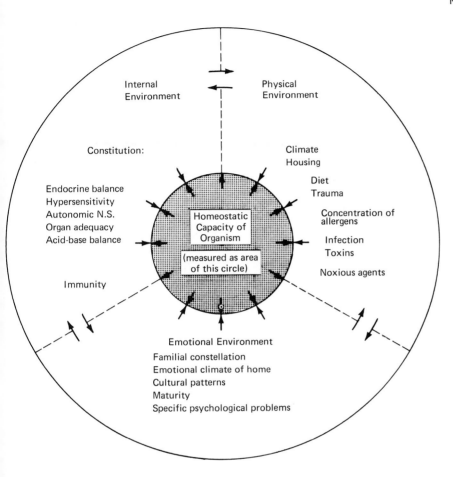

Internal
Environment

Physical
Environment

Constitution:

Endocrine balance
Hypersensitivity
Autonomic N.S.
Organ adequacy
Acid-base balance

Immunity

Climate
Housing

Diet
Trauma

Concentration of
allergens

Infection
Toxins

Noxious agents

Homeostatic
Capacity of
Organism

(measured as area
of this circle)

Emotional Environment
Familial constellation
Emotional climate of home
Cultural patterns
Maturity
Specific psychological problems

Figure 15-1 A conceptual model illustrating, in part, the interacting factors basic for an understanding of the patient. *(From J. B. Richmond and S. L. Lustman, "Total Health: A Conceptual Visual Aid," Journal of Medical Education, 29:23, 1954.)*

ments" may become altered in specific situations or disease states. The inner circle represents the homeostatic responses of the child to the three environments which influence his growth. It is hoped that the nursing student will find this guide useful in defining the multiplicity of factors operative in adjusting normal nutritional needs for therapeutic care. The nurse will need to begin by understanding *the nature of the disease or condition* affecting the child (particularly the hereditary aspects, such as an inborn error of metabolism) and *the principles of diet.*

Phenylketonuria: A Defect in Utilization Phenylketonuria (PKU) is an inborn error of metabolism resulting from a mutant autosomal recessive gene. The defective gene inhibits the synthesis of phenylalanine hydroxylase, which oxidizes phenylalanine (an essential amino acid) to tyrosine (another amino acid). Phenylalanine accumulates in the blood and its alternate metabolites, the phenylacids, are excreted in the urine. If the disorder is not treated, the rise in blood phenylalanine causes irreversible damage to the central nervous system with subsequent

mental retardation. The treatment is a low-phenylalanine diet to reduce the serum phenylalanine levels (maintained between 6 and 10 mg/100 ml). However, adequate amounts of phenylalanine must be provided for growth. Initially at 1-week intervals, blood levels, height, weight, and general development are closely monitored to ensure the efficiency of the diet.

Low-Phenylalanine Diet Natural protein contains 2 to 5 percent phenylalanine, so children with PKU need an artificial replacement for dietary protein. Special phenylalanine-restricted preparations, complete in all constituents except phenylalanine, are available. Lofenalac* is the most commonly used available preparation. However, the phenylalanine content of Lofenalac (1 cup contains 120 mg phenylalanine) is not likely to be sufficient to meet the demands of the infant's growth, and additional sources

* A feeding preparation made from hydrolyzed casein supplying dietary nitrogen as amino acids. It contains 0.60 to 0.1 percent phenylalanine and is supplemented with tyrosine (which becomes an essential amino acid for these patients), vitamins, iron, and other minerals. In normal dilution Lofenalac provides 20 kcal/oz.

must be provided. Whole milk or evaporated milk is added to the Lofenalac formula to meet the phenylalanine requirements. (The phenylalanine requirement for a child ranges from 65 to 90 mg/kg body weight during the newborn period and decreases to 20 to 25 mg/kg body weight by age 2 years.[70]) Phenylalanine deficiency leads to severe illness, with acidosis, hypoglycemia, extensive skin rash, microcytic anemia, and overwhelming infection.

Solid foods (cereals, fruit, and vegetables) may be introduced around the usual age (2½ to 3 months) and are added to the diet according to their calculated phenylalanine content. A useful measurement, where solid foods are concerned, is the *equivalent* (an amount of solid food containing 15 mg phenylalanine) for example, 1 cup applesauce is the equivalent of 15 mg phenylalanine. It is necessary that a balance be created between the essential amino acids in the milk substitute and sufficient phenylalanine from natural sources (fruits, vegetables, and cereals).

The diet is prescribed by the doctor according to the child's growth needs and his blood levels. It is calculated by a nutritionist, who determines the amount of formula and the number of solid food additions. Special low-protein flours and pastas are available and with sugar, honey, jams, and jellies help to provide calories and lend variety to the diet.

As yet, there is no agreement about the length of time the diet should be continued. Some suggest dietary control for the first 5 years of life, when the maximum brain growth takes place. More conservative schools suggest lifelong maintenance to prevent possible regression after termination of the diet.

Diet Adjustment by Age and Developmental Stage
In infants diagnosed before 6 weeks of age, the low-phenylalanine diet appears to prevent brain damage, provided that the diet is followed. Herein lies the challenge. The diet must be continuously adjusted to meet the increasing needs for protein and the proportionally lowered need for phenylalanine as the child grows. These adjustments must correlate with his age characteristics to normalize his food-related experiences and to prevent possible detrimental effects on his phenylalanine intake. For example:

Infant stage: The transition from bottle to baby foods to cup drinking may cause a temporary decline in food intake as the child acquires these new skills.
Toddler stage: New manipulative skills (self-feeding) may lead to dietary accidents because the child's greater mobility gives him access to forbidden foods. Decreasing growth leads to decrease in appetite and possible food refusals.

Preschool period: Increased independence leads to the possibility of snacking outside the house. Birthday parties and holidays become issues.
The school years: Peer group identification may lead the child to hide his special drink (Lofenalac) or bread to escape being different.

Frequent home visits by the public health nurse or nutritionist can be a source of support and provide an opportunity to view the interrelationships of the child's internal, physical, and emotional environments. The following areas should be explored:[71]

1 *Adequacy of present diet*
   a Typical meal patterns
   b Food likes and dislikes
   c Ability of family to provide and prepare an adequate diet
2 *Attitudes of family* (social, cultural, and emotional) which affect the ability of the parents to do the following:
   a Provide the recommended diet
   b Help the child enjoy eating
   c Help the child become independent in the feeding situation
3 *Special dietary needs*
   a Medical diet order (full understanding of aim)
   b Relationship of diet order to family food pattern
   c Availability of foods ordered and finances to purchase them
   d Methods of using foods
4 *Techniques of feeding*
   a Environment
   b Schedule
   c How the child is fed (utensils should be appropriate for child's use)
5 *Degree of independence*
   a Ability to feed self
   b Ability and readiness to chew and swallow

With the birth of a phenylketonuric child, parents face physical, emotional, and financial tension which in turn can affect the parent-child relationship and other family relationships. Furthermore, if it is believed to be through food that the infant forms his first basic relationship to the world, it seems reasonable to speculate that a special diet carries the risk of bringing about a negative adaptation to the very broad range of food-related learning experiences. As parents are helped to understand the dietary treatment of their child's condition and to view his behavior in relation to the developmental characteristics for his age, they will be able to recognize normal behavior and set consistent goals despite his medical problem.

It is hoped that this information will help create for the nursing student an awareness of the need for continuing assessment and adaptation of diet in the growing child and, as a consequence, will lessen the tendency to oversimplify diet to the detriment of the patient. Furthermore, it is this awareness that should lead the nurse to seek collaboration with the health care team (nutritionist or dietitian, doctor, social worker, and any other professionals), to ensure that all factors in the child's environment—physical, emotional, and internal—have been cared for.

REFERENCES

1 M. L. Manning, "The Psychodynamics of Dietetics," *Nursing Outlook*, April 1965, p. 57.
2 National Dairy Council, *A Source Book on Food Practices with Emphasis on Children and Adolescents*, 1968, p. 4.
3 "What Does 'Nutrition' Really Mean?" (commentary), *Nutrition Today*, 3(4):26, December 1968.
4 "Some Questions and Answers about Dietary Supplements," FDA Fact Sheet, U.S. Department of Health, Education, and Welfare, 1971.
5 C. H. Robinson, *Normal and Therapeutic Nutrition*, 14th ed., The Macmillan Company, New York, 1972, pp. 286–287.
6 "Food Labeling Regulations, The Official Summary," *Nutrition Today*, 8(1):14–15, January–February 1973.
7 R. E. Shank, "A Chink in our Armor," *Nutrition Today*, 5(2):5, summer 1970.
8 Department of Health, Education, and Welfare, *How Children Grow*, Division of Research Resources, National Institutes of Health, Bethesda, Md., June 1972, p. 12.
9 Ibid., p. 15.
10 Ibid., p. 17.
11 H. P. Martin, "Nutrition: Its Relationship to Children's Physical, Mental, and Emotional Development," *American Journal of Clinical Nutrition*, 26(7):767, July 1973.
12 I. J. Wolman, "Some Prominent Developments in Childhood Nutrition," *Clinical Pediatrics*, 12(2):74, February 1973.
13 Martin, op. cit., p. 770.
14 S. K. Livingston, "What Influences Malnutrition," *Journal of Nutrition Education*, summer 1971, pp. 18–26.
15 R. H. Barnes, "Nutrition and Man's Intellect and Behavior," *Federation Proceedings*, 30(4):1429–1433, July–August 1971.
16 F. B. Monckeberg, "Malnutrition and Mental Behavior," *Nutrition Reviews*, 27:191, 1969.
17 H. P. Chase and H. P. Martin, "Undernutrition and Child Development," *New England Journal of Medicine*, 282(17):933–939, April 23, 1970.
18 S. Champakam, "Kwashiorkor and Mental Development," *American Journal of Clinical Nutrition* 21(8):844–852, 1968.
19 ———, "Malnutrition and Mental Behavior," *Nutrition Reviews*, 27(7):191–193, 1969.
20 J. Cravioto and B. Robles, "Evolution of Adaptive and Motor Behavior during Rehabilitation from Kwashiorkor," *American Journal of Orthopsychiatry*, 35:449, 1965.
21 J. Hirsch and J. L. Knittle, "Cellularity of Obese and Nonobese Adipose Tissue," *Federation Proceedings*, 29(4):1516–1521, July–August 1970.
22 H. A. Guthrie, "Infant Feeding Practices," *American Journal of Clinical Nutrition*, 21:863, 1968.
23 "Salt in Infant Foods," *Nutrition Reviews*, 29(2):28, February 1971.
24 S. Innami and O. Mickelsen, "Nutritional Status—Japan," *Nutrition Reviews*, 27(10):277, October 1969.
25 "Salt in Infant Foods," op. cit., p. 30.
26 S. J. Fomon, *Infant Nutrition*, W. B. Saunders Company, Philadelphia, 1967, p. 95.
27 Council on Foods and Nutrition, "Iron in Enriched Wheat Flour, Farina, Bread, Buns, and Rolls," *Journal of the American Medical Association*, 220(6):13–17, May 8, 1972.
28 G. A. Goldsmith, "Iron Enrichment of Bread and Flour," *American Journal of Clinical Nutrition*, 26:131, February 1973.
29 G. A. Goldsmith, "The Experts Debate the Added Enrichment of Bread and Flour with Iron," *Nutrition Today*, 7(2):5, 6, and 9, March–April 1972.
30 H. Bruch, *Eating Disorders: Obesity, Anorexia Nervosa, and the Person Within*, Basic Books, Inc., New York, 1973, chaps. 4 and 14.
31 N. S. Wenkam, "Cultural Determinants of Nutritional Behavior," *Nutrition Program News*, U.S. Department of Agriculture, July–August 1969, p. 1.
32 H. B. Moore, "The Meaning of Food," *American Journal of Clinical Nutrition*, 5(1):79, January–February 1957.
33 R. J. Wolff, "Who Eats for Health?" *American Journal of Clinical Nutrition*, 26:443, April 1973.
34 S. J. Fomon, "Comments Concerning Skim Milk in Infant Feeding," *Maternal and Child Health Service*, Nov. 2, 1972, p. 3.
35 W. E. Laupus and M. J. Bennett, *Textbook of Pediatrics*, 9th ed., W. B. Saunders Company, Philadelphia, 1969, p. 130.
36 S. R. Williams, *Nutrition and Diet Therapy*, 2d ed., The C. V. Mosby Company, St. Louis, 1973, p. 15.
37 J. L. Lasser and M. K. Brush, "An Improved Ketogenic Diet for the Treatment of Epilepsy," *Journal of the American Dietetic Association*, 62(3):284, March 1973.
38 J. M. Signore, "Ketogenic Diet Containing Medium-Chain-Triglycerides," *Journal of the American Dental Association*, 62:3, March 1973, p. 286.
39 D. H. Calloway, "Recommended Dietary Allowances for Protein and Energy, 1973," *Journal of the American Dietetic Association*, 64(2):160, 1973.
40 Ibid., p. 161.
41 D. Erhard, "Nutrition Education for the 'Now' Generation," *Journal of Nutrition Education*, spring 1971, pp. 135–139.
42 U. D. Register and L. M. Sonnenberg, "The Vegetarian Diet," *Journal of the American Dietetic Association*, 62(3):253–261, 1973.
43 Fomon, "Comments Concerning Skim Milk in Infant Feeding," op. cit., pp. 1–6.
44 L. Anderson, M. Dibble, H. Mitchel, and H. Rynbergen, *Nutrition in Nursing*, J. B. Lippincott Company, Philadelphia, 1972, p. 139.
45 L. E. Holt, "Energy Requirements," in H. L. Barnett, *Pediatrics*, 15th ed., Meredith Corporation, New York, 1972, p. 129.
46 S. R. Ames, "The Joule—Unit of Energy," *Journal of the American Dietetic Association*, 57(5):34–39, November 1970.
47 J. G. Bieri, "Fat-soluble Vitamins in the Eighth Revision of The Recommended Dietary Allowances," *Journal of the American Dietetic Association*, 64(2):171, 1974.

48 O. A. Oswald, "Vitamin A Physiology," *Journal of the American Medical Association*, 214(6):34–39, Nov. 9, 1970.

49 R. L. Pike, and M. L. Brown, "Nutrition: Physiological Aspects," in *Nutrition: An Integrated Approach*, John Wiley & Sons, Inc., New York, 1967, p. 279.

50 J. G. Bieri, "Fat-soluble Vitamins in the Eighth Revision of the Recommended Dietary Allowances," *Journal of the American Dietetic Association*, 64(2):172–173, 1974.

51 Fomon, *Infant Nutrition*, op. cit., p. 126.

52 R. R. Streiff, "Folate Deficiency and Oral Contraceptives," *Journal of the American Medical Association*, 214(1):40, Oct. 5, 1970.

53 R. E. Hodges, "Nutrition and 'The Pill,' " *Journal of the American Dietetic Association*, 59(3):212–216, September 1971.

54 R. L. Pike, and M. L. Brown, "Nutrients in Foods," in *Nutrition: An Integrated Approach*, John Wiley & Sons, Inc., New York, 1967, pp. 363–364.

55 Roberta O'Grady, "Feeding Behavior in Infants," *American Journal of Nursing*, 71(4):736–739, April 1967.

56 S. J. Fomon, *Infant Nutrition*, op. cit., p. 5.

57 ——— "Nutrition in Oral Health: Research and Practice," *Dairy Council Digest*, 40:6, November–December 1969.

58 R. S. Illingsworth and J. Lester, "The Critical or Sensitive Periods, with Special Reference to Certain Feeding Problems in Infants and Children," *Journal of Pediatrics*, 65:839, 1964.

59 C. Woodruff, "The Role of Fresh Cow's Milk in Iron Deficiency Anemia," *American Journal of Disease in Childhood*, 124:18–23, July 1972.

60 W. T. Hughes and F. Falkner, "Infant Feeding Problems: A Practical Approach," *Clinical Pediatrics*, 3:65–68, February 1964.

61 R. S. Lourie et al., "Why Children Eat Things That Are Not Food," *Children*, 10(3):143–146, July–Aug. 1963.

62 "Highlights from the Ten State Nutrition Survey," *Nutrition Today*, 74:4–10, July–August 1972.

63 M. L. Johnson, B. S. Burke, and J. Mayer, "The Prevalence and Incidence of Obesity in a Cross-section of Elementary and Secondary School Children," *American Journal of Clinical Nutrition*, 4:231–238, May–June 1956.

64 M. E. Moore, A. J. Stunkard, and L. Sole, "Obesity, Social Class, and Mental Illness," *Journal of the American Medical Association*, 81:962–966, Sept. 15, 1962.

65 J. A. Spargo, F. P. Heald, and P. S. Pekos, "Adolescent Obesity," *Nutrition Today*, 1(4):2–8, December 1966.

66 "Drugs," *Dairy Council Digest*, 40:5, September–October 1969.

67 R. S. Goodhart and M. E. Shils, *Modern Nutrition in Health and Disease*, Lea & Febiger, Philadelphia, 1973, p. 978.

68 E. Newberger and R. Howard, "A Conceptual Approach to the Child with Exceptional Nutritional Requirements," *Clinical Pediatrics*, 12:456–467, August 1973.

69 J. B. Richmond and S. L. Lustman, "Total Health—A Conceptual Visual Aid," *Journal of Medical Education*, 29:25, May 1954.

70 L. E. Holt and S. E. Synderman, "The Amino Acid Requirements of Children," in W. L. Nyhan (ed.), *Amino Acid Metabolism and Genetic Variation*, McGraw-Hill Book Company, New York, 1967, pp. 381–390.

71 *Feeding Mentally Retarded Children* (pamphlet), U.S. Department of Health, Education, and Welfare, 1965.

BIBLIOGRAPHY

Anderson, L., Dibble, M. J., Mitchel, H. S., and Rynbergen, H. J.: *Nutrition in Nursing*, J. B. Lippincott Co., Philadelpha, 1972, chaps. 13–17 and 29.

Aykroyd, W. R.: "What Do We Mean by 'Nutrition'?" *Nutrition Today*, 7(6):30–31, November–December 1972.

Barnett, H. L.: *Pediatrics*, 15th ed., Meredith Press, New York, 1972, chap. 3.

Beal, V. A.: "On the Acceptance of Solid Foods, and Other Food Patterns, of Infants and Children," *Pediatrics*, 20:448, 456, September 1957.

Butterworth, C. E.: "Interaction of Nutrients with Oral Contraceptives and Other Drugs," *Journal of the American Dietetic Association*, 62(5):510–514, May 1973.

Cheek, D. B.: "Cellular Growth, Hormones, Nutrition and Time," *Pediatrics*, 41(1):30–43, part 1, January 1968.

Davis, Karen: "Adequacy of Infants' Diets," *American Journal of Clinical Nutrition*, 25:933–938, September 1972.

Donald, E. A., et al.: "Vitamin B_6 Requirement of Young Adult Women," *American Journal of Clinical Nutrition*, 24:1028–1041, September 1971.

Fomon, S. J.: *Prevention of Iron Deficiency Anemia in Infants and Children of Pre-school Age*, Public Health Service Publication 2085, U.S. Department of Health, Education, and Welfare, 1970.

———: "A Pediatrician Looks at Early Nutrition," *Bulletin of the New York Academy of Medicine*, 47:569–578, June 1971.

Food and Nutrition Board: *Recommended Dietary Allowances*, 7th ed., National Academy of Sciences, National Research Council, Washington, D.C., 1968.

Foster, S.: "Sickle Cell Anemia: Closing the Gap between Theory and Therapy," *American Journal of Nursing*, 71(10):1952–1956, October 1971.

Frankle, R., McGregor, B., Wylie, J., and McCann, M.: "Nutrition and Life Style, *Journal of the American Dietetic Association*, 63:269–273, September 1973.

Goodhart, R. S., and Shils, M. E.: *Modern Nutrition in Health and Disease*, 5th ed., Lea & Febiger, Philadelphia, 1973, chaps. 24 and 36.

Himsworth, H.: "What 'Nutrition' Really Means," *Nutrition Today*, 3(3):18–20, September 1968.

Hirting, D. C., and Drury, E. E.: "Vitamin E Content of Milk, Milk Products, and Simulated Milks: Relevance to Infant Nutrition," *American Journal of Clinical Nutrition*, 22(2):147–155, February 1969.

Huenemann, R. L.: "Interpretation of Nutritional Status" (commentary), *Journal of the American Dietetic Association*, 63(2):123–124, August 1973.

Illingsworth, R. S.: *The Development of the Infant and Young Child*, The Williams & Wilkins Company, Baltimore, 1972, chap. 6.

Infant Feeding Guide, for use by professional staff, Washington State Department of Social Health Services, Health Services Division, Local Health Services, Nutrition Unit, 1972.

Krause, M. V., and Hunscher, M. A.: *Food Nutrition and Diet Therapy*, 5th ed., W. B. Saunders Company, Philadelphia, chaps. 16 and 17.

McCann, M.: "Evaluation of Nutritional Status," *Pediatric Annals*, April 1973, pp. 67–76.

Moore, T.: "The Calories versus the Joule," *Journal of the American Dietetic Association,* 59(4):327-330, October 1971.

Nelson, W. E.: *Textbook of Pediatrics*, 9th ed., W. B. Saunders Company, Philadelphia, 1969, chaps. 2 and 3, pp. 1046–1051, 1260–1263, 757–758, 134, 844, 1499, and 1050–1052.

Newton, N.: "Psychologic Differences between Breast and Bottle Feeding," *American Journal of Clinical Nutrition*, 24:933–1002, August 1971.

Pike, R. L., and Brown, M. L.: *Nutrition; An Integrated Approach*, John Wiley & Sons, Inc., New York, chaps. 2–4, 12, and 15.

Pipes, Peggy: "Development of Feeding Behavior" (personal communication), Child Development Center, Seattle, Wash.

Robinson, C. H.: *Normal and Therapeutic Nutrition*, 14th ed., The Macmillan Company, New York, 1972, chaps. 21–24.

Scrimshaw, N. S.: "Nature of Protein Requirements," *Journal of the American Dietetic Association*, 54(2):94–101, February 1969.

Tappel, A. L.: "Vitamin E," *Nutrition Today*, 8:4–12, July–August 1973.

Van Itallie, T., and Campbell, R. G.: "Multidisciplinary Approach to the Problem of Obesity." *Journal of the American Dietetic Association*, 61:385–390, October 1972.

Williams, S. R.: *Nutrition and Diet Therapy*, 2d ed., The C. V. Mosby Company, St. Louis, 1973, chaps. 2–9, 18, and 19.

Wolff, O. H.: "Obesity in Childhood," in Gairdner, D. (ed.), *Recent Advances in Pediatrics*, Little, Brown and Company, Boston, 1965, chap. 9, pp. 216–233.

Ziegler, E. E., and Fomon, S. J.: "Fluid Intake, Renal Solute Load and Water Balance in Infancy," *Journal of Pediatrics*, 78(4):561–568, April 1971.

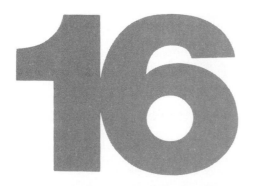

ACCIDENT PREVENTION

JUDY L. MOORE

Accidents are the largest cause of death or injury in childhood after the age of 1 year. Obviously, then, prevention of accidents is a major area of concern for pediatric health care professionals. Nurses can and should be assertive in promoting accident prevention, both in their professional role with children and families and in their citizen role in the community. Accident prevention can be thought of as a combination of safety consciousness and future-oriented awareness of children's developmental changes as they affect children's vulnerability to various accidents. This chapter deals with the scope of the problem of accidents and takes a development-based preventive approach to the common accidents at each age from birth through adolescence.

THE SCOPE OF THE PROBLEM

Statistics gathered for the 1970 White House Conference on Children report that 15,000 children under age 15 die from accidents each year in the United States and another 19,000,000 are injured severely enough to seek medical care or to restrict their usual activity. Two-thirds of the accidents involving children occur at home.[1]

When the accidental death rate for children between 1 and 4 years of age is compared with the other four leading causes of mortality in this age group, accidental death is by far the most prevalent (see Fig. 16-1). The percentage breakdown of accidents from these data is:

Motor vehicle accidents	33 percent
Fires and explosions	22 percent
Drowning	14 percent
Inhalation and ingestion	13 percent
Falls and similar accidents	12 percent
Poisoning	6 percent

The expense to society in general for accidents is untold in terms of numbers of missed school days, numbers of emergency room visits, and cost in dollars. The expense to the children and parents involved is more than money, time, and loss of education. It is difficult to assess the costs in psychologic trauma, permanent disfigurement, permanent disability, and death.

Safety as a social value is gaining momentum in the United States. The idea that accidents are "acts of God," just happen, or cannot be prevented is fading. But safety itself is expensive because it requires redesign of products, changes in housing and building codes, education of the public, and new legislation.[2] Most or all of these processes fre-

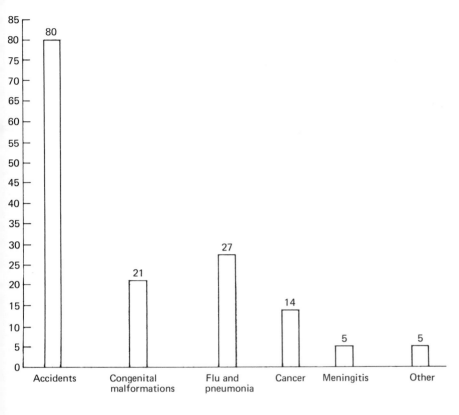

Figure 16-1 Deaths per 100,000 population for children ages 1 through 4 years. [*Adapted from Profiles of Children: White House Conference on Children 1970, Washington, D.C., U.S. Government Printing Office, p. 64* (1966 statistics).]

quently have not been undertaken until some disaster has made people aware of an unsafe condition that could be corrected, and of course, by that time it is too late for the earlier victims. For example, when reports appeared of the large number of children who had suffocated in unused refrigerators, the public concern was sufficient to precipitate neighborhood clean-ups and to eventuate in legislation making it illegal in many parts of the country to leave doors on discarded refrigerators. Similarly, government-imposed control forbidding the use of highly flammable fabrics for children's clothing followed public awareness that numerous children had been burned as they stood near open fireplaces or other sources of fire.

Accidents vary according to geographic location. Drownings have their highest incidence in areas where there are many lakes, rivers, seashores, and home swimming pools. Snow, ice, and furnaces present hazards in the North. Small-area heaters give rise to fires and asphyxiations in the South, where they are used infrequently and often not cared for properly. Lead poisoning is most common in the slum areas, where old lead paint peels from walls, furniture, and window ledges and is eaten by young children. Injuries from farm equipment and poison-ings from agricultural pesticides are obviously rural area problems.

Some childhood accidents are seasonal, such as drownings, hunting incidents, and firecracker injuries. In addition, there is evidence that children's accidents peak around holidays, weekends, and periods of family disorganization such as when parents are ill or have house guests. Similarly, the early morning hours when children are apt to be up before other family members and evenings or other fatigue periods are especially likely to be marked by accidents.

Accident proneness, primarily a popular (rather than scientific) term, refers to the alleged predisposition of some people toward involvement in accidents. Accident proneness generally is regarded as a psychologic phenomenon in which a person who has unresolved guilt feelings unconsciously manages to suffer repeated accidental injury in order to satisfy his wish for punishment and thereby relieve his guilt. It has been suggested that accident proneness is more apparent than real.[3] To establish incontrovertibly that accident proneness is a valid concept, it would be necessary to identify persons whose accident rate statistically exceeds the incidence of accidents among the general population.

The general population in this sense would need to be similar to the suspected accident prone group in terms of socioeconomic status, age, sex, and the other variables known to affect accident rates. Several investigations of this nature have yielded little or no support for the concept of accident proneness.[3, 4] Foote[3] suggests that the label "accident prone" has been much overused and should be applied only to a tiny minority if at all.

PARENTAL ROLES IN ACCIDENT PREVENTION

There are extremes of the continuum of accident prevention. At the one end is indifference to hazards, and at the other is total rigidity and overprotection. Neither extreme is healthy for growing, curious children. A good "rule of thumb" for parents is to provide rational *consistent* limits of safety with objects or situations that carry a substantial risk of injury but to otherwise give children freedom to explore, learn, and enjoy.

Consistency in this context may be defined as unwavering adherence to the same principles and regulations. Adults need to set firm limits on unsafe activities and act promptly and consistently to ensure that the rules are enforced. The specific limits that are set and the modes of enforcement vary from family to family.

Even within families different forms of discipline may appropriately be used to back up safety regulations, depending upon which disciplinarian or which child is involved or upon the seriousness of the particular hazard. Age-related developmental characteristics comprise a major basis for anticipating the types of accidents to which children are prone. Obviously, playing with matches is a hazardous temptation for preschoolers but not for infants, and instruction in bicycle safety is appropriate primarily for school-age children; the remainder of this chapter is focused on normative child development considerations such as these. In addition, *individual* characteristics require careful evaluation if prevention is to be geared effectively toward the needs of particular children and families. Behavioral traits such as general temperament, responsiveness to teaching rather than to authoritative decree, level of activity, attention span or task persistence, intelligence, and degree of impulsivity or caution are part of the nurse's appraisal of a particular child's accident prevention needs.[5] Family characteristics including availability of supervision for children, types of hazards which exist in the home or neighborhood, socioeconomic resources, disciplinary styles, and personality characteristics of parents also must be evaluated and utilized.

In all ages of childhood, preventing accidents is a fairly easy task in some areas and difficult in others. Prevention is greatly facilitated by utilization of knowledge about children's developmental characteristics. Young infants need protection. Toddlers and preschoolers require extensive supervision. As experienced parents know, it takes only a few seconds for a normal toddler to disappear; if he is out of sight and quiet, parents had better start looking for him quickly because he is probably "into something." But age-appropriate teaching becomes progressively feasible and effective in the toddler and preschool years. Particularly with young children, the substitution of permissible activities for unsafe ones is an extremely useful technique for avoiding injuries while at the same time minimizing frustration for all persons involved. School-age children and adolescents are without direct adult supervision much of the time, but have the experience and cognitive maturity to respond well to safety education and hence to "supervise" themselves. Children of all ages seek adult approval and do not often repeat activities that cause disapproval or punishment (unless their basic need for approbation is not being met in positive ways).

Perhaps the major difficulties in accident prevention are anticipating the almost endless variety of hazardous situations children may get into and deciding where to draw the line between that which constitutes play and other beneficial experience and that which carries too great a risk.

Discipline used to enforce safety rules must be firmly, promptly, and consistently applied whenever a child transgresses. The child who is old enough should be instructed to avoid dangers whenever they can be anticipated, and he should be made to understand exactly what is expected of him. In response to a dangerous childhood activity, it is extremely unwise for adults to ignore it, to be amused because it is cute or exciting, or to fail to respond because of being too tired or busy.

The examples set by parents and other persons older than the child have a strong influence on a child's safety attitudes and behavior. Adults must practice what they preach in all safety matters, for children will imitate them rather than behave as they have been told. Safety-conscious parents who practice good safety habits have an excellent chance of bringing up children whose records are relatively free from accidents.

A nurse can be instrumental in the prevention of

childhood accidents. He has many opportunities to do anticipatory teaching about child development as it affects accident-related behavior. Preventive teaching can be directed toward individuals or groups, children or adults. The identification of environmental hazards is appropriately part of the nurse's role as he works either with individuals or with groups and as he influences policy setting in institutions, communities, or broader settings.

ACCIDENT PREVENTION AT DIFFERENT AGES
Infants

Young babies are totally dependent on those around them to provide a safe environment. Since the infant has little mobility, he should be fairly easy to protect. But consider these hazards in his environment: pins, plastic bags, automobiles, infant seats, unrailed beds, sun, bathtubs filled with water, toys, fires, and careless siblings or adults. Infants are unable to remove themselves from or protect themselves against dangers that can come to them.

Pins Diaper pins should *always* be kept closed, whether or not they are in use. Ideally they should be stored in places out of reach of toddlers, but if a diaper pin does find its way to the mouth of an infant or toddler, it is better swallowed closed than open. A child with poor motor coordination and immature judgment can do less damage to himself or others if pins are closed.

Suffocation Infants who are too young to remove objects from their faces are potential candidates for suffocation. There is a small but real risk that a young infant placed prone on a pillow or very soft mattress may be unable to turn his head sufficiently to breathe; for this reason soft undersupports for babies are contraindicated. A more substantial suffocation hazard is plastic garment bags. Plastic bags are lightweight and are easily transported to the baby or his crib by immature siblings or even by gusts of wind. Plastic bags should be tied in knots and discarded.

Automobiles Automobiles present a danger to persons of all ages. For infants a reasonably safe practice is to have a car bed that can be securely strapped to the back seat by seat belts. Several automobile manufacturers and other companies presently market protective car seats that attach to the original car seat and, by means of chest and lap belts, provide secure seating for infants of all ages. If an infant

seat is used instead, it should be strapped in according to the method illustrated in Figure 16-2A. The arrangement shown in Figure 16-2B is unsatisfactory because in the event of a collision the baby is likely to be thrown forward.

Falls Falls are a common cause of accidental injury in infancy. A large number of families today use infant seats. Babies who cannot yet sit alone like to be propped in a semi-upright position to look around them, especially to watch their parents and siblings as they work or play. Infant seats must be placed on firm objects and away from edges, because it is possible for a wiggling baby to tip them over or for another person to knock them over accidentally. Toddlers or preschoolers occasionally reach to play with an insecurely propped baby, with unexpected results. The floor or playpen is probably the safest place to put a baby while in an infant seat.

Growth and development norms cite approximately 1 month to 6 weeks as the age at which a baby becomes able to turn over. But even newborns may squirm vigorously enough to move themselves along. This mobility makes it possible for a very young baby to move from the middle of a bed to the edge (and on to the floor) in a short period of time. The same hazard applies in regard to sofas, easy chairs, and various other places a busy parent might choose to place the baby unguarded for a few minutes.

A study of depth perception in infants showed that most human infants can discriminate depth as soon as they can crawl. However, their locomotor abilities are poorly developed, so that even though a baby may perceive the brink of a ledge he may fall over it while trying to crawl away from it.[6]

Malfunctioning crib sides should be repaired, tied securely, or replaced: if they fall, the baby is likely to fall too. It is good practice to always raise the crib side all the way up when the baby is in the crib. If the rail then accidentally falls, it will probably catch at the halfway mark and provide some measure of safety. If a rail kept at the halfway mark drops, there is no margin of protection.

Sunburn The benefits of fresh air and sunshine are widely known. Overexposure to sunshine, however, can cause serious illness or death, especially to babies. Sunbaths for 5 minutes at a time in the beginning are a safe practice. It should be remembered that sun rays through a window are just as potent as the sunshine outside.

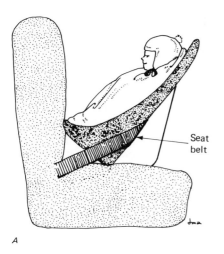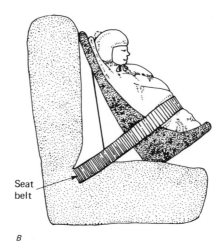

Figure 16-2. *A.* Proper positioning of infant seat in a car. In the event of front end collision the infant seat will be held securely by the seat belt and the child's head will be supported and protected by the back of the infant seat. *B.* Less satisfactory positioning of infant seat in a car. In the event of collision the infant seat may be tipped forward and the child's head and neck will be unprotected.

Water   Bathtime is a delightful play period for most babies, but unless babies are constantly firmly held, they are in grave danger of drowning, even in a shallow bath. It is a full time job to hold a slippery, wiggling baby while bathing him. Since he cannot hold his head up or control other movements well, one should never let go of him while he is in the water. When the phone or doorbell inevitably rings, a parent should either ignore it or wrap a towel around the baby and take him along to answer the call.

Toys   Toys should always be chosen with the child's developmental level of accident vulnerability in mind. For infants, who put everything in their mouths and have poor motor coordination, toys should have smooth edges and no small removable parts. Ingestion or aspiration of eye buttons, plastic or cloth tabs, or other parts of toys can cause serious consequences such as foreign bodies in the esophagus, stomach, or upper respiratory tract.

Ingestions   Even young infants sometimes swallow other harmful objects besides parts of toys. Some people believe that if one pill is good, two will be better. This attitude can lead to serious problems regarding the use of aspirin and other drugs. Parents or other caretakers of infants or children receiving medications need careful instruction in proper dosage and administration. Errors in the mixing of powdered or concentrated baby formulas also can result in electrolyte imbalance serious enough to require emergency treatment, and unsterile formula can produce illness in very young babies. Infants who creep or crawl need adequate protection from pesticide tablets and other inedible substances they may find on the floor.

Toddlers

When babies start crawling and walking, parents need to sharpen their wits and take a careful look at the environment from their child's point of view. It may be enlightening to get down on the floor and try to imagine what the world looks like to the child. After babies start crawling, it is usually only a short time before they begin pulling up on furniture, then walking around it while holding on, walking without support, and finally running. Add mobility to the normal curiosity of a child who is developing his sense of autonomy, and the potential danger is evident. Children at this age learn by trial and error, since they have few experiences on which to build. Adults should provide an environment in which the toddler can explore and manipulate things autonomously without unnecessary restrictions or risks to his safety.

Ingestions   Locking up medicines, poisons, cleaning materials, hydrocarbon solutions, and other dangerous substances that could be ingested or splashed on skin or eyes by a curious toddler is a practice to be strongly encouraged. If not actually kept under lock, these chemicals should at least be placed well out of reach (Fig. 16-3). Keeping medicines in a purse is definitely a hazard, as purses are attractive and accessible playthings. Poisonings from medicines carried in purses are common in young children. Manufacturers of drugs are increasing the use of safety packaging, although the different types of supposedly childproof bottle caps vary in their effectiveness.[7]

The practice of storing gasoline, kerosene, or other toxins in soft-drink bottles is to be stringently avoided. Toddlers and other young children asso-

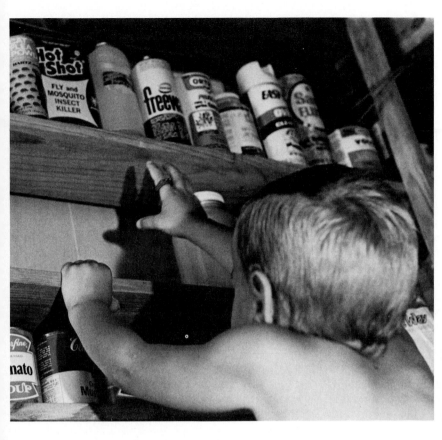

Figure 16-3 Poisons and caustics must be made inaccessible to children who are too young to be relied upon to use them safely. *(Photo courtesy of George Lazar.)*

ciate food containers with enjoyable edible substances, and many children have been seriously or fatally poisoned by ingesting toxic materials (for which young children have notoriously little taste discrimination) from soft-drink containers.

Recent studies support the theory that the ingestion of obviously nonedible chemicals may have a psychiatric basis. Children who receive adequate maternal attention and protection from harmful substances are less likely to ingest this material than children whose mothers are unable to afford a protective environment due to their own emotional needs. Thus the child may deliberately explore dangerous materials to receive negative attention from his mother. The mother's problems may not become apparent until she recounts the accident and her response to it or until her interactions with the child are observed by health-care personnel.

Climbing Toddlers climb. Climbing is very appealing to them and provides good exercise, learning opportunities, and a gratifying sense of accomplishment. Both indoors and out, this activity can present problems and anxieties for parents. Constant observation and assistance when needed, and the provision of safe things to climb on can prevent falls while still allowing the child the thrill and experience of climbing. Play-sets and jungle gyms are fun for children, whether they have their own or take a trip to the park for such experiences. On farms there are many fences and carts on which to climb and scramble.

Traffic Streets are extremely hazardous for toddlers. Children who are allowed to play outside in unfenced areas must be taught early not to go into roads or play at curbs. Both children and adults need to be cautioned about the possibility that someone may start up a parked car and back over a young child playing quietly in the driveway. Secure babyseats are required to prevent accidents for toddlers who are passengers in automobiles and to minimize distractions for the driver.

Water A few inches of water left in a bathtub can be lethal to curious toddlers, most of whom are very attracted to water play. All family members should make it a firm habit to empty tubs immediately after baths. Scalding is another hazard; young children have been seriously burned by turning on the hot water in an unsupervised moment in the tub.

Pools, ponds, lakes, rivers, creeks, drainage ditches, and water troughs are obviously dangerous. If these water hazards can possibly be fenced off or the play area fenced in, this precaution should be taken. Constant supervision is essential whenever toddlers are playing anywhere near water.

Miscellaneous Hazards A curious, fast-moving toddler can get into many kinds of trouble. For instance, matches, hot cooking utensils, irons, razors left on the edge of the tub or sink, scissors, knives, tools, burning candles, fireplaces, heaters, fans, broken glass, open wells, venetian blind cords, and open safety pins all provide the potential for a trip to the emergency room. Safety-conscious families try to prevent traumatic experiences for all concerned by keeping matches out of reach; turning pot handles to the back of the stove; never leaving a hot iron within reach; putting razors, scissors, knives, and burning candles out of reach; screening fireplaces, heaters, and fans; removing broken glass; covering open wells; and tying or cutting blind cords so that children cannot get their heads through the loops. The accident possibilities for toddlers are endless, so the best possible prevention at this age is close supervision.

Preschoolers

Preschool children continue to be vulnerable to the hazards of the toddler group, but it is easier to begin teaching safety habits to preschoolers. They like to imitate adult behavior and have active imaginations to assist their imitating. They show a sense of initiative and love to help their parents. If parents understand this and take advantage of it, the preschool years are the ideal time to enlist the child's participation in safety routines such as always letting the bath water out of the tub after bathing. Preschoolers can learn and remember how to handle scissors safely and why certain cleaning solutions are kept locked up or out of reach. A 3-, 4-, or 5-year-old begins to understand, with adults' help, why it is dangerous to cross streets. He is learning to move about daily in the world about him by asking "why?" His understanding of language is improving constantly and he soaks up information (including safety information) like a sponge.

Automobiles Automobile accidents are a principal cause of injury to children in this age group also.

Preschoolers tend to be too short to see comfortably out the window when they are seated in a car. They also like to be in the front seat with the driver. It is a good preventive habit never to allow small children to ride in the front seat of the car unless they are wearing safety belts or, preferably, are strapped into one of the commercially available car seats designed for use by children in either front or back seat. It is dangerous to let a child stand up in the front seat because in the event of a collision he may become a missile flying against the dashboard or window. If the driver swerves to avoid hitting something, the child can be thrown sideways. Injury resulting from falling against the gear shift lever is not uncommon and can be very serious.[8]

Falls from moving vehicles must be precluded by teaching children not to play with door handles and locks. Seat belts also obviously make such falls impossible.

Another chance for injury or death in an automobile arises when adults leave children in the car while they "run into the store for just a minute." A preschooler imitating his parents by pretending to drive can dislodge the car from its parked position and set it rolling out of control. Playing with the cigarette lighter is also dangerous. For these reasons children should *always* be taken with the parents when they leave the car even briefly.

Adventurousness The preschool child enjoys playing simple games such as hide and seek. The excitement of the game, in combination with the young child's inexperience and immature judgment, sometimes results in a disastrous choice of a hiding place. Children must be cautioned against climbing into or under cars, into drainage pipes and unsafe buildings, and down holes in the ground. All unused refrigerators, freezers, trunks, washing machines, and abandoned cars should have the door handles or hinges removed to prevent small children from crawling into them to hide and then being unable to get out when it is time to run to home base.

School-Age Children

Entrance to school modifies the child's daily living patterns, and consequently, the kinds of accidents to which he is vulnerable and his modes of dealing with hazards also change. As the degree of previous parental supervision progressively lessens, the school-age child receives safety information from teachers, life guards, policemen, firemen, nurses, other children, the media, and many other sources. His increasing cognitive maturity, including im-

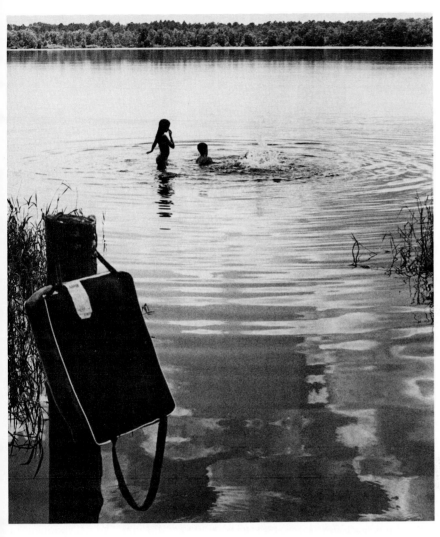

Figure 16-4 School-age children can be taught to swim, if they have not already learned, and to observe water safety rules. *(Photo courtesy of George Lazar.)*

proved ability to remember past experiences and anticipate probable outcomes of his actions, in combination with his usually strong sense of duty and his developing motor coordination, make him a good candidate for the safety instruction his new life-style requires.

Water School-age children can be taught how to avoid accidents in and around water. The following swimming rules should be explained and enforced as necessary.

1 Never call for help unless you really need it.
2 Always swim with another person, never alone, even in water that is familiar to you.

3 No ducking allowed.
4 Always know how deep the water is where you are diving.
5 Always have a rope, float, long stick, or life preserver handy to throw or hand out to someone who is in trouble in the water (Fig. 16-4).

Bicycles School-age children characteristically love bicycles. Teaching bicycle safety regulations is for this age group an extremely important area of accident prevention. The rules of the road for automobiles are the same for bicycles, and bicycle riders must also learn to drive defensively, which includes being aware that most cars have one or more blind spots from which drivers do not always see bicycles when they need to. Riding on busy or darkened streets and hitching rides by holding onto a moving vehicle are extremely dangerous, as is darting out from behind parked cars.

Carrying a passenger on a bicycle is hazardous. The incidence of injuries as a result of entangling a foot in the wheel spokes when riding on the handle bar, cross bar, or fender of a bicycle is unknown. The bicycle operator who has a passenger is likely to become distracted or to experience difficulty with balance.[9]

Firearms Gun accidents are common in the school-age period. Because they have good fine-motor coordination and know much more about what is going on around them than some parents think they do, children of this age are able to find and manipulate guns that are "hidden" about the house. The ammunition that may be in another place that parents think is safe is also accessible to the smart school-age child. Parents who have a gun should keep it under lock and put the key where children cannot obtain it. Children of this age can understand safety rules concerning guns and should be taught them without fail.

Climbing Most young boys and girls share a love for climbing trees. Adults should teach children how to climb in the safest possible way (Fig. 16-5). For instance, most children can understand that they should not climb out on dead or smaller limbs because they are the most likely to break. Tree houses may also help prevent falls from trees if they are sturdily constructed under adult supervision or assistance. Climbing electrical poles, water towers, and other obviously dangerous structures must be forbidden and the reasons for this limitation explained.

Adolescents

The adolescent is engaged in finding out who he is and in identifying his roles and status in relation to other people. Because of his great need to belong, his peers are very important to him. Striving for peer admiration leads to more accidents in this age group than probably any other single cause. An adolescent may do things that he knows are dangerous to avoid losing face or to gain prestige. Safety instruction and help in developing alternative ways of attaining self-esteem and peer acceptance are useful modes by which adults can help adolescents avoid accidents.

The need for peer approval and the age-typical rebellion against adults have led many adolescents to experiment with alcoholic beverages, drugs, and other dangerous substances and activities. Secret clubs and organizations often have various hazardous initiation rites than can lead to serious problems.

Accident prevention for adolescents presents special difficulties because these children are more independent and less supervised and because both adolescents and parents are usually trying to develop the young person's rights and skills in making his own decisions. The teen-ager may ask for help when he feels that he cannot deal with a situation or make a decision, but unasked-for advice may be rejected or counteracted because he feels a great need to establish independence. If a program of safety education has been carried on consistently throughout childhood, then the adolescent will have developed habits and acquired knowledge that will help him avoid serious trouble or potentially hazardous situations. Good safety habits originate in adult interactions with infants and culminate in the children becoming safety-conscious adults themselves.

Cultural Influences Not all accidents that befall adolescents are attributable to peer pressure or the striving for independence. The American culture as a whole has generally rewarded those who take risks.

> The risk taker—the explorer, the voyager, the medical researcher, the entrepreneur, the prize fighter and the bull fighter, the sports car racer, the test pilot—has always been endowed by society with heroic qualities, even when his risk taking is unsuccessful and he is maimed or killed.[2]

Competition is a related prominent feature of our society, and one concomitant is that injuries from sports accidents are quite prevalent.

Automobiles When teen-agers begin to drive, automobile accidents increase for them. Their lack of driving experience has a bearing on their higher accident rate. The automobile is important to youth because it represents freedom, both real and symbolic, from parental control and discipline. Driver education programs for adolescents have been very successful in minimizing driving accidents. Again, it is extremely important for parents to demonstrate safe practice, because parental example can be a strong influence on children's behavior.

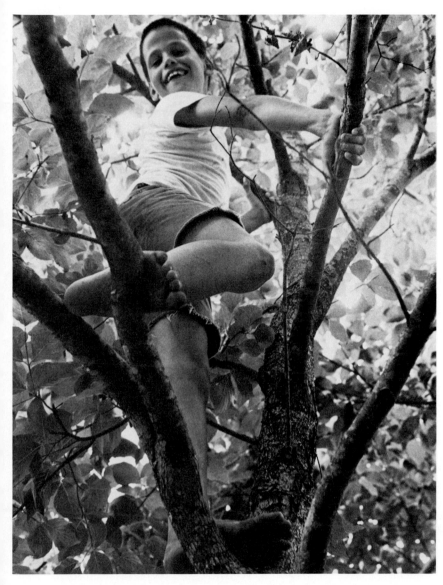

Figure 16-5 Safe climbing in trees includes avoiding slippery shoes and weak or dead limbs as well as keeping a secure hand hold. *(Photo courtesy of George Lazar.)*

Rapid Body Changes The adolescent growth spurt is normally accompanied by some degree of increased clumsiness. Growth and change of body proportion and strength create an unfamiliarity with one's physical apparatus and a rapidly outdated body image, so that teen-agers often do not accurately anticipate what may happen when they undertake some bodily activity. The arms and legs with which an adolescent approaches, for example, a sports endeavor, are in a sense not the same as those he used a few weeks earlier. Accidents are likely to occur in the course of his adaptation to his physical changes.

REFERENCES

1 *Profiles of Children: White House Conference on Children,* U.S. Government Printing Office, Washington, D.C., 1970.
2 W. Haddon, Jr., E. A. Suchman, and D. Klein, "Toward a Science of Accident Prevention," in *Accident Research*, Harper & Row, Publishers, Incorporated, New York, 1964, p. 7.
3 N. N. Foote, "Sociological Factors in Childhood Accidents," in W. Haddon, Jr., E. A. Suchman, and D. Klein (eds.), *Accident Research*, Harper & Row, Publishers, Incorporated, New York, 1964, p. 455.
4 H. Klonoff, "Head Injuries in Children: Predisposing Factors, Accident Conditions, Accident Proneness, and

Sequelae," *American Journal of Public Health*, 61:2405–2417, 1971.
5 A. P. Matheney, Anne M. Brown, and R. S. Wilson, "Assessment of Children's Behavior Characteristics—A Tool in Accident Prevention," *Clinical Pediatrics*, 11:437–439, 1972.
6 Eleanor J. Givson and R. D. Wal, "The Visual Cliff," *Scientific American*, 202(4):64–71, 1960.
7 A. K. Done, A. L. Jung, M. C. Wood, and M. R. Klauber, "Evaluations of Safety Packaging for the Protection of Children," *Pediatrics*, 48:613–628, 1971.
8 I. B. Pless, K. Roughmann, and Paula Algranati, "The Prevention of Injuries to Children in Automobiles," *Pediatrics*, 49:420–427, 1972.
9 Teresa Berry, F. D. Burg, and H. Kravits, "The Toddler As a Bicycle Passenger," *Pediatrics*, 49:443–436, 1972.

BIBLIOGRAPHY

Coleman, A. B., and Alpert, J. J. (eds.): "Poisoning in Children," *The Pediatric Clinics of North America*, 17(3):471–753, 1970.
Done, A. K.: "Poisoning from Common Household Products," *The Pediatric Clinics of North America*, 17:569–581, 1970.
Schaffer, H. R., Greenwood, Anna, and Parry, M. H.: "The Onset of Wariness," *Child Development*, 43:165–175. 1972.

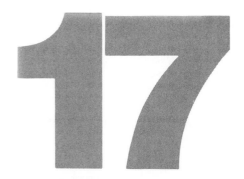

THE ROLE OF EXPERIENCE IN CHILD DEVELOPMENT

JUNE TRIPLETT

When a nurse interacts with a child at any given moment, he has already had many life experiences which have had an impact on his development. And, because each child is unique, he has determined to some extent what these experiences have been. It is the purpose of this chapter to examine some of these life experiences, how they can be predicted to affect and be affected by individual children, and how they determine a child's view of himself and his approach to learning. This is no simple task. It is easy to understand that a child from Uganda, Israel, or England might have life experiences different from those of a child from the United States, but there is a tendency to assume that the United States is a melting pot of ethnic groups and that most children share similar backgrounds. This assumption is exemplified in proverbs, regulations, policies, and unwritten behavioral expectations such as:

Children should be seen and not heard.
To be eligible for kindergarten, a child must have reached his fifth birthday prior to September 1.
A child must be at least 40 inches tall to register for swimming classes.
No hospital visitors under 14 years of age are allowed.
Spare the rod and spoil the child.
Soap is cheap. The least they (the poor) could do is to keep clean.
All children under 10 must have temperatures taken rectally.

And yet one has only to look at a group of children of the same age in a classroom, playground, or neighborhood to realize that there are marked differences in their size, agility, ability, approaches to new situations, or responses to stress. These differences are not accidental or unpredictable but are caused when a child with a particular genetic endowment begins to interact with his environment shortly after birth. The more positive this interaction is, the more likely it is that the child will achieve optimum development and become a healthy, happy, effective adult. Figure 17-1 illustrates some of the relationships which are examined in the next section.

The interaction between a child's innate capacities and his life experiences determines to a large extent how the child learns to cope with the stresses of growing up and how he views himself. The baby who is born healthy and has a variety of life experiences is likely to manage himself well in new situations and feel good about himself. The infant whose genetic endowment is impaired will need enriched life experiences if he is to achieve to the same extent. The highly able child who has insufficient stimulation and experiences may have trouble handling new learning because of his limited background.

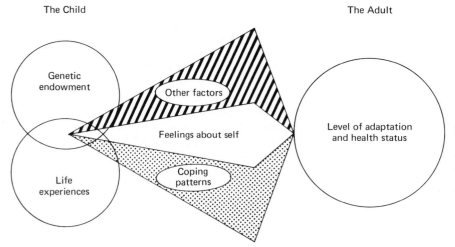

The Child

The Adult

Genetic endowment

Other factors

Feelings about self

Level of adaptation and health status

Coping patterns

Life experiences

Figure 17-1 The interaction between the child's genetic endowment and his life experiences provides opportunities for the child to learn coping patterns and develop self-esteem. How he feels about himself and how he copes with life help determine his level of adaptation as an adult.

It is plain to see that nursing has a responsibility to help provide adequate experiences for children and that nurses are frequently in a position of needing to know what a particular child's life experiences have been in order to plan nursing intervention, particularly when a child's coping mechanism breaks down or when he shows signs of a poor self-concept. It is helpful in these situations to understand the coping process in detail as well as the steps in developing a concept of self.

THE COPING PROCESS

Coping, as it is described by Murphy[1] and others, includes the ways people deal with new demands and with stressful experiences which cannot be handled by reflex or habit. The infant who reaches toward the stove and draws his hand away is not coping but has already learned through previous experience that stoves may be hot. If he finds the oven door down for the first time and thinks of a way to go around the table rather than passing close to the stove, he has learned to cope. Thus, there is an element of problem solving in coping. Coping is a process made up of steps taken to meet a challenge or to take advantage of an opportunity. It includes all the complex ways a child deals with reality as he sees it.[1]

Developmental Sequence of Coping

Coping begins very early, at least in an elementary form, when the infant learns to manage stimuli from the environment. If he so desires, he can turn his head away from or spit out the nipple by the time he is a month old. During the next few months he is in-

creasingly able to manage his own body to diminish, increase, or modulate stimulation for himself. He can kick the cradle gym, reach for objects, and indicate needs by selective crying. He also learns that he can get responses from others through his own efforts at smiling and laughing. He finds out that making an effort produces results. During the latter half of the first year, he continues to develop his capacity to differentiate between himself and his environment and to determine what forces he can and cannot control. He is already developing some characteristic coping patterns of moving away, against, or toward an object or person. For example, some young children become stiff and unyielding, refusing to have anything to do with new experiences. Others may become limp and passive and allow new experiences to overtake them without being involved in the process, while many see new experiences as challenges to be mastered.[1] To illustrate this process further, imagine a situation in which a toddler discovers his favorite toy out of reach on the counter. What are his choices at this moment of discovery? First he must decide whether he will try to get the toy or leave the scene. If he leaves, he may distract himself with another toy or console himself by a few minutes of thumb-sucking or crying. If he stays, he is faced with still more choices. He may try briefly to reach the toy, give up easily and leave, or continue to try new approaches to secure the object. If he is unsuccessful after a few attempts, he may seek help by crying angrily, by sobbing pitifully, or by seeking out someone and gesturing for the toy. Some children reject these choices and continue to seek a way to do it themselves.

As the child moves through toddlerhood and the early preschool years, many more demands for coping arise as he gains pleasure in mastering loco-motion, body functions, and language and begins his stubborn defense against adult pressure. Gradually, depending upon constitutional, experiential, and other factors, he develops his own characteristic coping style.

The process the child goes through when faced with a new experience is diagrammed briefly in Figure 17-2 and expanded in Figure 17-3.

Determinants of Coping Patterns

In general, coping is required when a child is faced with a new situation or set of circumstances. What he does and how he carries it out is dependent upon many factors within the particular situation and the individual child, and the interaction of all these determines the outcome of his coping efforts (see Fig. 17-3).

The Child   The child's innate capabilities and his life experiences again interact to determine how he will perceive and respond to a situation. More specifically, *his level of development* determines in part his ability to respond or the number of response choices he has. The baby who has not yet learned to grasp cannot get the new mobile on his crib but the school-age child may have many alternative approaches to securing a kite caught in a tree.

A child's response to new situations is also dependent upon his personality which developed through the interaction of his innate temperament and his environment. These differences in temperament are obvious to a skilled observer in a newborn nursery. Even at this young age, some infants are aggressive in their approach to sucking, some resist the routine imposed on them, and others adapt readily. These early behaviors have been classified and studied, and nine characteristics have emerged which help in understanding children's behavior. These include (1) the range and degree of the child's motor activity, (2) the regularity (rhythmicity) of his schedule, (3) his response to new objects or people, (4) his adaptability to change, (5) his sensitivity to stimuli, (6) the energy he puts into responses, (7) the general mood of the child (friendly, unfriendly, cheerful, cranky, etc.), (8) his distractibility, and (9) his attention span and persistence in an activity.[2] Using these characteristics as a base, it could be predicted that a youngster who typically responds slowly and carefully to new people and who resists change will have more difficulty adjusting to nursery school than one who views everyone as a friend and is highly adaptable to change.

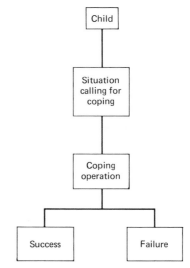

Figure 17-2   A child faced with a new situation selects a means of coping which may lead to success or failure.

The child's *perception* of the situation is an important determinant of his response to it. He may be so overwhelmed by the many stimuli reaching him that he cannot attend to any of them. Or he may focus on one aspect to the exclusion of others, thereby distorting his assessment of the situation and increasing the likelihood that his response to it will be inadequate.

Perception is closely related to the child's *memories* of other similar new experiences and his feelings related to these memories. The child who gets a great deal of pleasure from his accomplishments may recall how good he felt the last time he successfully coped with a new experience and enter into this one with enthusiasm. If he remembers earlier new experiences as painful or frustrating, these memories can negatively influence his perception of the new event.

The *resources* of the child are also an integral part of the coping process. Energy and stamina are important for mastering some tasks, just as coordination or intelligence are for others.

The *environmental supports* available to the child can make a difference too. Children have often indicated more willingness to undergo physical examinations or tests if they can draw on their parents for support. The adolescent uses the support of his peers to reinforce his decision making. The hospitalized child may be able to endure separation from his parents if provided with a familiar object from home.

The other major factor within the child is the presence of *defense mechanisms* and the ways they

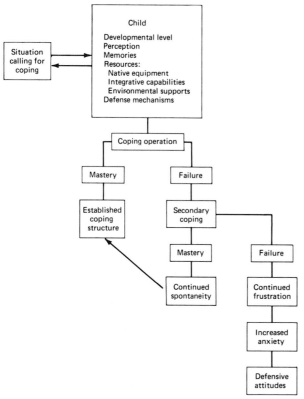

Figure 17-3 Many forces within the child and the situation determine how the child copes with a new situation, and his choice of action leads to successful coping or failure.

are customarily used. For example, if a child learns to suppress stimuli which are threatening, he is then able to focus on the part of the new experience which can be mastered. Defensive patterns become established between the child's second and fourth years.

It should be readily apparent by now that what a particular child brings to a new situation is highly complex and individual and becomes even more complex when the situation itself is examined.

The Situation   It has already been implied that situations requiring mastery may range from simple to complex. A first date is likely to require more skill in coping than a first experience in baby-sitting. Some situations have a high degree of inherent challenge or urgency, such as when someone needs mouth-to-mouth resuscitation. Others are basically gratifying, while some are threatening or challenging. The expression on a toddler's face the first time he stands alone is a perfect example of gratification through mastery. Many situations to which children are ex-

posed may present various combinations of challenge, gratification, frustration, or threat. For some children, learning to ride a bicycle can begin as a challenge but may provide a great deal of frustration before gratification is achieved.

The Coping Operation

What a particular child does to cope with a new situation depends then, on all the factors just reviewed. How the child takes action is also important. Does he characteristically let the environment shape him or does he actively shape the environment? Does he tackle the new experience confidently or expect to fail? When he manipulates adults to get the help he needs, does he do so ingratiatingly, coyly, or aggressively? Is he able to postpone gratification or must he experience it immediately?

It is also essential to look at the outcome of the child's coping efforts. If his efforts succeed, the steps he took become more firmly established in his coping structure. But what if his efforts are unsuccessful? Some children will impulsively try again; others stop to figure out where the first approach went wrong and modify it appropriately. If their secondary coping results in mastery, this too leads to an established coping structure. However, if a child fails after the first or second trial he may experience frustration leading to increased anxiety and the use of defense mechanisms to explain away his failures.[1] Obviously, too many failures in coping will cause the child to perceive himself as a failure or to fail repeatedly because he expects failure. Refer to Figure 17-3 for a summary of this discussion of the various steps in the coping process.

There is a close relationship between coping operations and self-esteem. Self-esteem and its development are examined in the following section.

THE DEVELOPMENT OF SELF-ESTEEM

A child's sense of self begins to develop early in life as he learns about his own body, his physical needs, and the gratification he feels when those needs are met. Anyone who has watched the 3- to 4-month-old infant's fascination as he visually examines his hands has had a glimpse of his efforts to determine what he is. At first he doesn't pay any attention to that which is not a part of himself, and for the first several months even his mother is not differentiated from himself. By 6 months he begins to separate his own identity from his mother's and to explore the world about him in terms of its impact on him. How objects feel, taste, smell, and sound and how they can be obtained, grasped, dropped, or thrown become paramount questions to which he seeks answers. He also begins to sense that there are some limits to his world and that there are some objects or people he cannot control.

Soon after his first birthday he becomes quite enamored with the idea that he can "do it myself," which also gives him an idea of who he is as a person. He looks for limits at the same time he is trying to be autonomous, and this struggle continues for many months. By the time he is 2, he loves himself very much and may be acutely aware that displeasing his parents makes him uncomfortable. He begins to dislike his unacceptable impulses and may even dislike himself, but only in terms of the external controls he has violated. Gradually he moves from learning who he is and how much of his life he can control to a period of actively seeking experiences. He takes the initiative in finding new activities, of trying out different roles—mother, father, baby, policeman, doctor, nurse, astronaut, etc. As he does these things, he also begins to compare himself with others—to learn about liking and being liked, approving and being approved of, failing and succeeding—and he gets an image of himself in these terms. In other words, the young child's concept of himself is a reflection of how he believes others (primarily his parents) feel about him. If he has failed to meet excessive demands placed on him, his self-esteem will be low, but it may also be low if his opportunities to achieve have been limited by overprotective parents or an unstimulating environment. Here, too, the relationship between coping mechanisms and self-esteem is very apparent. Some people believe that each time a child learns to cope with a new experience his ego is strengthened because he has successfully integrated a new set of relationships and added to his knowledge of the world and himself.

By the time a child enters kindergarten, his conscience has taken over many of the controls formerly exerted by parents; in fact, his conscience may exact better behavior than his parents require. It is at this age that children begin to establish their identity through doing, or what Erikson calls developing a sense of industry.[3] It is important to them to *produce*, and children between 6 and 9 will spend long periods of time on embroidery, carpentry, artistic endeavors, and the like. If they are helped to do at least some tasks well and receive recognition for accomplishments, they see themselves as worthwhile. Unfortunately when children start school they may also discover themselves being judged by the color of their skins or the clothes they are wearing rather than by what they can do. Such prejudice may then negatively affect their self-esteem.

Young school-age children begin to depend more on their peers' opinions of them than on their parents', and self-esteem tends to be more positive when the child has the freedom to interact with peers. Children learn through peer interactions to accept rules and regulations in games and other reasonable restrictions placed on them, and in so doing see themselves as reliable and worthwhile.

As the child moves into adolescence, he begins to look more closely at who he is and what he wants to be. If he is to become independent, he must alter his relationships with his parents and with his past. He has to give up his heroes or heroines and establish his own character and personality. His view of himself may include, separately or simultaneously, how he was, and how he is, and what he will be for each of many traits and characteristics. It is no wonder that the adolescent goes through a period of identity diffusion.[4] The adolescent relies on his peers to help him through this period, which is reminiscent of the struggle he went through as a 2-year-old. If he has been reasonably successful in coping with life to this point, he continues to seek opportunities to master new experiences.

RELEVANCE OF SELF-ESTEEM AND COPING PATTERNS TO LIFE EXPERIENCES

It should be clear by now that the numbers and kinds of experiences children encounter exert a great deal of influence on their development. It should also be apparent that these interactions of constitutional and experiential factors are extremely complex and require very careful assessment of each child prior to planning, implementing, and evaluating nursing intervention. Perhaps the following example will help in making these ideas more understandable.

During his weekly visit to a nursery school, a nurse watches David display a temper tantrum upon his mother's departure. Should the nurse be concerned? To answer this question, he draws on his knowledge of all children and recognizes that many children have temper tantrums. He also knows that tantrums are more common around the age of 2, and if he finds David to be in this age range, he may delay further investigation. If he finds that David is already 4, he will need to look at him more closely.

He then draws on his knowledge to consider a number of reasons why children have temper outbursts. These might include mental retardation or other reasons for a developmental delay, inability to express feelings verbally, low tolerance for frustration, imitation of the behavior of a favorite person, inability to delay gratification, a habitual response pattern to stress, or a typical way of responding to a new experience of separation.

The nurse's next step is to gather information which will support or refute these considerations. David's life experiences and his responses to them can be determined by observing him in a variety of settings and talking with the teachers and parents. The nurse may find, for example, that David has learned that his mother frequently will give in to his requests if he only threatens to have a tantrum. For David, having a tantrum was originally successful as a coping method and has now become a habitual response for getting his way.

Through this process of data collecting, many of the tentative explanations can be ruled out and decisions made about the kind of nursing intervention indicated. To carry out this assessment the nurse must also be knowledgeable about the kinds of experiences David can be expected to have had which are consistent with the environment in which he lives, his relationships with his parents, their approaches to child rearing, and any situational or developmental crises David may have encountered. Some typical life experiences which can be anticipated in various circumstances are presented in the next section, which is followed by a section on atypical experiences.

TYPICAL LIFE EXPERIENCES

This section focuses on the range of life experiences which can be expected of children who live in average or typical American families without major disruptions. On the surface at least, these families share many commonalities in their lifestyles, but closer scrutiny can reveal many subtle differences which can affect children's development. The early parent-child relationships which are established, the child-rearing practices the parents adopt, the child's place in his family, and his school and social experiences all contribute to his development, and each will be examined separately.

Early Parent-Child Relationships

When a healthy baby is born to a couple, it is generally assumed that the mother instinctively develops a close, warm relationship with her infant and that a similar relationship grows automatically, but more slowly, with the father. Fortunately, these assumptions are often true, but in a significant number of situations parenthood is experienced as a crisis. The way in which this crisis is resolved can greatly influence the parents' feeling toward the infant and affect his future development. Why is this so? Prospective parents have both conscious and unconscious expectations of what constitutes acceptable parental behavior. They may hope to imitate their own parents or may have strong negative feelings about how they were reared and plan to avoid certain practices. One or the other may have many ambivalent feelings and beliefs about parental roles, or their views may actually be in conflict.

Not only do couples have expectations of themselves as parents, but their families, friends, churches, and schools have standards by which they judge acceptable parental behavior (Fig. 17-4). Even before the baby's birth, then, the parents may be concerned about their ability to meet their own expectations and those that others hold for them.

Coupled with expectations of themselves, new parents frequently have preconceived ideas about what characteristics are desirable in a baby. Some may be glad for a baby of either sex as long as it is healthy. Others express a deep need for a boy to carry on the family name or to emulate the father's athletic prowess. Some mothers need a dainty, passive infant who responds to cuddling, while others enjoy the active, sturdy baby who appears ready to fight the world. When all these expectations coincide with the qualities of the baby, a healthy parent-child relationship is apt to develop, but the crisis of parenthood may well continue when there is a mismatch between expectations and outcomes. Many parents are able to resolve this conflict themselves if they have an understanding of how babies' innate temperaments differ.

Developing sensitivity to the changing needs of infants is also an essential part of the parenting process, and the groundwork for an ongoing, everchanging relationship is established early. Ideally, parents must be able to shift from providing complete care for a totally dependent infant to interacting with their grown child on equal terms as an adult. As the infant grows, they begin to translate their unconscious or conscious values and beliefs into behavioral expectations for their child. These expectations in turn influence the child-rearing practices they believe will meet their goals for the child and the kinds of experiences they will provide. If parents believe it important that their children be God-

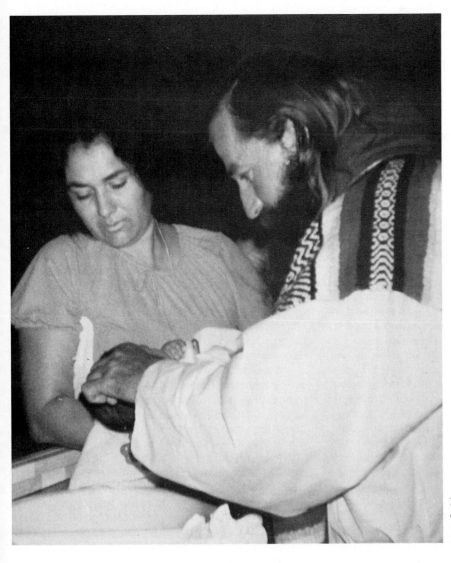

Figure 17-4 Early parent-child experiences, like later ones, reflect parents' expectations of themselves and of their child.

fearing or respectful of authority, or independent and creative, these beliefs influence their actions and their children's development.

Child-Rearing Practices

There are probably almost as many views of child rearing as there are parents rearing children—or professionals giving advice about child rearing. For this reason, it is difficult to categorize these approaches with any certainty as to their influence on a child's life experiences. Perhaps it might be helpful to think of child-rearing practices as being on a continuum ranging from restrictive to permissive while at the same time considering the *quality* of restric-

tiveness or permissiveness. For example, a parent can be permissive to the point of ignoring a child or can be judicious in using permissiveness to foster self-reliance. A restrictive parent can be literally abusive or can apply restrictions for the safety of the child. Within this continuum, an attempt will be made in this section to review the range of ways parents can contribute to their children's ability to cope and to the development of their self-concepts during successive age periods. The different behavioral expectations parents hold for their sons as compared with their expectations for daughters are also included.

Early infancy requires a great deal of giving on the part of the parents with relatively little in return.

The baby is totally dependent on adults to anticipate and meet his needs, and few parents make unrealistic demands on their babies during this period regardless of their beliefs about child rearing. This is the time for parents to become well acquainted with their baby, to assess his temperament, to find what actions excite or comfort him, and to provide him with opportunities to explore his body and immediate environment. If they meet his needs without causing him frequent or long periods of frustration, his basic sense of trust will develop and serve as a useful base for new learning. Although there may be some parents who find little personal satisfaction in caring for young infants, they are generally able to meet their infant's needs for this short, unrewarding period.

During the latter half of the first year there are many more opportunities for the infant to learn how to cope with his expanding environment and for his parents to employ specific child-rearing practices. Most parents enjoy watching the child's unique personality emerge, but they also start taking action to shape that personality to meet their expectations. Those parents who value curiosity are likely to put away dangerous or fragile items, put safety plugs in the electrical outlets, and let the infant crawl about unhampered by frequent "no-no's." They are child-centered in their permissiveness while providing some limits. Parents who see the child as an extension of themselves may begin to establish firm limits for acceptable behavior, since misbehavior is commonly seen as a reflection on their parenting abilities. These are the parents who expect the child to "just look" at all the objects rather than touching, tasting, or smelling them.

Some parents, primarily mothers, find it very difficult to allow the older infant's growing independence, but their reluctance is based on personal problems rather than their beliefs about child rearing. Some are happiest when they have someone totally dependent upon them, as it gives them a feeling of strength and security. Others cannot let go because they must be in control. For such a mother, the major fulfillment in motherhood is through controlling the behavior of her child.[5]

As the infant passes through toddlerhood, there are many times when parents can facilitate or impede their children's ability to cope. Again, the way they do this depends to some extent on whether their philosophy of child rearing is more inclined toward the permissive or the restrictive approach. When a situation arises which requires coping, parents can manipulate the *situation*, influence the *child* in a variety of ways, do both, or do nothing.

Assume that the situation is one in which the 3-year-old has been riding a tricycle for the first time and has just tipped it over. One parent may focus on the situation and right the tricycle before the child has a chance to try. Another might focus on comforting the child and blame the "naughty trike" for tipping over. Another may offer to help and, in so doing, make it easier for the child to accomplish the task. Still another could verbally suggest a way of picking up the trike, remind him of how he had managed in a similar situation, or give him support so that he could figure out a way to do it if he tried. Some parents might turn their backs to the situation, either out of lack of interest or in a deliberate move to allow the child to cope alone. The parent's response if the child is successful affects not only the youngster's future coping but his self-esteem as well. A comment that "it was a heavy trike to pick up by yourself" allows the child to make the inference that he is strong and that it is good to be strong. On the other hand, the remark "maybe next time you'll be more careful" will make the child feel less adequate. Obviously, remarks made if the child is unsuccessful in his efforts will have similar influence.

A child's coping repertoire can also be affected by the amount of sex-role stereotyping to which he is exposed. A girl's crying may be reinforced by her father, but the same man may not allow his son to cry. The preschool child who observes both parents doing the dishes together or sharing in the labor of harvesting a crop does not have to concern himself with whether a particular task is one for a man or a woman but simply considers that it is there for him to master. There are many subtle ways that the preschool child absorbs sex-role stereotypes, and these experiences produce attitudes that may unconsciously affect choices for years to come. One seldom sees a TV commercial in which a lively little girl gets so dirty that only brand X soap will remove the stains. Apparently only little boys get that dirty! When kindergarten or nursery school children tour the hospital or have a visit from a nurse or doctor, how many little boys wear nursing caps? In a coloring book to prepare children for a physical examination, only the boys wear a stethoscope and assume the physician's role. Each of these early memories may be called upon later when a child plans what he will do when he grows up.

As the child moves into school age, his intellectual growth makes it possible for him to cope with more complex problems—but again, his responses are dependent upon the influence exerted by his parents (and increasingly by others). It is particularly during this time that the parents may actively promote their expectations for the child's future. A mother who wants a genius may seize on school-related tasks as a means to this end and insist on perfection from the child and grade acceleration by the school. If she has a highly motivated intelligent child, she might succeed in her ambition, but if not, the child will have to devote energy to coping with an overly demanding parent rather than to other learning. There is some evidence that a child whose parents excessively value his accomplishments is likely to have grandiose ideas of what he is capable of achieving. Such a child would conceivably persist in a coping operation which had failed repeatedly without stopping to consider alternative approaches.[6]

Parents who restrict the range of experiences for their school-age child not only limit his opportunities for coping but may deny him the satisfaction which comes from developing a sense of industry. At the same time, parents who are too permissive do not help the child acquire respect for necessary rules and restrictions. In fact, parents who encourage autonomy in their children within clearly defined and enforced boundaries seem to foster higher self-esteem in the children than parents who set few limits on behavior or whose strict limit setting allows for no questioning.[7] The child whose parents are inconsistent in limit setting and enforcement is also apt to have difficulty in determining his own self-worth.

The sex stereotyping which began earlier can take on much more significance during the school years. Some parents are able to accept a high degree of sensitivity, tenderness, and compassion in a son and allow him to use withdrawal as a coping mechanism in situations calling for aggression and competition. Boys may be expected to be stoic following painful injuries, which limits their range of coping mechanisms for dealing with stress. Girls may be reinforced for using tears to get something from their fathers. The girl who insists on playing baseball long after other girls her age have lost interest in the sport or the boy who prefers cooking to competitive sports are both apt to receive pressure from parents and others to conform to sex-role norms. If they are still depending upon their parents' views of them to build their own self-esteem, such pressure could be damaging.

When adolescence begins, established coping patterns may break down as the youth adjusts to his rapidly changing body. Body contours which change rapidly or fail to change at the expected time can cause acute problems. Teasing, sarcasm, and bad jokes by family and friends can make minor problems into major ones. Ambivalent feelings of dependence and independence leave the adolescent *and* his family confused and frustrated. Parents who continue restrictive practices make the adolescent's need to break away from home even more critical. Couples who see their children's behavior as reflecting on them will probably continue to be less sensitive to their children's needs than to their own. On the other hand, parents who see themselves as worthwhile and who value their children for their intrinsic worth rather than for their behavior or appearance are able to provide their adolescents with the security they need during this period. One mother demonstrated her understanding of her daughter's need for a temporary escape from a difficult situation.

Lana was using delaying tactics instead of leaving for school and looked so dejected her mother pressed her for an explanation. Lana exploded with her unhappiness at school and ended with a comment that at times she just couldn't stand it. Her mother listened and finally said lightly, "Will you please tell me that you don't feel well so I can call the school to excuse you for the day?" With this remark, Lana relaxed, smiled, and for at least a little while felt close to her mother.

Studies of adolescents seem to bear out the idea mentioned earlier that children develop greater autonomy and self-confidence when parents maintain consistent limits while providing explanations for the limits and allowing adolescents to question them. Parents who serve as role models for reasonable independence and who promote positive identification based on love and respect for the child also contribute to the adolescent's responsible independence.[8]

The adolescent's rate of maturation also determines the amount of stress he has and how he copes with the many changes he is experiencing. Stress is apt to be minimal, for example, for the girl who is small, delicate in build, has a good figure, and begins menstruating as a seventh grader. Since these characteristics fit the stereotypic expectation held for girls by adults and peers, she has fewer concerns about her appearance and acceptance and knows that she "measures up" to expected standards. Girls who mature late do not appear to have as much stress as late maturing boys, probably because small size is seen as a desirable feminine characteristic.

Boys expect themselves to be tall and broad shouldered and to have adequate facial and body hair by the time they are 15. The boy who matures

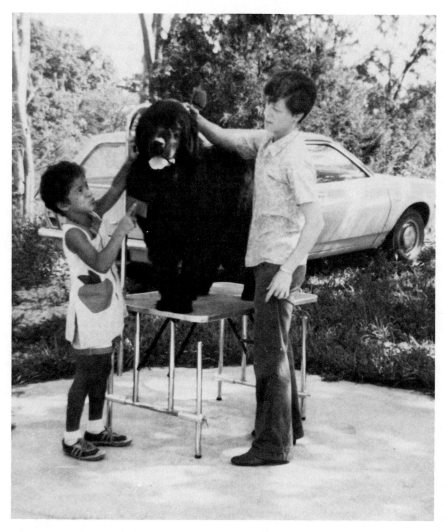

Figure 17-5 "When I'm 10, I can have my own dog to groom and show."

early is treated more maturely, which often makes for a good psychologic adjustment. The late-maturing boy may be at a disadvantage because he is treated according to his size rather than as his age or interests might dictate. As a result, these boys are unable to value themselves for their rugged physiques, so they try to excel in other ways. Many times they become more anxious and utilize attention-seeking behaviors such as clowning or playing practical jokes.[8]

In summary, the ways in which parents rear their children have a great deal of influence on the range and quality of experiences the children encounter (Fig. 17-5). How parental attitudes, values, and expectations are transmitted to children is also crucial to their developing concepts of self.

Sibling Relationships

Thus far, the emphasis has been on the child-rearing practices of the parents as they influence children's coping abilities and self-esteem. There are other life experiences which can be expected to affect a child's development. Two of these interrelated factors are the child's place in the family and his relationships with his siblings. Firstborn children tend to differ from later children in the family because they are provided rather exclusively with adult models with whom to identify. The oldest or only child takes the adults' high performance standards for his own. When he is puzzled, it is an adult to whom he goes for help, and he usually receives more logical and consistent explanations than he would receive from an older sibling. Some studies show that firstborn children tend to be more conscientious, more responsible, less aggressive, and more intellectually curious than children born later. Firstborns can expect support to be available from their parents as they learn to cope, since they are not competing with other siblings for attention. They are also reinforced for achievement and learn to gain satisfaction for it. On the other hand, because pressures for achievement have been high, firstborn children are likely to be anxious and oversensitive. Middle children in a family tend to be more socially gregarious than firstborn children and to seek physical demonstrations of affection. Youngest children have been found to be more striving and more defiant.[8]

The ways in which siblings affect each other's development depend upon sex and age differences. The firstborn child whose sibling is born after he has started school and when he is less dependent upon his parents will experience less hostility toward the baby than he would have at age 3. As a 3-year-old, he would have feared loss of "nurturance" from his parents since he was accustomed to their exclusive attention. Because young children tend to identify with an older child and imitate his behavior, girls who have older brothers tend to be more aggressive, ambitious, intellectually able, and "tomboyish" than girls with older sisters. When two siblings of the same sex are less than 2 years apart in age, they may strongly resemble one another with regard to their development. This is not as true when sex is different or when age differences are greater.[8]

The way he learns to interact with siblings provides a pattern of interaction for the child as his environment expands to the school and community. If he is powerless at home, he may expect and achieve powerlessness also with his peers.

Peer Relationships

When a child begins to spend periods of time with age-mates outside the home, he is exposed to the values and practices of others which may complement or conflict with those he has been learning at home. If parents have selected a nursery school or day care center on the basis of what they want it to do for the child, there will probably not be a wide divergence in philosophies between home, teachers, and playmates. The preschool child learns a great deal from his peers and finds out which of the behaviors he used at home are acceptable to the group. For example, children are not as tolerant as some adults when a 3-year-old continues to soil himself.

He is told in no uncertain terms about his odor and that his presence is unacceptable. Children in nursery school are exposed to a wide range of behaviors in peers and may lack the judgment to know which of these will be acceptable to parents. For example, slang, swear words, or aggressive behavior used at home by a dainty little girl may be extremely upsetting to her parents. Thus, conflict may arise which is potentially damaging to self-esteem.

In the preschool years it is still more important to the child to please his parents than his peers, but this gradually changes as he enters and progresses through the elementary grades. "All the boys do it" carries more weight than mother's "I don't want you to do it." Boys and girls engage in common activities the first year or two of school, but gradually the sexes segregate for most social activities. Clubs assume great importance during this time and many may have rules which restrict membership to the same sex. To be rejected by peers or to be excluded from a group can be extremely traumatic, and some children will go to great lengths to conform to group norms or to buy friendships. Others, of course, will see this rejection as congruent with their already low self-esteem and may withdraw even more from peer contact.

The child needs the opportunity to interact positively with a wide range of children in terms of religion, social class, ethnicity, or race if he is to develop a foundation for managing future interactions as an adult (Fig. 17-6). He may also need help from his parents not to stereotype people according to these various labels, since he will hear many stereotypic remarks.

By adolescence peer contacts again broaden to both sexes, although typically girls continue to have close relationships with girl friends more than boys do. If peer group norms differ widely from those of his family, the adolescent will have a great deal of conflict which is apt to be resolved in favor of the peer group. If he can adhere to group norms *and* maintain the love and acceptance of his parents simultaneously, he will be better able to establish his autonomy and see himself as worthwhile.

School Experiences

Starting school is often considered a crisis by the child and sometimes by the parents. The child is exposed to different expectations and must learn to share the teacher's attention with many others. Jimmy's situation illustrates one youngster's experience.

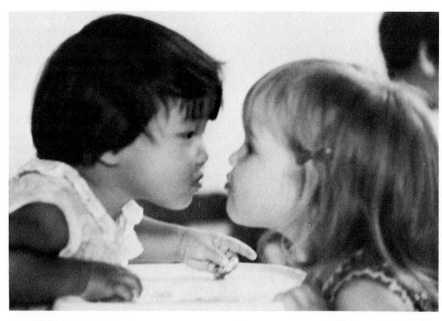

Figure 17-6 "Shall we be friends?"

Jimmy started first grade with a great deal of enthusiasm based partially on his own exuberant nature as well as on the experiences of his older siblings. Within a few weeks he began to change. He cried more readily and was reluctant to get up in the morning but could not explain what was wrong. A conference with his teacher revealed that Jimmy was improving in his ability to sit still but continued to bother his classmates with behavior such as tapping his pencil on their desks as he went by. He was having some difficulty following directions. As Jimmy began to bring written work home, his mother noted frowning faces drawn by his teacher on most of his papers, plus critical comments that he had made a poor choice of colors, that he had not used enough variety of colors, or that his work was not carefully done. For this teacher all trees had to be green, and animals had to be colored realistically to be acceptable. Jimmy was not used to being unacceptable, but neither was he able to contain his energies and stifle his creativity.

Conflict and unhappiness resulted, and eventually a change of schools rescued the youngster from failure. This change was made necessary because of a conflict between the personality of a child and the expectations of a teacher. In this instance, the mother was sensitive to her child's needs and took action to prevent further damage to his coping ability and self-esteem. For another child with a different personality, this same mother might well have supported the child to meet the teacher's expectations.

It can be seen that school experiences can have a tremendous impact on the child. In many instances this impact is highly positive. Children do receive a great deal of stimulation, and in many classrooms their creativity is fostered. The child is exposed to many new ways of solving problems, and when he is successful his self-esteem prospers. However, sex-role stereotyping can impose some limitations on learning. A mother conferring with her daughter's fifth grade teacher was shocked and angry when the teacher told her not to be concerned that Nan had not made a full year's progress in math scores. Since she was a girl, math would not be important to her anyway!

Questions are being raised as to the dangers of stressing success in school as prerequisite to a positive self-esteem. If one's ego grows only through mastery, then the child who is limited in his ability to master academic skills is penalized. Perhaps children have a right to fail if it means they have sought answers to complex questions and not found them, or if they have learned through their failures. The move to pass-fail grades in some colleges is an attempt to encourage students to take courses out of their field or even out of their depth without fear of failure. But perhaps it is too late for college-age people to function without the motivating force of doing well. There are no answers now to these ideas, but they are worth much thought and research if children are to achieve their potential as creative and capable adults.

Unfortunately, not all children escape tragedy and crises in their lives, and atypical life experiences can also influence children's development.

ATYPICAL LIFE EXPERIENCES

If parents could choose the kind of life they would want for their children, they would undoubtedly request an abundance of life's basic needs and pleasures and a minimum of stress. In reality, many families have life-styles which may or may not be of their own choosing and are beset by crises outside their control. Some of these life-styles and crises are examined in this section as to their influence on children's development. To do so requires some artificial categorization, since some events can be considered crises when they occur, but as adjustments are made, a change in life-style may result in satisfactory crisis resolution. For example, a car accident may create a crisis and leave an infant without parents, but if he is adopted quickly he may not experience his parents' death as a crisis. But his life-style may differ from the majority of his peers because he is adopted. This can reappear as a crisis for him at various points in development. For this reason, placement in an adoptive or foster home is included in the section on situational crises along with prematurity, congenital handicaps, chronic illness, and death of family members.

Differing Life-Styles

Although there are many life-styles that could be examined for their relevance to child development, only three are presented in any detail: those of single-parent families, families with stepparents, and families with low incomes.

Single-Parent Families   It is generally estimated that 1 of every 15 children in this country lives with only one parent. This figure includes (1) children whose natural parents were not married and who live with the mother or father, (2) an increasing number of children who have been legally adopted into a one-parent household, and (3) children who have lost one parent through death, desertion, or divorce. In addition there are those children who live with one parent during temporary separations due to military assignments, imprisonments, prolonged hospitalization, etc. The effect of living in a one-parent family is emphasized in this section; children's responses to adoption, death, and chronic illness of a family member will be discussed later in this chapter.

An absent parent can evoke special needs in children. As they pass through the developmental stages which require them to identify with first one parent and later the other, one or the other is not available to them. Without such experiences, the children's understanding of male and female roles may not be complete. The presence of two parents also gives the child more choices of coping strategies as he observes the different ways his parents cope. Two persons can provide more support to him as he grows and can probably provide him with a wider variety of learning experiences. Single parents who are overburdened with job and family responsibilities and seldom get a respite from these demands may simply not have the energy and patience to foster their children's learning. It is also easy to expect opposite-sex children to assume the responsibilities of the missing parent before they are developmentally ready. Failure to live up to these unrealistic expectations could negatively afffect such children's self-esteem.

The reason for a child's one-parent status makes a difference in the minds of many people. It is still true that children who have lost a parent through death are more likely to receive sympathy and support from the community than those whose parents have been divorced. Traditionally, the single woman who has kept her child has encountered a great deal of prejudice and discrimination which has often carried over to the child. Both fictional and biographic literature portray many instances where children were abused, their engagements were terminated, and other various forms of retribution were employed on the victims because of their illegitimate status. Fortunately, these attitudes are changing, and children growing up in these situations today are less apt to be penalized. There are still people, however, who attribute a girl's growing interest in boys to the fact that she is "turning out just like her mother." Since single-parent adoptions are still relatively uncommon, they may be treated either with suspicion or with recognition for the person's altruism.

When a child loses a parent through *divorce*, its effect on him will vary according to his age and circumstances. The young child who soon forgets may only have to face the usual problem of having one parent, but divorce can have a tremendous impact on somewhat older children. The following situation exemplifies this point.

Luann was in kindergarten when the divorce was finalized and her father moved out of the state.

She was too young to understand the concept of divorce even though her mother tried repeatedly to explain it to her. She talked a great deal about how her life used to be. "There used to be four people in our family . . . my daddy use to take me to the park, we used to live in a different house . . . we had a dog before that I could play with, my mommy doesn't have time to play with me anymore." She also evidenced some magical thinking typical of her age group when she reported that her father would return to his family *if* she made her bed every day and *always* picked up her toys. What will it do to this child's feelings of guilt when her father does not return? Will she then see herself as bad?

Luann was fortunate in having a capable mother who sought help for her daughter, but not all children receive this help.

Eddie's mother was very bitter toward his father and had generalized this bitterness to all men. She was beginning to show some favoritism toward Eddie's sister and had unreasonably high behavioral expectations for Eddie. Eddie had learned to cope by being excessively neat and well organized and by allowing his hostility to show only when wearing a policeman's hat at Head Start. Without intervention, he may limit his learning experiences to those which are not potentially conflictual with his mother's expectations, or at some point he may give up hope of pleasing his mother and take on her tendency to equate maleness with bad behavior and just be bad.

Another preschool reaction to divorce which can upset parents is apparent unconcern at the loss. The enormity of this disruption can be so great in the child's mind that he denies that it has happened and makes no overt changes in his behavior.

As the child learns to think abstractly, he is more capable of understanding the concept of divorce. He has by then passed the point of viewing both parents as infallible, which allows him to assign blame for the divorce to one or the other parent and to show a great deal of hostility, often toward the remaining parent. Thus, with increasing age the child moves from seeing himself as responsible for the divorce to seeing someone else as responsible and blaming that person in the same way he blamed himself earlier. These youngsters can often profit from talking with an objective outsider about their situations and feelings.

It was mentioned earlier that children living in one-parent families *may* have special problems which arise from their situations. These problems may not differ in degree from those of children whose fathers are away from home a great deal or who pay little attention to them. Many of the problems may be prevented or ameliorated by providing substitute experiences for the children involved. The Parents Without Partners organization provides this opportunity in some communities, and in others volunteer organizations such as Big Brothers of America fill this need. A male relative or neighbor can be used to provide a boy with activities his mother chooses not to engage in, such as hunting, fishing, or competitive sports, and a male teacher for a fatherless girl may help orient her to a man's view of the world. The same kinds of arrangements can be made for children where the mother is absent.

Stepparents Not all single-parent family units remain so throughout the child's growing years. As the divorce rate increases, so does the incidence of children with stepparents. For many children, the new parent brings all or most of the missing ingredients to their lives, and thus normalcy is restored. For others, there are varying periods of additional disruptions which may or may not end in satisfactory adjustment. Again, folklore, literature, and TV may provide children with expectations of wickedness from stepparents or may foster the self-fulfilling prophecy of emotional neglect of children as a parent moves in and out of marriages. Stepparents themselves are aware of the hazards they face and may try too hard to replace the former parent. In all probability, the disruption of the child's development comes from his channeling energy away from seeking and mastering new experiences and devoting his attention to coping with the stress of the adjustment process. The child's self-concept may also suffer if he perceives a stepbrother or half-sister as more valuable to his parents than he.

Life-Styles of the Poor Much has been written in recent years about the life-styles of low-income families, both in terms of identifying differences in child-rearing patterns and in warning professional workers not to stereotype the poor by expecting markedly different approaches to child rearing than such approaches in more affluent families. This warning is well founded, but at the same time it is important to be aware of *potential* differences. It is not possible to detail many of these differences here, but a few of them that can have profound influence on children's development can be highlighted. Among these are limited learning experiences during infancy and the preschool years, delayed language development, and inadequate socialization experiences to facilitate the school-age child's moving into the "foreign" culture of middle-class schools.

All three factors may be related and in part can be accounted for by the same reasons. Parents with low incomes are often unaware of children's developmental needs; they are frequently faced with many simultaneous and urgent demands on their time, energy, and other resources; many have so many unfulfilled needs of their own that they cannot attend to their children's needs; and they are frequently oriented in time to the present, which precludes provision for children's future development. It can also be difficult for someone who did not experience adequate mothering or the kinds of enculturation that lead to success in the societal mainstream to provide it to a child. One mother who grew up in an institution constantly referred back to this experience with the words, "I never had a mother so I don't know how to help my children do that." It should be emphasized, however, that most parents, regardless of social class, want to do what is best for their children. Many of the federally funded programs in the last decade, such as Head Start, Home Start, and Health Start, were designed to meet limitations identified in lower-class families, and thousands of parents have taken advantage of the offerings.

Some of the preliminary reports from Home Start programs indicate accelerated learning in the infants and increase IQ scores in the participating mothers. Similar results are being reported for many of the other programs. Since "intelligence" tests are primarily a measure of the ability to use middle-class problem-solving and language skills, these IQ elevations are probably far more a reflection of middle-class enculturation than of any fundamental change in innate ability. To the extent that this IQ increase is long-lasting, however (and the permanency of this change so far remains questionable), it may facilitate children's chances of success in school and of ultimately escaping poverty.

The poor may not be able to buy materials or take advantage of experiences advocated for furthering child development. What is more important is that they do not always know how to utilize existing opportunities to teach their children. For instance, there are many items in an impoverished household which have different textures or make various sounds from which an infant can learn. Plastic pants feel different from cloth diapers; a baby bottle used for pounding sounds different from a spoon. (Awareness of these differences sets the stage for discriminating later between the superficially similar numerals 2 and 7 or the letters *p* and *b*, with which poverty children frequently have trouble in school.) But for these early discrimination experiences to be meaningful, parents need to supply words and encourage curiosity, and they frequently do not do this. Parents and older siblings can help the toddler and preschooler begin to grasp concepts of numbers, color, and size. Does he want *one* or *two* pieces of candy or can he count the people in the room? Daddy's shirt is *bigger* than his, but his shirt is bigger than the baby's. The cans of fruits and vegetables can be used to teach size and, for the somewhat older child, can be matched according to pictures on the labels. Socks can be matched for color, and the color of items of clothing can be named when dressing the child. These suggestions may sound too simple, since many parents do these things almost instinctively, but for some low-income parents such actions do not come naturally. In part this socioeconomic difference can be accounted for by how parents themselves have learned to use and transmit language skills. Children learn language from their parents, but their attempts at language must be heard and reinforced. One mother thrust her 2-year-old on the examining table at the well-baby clinic with the words, "She won't talk at all." Even in the strange clinic setting, Theresa used a great deal of jargon as well as several distinguishable words which she repeated after the examiner. This mother had never stopped to listen to her daughter's speech. Not only do educationally and economically deprived parents often fail to listen, they also characteristically do not direct much speech to the children. Their own limited education and low socioeconomic life experiences are reflected in a smaller vocabulary which, in turn, limits the words the children hear. Many parents are apt to give instructions or reply to questions with a gesture or a very short response rather than with an explanation. The speech heard by these children differs in quality and quantity from that heard by middle-class children. In addition, it is less likely that speech errors will be corrected or that appropriate responses will be rewarded. Neither is the child from such a home apt to learn to listen to others. Instead he pays attention to the person talking and tries to figure out his mood rather than listening to what is being said. Often children and adults do not expect to be heard unless they yell—therefore, everyone yells. As a result, the noise-to-signal ratio is slight, and hearing discrimination is not well developed. Also, poverty children may not learn to come to adults for help or approval, which again limits their learning at home and particularly in school.

It should be apparent that children from low-income homes are likely to have fewer successful experiences on which to draw when faced with a new learning opportunity, nor are they apt to develop a wide range of coping skills. In addition, poor children have had many experiences in coping which are not particularly helpful to them when they must move into the middle-class society of the schools. The very young school child may have learned to manage himself in a street society and to fend for himself for some of his meals and personal needs. He may already have the responsibility of caring for his younger siblings. Unfortunately, these coping skills are not too helpful in the eyes of a middle-class teacher.

Sally's experiences in growing up in poverty might illustrate some of the problems these children face in school as children and adolescents:

Sally grew up in a small university city where there were relatively few low-income families. She confided one day that "the kids in school don't like me very good," and in response to questions explained that her clothes weren't as nice and her house wasn't very good either. Sally depended on clothing given to the family and selected those items which came closest to fitting. Her mother did not know how to alter them to fit, nor did she think to sew on buttons—if there were any available to sew on. Sally had no help in learning how to enhance her appearance to increase her acceptability to middle-class age-mates and teachers, nor was there a mirror in the house to reflect her image. There were no sheets, limited bedding, and no pajamas, so all the children slept in their clothes.

When Sally was about 12, she announced that she had finally figured out that her dresses would look better if she didn't sleep in them. There were no hangers or hooks to hang up a dress, but at least it didn't pick up the odor of the wet bed. About the same time, Sally's sister, who was enrolled in the junior high home economics program, was suspended from school until she could bring the money to purchase needed sewing supplies. Thus, even learning how to take care of clothes was curtailed.

Sally's clothes were washed regularly, but with insufficient soap and inadequate rinsing. They quickly became discolored under this treatment and appeared dirty. Sally had been sent home from school several times with instructions to clean up, but under the circumstances there was little she could do to appear cleaner. Thus, she was shamed by the teacher and ignored or teased by her peers. She had no recourse but to expect rejection and failure.

Situational Crises

Many families go through stressful events which cause temporary disruptions in family relationships and which can favorably or unfavorably influence the child's development. Some families become even more cohesive under stress. When a child contributes to resolving the crisis, he can gain in skill and self-assurance. When the crisis is too severe for the family's resources or when the child himself precipitates the crisis, he is bound to be affected. Although crisis has been defined in many ways, most definitions include mention of a disruption or change which requires some adjustment on the part of the family if they are to cope with the disruption and return to their former level of functioning. In many instances a crisis is short-lived, but in others crisis may be a chronic state.

In the material which follows, prematurity is considered first as a short-term crisis. The placement of children in foster or adoptive homes, chronic illness or disability, and death of family members are crises when they first occur. Even though the family may move toward resolving the immediate crisis, there will be certain points in a child's development when the crisis recurs, as will be explained more fully later.

Prematurity and Congenital Malformations It was pointed out earlier that parenthood is often viewed as a crisis when the newborn is full-term and healthy. If difficulties arise even in normal situations, it is obvious that problems can be anticipated if the baby is born prematurely or with handicaps. Prematurity and congenital malformations as they may affect subsequent experiences and development of children and families are discussed in Chapter 23.

Congenital and Acquired Handicaps When an infant has congenital anomalies or when he acquires a defect later in life, the potential is high for additional problems. Not only may there be a prolonged hospitalization; but there may be a question of whether he should be placed in an institution or returned to his own home. If he goes home, the parents are constantly faced with visible reminders of their child's difference. In all probability he will require expensive treatment, making many extra demands on the parents' resources. How the parents cope with these demands will greatly influence how the child feels about himself and how he copes with new experiences. Typical reactions range from denying that a handicap exists to an intense overprotectiveness, with most parents falling somewhere in between.

The denial reaction is exemplified in an autobiography of a girl with cerebral palsy. Ayrault[9] recalls that she was expected to achieve as though she had no handicap, and little recognition was given her when she did achieve against tremendous odds. She accomplished a great deal at a time when people with cerebral palsy were expected to remain out of sight, and certainly her coping style was very effective. At the same time, her book conveys some feelings of bitterness toward her parents and perhaps some self-doubt about her value to them.[9] In contrast, Killilea's[10] portrayal of her daughter's development vividly points out that Karen was an important and valued member of the family regardless of what she could and could not accomplish.

There is a tendency on the part of many parents to limit the life experiences of the handicapped child. They are less likely to be taken shopping or on special outings. If a child is not mobile, his experience may be restricted to his immediate environment. Not only does this limit the child in his learning about things, it may also protect him from outsiders who view him differently from his family. One mother of a severely burned child with disfiguring scars said she made sure her daughter went somewhere outside the neighborhood regularly, as she had to learn to cope with the stares and questions of others. She also helped the child to cope with these experiences and conveyed her love and concern to the child. Without such support, youngsters can see themselves as without value. As an adolescent, Tom had stoically coped with his scarred face and body for many years, but when a nurse placed her hand on his arm in a gesture of concern, his façade crumbled as he told her that he viewed himself as repulsive because people avoided touching him.

It seems, then, that if handicapped children are provided with a wide range of learning experiences, learn to view their assets and liabilities realistically, and are valued for what they are rather than for what they can achieve, they will learn to cope and achieve in ways similar to their nonhandicapped peers.

Chronic Illness in a Family Member Any disabling chronic illness in a parent or an illness which has many exacerbations and remissions can produce both short- and long-term disruptions with which a child must cope. His method of coping is, of course, dependent on many factors including his age, the severity of the stress, and the help available to him. Using mental illness of either parent as an example, several points will be considered. When a mentally ill mother is maintained at home, she may be unable to fulfill expectations associated with her maternal role. She may be emotionally labile and inconsistent in interactions with family members and may demand nurturance rather than providing it. If it is the father who is ill at home, his wife may be so overwhelmed with responsibilities and financial worries that she is limited in the extent to which she can meet her children's needs.

Looking more specifically at age, even the young infant can be seriously affected if his mother is severely ill. She may give meticulous physical care, but unless the baby can sense her love and can trust her to meet his needs, he will probably not prosper. As the baby grows into toddlerhood and begins learning through imitation, he will mimic both normal and abnormal behavior. He frequently will not receive the help he needs to master the developmental tasks for his age even though he may, through inattention of parents, have the freedom to develop autonomy. It may be difficult for him to develop a positive sense of self if his mother's interaction with him is minimal, inconsistent, or contradictory. Intermittent hospitalization of the mother during this period can result in separation anxiety and fears of abandonment for the child.

As the child learns to communicate through language, he may hear ideas expressed by the mentally ill parent which he has no way of knowing are not realistic. The preschooler normally has difficulty in separating reality from fantasy, and to hear and observe abnormal ideas and behaviors is doubly confusing. He is likely to absorb some of the parent's distorted means of coping with new situations, again not knowing that they are inappropriate in healthy people.

The stigma of mental illness may affect the preschool child through his playmates, but it assumes even greater significance to the school-age child, who depends so heavily on being accepted by his peers. By this age the child may be taking on more responsibilities toward the ill parent and may try to limit the parent's bizarre behavior. Assuming responsibilities beyond his age at home and trying to maintain normal contacts with peers can be a tremendous burden for a child.[11] If the parent's behavior exposes him to ridicule by his peers, he may come to reject or resent the ill parent and then feel guilty for doing so.

With the development of causal thinking, the older school child begins to look for possible reasons for the parent's behavior. He may question his own responsibility in causing the problem or wonder if he has the same defect. This line of questioning becomes even more apparent in the adolescent, who is trying to establish his identity and has some knowledge of genetics. Many of the earlier problems also assume increased importance during this period, particularly if the illness interferes with peer relationships. It is obvious from this brief overview that children who live in a home with a mentally ill parent, especially the mother, are highly vulnerable and in need of outside support and assistance.

The extent to which other disabling illnesses in the family have similar effects depends on the illness and the degree to which it consumes the energy and attention of the parents and children. Parents have been known to devote the bulk of their resources to a severely retarded child or one with a chronic illness like cystic fibrosis to the detriment of normal siblings, but this is not often the case. Studies have shown that siblings are not adversely affected by the presence of a retarded sibling as long as parents show love and attention to all the children, and this is probably true for other handicaps as well.

Death of a Family Member   Anyone who has had an experience with death in a family with young children has been faced with the problems of what to tell them, how much they should be included in the grieving process, and just what their understanding of death is. For example, when 5-year-old Pamela was told of her mother's death, relatives were shocked when she queried whether her father would marry again. Such a question would not come as a surprise to those who are knowledgeable about the preschooler's concept of death. For them, death is temporary. They "shoot" a playmate who falls dramatically and then rises to shoot in return. Or they watch TV characters die on one show and return on another, so that there is no need for concern on the part of the child who has had no previous experience with actual death. Pamela's response might also be explained on the basis that she had already acquired the concept of permanence and was so overwhelmed at the enormity of her loss that she had to deny it, or she may have been indirectly expressing concern about who would take care of her.

Children of Pamela's age and beyond often feel responsible for a parent's death. As long as they believe in magical thinking it is easy to assume that their earlier angry wish for the parent to drop dead had come true. They may then see themselves as bad and deserving of punishment.

Another related problem for children of late preschool and early school age is the confusion in their thinking regarding illness as a punishment for mis-

behavior. If the parent was ill before death, then the child fears his misbehavior could have caused the illness which led to death. By the time the child is 10, he has usually grasped the concept of death as final and inevitable for everyone and usually can understand cause-and-effect relationships. He can devote his energies to coping realistically with the situation and does not sustain damage to his self-esteem by unreasonable feelings of responsibility and guilt.

The explanations children receive during this period can relieve much of their guilt and assure them that they will be taken care of in spite of the parent's death. It should not be assumed that the effects of a parent's death disappear when the acute grief and mourning have passed. Grief can reappear when a father figure is needed to participate in Cub Scout activities or when a mother-daughter banquet is scheduled. Children need help in coping with these as well as earlier experiences.

Feelings of guilt and responsibility are also common reactions when a sibling dies. In a study[12] of 58 children between 2½ and 14 years old who had experienced the death of a sibling, it was found that half of the children felt responsible for the sibling's death. They dwelled on the nasty things they had done to him prior to his death, believed that they should enjoy nothing, and felt they deserved the worst. If their general functioning deteriorated, especially in school, they felt all the more depressed and useless. It was also found that many of the siblings had distorted concepts of illness, death, medical care, hospitalization, and religion. The deaths of siblings frequently precipitated fears of their own imminent deaths, and these fears were reinforced by their parents' restrictiveness and overprotection.[12] Such overprotection limits the child's ability to master new experiences and to think well of himself.

Even in families in which there are few overtones of guilt, there may be a major disruption of family functioning as the remaining members adjust to new role relationships. If, for example, a sibling is expected to fulfill his parents' expectations of his deceased brother, he may be unable or unwilling to do so. In this event, he may continue to experience adverse effects from his brother's death. Here, too, outside intervention is often indicated.

Foster Home Placement   Placement in a foster home is usually a temporary measure until a child can return to his own home or be placed for adoption. When children are not considered adoptable, they may remain in foster homes and develop the same kinds of relationships with foster parents as with adoptive parents. It also happens that children are moved frequently from one foster home to another, with disastrous results to their self-concepts.

Since placement is often on an emergency basis, foster parents are called upon to meet extraordinary needs of children in their care. Such children may have been neglected or abused, or may have suffered the loss of both parents; or this may be one more in a series of placements. It stands to reason that these children feel abandoned by their parents and may fear abandonment by the foster parents as well. If the children feel they have precipitated the abandonment by their behavior, they may test the foster parents to their limits—as if to rule out or verify their worth for themselves. Children who remember their previous homes tend to emphasize the good things which happened and blame themselves for deserving the beatings or neglect. Even though they may have more material advantages in the foster home, when given a choice they frequently elect to return to their original homes. For these reasons, before considering permanent removal of children from their own homes, every effort should be made to make those homes safe and beneficial for the children.

Fortunately, there has been more emphasis recently for periodically reviewing the status of children in foster homes to determine potential for adoptive placement. Many children with mixed racial backgrounds or with physical defects who were formerly considered unadoptable are now being placed.[13] This trend will probably continue as fewer infants are released for adoption. For many of these children, being placed in an adoptive home or being adopted by the foster parents means that they are lovable and have a valuable place in the world. In all probability, however, they will continue to need extra help from their new parents and perhaps professionals if they are to cope with life successfully.

Adoption Children who are placed in adoptive homes as infants are probably not aware of any crisis even though adoption is usually considered as such by the parents. The crises for the child are more likely to occur at different stages in his development, depending in part on when and how he is told about his adoption. Children may need help in understanding that they were in no way responsible for the placement decision. Unless this is done, children may believe that their parents gave them up because they were not lovable. The child who grows up knowing he was "chosen" may not experience a crisis until he discovers that he is different from his peers and that such differences are not always tolerated. Being different by virtue of adoption loses some of

its importance for a time, but usually reappears with adolescence. When the adolescent is struggling to learn his adult identity, he may find it very difficult not to know who his natural parents were. If he becomes too absorbed in this quest, he may have insufficient energy to meet other demands.

In addition to the preceding problems, the child who is placed for adoption later in life may experience other difficulties. If he remembers his own home, he may, like the foster child, feel that it was his own behavior which precipitated his removal and may continue to be burdened with shame or guilt. He, too, may fear abandonment, particularly if his adoptive parents tease him or threaten to send him "back where he came from."

On the other hand, periods of crisis may be no greater for the adopted child than for any other. Most children, whether they are natural-born or adopted, fantasize to some extent that they truly belong with someone else who is either more famous, wealthier, or more ideal than their present parents. As in so many other situations, the parents' ability to meet the needs of their children is the crucial point. Their motives for adoption and the social acceptance of adoption in their community also exert some influence.

Maltreated Children

Unfortunately, not all parents are able to meet their children's basic physical needs, let alone their psychosocial needs. If adults did not have their own needs met as children or if the stresses they face are too severe for their own coping abilities, their children may suffer. Some sustain at least temporary damage because they are deprived—deprived of love from parent figures, of basic nutrients, of the stimulation necessary for growth, or of parental attention and concern. Others are physically and psychologically battered. But the binding force which links all these conditions together is the inadequacy of the parents to meet the responsibilities of parenthood.

The effects of some of the more obvious problems on children's development will be examined in detail. Failure to thrive, neglect, and maternal deprivation will be considered together under child abuse, although in actuality overt child abuse may be an extension or extreme manifestation of one of the other conditions.

Failure to Thrive and Neglect In recent years the phrase *failure to thrive* has been used to denote a psychosocial disruption in the child's life which manifests itself in growth failure, malnutrition, and a delay in motor and social development.[14] In earlier literature, failure to thrive was used as a presenting symptom which required an extensive differential diagnosis to arrive at a cause for the child's condition. Thus, it becomes important in reviewing literature to make sure of the author's intent in using the words. Since there are a number of physical conditions which can cause a child not to thrive, it is crucial that an infant's condition not be attributed to a psychosocial disruption without substantiating evidence.

The infant or child who is admitted to the hospital for failure to thrive has not been able to establish a sense of trust in his caretakers. He appears unusually solemn and watchful and may resist physical contact as though he had had no previous experience with being cuddled. His failure to gain weight may be caused by an actual lack of food due to starvation or neglect, may reflect a severe eating problem in which the mother repeatedly but unsuccessfully tried to feed the child, or may indicate failure to gain based on a lack of love. Several early studies on maternal deprivation pointed out the high mortality rates among institutionalized infants whose physical needs were well met but who lacked a consistent, warm mother figure. This kind of deprivation still happens in homes in which love is lacking. It is easy to see how the coping ability of these children would be affected by a lack of nurturance. There is some evidence to suggest that the intelligence of children is diminished by malnutrition. Certainly they have less energy and stamina to devote to coping. If smiling and cooing bring no recognition and crying is ignored, these methods of controlling the environment are discarded and probably replaced by hopelessness. Without memories of successful experiences and without support from parents in meeting new experiences, the child has no choice but to give up. The child's view of himself also suffers if he does not experience love or have success in coping with his environment. This dismal picture of the child's future can be altered when he is admitted to the hospital for treatment and when parents are given assistance in meeting their responsibilities. In one follow-up study of 40 children without physical cause for their failure to thrive, about one-third of the children from the more favorable homes had recovered, although 16 of the 40 children remained below the third percentile in height and/or weight.[14] No definition was included of what constituted a favorable home.

There is little doubt that infants who fail to thrive (when physical causes have been ruled out) have

been neglected. It is much harder to define neglect in other situations. For instance, the child who is malnourished may be neglected, or he may have been receiving more than his share of the limited food available. The preschooler in the lower-class home may be neglected in terms of intellectual stimulation, but perhaps no more so than the upper-class child who is provided with material things but is neglected insofar as love and attention are concerned. Usually when a child is referred to as neglected, assumptions are made that he is from a poor home and does not receive adequate protection and care. Sometimes the inference is also made that there has been a deliberate withholding of life's necessities by the parents and that such parents do not deserve to keep their children. Certainly there are parents who do not want their children or who are totally unable to meet a child's needs, but they are in a minority. The majority desires to be good parents, but their lives are so disorganized and so prone to crises that their good intentions fail miserably. These are the people at the end of the poverty continuum, and much of the earlier discussion about low-income life-styles applies here. It is probable that children from these homes rapidly learn survival techniques at an early age, but once these are learned, there is little incentive or energy to learn new approaches or to broaden opportunities for mastery. Thus, coping skills frequently are highly developed in some areas and lacking in others. It is possible for a socially isolated child with no standards of comparison to view himself positively if he gets recognition from family members for his contributions to the family's survival. He may not realize until he starts school how "neglected" he has really been. In this case, he may have developed a sense of trust in his parents upon which he can build in the school setting. It is more likely however, that he will grow up without trust in adults, will have difficulty in meeting his developmental tasks, and will have been conditioned for failure.

Child Abuse Although state laws and definitions vary, the abused or battered child is generally considered to be one who has sustained a nonaccidental injury through acts or omissions by the parents or legal guardians. For a significant number of children (5 to 27 percent in various studies), abuse results in death. Permanent physical disability and mental retardation are often the sequelae of abuse for others. Aftereffects are less serious for some children but still apparent. Many children who are abused are also malnourished, either from deliberate starvation or from their inability to gain weight during periods of high stress. Still others may bear no physical signs of abuse but may have a noticeable delay in language and may have learned behaviors which interfere with development. Some young children who are expected to gratify their parents' needs quickly learn that they cannot expect to have their own needs met. Helfer[15] relates a graphic example of this phenomenon.

> Shortly before I left Denver to assume my present position in New York, I was in Judge Delaney's court testifying in a case of child abuse. The judge was talking to the mother and father in his usual reassuring manner. During the conversation the 20-month-old child in question was walking about the courtroom and tripped and fell. She had a mild bump on the arm and started to cry. There was not one flicker of interest from the mother and father, nor even any sign that they heard the child's cry. The social worker came from the back of the court, picked up the child, and comforted her. Within a very few moments the child was quiet. A few minutes later Judge Delaney said something to the mother that upset her, and she began to cry. Within seconds the 20-month-old child was over to her mother trying to get her to calm down. She was essentially taking over the role of the mother.
> Observing this little girl deal with her mother's stress made one realize that she, in her short 20 months of life, had learned what she had to do to keep from getting injured. She, if you will, had developed her own "plan for protection." Her actions not only protected her but they also calmed her mother.[15]

Descriptions of abused children as they are seen in the hospital can be used to infer effects of abuse. These children cry less than expected and do not expect support or comfort from their parents. They form surface relationships with people and seem to be searching for tangible evidences of concern, such as food or small gifts. They show apprehension when other children cry and may exhibit fear of physical contact. Without intervention, these children are believed to become adults who rely on violence as their approach to problem solving. Not only are they more prone to assault and murder others, but they also tend to become abusing parents.[16]

With intervention, the course of development for abused children is somewhat more favorable, although the aftereffects of abuse have not been subjected to much scrutiny. Martin[16] found that after several months or years of intervention the typical child tended to relate superficially and indiscriminately to adults and to be solicitous and agreeable. He responded well to praise, controls, and limits, but sought clues from adults for their reactions to his behavior. He did not trust himself to monitor his own behavior, nor did he find it easy to develop deep trusting relationships with significant others. These characteristics probably persist into adulthood. As yet, there is no documentation on whether these abused children who received professional help will become abusing parents.

Within the past few years, attention to problems of child abuse has broadened to focus on morbidity as well as mortality and on the abusing parents as well as the children. If physical or emotional battering is to be prevented, it is imperative that nurses work with others to identify situations in which the potential for abuse is high and to discover the underlying problems and work toward their solution. Unfortunately, this is not easy. Parents who batter their children are found in all social classes and in homes in which nurses or other professional workers do not visit routinely. Nonetheless, parents who are likely to abuse children have certain characteristics which can alert the nurse to possible danger. Helfer[15] says that abusing a child requires the presence of three characteristics: (1) potential for abuse is present in the parents, (2) the child has special traits or for a variety of reasons is vulnerable to abuse, and (3) a number of crises have occurred, creating high stress levels in the parents. Each of these needs further elaboration to make them applicable for nursing.

Parents who have the potential for child abuse frequently can be identified by their personal history. One or both parents often were abused as children because they were unable to meet their own parents' needs. As a result, they did not experience the love and nurture needed, nor did they learn to give or accept help from others. Thus, they tend to be isolated, lonely adults who were attracted to each other as they searched for a loving parent figure. (In some instances the spouse was not abused as a child but is a highly passive individual who allows the abuse to occur.) As parents, they do not know how to nurture an infant and are unable to ask for help in learning these skills. Such parents have unrealistic expectations of the infant. They desperately want the infant to meet their unfulfilled needs for mothering; this leads to feelings of further rejection when the infant cannot do so. Thus, the mother who expresses strong negative feelings toward the infant who cries too much, is messy while eating, or resists too early attempts at toilet training may be giving the nurse clues that her level of stress is uncomfortably high.

The infant or child who is the recipient of abuse may be the only child in the family to experience such treatment. This is believed to occur because there is something different about the child which increases his vulnerability. The pregnancy or delivery may have been particularly uncomfortable, or if he were premature, the mother may have had little opportunity to establish a relationship with him. She might, for example, blame the infant for coming too early and causing extra expense. Or the infant may be of a different temperament from other siblings, thus creating problems in management. For whatever reason, when a particular child is unable to meet the expectations of one or both parents, the second necessary condition for battering has been met.

The third condition of a crisis or a series of small crises happens periodically to all parents, but in most instances of high stress, parents have learned to call for help from relatives, neighbors, or close friends. Without this source of support or relief, the abusing parent takes out frustration on the child who has been unable to meet the parent's needs.

Early attempts to break this cycle have focused on situations in which abuse has already occurred; legal, social, and medical interventive actions have been primarily punitive. Removing the abused child from the home and jailing the offending parent has been the primary recourse in many communities. Intensive psychotherapy has sometimes been effective but is too expensive to be practical. More recently, efforts are being made to break down the wall of isolation surrounding abusive parents in order to make help more readily available. Parents are being mothered by specially trained aides from the community and are also forming Parents Anonymous groups similar to Alcoholics Anonymous. Professional input into the organizations from a variety of disciplines, including nursing, helps parents identify factors which can lead to abuse. As parents' needs are met by outsiders and they learn to call on someone for help during crises, they are able to avoid further episodes of abuse. It is estimated that, if this kind of help were generally available, 80 percent of the homes in which battering has occurred could be made safe for the children.

While homes are being made safe for the return of abused children who are temporarily in foster homes, foster parents may need encouragement and support in allowing the abused child to regress to the point that he can experience a loving mother-child relationship before he can learn more age-appropriate developmental tasks. This is a relatively new area of scientific concern and much remains to be learned about helping children recover from the long-term effects of abuse.

There is also an urgent need for programs which focus on identifying vulnerable children before abuse has occurred. Certainly the community health nurse is in a position to identify families in which there is a history of abuse in one or both parents, a pattern of social isolation, and unrealistic expectations of the child. Whether frequent nursing visits or attempts to involve the parents in meaningful interactions with others can prevent abuse is yet to be demonstrated.

NURSING MANAGEMENT

Nurses find themselves in a variety of situations and roles in which they can contribute to the well-being of children: clinical specialist, community health nurse, pediatric nurse practitioner, school nurse, neighbor, relative, or parent. The form of intervention will vary with the particular nurse and the situation, but many of the steps in the process will be similar. In many instances the nurse will be faced with situations which *may* require nursing intervention. The first step is to determine whether nursing intervention is needed and, if it is, whether he should intervene in the situation itself, with the involved child, his parents, or significant others. He must then make decisions about what needs to be accomplished, the form nursing intervention should take, and how he will evaluate its outcome. These are familiar steps and should require only brief elaboration.

Fortunately for the nurse, the need for his intervention is frequently obvious. The child admitted to the hospital with pneumonia, the toddler without any immunizations, the mother whose 14-month-old is refusing solid foods, the neighbor's child with an elevated temperature, and the child who has been abused all need nursing knowledge and skills. But what of the child whose parents were just divorced or the children in the hospital waiting room whose sibling has just died or the adolescent who gets sick each time an examination is scheduled? To decide whether nursing intervention is needed in these situations, there are several questions the nurse can ask himself. What is likely to happen in the situation or to the child and family without intervention? Are there actions which, if taken, could modify the outcome? Are these actions feasible in terms of available resources (time, skill, knowledge, cost, motivation, etc.) of the nurse, child, and family?

It may well be that the nurse cannot answer these questions unless he intervenes sufficiently to gather more data. This data collection process is also necessary if he decides that intervention is indicated and then enters into more specific assessment. Assessment is a process through which the nurse sorts through the possibilities to discover the actual situation. It is a series of steps in which he selects from his knowledge the information which might be useful in a given situation, gradually becoming more discriminating with each step. It could be compared to passing a solution through a series of screens or filters, each one a little finer than the one before. An example of these ''screens'' follows and is illustrated in Figure 17-7.

When a community health nurse interacts with a family for the first time, he brings a body of knowledge about people, health, and disease. When he finds that this particular white family unit consists of a graduate student husband, a pregnant working wife, and 2-year-old Julie, he can focus on his knowledge of student couples, pregnancy, infancy, and early childhood. As he gets to know the family, he may find that their primary concern is Julie's refusal to be toilet trained. Next he draws on his knowledge of the toilet training process, of the associated problems, and of what can be done about them. He is then ready to find out how this information applies to Julie and her parents.

To accomplish this screening, the nurse must be able to establish a relationship with the family and to obtain pertinent information through interviewing and appropriate assessment skills. Unless he does this, he may spend time offering solutions to problems which, in the parents' minds, do not exist. The nurse's knowledge helps him decide what to look for, but he must also be able to determine the extent to which this family is similar to and different from other families in general. Sometimes he must evaluate each family member and then the family as a whole, since family structure and role expectations can vary so greatly.

The nurse may also apply the same process when he wants to assess a situation rather than a specific child or family. For example, if a clinical specialist notes that children are crying excessively following ear, nose, or throat surgery, he might question whether nursing intervention is needed. He finds supporting evidence in the literature that too much stress following surgery can impede healing and cause long-lasting psychologic damage. He then explores the situation sufficiently to find out that excessive crying occurs at times when parents are not allowed to be present, such as during meals and at

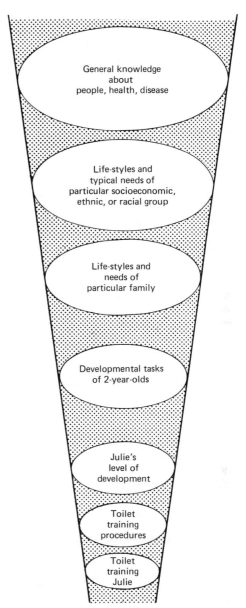

Figure 17-7 The nurse uses a series of screens to determine how a particular family is similar to and different from families in general.

bedtime. Parents are excluded at these times by unit policy. If children's crying is to be lessened, nursing intervention should logically focus on the situation rather than on the children and their parents. Should he intervene? He has already established that the existing policy is probably harmful and that crying would be diminished if parents were allowed to remain with their children. The third question asked earlier is the crucial one. Does the nurse have the resources to intervene successfully? In this situation resources might include his formal authority to act, his power or influence, his memories of previous interventions, and the degree of stamina it might require to effect the change. He might then consider the people who could be expected to support the change and the possible consequences to others if the change were made. For example, if parents were allowed to stay against the will of some nurses, might those nurses be punitive in their attitudes toward the parents?

In order for a nurse to make decisions about nursing intervention, a wide range of approaches must be available. Approaches must be selected which are *acceptable to the family* and can be understood and used by them. Perhaps a slum mother who has not responded to clinic appointments based on the child's needs for immunizations would take her child to the clinic if she knew it would give her a chance to socialize with other mothers. Expectations of a group as to its members' behaviors can also be used as a motivating force.

The nurse also needs to set goals which are within reach of the people involved and which can provide opportunities for positive reinforcement. Without these goals, success is unlikely and evaluation of intervention is difficult.

REFERENCES

1 Lois B. Murphy, *The Widening World of Childhood*, Basic Books, Inc., New York, 1962.
2 A. Thomas, Stella Chase, and H. G. Birch, "The Origin of Personality," *Scientific American*, 8:102–109, 1970.
3 E. H. Erikson, *Childhood and Society*, 2d ed., W. W. Norton & Company, Inc., 1963, pp. 259–260.
4 Eileen Tiedt, "The Adolescent in the Hospital," *Nursing Forum*, 11(2):120, 1972.
5 Fredelle Maynard, "The Many Faces of Motherhood," *Woman's Day*, 1:109–110, 1972.
6 B. R. McCandless, *Children*, 2d ed., Holt, Rinehart & Winston, Inc., New York, 1967, p. 270.
7 S. Coopersmith, *The Antecedents of Self Esteem*, W. H. Freeman and Company, San Francisco, 1967.
8 P. H. Mussen, J. J. Conger, and J. Kagan, *Child Development and Personality*, 3d ed., Harper & Row, Publishers, Incorporated, New York, 1969.
9 Evelyn Ayrault, *Take One Step*, Modern Literary Editions Publishing Company, New York, 1963.
10 Marie Killilea, *Karen*, Dell Publishing Company, New York, 1952.
11 Elizabeth Rice et al., *Children of Mentally Ill Parents*, Behavioral Publications, New York, 1971.
12 A. C. Cain, Irene Fast, and Mary Erickson, "Children's Disturbed Reactions to Death of a Sibling," *American Journal of Orthopsychiatry*, 34(7):741–752, 1964.
13 Ursula M. Gallagher, "Adoption in a Changing Society," *Children Today*, 1(5):2–6, 1972.
14 H. H. Glaser et al., "Physical and Psychological Development of Children with Early Failure to Thrive," *Journal of Pediatrics*, 73:690, 1968.
15 R. E. Helfer, "A Plan for Protection: The Child-Abuse Center," *Child Welfare*, 49(9):486, 1970.
16 H. Martin, "The Child and His Development," in G. H. Kempe and R. E. Helfer (eds.), *The Battered Child and His Family*, J. B. Lippincott Company, Philadelphia, 1972, p. 104.

BIBLIOGRAPHY

Ansfield, J.: *The Adopted Child*, Charles C Thomas, Publisher, Springfield, Ill., 1971.
Barnard, Kathryn E., and Powell, Marcene L.: *Teaching the Mentally Retarded Child*, The C. V. Mosby Company, St. Louis, 1972.
Erikson, E. H.: *Identity, Youth and Crisis*, W. W. Norton & Company, Inc., New York, 1968.
Fraiberg, Selma: *The Magic Years*, Charles Scribner & Sons, New York, 1959.
Ginott, H.: *Between Parent and Child*, The Macmillan Company, New York, 1969.
———: *Between Parent and Teenager*, The Macmillan Company, New York, 1969.
Gordon, T.: *Parent Effectiveness Training*, Peter H. Wyden, Inc., Publisher, New York, 1970.
Grollman, E.: *Explaining Divorce to Children*, Beacon Press, Boston, 1969.
Helfer, R. E., and Kempe, G. H.: *The Battered Child*, The University of Chicago Press, Chicago, 1968.
Howe, Florence: "Sexual Stereotypes Start Early," *Saturday Review*, 76(82):92–94, Oct. 16, 1971.
Kempe, C. H. and Helfer, R. E.: *Helping the Battered Child and His Family*, J. B. Lippincott Company, Philadelphia, 1972.
LeMasters, E. E.: *Parents in Modern America A. Sociological Analysis*, The Dorsey Press, Homewood, Ill., 1970.
Parad, H. J.: *Crisis Intervention*, Family Service Association of America, New York, 1965.
Tiedt, Eileen: "The Adolescent in the Hospital," *Nursing Forum*, 11(2):120, 1972.

18

CULTURAL INFLUENCES ON DEVELOPMENT

ALICE H. MURPHREE

Part of man's adaptation, including his health and child-rearing practices, involves social organization, or the ways people arrange themselves in groups to meet their needs. One of the universal groupings within social organization is the family. The behavioral relationships between individuals in families and between families and other individuals or groups, such as providers of health care, are based on what they believe is the best way to accomplish their goals and to utilize the means at their disposal. The way people view their health or the lack of it, their definition of illness, their behavior in relation to an illness, their health- and treatment-related activities before arrival at the clinical setting, their expectations and fears, their responses to the setting and its personnel, and their actions after they leave are all directly related to their cultural background.

Culture can be defined as "the symbolically transmitted, learned behavior that people use or have used to adapt to their environment." Culture stands in interactional relationship to such factors as the social organization, religion, folklore, the educational system, and the economy. This chapter stresses *cultural relativity*, a concept most applicable to the successful delivery of health care. This anthropologic concept can be translated into nursing practice as the following: "Human behavior is at least in part the product of the various cultural settings in which it occurs." In other words, patients do not come to the clinical setting from a vacuum.

THE FAMILY, ITS FUNCTIONS, AND ITS ETHNIC VARIATIONS
Definition of Family

For the purposes of this discussion, the social and biologic unit known as a family is defined as "A socially organized group of two or more individuals of either or both sexes, including either adults or adults and children, functioning together to meet at least some portion of the basic human needs." Anthropologists have long recognized and studied the family in relation to kinship, social organization, culture and personality, rites of passage, socialization processes, marriage institutions, and the like. In this instance, however, only that portion of the above definition which specifically includes children in relation to health care will be considered.

Types of Families

Despite such problems involved with the validity of research on marriage and the family as pointed out by Tavuchis,[1] there are definite bodies of information about the family as an institution. One concerns the types of family known. The simplest form, which comes most readily to mind for persons in Western culture, particularly in the United States, is the nuclear family.

The Nuclear Family Middle-class Americans typically envision the nuclear family as consisting of one mother and one father, married (by some socially acceptable ritual), and one or more children—preferably at least one boy and one girl. Certainly, this seems to be the ideal presented in the American media. However, Jessie Bernard has this to say:

> For many years researchers had spoken of "broken homes" or "broken families" as though intact homes were the norm. Only recently has it become clear that for a considerable proportion of the population, Negro or white, the female-headed family is a standard phenomenon—culturally acceptable, if not prescribed or preferred. Thus, at any given time—say, during the taking of the 1960 census—over half (50.9 percent) of all the nonwhite families with incomes under $2,000 in central cities were headed by women. Over a given period, a considerably larger proportion of women will find themselves, at some time or another, the heads of families. These families are poor because they have women as heads; and, conversely, they probably have women as heads because they are poor.[2]

Obviously, also, some proportion of the divorced, deserted, widowed, or even never-married *males* are the only parents in a nuclear family, for whatever period of time. Miller presents additional perspective:

> Anthropologists have even argued that the nuclear family is not the basic and elementary social unit of mankind. In primitive tribes the male accompanying a mother and an infant is not necessarily the child's father, and in some such groups the concept of individual biological fatherhood does not exist. Nevertheless no one denies the significance of the mother-child bond or the necessity for a father figure in a child's life.[3]

To add to this complexity, there are also a great number of children who are in the custody of grandparents, aunts, uncles, older siblings, foster parents, or other parent surrogate figures. Thus the safest way to define the nuclear family is to say that it is that adult(s)-child(ren) group which acknowledges

itself to be in parent-child relationship. While it is widely recognized that the basic family unit could be the mother-child dyad, for present purposes the nuclear family itself will be considered the basic unit, regardless of the kinship bonds, genders, or number of parents which compose it.

The Extended Family Nuclear families can be combined to make various family types. The extended family is one such variation. An extended family arrangement may be vertical across generations to include parents, children, and grandchildren as a closely knit social unit; or it may extend horizontally to include siblings, their spouses, and their children. In comparison with the tightly knit and relatively isolated parent-child nuclear family, extended families have obvious additional relational complexities as the family members go about meeting their needs within the family context.

Polygamous Families Among those peoples who recognize marriage forms different from Western culture's one-spouse ideal of monogamy, *polygamy* (multiple spouses) can produce other variations of family organization. An important point, however, is that in practice, where the household head (or family head) assumes economic responsibility, any multiple household arrangement is a direct function of the individual household head's economic position. In other words, usually only wealthier persons can support more than one nuclear family.

In *polygyny*, in which one man has several wives, the entire group may be housed together, with children generally the joint responsibility of the wives; or each wife and her children may be housed separately with the husband/father rotating his visits among households. This family form has been acceptable, for example, among many Near Eastern, African, and Pacific Island peoples. With the rarer *polyandry*, in which a woman has more than one husband, the men may be considered joint fathers for all children or the senior husband may be given that role.

Other Variations Another type of family arrangement known in Mediterranean and Latin American cultures and elsewhere could be termed the second household. Here a nuclear family of the male's mistress and her children may be socially, if not legally or religiously, recognized. Where such institutions are recognized, the family dynamics and internal relationships may be somewhat similar to those of polygyny.

Still another type is the one-parent family, considered by some to be the typical family form among lower-income blacks in the United States. This form may encompass either one adult and several children or several adults and their respective offspring. Spouses or lovers, socially and legally recognized or not, may be intermittently present in the household. Incidentally, depending on kinship status among the adults, some such multiple-parent households could be considered forms of either horizontal or vertical extended families.

As mentioned earlier, the Western ideal generally remains monogamy. But as has been aptly observed, the marriage practices of Western culture tend actually to be *serial* monogamy. Few adults are unfamiliar with the "yours, mine, and ours" jokes concerning children in a household in which one or both spouses are remarried. And the child with "two sets of parents" is a common occurrence in many settings, particularly among the middle-class whites in the United States.

Other variations of family and child-rearing arrangements are found in the many communal and communistic societies. Mormons, Oneidans, the Hutterites,[4] and similar utopian groups in the United States have utilized such concepts as multiple spouses and group responsibility for children. One of the more prominent movements of this type in the contemporary world is the kibbutz[5] in Israel. In these communes the principle "from each according to his ability and to each according to his needs" predominates. The children are reared in age groups by specially trained personnel, and the group as a whole assumes responsibility for all children. During the early days of the kibbutz movement, when both economic and physical existence hung in the balance, the best each commune had to offer went to the children. Typically, once past weaning, the child and parents visited only at specifically arranged times. Biologic parenthood was recognized, but many of what Western culture considers parental responsibilities were assumed by the group.

A final and as yet somewhat unpredictable social phenomenon concerning the family institution and its impact on children is visible to those who observe groups of contemporary young people. The counterculture, or street culture, seen where young adults congregate, as around academic settings, obviously has been producing children (Fig. 18-1). Some of these offspring are entering both the free schools and the public school system. They can be seen in the hippie ghettos and hitchhiking with the adults. The conscious effort to create new life-styles within the counterculture groups must have impact on the children growing up there. As yet, few research results have reached print, but the few available[6,7] may form the basis of interesting hypotheses concerning the children and their health care.

The important point here is that the child seen clinically is usually accompanied by a family member or members. However, there is no guarantee that the adults present are the biologic parents, and the family milieu may be one other than that so frequently envisioned by persons from the middle-class culture.

Functions of the Family

Whatever the family type or form, certain functions usually are performed by all families. Many of these functions are related to the fact that the human infant requires such an extended portion of its lifetime to attain maturity and must be protected during this time of vulnerability.

It seems pertinent, in this context, to reemphasize the earlier statement that males, as well as females, may be parents in one-parent nuclear families. Historically, the nursing infant deprived of his mother or her lactating ability usually required the services of a wet nurse to breast-feed him. It may be noted that, depending on the place and time in history, a female's ability to lactate was not the only consideration in utilizing her as a wet nurse. Certain social or moral characteristics were also considered to be important. According to Thomas Raynalde,[8] in sixteenth-century England, along with such desirable attributes as being neither too fat nor too lean and having delivered a "man chylde" at least 2 months previously, the ideal wet nurse should be "good and honest of conversation, neither too sad or forlorn, too hasty or ireful, too fearful or timorous, not too light and wanton." Such considerations seem to indicate an awareness of the effects of the mothering individual's personality on the child. However, it was implied that personal characteristics were transmitted to the child directly through the milk, not through the psychologic dynamics currently recognized.

Obviously, twentieth-century technology has replaced the wet nurse by creating the bottle and formula. Contemporary children can be nursed by bottle, and thus the presence of a female is no longer necessary, at least not for physical survival.

Most of the basic human needs of the other family members are met within the family setting also. Such human requirements as adult sex needs, sustenance, protection from the elements, physical well-being (health), and the need for affection are family functions to a considerable extent. The family

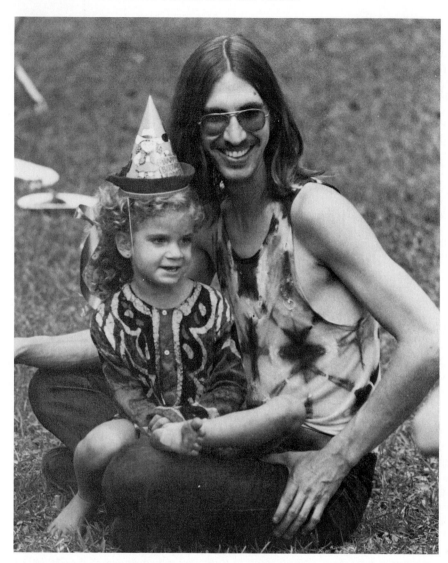

Figure 18-1 Every subculture has its own characteristic ways of dealing with children, as well as its own overall system of values, to which children are enculturated. *(Photo courtesy of George Lazar.)*

is the immediate group with whom all its members identify, and certainly not all the attention focuses on the children.

Usually the young are produced, physically nourished, and protected within the family framework, thus contributing to the perpetuation of the larger group. The processes of psychobiologic growth and development and of socialization occur under the massive influence of the family. It is originally in the family that the children absorb or are consciously taught the language, beliefs, value system, and other mores (including those concerning health) of the culture to which the adults belong.

CHILDREN IN THE FAMILY

No matter what the family structure, it is most usually in a family setting that children are tended through their nurturing period. It is therefore appropriate here to consider certain aspects of the child in the family.

The Value of Children to the Family

In more complex societies, the degree to which children are wanted seems to vary in cycles whose time span depends, among other sociocultural vari-

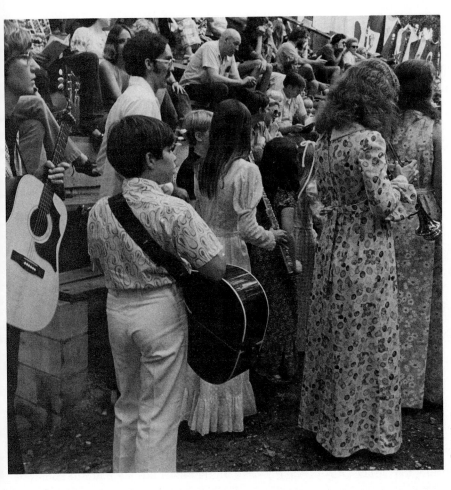

Figure 18-2 Many skills and values are transmitted within the subcultures of childhood. *(Photo courtesy of George Lazar.)*

ables, on the economy. Sometimes such cycles are as short as a generation and at others they may last for a century. When conditions are right for large families, children are so highly valued that a woman's fecundity may be a major qualification contributing to her desirability as a marriage partner or as a member of the husband's extended family. Without going into the sexist chauvinism of this concept, it is important to bear in mind that such conditions directly affect whether a child is socialized in an all-adult, one-child setting or a several-adult, many-children environment. Whichever situation obtains, there obviously are vital psychologic and physical consequences for the child.

Relationships Experienced by Children in the Family

In the family setting the child learns the acceptable behavior patterns peculiar to his culture. One such pattern is that associated with child-to-child relationships, one of the foundations for lifelong modes of interpersonal relations. If the larger social group is one in which young children are the responsibility of older children, the child learns child-child relationships well and early.

In many societies, unlike our middle-class Western culture, the entire child group and its activities are in some measure separated from the adults for many of the waking hours. Overt sexual games and other expressions of observed adult behavior are emulated by the children, and this is considered natural and normal by the group. In such groups, the younger children may learn their future adult roles by observing and participating with older brothers, sisters, cousins, and others rather than by directly observing adults. The children who grow up in children's groups without a lot of contact with adults may well have the feeling that they as a group

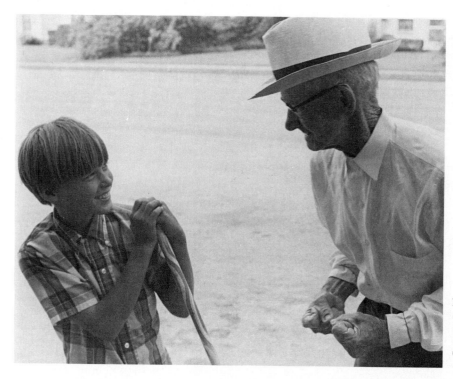

Figure 18-3 Children who have opportunities to interact with older people have access to a great deal of enrichment. *(Photo courtesy of George Lazar.)*

are significant and relevant to one another, and they characteristically feel a strong sense of group identity (Fig. 18-2).

In contemporary Western society, by contrast, many children may have only one sibling or none. This situation frequently results in the adults' deliberately setting up an environment in which the young child is introduced to experiences of getting along with other children. Some of the settings consciously created for such purposes are nursery schools, day care centers, adult-generated neighborhood play groups, and the like.

Another set of family relationships available to the child is that between the child and adult. It is from the adults of the family, whether they are biologic parents or others performing the nurturing function, that the child learns acceptable behavior for children vis-à-vis adults. For instance, if the cultural setting is one in which children are an economic burden (as in low-income situations), the child may learn to compensate the family in whatever ways are available. He may become a contributor to the family income or work force at an early age through chores, salaried jobs, or some other means; or he may learn to stay as isolated from adults as possible. On the other hand, if the cultural setting is one in which children are highly valued and are not too great an economic liability, the child may learn

early of many pleasant consequences of the adult-child relationship. The cultural mores—concerning loving reverence for age, for instance—may be imparted through such relationships (Fig. 18-3).

The third set of relationships to which children are exposed in the family are the adult-to-adult relationships. The ways in which various groups of adult men and women appropriately interact may become clear. Such groupings combine in multiple ways based on age, sex, and social relation. In the relatively intimate, typical Western family setting, the child may observe and internalize the ways his parents relate to one another, how they interact with their parents or other older relatives, how they socialize with their friends and neighbors, and how they express their social status with employers or employees. The entire set of relationships available to the child in the family setting is grist for the socialization mill.

Children's Roles in the Family

Finally, in considering aspects of childhood in relation to the institution of family, it seems of value to include some of the roles played or functions fulfilled by children in the family setting. One such role is that of messenger. For instance, in some of the Latin-American cultures when neighboring adults are in one another's debt, because of adult discomfort, a child may be sent to borrow needed household material. Or, because it is inappropriate for women to be seen too frequently away from their households unescorted, a child may be sent to seek information or to make a forgotten purchase at the market. Examples of this, particularly among the poorer families, are found among Oscar Lewis' writings.[9, 10]

In our culture too, the child often plays the role of messenger or errand performer. In rural farm families the younger children may be sent to take water or food to the adults working in the fields. Nonrural children are often dispatched on errands both within and outside the house. This role may enhance the child's self-esteem because he may feel he is making a valuable contribution to the family. Another familiar image is that of the child who is put in the role of messenger between quarreling parents with such requests as, "Tell your father I would like some more meat, please," or "Tell your mother I am taking the car." It is doubtful that the dynamics involved in this kind of go-between role do much more than make the child uncomfortable.

Another role or function for children in the family setting is that of ego extension for the adults. At least where children are felt to reflect the training and characteristics of the adults with whom they were associated during maturation, the way a child "turns out" is taken as a measure of success in child rearing. As such, a "good" or "bad" child (concepts always culturally defined and varying widely among cultures) is a source of pride or shame to both the child and the adult. In some other societies such relationships may not be recognized, and each individual child or adult may be seen as the product of fate's whim, the decree of the gods, or some other supernatural influence.

In our society, where good health very often is recognized as some mark of morality and illness is seen as punishment, the following incident perhaps serves to illustrate the way in which children may function as ego extensions.

In the course of anthropologic field work a household interview was being conducted in a black home in the South. The mother was reporting the names, ages, and general health of her several children present in the room. It was winter and the children had colds and symptoms of other infectious diseases.

Having completed the report on the children in the room, the mother opened a door into the next room and proudly announced that this was the baby and that he was well. She explained that she felt the need to "always have one well child—the baby." As long as the child remained an infant and could be kept relatively isolated from older children and their frequent infections, she could keep the baby well. This woman implied that she felt a certain sense of virtue in being able to keep at least the youngest child well. This situation also suggests a tentative explanation for some of the resistance encountered in trying to implement family planning programs. This woman seemed to feel that she had to keep a baby in the house in order to have one well child in her family and hence to demonstrate her mothering ability and deservingness.

In societies in which social status is both ascribed and achieved, a child's future upward social mobility may well be among his parents' fondest hopes. Conversely, an offspring's fall in status may constitute one of the parents' greatest fears. This is particularly true in Western culture, where financial success is seen as an expression of social and moral worth. In short, the child may be burdened with many of the adults' aspirations and probably will have internalized these values during the process of maturation. Obviously, when the parental values are rejected, as in the rapidly changing contemporary society, much emotional stress is produced for both child and parent.

The child may serve as the recipient of another's love, thus participating in the satisfaction of the human need for emotional ties. The psychologic dynamics associated with "mother love" have been exhaustively reported in the literature. It is also true that the individual child may also perform this affect-recipient function for siblings, despite the prevalent literature concerning sibling rivalry. It is noteworthy that some recent research has indicated that males may feel urged to procreate not only to demonstrate their virility but to satisfy a need for begetting and loving children (Fig. 18-4). Divorced or separated males have reported a real feeling of emotional loss after separation from their children.

Children also serve the function of contributing to the family's well-being through productive labor, although not as much in contemporary middle-class Western culture as elsewhere. In the recent past, when farm families were more numerous than now, the child performed valuable productive labor as soon as he passed the toddler stage. At first this labor may have been limited to chores in the vicinity of the house or barnyard, but with increased physical strength the children regularly went into the fields to participate in the farming operations.

In fact, in many rural agricultural areas, children

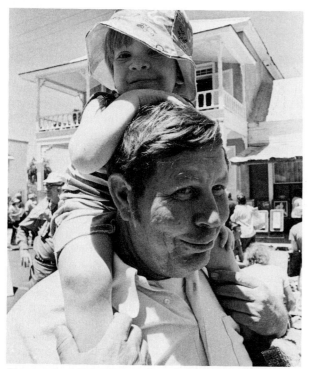

Figure 18-4 Although mother's relationships with children have received the greater professional attention, interactions between fathers and children seem to be major developmental influences for both participants. *(Photo courtesy of George Lazar.)*

were permitted only limited schooling because they were kept at home to work during planting and harvesting periods. In parts of the United States the school calendars are still predicated on the seasonal labor demands of whatever crops are produced locally. This scheduling came about in an effort to alleviate some of the educational inadequacies experienced by rural children as well as to facilitate agricultural production. The children of migrant agricultural workers frequently labor in the fields with the adults to augment the adults' productivity. Where the pay is based on the amount an individual harvests or cultivates, the child's economic contribution to the family can be significant, particularly at low pay rates. Similarly, young girls in Cuban and Puerto Rican families in New York often work with the older females doing piece-work sewing that is part of the home production in the garment industry.

A final illustration of the types of roles that children may perform in the family concerns ritual. For all peoples, rituals express and reinforce cultural values to a greater or lesser degree, and much ritual is centered upon or performed by children. For many, the naming of the child is one of the most important events of a whole lifetime and is associated with a multitude of social and religious considerations. In Western society, this event frequently is celebrated with a religious ritual known among gentiles as baptism or christening. Sometimes the unnamed or unbaptized child is not recognized as a real person, and in rural Greece such a child may be looked upon as a monster or as having supernatural powers.[11] Depending on the religious fervor and predilections of the family, this naming ritual will be of greater or lesser intensity for the whole group.

Later in the child's life there may be some ritualistic recognition of development and changing status, such as confirmation or Bar Mitzvah, as the child moves from childhood to adolescence. In middle- and lower-class Western society generally, childhood ritualistically ends with the marriage ceremony, whether civil or religious. It seems that the upper-class practice of debut, or presentation of the eligible young daughter to the social group before marriage, is falling into disuse.

Other types of rituals function to intensify group solidarity or group mores. For example, the ritual surrounding a formal banquet expresses the felt importance of the occasion and the participants, the importance of their ability to behave properly as expected, their social position, and the like. A simpler ritual may surround the eating of meals in the family setting or the bedtime ceremonies in some families. And of course many children's games are most ritualistic, for example, choosing up sides, skipping rope, and playing jacks or mumbly-peg. Thus, through the child's participation in rituals the socialization process is enhanced—that which the family (and the larger group) considers important and valuable is taught and internalized.

Consider for a moment the ritualistic behavior on the part of the staff in the clinical setting as experienced by the sick child and the family. The regular, ceremonial way in which medications are administered, diagnostic and treatment procedures are performed, patients are visited by physicians, housekeeping chores are accomplished, and the (to the uninitiated) mysterious paraphernalia involved in such activities all make up a most impressive set of rituals. Some rituals of the clinical setting may be more emotionally rewarding to the staff than to the patients, particularly children. The sick child may be the focus of many ritualistic procedures in the clinical setting, but the impact may be in startling contrast to any rituals previously experienced in the family setting. And the values, not to mention frustrations and fears, which are internalized may contribute greatly to lifelong attitudes concerning health, illness, and treatment.

HEALTH AND THE FAMILY

Due in part to the long dependency period for the human young, it is in the family milieu that the child initially experiences illness and the overall cultural attitudes surrounding it. Here are first transmitted the perceptions defining illness and the appropriate behavior concerning health and illness. If the family is part of a group which endemically suffers malnutrition, for instance, the manifestations of that condition may be so common as to escape recognition as a complaint. If, on the other hand, the family is part of a group that considers that preventive practices such as prophylactic dental care and regular immunizations are appropriate, this is among the first internalizations concerning health. As another example, for many in the rural South (as well as in other warm climates) childhood impetigo is sufficiently common that it may not receive prompt or any clinical treatment. It may be viewed as something all children have and that goes away "if they don't scratch too much." That serious cardiac or renal damage may result from a streptococcal infection is unknown and unfeared, and the most conscientious of adults may be inclined to ignore impetigo.

Not all attitudes concerning the feeding of children are those typical of the middle class. The middle-class ideal is that the family diet is to be "good," meaning healthful and appealing, and that obesity has a negative value. In other cultural settings, attitudes about the amount of food consumed and consequent body configurations are not the same. The following description is a case in point.

Food has an emotional and social significance in rural Greece that it does not have in northern Europe or the United States. The mother feeds the baby (overfeeds it, to our way of thinking) so that it can grow fat and thereby have the strength to withstand the inevitable challenge of illness. Giving food is a communication of love, a way of building a relationship, warding off anxiety, doing magic for building power to withstand future evils, and making children, friends, and guests feel wanted, at home, and protected. People are proud of how much they can eat.[12]

A somewhat similar situation appears in the rural South. A "stout" (meaning big, strong, sturdy, and only incidentally fat) child is admired and is often the source of pride for adults in the family. From the clinical point of view, many of these children are obese and potentially subject to the diseases associated with obesity. While the rural Southern diet is admittedly heavy in carbohydrates, there appear to be other cultural values involved also. Stout children are often seen as an indication of parents' merit in that they must have worked hard, been good providers, and adhered to other Protestant ethics.

If the family belongs to one of the Mediterranean or Latin-American cultures, it is common to accept "the evil eye" as a cause for some illnesses or physical and psychologic conditions. Infants and small children are considered particularly susceptible. The child learns under what conditions the evil eye is operant and what to do for protection, whether this involves wearing an amulet or avoiding particular people and situations. The phenomenon of the evil eye is similarly acknowledged among many African and Caribbean cultures and hence is not unknown by American blacks and, possibly from this source also, by whites.

It is in the family that the child also learns what procedural steps are undertaken at times of illness. Usually, adult females have the responsibility for deciding who is sick, whether or not to initiate treatment, and what kind. In many Western cultures, for instance, the female begins treatment at home with patent medicines, remnants of previously prescribed medications, or a folk remedy. She may seek advice from older females, either within or outside the extended family, and may willingly follow such advice. Another possible option is to take counsel with the local pharmacist. If the symptoms disappear during this process, the illness may be considered cured and the treatment stopped. On the other hand, persistent symptoms may ultimately result in seeking a physician's care. Such extramedical practices are common even in middle-class American families where medical attention is regularly sought.

In our culture the decision to seek and accept clinical care is usually made in the immediate family. As Foster points out, such is not the case everywhere.

In middle-class society in the United States the physician's recommendation that an appendix be removed probably will mean consultation with the patient's spouse, but it is not the occasion for a big family council meeting. . . . Public health personnel working in intercultural programs have found that even in small families a patient often is not free to make decisions that are taken for granted in Western countries. Bailey points out how, among the Navaho, the decision to enter a hospital is reached only after a family conference: A woman and her husband alone are not free to exercise their discretion in this regard. Margaret Clark found exactly the same situation in the Spanish-speaking Mexican enclave of Sal Si Puedes in San Jose, California: Hospitalization is a grave and serious step, a family and not an individual problem.[13]

With respect to folk beliefs and practices as contrasted with scientific clinical practices, research clearly shows folk beliefs in most groups, if not all.[14, 15] The child learns from his family members not only the subject matter of these beliefs but from whom the associated secrets are to be learned. Among some groups in both rural and urban United States there is a widespread belief in hexing, voodoo, and conjuring. The beliefs concern health as well as other aspects of living. Many people are firmly convinced that birth abnormalities (less impairing ones being termed, significantly, birthmarks) can be caused by the behavior of the pregnant woman or those around her. In other words, it is believed that a woman can "mark" her baby. Children are likely to learn and share the many folk beliefs specific to their cultural background.

For some families, religious support of some kind may be utilized either simultaneously with or in place of any part of the treatment process, even the ultimate one of seeking clinical treatment. It is important for the nurse to be aware that clinical procedures and folk or religious healing practices often are not felt to be mutually exclusive; therefore it is possible that the family may be implementing certain folk or religious healing practices while a child is being seen by a physician or is hospitalized. Such decisions are culturally based and determined by many factors including type of treatment resources available and acceptable, economic cost, knowledge about the cause of disease, and religious attitudes and practices concerning illness.

The child experiences not only his own illnesses and their results, but also the illnesses of other children and adults in his family. The family's response to such events also becomes part of his knowledge and attitudes toward illness, the family, and the child's place in it. For the pediatric patient, then, although it may be his first experience with a health problem, his behavioral responses will be predicated on the way health, illness, and treatment were perceived in the family setting.

Of particular importance is the fact that the majority of health professionals come from backgrounds that are stereotypically middle-class. The phenomenon of *ethnocentricity* is almost universal. In simplified terms, ethnocentricity refers to the unconscious assumption that "everyone is like me," or "my way is everyone's way and, if not, it should be." The resultant narrow stance from which judgments and decisions are made is a very hazardous one for health professionals. Patients are not all of the middle class and therefore are neither all alike nor all like the professional.

To be able to most appropriately and efficiently interact with patients in diagnosis, treatment, and care, health professionals benefit from an acute and continuing awareness of the following fact: *The cultural variations of disparate class, family, and ethnic backgrounds create an extreme diversity in beliefs and attitudes, with as many such diversities relating to health as to any other human interest.*

REFERENCES

1 N. Tavuchis, "The Analysis of Family Roles," in Katherine Elliott (ed.), *The Family and Its Future*, J. & A. Churchill, Ltd., London, 1970.
2 Jessie Bernard, *Marriage and Family among Negroes*, Prentice-Hall, Inc., Englewood Cliffs, N.J., 1966, p. 41.
3 D. Miller, "Parental Responsibility for Adolescent Maturity," in Katherine Elliott (ed.), *The Family and Its Future*, J. & A. Churchill, Ltd, London, 1970. p. 25.
4 J. A. Hostetler and Gertrude E. Huntington, "The Hutterites in North America," in George and Louise Spindler (eds.), *Case Studies in Cultural Anthropology*, Holt, Rinehart & Winston, Inc., New York, 1967.
5 M. E. Spiro, *Kibbutz: Venture in Utopia*, Dehocken, New York, 1956.
6 W. L. Partridge, "The Hippie Ghetto, The Natural History of a Subculture," in George and Louise Spindler (eds.), *Case Studies in Cultural Anthropology*, Holt, Rinehart & Winston, Inc., New York, 1973.
7 B. J. Wallace, "Rural Hippie Communes: An Experiment in Cultural Change," in J. B. Aceves (ed.), *Southern Anthropological Society Proceedings*, no. 6, University of Georgia Press, Athens, 1972.
8 T. Raynalde, *The Byrthe of Mankind*, London, 1540. Excerpted in Logan Clendening, *Source Book of Medical History*, Dover Publications, New York, 1960, p. 179.
9 O. Lewis, *La Vida*, First Vintage Books Edition, February, 1968, Alfred A. Knopf, Inc., and Random House, Inc., New York.
10 O. Lewis, *A Death in the Sanchez Family*, Vantage Books, A Division of Random House, New York, 1970.
11 R. and Eva Blum, *Health and Healing in Rural Greece*, Stanford University Press, Calif., 1965.
12 Ibid., p. 108.

13 G. M. Foster, *Traditional Societies and Technological Change*, 2d ed., Harper & Row, Publishers, Incorporated, New York, 1973, pp. 118 and 119.
14 Alice H. Murphree, "A Functional Analysis of Southern Folk Beliefs Concerning Birth," *American Journal of Obstetrics and Gynecology*, vol. 102, no. 1, September 1968.
15 Alice H. Murphree and M. V. Barrow, "Physician Dependence, Self-treatment Practices, and Folk Remedies in a Rural Area," *Southern Medical Journal*, vol. 63, no. 4, April 1970.

BIBLIOGRAPHY

Alland, A.: *Adaptation in Cultural Evolution, An Approach to Medical Anthropology*, Columbia University Press, New York, 1970.
Anderson, Margaret: *The Children of the South*, Dell Publishing Company, New York, 1966.
Carden, M. L.: *Oneida: Community to Modern Corporation*, Johns Hopkins Press, Baltimore, 1969.
Clark, Margaret: *Health in the Mexican American Culture*, University of California Press, Berkeley, 1959.
Dubos, Renee: *Man Adapting*, Yale University Press, New Haven, 1965, chaps. IX, "Changing Patterns of Disease"; XII, "Hippocrates in Modern Dress; and XVI, "Medicine Adapting."
————: *Man, Medicine and Environment*, New American Library, New York, 1968, chaps. 2–6.
Eaton, J.: "Folk Obstetrics and Pediatrics Meet the M.D." in E. Jaco (ed.), *Patients, Physicians, and Illness*, Free Press, Glenco, Ill., 1958, pp. 207–221.
Kunkel, P., and Kennard, Sara Sue: *Spout Spring–A Black Community*, in George and Louise Spindler (eds.), *Case Studies in Cultural Anthropology*, Holt, Rinehart & Winston, Inc., New York, 1971.
Naegle, K. D.: *Health and Healing*, Elaine Cumming (ed.) Jossey Bass, Inc., San Francisco, 1970.
Weaver, T. (ed): *To See Ourselves, Anthropology and Modern Social Issues*, part 4, "Race and Racism," part 5, "Poverty and Culture," and "Early Childhood Intervention: The Social Science Base of Institutional Racism" by Stephen S. Raratz and Joan C. Parats, part 6, Scott, Foresman and Company, Glenview, Ill., 1973.

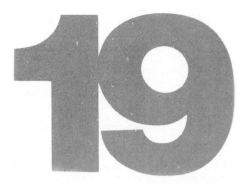

FETAL MALFORMATIONS

GLADYS M. SCIPIEN

Before the birth of their child, parents fantasize about his sex and appearance and about the pleasures the new family member will bring. A normal neonate—pink, randomly moving all his extremities, crying vigorously, and assessed as healthy—is looked upon by most parents as an endless wonder and a delightful human being. With the birth of a deformed infant, however, hopes and expectations are destroyed. Anger, guilt, frustration, and hostility replace the joyous relief that usually accompanies birth. When parents and other family members learn that the baby has a birth defect, the family is thrown into crisis.

Professional nursing activities vis-à-vis fetal malformations span a broad range. Nurses are involved in *teaching* for preconceptional and prenatal prevention of deformities, in *identifying* babies and children who have malformations, in *promoting* and *participating in* treatment, and in *helping* afflicted children and their families cope with their special problems. Nurses work with or in behalf of birth defective children and their parents in virtually unlimited settings, including prenatal and maternity care units, newborn nurseries for both high-risk and apparently well babies, most types of pediatric medical and surgical units, rehabilitation centers, schools, centers for the mentally retarded, and homes. This chapter presents general information and principles about birth defects and nursing of affected children and families. The discussion of specific defects is deferred to the appropriate chapter in Part 4.

Fetal malformations are congenital anomalies of body structure or function which are present at birth and which result from a deleterious influence on the embryo or fetus at an early stage of development. Some defects are insignificant, while others involve major organs and may be incompatible with life. Between these extremes are many deviations from the normal which can be partially or totally corrected through skillful surgical intervention or concerted rehabilitative efforts. It is important to understand that not all birth defects are obvious at birth. For example, mental retardation, inborn errors of metabolism, and certain types of congenital heart disease are not immediately apparent. They may become evident as growth and development progress.

THE SCOPE OF THE PROBLEM

Birth defects constitute a major health problem, for approximately 250,000 newborns delivered each year in the United States will eventually develop symptoms of some fetal malformation. In addition, there is a pronounced tendency for defective fetuses to be spontaneously aborted or stillborn, and fetal malformations are believed to cause about 500,000 such deaths each year. Birth defects are the second leading cause of death in infancy.[1]

In spite of the large numbers of people involved and the sophisticated diagnostic methods available in many settings, it is impossible to determine the exact incidence of congenital anomalies. Defects which produce no signs or symptoms may go undetected indefinitely. The reported incidence of malformations varies with the diagnostic capabilities of health care workers who examine children. Racial and geographic variations in type and incidence of defect add to the difficulties in assessing the overall frequency of fetal malformations. It seems that identifying an increase or decrease in the number of cases of a particular anomaly would be useful, as would a determination of the reasons for its changing prevalence. Cataloging the types of defects found in rural as compared to urban settings might facilitate the identification of local causative factors. Parental age, parity, and other factors which are known or believed to have a teratogenic (anomaly-producing) influence are being investigated.

No statistics can express the emotional costs experienced by affected children and their family members at the time of diagnosis and during the often prolonged and uncertain treatment, nor can they describe the physical and mental handicaps with which some children survive. The birth of a child always imposes changes upon the family (see Chap. 8), but the impact is especially forceful when the newborn has some kind of congenital anomaly. Clearly, fetal malformations affect a staggering number of children and families each year. In addition, enormous monetary and health manpower expenditures are involved in the innumerable diagnostic measures and surgical procedures which are performed, the repeated hospitalizations which are required, and the rehabilitative services to afflicted infants and children as they strive to survive and to overcome a multiplicity of handicapping conditions. Each year children with birth defects spend approximately 6 million days in hospitals at a cost in excess of 180 million dollars.

Although many birth defect victims experience recurring medical or surgical difficulties, their survival rate and rehabilitative potential have improved remarkably in the last 12 to 15 years, with the result that great numbers of these infants and children can live useful, productive lives. The demands and challenges for nurses and other health-team mem-

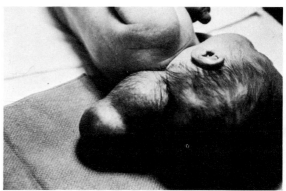

Figure 19-1 Occipital encephalocele. An example of a neural tube defect.

bers who work with birth defective children and families are overwhelming at times, but the overall rewards and satisfaction experienced can be most gratifying.

TYPES OF MALFORMATIONS

Intrauterine growth deviations may be simple or complex and hence are divided into two large categories. An anomaly which affects anatomic structure and threatens survival of the neonate is called a *major defect*. Transposition of the great vessels of the heart is an example, as is a neural tube defect such as encephalocele (Fig. 19-1). There are some severe anomalies which are incompatible with life despite present-day treatment; for example, anencephaly is usually fatal soon after delivery. Medical or surgical intervention improves the high-risk status of birth defective neonates, but the extent of the defect, the organ or organs involved, and the time interval between delivery and repair may be contributing factors to residual handicapping conditions.

There are many conditions which have a congenital basis and which, although present at the time of birth, may not become evident until later in infancy, early childhood, adolescence, or possibly even adulthood. Examples of anomalies which are not likely to be detected at birth are congenital hip and color blindness. Defects which are not life-threatening are classified as *minor defects*. Such a categorization does not mean that identifying or recording their presence is unimportant. On the contrary, such notations are most important, for minor anomalies, in addition to requiring therapeutic intervention to permit the best possible development of the affected child, may also be indicative of other, internal malformations not previously diagnosed.

THE INTERDISCIPLINARY TEAM IN HEALTH-CARE DELIVERY

The greatly improved prognosis of newborns with fetal malformations is primarily due to two factors which have had a phenomenal impact not only on survival but also on the involved child's eventual productivity. The first of these factors was the institution of the interdisciplinary team approach in health care delivery. The second was the recognition of the interaction of the financial, social, and psychologic problems which are associated with handicapping conditions.

When congenital defects cause chronic handicap or disability, as is often the case, intensive supportive health care is necessary over a period of years. An interdisciplinary team approach is essential if the child and his family are to receive the comprehensive care that can support maximum rehabilitation and optimum health maintenance. Physiotherapists, physicians of several specialties, prosthetists, nutritionists, social workers, special educators, and representatives of crippled children's and family services groups, among still others, have the expertise to provide the services appropriate. An important feature of the team is that its members change as patient needs change. For example, as a youngster nears school age a teacher usually becomes an integral part of the group.

It is the responsibility of the team to assess the needs of the child and family members and to provide for those needs as thoroughly as resources permit. Effective communication is imperative, both among the members of the team and between the professionals and the family. The team must be sensitive to what the mother and father are experiencing. They must also be sensitive to one another's needs, for these are situations in which one team member derives needed support from another in their joint endeavor to help the family.

As the team works together, the coordinator role is assumed as needed among the several members. For example, in one family or at a particular time the coordinator may be a physician; in another instance it may be a nurse, social worker, psychologist, or some other person.

A nurse is in a most enviable position, for he gives direct care to the patient and therefore has extensive contact with the child and the parents in addition to collaborating with others on the health team. If he is to be an effective professional and if he is to use his unique skills for the patient's greatest advantage, he must be an active team participant.

The knowledge he gains from working so closely with the family frequently makes it appropriate that he be the person who coordinates the team's activities. The interdisciplinary approach to health care delivery assures a patient of the highest quality of professional services.

CAUSES OF FETAL MALFORMATIONS

According to the National Foundation—March of Dimes, an organization committed to an investigation of birth defects, several factors are known to produce malformations of the developing fetus. About 20 percent of the known deviations occur as a result of environmental influences on the fetus. Another 20 percent can be traced to genetic traits in one or both parents. The remaining 60 percent appear to be caused by an interaction of the environmental and hereditary influences. Most human malformations, then, are due to a combination of internal factors present in the fertilized egg and external factors which may affect its growth in utero.

It is the environmental influences which have been the major focus of nurses' and most other health professionals' attention. These external influences are controllable in many instances so that birth defects can be prevented, and sometimes the preventive measure is as simple as prenatal counseling about the use of medications or protecting oneself and susceptible others from avoidable X-irradiation. The three main groups of environmental teratogens are viruses, drugs, and radiation. Ironically, these three pose little or no threat to the pregnant woman but can have devastating effects on her unborn child.

Viruses

Before discussing some facts related to viruses and birth defects, it is important to make a distinction between a congenital *disease* caused by a persistent fetal infection and a congenital *malformation* which may result from the teratogenic action of the infectious organism. An infant born with an infection may or may not be malformed. Whether or not a prenatal infection produces deformities depends upon the nature of the infectious organism, the developmental stage of the embryo or fetus at the time it is exposed to the organism (see Chaps. 8 and 20), other factors such as the mother's antibody titer, and probably still other variables not yet understood. In the case of a baby who is both infected and anomalous, the malformation, of course, may or may not be related to his infection. Finally, an infant with a birth defect due to an infectious organism may or may not have the infection at the time of birth.

The classic example of a prenatal infection which is known to cause fetal malformations is rubella. The initial discovery of the teratogenic potential of viruses was an outgrowth of a rubella epidemic. An Australian, Gregg, reported in 1941 his observation that large numbers of women exposed to rubella early in their pregnancies delivered anomalous infants. In 1964 when the rubella epidemic swept across the United States, about 30,000 fetal deaths and 20,000 live births of congenitally malformed infants were attributed to rubella during pregnancy. The incidence and type of anomaly depended upon the gestational age of the fetus at the time of the maternal infection. The earlier the mother contracted the disease, the greater the likelihood that her baby would be affected. About 50 percent of the mothers infected in the first month of pregnancy produced infants with abnormalities, as did about 22 percent of those who contracted the virus during the second month and 7 percent who were infected during the third month.[2] These women delivered babies with congenital cataracts, deafness, congenital heart disease, and developmental brain disfunctions such as mental retardation.

Since 1962, when it became possible to isolate the rubella virus, it has become know that infants of women who had rubella during pregnancy carry and can transmit the virus for perhaps as long as 12 to 14 months after birth. Such babies are a source of rubella infection for all nonimmune persons with whom they come in contact. This fact has obvious implications for all females of childbearing age, including nursing personnel who care for these babies during hospitalization.

The rubella virus's capacity to produce birth defects has been established beyond question. Yet to be proved or disproved is the hypothesis of some investigators that infants conceived 1 year or more after maternal infection with rubella can be born with anomalies.[3] The possibility of a maternal carrier state has prompted some physicians to advise women not to become pregnant for about 18 months after exposure to rubella.

As a result of research demonstrating that the reinfection rate for rubella is higher in adults than in children, the question has arisen as to whether immunity produced by infection with this virus is lifelong. Of particular concern are pregnant women who had childhood rubella, who have low levels of serum antibodies to the virus, and who come in contact with currently infected persons. Reinfection

of those women could be potentially hazardous to the fetus.[4]

Another virus which appears to distort fetal development is cytomegalovirus. In crossing the placental barrier it initiates a chronic infection in the fetus. Some obstetric investigators believe that fetal infection occurs regardless of the trimester of pregnancy in which the mother contracts the virus. Common deviations known to result from cytomegalovirus infection include microcephaly, hydrocephaly, chorioretinitis with microphthalmia and blindness, mental retardation and other kinds of cerebral dysfunction, and visceral and skeletal malformations. Current evidence suggests that the prevalence of undiagnosed cytomegalovirus infection is much greater than previously realized, and there is reason to believe that this virus may eventually be shown to be responsible for a substantial number of births of anomalous babies. Other viruses are suspected of producing fetal malformations, but the whole area of viruses as teratogens is still incompletely understood.

Drugs

Drugs, taken alone or in combination, are known to account for a small percentage of infants born with fetal malformations. Several specific drugs have been proven to be teratogenic; others have been heavily implicated, and drugs in general are felt to carry such a potential for damaging the embryo or fetus (possible production of birth defects is only one of the hazards) that their use during pregnancy is strongly discouraged.

The teratogenic potential of drugs became known after the birth, in 1961 and 1962, of thousands of German infants with gross abnormalities of the extremities. The deformity or absence of limbs (phocomelia), occurred in practically all offspring of women who had used the sedative thalidomide during the early part of their pregnancies (Fig. 19-2). Subsequent investigations showed conclusively a cause-and-effect relationship between maternal use of the sedative and fetal development of deformities. With the aim of avoiding another such tragedy, the United States Food and Drug Administration tightened its regulations regarding the release of new drugs for human use. The thalidomide experience clearly demonstrated the dangers of medicines during pregnancy.

Certain anticonvulsant medications are suspected of being teratogenic because of repeated instances of cleft lip or palate, or both, seen in in-

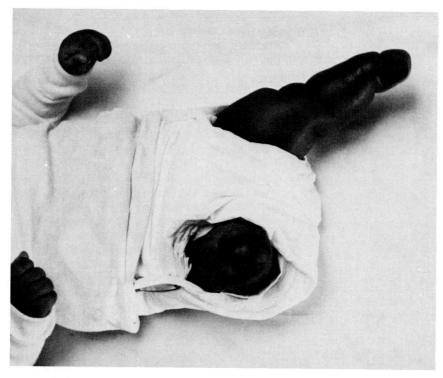

Figure 19-2 A child with phocomelia.

fants whose epileptic mothers took specific medications during their pregnancies.[5] Some newborns also demonstrated cardiac anomalies, in addition to facial defects. But since many women receive these medications during pregnancy without ill effect, controlled investigations are needed before anticonvulsant drugs suspected of damaging fetuses can be positively identified.

Some other pharmaceutical products which also may have potential teratogenic properties when given to pregnant women in the first trimester include diethylstilbesterol and ergonovine maleate.[6,7] Aminopterin, a folic acid antagonist used in the treatment of cancer, has resulted in severe skeletal malformations in the offspring of research animals.[8]

In today's drug culture, a word should be said about the use of hallucinogenic substances in pregnancy and the attendant danger of a malformed infant. Several drugs are being investigated, and in some instances the results have already been published. There are conflicts regarding the conclusions reached. For example, Zellweger reported chromatid breaks in peripheral white blood cells of lysergic acid diethylamide (LSD) users, and when these pregnant women delivered, their neonates demonstrated anomalies of the lower extremeties.[9]

On the other hand, Gardner collected data which revealed no damage to the chromosomes of mothers who admitted using LSD and who also delivered infants with abnormalities.[10] Bloom suggests that "street" LSD may contain one or more contaminants which could be responsible for chromosomal breakage, in addition to factors thus far unknown which might be related to drug use.[11] Another investigator has reported the presence of cyanotic heart disease in the offspring of women who used LSD early in pregnancy.[12] It is apparent that more extensive study is needed before the question of teratogenic properties of LSD or other hallucinogens can be answered. Knowledge about a possible relationship between amphetamine use and birth defects is similarly inconclusive at this time. There is evidence that at least some of the amphetamines may be associated with cardiac anomalies in human offspring.[13]

The teratogenic properties of drugs are difficult to assess. It appears that a drug with an inherent potential to produce congenital malformations may nevertheless not do so unless other conditions are present, such as perhaps a hereditary predisposition on the part of the developing child to respond to that chemical influence.

Radiation

Studies relating radiation and fetal impairment have shown beyond any doubt that radiation causes birth defects. Unfortunately, the greatest amount of damage occurs before the sixth week of embryonic life, which often is before the pregnancy is suspected. The earlier the exposure, the more extensive is the fetal damage. Exposure at later gestational stages may result in less apparent deviations.

Some common disorders which may be seen in neonates irradiated during development include midline malformations of the central nervous system (such as spina bifida, meningomyelocele, anencephaly, and microcephaly,) cataracts, and mental retardation.

The risk of fetal damage should always be considered when radiologic studies are being conducted on pregnant or possibly pregnant females. It would appear to be particularly dangerous, for example, to do radioisotope studies on a woman in the last half of her menstrual cycle because of the possibility of a pregnancy. If radiologic studies are unavoidable, then a physician should advise the woman of the possibility that fetal damage may result. In each instance, the right of the woman to have an abortion should be respected.

Frequently nurses in pediatrics accompany youngsters to radiology for diagnostic studies. Although nurses are most helpful in supporting the child and hence in obtaining the necessary roentgenograms, care should be taken (by having them wear a lead apron or stand behind a lead screen) that they are protected from possible radiation exposure.

Atmospheric or environmental radiocontamination also contributes to the risk of fetal deviations. This is a frustrating area of concern, for there is very little human control over contamination which occurs after nuclear accidents or the testing of nuclear weapons. The disastrous effects of radiocontamination were dramatically documented by the atomic bombing of Nagasaki and Hiroshima.

It has been said with respect to viruses and drugs that the majority of fetal malformations cannot be simplistically attributed to a single cause; this is also true of radiation. The dangers of large doses of radiation to the embryo are known, but the effects of smaller doses are not known conclusively.

GENETIC COUNSELING

Persons who have hereditary disorders, who come from families in which someone else has some inherited defect, or who have previously produced a child with a congenital anomaly generally have a higher than usual probability of producing a congenitally defective child. For some disorders it is possible to calculate the risk of transmitting the defect to subsequently conceived children. Prospective parents should have access to genetic counseling to give them information upon which to make a decision about whether to have their own children or adopt, or whether to continue or terminate an existing pregnancy. Likewise, genetic counseling should be made available to the affected individual and his siblings as they approach marriage and parenthood. On occasion, other relatives also desire such information.

A positive diagnosis of hereditary disorder must be established before counseling is begun. An extensive family history in pedigree form is essential. Attention is also given to environmental influences which may explain the presence of the defect. Physical examinations on all family members are usually required, but karyotype studies are not done routinely before the initial counseling session. Once the genetic evaluation has been completed, the couple is referred for counseling. Whether the counseling is conducted at one of more than 200 centers listed by the National Foundation—March of Dimes or in the office of a physician depends entirely on the availability of resources within a community.

It is important to remember that genetic advice should not be given too soon after the birth of a deformed infant, for parents' response to the birth may interfere with their understanding of what is said. Timing, therefore, is a most important variable. Any information which is given should be geared also to the educational background of the persons involved. The facts being shared are difficult for many parents to comprehend, even under the best circumstances, and when unfamiliar terminology is used, greater confusion results.

Although there is a dilemma regarding the credentials of the counselor or the number of sessions necessary, some generalizations can be made. The strongest motivator for seeking advice and using it is the physician who makes the diagnosis and cares for the patient, but many doctors are not involved in or concerned with counseling.[14] Genetic counselors who ultimately work with families are generally unknown to the parents who seek their services. This fact alone produces some apprehension which, when coupled with the topic to be discussed, commonly results in a high level of anxiety.

More than one counseling session is advantageous, for parents may be confused and overwhelmed by the information they receive at the initial conference. A second visit provides an opportunity to discuss anxieties, fears, and feelings of guilt which the parents were reluctant to verbalize previously. The second session allows the counselor to assess parental interpretation and understanding of the information given at the earlier meeting. Such a visit also provides an opportunity for identifying social welfare and volunteer agencies which may assist and support families in adjusting to the chronic disability of their child.

Several options are available to parents who have been counseled. There are several alternatives they may wish to explore, especially if the risk of having a defective child is high and the malformation is serious. If they decide to have no children, contraception is one option; sterilization is another. Adoption is a possibility if there is a desire to increase the family.

Occasionally parents elect to take the risk of pregnancy. In those cases a transabdominal amniocentesis can be performed before the 14th week of gestation for the management of genetic high-risk patients. This procedure makes it possible to diagnose some abnormalities early in pregnancy; however, a woman may be faced with making a decision about abortion if a defect or an inborn error of metabolism is discovered. At the present time, chromosomal disorders as well as metabolic errors such as galactosemia, glycogen storage disease, maple sugar urine disease, Tay-Sachs disease, Hurler's syndrome, Niemann-Pick disease, and Hunter's syndrome can be diagnosed by amniocentesis.

Genetic Counseling and the Nurse

When a deformed baby is born, the nurse is one professional who has contact with the infant as well as the parents. After the initial shock and disbelief, parents have many questions to ask. It is very important for them to talk with someone who is comfortable in discussing their baby's anomaly. They need to verbalize their fears and apprehensions with someone who understands.

Although parents are familiar with physicians and other health professionals, meeting with a genetic counselor will be a new experience for them. They may need some assistance in formulating appropriate questions. It may be difficult to identify specific areas which are of greatest concern to them and their family. A nurse can help them know what to anticipate and lower their anxiety level and make the counseling a better experience.

Attending the counseling session helps the nurse to be maximally effective as a liaison between the genetic counselor and the family. Hearing what is said to the parents facilitates the nurse's reiteration of the information which the counselor gives the parents. Questions can be answered more adequately, and elaborating on the information given can be done more easily. A nurse can recognize the need for additional counseling conferences and can direct parents to family planning centers, adoption agencies, or social welfare organizations.

The way in which parents make use of the information they are given is a personal determination they must make without professional intervention. The decision not to have children, to terminate a pregnancy, or to risk having an anomalous baby is usually a difficult one. Nurses can assist by referring parents or prospective parents for genetic counseling and by helping them collect and interpret information upon which to base their decision. Genetic counseling is expensive and its use is primarily confined to those who can afford it, but nursing can be instrumental in identifying those families found in the hospital or community who need the service and to whom it should be offered.

Currently nursing involvement in genetics and genetic counseling is limited. But the scope of the problem is immense, as are the implications for nursing. Hopefully a better understanding of fetal malformations and of their consequences will precipitate a greater number of referrals to geneticists and genetic counseling centers as well as more active nursing participation in this emerging field of specialization. A nurse has the education, the experience, and the contact with involved persons to make a substantial contribution in decreasing the number of babies born with fetal malformations or impaired intellect.

THE NURSE AND INTERHOSPITAL TRANSPORTATION

Early identification of the health problems of an infant with fetal malformations increases his chance for survival. The nurse in assessing, monitoring, and evaluating the neonate is in the position to detect an anomaly early. Observation of the newborn in a nursery should be done conscientiously, for as the infant adjusts to his new, external environment, problems in adaptation may become apparent and birth defects may be identified.

Some newborns with birth defects are critically ill. They may need to be transported to medical centers or to specialized pediatric hospitals where highly sophisticated diagnostic procedures and techniques can be performed and where the expensive, complex equipment imperative for survival is available. Skilled health team members at these centers have the knowledge and expertise essential for dealing with the very special problems of an acutely ill neonate. When a newborn needs to be transferred, consideration of his physical status, of the equipment of the transporting vehicle, and of the coordination of administrative details between the hospitals contributes to the safety and efficiency with which the transfer is completed. Transfer has become relatively common, and some states now support neonatal programs designed to transfer infants safely in specially equipped helicopters, airplanes, or ambulances.

The Physical Status of the Infant

When an acutely ill infant is to be transferred, provision should be made to ensure that the trip will be safe and that there will be no appreciable deterioration of the infant's condition. It is especially important to prevent or immediately recognize hypoxia, hypoglycemia, hypothermia, and aspiration, since all may contribute to the patient's demise.

Because of their high metabolic rate, newborns are susceptible to hypoglycemia, especially if they are not fed by mouth during the first few hours of life. The symptoms of hypoglycemia (see Chap. 20) should be familiar to all professionals who work with newborns. Some physicians start a 10 percent glucose intravenous solution to prevent the occurrence of hypoglycemia during transport.

Hypoxia must be prevented. Oxygen, if necessary, should be administered by mask, incubator, or assisted ventilation. Transporting a newborn with an endotracheal tube in place is particularly difficult; the tube may be dislodged in the course of moving, resulting in further distress. Adequate oxygenation decreases neonatal stress and prevents cerebral damage which may impair intellectual function.

Hypothermia is a major hazard to the neonate. The thermoregulatory mechanism of his central nervous system is immature, and unless he is protected against loss of body heat, he tends to assume the environmental temperature. Even moderate hypothermia is poorly tolerated by the newborn. The best means of ensuring temperature maintenance is a heated incubator with its own self-contained power pack or a warming unit for automotive currents. Blankets with an inner layer of aluminum foil are also effective in reducing heat loss.

Positioning remains an important measure for preventing aspiration. The baby should be kept on either side or on his abdomen in the process of being transported. As always, the patient's physical problem dictates which is the best position for him. If the newborn has a tracheoesophageal fistula, for example, he must be kept in a sitting position to decrease the possibility of aspiration and the development of pneumonia which would require postponement of surgery. Similarly, an infant with an omphalocele (Fig. 19-3) is kept on his back with his head to the side.

On occasion, intravenous fluid therapy is begun before the infant leaves the hospital. The infusion site should be chosen carefully. A scalp vein appears to be most suitable, for there is no interference when the body position is adjusted. The baby also is allowed freedom to move his head from side to side without the danger of infiltration, which is not the case if the site is in an extremity.

The Transporting Vehicle

Several hours of travel may be required for interhospital transport when an ambulance is used; therefore, the ambulance must be adequately equipped for safe transfer, and all the equipment must be in working order. There must be an adequate supply of oxygen, including supplemental tanks for use in case the vehicle is delayed by mechanical difficulty. A warming unit for automotive currents as well as a suction apparatus should be in working order. No ambulance should be used unless it has adequate equipment to handle routine and emergency situations which might arise during transport.

Nursing Management

All pertinent information should accompany the infant as he goes from one hospital to another. A nurse who accompanies the baby shares with the receiving health team members what has transpired since birth. The report should include the maternal history, the infant's status at delivery (including his Apgar score), and his behavior in the nursery. The data accumulated up to the time the baby is received in the referral hospital will serve as a baseline against which to assess his subsequent status.

If it is not possible for a nurse to accompany the patient, a set of written notes, complete in every detail, should identify problems, report observations, and state the sequence of pertinent events. Another alternative, which is more personal and more informative, is a telephone conversation with the head

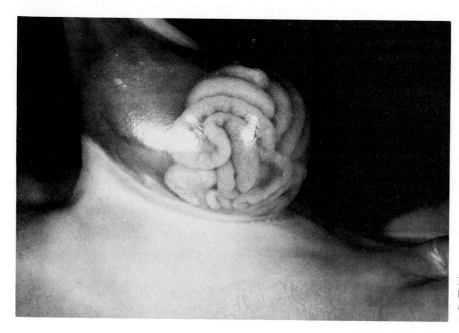

Figure 19-3 Omphalocele. Portions of the bowel and liver are herniated through the umbilicus.

nurse of the pediatric ward to which the patient will be admitted. The nursing assessment with its observations and evaluations is usually graciously and appreciably accepted by those who will be responsible for caring for the baby. A phone report informs the nurses at the receiving station of the baby's status at the beginning of transport, and it also allows them time to assemble equipment they will need for him.

Often in the hurried arrangements for interhospital transport, legal consent forms and signatures for required surgery are overlooked. Consequently, surgery will have to be postponed until permission for the procedure is obtained. If the father accompanies the baby there is no problem, but there are situations in which he elects to remain with his wife. On those occasions, arrangements for telegram permissions or other legal forms acceptable to the receiving hospital will need to be made.

The transfer of a critically ill newborn involves the combined, coordinated efforts of many people in two health care facilities. Transfer needs to be done without delay and without needless administrative impediments. Although the ambulance or helicopter ride has a traumatizing effect on any neonate, whether it contributes to a deteriorating health status in the case of an ill newborn depends on the professional forethought in planning the move.

Parents whose infants are moved to referral centers are forced to accept separation almost im-

mediately after birth. Also, they may have to travel long distances to see their infants. Both factors preclude early or frequent contact with their baby. The personnel of obstetric units as well as the receiving hospitals need to be aware of the psychologic and emotional impact on the parents of these children.

REFERENCES

1 Victoria P. Coffey, "Monitoring of Congenital Defects," *Journal of the Irish Medical Association*, 66(5):131–134, March 10, 1973.
2 L. W. Catalano and J. Sever, "The Role of Viruses As Causes of Congenital Defects," *Annual Review of Microbiology*, 25:270, 1971.
3 S. A. Plotkin and W. J. Mellman, "Rubella in the Distant Past As a Possible Cause of Congenital Malformations," *American Journal of Obstetrics and Gynecology*, 108(3):387, Oct. 1, 1971.
4 R. L. Northrup, "Rubella Reinfection during Early Pregnancy," *Obstetrics and Gynecology*, 39(4):524–526, April 1972.
5 J. Wilson, "Present Status of Drugs As Teratogens in Man," *Teratology*, 7(1):7, February 1973.
6 B. MacMahon, "Etiology of Congenital Defects," *New England Journal of Medicine*, 287(10):514, Sept. 7, 1972.
7 T. David, "Nature of Etiology of the Poland Anomaly," *New England Journal of Medicine*, 287(10):487–489, Sept. 7, 1972.
8 J. Warkany, *Congenital Malformations*, Year Book Medical Publishers, Inc., Chicago, 1971, p. 96.
9 H. Zellweger et al., "Is Lysergic Acid Diethylamide

(LSD) a Teratogen?'' *Lancet*, no. 7525, p. 1066, Nov. 18, 1967.

10 L. Gardner et al., ''Deformities in a Child Whose Mother Took LSD,'' *Lancet*, no. 7659, p. 1290, June 13, 1970.

11 A. D. Bloom, ''Induced Chromosomal Aberrations—Biological and Clinical Significance,'' *Journal of Pediatrics*, 81(1):1–8, July 1972.

12 V. Pilapil, R. A. Hays, and O. E. Ehrhardt, ''LSD and Cyanotic Heart Disease,'' *Journal of the American*

Medical Women's Association, 28(3):131–132, March 1973.

13 J. T. Nora et al., ''Dexamphetamine: A Possible Trigger in Cardiovascular Malformations,'' *Lancet*, no. 7659, p. 1290, June 13, 1970.

14 Claire O. Leonard, G. Chase, and B. Childs, ''Genetic Counseling: A Consumer's View,'' *New England Journal of Medicine*, 287(9):433, Aug. 31, 1972.

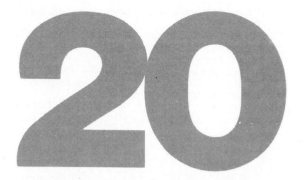

THE HIGH-RISK INFANT AND FAMILY

JULIA R. St. PETERY

The high-risk infant is a newborn who has a higher than average chance of perinatal morbidity or mortality because of predisposing maternal, obstetric, or maturational conditions. Threats to the newborn can also be classified into antepartum, intrapartum, and postpartum factors, according to when they occur in relation to birth. These risk-producing conditions are numerous and diverse. They may be related, such as maternal diabetes and prematurity, or unrelated, such as maternal drug addiction and breech birth. Indeed, many babies born under one or more of these ominous conditions turn out to be healthy, unaffected infants. Conversely, even the best planned pregnancies, with good prenatal care and an uncomplicated delivery, may produce a seriously ill or defective baby.

The common characteristic among the conditions discussed in this chapter is the empirically observed and statistically significant correlation they share with an increase in infant morbidity and mortality. In the cumulative experience of obstetrics and pediatrics, these conditions have come to be recognized as *absolute red flags*, signaling danger to the newborn. These flags are never to be ignored, but must always alert physician and nurse to the special needs of these babies.

With the increased recognition of these perinatal hazards, there has been a rise in the number of referral centers having both obstetric facilities for the complex delivery and intensive care nursery for the baby delivered. The recent and rapid development of neonatology is partly due to growing awareness that sick newborns require a very specialized and continuous care system. The professional who chooses the intensive care nursery must have many specialized skills, including resuscitation, suctioning, operative technique, and equipment operation. Above all, nursery personnel must daily polish a keen power of observation, for anticipation often leads to an early diagnosis which may be the deciding factor in the life of the sickly newborn. Professional nursery personnel also bear the responsibility of keeping abreast of a vastly broad and rapidly progressing flood of knowledge, and of selecting those technical advances best utilized in a particular nursery. With this combination of specialized nursing, up-to-date neonatology, and the best of technology, the intensive care nursery is becoming the only place for the high-risk infant. Such an infant should therefore be delivered in or rapidly transported to a hospital with such a facility.

Before discussing high-risk conditions in detail, it is necessary to define certain terms. As the field of neonatology grows, even basic terms are constantly being expanded and revised. However, for the ensuing discussion, definitions will be as follows:

fetal death the death of the fetus before it is delivered, regardless of its gestational age
immature infant a liveborn premature infant with a birth weight of less than 1,000 Gm (2 lb, 3 oz)
infant mortality the death of an infant within the first year of life
low-birth-weight infant a liveborn infant of less than 2,500 Gm (5 lb, 8 oz), regardless of gestational age
neonatal death the death of an infant within the first 28 days of life
perinatal mortality the combined fetal and neonatal deaths resulting from gestations of 28 weeks or longer
premature infant (also called **preterm infant**) a liveborn infant with a gestational age of less than 37 weeks, regardless of birth weight

The predisposing factors included here are by no means all-inclusive; this chapter is meant to serve merely as an introduction and guide. One of the major areas omitted is that of congenital malformations, which are discussed in Chapter 19 and Part 4.

ANTENATAL FACTORS

Even before pregnancy begins, there are factors that statistically threaten the baby. These include the mother's social and economic background, her age, and her previous obstetric history.

Socioeconomic Factors

There is much evidence that the socially and economically deprived are far more likely to have high-risk babies. This is partially explained in their isolation from adequate prenatal care, which could otherwise diagnose and correct or ameliorate problems in pregnancies. One of the major skeletons in the American health care closet is the sorely wanting health needs of the core cities and rural poor. Even with inroads into these areas, the unborn fetus, unseen and unheard, is likely to be given low priority for diagnostic and preventive care.

In addition to lack of antenatal care, poverty predisposes to malnutrition. Animal studies demonstrate that various forms of maternal malnutrition result in fetal loss (abortion) and lowered birth weights. The evidence in human beings is somewhat confusing, for much data of the past has supported the statement that ". . . the human fetus seems to be largely protected from the deleterious effects of maternal malnutrition."[1] However, there is little doubt that fetal loss and low birth weight are greatly increased in impoverished populations, and it has long

been assumed that malnutrition was the causative factor. This is best exemplified by the severe protein-calorie deficiencies seen in underdeveloped countries, where women with this form of malnutrition have been shown to have increased rates of fetal wastage and low-birth-weight newborns.[2]

Recently great interest has focused on the effect of maternal malnutrition on the growth of the fetal brain, since studies have revealed a lowered intellectual achievement in a significant fraction of low-birth-weight babies. In human beings, the brain is thought to undergo its most rapid growth during the last trimester of pregnancy and up to about the second year of life.[3] It is postulated that because the brain has intensified needs during this rapid growth it is much more susceptible to deprivation of nutrients and thus may suffer indelible retardation if deprived within this period.

An awareness that there may also be more subtle aspects of undernutrition has led many American obstetricians to lessen their restrictions on weight gain in pregnant women, since very small or negative weight gains have been associated with an increase in fetal loss and complications. Likewise, an interest has arisen in the diet of the pregnant teenager, for it may be deficient because of poverty or poor food habits or because this young mother is still growing herself and must support her own growth as well as that of the rapidly growing fetus. Concern has also evolved for the diets of women before they ever become pregnant, for pre-pregnancy diet affects gestational food habits and the mother's metabolic reserves.

While researchers try to clarify the precise mechanisms by which maternal undernutrition affects the fetus, the education toward and provision for adequate prenatal diet are doubtlessly of extreme importance.

National and racial origins are influential. The northern European countries lead the world with the lowest rates of infant mortality. The United States has placed surprisingly far behind (fourteenth place) in recent years, which is especially distressing to those who view infant mortality as an accurate index of a society's general well-being. Shapiro attributes these high rates to recent increases in birth rates among very young mothers and mothers of very high parity, and especially to an increase in nonwhite premature births.[4] In contrast, the Japanese have an excellent rate, even Japanese living in the United States. Blacks and American Indians suffer the highest infant mortality rates in the United States; this is no doubt a reflection of their economic deprivation and its incumbent penalties.

The occupation of the father has been shown to correlate with pregnancy outcome; the higher the father's income, the less likely a perinatal disaster. Especially at risk are those pregnancies without an identified father, for these most often represent the unplanned and illegitimate pregnancies, which are highest among the poor and the young.

Age of the Mother

The reproductive years, physiologically demarcated by ovulation, are heralded by menarche and dismissed with menopause. Most babies are born to mothers between 20 and 30 years of age. Because of irregular ovulation at the beginning and end of the reproductive span, the earliest and latest years are relatively sterile. However, it is also then, before approximately age 16 and after 40, that one sees a great increase in maternal complications. The very young mother is known to have a higher incidence of toxemia and illegitimate and low-birth-weight babies. The rate of neonatal mortality is highest in mothers under 19 years, next highest in mothers over 35 years, and lowest in mothers 25 to 30 years old.

Previous Obstetric History

For the nurse as well as for the physician, the most important factor in the previous obstetric history of the mother is prior fetal loss. As the number of prior stillbirths increases, so does the chance of another subsequent perinatal loss. A woman who has had three or more prior fetal deaths has about one chance in three of another perinatal loss. This repetitive loss might be expected in maternal diabetes or severe Rh isoimmunization, but the cause is obscure in many cases. Among the causes sought in such women are the following:

1 Uterine tumors (myomas, fibroids)
2 Developmental uterine anomalies (bicornuate uterus)
3 Incompetent cervix
4 Dietary deficiencies

If found, some of these etiologic conditions can be remedied.

Maternal Disorders

Once conceived, the fetus is a captive to the maternal milieu. If the milieu is abnormal, the growth and very existence of the fetus are challenged. The alteration of maternal physiology may be permanent, as in diabetes or heart disease. It may be peculiar to pregnancy, as with toxemia. Then again, it may represent a transient noxious agent, such as an infection, which happens to affect mother and therefore baby at an inopportune time. Most systemic maternal afflictions affect the baby as well.

Maternal Diabetes Mellitus Prior to the advent of insulin in the 1920s, most diabetic women did not reproduce. Today, with appropriate management, many diabetics give birth. Although diabetic mothers have essentially the same low maternal mortality as other women, their offspring still suffer a high perinatal mortality of 10 to 30 percent. The diabetic mother may be a growth-onset, insulin-dependent diabetic (also known as a juvenile diabetic), or merely a mild, asymptomatic gestational diabetic, whose glucose tolerance is normal between pregnancies. The severity of the maternal diabetes appears to greatly increase the number of stillbirths but not the outcome of the liveborn infants. That is, insulin-dependent diabetics are more likely to have stillbirths than their gestational diabetic sisters, but the liveborn babies of both groups are subject to similar problems. White has classified maternal diabetes into stages of severity and related these categories to the chances of fetal salvage.[5]

No one knows for sure why diabetics' babies die in utero. Some investigators feel that maternal ketoacidosis is the cause. It is also known that diabetic mothers have a greatly increased incidence of toxemia with all its complications, including stillbirths. The risk of intrauterine death is especially elevated in the last few weeks of gestation, possibly because of placental dysfunction, or the inability of a normal placenta to adequately service the often-large fetus. Because of increasing risk as term is approached, most diabetics are electively delivered at 36 to 38 weeks of gestation. Many diabetic mothers are now followed with serial urinary estriol levels, particularly in the last trimester. A falling level of this fetoplacental metabolite is considered evidence of fetal distress and an indication for prompt delivery. Delivery is frequently by cesarean section because of previous sections, a large baby (see below), or a cervix that is unfavorable for labor induction.

If intrauterine death is prevented, the diabetic progeny is still at increased risk. The majority are larger than average for their gestational age. Their largeness, termed *macrosomia* ("big body"), is thought to be partially secondary to maternal hyperglycemia. The typical baby of a diabetic mother is big, fat, plethoric, and balloon-cheeked (Fig. 20-1). Macrosomia may contribute to dystocia, difficult delivery, and resultant trauma such as intracranial

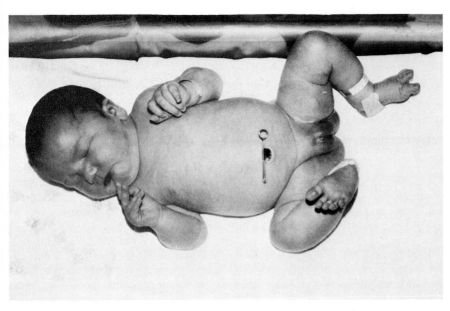

Figure 20-1 White female newborn of a diabetic mother. Born after 40 weeks' gestation, the baby weighed 10 lb, 3 oz. Notice the characteristic fat and plethora. The round, unmolded head is typical of infants delivered by cesarean section.

hemorrhage. The actual maturity of the infant correlates with gestational age rather than with birth weight. These babies, large though delivered early, are often referred to as "oversized premies."

In the first few days of life, the diabetic offspring is subject to several problems, including respiratory distress syndrome (RDS), hypocalcemia, and hyperbilirubinemia. The higher incidence of respiratory distress (discussed later in this chapter under the section on "Special Problems of Preterm Infants") may well relate to premature delivery and increased frequency of cesarean section, both of which predispose to respiratory distress syndrome. Even without classic RDS, diabetic progeny often have transient tachypnea in the first 3 days of life. The treatment and nursing care for RDS in these babies is essentially the same as for other newborns with the syndrome and is presented in Chapter 33.

Hypoglycemia, defined as a blood sugar level below 30 mg/100 ml, probably occurs in more than half of diabetic progeny. It is presumed to be secondary to maternal hyperinsulinism and/or fetal pancreatic overgrowth in response to maternal hyperglycemia. The nurse should assess for symptoms of hypoglycemia, which include jitteriness, tremors, cyanosis, and/or seizures, and which appear within the first 24 hours of life. Many nurseries try to prevent hypoglycemia by beginning oral feedings earlier and giving them more frequently to these babies. Once the infant is symptomatic or the blood sugar is less than 30 mg/100 ml, intravenous glucose is considered the best therapy. Prompt recognition of symptoms and institution of treatment are necessary because the brain requires glucose for its metabolism and may sustain permanent damage if deprived.

Hypocalcemia produces symptoms such as jitteriness, tremors, convulsions, and apnea. It usually responds to treatment with calcium salts (gluconate or lactate), given intravenously in a 10 percent solution for immediate therapy and orally in a 5 percent solution for long-term maintenance.

The hyperbilirubinemia of diabetic progeny is thought to be due to liver immaturity or inability to conjugate bilirubin; it occurs at 5 to 7 days of life, which is slightly later than the physiologic jaundice of full-term newborns. Like other plethoric babies, infants of diabetics probably present to their livers an increased load of hemoglobin breakdown products, namely, bilirubin. Since brain cells of the newborn may be permanently damaged by accumulations of this pigment, early recognition of jaundice and prompt treatment to reduce the bilirubin level are extremely important. Therapy may begin with phototherapy, but exchange transfusion is indicated if the bilirubin exceeds 20 mg/100 ml. (Phototherapy requires the constant use of eye patches to protect the child's eyes from injury by exposure to the light. The light can be turned off and the eye coverings removed for short parental visits.)

Toxemia Toxemia is a disorder of pregnancy which places both the pregnant or postpartum woman and her baby in jeopardy. It may occur any time between the 24th week of gestation and 2 weeks postpartum. Toxemia is a syndrome occurring in two major forms: preeclampsia and eclampsia. *Preeclampsia* includes high blood pressure, generalized edema, and proteinuria; if convulsions and/or coma also occur, it is termed *eclampsia*. Although peculiar to the pregnant or puerperal woman, toxemia exists much more frequently under certain conditions, including the following:

1 Primiparity (three times more often than in multiparity)
2 Underlying chronic hypertension or renal disease
3 Diabetes mellitus
4 Low socioeconomic background
5 Multiple births

Toxemia in the United States occurs as pre-eclampsia in approximately 6 to 7 percent of all pregnancies, and as eclampsia in less than 1 percent. It remains, along with hemorrhage and infection, a major cause of maternal mortality. According to Cavanagh and Talisman,[6] "Although largely preventable, toxemia of pregnancy is at present listed as the main single cause of maternal death in the United States. In this country, about 400 women and 30,000 babies are lost annually from this cause."

Because the exact cause of toxemia is unknown, antepartum treatment is directed at alleviating the symptoms by diet, salt restriction, bed rest, and antihypertensive and anticonvulsant medications. (Women treated at home require prompt referral to the community health nurse.) However, delivery itself is considered the only "cure" to stop the disease process. For this reason, preterm deliveries, either by spontaneous labor or by induction or cesarean section, are quite common in toxemic mothers.

The effects of toxemia on the baby are varied. Toxemia is thought of as a vascular disease, and in more severe forms leads to placental insufficiency and resultant chronic fetal distress and hypoxia. Compared to nontoxic mothers, the perinatal mortality is two to three times higher in preeclamptics and 40 times higher in eclamptics. This elevated mortality is mostly due to an increase in stillbirths, presumably from intrauterine hypoxia. The above-mentioned necessity for therapeutic preterm delivery adds to the hazards of prematurity. In addition, toxemia is also associated with placental abruption, with its own increased perinatal mortality and prematurity. The liveborn toxemic baby is often shorter and lighter than average for its gestational age and may be a classic malnourished "small-for-dates" baby. This newborn may be asphyxiated. He may also suffer effects from prenatally administered drugs aimed at controlling the mother's hypertension and seizures. These drugs include magnesium sulfate, paraldehyde, and barbiturates, which are known to cause lethargy and respiratory depression in the baby. In the nursery, the infant may also experience hypoglycemia. As for long-term prognosis, there are some follow-up studies which suggest that these babies have an inordinately high rate of physical and mental abnormalities in later life.

Narcotic Addiction With the increase in drug abuse in recent years, it is not surprising that the incidence of neonatal narcotic addiction has risen. Although many drugs are abused, heroin is the most common addicting drug causing symptoms in neonates. Heroin-addicted mothers who are on methadone maintenance programs are also at the same risk of giving birth to an addicted baby.

Heroin and methadone rapidly cross the placenta and thereby lead to fetal addiction. Since delivery literally severs the baby from his source, he is then in danger of developing the withdrawal syndrome.

Most of the symptoms of neonatal withdrawal occur within the first 4 days of life and include the following:

1 Hyperirritability (general increase in activity and responsiveness)
2 Coarse tremors
3 Shrill, high-pitched cry
4 Sneezing
5 Sweating
6 Vomiting and diarrhea
7 Ravenous appetite
8 Abrasions (from rubbing skin on sheets)

Clearly, some of the symptoms may suggest other causes, such as central nervous system damage, hypoglycemia, or hypocalcemia. All such symptoms require immediate diagnostic investigation.

Not all babies of addicted mothers will develop the withdrawal syndrome. Zelson et al. have shown a relationship between the nature of the mother's habit and the incidence of neonatal withdrawal:[7]

1 The incidence of withdrawal symptoms increases with the duration of the mother's habit; that is, the longer the mother has been addicted, the more likely the baby is to show withdrawal.
2 The incidence of withdrawal symptoms increases with the dose of heroin; the more the mother requires, the more likely her infant is to demonstrate the syndrome.

Without treatment, the symptoms previously mentioned progress to seizures, apnea, fever, dehydration, circulatory collapse, and death. In the era before treatment was known, the mortality of addicted babies was very high. Early therapy was replacement with paragoric or morphine, followed by gradual withdrawal. More recently, phenobarbital, chlorpromazine (Thorazine), and diazepam (Valium) are being used (separately) with good results. Diazepam must be used with caution in the newborn because it may displace bilirubin from albumin and thereby exacerbate hyperbilirubinemia. Other general supportive therapy includes admission to an intensive care nursery for close observation; quiet and darkened surroundings to decrease sensory stimulation and its attendant risk of seizures; and intravenous fluids if oral feedings are not tolerated. With treatment, the withdrawal symptoms decrease rapidly within 24 hours and usually disappear by 4 days.

Most addicted babies recover. But immaturity and low birth weight, the most common physical characteristics of addicts' babies, extract their usual high tolls. In Zelson's series of 384 babies, 49 percent were under 2,500 Gm (5 lb, 8 oz).[8] The babies who do not die of immaturity or unrelated complications have no evidence of increased physical handicaps. Although a great deal of interest and speculation has been focused on chromosomal breaks in users of *psychotropic* drugs, most series of *narcotic* addicts' babies show no increased rate of congenital anomalies above the general population. After these babies are discharged from the nursery, their fate is probably related to the sociocultural situation to which their mothers return.

Maternal-Fetal Blood Group Incompatibilities   If a fetus possesses red blood cell antigen which the mother does not possess, the escape of fetal red blood cells into the maternal circulation will cause the mother to produce antibodies against that fetal antigen. This process is the *isoimmunization* of the mother against her fetus. If the maternal antibodies cross the placenta in large enough numbers, they attach to the fetal red blood cell antigens and destroy the cells. The destruction of fetal red blood cells leads to increased fetal bone marrow production of young red blood cells, known as erythroblasts. From this pathophysiology is derived the term *erythroblastosis fetalis*, which is the most common cause of *hemolytic disease of the newborn*. The commonest cause of erythroblastosis fetalis is ABO incompatibility, but the most severe forms of the disease result from Rh incompatibility. Less than 2 percent of cases are due to minor blood factors such as Kell, E, and c.

The blood group incompatibilities and their diagnosis and therapy are discussed in Chapter 35.

While Rh isoimmunization has long been a major source of high-risk infants, the recent introduction of anti-D gamma globulin has so far been highly successful in preventing sensitization of unsensitized Rh negative mothers, and hopefully will reduce Rh disease to a rarity. ABO incompatibility, for which no prevention is yet available, fortunately is usually mild or amenable to therapy.

Infections   As already said, whatever threatens the mother threatens the baby. Microbes, including viruses, bacteria, and protozoans, by infecting the pregnant mother, may infect the fetus. However, a maternal infection does not necessarily mean that the fetus will also be infected. The two most frequent routes of fetal infection are across the placenta and through the mother's birth canal. Transplacental infection may occur if the microbe is circulating in the mother's blood, as in the case of rubella, cytomegalovirus (CMV), or syphilis. Also, if the mother has an infected genital tract, then after the rupture of membranes and during labor and delivery the fetus is intimately exposed to infected tissues, as with *Neisseria gonorrhoeae* and herpesvirus hominis. Thus, fetal infection may occur at any point in gestation or during its termination.

If fetal infection occurs early in gestation, there may be teratogenic (birth defect–producing) effects on the fetus, resulting in abnormal tissue development. During organogenesis, infection may stunt or cause inflammation of the organs. Because embryonic organs differentiate at varying points in gestation, the exact time of a teratogenic microbial infection may be critical in determining what organ is damaged. In general, the earlier the fetus is infected, the more severe the consequences. Most, if not all, known transplacental infections are thought to cause an increase in spontaneous abortions, stillbirths, low birth weights, and deformed or ill neonates. Those babies who are liveborn may have malformations or inflammation in any organ system, but the central nervous system (CNS) appears to bear the brunt of most infections. CNS manifestations may include microcephaly, hydrocephalus, cerebral calcifications, mental retardation, and seizures. The other organ frequently involved is the liver, with a varying picture of hepatomegaly, hepatitis, jaundice, and abnormal bleeding tendencies. These consequences are often amazingly similar, whether the infecting agent is viral (as in rubella, CMV, or herpes), bacterial (syphilis), or protozoan (*Toxoplasma*). Most of the infections contracted from the birth canal are bacterial (a notable exception is herpesvirus hominis) and affect the baby either by direct contact, as the eyes in gonorrhea, or systemically, as in aspiration pneumonia, sepsis, and meningitis. Localized infections of the skin and eyes are usually inconsequential if treated promptly. However, the systemic infections are much more difficult to control and have a much higher morbidity and mortality.

In general, all these recognized (and probably many more as yet unrecognized) infections have the terrible potential to kill or maim the fetus or neonate. Even the survivors have a statistically high chance of serious lifelong sequelae such as brain damage, blindness, or deafness. At present, there is little hope of reversing these disease processes. Prompt recognition, often by a nurse, and treatment of the maternal infection, as in syphilis, may allay fetal disease. However, all too often the infection in the mother is subclinical or undiagnosed. Even if diagnosed, no "cure" may exist. Clearly, preventing the infection in the mother is the logical goal. A notable example is vaccination against rubella—not merely to prevent the mild childhood disease but to prevent an infected child from infecting pregnant women. Also, if rubella vaccine immunity proves lasting, the protected little girls may become protected mothers during their reproductive years.

Much remains to be learned about these infections before a simple injection prevents them all; such is the task of concerned biologists, obstetricians, and neonatologists.

Rubella   Rubella virus, the causative agent of German measles, is also the cause of the congenital rubella syndrome. At present, it is the prototype of intrauterine viral infections. The door to our present knowledge was opened in 1941 when Gregg, an Australian ophthalmologist, first observed and reported the relationship between congenital cataracts and the occurrence of rubella in the mother's early pregnancy.

German measles is a common and innocuous exanthem of childhood, and only 15 to 20 percent of adults are not immune. However, as in other intrauterine infections, it is this nonimmune pregnant population which is at risk, because a primary infection and viremia of the mother may well lead to transplacental fetal infection.

With the finding of the technologic tools of virus isolation and serologic identification of rubella, the huge pool of data available in the unfortunate epidemic of 1964 threw much light on the pathogenesis of congenital rubella. It made clear that the timing of maternal infection is critical, and the highest rate of anomalies occurs when the mother contracts rubella in the first 8 weeks of pregnancy. The virus appears to have teratogenic powers as late as 16 to 18 weeks of gestation, but in general, the earlier the infection, the more severe and numerous the congenital defects. It is in the first trimester that organogenesis is most active. The virus appears to slow down the division of infected cells, thereby reducing the total number of cells in a given organ. This underdevelopment of cells is reflected in the high incidence of low-birth-weight babies manifesting this syndrome. Like other intrauterine infections, rubella presents a wide spectrum of clinical manifestations, including abortion, stillbirth, affected baby, or normal newborn.

One can divide the congenital rubella syndrome into the transient neonatal findings and the lasting stigmas of organ anomalies. At birth, these babies are classically of low birth weight, and may develop jaundice, petechiae, anemia, thrombocytopenia, and hepatosplenomegaly. The more lasting imprints of congenital rubella infection may be present at birth or appear later. Any baby may have any combination of anomalies, including the following:

Eyes: chorioretinitis, cataracts, glaucoma, microphthalmia
Heart: patent ductus arteriosus, pulmonary artery stenosis and coarctations, ventricular septal defect, atrial septal defect
Central nervous system: microcephaly, seizures, mental retardation
Ear: nerve deafness
Liver: hepatitis

Plainly, many of these problems can be life-threatening. Some infants succumb to bleeding diatheses in the nursery; others die of the complications of their defects. In general, of those babies with thrombocytopenia, one-third die in the first year of life. This statistic reflects the large toll rubella extracts. Those babies who survive may only manifest deafness, but many will have varying degrees of mental retardation and central nervous system damage.

The treatment of the baby is purely symptomatic or aimed at correcting the specific defect, such as cataract removal or cardiac surgery. Rubella babies are usually isolated in the hospital, since they may excrete the virus for months, thus acting as a potential source for more infections. There is no known medicinal redemption for the damage already done. Presently, the hope is in the prevention of this disease by immunizing the population against rubella, as previously stated.

Cytomegalovirus   Cytomegalovirus (CMV) is a DNA virus related to herpes, and it causes cytomegalic inclusion disease (CID). This infection is usually mild or inapparent in older children and adults but, like some other viral agents, wreaks havoc on the developing fetus. A majority of adults have antibodies to CMV; those women who do not are at risk of primary infection, which may include viremia and therefore transplacental transmission to the fetus. Although acquired CID may manifest itself in the adult as hepatitis or respiratory illness, it most often is subclinical and goes unnoticed. This fact has made it difficult to identify exposed pregnant women. Recently, prospective serologic studies in pregnant populations have helped pinpoint the time of maternal seroconversion and therefore the time of risk of transplacental infection.[9]

Infected babies are frequently born preterm and are often of low birth weight or small for gestational age. As in other intrauterine infections, there is a spectrum of clinical manifestations, ranging from normal to severely affected babies. The classic neonate may be indistinguishable from a baby infected with rubella or toxoplasmosis. He frequently presents with rapidly progressive jaundice, petechiae, hepatosplenomegaly, dyspnea, and convulsions. Those with severe disease often die within the first 2 weeks of life. Although a few survive, most of the surviving babies develop microcephaly or hydrocephalus, mental retardation, spasticity, blindness, and chronic liver disease.

Although no specific therapy is known, 5-iodo-2'-deoxyuridine (5-IDU) has been used with some clinical improvement. As with rubella, infected infants shed the virus and thus may infect other infants or pregnant nursery personnel. Obviously, identification of the susceptible female, with the aim of preventing the birth of affected children, will become important in the future.

Although relatively little is known about CID, Monif has said that ". . . in terms of neonatal morbidity and mortality resulting from a viral agent, infection with cytomegalovirus may be second only to rubella virus in importance."[10]

Herpes Herpesvirus hominis (HVH), a large DNA virus, is most often manifested in the form of "cold sores" or "fever blisters." Indeed, most adults have experienced one or more mild or subclinical infections by this virus. Those previously infected have circulating antibodies against the virus.

However, the neonate of a mother who has never had the infection has received no protective antibodies from the nonimmune mother. Besides the mouth, lips, conjunctiva, and other sites, the genital tract of the male or female may be a site of herpes infection. If the mother experiences her first herpetic vulvovaginitis and/or cervicitis near the time of delivery, the baby is exposed to a large inoculum of virus in the birth canal during labor and delivery. Less commonly, the baby may acquire the virus transplacentally during maternal viremia.

The baby infected with herpes usually appears normal at birth; disease at birth occurs only in the rarer transplacental infections, or possibly through a chronically leaking membrane. The incubation period of 6 to 7 days is reflected in the observed onset of neonatal herpes at 4 to 8 days of life. Scattered skin vesicles may occur. The infant may first become lethargic, feed poorly, and have fluctuating temperatures; then he may rapidly develop jaundice, dyspnea, cyanosis, petechiae, and hepatosplenomegaly as the virus disseminates destructively through most organs of the nonimmune infant. This progression of clinical signs frequently terminates with apnea, massive hemorrhage, shock, or seizures. Miller et al. reported bleeding in 40 percent of 55 cases of fatal neonatal HVH infections.[11] At present, death is the usual consequence. Those who recover may manifest severe central nervous system damage and blindness from retinal involvement. A few babies escape unscathed, with subsequently normal growth and development.[12]

At present there is no proved effective treatment. Because 5-iodo-2'-deoxyuridine (5-IDU) has been successful in other forms of herpetic disease, it is being tried in neonatal herpes. The same is true for the use of gamma globulin in an attempt to replace the newborn's missing antibodies. Prophylactic cesarean section delivery is recommended for babies whose mothers have known genital herpes, in an attempt to prevent the baby's contracting the virus from the birth canal. Obviously cesarean section would appear futile in long-ruptured membranes or transplacental infection.

Babies from herpetic mothers are usually isolated to prevent the spread to other susceptible persons, notably other newborns. Only time and experience with 5-IDU, selected cesarean sections, gamma globulin, and newer drugs will tell whether medicine is approaching an effective way of treating, or preventing, this neonatal catastrophy.

Toxoplasmosis Toxoplasmosis is an infection caused by *Toxoplasma gondii*, an obligate intracellular protozoan. It is crescent-shaped and slightly smaller than the normal human red blood cell. Toxoplasma is by no means limited to humans; in fact, this organism has been found in many animals throughout the world, including chickens, ducks, dogs, cats, and horses. Toxoplasmosis has been contracted by humans who eat raw or undercooked meat.

The infection may be acquired or congenital. Approximately one-third of all adults are immune, thus leaving two-thirds of adult women susceptible during pregnancy. Immunity or disease may be diagnosed by demonstration of Sabin-Feldman dye test antibody titers. The acquired infection is often mild, and thus may go undiagnosed in the pregnant woman. Rarely, the acquired disease may be acute and fatal, with rash, pneumonia, myocarditis, or encephalitis. It may also be subacute with fever and lymphadenopathy.

The organism crosses the placenta during primary maternal infection; the significance of the time in gestation is not known. Infection of the fetus notably includes destruction of nervous tissue, although many tissues may be involved. The congenital syndrome classically includes chorioretinitis, intracerebral calcifications, and hydrocephalus or microcephaly. The congenital form may present in the newborn as jaundice, petechiae, hepatosplenomegaly, meningoencephalitis, or seizures. Or, the disease may not be suspected until delayed psychomotor development, abnormal head size, or seizures lead to the diagnostic workup. The prognosis for affected infants is generally grim, with a high incidence of mental retardation.

Acquired toxoplasmosis has been treated in recent years with a combination of pyrimethamine (Daraprim) and a sulfonamide. One wonders whether this therapy could be given to the infected pregnant mother to prevent the congenital disease. Griffith has summarized the present state of therapy during pregnancy; since the combination therapy is known to be teratogenic, it is thought to be contraindicated in the first trimester.[13] However, it is probably safe and indicated in later pregnancy. Griffith goes on to say that asymptomatic but infected infants should be treated in the hope of preventing delayed sequelae. It must be kept in mind that sulfa compounds in the last trimester of pregnancy and in the neonatal period must be used with extreme caution.

As for prevention, the evidence of contraction from cats, undercooked meat, and infected patients makes it obvious that pregnant women should be cautioned to avoid handling cats or their litter boxes, to avoid undercooked meat, and to avoid contact with known patients.

Syphilis *Treponema pallidum*, a spirochete of ill repute, is the cause of syphilis. More than 30 years ago, in the prepenicillin era, maternal syphilis was a major cause of stillbirths, prematurity, and neonatal infections. With penicillin, the incidence of syphilis decreased and the congenital infection was rarely seen. However, the soaring rates of venereal disease in recent years have effected an increase in the number of congenital cases.

Unlike some infections, syphilis elicits an antibody response, but this does not protect against repeated reinfections. Because the active infection in women may be missed with the primary chancre often hidden in the genital tract, prenatal detection of syphilis is usually accomplished by serologic testing (STS, VDRL) of all pregnant women. This testing will miss those women who become infected after the serology or those infected so recently that antibodies have not appeared. *Treponema* does not appear to cross the placenta generally until after the fourth month of gestation. Treatment of the mother with adequate doses of penicillin will usually prevent the congenital illness since penicillin readily crosses the placenta.

Although congenital syphilis can cause stillbirths and prematurity, the liveborn syphilitic baby is usually normal at birth. The first evidence of disease may be jaundice, as late as 2 weeks of life, accompanied by anemia and hepatosplenomegaly. After 2 weeks, the baby may begin to demonstrate "snuffles" (persistent rhinorrhea), a coppery rash, mucous patches, condylomas, and pseudoparalysis from bone inflammation. If undetected or untreated, the infant may go on in later life to manifest more permanent and severe somatic stigmas of congenital syphilis, such as deformed teeth, bones, nose, and joints and central nervous system syphilis.

The treatment of the infected newborn is simple and effective: intramuscular penicillin for 10 days or one long-acting penicillin injection. Because the maternal antibodies cross the placenta, the baby of a previously infected mother may have a positive serology without being infected. The question then arises as to whether the baby should be treated. Close follow-up for onset of signs and documentation of a falling serologic titer is the ideal procedure, but a far more pragmatic approach is the simple administration of one dose of long-acting penicillin in the nursery. The use of long-acting penicillin eliminates the possibility of missing the disease with poor follow-up.

Plainly, the prevention of congenital syphilis is the prevention of maternal syphilis, a problem fraught with social and moral implications. However, the more frequent and thorough the prenatal care, the less likely maternal disease will go undetected and untreated. This is but another reason that high quality prenatal care, especially to those who might not seek it out, is so very important in reducing perinatal morbidity and mortality.

(Sepsis and ophthalmia neonatorum are discussed here because, although postnatal in occurrence, they are frequently a consequence of maternal infection.)

Sepsis   Sepsis is a Greek term meaning "decay" or "putrefaction." Sepsis neonatorum is clinically defined as bacterial infection of infants in the first 30 days of life as demonstrated by culturing the organism from the infant's blood. Before the advent of antibiotics, sepsis of the newborn was almost always fatal. Even with effective antibiotics, sepsis continues to be an important cause of neonatal morbidity and mortality. It is estimated to occur in approximately 1 out of every 1,000 live births, but in the subpopulation of low-birth-weight infants the rate is about four times higher.

In addition to low birth weight, other predisposing factors include premature and prolonged rupture of the amniotic membranes, infection of the amniotic fluid before or after rupture of the membranes, prolonged and difficult labor, instrumental deliveries, maternal toxemia, and bleeding. Although full-term, normal newborns can develop the disease, it is far more likely and earlier in onset in the newborn already under stress. Sepsis is also more common in babies with major congenital anomalies, particularly of the genitourinary, gastrointestinal, or central nervous system. This is especially true if surgery is required in the newborn period. It has also been observed that more males than females have neonatal sepsis.

The agents responsible for sepsis are unlimited, but usually reflect the flora of the mother's genital tract (group B beta-hemolytic streptococci), the mother's perineum (gram-negative rods), the nursery personnel's hands and respiratory tract (*Staphylococcus*), and the contaminants of nursery equipment (*Pseudomonas*). The importance of nosocomial (hospital-acquired) infections cannot be overemphasized; the seemingly laborious attention paid to aseptic technique in all aspects of nursery care, even the time-consuming handwashing, has been shown to effectively reduce the rates of infection.[9] Also, those organisms carried by nursery staff are likely to be resistant to the usual antibiotics and antibacterial solutions used frequently in the nursery.

The prevalence of certain organisms as leading causes of sepsis has changed over the past 30 years from group A beta-hemolytic streptococci to staphylococci to gram-negative organisms (primarily *Escherichia coli* and *Klebsiella*), with the most recently emerging leader being group B beta-hemolytic streptococci. (A recent review of group B streptococcal infections of the neonate is available.[14-17]) The changing patterns of pathogens have paralleled the discovery and use of newer antibiotics; how these two phenomena are related is uncertain but often conjectured.

The baby may acquire the organism in various ways. One obvious but uncommon route is transplacental, as with *Listeria monocytogenes*. Another apparent route is via infected amniotic fluid, which the fetus, if hypoxic, may gulp and aspirate (with subsequent pneumonitis) or swallow (with gastrointestinal inoculation with the infective organism). Acquisition after birth usually depends on which organisms colonize the baby first. Most infants are sterile at birth, but rapidly acquire colonies of bacteria, which all persons carry about on their skin and mucous membranes and in their respiratory and gastrointestinal tracts. Occasionally a localized infection, at the umbilical stump or the site of an intravenous catheter, may be identified as the offending source.

The symptoms of neonatal sepsis are myriad but often begin with poor feeding, nonspecific respiratory changes, or lethargy in a previously vigorous infant. There is justification for suspecting sepsis in any baby noted by nurses or mother to be "just not doing well." Other symptoms may include pallor, jaundice, vomiting, diarrhea, hypothermia, hyperthermia, or disseminated intravascular coagulation. Complications or frequent concurrent infections include meningitis, pneumonia, and urinary tract infections, and symptoms may reflect the pathology of those processes.

Once suspected, a rapid and complete investigation must be made to elucidate a nonbacterial cause, such as CID, rubella, or gastrointestinal obstruction. Tests for the diagnosis of sepsis include cultures of blood, spinal fluid, and urine. In the case of prolonged rupture of membranes or obviously infected amniotic fluid, cultures of the baby's skin, gastric aspirate, or external ear canal immediately after birth may yield the organism. Treatment of sepsis in the newborn should begin as soon as cultures are collected and other causes ruled out, since sepsis is often fulminant and fatal. Initial antibiotics are selected to provide the broadest possible protection until the exact organism and its sensitivities are known. The knowledge of a particular nursery's usual offenders and their antibiotic susceptibility in that given hospital is necessary for drug selection. At present, most initial regimens include penicillin or ampicillin and either kanamycin or gentamicin. Penicillin covers group B streptococci, ampicillin also combats some *Proteus* organisms and *E. coli*, and kanamycin and gentamicin usually cover *Klebsiella* and *Pseudomonas* organisms. The emergence of resistant strains of organisms is a constant threat, and pharmaceutical research has to run hard to keep up with the bacteria's ability to mutate. Once the organism is cultured, parenteral therapy with the proper antibiotic is usually continued for at least 10 days. In addition, supportive measures are important, such as close observation, fluid and caloric maintenance; and antishock procedures should be performed when indicated.

Ophthalmia neonatorum   Ophthalmia neonatorum is the gonococcal infection of the neonate's eyes and is acquired as he passes through an infected birth canal during labor. The term usually refers to conjunctivitis, although deeper and more severe infections may occur. In 1881, Credé first introduced silver nitrate drops as a prophylaxis against gonococcal ophthalmitis of newborns. Prior to that time, the infection was a leading cause of blindness. With the introduction of penicillin in the 1940s, maternal gonorrhea, the source of the baby's infection, dropped. This, combined with the routine use of prophylactic drops, resulted in very few cases being seen. However, with the recent rise in veneral disease, case reports are increasing. Because a 1 percent solution of silver nitrate ($AgNO_3$) causes a chemical conjunctivitis, other prophylactic measures, such as various antibiotic ointments, have been developed. Nevertheless, the chemical conjunctivitis is usually harmless, and silver nitrate remains widely used and effective.

Bacterial conjunctivitis from the gonococcus or other birth-acquired organisms usually occurs 2 to 5 days after birth, whereas chemical conjunctivitis occurs in the first 24 hours. Signs of bacterial disease include puffy eyelids, reddened conjunctiva, and purulent discharge from one or both eyes. Causative organisms include the gonococcus, staphylococcus, pneumococcus, and pseudomonas. These infections are generally rapidly responsive to topical therapy, such as neomycin and bacitracin. However, because the gonococcus can quickly destroy the entire eye, systemic penicillin is added. Similarly, because pseudomonas may rapidly invade the globe and bloodstream, particularly in preterm babies, parenteral antibiotics are instituted along with topical therapy. Isolation of the affected baby is the best policy, regardless of the organism.

Prevention of gonococcal ophthalmia would ideally include identification of the infected mother prior to delivery, as by screening vaginal cultures late in pregnancy. At present, proper instillation of silver nitrate drops or other antibacterial agent is the best prophylaxis. Meanwhile, close observation by nursery personnel and prompt reporting of all signs of conjunctivitis is essential if the risk of permanent loss of vision is to be avoided.

Miscellaneous Maternal Afflictions   Any affliction of the mother is a potential threat to the fetus. The pregnant woman may have any chronic or acute coincidental illness, which may or may not affect her infant. A few of the problems will be subsequently mentioned, but many others exist.

Maternal heart disease   Although only 1 to 2 percent of all pregnant women have organic heart disease, it remains a significant cause of maternal mortality. Most obstetric literature divides the causes as follows:

85–90%	rheumatic heart disease
5–10%	congenital defects
0– 5%	heart disease secondary to hypertension, thyroid, and coronary artery disease.

These figures are changing, which probably reflects that with better care and corrective surgery, females with congenital heart disease are surviving to reproduce. Also, there has been a steady decrease in the incidence of acute rheumatic fever in recent years.

The outcome of the individual pregnancy depends on the severity of the heart lesion, the maternal age, and the cardiac reserve of the mother. In general, the more severe the lesion and the older the mother, the less the cardiac reserve. This reserve is very important, because pregnancy normally alters body fluid and hemodynamic physiology. The expanded plasma volume, increased cardiac output, and faster heart rate place demands on the mother's heart. If the heart has insufficient reserve to meet these new stresses, congestive heart failure will occur, with serious fetal hypoxia and serious maternal consequences if uncorrected. Community or clinic nurses have a responsible role in the early detection of congestive failure and in seeing that the patient obtains immediate treatment. If heart failure or severe cyanosis exists before conception, spontaneous abortion or fetal death usually occurs. Fortunately, most women with heart disease have adequate cardiac reserve, if managed meticulously by the obstetrician and cardiologist throughout gestation. Their babies, if liveborn, are usually normal.

Maternal cigarette smoking Smoking mothers generally have smaller babies than nonsmoking women. Nurses can educate and encourage pregnant women to stop or decrease their smoking. The more cigarettes the mother smokes, the lower the birth weight tends to be. There is probably no shortening of pregnancy; the lower birth weights have been postulated to result from diminished uterine blood flow secondary to effects of nicotine on blood vessels. There appears to be no difference in perinatal mortality between infants of smokers and nonsmokers.

Maternal renal disease The rate of asymptomatic bacteriuria is increased during pregnancy. This is thought to be secondary to urinary stasis and ureteral dilatation as the gravid uterus crowds the pelvis. However, there is much debate over whether or not asymptomatic bacteriuria is associated with premature labor and increased perinatal loss. Acute pyelonephritis is known to raise fetal morbidity and mortality. Chronic renal disease complicates pregnancy only if renal function is lowered or hypertension exists. In these instances, premature labor and toxemia appear to occur more often than usual.

Maternal anemia In normal pregnancies the plasma volume expands more than the red blood cell mass, with a resultant mild drop in hemoglobin concentration. Also, the growing fetus normally extracts relatively large amounts of iron from the mother, predisposing to maternal iron deficiency. Only severe anemia appears to affect the fetus; this effect is thought to be mediated through chronic intrauterine hypoxia, since the maternal circulation in this circumstance has a diminished red blood cell mass to deliver oxygen to the placenta.

Anemia in pregnancy is most commonly due to iron deficiency. This is usually readily responsive to oral iron supplementation and dietary instruction. Megaloblastic anemia, resulting from folic acid deficiency, is less common. There has been some evidence suggesting a relationship between folate deficiency and abruptio placentae. Folate deficiency, like iron deficiency, is easily preventable by oral prenatal supplements.

The hemoglobinopathies, although relatively infrequent, pose more serious consequences. The major hemoglobinopathy in this country is homozygous S hemoglobin, or sickle cell disease. Those females who survive to reach childbearing age usually have a very difficult pregnancy, with a marked increased in anemia, painful crises, and infections. Although most patients survive their pregnancies, the fetal wastage is very high, with up to 50 percent

of pregnancies resulting in fetal death or prematurity.

INTRAPARTAL FACTORS

Intrapartal factors refer to circumstances occurring during the period of labor and delivery. For the most part, these are obstetric complications, including difficult labor, presentations other than vertex, operative delivery, and accidents of the placenta and umbilical cord. Multiple births, most commonly twins, may have antepartal complications but also pose hazardous entry problems. These complications of delivery may result in direct trauma to the infant, such as fractures or hemorrhages. Another type of insult to the baby is distortion of his blood supply, leading to hypoxia, which then results in metabolic derangements that can maim and kill the baby. Any baby who is the product of an abnormal labor and/or delivery must be considered at high risk, and should be given rapid nursing and medical assessment and special observation even if no specific therapy is indicated.

The analgesic and anesthetic drugs given to the mother during labor and delivery may cross the placenta rapidly and effectively sedate the baby. The chance of this occurrence depends on the particular drug(s) used, the route, the doses, and the time interval before delivery. The affected baby may be just slightly drowsy or may be completely apneic and in need of immediate respiratory assistance. This baby must be watched until the drug effect is gone.

To understand how these intrapartal factors manifest themselves in the infant, one must be able to distinguish the normal from the abnormal appearance of the newborn in the delivery suite. Everyone is acquainted with the healthiness of a lustily crying, pink, wiggly neonate. (The reader is referred to Chap. 9 for a detailed description of the normal newborn.) The baby who is not so vigorous is described as "depressed." The depressed baby may represent inadequate respiration, central nervous system damage, circulatory failure, or asphyxia. The most renowned method of quantitating the state of the newborn was formulated by Dr. Virginia Apgar and is based on a scoring system of 0 to 10 points[18] (see Chap. 9 for details). Most healthy newborns score from 7 to 10: babies scoring 4 to 6 points usually require some gentle stimulation and assistance, and babies with 3 or fewer points are in dire need of immediate resuscitation. Although the original Apgar system has been modified innumerable times, it remains a basic tool for rapid assessment of the newborn.

Fetal Distress

Fetal distress refers to the few clinical signs presently known which suggest that the fetus is in danger. The two classic signs are fetal bradycardia (heart rate less than 100 beats per minute) and passage of meconium prior to birth in a nonbreech presentation. Other suggestive signs include fetal tachycardia (heart rate over 200 beats per minute) and marked fetal thrashing. There are many causes of fetal distress, but most are mediated through dysfunction of the cord or placenta, resulting in fetal asphyxia which is manifest as fetal distress.

Asphyxia is defined as hypoxia (diminished O_2), hypercapnea (elevated CO_2), and acidosis (lowered pH), and is best measured by blood gas determinations. Asphyxia represents the metabolic disturbances of the suffocated baby. The asphyxiated newborn is limp, pale, and poorly responsive. *Asphyxia neonatorum* is a spectrum and may be mild or severe. Mild or partial asphyxia is probably a part of every normal delivery. Indeed, the asphyxia induced by delivery may be part of the stimulus for the initiation of breathing. Most babies respond to this stimulus, breathe, and thereby elevate their O_2, diminish their CO_2, and eventually correct their acidosis. However, the very small, weak, damaged, or severely suffocated baby may not be able to respond adequately, and may die without resuscitation.

The most obvious and foremost aim of therapy is the immediate establishment of an adequate airway and gas exchange. This is usually performed with an infant resuscitation unit in the delivery room by an obstetrician, pediatrician, or anesthesiologist. These critical minutes for the baby certainly merit the most experienced operator available. The baby's nose and oropharynx are first cleared of secretions by suctioning. A mouthpiece or endotracheal tube is inserted, and insufflation is provided by mouth-to-mouth breathing, mouth-to-tube breathing, or a positive pressure apparatus. The resuscitator's assistant monitors the infant's apical heart rate with a stethoscope, tapping his finger in rhythm with the infant's heartbeat. Once adequate gas exchange occurs, the heart rate usually accelerates; if the heart rate remains very low or undetectable, ventilation is inadequate or severe acidosis prevails. External cardiac massage then becomes necessary. Intravenous administration of buffer solutions (sodium bicarbonate or THAM) may be necessary to correct profound acidosis. Supplemental oxygen may help restore the baby's oxygenation, but is no substitute for adequate gas exchange and circulatory assistance.

The concern over asphyxia is far more than the immediate prevention of death; asphyxia is thought to be a major cause of intracranial hemorrhage, hypoxic brain damage, and perhaps lung hypoperfusion. Therefore, the baby who survives the initial insults may later show manifestations of such brain damage as cerebral palsy, mental retardation, and learning defects. In addition, the hypoxic fetus may gasp during delivery, with the dire consequence of aspirating amniotic fluid, which may contain meconium and/or infective organisms. Aspiration pneumonia results and is often severe and difficult to treat.

Placental Accidents

The placenta is the fetal organ of respiration and excretion, serving as lungs and kidney. It is also the source of fetal nutrition. It is a complex network of tiny vascular interfacings, allowing intimate but indirect contact of maternal and fetal circulations. The myriad invaginations of tissue create increased surface areas, much larger than the apparent placental circular area. To this larger interface the maternal blood brings necessary nutrients, such as glucose and oxygen, which pass through the placental membranes into the fetal circulation. Likewise, the fetal blood transfers its metabolic by-products such as CO_2 into the maternal circulation for clearance by maternal lung and kidney.

The placenta is normally delivered within ½ hour following the baby; detachment from the uterine wall actually occurs within 1 to 5 minutes after delivery. Because before birth the fetus has no other source of oxygen or glucose, any loss of placental function threatens these life-sustaining supplies. If the placenta comes loose before the baby is born, hypoxia quickly ensues, producing asphyxia and cellular level damage. Also, abnormal separation of the highly vascular placental tissues may lead to serious maternal and/or fetal bleeding. Obviously, the degree of placental malfunction ranges from trifling to life-threatening. The two major placental problems are premature detachment (placenta abruptio) and abnormally low implantation in the uterus (placenta previa). Gross structural abnormalities of the placenta, such as hemangiomas or massive infarctions, are relatively rare and manifest themselves in long-term fetal malnutrition and runting.

Placenta Abruptio Placenta abruptio is the premature separation of the placenta from the uterus.

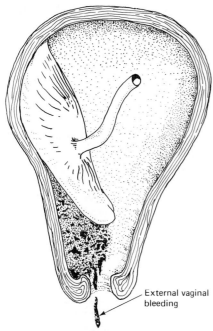

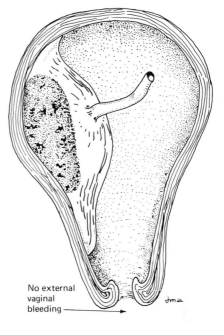

Figure 20-2 Placenta abruptio, *marginal* type, which represents about 80 percent of all cases. The prognosis is better than for the central type.

Figure 20-3 Placenta abruptio, *central* type, which represents about 20 percent of all cases.

It is estimated to occur in 1 out of every 100 to 200 deliveries. There are two types of separation. The most common type accounts for about 80 percent of cases and is *marginal*; a margin of the placenta detaches and leads to observable external vaginal bleeding. The blood from the separated margins usually easily escapes around the presenting fetal part and passes through the vaginal vault and is observed perineally (Fig. 20-2). This bleeding is relatively painless. The less common placental abruption is *central*, accounting for about 20 percent of cases. The placental margins remain attached, with detachment and bleeding occurring centrally. The blood cannot escape the intact margins, and builds up in a hidden pool, which is usually very painful (Fig. 20-3). Central abruption is more dangerous to mother and fetus; large amounts of blood may be lost into the hidden pool before the condition is recognized.

The actual cause of abruption is not known, but the predisposing factors include maternal hypertension (and therefore toxemia), increasing maternal age, increasing parity, and short umbilical cord.

The consequences are obviously dependent on the degree of detachment and the obstetric management. The maternal mortality is less than 1 percent, but the perinatal mortality is high, estimated to range from 30 to 80 percent. The baby usually dies of asphyxia; if he survives, it is probable that he will have hypoxic brain damage. Also, the survival of the liveborn babies is poorer because of the increased incidence of prematurity. When the mother's life is threatened by abruption, the obstetrician has no choice but to deliver the baby as soon as possible, regardless of its state of maturity.

Placenta Previa   Placenta previa is implantation low in the uterus such that the placenta is near or overlies the internal cervical os. Thus, during labor and delivery the placenta is in the way of the presenting fetal part (see Fig. 20-4). Placenta previa is estimated to occur in approximately 1 of every 200 pregnancies.

Various classifications are based on how much of the placenta actually overlies the internal os. The more os covered, the more hazardous the condition. Because the os dilates during normal labor, the degree of previa is most significant if considered in terms of a fully dilated (10 cm) cervical os. One classification is as follows:

1   **Total**   the placenta completely covers the internal os in an estimated 20 percent of all cases.
2   **Partial**   the placenta partially covers the internal os in approximately 30 percent of all cases.

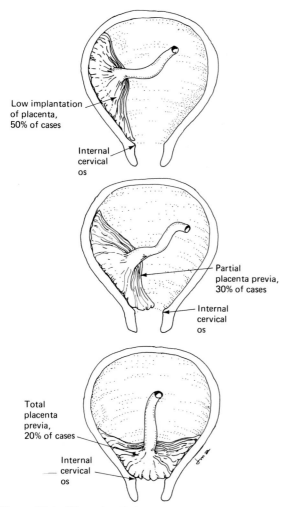

Low implantation
of placenta,
50% of cases

Internal
cervical
os

Partial
placenta previa,
30% of cases

Internal
cervical
os

Total
placenta
previa,
20% of cases

Internal
cervical
os

Figure 20-4 Placenta previa.

3 Low implantation the placenta is adjacent to but not over the internal os in the remaining 50 percent of cases of placenta previa.

The cause of placenta previa is unknown, but it is statistically associated with increasing parity, advanced maternal age, and a rapid succession of pregnancies. Placenta previa should be suspected in any case of painless, bright red vaginal bleeding in the last trimester. If the bleeding is minimal and the baby is premature, placental localization is attempted, frequently by isotopic placentography (placental scan); once diagnosed, labor is delayed as long as feasible and elective section is done when the baby is judged mature enough. If bleeding is heavy or the baby is full term size, a careful vaginal examination is performed in a double setup; that is, in a prepared operating room so that immediate

cesarean section can be done if previa is found, since the hemorrhage secondary to examination may be massive. Cesarean section remains the choice method of delivery for most cases of placenta previa.

Although maternal mortality has decreased to 1 percent, perinatal mortality is still about 20 percent. This high perinatal mortality is related to an increased occurrence of prematurity, prolapse of cord, hypoxia, and fetal blood loss through the placenta. Therefore, the infant delivered from a placenta previa must often be watched not only for routine premature care but also for signs of uncorrected asphyxia (apnea, bradycardia), and blood loss (pallor, diminishing blood pressure, tachycardia, and lethargy).

Prolapsed Cord

Prolapse of the umbilical cord occurs when the membranes are ruptured and a segment of the umbilical cord lies ahead of the presenting fetal part in the birth canal. This accident occurs in approximately 1 of every 200 to 300 deliveries. It usually occurs when the presenting fetal part does not fit snugly into the bony pelvis, thus leaving room for the cord to slip down. This misfit of the fetal part occurs in such circumstances as (1) prematurity (small baby in a relatively big space), (2) nonvertex presentations (foot or shoulder), and (3) contracted pelvis (fetal part cannot descend).

The problem to the fetus is clear: the cord is compressed between the presenting fetal part and pelvic structures, causing fetal hypoxia (Fig. 20-5). The diagnosis is usually made by palpation of the cord on vaginal examination. If the cord is pulsative, management usually includes immediate knee-chest or Trendelenburg position of the mother to relieve the pressure on the cord while preparations are made for immediate abdominal delivery. However, many of these babies are dead before delivery, and perinatal mortality is estimated at 30 to 35 percent. Those who survive are subject to hypoxia, asphyxia, and prematurity, with all their possible sequelae.

Dystocia

Dystocia is defined in present-day obstetrics simply as "difficult labor." The word itself is derived from the Greek word stems for difficult (*dys*) and birth (*tokos*). Although there are many causes of difficult labor, most fall under one of the following three categories: (1) uterine dysfunction, (2) fetal malposition or malformation, or (3) inadequate bony pelvis.

Thinking simplistically, labor is the expulsion of an object through a passage. If the expulsive force is insufficient, the object will not pass; if the object is too big or misshapen, it will not pass; if the passage is too small or distorted, the object will not pass. In any individual patient, one, two, or all three problems may exist.

Uterine dysfunction, or insufficient uterine force, is also called uterine inertia. It most often refers to diminished or poorly coordinated uterine contractility; less commonly it is caused by hypercontractility or abnormal uterine rings. If the other categories of dystocia are ruled out, namely, inadequate pelvis or fetal malposition, hypocontractility frequently responds to oxytocin stimulation. If not, cesarean section is the safest delivery.

Abnormalities of the bony pelvis are most commonly deviant shapes and sizes. If the pelvis is flattened or shortened in any diameter, it may or may not permit a normal-sized fetus to pass. This condition is commonly termed "contracted pelvis." If digital vaginal examination is not diagnostic, x-ray pelvimetry provides an accurate way of measuring the various diameters of the pelvis and fetal head. CPD (cephalopelvic disproportion) means that the head is too big for the pelvis or the pelvis too small for the head. When true pelvic contraction or CPD is diagnosed, abdominal delivery is the only choice.

The fetus most often impedes delivery by malposition or malpresentation, but occasionally by excessive size or congenital malformations. The most common presentation is the vertex, and the most common position is occiput anterior; any other presentation or position is prone to prolong labor. Fetal weight greater than 4,000 Gm (8¾ lb) is not infrequently associated with difficult labor and delivery. Fetal malformations, such as hydrocephalus, may rarely cause dystocia.

Only a superficial overview of dystocia has been presented here; each cause carries its own management and perinatal risks. The major significance of dystocia to the baby is that prolonged labor, which almost always accompanies a difficult labor, is definitely associated with an increased perinatal loss. In general, total labor lasting longer than 20 hours or a second stage exceeding 2 hours defines prolongation. Fortunately, cesarean section offers a relatively innocuous escape route when vaginal delivery is not feasible. Obviously, the earlier that decision is reached, the better for the baby.

Nonvertex Presentations

Nonvertex presentations include any presentation that is not the vertex of the fetal head, such as

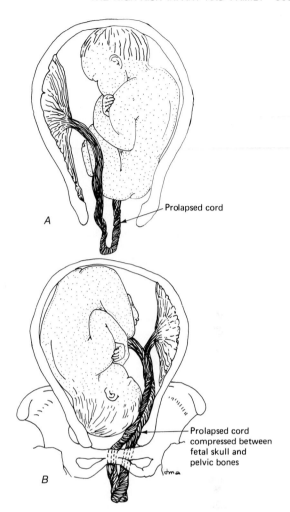

Figure 20-5 Prolapse of the umbilical cord. *A.* In a breech presentation. *B.* In a vertex presentation.

breech, brow, face, and shoulder. Only breech is statistically a common occurrence. However, any abnormal presentation must be considered an added risk to the fetus. Breech will be discussed because of its frequent occurrence.

In the breech presentation the buttocks or one or both feet comprise the presenting fetal part. There are three types. *Frank* breech occurs when the legs are fully extended up over the fetal abdomen and thorax. In *complete* breech, both legs are flexed and folded against the fetal abdomen. *Footling* breech indicates that one or both feet have dropped down below the fetus and thus present before the buttocks.

Breech presentation occurs in approximately 3 to 4 percent of all deliveries, but the more premature the fetus is, the higher the incidence. Before 30 weeks of gestation, almost 25 percent of fetuses are breech. The decreasing incidence of breech birth as term is approached is thought to be related to the fact that in early gestation the fetus is relatively small and turns easily within its uterine confines. After 30 to 32 weeks, the rapidly growing fetus begins to crowd the uterus and pelvic structures and adapts to the most easily fitting position, which is usually head down. Thus, the most common predisposing (but not causative) factor in breech presentation is prematurity. In multiple gestations such as twins, one fetus is frequently breech. Other factors are debatable and include multiparity, contracted pelvis, and fetal anomalies such as anencephaly.

The complications of breech delivery are very significant, and result in an increased perinatal mortality of five to six times that for vertex deliveries. Prematurity and its problems account for many breech deaths. Overall, regardless of fetal weight, the most common cause of death is tentorial tearing with intracranial bleeding. This bleeding usually results from traumatic extraction of the aftercoming head. Unlike the hours and days of molding that goes on in vertex presentations, the head of the breech baby must rapidly adapt its shape to pass through the pelvis. In addition, asphyxia easily transpires once the fetal head is in the pelvis, since the head is firm and may press on and occlude the umbilical cord. Piper or other special forceps are frequently used to safely deliver the head. Cord prolapse also occurs more often in breech births.

There is no proven way to prevent breech presentation. Abdominal manipulation (external version) may convert a breech position to a vertex presentation, but it does carry a small risk to the fetus. The most important factor is the early decision as to whether or not vaginal delivery is safe; if not, cesarean section is indicated. Approximately 10 percent of all breeches are delivered by cesarean section. Indeed, liberal use of abdominal delivery is a way of reducing some of the perinatal loss. In addition, some authorities strongly suggest that a second expert attendant be present to assist with the aftercoming head and possible infant resuscitation.

Obstetric Forceps

Obstetric forceps are variations of curved blades which are applied to the fetal head to provide traction and extension. In the past, forceps were destructive instruments to remove a dead or dying fetus from the mother who would otherwise also die. Today, forceps are used mainly to ensure a safe and slightly hastened passage for the baby. An oversim-plified version of the modern classification of forceps operations is as follows:

1 **Outlet forceps** (low forceps) head engaged (past the pelvic inlet), skull on the perineum, sagittal suture in the anteroposterior diameter of the pelvis.
2 **Midforceps** head engaged but skull not on the perineum; if any rotation is required, a midforceps procedure is performed.
3 **High forceps** head not yet engaged; almost never justified.

The maternal indications for forceps include exhaustion and systemic disease such as heart disease which limits the mother's reserve. Fetal indications include fetal distress, rotational arrests (occiput posterior or transverse), and the aftercoming head of the breech baby. Regardless of the indications, however, certain prerequisites exist before forceps deliveries can be performed, including full cervical dilatation, an engaged head, and no pelvic contraction. If the prerequisites cannot be met, oxytocic stimulation or cesarean section offer alternatives.

Most forceps deliveries today are elective outlet (low) forceps, which carry almost no risk to the fetus. The risk of midforceps is mostly undue force on the fetal head with subsequent intracranial hemorrhage; this risk rises with the height of the head above the perineum. Occasionally a facial nerve palsy may result from forceps pressure over the mandibular ramus, but fortunately most of these palsies resolve in the first few days of life.

Cesarean Section

Only in this century has cesarean section become a safe procedure; previously, infection and hemorrhage claimed most mothers. This procedure is presently performed in 5 to 8 percent of all deliveries in the United States. The two major categories of cesarean sections are repeat and primary. Each accounts for about one-half of the total.

Repeat sections are done for women who have had a previous cesarean section. There is a small but real (1 percent) risk that if labor is allowed the uterus will rupture at the site of the scar left by the earlier section. For this reason, most obstetricians elect to deliver all subsequent pregnancies abdominally. Repeat sections carry a relatively low risk to the fetus, but it is about twice as high as vaginal delivery. This is usually because the baby is not infrequently smaller than calculated; also, section babies have an elevated incidence of the respiratory distress syndrome, and the mother's anesthesia may depress the baby.

Primary sections are done because of numerous complications which threaten the mother and/or baby. The most common indication is dystocia, whether due to cephalopelvic disproportion, mal-presentation, or uterine dysfunction. Other indications for primary section include placental accidents, fetal distress, toxemia, and maternal diabetes. Obviously, babies born by primary section are placed at risk by whatever condition necessitated the abdominal delivery. Add to this the problems encountered by babies born abdominally rather than vaginally, and it is not difficult to understand why these infants have a high rate of perinatal loss. However, with modern techniques, cesarean section often salvages more babies than it harms and should always be performed when vaginal delivery may injure mother and/or baby.

Section babies, even when apparently well, are frequently placed in incubators for a period of observation. Nurses should watch for respiratory distress, depression secondary to anesthesia, and any other specific problems made likely by the reasons for the cesarean delivery.

Twinning

Twinning occurs in 1 out of every 80 to 90 pregnancies; triplets and higher multiples are rarer. Multiple pregnancy is more common in the black than white race and in older women. An increased incidence of multiple births has been noted in women taking fertility drugs such as clomiphene, since the drugs stimulate ovulation and may result in multiple ovulations at one time. Approximately two-thirds of twins are dizygotic, or fraternal, and represent two different ova and two different sperm. The remaining one-third are monozygotic, or identical, representing one ovum and one sperm. The following discussion of twins applies in general to any multiple gestation, since the problems are similar.

In general, twins have a perinatal mortality that is two to three times higher than that in single births. The major factor contributing to this increased loss is premature labor. Estimates range from 30 to 80 percent being delivered preterm. This early labor, combined with the constant competition between twins for intrauterine space and nutrition, results in approximately one-half of all twins weighing less than 2,500 Gm (5½ lb). Babson has stated that "multiple pregnancies account for more undergrown neonates than any other known cause."[19] The gravity of this situation is complicated in that close to 50 percent of all twins are not diagnosed until labor

and delivery. This late diagnosis is tragic, since it has been well demonstrated that restricted activity, especially bed rest, can often delay the premature labor of these women. Since most pregnant women are encouraged to exercise freely, the detection of twins in prenatal visits becomes imperative.

The next most common problem is delivering the second twin safely. Whereas the first twin usually presents in a routine manner, the second twin is often malpositioned. While awaiting uterine contractions to realign the second twin, there is a risk of premature separation of its placenta and prolapse of its cord. Because of these problems, obstetricians often must resort to forceps or version to hasten delivery, in an attempt to prevent fetal hypoxia. The fact that only half of twins are diagnosed before labor is again an obvious problem, since expectant management of twin delivery, especially with providing double supplies of resuscitation equipment and personnel, would be very desirable.

The other problems of twinning include increased rates of toxemia, maternal anemia, placenta previa, and hydramnios. If monozygotic twins share a single amniotic sac, they risk entanglement of their cords, which can result in death of one or both fetuses. Also, monozygotic twins may have vascular connections in their placental mass, with twin-to-twin transfusions resulting in one large, plethoric twin and another small, anemic twin.

Thus, although twins are a source of perinatal problems, they also provide an excellent opportunity for prevention of such problems. Early diagnosis is the key factor, and only high-quality, frequent prenatal care can do that. This early detection will allow for adequate bed rest to prevent premature labor, judicious and expectant management of labor and delivery, and dietary management to guard against toxemia and anemia. With regard to bed rest, Cavanagh has put it so well: "Bed rest at home does not carry the financial burden of hospitalization, and may go a long way to reducing the bills for care in the prematurity nursery."[20]

POSTPARTUM FACTORS
Maturation

Once the baby is born, the decisive factors in its chances for survival are its gestational age and birth weight. In previous years, birth weight alone determined prematurity, for any baby below 2,500 Gm (5½ lb) was defined as "premature." Indeed, low birth weight is very significant, for while low-birth-weight babies account for only 7 to 10 percent of live births, they account for two-thirds or more of neonatal deaths. Their neonatal mortality is more than 20 times higher than babies weighing more than 2,500 Gm. However, recently it has become apparent that weight is not the only determinant of survival. Because maternal menstrual histories notoriously do not pinpoint conception, estimated menstrual age is an inaccurate measure. In the past 5 to 10 years, rather accurate methods have been developed for assessing each baby on its physical appearance and neurologic status as to its true gestational age. This is possible because, regardless of most intrauterine conditions, certain patterns of physical and neurologic development occur in a precise chronologic sequence.

Because of the growing awareness of the importance of gestational age, many neonatal centers now include accurate recording of it on all admissions. Some nurseries utilize a checklist to ensure standardized descriptions. Some of the physical characteristics used in assessing gestational age are the following:

Characteristic	Less than 37 weeks	40 weeks
Skin	Thin, red, lanugo present	Thick, pale pink
Hair	Fuzzy	Silky, each hair seen
Ear cartilage	Pliable	Stiff
Breast tissue	Not palpable or less than 3 mm (0.12 in.)	5–7 mm (0.20–0.28 in.)
External genitalia, male	Testes undescended or in canals	Testes descended
Soles	1–2 creases on anterior sole only	Creases present over entire sole

Lubchenco[21] and others have revealed the relevance of gestational age and birth weight to estimating neonatal mortality risks. In general, the older the gestational age, the better the chance of survival. This assessment of survival chances has paralleled the recognition of two major categories of low-birth-weight babies, namely, the truly *premature* or preterm baby, and the baby who is *small for gestational age*, whatever that age may be. This recognition is reflected in changing definitions, as previously listed at the beginning of this chapter. The low-birth-weight infant is any weighing less than 2,500 Gm (5 lb, 8 oz). The preterm is any baby born before 37 weeks of gestation. The SGA (small-for-gestational-age) baby is any infant weighing less than two standard deviations below the mean weight for his given gestational age.

The importance of gestational age is related to the simple fact that the longer the gestation, the more mature the various organ systems will be. Much of the loss from prematurity is simply that the fetus is not ready to function independently of the uterus. Those organs which work in utero—for example, the heart—cause little difficulty. But those whose work initiates with birth, such as the lungs and digestive tract, may not be ready if birth is too early.

Preterm Infants

The truly preterm infant is one of less than 37 weeks' gestation. There are many causes of premature labor, several of which have already been mentioned in this chapter. These include twinning, placental accidents, and premature rupture of the membranes. However, frequently the cause of premature labor remains cryptic. Iatrogenic causes of preterm birth must not be forgotten, such as ill-timed repeat sections and early delivery of diabetic mothers and Rh-isoimmunized babies. Obviously, the risks of prematurity must be weighed against the risks of the disease itself.

Appearance and Activity In appearance, the premature infant is scrawny from underdeveloped subcutaneous tissue, is thin-skinned, and has prominent eyes and a relatively large head. After several days of life, the soft, malleable head may assume an elongated shape in the sagittal plane from resting on one side or the other. In contrast to the term baby's normal state of flexed extremities, the preterm infant's extremities are skinny, have less muscle tone, and often lie extended or scarf-like wherever they are placed (Figs. 20-6 and 20-7). General activity is more feeble, and the cry is weaker. The preterm infant may suck, but often his suck is ineffective and not coordinated with swallowing. This difficulty has led to the widespread use of gavaging, or feeding via a soft tube introduced through the nose or mouth into the stomach. Also, because of the underdeveloped swallowing reflex, the premature infant may aspirate secretions or liquids from his nose or oropharynx; thus adequate suction must always be kept near the baby's bed. The central nervous system centers for respiration are underdeveloped, which results in periodic (irregular) breathing and apneic episodes. Various alarm devices have been made which respond to irregular breathing and thus alert the nursing staff, but these serve only to augment expert observations.

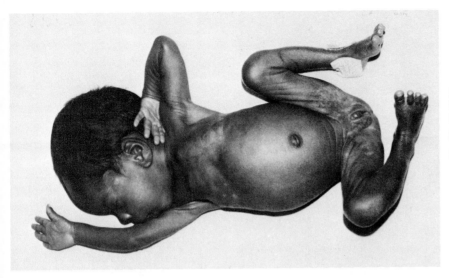

Figure 20-6 Premature black female. Birth weight was 1,300 Gm (2 lb, 14 oz) at estimated gestational age of 32 weeks. The photograph was taken at 38 days of age; weight was 1,415 Gm (3 lb, 1½ oz). Note the thinness of the skin. Absence of subcutaneous fat is especially noticeable in thigh folds, labia majora, and over the ribs. The open hands and scarf-like, "draped" position denote the diminished muscle tone of the premature infant.

Care of the Preterm Infant The routine care of the preterm infant varies from nursery to nursery, but the basic premises are the same. In general, the policies attempt to attend the same needs that the intrauterine environment provided, namely a safe, stable environment and adequate nutrition.

Temperature control The newborn usually comes from a warm (37°C, or 98.6°F) uterus to a much colder, drafty delivery suite; this is to the comfort of the mother and her attendants, but to the possible detriment of the baby. In addition, the wet newborn expends considerable energy in evaporation. The preterm baby has less subcutaneous fat to act as insulation and lower body stores of metabolic energy to replace these losses to evaporation and cooling. Therefore, the rapid drying and warming of the newborn preterm is very important in conserving the infant's energy. This carries over to the nursery, where the preterm continues to be poorly insulated and may be unable to take adequate oral supplies of caloric energy. The preterm infant, because of his poor insulation, is essentially a poikilotherm, taking on the temperature of his environment. Thus, most nurseries utilize various incubators or radiant-heat units to supply a constant environmental temperature to the baby. Thermoneutrality, in which the temperature of the baby's environment is neither higher nor lower than his normal body temperature, requires the least energy from the infant.

The various incubators also preclude the necessity for clothing other than diapers. Keeping the baby undressed is advantageous in that it allows the nurse much more complete observation of the infant from a distance, so that breathing patterns, abdominal contour, skin color, and movement may be easily observed. The importance of temperature control must be remembered when procedures such as weighing, measuring, bathing, or diagnostic tasks must be performed. Any that cannot be done within the confines of controlled temperature must be done rapidly with great attention to maintaining the baby's temperature.

Feeding The caloric requirements of the preterm infant are high in order for it to maintain the rapid growth appropriate for its stage of development. These approach 120 cal/kg body weight per day. Many preterm infants cannot adequately suck this amount so gavage is done. To reduce the volume of required calories to a size tolerated by the baby's immature gut, special formulas with concentrations of 24 and 26 cal/oz have been developed and used. If gavage is unsafe, as in infants requiring assisted ventilation, temporary fluid and caloric requirements may best be augmented with intravenous fluids including dextrose. Unless the more sophisticated techniques and solutions of total intravenous alimentation are used, IV dextrose is inadequate for long-term caloric supply. Regardless of the route, nurseries are increasingly feeding small babies earlier and earlier to refurbish their very limited energy stores.

Bathing In most nurseries, nurses or personnel supervised by nurses routinely bathe babies daily. This procedure is more than mere homage to cultural customs; it allows removal of many potentially

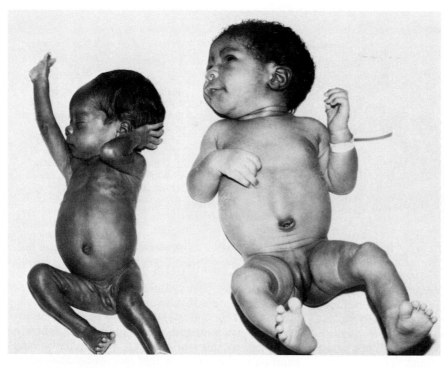

Figure 20-7 The same premature infant pictured in Figure 20-6 is shown with a 2-day-old black female born at 40 weeks' gestation and weighing 3,140 Gm (6 lb, 14 oz) at birth. This comparison demonstrates the full-term infant's characteristically greater muscle tone, darker genital pigmentation, curlier hair, more subcutaneous fat (including the genital region where the labia majora cover the clitoris), sole creases, and open, mature eyes (as contrasted to the bird-like lids of the premature infant).

pathogenic bacteria from the skin, especially from around the umbilicus and eyes. It also permits a close examination of the infant's external anatomy, which may reveal jaundice, respiratory distress, early infections such as omphalitis or conjunctivitis, and other problems such as bullae or vesicles. The soap or antibacterial used for bathing has been hotly debated since the Federal Drug Administration in December 1971 announced that 3 percent hexachlorophene should not be routinely used because of possible central nervous system toxicity. Some authorities recommend the use of plain tap water with or without a mild soap. Regardless, the practice of daily bathing remains a good one.

Meaurements Many measurements go into the care and ongoing assessment of a preterm baby's growth. Vital signs, such as temperature, heart rate, respiratory rate, and blood pressure, are indicators of the infant's physiologic status, and abnormal values are frequently the cue that something is amiss. Daily weights must be accurate, for infections may present in preterm infants as merely poor weight gain. Daily head circumference may reflect the too-rapid rise seen in meningitis, intracranial bleed, or hydrocephalus. Thus, seemingly routine and tedious measurements may offer valuable parameters for assessing the baby's well-being.

Special Problems of Preterm Infants The problems to which preterm infants are particularly susceptible include respiratory distress, hyperbilirubinemia, infection, and anemia. Each of these areas has been covered more completely in other sections of this book, and is only briefly mentioned here.

Respiratory distress Idiopathic respiratory distress syndrome (RDS), or hyalin membrane disease (HMD), is almost exclusively a disease of preterm infants. It is thought to be due to a deficiency of pulmonary surfactant, a substance which helps the air sacs to remain open after initial inflation. The syndrome presents as grunting, elevated respiratory rate, cyanosis and retractions within the first few hours of life. Therapy is still primarily supportive and includes judicious titration of inhaled oxygen, assisted ventilation when necessary, and buffer correction of acidosis. New methods of maintaining open alveoli include continuous positive airway pressure and continuous negative extrathoracic pressure. An even more exciting development has been the recent finding that treatment of mothers with steroids (usually betamethasone) for 24 hours prior to delivery in selected cases appears to stimulate rapid maturation of lung surfactant, and thereby decrease the incidence and severity of HMD in the infants.[22] Much work remains to be done to substantiate this observation, but it offers hope of prevention.

Other respiratory ills afflict the immature baby, including pulmonary hemorrhage, pneumonia, oxygen toxicity, and pneumothorax. Frequently these entities are complications of idiopathic respiratory distress syndrome. RDS and the nursing care of afflicted infants are presented in detail in Chapter 33.

Hyperbilirubinemia   Hyperbilirubinemia of the preterm infant is similar to that of the term newborn in regard to its origins, but its consequences tend to be more dangerous. Like any newborn, he may suffer from Rh or ABO incompatibility. More often, however, his hyperbilirubinemia reflects the immaturity of his liver, and its inability to conjugate and excrete the bilirubin presented to his system. This is the same mechanism responsible for the physiologic jaundice of term newborns. However, the dangers of hyperbilirubinemia, regardless of the cause, are increased in the preterm infant, because the brain damage (*kernicterus*) caused by excess bilirubin appears to occur at lower blood bilirubin levels in the preterm infant. This is possibly due to several factors. For one, the preterm infant often has less serum albumin to bind the bilirubin and render it harmless to the tissues. Also, the preterm infant is more likely to be acidotic, which appears to enhance the passage of bilirubin into the central nervous system. The inherent susceptibility of the immature brain itself to bilirubin staining is unquantitated. Because the preterm infant is injured by lower levels of bilirubin, exchange transfusion is recommended at levels below the standard 20 mg/100 ml; some authorities suggest exchange at values as low as 12 mg/100 ml.

Other efforts to reduce or prevent hyperbilirubinemia include phototherapy and early feeding or hydration. Phototherapy, which transforms bilirubin in the skin into harmless by-products, is frequently a useful adjunct in preventing the need for exchange transfusion. Since the infant's eyes must be patched to protect them from the blue spectrum lights, attendants must periodically remove the patches and check the eyes for signs of conjunctivitis or deeper infections. Early feedings and hydration are believed to aid the infant in removing bilirubin products from his gastrointestinal tract.

Infection   The discussion of neonatal sepsis is presented earlier in this chapter, and suffices for most of the basic information. The preterm infant appears more susceptible to infections, both localized and systemic, than the term baby. This has been attributed to the general immaturity of his immune system. All newborns receive some IgG globulins transplacentally from their mothers, but this is a time-related occurrence, so that the premature infant has lower levels. Also, other conditions which predispose to neonatal infections, such as premature rupture of the membranes and maternal hemorrhage, occur more frequently in prematurity. The diagnosis and treatment of infections are essentially the same in preterm and term babies; the major difference is a heightened suspicion of preterm infants, in whom presenting signs are often very subtle.

Anemia   The anemia of prematurity is an exaggeration of the so-called "physiologic anemia" of full-term infants. All newborns manifest a gradual drop in their hemoglobin levels for the first 6 to 12 weeks of life. It is thought that the bone marrow halts production of red blood cells in response to the elevated oxygenation of extrauterine respiration. At 6 to 12 weeks, the bone marrow responds to the lowered hemoglobin level and begins to manufacture red blood cells again. Thus, the anemia usually disappears spontaneously. The problem with premature infants is that their total body iron stores and red blood cell mass are small compared to term babies, and as the premature grows rapidly in the first 2 months, he dilutes his red blood cells more than the term infant does. Only rarely does the hemoglobin level fall low enough to require a transfusion. Oral iron supplement is thought to be poorly utilized during the first 2 or 3 months of life, but its availability is important once the bone marrow starts up again. Most authorities agree that iron-fortified formulas or iron supplement to breast milk is the safest way of assuring the premature an adequate iron source.

Prognosis   The prognosis for preterm infants is varied. In general, the lower the birth weight, the more likely it is that the infant will have serious sequelae. Compared to term babies, preterm infants have a much higher incidence of mental retardation, learning disorders, and neurologic handicaps such as seizures, deafness, blindness, and cerebral palsy. The fact that a high percentage of preterm infants come from and therefore return to impoverished families compounds the handicaps that these children bear.

Recent evidence shows the importance of close bodily contact between mother and child to allow "bonding" (discussed in depth in Chaps. 23 and 24), which results in appropriate mothering behavior. The ill or incubated preterm infant may be isolated from his mother for days or even months. Recognition of the importance of bonding has led nurseries to allow and encourage mothers (and fathers) of hospitalized newborns to hold and care for their infant whenever possible. Delaying the parents' interaction with their new baby may lead to continued abnormal parenting behavior. Indeed, there is evidence of increased child battering among preterm babies.[23]

Teaching the mother or her surrogate to properly feed and care for the preterm infant also allows earlier discharge from the nursery. In fact, many nurseries are lowering their discharge weights to unprecedented levels with good results.

The Small-for-Gestational-Age Infant

The small-for-gestational-age (SGA) or small-for-dates (SFD) infant is defined as any newborn whose birth weight is less than the 3d percentile or less than two standard deviations below the weight expected for his gestational age. The SGA baby has also been referred to as *dysmature* or *pseudomature*. The term *intrauterine growth retardation* (IGR) is frequently used to denote the process which results in the SGA infant.

It is estimated that 1 out of every 3 low-birth-weight babies is truly small for gestational age; the remaining two-thirds are appropriately sized for their gestational age. Since the incidence of low-birth-weight infants is approximately 8 to 10 percent of live births, depending on the maternity population, the SGA infant is expected in at least 3 of every 100 births. Because these infants may have special problems, the early recognition of the SGA newborn becomes mandatory for proper nursery management.

The cause of intrauterine growth retardation is identified in only a small percentage of undergrown newborns. The most clearly defined causes are fetal chromosomal abnormalities and fetal infections. A much larger and more speculative group involves inadequate fetal nourishment from maternal malnourishment, vascular insufficiency, or uterine crowding. It must also be noted that infants with major congenital anomalies, even when not associated with aberrant chromosomes or infections, are often growth-retarded at birth. It is as if whatever noxious agent brought on the anomaly likewise distorted the general fetal growth.

The more commonly identified chromosomal aberrations associated with intrauterine growth retardation include the trisomies D, E, and G (Down's syndrome) as well as chromosomal deletions such as XO (Turner's) syndrome and cri-du-chat syndrome. Because chromosomes contain the genetic material which dictates and regulates growth and development, it follows that abnormalities of the

chromosomes may lead to deranged fetal growth. Thus, any SGA baby should be examined for physical characteristics of chromosomal syndromes.

Almost all presently recognized intrauterine infections may cause intrauterine growth failure. These infections have been discussed previously in this chapter and include rubella, cytomegalovirus, and toxoplasmosis. Rubella virus has been shown to actually arrest the cellular division of infected embryonic tissue. Presumably other infective agents might likewise disorder cellular, and therefore fetal, growth.

Unlike the above-mentioned genetically abnormal or microbe-infected babies, most SGA infants have no readily identifiable cause. These infants appear truly malnourished, and presumably represent an inadequate transport of nutrients from the mother to the fetus. The condition of these babies has been variously referred to as fetal malnutrition, intrauterine malnutrition, chronic fetal distress, and chronic placental insufficiency.

The mother's ability to supply metabolic material to the fetus may be curtailed for various reasons. If the mother's own oxygenation is subnormal, her capacity to adequately oxygenate her fetus is hampered. This point is demonstrated in the higher incidence of undergrown newborns in women with cyanotic heart disease and in women living under the hypoxic conditions at high altitudes. Likewise, maternal starvation limits the quality of nutrient flow to the fetus, resulting in poor fetal growth. Maternal malnutrition as a cause of fetal stunting has been most lucidly demonstrated in animal studies; parallels in humans are more difficult to substantiate. One human example is true maternal protein-calorie deficiency (most often seen in underdeveloped countries), which leads to a high rate of abortions, stillbirths, and undergrown newborns. The more subtle effects of less severe human maternal malnutrition remain to be fully defined. Another disorder inherent in the mother is diminished vascular supply to the uterus. Severe toxemia, diabetic vascular disease, and other forms of maternal hypertension result in vascular constriction and insufficiency, thereby limiting the quantity of nutrient flow to the placental interface for fetal nourishment.

Certain structural defects in the intrauterine environment may retard fetal nutrition. Twins or other multiple births are frequently SGA as well as preterm infants; their diminished growth appears to result directly from competition for limited space and nourishment in the crowded uterus. Lesions of the placenta such as hemangiomas and infarctions do occur but are rarely extensive enough to limit

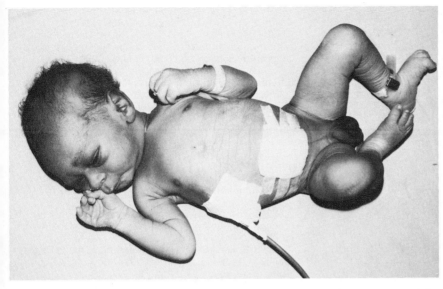

Figure 20-8 Postmature black male born at 43 weeks' gestation and weighing 2,840 Gm (6 lb, 4 oz), 2 days old when photographed. Note the diminished subcutaneous fat, cracked skin (especially noticeable over the upper abdomen and hands), long nails which extend beyond the ends of the fingers, heavy genital pigment, sole creases, and curly hair, which distinguish the postmature infant from the premature. The chest tube is for treatment of pneumothorax, which is often seen in postmature infants following meconium aspiration before birth or resuscitation at delivery.

fetal growth. In contrast to the usual situation of two umbilical arteries, a single umbilical artery is thought by some authorities to be associated with intrauterine growth retardation; presumably, reduced arterial flow directly results in diminution of nutritional supply to the fetus.

Description and Care The classic SGA infant is described as long and skinny with relatively large head, hands, and feet. His skin is loose, dry, and occasionally cracked. The hair is sparse and the umbilical cord is thin. If close to term in age, as is the usual case, the baby may have the physical characteristics appropriate for that gestational age, including sole creases, firm skull bones, and stiff ear cartilage. If not ill, he is more vigorous, active, and hungry than expected for his weight. In general, increasingly severe fetal malnutrition first retards weight, then length, then head circumference. Because of long-standing malnutrition, the SGA baby has an undersized liver, lowered metabolic supplies, and diminished subcutaneous tissue. As a result of these lowered energy resources and poor insulation, he is particularly prone to hypoglycemia, especially in the first 2 days of life. Close observation and serial blood sugars may identify this problem. However, many nurseries try to prevent hypoglycemia by beginning early feedings or intravenous glucose in the first few hours of life. In addition, every effort should be made to prevent inordinate cooling of the baby, since cooling consumes much of the infant's already inadequate energy stores and thus leads to hypoglycemia.

The malnourished neonate also has an elevated incidence of asphyxia neonatorum, and subsequently often requires resuscitation and metabolic correction. Intrauterine malnutrition results in lessened metabolic stores, thereby lowering the ability of the fetus to withstand the metabolic stresses of labor and delivery; the final expression of this inability is asphyxia. Close observation is needed for the unexpected apnea which may occur after resuscitation of these infants.

The prognosis for the SGA baby varies. If his smallness is associated with chromosomal aberrations, major congenital anomalies, or severe intrauterine infections, morbidity is marked and mortality is high. Otherwise, the SGA infant is thought to have a higher incidence of long-range sequelae, such as learning and behavior disorders and diminished adult stature. The lowered intellectual achievement is thought possibly to be due to fetal malnutrition during the peak intrauterine brain growth spurt during the last trimester of pregnancy, thus impairing critical brain development. Obviously, when the cause of intrauterine growth retardation is so frequently unknown, the ability to predict the individual infant's outcome is very limited. Like other high-risk babies, this child's prognosis is dependent upon the availability of good perinatal and neonatal medical and nursing care and upon the adequacy of family and community resources after he leaves the hospital.

Postmaturity

The postmature infant is one whose gestation is 42 weeks or longer and who shows signs of intrauterine weight loss and dehydration. The mechanisms that initiate normal labor are poorly understood; why labor is occasionally delayed past term is even less clear. However, it is known that the longer the gestation goes beyond 40 weeks, the higher the fetal morbidity and mortality.

The postmature infant is classically long, thin, with loose wrinkled skin that is often stained greenish-yellow and cracking. The nails are long and the skull firm. His wide-eyed alertness is more like that of a 2- or 3-week-old infant than that of a newborn (Fig. 20-8). Like SGA infants, these babies appear to suffer intrauterine malnutrition and hypoxia and frequently require resuscitation at birth. They are particularly prone to meconium aspiration, pulmonary hemorrhage, and hypoglycemia. Again like SGA infants, they appear to benefit from early feedings or intravenous glucose to avoid adding to their metabolic stress. Unless they suffer hypoxic damage or neonatal problems, their outlook is reasonable.

REFERENCES

1 C. M. Drillien, "The Small-for-Date Infant: Etiology and Prognosis," *Pediatric Clinics of North America*, 17(1):9, February 1970.
2 Sohan L. Manocha, *Malnutrition and Retarded Human Development*, Charles C Thomas, Publisher, Springfield, Ill., 1972, p. 174.
3 J. Dobbing, "Vulnerable Periods of Brain Development," in *Lipids, Malnutrition, and the Developing Brain*, Associated Scientific Publishers, Amsterdam, 1972, p. 12.
4 S. Shapiro et al., *Infant, Perinatal, Maternal, and Childhood Mortality in the United States*, Harvard University Press, Cambridge, Mass., 1968, p. 134.
5 Priscilla White, "Pregnancy and Diabetes," in A. Marble et al. (eds.), *Joslin's Diabetes Mellitus*, Lea & Febiger, Philadelphia, 1971, pp. 581–598.
6 D. Cavanagh and M. R. Talisman, *Prematurity and the Obstetrician*, Appleton-Century-Crofts, New York, 1969, p. 179.
7 C. Zelson et al., "Neonatal Narcotic Addiction: 10 Year Observation," *Pediatrics*, 48(2):178, August 1971.
8 Ibid.
9 G. R. G. Monif et al., "The Correlation of Maternal Cytomegalovirus Infection during Varying Stages in Gestation with Neonatal Involvement," *Journal of Pediatrics*, 80:17, January 1972.
10 G. R. G. Monif, *Viral Infections of the Human Fetus*, Macmillan & Co., Ltd., London, 1969, p. 73.
11 D. R. Miller et al., "Fatal Disseminated Herpes Simplex Virus Infection and Hemorrhage in the Neonate," *Journal of Pediatrics*, 76:409, March 1970.
12 D. E. Torphy et al., "Herpes Simplex Virus Infection in Infants: A Spectrum of Disease," *Journal of Pediatrics*, 76:405, March 1970.
13 Elizabeth L. Griffith, "The Treatment of Toxoplasmosis during Pregnancy," *Journal of the American Medical Women's Association*, 28:140, March 1973.
14 G. H. McCracken, "Group B Streptococci: The New Challenge in Neonatal Infections," *Journal of Pediatrics*, 82(4):703–706, April 1973.
15 R. A. Franciosi, "Group B Streptococcal Neonatal and Infant Infections," *Journal of Pediatrics*, 82(4):707–718, 1973.
16 Leslie L. Barton, "Group B Beta Hemolytic Streptococcal Meningitis in Infants," *Journal of Pediatrics*, 82(4):719–723, 1973.
17 Carol J. Baker, "Suppurative Meningitis Due to Streptococci of Lancefield Group B: A Study of 33 Infants," *Journal of Pediatrics*, 82(4):724–729, 1973.
18 Virginia Apgar, "A Proposal for a New Method of Evaluation of the Newborn Infant," *Current Researches in Anesthesia and Analgesia*, 32:260, July–August 1953.
19 S. G. Babson and R. C. Benson, *Management of High-Risk Pregnancy and Intensive Care of the Neonate*, The C. V. Mosby Company, St. Louis, 1971, p. 40.
20 Cavanagh and Talisman, op. cit., pp. 131–132.
21 Lula O. Lubchenco, "Neonatal Mortality Rate: Relationship to Birth Weight and Gestational Age," *Journal of Pediatrics*, 81(4):814–822, October 1972.
22 Mary Ellen Avery, "Prevention of Hyaline Membrane Disease," *Pediatrics*, 50:513, October 1972.
23 Leo Stern, "Prematurity As a Factor in Child Abuse," *Hospital Practice,* 8:117, May 1973.

BIBLIOGRAPHY

Abramson, H.: *Symposium on the Functional Physiopathology of the Fetus and Neonate*, The C. V. Mosby Company, St. Louis, 1971.
———: *Resuscitation of the Newborn Infant*, The C. V. Mosby Company, St. Louis, 1973.
Korones, S. B.: *High Risk Newborn Infants: The Basis for Intensive Nursing Care*, The C. V. Mosby Company, St. Louis, 1972.
Perinatal Factors Affecting Human Development, World Health Organization, Washington, D.C., 1969.
Pierog, Sophis H., and Ferrara, A.: *Approach to the Medical Care of the Sick Newborn*, The C. V. Mosby Company, St. Louis, 1971.

21

THE MENTALLY RETARDED CHILD

AMANDA SIRMON BAKER and
PAULINE HINTON BARTON

Mental deficiency refers to subaverage general intellectual functioning which originates during the developmental period and is associated with impairment in adaptive behavior.[1] This is the official definition of mental retardation adopted in 1958 by the American Association on Mental Deficiency. Mental retardation is one of the most serious handicapping conditions in the United States. It is a major health, social, and economic problem which denies afflicted persons the opportunity to compete academically or vocationally or to be accepted socially. The stigma of mental retardation prevents the retarded person from being treated as an equal by society and even robs him of the right to determine his own destiny.[2]

The following facts illustrate the extent of the problem. Between 100,000 and 200,000 babies born each year in the United States are mentally retarded. The causes of retardation can be identified in approximately one-fourth of the cases; in the remaining cases inadequacies in prenatal and perinatal care, nutrition, child rearing, and social and environmental opportunities are suspected as causes. Statistics show that in 1970 more than 6 million people in the United States were retarded. About 2½ million were under the age of 20. Of those under 20, approximately 75 percent were mildly retarded (educable); 15 percent were moderately retarded (trainable); 8 percent were severely retarded (some trainable); and 2 percent were profoundly retarded (unable to care for themselves).[3]

Mentally retarded children are, first of all, children with the same basic needs as all other children. They are found in all segments of society. The multiple and complex problems which they present demand the attention and services of the health disciplines, of educators, and of other helping professions. Each discipline contributes unique as well as shared knowledge and skills to the study and solution of these problems. Nursing has major responsibilities in the areas of prevention, case finding, and management.

The nursing knowledge and skills that are basic to the nursing care of normal children are also utilized in the case of the retarded. However, the nurse who effectively uses his knowledge of growth and development in assessing the developmental needs of a normal 18-month-old toddler may become frustrated in planning care for a 6- or 8-year-old toddler. Yet, the process is the same: after an assessment of the child's functional level of development, goals are defined and implemented which help him achieve the next developmental tasks. In order to do this, the nurse must be able to think about children in

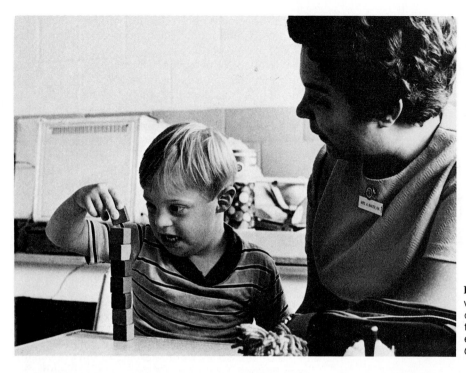

Figure 21-1 Nursing intervention to promote growth and development begins with a thorough developmental evaluation. *(Photo courtesy of George Lazar.)*

terms of their *functional level* rather than their *chronologic age* (Fig. 21-1).

SOCIETAL ATTITUDES TOWARD THE RETARDED

Factual knowledge and skill in working with children do not ensure that a nurse will be able to work effectively with retarded children and their families. The nurse may first need to work through his own feelings about defective or handicapped persons, for nurses as well as other professionals are caught in a cultural dilemma. Nurses reflect the cultural tendency to value intellectual capacity and achievement and to feel threatened by persons who are defective in this area. One of the sad truths of our culture is the tendency to cast out the weak, the deformed, and other helpless members. The authors contend that, regardless of the theoretical knowledge available to nurses and regardless of their assessment skills or their techniques for improving retarded persons' performance, the nursing needs of retarded children and their families will not be met unless underlying societal attitudes are changed.

During the last decade, Americans discovered that the Scandinavian countries were much further advanced in the care, education, and rehabilitation of the mentally retarded than the United States. In an effort to close the gap between American and Scandinavian services, attempts were made to replicate the Scandinavian model in various parts of the United States. In spite of these efforts, there were no resultant major changes in the care and rehabilitation of the retarded in this country. Lippman's[4] study of attitudes toward mental retardation in several European countries may explain why progress has been slower in the United States. He found that, especially in the Scandinavian countries, public leaders and people working with the retarded expressed attitudes and expectations that were markedly different from those in the United States. The Europeans expressed a philosophy which recognized the ultimate dignity of the individual. There was respect for the potential of each person, a conviction by professionals that the retarded can be helped, and acceptance of the social responsibility for providing adequate services.

Nursing can play a vital role in helping to modify existing attitudes toward retardation. Nurses can accept responsibility for teaching other members of the health team, including other professionals, and can initiate and support community educational and service programs. They can demonstrate to the child, his family, and his neighbors their concerns and respect for the dignity and potential of the deviant child. However, as a first step they must individually work through their own feelings about the retarded. This is not an easy or comfortable process. It involves an honest appraisal of personal attitudes and defenses which are used to avoid personal involvement in the care of retarded children and their families. Before the nurse denies having prejudices and negative feelings about the deviant child, he should ask himself such questions as:

1   What is my first reaction when I am told that a child is mentally retarded?
2   Do I tend to agree with the professional or family member who advises the mother to institutionalize her newborn mongoloid child before she becomes too emotionally involved?
3   What are my feelings about caring for a 6-year-old who is not toilet trained?
4   Can I warmly touch or embrace a child with grotesque physical features?
5   Do I believe that retarded persons can really be helped?

This personal assessment must be followed by experiences in working with retarded children—experiences that develop the ability to react to each child in terms of his individual needs and potential rather than in terms of his physical features or level of functioning.

THE NURSE AS THE CHILD'S ADVOCATE

A problem as complex as mental retardation calls for a large team of specialists from nursing, medicine, physical therapy, speech therapy, psychology, occupational therapy, and social work. The number of persons who work with any one child varies, depending on the child's specific problems and level of functioning. All share the common goal of helping the child achieve his maximum potential. But the size of the team and the child's widely varying problems can lead to fragmentation, with each group focusing on a particular problem and using specialized approaches to management.

The old saying that the sum of the parts is less than the whole is never truer than in the care of the retarded. Speech training, teaching of self-help skills, correction of physical defects, and the other facets of treatment are each important in promoting development. Yet if the child is to attain his potential, each special service must be incorporated into one overall plan which provides for the total spectrum of his developmental needs. It is often appropriate that the nurse be primarily responsible for constructing and overseeing this plan. The nurse thus becomes the advocate of "the whole child."

As advocate, the nurse not only works directly with the child but also acts in the child's behalf by his professional interactions with the other members of the team. Parents, for example, are very important members of the team and may need help understanding the goals and approaches of the many specialists and in developing and carrying out a plan of daily care that meets the needs of both child and family. The nurse may need to help a family acquire the necessary services that are available to help them. In some cases, the child's behavior or level of functioning may prevent his being accepted into available programs. Nursing efforts must then be focused on helping the child develop the behaviors that make him eligible for specific programs.

Nurses work in similar ways with cottage parents or caretakers in residential centers. Residential treatment is usually less effective than it might be because caretakers are not made aware of the professionals' plans or are not shown what they can do to assist. All too often cottage parents have little idea what happens when they send a child to the clinic, to occupational therapy, or to other specialty areas, and consequently they fail to utilize and provide practice in the cottage for the new skills being developed in these special programs. Some children are denied access to schools or to other services because cottage parents do not effectively help them overcome poor attention span, hyperactivity, incontinence, or inability to relate to an adult. Such was the plight of the institutionalized child in the following case history before a nurse assumed the role of advocate.

Judy was admitted to a large institution at age 4 with a diagnosis of deafness and mental retardation due to her mother's rubella during the first trimester of pregnancy. Reasons given for the child's institutionalization were extreme hyperactivity and destructive behavior with which her parents were no longer able to cope. Her hyperactivity, poor attention span, and deafness made accurate mental assessment impossible.

This same behavior in the institution led to Judy's being kept in bed most of the time because she fought with other children, tore up toys, and tried to run away. For the next 4 years, Judy remained "caged" except for infrequent opportunities to run around the play room. During this time she did learn to feed herself but had to be fastened in the chair to sit still long enough to eat. Her hyperactivity and destructiveness prevented her from being included in any of the training programs. The staff said that they did not have time to give her the individual attention she required.

When Judy was 8 years old, her cottage was chosen as a laboratory for nursing students. A graduate student in pediatric nursing worked with her intensively for the first 3 months, followed by junior students who rotated through the cottage for 2-week periods.

Initial nursing goals were directed toward helping Judy develop basic trust, relate to children and adults, and learn to play with toys. Beginning approaches included holding, cuddling, and vigorous physical activity. As Judy learned to relate to the students, she began to develop an interest in toys and to initiate contacts with adults. Six months later she was out of bed most of the day, engaged in quiet play for as long as 30 minutes, and rarely expressed aggression toward other children.

Special education and speech therapy consultants felt Judy was now ready to begin learning basic sign language, so this became a major goal for nursing students and cottage parents. She now understands and responds to simple signs such as those for "let's eat," "sit down," "go for a walk," "good," and "no." Now, at the end of the first year of the program, nursing goals are directed toward increasing her communication skills, her ability to participate in groups, and her self-help skills. These skills will enable her to participate in deaf education and make it possible to include her in other specialty programs as well as the general cottage activities.

As other specialty groups become more involved in Judy's care, nursing objectives will focus more on interdisciplinary communication while continuing to promote an environment which is conducive to the attainment of her maximum potential. Her progress during 1 year, after virtual isolation for 4 years, raises the question of whether institutionalization would have been necessary if her parents had received the support, guidance, and information they needed from the time the initial diagnosis was made.

THE RETARDED CHILD IN THE HOME

The retarded child has the same basic need as any other child to have an environment that provides experiences which give him a concept of himself as loved, wanted, valued, and respected. Children behave in terms of their perceptions of themselves, whether positive or negative, and society will tend to evaluate them *in terms of their behavior*. In order to provide a self-enhancing environment for their child, parents must have experiences which enhance their feelings of adequacy as parents.

Parental Reactions to Diagnosis

Parental reactions to mental retardation in their child vary widely. The degree and kinds of responses are influenced by such things as social class, marital relationships, attitudes toward deviance, past experiences, and parental aspirations. Despite the wide range of reactions described in the literature, some are found to be more prevalent than others—guilt, ambivalence, disappointment, frustration, anger, shame, and sorrow.

Solnit and Stark[5] have used the mourning process as a model for understanding the depressed reactions of mothers who have given birth to a defective child. Psychologic preparation during pregnancy includes both anticipation of a perfect child and fear of a damaged one. Thus, the birth of a defective child represents the loss of the desired child and the realization of the mother's fears. The initial phase of the mourning process is one of numbness and denial. This reaction is followed by a dawning awareness of the disappointment and loss, which is accompanied by affective and physical symptoms. In the last phase, the intense re-experiencing of the memories and expectations gradually reduce the strength of the wish for the idealized child.

Whether the realization that the child is mentally retarded occurs soon after birth or much later, parents almost invariably react with a profound sense of shock.[6] Their dreams of the future for their child are shattered and their own feelings of adequacy are threatened. Preoccupied with their own sorrow and grief, many withdraw from others for a time. Just as the mourning of the death of a loved one serves a useful purpose, mourning as a response to retardation in their child allows parents to work through their grief, face their problems, and emerge with attitudes and plans which will enable them to focus on the child's needs.

It is a mistake to try to interrupt this grief process too quickly with reassurances and advice. All too often while parents are still in the initial phase of disbelief or denial, they are pressured by presumably well-meaning family and professionals to make decisions about institutional placement. It is equally unwise to offer false hopes of cure or other unrealistic improvement through special medical or educational programs.

Parents need an atmosphere which allows them to feel, think, and talk about their feelings and their reactions to their child's retardation and encourages them to raise questions, doubts, and fears. One of the greatest obstacles is the anxiety which the child's condition may arouse in the nurse and other professionals. The nurse may try to reduce his own anxiety by avoiding the situation and rationalizing that the physician will talk with the family about their problems. The difficulty with this approach is that the physician and others may have similar anxieties

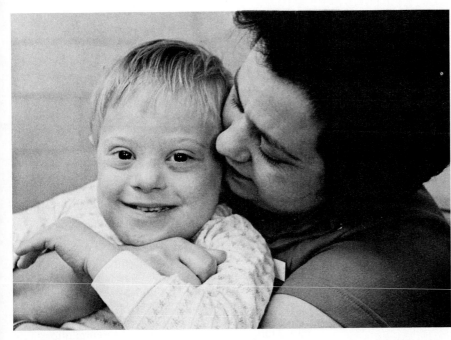

Figure 21-2 The way the nurse interacts with a child conveys to the child, his parents, and others her acceptance and re- *spect for the child. (Photo courtesy of George Lazar.)*

and defenses; as a result, the family may receive help from no one.

There is a difference in the typical grief reactions of parents of retarded children and those mourning the loss of a child through death. Parents struggling with a diagnosis of retardation have no time to work through the loss of the desired child before there is a demand to invest the new and handicapped child as a love object. There will be painful reminders of this loss as they watch children of comparable age at the commencement of school, adolescence, and maturity. Thus, residues of grief and distress may remain.[7]

Nursing care should be based upon a careful assessment of the family, including the stage of the parents' grief reaction. Parents cannot be expected to make decisions and long-term plans for the child while they are still in the initial phase of disbelief. However, they *are* faced with providing day-to-day care for the child. The focus of nursing should be on helping parents work through their feelings and provide immediate care for the child. The way in which the nurse handles and cares for the child can help promote positive feelings, for the parents' reactions are influenced by the reactions of other people (Fig. 21-2). It is difficult to have positive feelings when others seem repelled by the child's handicap. The nurse's posture, expression, and tone of voice as he cuddles, holds, or talks to the child can say to parents, "Your child is to me an individual with the potential for growth whom I can enjoy, value, and care

for." Unless the nurse accepts the child and does in fact view him as an individual with the right to develop to his fullest, still unrealized potential, he will not be able to convey this message convincingly.

For the majority of mentally retarded children, the diagnosis is not made in early infancy. The public health nurse is often the only professional who has an opportunity to discover developmental problems of young children that might otherwise go undetected until the child reaches school age.

At whatever age the diagnosis is made, many of the preceding comments apply. However, unless retardation is noted at birth, attachment between the parents and child proceeds without knowledge that the child is retarded. Some parents may close their minds to limitations that are apparent to everyone else. They are so eager to convince themselves of their child's normality that they focus on one or two things that he does well and ignore all areas in which he performs poorly. This denial may cause the parents to delay having the child checked by a physician. In fact, it is questionable whether they would profit from having the child evaluated while they are still denying the problem.

The answer to assisting parents in recognizing and accepting the diagnosis of mental retardation, cerebral palsy, or other handicapping condition lies not so much in careful preparation for telling them that the child is handicapped but more in planning experiences that will help them develop their own awareness of the problem, which can be further interpreted, confirmed, and validated by the professional.[9]

Recognizing and admitting that the child has a problem can be a turning point in the parents' ability to cope. They will need an opportunity to express their fears and anxieties in order to move on to looking at their problems more objectively. At this point they are ready for professional help and guidance in learning how to work with their child.

Promoting the Retarded Child's Growth and Development

Enhancing Parental Effectiveness Most persons learning to be parents find role models in their own parents, neighbors, or what they read or see on television. Parents of retarded children usually have no role models. They may have few guidelines for helping their child with simple skills which other children seem to learn automatically.

Yet the retarded child goes through the same stages of development as other children until he reaches his developmental limits. The primary differences are in the rate of growth, the level which he eventually achieves, and the amount of help he may need in achieving developmental tasks. Watching the development of a retarded child might be compared to watching a slow-motion film. Slow motion reveals that *small component parts* make up a single movement which happened so rapidly that only the gross action was otherwise noticeable. For example, applying the analogy to the task of self-feeding, Barnard and Powell[10] have identified 18 separate actions that a child goes through when feeding himself.

Nurses as well as parents may become discouraged and give up trying to teach a retarded child because they cannot see progress toward larger tasks, such as self-feeding, dressing, or toileting. But if they will break these larger tasks down into the component behaviors, the progress the child is making becomes more visible and can be more accurately evaluated. Parents thereby receive reinforcement for their effort, and the child's progressive experiences help him continue to advance.

The type of experience that is appropriate for any child—retarded or not—depends upon developmental readiness. For example, until a child is able to reach for an object, grasp it, and lift it to his mouth, he is not ready to use a spoon. Nurses, using their knowledge of child development, can help

parents learn to read the signs of a child's readiness and to act on them. If parents miss developmental cues the child gives them, they may fail to provide needed experiences or stimulation. The child then fails to acquire the skills of which he is capable. If parents misinterpret cues, they may expect achievements which the child is not developmentally able to produce. The parents then become disappointed and frustrated, and the child is subjected to failure which can further threaten his sense of adequacy and security. It is especially important that the parents of *retarded* children learn to read cues which tell them a child is developing the component parts of a task and when he is ready for help in putting these parts together.

Enhancing the Child's Self-Esteem The child's self-concept is a potent factor influencing what he will become and how well he will be able to use the abilities he does possess. Through his interactions with others, including his family members, he learns what to expect of the world and what the world expects of him. The reactions of society and the limitations imposed by his handicap increase the likelihood that the retarded child will experience failure and rejection. However, it is possible to provide satisfying experiences which lead the child to view himself as adequate and secure, as being loved and as being able to do what is expected of him. If his background experiences are deprived, harsh, or inconsistent, he will have either confused or negative views of himself and of the world.

To develop an adequate self-concept, the retarded child has the same needs in terms of his physical and interpersonal worlds as the normal child. The age at which he is ready for certain experiences may vary from the normal and depends on his level of functioning (Fig. 21-3). An overall goal which requires special attention is helping him develop skills that promote independent behavior and adjustment to his peer group in the home and the school. Both the child and the parents receive positive reinforcement for their efforts if the child can learn self-help skills such as self-feeding, dressing, and toileting. Barnard and Powell[9, 10] provide comprehensive guidelines for the use of behavior modification techniques in teaching self-help skills.

Play Promotes Development Play activities can be effectively used in helping the child develop the component behavior required for a larger task. For example, play with blocks, stack toys, puzzles, pots and pans, and wooden beads can help a child develop the eye-hand coordination that is prerequisite

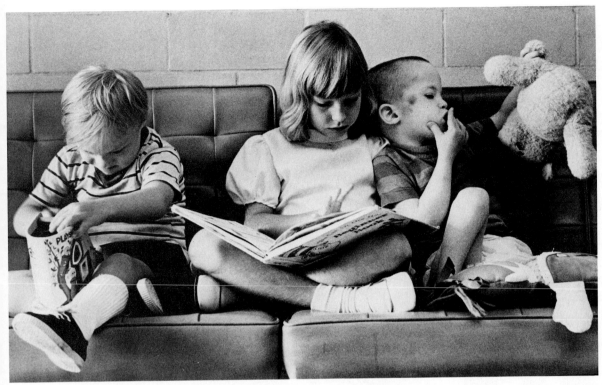

Figure 21-3 These children are all 7 years old, but their levels of functioning are very different. Each has the right to experiences that will help him develop to his maximum potential. *(Photo courtesy of George Lazar.)*

to the mastery of self-help skills. Special dolls or old clothing can be used in play to promote skill in tying, buttoning, snapping, and zipping.

Play can also be used to help the child prepare for eventual entry into school. Well-chosen play activities lengthen his attention span, increase his ability to accept limitations, and give him practice in group participation. These are factors which contribute to his ability to adjust to the demands and limitations of the school and to become accepted by his peer group. The better the child is able to conform to the accepted behavior patterns of his group, the less likely he is to be subjected to the ridicule and teasing which is so often the lot of the child who is different. The more the child is accepted by his peer group, the more likely he is to develop a concept of himself as adequate, liked, and respected (Fig. 21-4).

STRESS IN THE FAMILY

Variations in families, children, and communities, and all the many combinations in which they interact, make it impossible to draw any sweeping generalization about stress in the family of a retarded child.

Parents vary in their ability to accept and care for the child. Communities vary in their acceptance and in resources available. However, whatever the severity of the child's handicap or the family or community situation, significant and long-lasting effects on the lives of family members are to be expected. This is true even of the child whose parents are no more intelligent than he is. He may not be considered a deviant within the family. Yet the demands and expectations of the school and community may create even more problems for the already deprived family.[11]

Neither the child nor the family can escape the rejection which still exists in society and discourages families from social contacts. Neighbors may complain about the retarded child's behavior and refuse to let their children play with him. Many parents tend to withdraw from social activities. This withdrawal does not help substantially, for they cannot escape from the emotional hurt. They need to be drawn into more active social relationships. Parent organizations such as the American Association for Retarded Citizens can be especially helpful, as can church and civic groups.

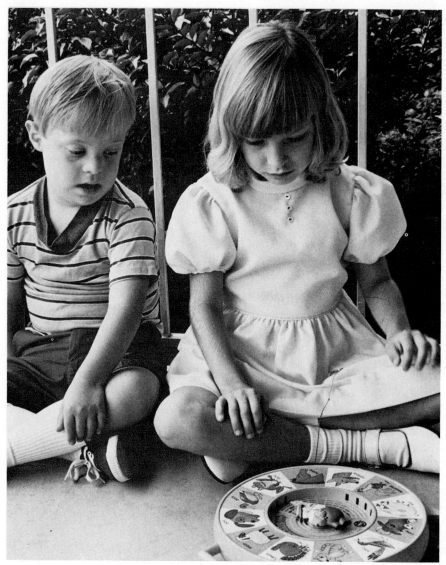

Figure 21-4 All children need friends and play experiences to develop their skills and promote a favorable self-concept. *(Photo courtesy of George Lazar.)*

There are many other problems which the family may have to face. Some children require nursing care around the clock and constant protection from common dangers. Just the simple routines of daily care of a severely handicapped child easily become burdens from which the family cannot escape. Baby-sitters may refuse to keep the child. As a consequence, the health of the mother, who usually bears the brunt of care, may be seriously affected. The financial cost of care can be a severe strain on the budget. The problem, which is already great, is increased by the tendency of many families to go from physician to physician and even to faith healers, seeking a cure for the child. The mother is often unable to work outside the home and contribute to the family income.

Parents and professionals tend to worry about the effect of the retarded child on normal siblings. There is a chance that other children in the family will become the target for high parental aspirations to compensate for their disappointment in the retarded child. Siblings also may be deprived of attention because parents are overwhelmed and overly involved in the care of the retarded child. The degree and type of effects on siblings are influenced to a large degree by the ability of parents to individualize their children, to give to each according to his needs, and to integrate the retarded child into the family as a valued and contributing member.

Some comments of two students to one of the authors illustrate the differing reactions of siblings and some of the factors responsible for them. One said:

I want help in getting my sister committed to an institution. She's pretty bright—can do housework and works especially well with young children. But she still needs someone to look after her. My parents are in poor health and soon she will be my responsibility. I resent her too much to have her with me. My mother spent all her time caring for her and all of our money going all over the country trying to help her. She didn't profit from any of it and now I am having to work to put myself through school. I've always had to sacrifice for her.

In contrast, the second student commented:

Dody has fit into our family and seldom caused any of our needs not to be met. She has her friends, participates in recreational activities, and helps with household chores as do the rest of us. My mother took most of the responsibility for teaching and disciplining. She received stimulation not only from our parents but from me, our two younger sisters, and our friends. We were encouraged to give her approval for the things that she did well and ignore her failures. I do not feel that we have been damaged by having a retarded sister. We have all learned to deal and cope with Dody and she has received a lot more from us in the way of education and love than she could have received anywhere else.

The nurse is concerned with promoting the well-being of all family members. Any plan of care must consider the needs of the retarded child in relation to the needs of the parents and the normal siblings.

THE MENTALLY RETARDED CHILD IN AN INSTITUTION

Our society has traditionally utilized institutions for the retarded to isolate deviant persons and to provide primarily custodial rather than habilitative care. The concept that institutional services could more appropriately aim at developing retarded persons into the most they are capable of becoming has not in the past been a popularly held expecta-tion. Emphasis on habilitation and money for institutional improvements began in the 1960s, after President Kennedy's interest in mental retardation gained publicity.

Nursing has just begun to develop its role as a leader in the residential care of the retarded. The majority of nurses who work in this area are in administrative positions or work only in the institutions' hospitals, concentrating on care for the acutely ill. Too many nurses still regard care of the retarded as being primarily custodial and are not involved in programs to meet developmental needs.

The authors believe strongly that society should make *community* care available for these handicapped members and provide emotional and financial support to families in order to make this possible. Until this goal is reached, however, there will be children in institutions for the mentally retarded, and nurses can provide an important service by accepting their responsibility for this population of patients and contributing their unique professional knowledge and skills.

One of the common inadequacies of institutions is the necessity to group persons for economy of care. This grouping often destroys the individual's identity and allows those responsible for his care to view him as a part of a group rather than as an individual human being with personal needs and desires, similar to others, but also unique. There can be warm and tender physical care given in institutions, but extreme social and emotional deprivation can exist at the same time. The "herding" phenomenon is evident in the following daily schedule for one cottage in one of the better state institutions. There are about 45 children, whose ages range from 3 to 14 years. Their levels of functioning range from infant to preschool. Six or seven personnel are available to give care.

6:00 A.M.   Bath and bed change. Only those children who are ambulatory are allowed out of bed. They roam aimlessly around, playing by themselves or with each other. Toys are not available. Cottage parents are busy with baths, which must be finished before breakfast.

8:00 A.M.   Breakfast is served. Children who can feed themselves or who are in the training program for self-feeding sit at tables to eat. The other children are fed in their cribs. Those who are still on bottles must hold them for themselves—no one has time to cuddle and interact with them during the meal. Children on pureed or regular diets are fed as rapidly as possible. Those who are unable to sit alone are fed lying down

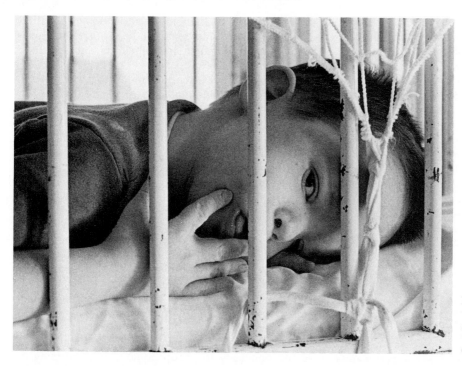

Figure 21-5 Lack of stimulation results in boredom, apathy, and loneliness as well as failure to develop. *(Photo courtesy of George Lazar.)*

rather than being propped upright. After the meal is finished, teeth are brushed and mouths rinsed.

9:30 to 11:00 A.M. After all have eaten, the children are cleaned up from breakfast, diapers are changed, and those who can move around in some fashion are placed on the floor to play. Toys are brought out, if they are available, and if cottage parents see toys and play as being important. A few of the children are dressed and sent to various activities, such as occupational therapy, speech therapy, or medical appointments.

11:00 A.M. to 12:00 noon Children are placed back in their cribs and cleaned up for lunch. Toys are removed if any have been out.

12:00 noon to 1:30 P.M. Lunch is served. The breakfast procedure is repeated.

1:30 to 3:00 P.M. Children remain in their cribs for rest period.

3:00 to 4:00 P.M. Ambulatory children are out of cribs. Some nonambulatory children may also be allowed out of bed, depending on which of the cottage parents are working that day.

4:00 to 6:00 P.M. Baths are given, night clothes are put on, and everything is made ready for supper and bedtime.

6:00 P.M. Supper is served.

7:00 to 8:00 P.M. Children are put to bed for the night. Many have been out of bed *only for baths* that day.

The monotonous routine begins again the next day at 6:00 A.M. Little or no developmental progress occurs in most children who pass their days this way (Fig. 21-5). The assumption is often made—but it is unjustifiable—that the lack of learning and growth results from limitations intrinsic in the retarded child. In such an impoverished setting, from what learning experiences might he learn? From what stimulation could he grow? Children with *normal* intelligence require experience and stimulation for their proper development; intellectually deficient children can hardly be expected to thrive on less (Fig. 21-6).

It is not useful to place blame for this experiential impoverishment on cottage parents. They are responsible for keeping the cottage clean and the children fed and clean. It is hard physical labor and often is on a low salary scale. There never seem to be enough personnel available to get everything done without hurrying.

Responsibility for the care, or lack of it, lies instead with those who set policies, decide priorities, and allocate funds. Nurses have the knowledge of growth and development and the management skills to assume leadership in planning, policy making, and priority setting as well as in implementing programs of care for the retarded. Many of the other disciplines concentrate primarily on one area: speech therapy, physical therapy, or education. Other specialized groups deal with legislative and public education aspects of programs. Nursing is the one discipline whose "target" is the child and family as a whole.

Programs to Stimulate the Retarded Child's Growth and Development

Custodial care, even at its best, has only the limited aims of hygiene, health maintenance, and protection. It is not designed to improve human competence. Almost all retarded children *can* develop some interpersonal skills and some independence in daily living activities, but these social and self-maintenance abilities require individually tailored programs of training and practice.

These individually prescribed programs need to be based on theories of growth and development, including learning. Erikson[12] describes the developmental tasks of the stages of development. The Robinsons[7] and others explicate Piaget's descriptions of the stages of cognitive development. Gordon[13] describes the child as a whole which is greater than the sum of its parts. These concepts can be used to identify the stage of development or level of functioning of an individual retarded child and to provide the experiences which he needs at that particular stage. For example, developmentally appropriate infancy sensorimotor learning experiences can be prescribed for the child who is still functioning as an infant even though his chronologic age might be 10 or 11 years. He can also be provided the interpersonal setting in which he can develop a one-to-one relationship, which is one of the prerequisites to establishing a sense of trust. Piaget's theory of intelligence as it pertains to mental retardation is presented well in Robinson and Robinson.[7] Spectacular advances occur in the development of individual children as a direct result of care planned by nurses and based on these theories, although change comes more gradually for some.

Bron is 13 years old chronologically but developmentally a young infant. He was admitted to an institution when only 18 months old, with almost no social or medical history given. His mother said he did not like to be touched and that he had epileptic seizures. He was started on medication to control the seizures, but the "flailing out" movement of his extremities continued when he was touched. Before long, the message got around—"Bron doesn't like to be touched"—and so he was very seldom touched except to be bathed and to have diapers changed. He was even fed lying down, with a minimum of contact. He learned to move around on his back on the floor by

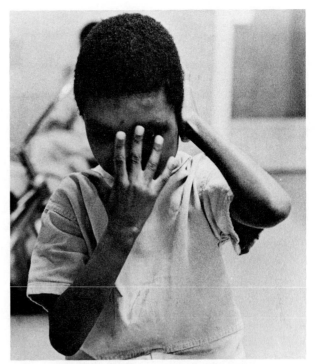

Figure 21-6 This boy finds ways for self-stimulation in an environment which fails to provide visual and tactile experiences. *(Photo courtesy of George Lazar.)*

pushing with his feet and lifting his hips, but he never crawled or pulled up. His head control was very poor, and he even was unable to sit up without support. He did not smile or laugh and seldom responded when his name was called.

When Bron was 12 years old, nursing students and occupational therapy students included him in their developmental programs. He was cuddled and caressed despite his protests, in order to desensitize him to touch. He was placed in a "relaxer" chair for sitting; toys were provided to increase fine motor skills and eye-hand coordination; he was played with, talked to, praised for just "being" and for each small accomplishment; he was rocked and exercised on a large beach ball to improve kinesthesia and equilibrium. He was taken for rides in a wheelchair and taken outside for sunbaths and play. In less than 1 year, Bron was a different child. He began to smile, then laugh. He learned to hold his head up and play with many types of toys. He began to sit alone and push up to a standing position when his feet touched the floor. His eye-hand coordination improved tremendously. He began to reach out and explore his environment. He truly became an inquisitive and developing infant.

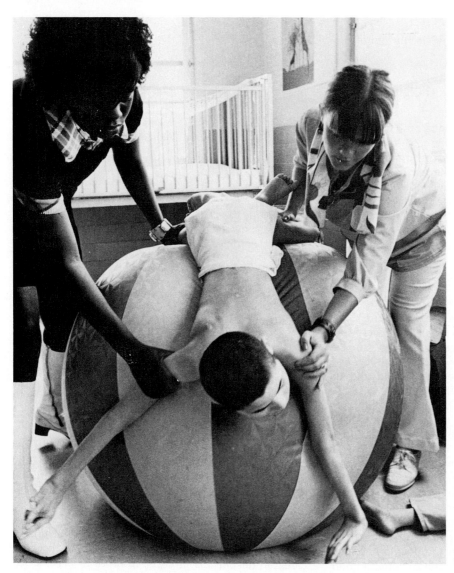

Figure 21-7 A large beach ball can be used as a substitute for the kinesthetic sensations of swinging and rocking. *(Photo courtesy of George Lazar.)*

Bron's developmental program had consisted of activities appropriate for an infant—those things which a mother does for and with her baby. It takes a little improvising to provide these for a large 12-year-old infant (Fig. 21-7). The beach ball was substituted for the swinging and rocking of being carried, the wheelchair was substituted for stroller, the relaxer chair for highchair, etc. The individual attention was provided by several different people, all following and updating goals and orders written by nursing students. The cottage parents were involved in the developmental program and are as thrilled as anyone with the progress Bron and others are making. The most recent new order is for Bron to begin using a

spoon and gradually learn to feed himself. Bron and his advocates are working on it.

THE CHILD WITH MULTIPLE HANDICAPS

Children who are born with one defect have problems, but more than one defect compounds the situation. The child with both mental and physical handicaps is especially unfortunate and requires costly intensive and extensive therapy from a variety of disciplines if he is to have an opportunity to develop (Fig. 21-8).

The child who is deaf or blind or both may become retarded as a result of limited learning experiences. This child needs more varied learning opportunities than does the child who is receiving messages through both vision and hearing. It is difficult for the child who is deaf at birth (prelingual deafness) to have any real conception of language. His development of communication, either oral language signs or finger spelling, is a long, tedious process. Communication is accomplished through play and close relationships with significant others. If these opportunities are denied the deaf child, his chances of reaching his potential are practically nonexistent. The blind child receives auditory messages, but unless he has the opportunity to develop a basic sense of trust (the developmental task of infancy) and can explore the world around him, he may well become withdrawn and fearful and hence not develop to his potential.

The child who has orthopedic handicaps which restrict his gross motor and fine motor adaptive skills has his world reduced to his immediate area unless someone helps him to move about and to explore and learn. The child with cerebral palsy is a good example of a child who might very well have been born with normal intellectual potential but who is so handicapped in other ways that he often never reaches his potential.

The child who has an unusual or unpleasant appearance is particularly handicapped in our society, where there is such emphasis on physical beauty. He may be shunned by others who are shocked at his appearance and do not know how to relate to him. He may well develop a negative self-concept and may not attempt to succeed in areas where he has to interact with others. If his learning ability also is impaired, many more opportunities are closed to him.

Children with multiple handicaps need a great deal of individual attention, concentrated therapy, and many special learning opportunities if they are to develop. Most of our institutions for the retarded do not offer this quality of care. These services must be provided in the community and made available regardless of the financial status of the family. If the child is placed in an institution and does not receive the many-faceted activities and relationships essential to his growth and development, he becomes more seriously handicapped and truly does become retarded in many ways and often totally dependent on others for his care.

THE RETARDED CHILD IN THE HOSPITAL

Toni, a petite 6-year-old resident of a large state institution, was admitted to a city hospital for eye surgery. No attempt was made by the nursing staff to

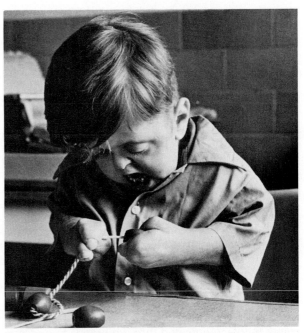

Figure 21-8 The child with multiple handicaps needs opportunities to develop. Intellectual potential may not be achieved because of the many physical handicaps and the adverse reactions of others. *(Photo courtesy of George Lazar.)*

assess her development or to prepare her for surgery. She was placed in a room alone with a net over her crib. After surgery, while still reacting from the anesthesia, she pulled off her eye bandages. No attempt was made to readjust her arm restraints, and one staff member commented that they would never be able to keep bandages on her. What happened? Why did Toni receive such inadequate nursing care? The answer probably lies in the fact that she was admitted to the hospital with the label "mentally retarded." There was believed to be no need to assess her development, for she was already diagnosed retarded. She must have a crib net—a retarded child might fall out of bed or run away. Why prepare her for surgery? A retarded child would not understand.

Astute observations or standardized testing would have shown Toni was functioning at the 4-year age level. Her language development alone should have been sufficient answer to one nurse's question, "Is she severely retarded?" At the institution, Toni had been prepared for and understood the reason for her hospitalization. She did not need a net over her crib. Since she did not have parents with her and was accustomed to sleeping in the room with a group of girls, she would probably have felt more secure in the room with another child. She needed specific information about the experiences which she would have before and after surgery. She could understand simple, concrete explanations. Play, which is her natural medium of expression, would have been particularly helpful in preparing her for surgery. Play experience of having her eyes bandaged before surgery might have reduced the trauma of waking up and being unable to see. Through play she could have worked through some of her feelings about her hospital experiences. What Toni needed was nursing care based on a thorough evaluation of all pertinent data available through written records, developmental testing, play interview, child's verbalizations, and observation of her behavior.

Nursing care that promotes effective nurse-child communication must be based upon an evaluation of the child's functional level of development. This is true for all children but especially so for the child with a wide discrepancy between his functional and chronologic ages. Acceptance, values, and information which the nurse wishes to convey to the child must be communicated through language and nonverbal behavior appropriate to the child's cognitive level. For example, preparation for surgery for a 10-year-old who is functioning at the 3-year age level must be geared at a level which a 3-year-old can understand. The retarded older adolescent or adult who can only think concretely cannot understand abstract reasoning. His teaching must be in terms of concrete objects and situations which have meaning for him.

Hospitalization can be a growth-promoting experience for the child and his parents. If the child receives the support and help which he needs to cope with his experiences, his sense of adequacy is enhanced. It may be the first opportunity which parents have had to talk about their feelings and seek professionals' answers to their questions. Their confidence in their parenting abilities can be increased if nurses follow through with training programs which have already been initiated by parents and support and reinforce the parents' effective actions. Long-term goals for the child can be developed during hospitalization by the nurse and his colleagues and the parents, and appropriate referrals can be made to ensure continued follow-through.

Expert nursing intervention is especially needed for the child who is admitted to the hospital from an institution. In all likelihood, little information about him will be available, so the nursing plan must be based primarily on an evaluation done in the hospital situation. Preparation for hospitalization is usually limited or nonexistent. Very few institutional resi-

dents will be visited by parents or persons they know. Nursing intervention must ensure that these children, no less than other patients, receive the comfort, support, and teaching that give them as much security as possible in a strange and unfamiliar setting.

The nurse also has an opportunity to influence the attitudes of other hospitalized children and their parents. Through the play program and other planned experiences, children may have valuable opportunities to begin to understand and accept others who differ from them. Parent attitudes can be beneficially modified by observing the nurse's reactions to the retarded child, having an opportunity to talk about retardation, and receiving factual information which can correct misconceptions they may have about mental retardation.

SPECIAL HEALTH PROBLEMS

Health professionals too often focus on the fact that a child is mentally retarded and then attribute any unusual symptoms or behavior to this fact, failing to look at the overall health status of the child. Retarded children often have lowered resistance to illness and need frequent medical and nursing care. Many also have congenital defects, such as a cleft palate or heart defects, which create special health needs.

These children are as varied and as individual in their health care requirements as any group of children, but there are generalizations which can be made. The child who is mongoloid might very well have cardiac problems and will be more susceptible than most to upper respiratory tract infections. The child with cerebral palsy may have difficulty swallowing and may be susceptible to aspiration pneumonia. Children who are not active and who eat poorly may become constipated easily. The child who is in the inquisitive stage of exploration (regardless of chronologic age) may put poisonous or other dangerous substances in his mouth or may injure himself in other ways.

Dental care or its absence can affect the child's health and development. Poor dentition can be due to many factors, such as malformation of the jaw and dental structures, lack of stimulation from chewing, inadequate cleaning of the teeth and gums, infrequent dental care, and the side effects of medications. The resulting unattractive mouth hampers not only the child's physical well-being but also his acceptance by others.

Lack of exercise, sunshine, and fresh air can compound a child's physical problems. Contractures develop from positions maintained too long; vitamin D deficiency results from underexposure to sunshine. Poor appetite and general malaise also often result from these insufficiencies. The child who is mentally retarded has the same basic needs as the normal child but may require care and assistance for a longer period of time to meet these needs.

A trusting relationship between the child, his parents, physician, and nurse is invaluable. The family may need help in obtaining medical care and financial assistance. The nurse can help by referring the family to the proper agency and by following up on the referral.

CLASSIFICATION

There are many systems for classifying mental retardation. Classification according to causative factors (infection, intoxication, trauma, etc.) is often used in medical and nursing literature. In a considerable percentage of cases the cause is not known; therefore, no specific diagnosis is possible except that of "mental retardation, causes unknown."

Rather than being derived primarily from causative factors, the following classification is based on the development of the child when the condition occurred. Only the most common conditions will be outlined here.

I Prenatal period
  A Chromosome anomalies
    1 Down's syndrome (trisomy 21)
    2 Klinefelter's syndrome
  B Errors of metabolism
    1 Phenylketonuria (PKU)
    2 Hypothyroidism (cretinism)
    3 Hurler's disease (gargoylism)
  C Malformation of the cranium
    1 Microcephaly
    2 Hydrocephaly
  D Maternal factors
    1 Rubella (German measles)
    2 Some other viral illnesses of mother
    3 Syphilis
    4 Anoxia
    5 Blood type incompatibility
    6 Malnutrition
    7 Toxemia
II Neonatal or perinatal period
  A Anoxia
  B Intracranial hemorrhage
  C Birth injury
  D Kernicterus
  E Prematurity

III Postnatal period
  A Infections
    1 Meningitis
    2 Encephalitis
  B Poisoning
    1 Insecticides
    2 Medications
    3 Lead
  C Degenerative disease
    1 Tay-Sachs disease
    2 Huntington's chorea
    3 Niemann-Pick disease
  D Physical injury
    1 Head injury
    2 Asphyxia
    3 Hyperpyrexia
  E Brain tumors
  F Social and cultural factors
    1 Deprivation
    2 Emotional disturbance
    3 Nutritional deficiency

Knowing the cause of the retardation or the period when it apparently occurred tells us *generally* what to expect in terms of behavior and potential. These expectations, however, cannot safely be assumed to be *absolute*. Each child is very much an individual and is as different from others with the same diagnosis as he is similar to them.

The IQ (intelligence quotient) score has been and is being misused and overused to conveniently separate retarded persons into three major categories:

1 Those with and IQ between 50 and 75 are referred to as the educable mentally retarded (EMR). These children function well in special education classes in public school and in general classrooms with understanding teachers. As adults they are usually employed in unskilled or semiskilled jobs and are extremely affected by the economic status of the society. When jobs are scarce, these persons are often considered expendable by employers. Aside from their precarious socioeconomic status, they usually blend in well with society and function independently as adults, although in times of crisis they may require assistance from social agencies. These people might not be considered retarded in a less complex society than ours, and in fact, function well in some segments of American society.

2 Those with an IQ between 25 and 50 are referred to as the trainable mentally retarded (TMR). These children rarely learn to read and write but can learn self-help skills, social skills, and simple job skills which will enable them to care for their own personal needs. They can learn to feed themselves, dress themselves, and care for their own hygiene and toileting needs. Such social skills as acceptable behavior, table manners, and speech or other means of communication can be learned and are necessary to function in our society. Job skills such as housekeeping, gardening, animal care, and other manual activities can be taught to these people and will help them become valuable members of society. As children and adults the trainable mentally retarded require assistance and usually function best in sheltered workshops and the home environment.

3 Those with an IQ between 0 and 25 are referred to as custodial, profoundly, or severely retarded. These children require help with most functions of daily living. They must be fed, bathed, and cared for by others. They function as infants or toddlers and require the same care and protection. These children can learn, but their tasks are those of infancy: to sit, to stand, and to relate to others. Some can learn to feed themselves with assistance. They can learn to play with toys and with other children. These children require continued care and protection as adults, either in the home environment or in an institution.

Intelligence tests do not measure intelligence or potential; they measure achievement. They are reasonably accurate for the large numbers of persons around the average, or mean, of the population but are not accurate for those who function at the extremes, either above or below average. They yield especially imprecise measurements of those persons with impaired motor coordination or impaired speech development, since performance on most of these tests requires use of motor skills and written or spoken language. Therefore, IQ scores cannot accurately be used as the sole diagnostic criterion by which a child is placed in any special program. Used in conjunction with other evaluations, IQ scores can be helpful in assessing and planning for retarded children. Periodic evaluations are essential to coordinate programs with the child's development.

Rather than relying heavily on the syndrome classification or the IQ categories, nurses and others will find it helpful to concentrate instead on the approximate age level at which the child is functioning and to develop objectives and goals to meet the developmental needs of that particular level. These age levels may vary for different activities within a single child; for example, he may be functioning at approximately age 3 years in gross motor activities and need

opportunities to perfect the skills of riding a tricycle, bouncing and catching a ball, running, etc., and yet may still be functioning at the 1-year age level in personal-social skills such as dressing, eating, and toilet training. The Denver Developmental Screening Test (DDST), described in Chapter 2, is helpful for indicating areas in which the child needs assistance. Growth and developmental needs, rather than the chronologic age and the developmental lag which exists, are the basis for program planning. Treating a child as though there were no hope for improvement and expecting nothing to happen often produce a self-fulfilling prophecy. Purkey[14] describes the effect of self-concept on school achievement; this can well apply to achievement in any area of living. Expectations must be realistic, however, so that the child will experience success and therefore feel successful. For example, instead of expecting a child to be independent enough at age 5 to attend kindergarten and being disappointed because he is not, it is more realistic and more constructive to be pleased that he is learning to feed and dress himself and is showing progress toward *becoming* independent.

Each child is an individual with various strengths and weaknesses. Nursing activities should build on his strengths and help him to overcome his liabilities or adapt to the limits they impose so that he can live his life to the fullest and achieve his potential, however great or small that might be.

REFERENCES

1 R. Heber (ed.), "A Manual on Terminology and Classification in Mental Retardation," Monograph suppl., *American Journal of Mental Deficiency*, 64(2):3, 1958.
2 L. T. Taft, "Mental Retardation: An Overview," *Pediatric Annals*, 2(7):10–24, July 1973.
3 *Profiles of Children: White House Conference on Children*, U.S. Government Printing Office, Washington, D.C., 1970.
4 L. D. Lippman, *Attitudes toward the Handicapped*, Charles C Thomas, Publisher, Springfield, Ill., 1972.
5 A. Solnit and M. Stark, "Mourning and the Birth of a Defective Child," in F. J. Menolascine (ed.), *Psychiatric Aspects of the Diagnosis and Treatment of Mental Retardation*, Special Child Publications, Seattle, Wash.
6 Ibid., p. 509.
7 H. B. Robinson and Nancy M. Robinson, *The Mentally Retarded Child: A Psychological Approach*, McGraw-Hill Book Company, New York, 1965.
8 R. D. Freeman, "Psychological Management of the Retarded Child and the Family," *Pediatric Annals*, 2(7):53–58, July 1973.
9 Kathryn E. Barnard and Marcene L. Powell, *Teaching the Mentally Retarded Child*, The C. V. Mosby Company, St. Louis, 1972, p. 27.
10 Ibid., p. 97.
11 M. J. Begab, "Mental Retardation and Family Stress," in F. J. Menolascino (ed.), *Psychiatric Aspects of the*

Diagnosis and Treatment of Mental Retardation, Special Child Publications, Seattle, Wash., 1971, pp. 128–143.

12 E. H. Erikson, *Childhood and Society*, 2d ed., W. W. Norton & Company, Inc., New York, 1963.

13 I. Gordon, *Human Development: From Birth through Adolescence*, Harper & Brothers, New York, 1962.

14 W. W. Purkey, *Self-concept and School Achievement*, Prentice-Hall, Englewood Cliffs, N.J., 1970.

BIBLIOGRAPHY

Adams, Margaret: *Mental Retardation and Its Social Dimensions*, Columbia University Press, New York, 1971.

Alpern, G. D., and Boll, T. J. (eds.): *Education and the Care of Moderately and Severely Retarded Children*, Special Child Publications, Seattle, 1971.

Blatt, B.: *Exodus from Pandemonium*, Allyn and Bacon, Inc., Boston, 1970.

———, and Kaplin, F.: *Christmas in Purgatory: A Photographic Essay on Mental Retardation*, Allyn and Bacon, Inc., Boston, 1966.

Farber, B.: *Mental Retardation: Its Social Context and Social Consequences*, Houghton Mifflin Company, Boston, 1968.

Grossman, Frances K.: *Brothers and Sisters of Retarded Children*, Syracuse University Press, New York, 1972.

Haynes, Una: *A Developmental Approach to Casefinding*, United States Department of Health, Education, and Welfare, Washington, D.C., 1967.

Hurley, R. L.: *Poverty and Mental Retardation: A Causal Relationship*, Vintage Books, Random House, Inc., New York, 1969.

Koch, R., and Dobson, J. C.: *The Mentally Retarded Child and His Family*, Bruner/Mazel, New York, 1971.

Leland, H., and Smith, D. E.: *Play Therapy with Mentally Subnormal Children*, Grune & Stratton, Inc., New York, 1965.

Schild, Sylvia: "The Family of the Retarded Child," in Koch, R., and Dobson, J. C. (eds.), *The Mentally Retarded Child and His Family*, Brunner/Mazel, New York, 1971, pp. 431–442.

Scipien, Gladys, and Wildoner, Marie: "A Study of the Concerns of Nurses Regarding Institutionalizing Mentally Retarded Children," *A.N.A. Clinical Sessions*, pp. 149–155, 1970.

Steele, Shirley (ed.): *Nursing Care of the Child with Long Term Illness*, Appleton-Century-Crofts, New York, 1971.

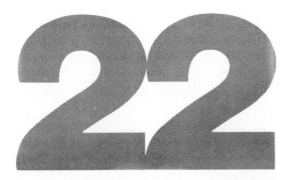

THE EMOTIONALLY DISTURBED CHILD

DORRIS BROOKS PAYNE

Deedle-deedle-deedledeedledeedle
Tweedle tweedle deedle deedle dum
Dumb Dumb Dumb Dumb
Dope Dope Dope Dope Dope
Nonononononononononono
Dumbdumbdumbdumbdumb
Deedledum deedledum dumdeedle
Deedledeedledeedledeedledeedle
(Susan, age 12)

This chapter identifies some of the emotional disturbances of childhood, describes the behaviors displayed, and suggests possible nursing interventions. Piaget's cognitive and affective stages comprise the theoretical framework for intervention, and transactional analysis and reality therapy provide the processes for intervention.

The chronologic age of a child gives insufficient data with which to work. It is not possible to evaluate development by age alone, and behavior which may be considered "normal" at one stage of development may be considered "disturbed" at another stage.

Many approaches are used in working with disturbed children within the parameters of various theoretical frameworks. Psychoanalysis probes to uncover past experiences that are thought to be affecting present behavior. Family and group therapy attempt to deal with the sociocultural factors involved. Physicochemical treatments may be used to control organic and metabolic factors. Behavior therapy, based on stimulus-response theory, uses learning techniques to alter unacceptable learned behaviors. Play therapy and other projective techniques are often useful methods which help to reveal the child's perceptions and feelings and which can be a mode of treatment as well.

No approach is effective with all children. Each approach is successful with some children. However, the basic logic of Piaget and the basic humanity of Berne and Glaser have been most helpful in dealing with emotionally disturbed children of all ages.

TYPES OF EMOTIONAL DISTURBANCE

There is not just one single definition of an emotionally disturbed child. Most definitions in the literature do have certain similarities. In one way or another they say an emotionally disturbed child does not perceive reality accurately, does not control his impulses well, and does not form satisfying interpersonal relationships. He may or may not have trouble learning. He may have trouble with perception, impulse control, relationships, any two of these areas or all three of them.[1,2]

Just as there is not one definition of emotional disturbance, there is not just one cause. Emotional disturbance, however, certainly implies interference in development. This interference may have been genetic, perinatal, social, physiologic, or psychologic or may involve any combination of them. There is probably not just a single cause for any specific individual. Some children have greater stress tolerance and can withstand more environmental crises than other children. Some environments are less stress-inducing than others and can support the successful development of intrinsically vulnerable children. Children can grow and develop in any environment. Children can also fail to develop in any environment.

Some 10 to 20 percent of the children and young people in the United States suffer from emotional problems ranging from superficial conflicts to psychotic episodes.[3] The extent and severity of an emotional disturbance depends upon the interaction of child, family, and environment at a given time, in a given place.

Emotional disorders are commonly grouped into such categories as the following:

1 Developmental: feeding problems, sleeping problems, mourning, separation anxiety, depression, sexual deviation
2 Neurotic: school phobia, bed-wetting, hysteria
3 Psychogenic: asthma, colitis, obesity
4 Psychotic: schizophrenia, autism
5 Antisocial: delinquency, drug abuse, violence

These categories reflect the descriptions of emotionally disturbed behavior: poor perception of reality, poor impulse control, and unsatisfactory interpersonal relationships.

Organic disturbances that require organic treatment are not included in this chapter. Disturbed behavior may have an organic basis and still respond to interpersonal therapy. Mental retardation is not included because the mentally retarded child has problems which differ from those of the emotionally disturbed child.

No categories are found for the child who suffers from the effects of poverty, for the child victim of discrimination (by race, sex, size, or any other variable), or for the abused child. Any of these children can suffer severe emotional turmoil. Indeed the abused child has deep psychologic wounds long after his body has healed. He may not display pathologic behaviors until years later.

DISTURBED BEHAVIOR

Every child occasionally displays disturbed behavior, as do the adults around him. No one unusual behavior need be seen as evidence that a child is emotionally disturbed. Any behavior is appropriate at some stage of development. A baby wets the bed frequently and a 6-year-old may wet the bed at times without being considered neurotic, but a 15-year-old who wets the bed has a problem. If a 4-year-old has an imaginary friend, it is only a developmental stage. A 10-year-old boy with a friend of the same sex is a "latency-age child" and not a homosexual. A 15-year-old girl with a boyfriend is a normal adolescent, not a sexual delinquent. Tantrums, aggressive acts, and sexual experimentation all may occur at any age. No behavior is, in and of itself, disturbed.

But whenever behaviors indicate poor perception of the world—extreme withdrawal, autism, suicide attempts—they may be considered disturbed. Poor control of impulses—stealing, violence, vandalism, promiscuity—indicates disturbed behavior. And whenever behaviors show evidence of poor interpersonal relationships—withdrawal, inability to communicate, poor self-concept, inability to evaluate self—they may be considered disturbed.

But all things are relative. One extreme behavior (withdrawal or aggression, for instance) will interfere with a child's ability to function to a greater degree than three or four lesser problems, such as nail-biting, overeating, and nightmares. Duration is a contributing factor, too. If several areas are involved over a period of time, the child's ability to function will be impaired.

The existence of seemingly problematic behavior is suggestive but not conclusive. It is not possible to make a nursing diagnosis and plan interventions on the basis of one apparently disturbed behavior, or even on the basis of many such behaviors. Behavior cannot be understood unless it is viewed within the framework of the child's family, culture, and developmental stage.

DEVELOPMENTAL STAGES

Piaget[4–6] has described specific stages in cognitive development from birth to maturity (see Chapter 7). Infants exist in a sensorimotor world—a world of action, not ideas. Babies develop a recognition that objects are permanent. When mother goes out of sight, she does not disappear into smoke. An infant learns that mother returns, that his big toe is always on his foot, and that his thumb is as near as his hand. Without a sense of object permanency, the child could not develop interpersonal relationships. Who can become closely involved with objects that do not return?

Babies show a certain knowledge of space, time, and causality—in action, not in thought. The child has space to turn in, to play in. There is a time when it is dark and no one plays with him, when everyone is quiet. His crying brings someone to him—whether or not it is dark and everyone else is quiet.

He is very powerful. He is all action. By 1½ years he acts differently at different times of the day, travels as far in space as he can, and is aware that his actions cause pleasure and displeasure, bringing reward and punishment.

He is now ready to learn language, to begin understanding symbols. He can find his way back and forth in out-of-the way spaces but cannot tell you how to get there. The toddler and preschooler cannot yet understand that things may look the same and still be different (two glasses of different sizes half full of liquid) or that things may look different and still be the same (equal amounts of clay in different shapes). At this age magical thinking is common: if he misbehaves, the sun will go down and it will be dark—and he does misbehave, and the sun goes down, and it is dark. The trees and the flowers can talk to him and help him if he needs help. He can step on a crack and break his mother's back. He does not believe anything is accidental. Therefore, if he is hurt, it must be because he is a bad boy; if he is rewarded, he must be a good boy.

It is only by 7 or 8 that a child can manipulate objects in such ways as classifying them or arranging them in order by size. He is beginning to understand cause and effect, and then only when dealing with concrete objects. He can tell time, but still does not have a full understanding of how long a day is. Every day may have 24 hours, but some days are longer than others and some hours seem longer than others. Space around him is increasing; his world is widening. He still has trouble mentally visualizing something not within his range of vision.

By 11 or 12, the child has increased his thinking skills immeasurably. He can understand relationships in time and space. He knows that today is tomorrow's yesterday, that wishing does not make it so, that he may be hurt whether he is good or bad.

Of course no behavior is purely cognitive. Affect is always involved. No behavior is purely affective either. All behaviors are a combination of thinking and feeling, and one does not cause the other.[7] In infancy, a lack of maternal feeling can be accompanied by retardation of thinking, but one is not the cause of the other. Feeling is necessary for thinking

to develop but does not produce it. In early childhood feelings cannot be generalized any more than thinking can. Moral values are based upon obedience to authority, and when the authority is not there the moral value may not be either. By 7 or 8, children are beginning to understand transactions. Their moral feelings are now based more on justice between their peers and are less dependent upon adult authority. By the time children have developed the ability to think abstractly, to see possibilities, they have also expanded the content areas of their abstract feelings: they have feelings not only for adults and peers, but for country, ideals, humanity, and religion.

A child's ideas about space, time, causality, and moral values are dependent upon his developmental stage. The world of ideas and feelings grows greater with age, just as the physical world and the space around one increase with age.

The disturbed child has interference with his thinking and/or feeling development. His world shrinks and he shrinks with it. He may lose only a little space but much time, and become all sensorimotor again. He may lose his feeling but not his thinking and become withdrawn and uncommunicative. He may lose his thinking but not his feeling and develop learning disorders. He may lose a little time and much space and become aggressive and frustrated.

To *understand* the disturbed child, it is necessary to first understand the ordinary well-adjusted child. To *help* the disturbed child develop to his fullest, it is necessary to know how interpersonal relationships can help and how they can be facilitated.

REALITY THERAPY

Reality therapy stresses the fact that all disturbed people have two things in common: they cannot meet their basic needs and they refuse to face reality.[8]

No child can meet his needs alone, but has to be involved with at least one other person to develop adequately. When the significant person in a child's life no longer is there, the child begins losing touch with reality. As the child grows older, his world becomes larger. Even though his mother may be away, he knows she is there. A younger child's world is much smaller, and the important people in his life need to be closer to him. A baby's world is quite constricted, and separations involving only short times and close spaces can be crippling.

Reality therapy focuses upon two of the basic

needs: the need for love and the need to feel worth-while.

Children may be given love and yet be made to feel worthless. The needs vary with age. A baby needs love; he does not usually feel worthwhile or worthless. An adolescent needs love, but he needs to feel worthwhile even more.

When essential needs cannot be fulfilled in the usual ways, children may adopt alternative methods of dealing with them. The antisocial child attempts to meet his needs for love and self-worth at the expense of others. The psychotic child deals with these needs at the expense of self.

To help with reality therapy it is necessary to become involved, to establish a relationship with the child. It is necessary to be responsible and reality oriented. It is necessary that the helping person have his own needs met, and that they be met by someone other than the child involved.

The first lesson is that everyone is responsible for his own behavior. This is reality. If parents can be helped to become more responsible in handling the child, no one will suffer. Children do not long resent responsible parents who can face reality. Sometimes they may even love them.

TRANSACTIONAL ANALYSIS

Games People Play,[9] a best seller in the sixties, introduced the American family to transactional analysis. Only an extremely obtuse person did not recognize himself and his favorite game.

A premise of transactional analysis is that every individual can speak with one of three voices—the Parent, the Child, or the Adult. Parent, Child, and Adult are the three psychologic "inner persons"—more technically, the three ego states—of which every person is composed. The Parent ego is a collection of *authoritative* attitudes, feelings, and behavior patterns which the growing person has observed in his own parents and parent substitutes. Hence, the Parent is the voice of blame-setting, of judgment, of prejudice, of arbitrary enforcement of nonrational rules. The Parent also nurtures and protects (and overprotects).

The Child ego state is a composite of remnants from one's own childhood, including insistence upon prompt gratification, fantasy, spontaneity, fun, irrational fears, and sulkiness. The Child is the voice of anger, reaction, creativity, curiosity, and prelogical thinking.

The Adult is a collection of feelings, behaviors, and attitudes which are mature and appropriate in relation to the circumstances in which the person finds himself. The Adult deals with reality. The Adult is open-minded, rational, organized, practical, objective, and intelligent. The Adult ego is the voice of reality, reason, probability, and abstraction.

Children spend much time and energy testing the truth and reliability of what their parents say. Those who find their parents are in tune with reality and not "playing games" are the fortunate ones. When a child knows, for example, that fire does burn, cars are powerful, and dogs do bite, he can use his energy for creative, constructive, and pleasurable pursuits. A child who is forever testing has no energy left for other pursuits. He has trouble developing his inner Adult ego and continues to be a battlefield for the constant struggle of Child against Parent. When the data from the parent conflict with reality, the child will be torn between the parent and the slowly developing Adult within him. If he fears the parent, he will deny the reality.[10]

The Child ego has the desire to be creative. He wants to create but does not quite know how. The Adult ego adds the *ability* to create to the Child's desire and builds, writes, and plays. When the Adult has not developed, creativity suffers. When the Child accepts Parent above reality, the Adult cannot develop, for the Parent cannot be tested or questioned. The Adult gives up, and the Child ceases to question.

In just such a way is prejudice born. In such a way are fanatics developed. When it is dangerous to question the Parent, or when Parent information is not only internalized but externalized as true, then no amount of Adult logic will change the unrealistic beliefs. Only convincing the Adult ego that it is not dangerous to question the Parent will help change the prejudice, the fanaticism.

Harris, in his guide to transactional analysis,[11] describes four possible situational relationships between the individual and the person with whom he interacts.

He can consider himself to be "all right" or "not all right" depending upon the responses (the "stroking" or "not-stroking") of the other.[11] He can also view the other as all right or not all right. The four positions are, therefore, (1) both all right, (2) both not all right, (3) and (4), one all right and one not all right. The individual does not travel back and forth among the positions. By preschool age, he has already chosen his niche in one of three: (1) I'm not all right, you're all right, (2) I'm not all right, you're not all right, (3) I'm all right, you're not all right. He stays there until he deliberately develops the fourth position—I'm all right, you're all right—as an adult.

Babies need stroking to grow. The parent, being powerful, is always right. So the first position of every child is that he is not all right but his parents are.

Some children consolidate in this position and live out their lives fulfilling the prophecy. They may become masochistic or sycophantic and find others to reinforce their feelings of inferiority. They may fight their way through life trying to prove not that they are all right but they are just as bad as everyone thinks. Ultimately the position can end in suicide or commitment to an institution.

During the second year of life, much of the stroking ceases. The child is on his own. Without stroking, his inner Adult ego gives up and does not develop. As the child grows older, he may withdraw and try to return to the infancy in which he was taken care of and stroked. He develops the position that he is not all right and everyone else is not all right. This position may also end in commitment to an institution for if no one is all right, there is no hope and the despair is overwhelming.

The autistic child may begin life in this position. He does not accept or register stroking as an infant, and from the beginning he thinks he is not all right and his parents are not all right. Since the Adult ego does not develop without stroking, the autistic child is unborn, as it were.

The abused child has a different beginning. He learns early in life that his parents (and others in general) are not all right. But he is not hurt when away from them, so *he* must be all right. This position of "I'm all right but no one else is" is a basically psychopathic approach.

Just as thinking everyone else is all right but I'm not may end in suicide, the position that I'm all right but the world is not all right may lead to murder.

Everyone gets into one of these positions and is firmly ensconced therein by the age of 3 or 4. Most remain in the first position, feeling inadequate and inferior to all others: I'm not all right but everyone else is. Some of the children in this group may be emotionally disturbed.

Children who choose the second or third position will be emotionally disturbed and very difficult to help. Both of these groups believe no one else is all right, including of course, the professionals who would help them.

The first three positions are not deliberate and are reactive in nature. Only the fourth position—I'm all right and so are others—is deliberately developed and is based on actions rather than reactions. It doesn't develop overnight. But it is possible to realize when the "inferior Child" ego or the "superior Parent" ego within is speaking and to help the Adult ego mature and speak out more often.

An interaction between two persons is called a *transaction*. Since any of the three ego states within an individual may speak out to another person, and since the person spoken to likewise has three "receivers," in every transaction one party speaks as either Parent, Adult, or Child, and the other responds are either Parent, Adult, or Child.

Without an Adult component, satisfying interpersonal relationships founder and may cease to exist. When two people relate as Child to Child, there is no one to give—both wish to take. If most of the interpersonal interactions are actually for the purpose of obtaining strokes, a Child-to-Child relationship will not survive long.

Any relationship between the Child and Parent, Child and Adult, Adult and Parent, or Adult and Adult may go on forever if neither member tires of it. However, if, for example, one is relating as Child to Parent and the other member is relating in any other way, such as Adult to Adult, trouble may result.

Developing the Adult ego takes much energy and conscious effort. Every time the individual recognizes that it is his Child or Parent ego who is speaking, he helps to control them and strengthens his Adult ego. When the feelings are aroused, the Child is about to burst forth. When the prejudices and value judgments are expressed, the Parent is speaking. Recognizing the Parent and Child helps to control them and let the Adult ego grow.

Failure to recognize the Parent and Child egos may lead to control of a portion of the Adult ego by one or the other. When the Parent controls the Adult, unreasonable prejudices are expressed and upheld against all reality. The control of the Adult ego by the Child ego may allow inappropriate feelings to be externalized as delusions or hallucinations.

Sometimes Parent, Child, or Adult ego will be completely blocked out. When the Child is nonfunctional, the individual is unable to play or have any fun. When the Parent is nonfunctional, the individual expresses no guilt, shame, remorse in any situation; he is a psychopath. When the Adult is nonfunctional, the individual is psychotic. He is out of touch with reality. (Susan's poem, quoted at the beginning of the chapter, is an example of Parent-Child conflict without Adult mediation.)

When the Parent input in infancy is very inconsistent, the beginning Adult cannot make sense out of cause and effect and may stop trying. The Adult ego cannot control either the Child or the Parent, and each one takes over at intervals. This is the manic-depressive personality. Madly fluctuating Parent-Child mood swings are extreme. The Child takes over in the manic phase, the Parent in the depressive.

In between the swings there may be a time of stability when the Adult ego is in charge.

Children need not become one-sided in their Parent-Child-Adult behavior. It is possible to help a child recognize which part of him is speaking. Even retarded children have been involved in transactional groups with amazing results.[12] Uncontrollable tantrums can be managed (once the child has learned the transactional terms) by merely asking, "who is speaking?" The child, once he knows enough to answer, "Child," also knows enough to calm down after he has identified the problem. It may take only a few minutes.

The children who think everyone else is not all right can also be helped. It just takes a little longer.

NURSING MANAGEMENT

Children respond to many different types of intervention. The nurse has to choose the means best suited to an individual child, yet the means with which he, as a professional, is most comfortable.

Play is effective with many children, especially young and nonverbal children, but can become merely an approved way of acting-out instead of a constructive means of expression or an effective developmental tool. The principles and practice of play therapy are explicated by Axline.[13] Play as a projective technique by which the child reveals his feelings and can be helped to deal with them is touched upon in Chapter 7. Poetry, art, music, and flowers are ways of reaching children who can respond to nonhuman entities but cannot yet form close relationships with other human beings.

Each of these forms of expression, of sublimation, requires discipline as well as emotion. None of the forms can withstand total emotional disruption. Generally, the greater the sublimation, the better the artistic creation. Raw emotion and expression in art show unsuccessful sublimation of aggressive and other urges. Kramer[14] says the quality of the finished product is one measure of successful intervention.

Susan and Jason were two children who could respond to poetry and art before they could form a close relationship with another human.

Susan was an apparently schizophrenic child of 12. She communicated by writing poetry. She formed relationships with no one. She talked very little and then only to inanimate objects. Her Adult had never been allowed to develop, and her Child and Parent were constantly at war. She knew there was something wrong with her but comforted herself with the thought that no one else was all right either.

Poetry was the way to reach her. But poetry can serve as a form of sublimation or merely as a way of acting out. Susan used it to act out. No one could understand what she wrote, and this reaffirmed her belief that something was wrong with everybody else. Her poetry needed to be channeled, to be organized. It needed to serve as a creative expression, a bridge to the outside, until she felt safe enough to face the world.

It was never necessary to analyze Susan's poetry for content, for hidden meanings. Poetry is always symbolic. It is abstract. It is expressive. If Susan could deal in symbols and abstractions in this form, why not in other forms?

At first it was enough for Susan just to stay within sight. Gradually, when she found she could depend upon someone, she moved closer. She did not speak. She wrote and wrote. Always her nurses maintained their one-sided conversation with her, about promises to be kept, reality to be reinforced. If a promise was for something good, like more paper and pencils for writing, or a walk in the garden, Susan was happy when the promise was kept. However, reality is never just good things. Sometimes the promises were for unpleasant things—no dessert for dinner because she had thrown hers on the floor the night before, no walk in the garden because she had run away and hidden and was not found until after dark.

But her paper and pencils and poetry were never taken away. Writing was her only constructive means of expression. Poetry was to become her way to face reality, to assume responsibility for her behavior, to develop her Adult ego.

In the early communication, the poetry was little more than the "deedle-deedle-dum." "That's your Child talking, Susan." "That's your Parent." "I can't understand them too well. I'd like to understand them, Susan." "You have such a rhythm, such a way with words, Susan." "Don't you want me to understand them?"

And on went the months. Then one day Susan pushed a poem forward saying, "Here"—the only word she used in speech.

War is war and peace is peace.
War is all. Peace is all.
War and Peace are mixed up.
Which is which?
War? War? War? Peace? Peace?
Deedle-deedle-dum.

"Susan, I think I can even understand deedle-deedle-dum now. Your Adult is growing." Susan came closer to a smile than at any time in the past 6 months.

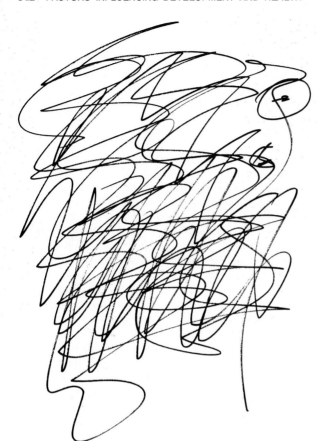

Figure 22-1 Jason: The Sea.

From that day on Susan improved rapidly. She began identifying her own Child or Parent. She took more responsibility for her own behavior. She continued to write.

But now we could talk because Susan would begin answering me and then begin initiating the conversation. It was a peak day when Susan gave me a poem and asked, "Does this make sense? Can you understand it? Or is it just the silly Child again?"

Questions

If the fog comes in on little
   cat feet, is that
Just on the ground? Or is
   it also
In the mind?
Does the fog come so quietly
   and softly that
You never know it's here
Until you no longer see the
   world?
Or can you push the fog away?

Can you see through it? Beyond it?
   Around it?
If we can make the rain,
   can we make the fog?
If we can stop the rain,
   can we stop the fog?
Or does it come so quietly on
   its little cat feet that
You don't know it's here
   Until it's too late?
Is it ever too late? To see
   the fog?
To know the fog? To walk
   through the fog?

Exactly 1 year, 3 months, and 22 days had passed between "Deedle-deedle-deedle" and "Questions."

Jason was 10 years old and had problems at school and at home. He was handsome and quite charming, but the charm disappeared into violence or withdrawal when he could not have his own way.

His parents encouraged "self-expression" and Jason expressed himself with abandon—or at least he expressed his Child ego. However, when his parents were tired or angry, they also expressed their Child side and it was then that Jason withdrew.

He was difficult to work with because he did alternate so violently in overt behavior. He had never been asked to look at his behavior before or to take the responsibility for it.

"Jason, your Child tells you to fight with your sister, your Parent tells you to feel guilty about it. How about your Adult? You can't always blame your behavior on your Child or your Parent. Let's just see what was going on here a minute ago."

And Jason began to identify his behavior, to face the reality of his behavior.

Although a bright boy, Jason could not yet handle abstract thinking. He was extremely concrete and needed to see and touch things before he could "think" about them.

He enjoyed art and working with his hands. His very first paintings were angry smears. Jason was "feeling" more than "thinking," and art served as an outlet for his excessive energy and aggression (Fig. 22-1).

It was not enough that Jason could act out his anger and hurt. It was necessary to give his expression some form, some meaning. But he was not yet ready.

At first he would insist that a multicolored smear was "mountains," "seashore," "a zoo." He became more adept at identifying his behavior. When he wanted to hit sister, he could identify his Child. He was usually quick to add, "But my Parent doesn't have to put me in the corner because I *didn't* hit her— and anybody could *want* to. That's no crime."

One morning Jason painted his usual picture. "Do you know what that is?" he demanded, thrusting it forward. "No." "It's a mess!" he said and tore it up with uncontrolled glee. "Now let's get down to business," he seemed to speak to himself more than to me.

Taking three felt-tipped pens and a sheet of white paper (with a border), he drew a car, a train, and a bicycle (Fig. 22-2). The train did not run on tracks and the car and bicycle were not on a road. All three were out in a field. The bicycle had no rider, the train no engineer, the car no driver. The train resembled a caterpillar. The car did not seem to face in either direction, although the steering wheel did give a clue.

If the drawing were to be analyzed for phallic symbolism, there would be no difficulty finding it. But Jason could explain more important things than sexual meanings. "They can all travel anyplace. They're free. There's nobody riding them all the time. They can just go anyplace they want to."

"We could talk about people riding you, Jason, but let's talk about freedom—and reality. Bicycles and cars and trains don't go anywhere unless someone moves them. Trains need some kind of tracks to run on. If you drive your car across a field, you'll probably have a repair bill. There is no absolute freedom, Jason. We all have some. Nobody has it all. That's reality, Jason."

"I don't like tracks."

"Lots of people don't. And that's one of the best things about pictures, Jason. You can draw trains without tracks if you want to and people will know how you feel. You won't have to act out. You can do it on paper."

"That's not enough yet." And Jason turned and walked away to stand, staring out the window.

And it wasn't enough. For more than 8 months Jason continued to have his outbursts of aggression and his episodes of withdrawal. But he became more and more aware of his behavior and better able to identify it.

"You know something?" he stopped painting to ask. "The more you fight to be free, the more everybody ties you down. How can you ever get free?"

We talked about freedom and individual needs and individual differences. Jason decided that perhaps he didn't want complete freedom after all, he just wanted to be himself.

"Now, all I have to do is figure out who 'myself' is." He went back to work on his painting. During the next hour he tore up three different pictures. But he

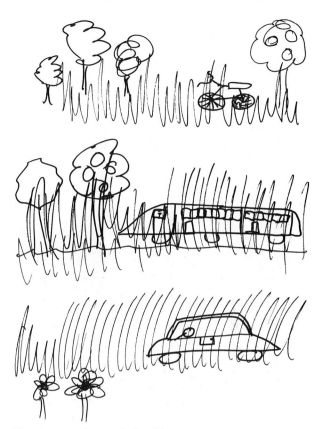

Figure 22-2   Jason: Going Places.

tore them up, not with aggression and tantrums, not in helpless frustration, but as a dissatisfied adult— still in control, still searching.

The process continued for 2 days. Jason could not express what he wished to express. On the third morning, we decided the Art Institute would be a welcome break. Jason had been there before and never failed to enjoy it. Usually he chattered nonstop, asking questions, commenting on likes and dislikes. On this particular morning he was very quiet. He seemed to be absorbing and mentally sorting every exhibit he saw. It was a tiring day and late in the afternoon when he returned to his room.

Within an hour Jason was back at my side with a completed picture (Fig. 22-3). He had used mostly black and white with touches of yellow, green, blue, and red. A yellow sunburst effect in the upper left corner was opposed by a solid red square in the lower right corner. All lines and borders were black. The diagonal black line crossing from the lower left corner to the upper right corner was bordered by a green line on either side with blue lines edging the outer side of the green. It was a beautiful picture.

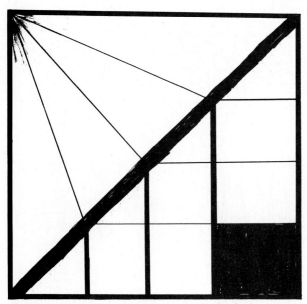

Figure 22-3 Jason: Freedom.

"Do you know what? It's really the tracks and the roads that are free because once they're laid out and know where they're going, they just go there whether anybody rides them or not." He took a pencil from his shirt pocket. Across the bottom of his picture he wrote "Freedom."

Jason had discovered himself and his freedom. His freedom was not everybody's, but it was his. And in less than a month he was ready to go home.

When he left, he gave me the picture and said, "Now we both have freedom." Jason was no longer a concrete-thinking little boy with behavior problems. He was an artist with a developing Adult ego.

REFERENCES

1 S. J. Harrison and J. F. McDermott, *Childhood Psychopathology*, International Universities Press, Inc., New York, 1972.
2 Report of the Joint Commission on Mental Health of Children, *Crisis in Child Mental Health: Challenge for the 1970's*, Harper & Row, Publishers, Incorporated, New York, 1970.
3 Ibid., p. 257.
4 J. Piaget, *The Child's Conception of Physical Causality*, Kegan Paul, Trench, Trubner & Co., Ltd., London, 1951.
5 J. Piaget, *The Origins of Intelligence in Children*, International Universities Press, Inc., New York, 1952.
6 J. Piaget, *The Construction of Reality in the Child*, Basic Books, Inc., New York, 1954.
7 J. Piaget, "The Relation of Affectivity to Intelligence in the Mental Development of the Child," *Bulletin of the Menninger Clinic*, 26:129–137, 1962.
8 W. Glasser, *Reality Therapy*, Harper & Row, Publishers, Incorporated, New York, 1965.
9 E. Berne, *Games People Play*, Grove Press, Inc., New York, 1964.
10 Muriel James and Dorothy Jongeward, *Born to Win: Transactional Analysis with Gestalt Experiments*, Addison-Wesley Publishing Company, Inc., Reading, Mass., 1971.
11 T. A. Harris, *I'm OK—You're OK*, Harper & Row, Publishers, Incorporated, New York, 1967.
12 Ibid., p. 173.
13 Virginia M. Axline, *Play Therapy*, Ballantine Books, Inc., New York, 1969.
14 Edith Kramer, *Arts As Therapy with Children*, Schocken Books, New York, 1971.

BIBLIOGRAPHY

Almy, Millie: *Young Children's Thinking*, Teachers College Press, Columbia University, New York, 1966.
Anthony, E. J., and Benedek, Therese (eds.): *Parenthood, Its Psychology and Psychopathology*, Little, Brown and Company, Boston, 1970.
Berkovitz, I. H.: *Adolescents Grow in Groups*, Brunner/Mazel, New York, 1972.
Chapman, A. H.: *The Games Children Play*, Berkley Publishing Corporation, New York, 1971.
Ekstein, R.: *Children of Time and Space, of Action and Impulse,* Appleton-Century-Crofts, New York, 1966.
Fagan, Joen, and Shepherd, Irma L. (eds.): *Gestalt Therapy Now*, Harper & Row, Publishers, Incorporated, New York, 1971.
Fagin, Claire: *Nursing in Child Psychiatry*, The C. V. Mosby Company, St. Louis, 1972.
Foster, Genevieve W. (with Karen D. Vander Ven, Eleanore R. Kroner, Nancy T. Carbonara, and George M. Cohen): *Child Care Work with Emotionally Disturbed Children*, University of Pittsburgh Press, Pittsburgh, 1972.
Freedman, A., and Kaplan, H. (eds.): *The Child: His Psychological and Cultural Development*, vol. 1: *Normal Development and Psychological Assessment* and vol. 2: *The Major Psychological Disorders and Their Treatment*, Atheneum Publishers, New York, 1972.
Gardner, W., and Moriarty, Alice: *Personality Development at Preadolescence*, University of Washington Press, Seattle, 1968.
Holmes, D., Holmes, Monica, and Appignanesi, Lisa: *The Language of Trust,* Science House, Inc., New York, 1971.
Kessler, Jane: *Psychopathology of Childhood*, Prentice-Hall, Inc., Englewood Cliffs, N.J., 1966.
Muller, P.: *The Tasks of Childhood*, McGraw-Hill Book Company, New York, 1969.
Rubin, E. Z., Braun, Jean S., Beck, Gayle R., and Llorens, Lela A.: *Cognitive Perceptual Motor Dysfunction*, Wayne State University Press, Detroit, 1972.
Satir, Virginia: *Peoplemaking*, Science and Behavior Books, Inc., Palo Alto, Calif., 1972.
Thomas, A., Chess, Stella, and Birch, H. G.: *Temperament and Behavior Disorders in Children*, New York University Press, New York, 1968.
Winnicott, D. W.: *Therapeutic Consultations in Child Psychiatry*, Basic Books, Inc., New York, 1971.
Wolff, Sula: *Children under Stress*, Allen Lane The Penguin Press, London, 1969.
Wolman, B.: *Children without Childhood*, Grune & Stratton, Inc., New York, 1970.

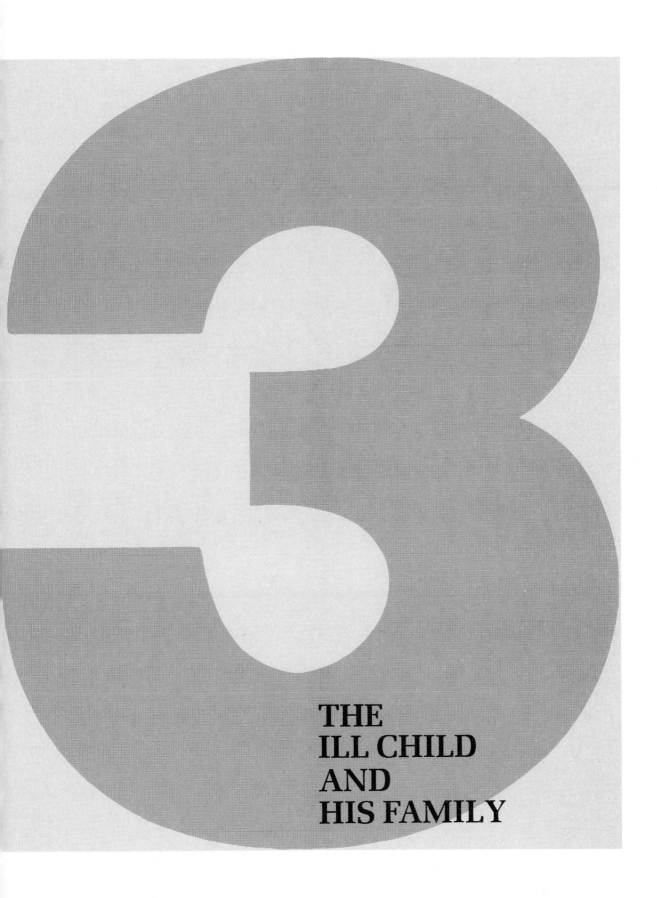

3

**THE
ILL CHILD
AND
HIS FAMILY**

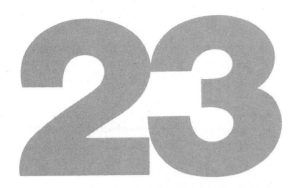

23

EFFECTS OF ILLNESS ON THE NEONATE

DOROTHY HALL

DEVELOPMENT OF MOTHERING

A crucial factor in the establishment of healthy family-child relationships is the development of mothering when a new baby enters the family. Maternal love has some acquired components and is not an altogether innate entity. It is acquired over a period of time, based on the relationship between the mother and her baby.[1] The development of mothering, then, has some identifiable components which are of help to the nurse in promoting a healthy family-neonate relationship. Nursing care given to the neonate cannot be separated from care given to the family, especially care given to the baby's mother.

Since the neonate is so dependent on his mother to meet his needs, a strong bond between mother and infant must be established if the neonate is to survive. Here are the steps which occur in attachment of the mother to her infant:[2]

Planning the pregnancy
Confirming the pregnancy
Feeling fetal movement
Giving birth
Seeing the baby
Touching the baby
Caretaking

leads to bonding

All these steps are essential elements in the development of healthy mother-infant relationships. The first four steps are discussed in Chapter 8.

Seeing the Baby

The importance of parents seeing their infant as soon as possible after delivery cannot be overstated. As more clinical studies are done, it becomes clear that seeing the baby means more than just viewing him through the nursery window. Klaus et al.[3] found mothers to be extremely interested in the eyes of their infants, with a great deal of time spent in the "en face" position. Figure 23-1 illustrates the en face posture. This finding is significant in light of the studies by Robson,[4] who identified eye-to-eye contact between the mother and her infant as an extremely important behavior in the development of the attachment between them. This early eye-to-eye contact is suggested by Robson to be a releaser of caretaking responses in mothers.[5]

Touching the Baby

After the parents have seen their baby, the next important step in attachment is to touch him. Rubin[6] and Klaus et al.[7] have studied maternal behavior and have identified an orderly progression of steps

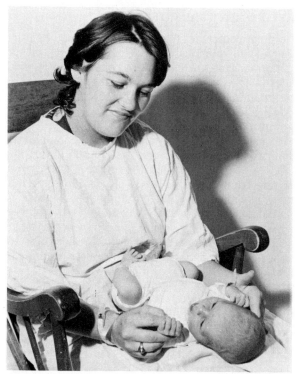

Figure 23-1 Palm contact with mother and baby in the "en face" posture.

in the touching process. The first contacts of the mother with her infant begin with fingertip touch. The first contacts are exploratory gestures. From fingertip exploration, the mother progresses to palm contact, then to full hand and arm touch as her involvement with her baby increases.[8] Figures 23-1 to 23-3 illustrate the progression of touch. Touching her baby is one way in which the mother identifies the child as hers and then begins her caretaking role.

Caretaking

What might be considered the final step in the development of mothering ability is the caretaking or nurturing role. Caretaking begins when a commitment is made to the infant, with seeing and touching as necessary precursors. This role is learned, requiring practice and guidance for the mother. Demonstration by the nurse of caretaking skills such as formula preparation and bathing and dressing the baby should be provided as well as opportunity for return demonstration by the mother. The mother should be encouraged by the nursing staff about her ability and skill in feeding, diapering, and handling of her baby. Rapport between the new mother and the nursery and postpartum nurses should be established so the mother will feel free to ask questions and seek guidance in her caretaking role.

EFFECTS OF PREMATURITY OR ILLNESS ON DEVELOPMENT OF FAMILY-NEONATE RELATIONSHIP
Effects of Prematurity or Illness on Development of Mothering

More often than not, the premature or ill neonate is separated from his parents very shortly after being born. He is put in an incubator in a special care nursery or perhaps even in a different hospital. The development of mothering in the three phases outlined is contingent upon close contact between mother and her baby. Seeing, touching, and caretaking are delayed or interrupted when separation occurs.

Maternal-neonate separation, then, may prevent or seriously impair the formation of an attachment between the mother and her child. If this separation occurs, the mother may never develop her ability to care for her infant. If some degree of attachment does develop, the mother may still feel uncomfortable with her caretaking ability, a fact which may further jeopardize this vital attachment.

Effects of Maternal-Neonate Separation

If an attachment between mother and neonate is not formed, it is easily understood that the infant who is dependent on his mother for nurturing and sustenance may be in jeopardy. Spitz[9] and Bowlby[10] have identified and described the effects of long-term maternal deprivation on the infant in terms of damage in the development of affection. More recently other studies have demonstrated evidence that maternal-infant separation contributes to possible rejection, neglect, and battering.[11, 12] Many times the child at risk for battering is one who is seen as somehow different by his parents.[13-15] A premature baby, a baby with a congenital anomaly, or an ill neonate obviously may be seen as "not normal" or as "different" by his parents. Further isolating this baby from his parents may be interpreted by them as evidence that their baby is indeed different. In such an instance the potential for neglect or battering is very real.

Summarizing the effects of mother-neonatal separation will identify these significant facts:

1 The formation of a mother-infant attachment is in jeopardy when mother and baby are separated.
2 If an attachment is not formed, the mother cannot develop her ability to love and care for her new baby.
3 If an attachment is not formed and the mother does not develop her ability to love and care for her baby, the baby's emotional and physical well-being are at risk.

Nursing Assessment and Intervention in Family-Neonate Separation

Once the effects of maternal-neonate-family separation are understood, the nurse can assess the existing relationship and plan accordingly to keep separation at a minimum.

Opportunity must be provided for continuing contact between the parents and the new baby. Provision for this contact means liberal visiting hours in special care nurseries. Parents need to spend time in close contact with their baby. They can wash their hands, gown properly, and go into the nursery to claim the baby as their own, not as a stranger they view through glass windows. Once in the nursery, provision should be made for the mother to establish eye-to-eye contact. If the infant is receiving phototherapy for hyperbilirubinemia, little harm will be done, and there is much benefit for both mother and baby, if he is taken out from under the light and put in his mother's arms for a few minutes with his eyes uncovered. At the same time, the nurse should explain to the parents why the baby is receiving phototherapy and why his eyes are covered.

If the baby is receiving oxygen, is too small to be taken out of the incubator, is requiring assisted ventilation, or cannot be picked up and held by his parents for another reason, opportunity can and should be provided for the parents to see, establish eye-to-eye contact with, and touch their baby (see Fig. 23-4). Any equipment necessary in the care of the infant or any special procedures must be explained and reexplained many times so that parents understand what is being done and why. Such explanations will take away some of the parents' feelings of isolation and strangeness about their baby.

If the baby's physical condition is such that the parents can get involved in caretaking, they should be allowed and encouraged to do so if they are ready. For example, a premature who maintains his temperature for short periods of time out of an incubator can be wrapped in warm blankets and held by his mother for feedings. The mother not only gains close physical contact with her baby, but also gains practice in feeding him. Praise for

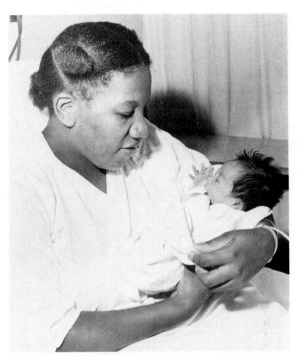

Figure 23-2 Fingertip touching.

mothering tasks should be given when appropriate. Growing confidence in her ability to care for her baby will help the mother see her baby as an infant whose needs she can meet.

Little has been written about sibling-neonate separation and its effects on the new baby's brothers and sisters at home. It is rather difficult for a child to envision a new baby whom he has not seen. Helping the parents explain to siblings why the baby cannot come home or about the illness of the baby is an important aspect of nursing care. Snapshots of the baby will help siblings identify the new baby as "theirs" and may help prevent sibling rivalry when the baby arrives home.

If the neonate has a congenital anomaly or a life-threatening illness, this situation must be dealt with by parents as well as siblings. Children will draw a conclusion on their own if information is withheld. Just as it is important for the parents to see and touch their baby so that they can see what the baby's real condition is, the siblings need to know what is going on with regard to the baby. They need to be told about the baby in terms they can understand. They may be told about a premature infant, that the baby is very small and has to be kept very warm in his own special room (i.e., the incubator), and that he has to be fed special food to help him

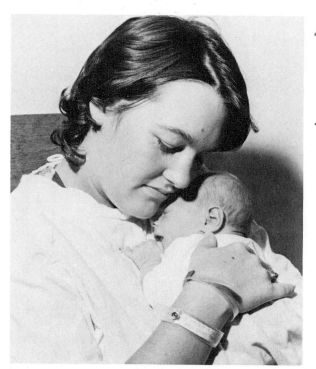

Figure 23-3 Full hand and arm touch.

grow before he can come home. Pictures taken at intervals will help siblings see that the baby is "getting big." In the instance of an anomaly or very serious illness, care should be taken to point out to siblings that neither the parents nor they are to blame for the baby's being sick. This is particularly important in the case of a child 2 to 5 years of age because this is the age of egocentric thinking[16] when a child is likely to interpret whatever happens as somehow due to his actions or thoughts. If the newborn is seriously ill, the siblings need to know about the baby's illness. If the baby does not survive and the siblings have not been told about the illness, they may fear that they, too, may die. If they *know* that the baby was ill when he died, they are not as likely to transfer their fear of death to themselves, since they are healthy, not sick as the baby was.

Psychologic Tasks of the Family

Kaplan and Mason[17] identified four psychologic tasks essential to the development of a healthy mother-infant relationship in the birth of a premature infant. The first task is that of "preparation for a possible loss of the child whose life is in jeopardy." It involves maintaining hope that the baby will sur-

vive, but at the same time preparing for his death. In the second task the mother "must face and acknowledge her maternal failure to deliver a normal full-term baby."[18] These first two tasks are accomplished in the first few days after delivery. During the ensuing weeks while the baby remains in the hospital, the third and fourth tasks are accomplished. The third is the resumption of the process of relating to the baby which had previously been interrupted."[19] In performing this task, the mother begins to recover some of the hopes of her pregnancy. Usually there comes a time when the mother believes the baby will survive, and she begins getting ready for the baby at home and seeking information about how to care for him. In the fourth task the mother must come to understand how a premature baby differs from a normal baby in terms of its special needs and growth patterns."[20] She needs to understand his special needs and characteristics, but she must also come to understand that these needs are temporary and that he will catch up, in time, with the normal full-term infant.

In the mothers studied, Kaplan and Mason identified good outcomes as ones in which the mothers accomplished the four tasks outlined and saw their babies as "potentially normal," gave "realistic care," and gained satisfaction from the care given.[21]

While these four tasks have not been identified in neonates with congenital anomalies or critically ill neonates, it would seem feasible that similar tasks would be necessary for healthy maternal-neonate relationships to develop.

Nursing intervention, then, should be aimed at helping the mother achieve these tasks. The mother must be helped to realize that her child may be in jeopardy; she must be helped in the process of anticipatory grief if she is to successfully accomplish the first task. Helping her verbalize her concern, permitting and encouraging her to cry, and recognizing and helping her recognize that feelings of depression are normal should be intrinsic elements of care given to this mother. Verbalized feelings of depression and outward signs of depression are indications that the first two tasks are being dealt with.

Once the first two tasks are accomplished and the third one, resuming a relationship with the baby, is begun, the nurse can encourage parental visitation to the nursery. Encouraging signs and indications of individuality should be relayed to the mother. Reports of steady weight gain, increase in the amount of formula the baby is taking, and increased activity give cues to the parents to begin the resumption of their relationship with their baby. Being avail-

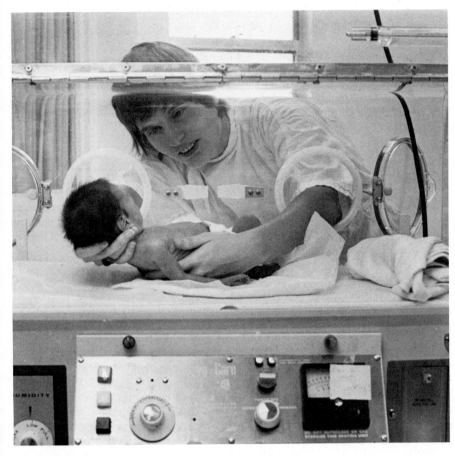

Figure 23-4   Mother getting acquainted with her premature baby.

able to answer parental questions regarding care of the baby and items needed for care at home is important in assisting parents with the third task.

Assisting parents with the accomplishment of the fourth task involves teaching them the special needs of the neonate. Just as important is helping them learn the "how-to" of caring for their baby. Encouraging visitation to the nursery and parental participation in feeding, diapering, and other aspects of care gives parents confidence in their ability to cope with their baby's needs and eliminates the parent-neonate separation which is so hazardous to the baby's well-being. Encouragement and praise in parental caretaking ability is as much a part of nursing intervention as is seeing that the baby is weighed and fed. While pointing out the special needs of their baby and helping parents plan for these needs, nurses must also help the parents understand that with time, proper care, and love their premature baby will probably catch up to his full-term friends. Remember, the battered child is most often a baby who is seen as different by his parents—nursing must anticipate and prevent this feeling.

EFFECTS OF PREMATURITY OR ILLNESS ON THE NEONATE
Sensory Deprivation

Premature and ill neonates experience sensory deprivations because frequently they are housed in incubators which limit the amount of stimulation. Until recent years, these babies were cared for almost entirely in their incubators, thus being deprived of cuddling and handling as well as visual stimulation. Scarr-Salapatek and Williams[22] and Wright[23] report findings which show that premature infants are vulnerable to developmental delays, especially if they remain in an environment which provides minimal sensory-motor stimulation. Their studies, which provided visual, tactile, and kinesthetic stimulation for premature infants in the nursery period, also show that early sensory stimulation is effective in promoting behavioral development.

Sensory Bombardment

Along with sensory-motor deprivation, the potential for sensory bombardment exists in the nursery setting for the premature and ill neonate. The infant cared for in an incubator is subjected to the constant noise of the incubator motor and possibly to the constant "beeping" of cardiac monitors. At the same time, he is in a brightly lighted nursery 24 hours a day. If he requires a ventilator, he hears its continual click. Little has been written regarding the effects of these types of sensory bombardment on the infant; however, sensory input of this kind precludes input of other stimuli and may thus be detrimental. For instance, the baby who hears the noise of the incubator motor 24 hours a day is the baby who is not being taken out of it to be held, cuddled, and talked to.

Nursing Assessment and Intervention

Nursing intervention to provide appropriate sensory-motor stimulation depends on identification of the area of deprivation or overstimulation. The baby in an incubator, condition permitting, should be taken out at intervals, wrapped up to keep him warm, and held. Feeding time is a good time to hold and rock him.[24] This gives the baby kinesthetic stimulation, rocking, as well as tactile input from being held. Walking around the nursery with the baby provides patterned visual stimulation. Auditory stimulation is provided by talking to the baby and providing a source of intermittent music. Babies receiving phototherapy receive additional stimulation when their eye patches are removed. Like babies in incubators, they need to be rocked, cuddled, and exposed to visual stimulation. Babies who cannot be taken out of incubators can receive kinesthetic and tactile stimulation by being touched and rocked back and forth in the incubator. Visual stimulation can be provided by hanging a toy such as a brightly colored bird or butterfly in the incubator.

Parents are important in providing sensory stimulation for their infants. They should be told why stimulation is important and how they can provide it at the hospital and at home. Parental visitation in the nursery needs to be encouraged so that they can touch, hold, and rock their baby. They need to be told that talking to their baby is important to his development. Parents and siblings can be shown how to make mobiles for the crib by suspending brightly colored magazine pictures on clothes hangers. Pamphlets explaining the importance of infant stimulation to parents as well as modes of stimulation are available.[25-27]

NEEDS OF THE PREMATURE OR ILL NEONATE
Development of Trust

Meeting the needs of the neonate is said by Erikson to be the prerequisite for the development of *basic trust*, the major developmental task of infancy. The nurse and family can assist the hospitalized neonate toward trust by providing physical comforts and consistent care. Development of basic trust is discussed more fully in Chapter 10.

Need for Individuality and "Tender Loving Care"

In addition to the premature or ill neonate's need for appropriate physical care, a healthy family-infant relationship and environmental stimulation, the need to promote his individuality is a vital part of his nursing care. Each baby in the nursery *is* an individual, and nursing should take his individual needs into account. If the baby's condition permits, he should be allowed to establish his own schedule for feeding. For example, most premature babies who are not acutely ill will wake hungry and crying at two-to-three hour intervals. Once their schedules are known, they then can be fed without being awakened from sleep. Involving parents in helping maintain their baby's individuality also promotes a healthy parent-child relationship. Baby clothes brought in from home and worn by the babies in the nursery help parents claim the child as their own and identify the child as an individual.

Babies need a great deal of tender loving care. Involving parents in this aspect of care is vital. Encouraging parents to make frequent visits to the nursery to see, feed, and hold their baby provides not only affection but sensory-motor stimulation and helps cement a healthy family-infant relationship.

Allowing the same nurse on each shift to care for a given baby provides continuity of care for that baby. In addition, the nurse can become a "mother surrogate" in those instances when parents cannot come for daily visits. In so doing, she can assess the neonate's needs for individuality on an ongoing basis and provide continuity of warmth and caring. Gentle handling, holding, rocking babies for feedings, and holding them after painful procedures are ways to provide this warmth and caring.

SUMMARY

The effects of illness on the neonate are intertwined with the effects of family-neonate separation and sensory-motor deprivation. The nursing care of the premature and ill neonate should aim at minimizing separation from the parents and environmental deprivation. Meeting the infant's needs for individuality and tender loving care should also be an integral part of planned care. Whenever possible involving parents in the care of their baby helps meet both the family's need for contact with their baby and the baby's need to belong to his family, thus helping minimize the detrimental developmental effects of illness on the neonate and on the family.

REFERENCES

1 D. Levy, "Problems in Determining Maternal Attitudes Toward Newborn Infants," *Psychiatry*, 15:273–286, August 1952.

2 M. Klaus and J. Kennell, "Mothers Separated from Their Newborn Infants," *Pediatric Clinics of North America*, 4:1020, November 1970. Reprinted with permission.

3 ——, ——, N. Plumb, and S. Zuehlke, "Human Maternal Behavior at the First Contact with the Young," *Pediatrics*, 46:187–92, August 1970.

4 K. Robson, "The Role of Eye-to-Eye Contact in Maternal-Infant Attachment," *Journal of Child Psychology and Psychiatry and Applied Disciplines*, 8(1):13–25, 1967.

5 Ibid.

6 Reva Rubin, "Maternal Touch," *Nursing Outlook*, 11:828–31, November 1963.

7 M. Klaus, J. Kennell, N. Plumb, and S. Zuehlke, op. cit.

8 Reva Rubin, op. cit.

9 R. Spitz, *The First Year of Life*, International Universities Press, Inc., New York, pp. 267–284, 1965.

10 J. Bowlby, *Maternal Care and Mental Health*, World Health Organization Monograph Series, Geneva no. 2, pp. 15–45, 1951.

11 L. Stern, "Prematurity as a Factor in Child Abuse," *Hospital Practice*, 8:117–123, May 1973.

12 M. Klein and L. Stern, "Low Birth Weight and the Battered Child Syndrome," *American Journal of Diseases of Children*, 122:15–18, 1971.

13 B. F. Steele and C. B. Pollock, in R. E. Helfer and C. H. Kemp (eds.), *The Battered Child*, The University of Chicago Press, pp. 28–35, 1968.

14 L. Stern, op. cit.

15 M. Klein and L. Stern, op. cit.

16 J. Piaget and B. Inhelder, *The Psychology of the Child*, Basic Books, Inc., Publishers, New York, 1969.

17 D. Kaplan and E. Mason, "Maternal Reactions to Premature Birth Viewed as an Acute Emotional Disorder," *The American Journal of Orthopsychiatry*, 30:543–45, July 1960.

18 Ibid., p. 543.

19 Ibid., pp. 543–544.

20 Ibid., p. 544.

21 Ibid., p. 545.

22 S. Scarr-Salapatek, "The Effects of Early Stimulation on Low-Birth Weight Infants," *Child Development*, 44:94–101, 1973.

23 L. Wright, "The Theoretical and Research Base for a Program of Early Stimulation Care and Training of Premature Infants," in J. Hellmuth (ed.), *Exceptional Infant*, vol. 2, Brunner Mazel Inc., New York, pp. 296–304, 1971.

24 A. Kulka, C. Fry, and F. J. Goldstein, "Kinesthetic Needs in Infancy," *The American Journal of Orthopsychiatry*, 30:562–71, July 1960.

25 P. E. Haiman and J. Myerberg, *Keep Babies Busy*, The Press of Case Western Reserve University, Cleveland 1972.

26 ——, and ——, *Soul Mother*, The Press of Case Western Reserve University, Cleveland 1972.

27 J. I. Gordon and J. R. Lalley, *Intellectual Stimulation for Infants and Toddlers*, University of Florida, Gainesville, 1967.

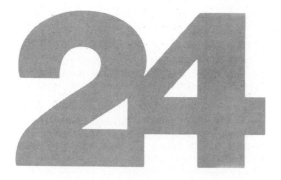

EFFECTS OF ILLNESS ON THE INFANT

FLORENCE BRIGHT ROBERTS

After the initial flurry of excitement over the arrival of a new baby and all the visitors have come and gone, the family settles down to the very real task of incorporating its newest member into the household routine (Fig. 24-1). The parents begin in earnest now the work of establishing mutuality with the baby. Because the mother is traditionally the primary caretaker, it is she who develops the greatest degree of mutuality with the infant, and hence it is in reference to the mother-child relationship that the child's development is usually discussed. It should be noted here, however, that more and more fathers are participating in the care of their infants, and qualities once thought to be exclusive to the mother-child relationship are also present in many father-child relationships.

THE PERIOD OF EARLY INFANCY
(1 TO 4 MONTHS)
Establishment of Mutuality

Mutuality is that special interaction through which the mother (or other caretaker) learns to identify and meet the infant's needs and from which she gains a deep sense of satisfaction. In turn, the infant learns to communicate his needs and to trust his mother to meet them. Through the establishment of mutuality the baby accomplishes the most important task of infancy—the development of a basic sense of trust.

The establishment of mutuality is not easy, however. The mother is recovering from the pregnancy and birth of her infant and has urgent needs of her own, particularly the need for rest. Her periods of rest and sleep may be interrupted for several weeks or more until the baby has established a predictable routine. Just as the mother becomes used to the baby's routine, he changes it. For instance, he may begin sleeping from 10:00 to 12:00 every morning and from 2:00 to 4:00 in the afternoon. When the mother identifies this pattern, she may plan activities or rest for herself during those hours. About the time she gets a schedule established, however, the baby will begin to be awake from 10:00 to 12:00 and sleep from 12:30 to 3:00, so that the mother must constantly readapt herself to the changing needs of her young infant. Frequent adjustments of this sort are very difficult for a mother, especially a first-time mother. A new mother will feel considerable frustration in those early weeks and may become very angry with her baby. If she does not recognize her anger as a normal response, she may become guilt ridden, suffer considerable damage to her self-esteem, and perhaps begin a cycle of guilt-ridden submission to the demands of the child, which can

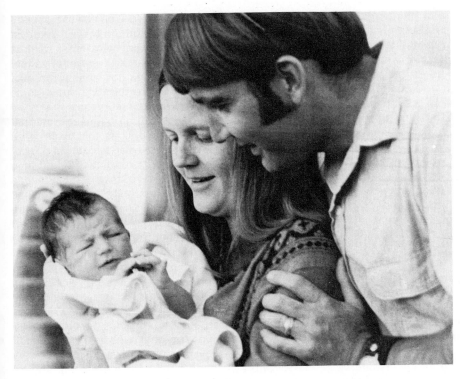

Figure 24-1 Following the initial excitement over a new baby, the family settles down to the task of incorporating its newest member into the household. *(Photo courtesy of Penelope Peirce.)*

lead only to the development of an unhealthy mother-child relationship.

The care of a normal infant is frustrating enough; the care of a handicapped or sick one is more difficult because the baby requires more care, he may not be able to be satisfied as readily, and the rewards of the mother's efforts may not be the development of a normal, healthy baby. In addition, the mother of a handicapped or ill baby often feels so guilty and angry that she has great difficulty establishing closeness with him and consequently has trouble sensing his needs.

Empathic Perception

One tool which a mother and infant use to establish and maintain the relationship of mutuality is called *empathic perception*, an unconscious awareness of each other that facilitates the development of communication between them.[1] Neither the mother nor the infant is consciously aware of the signals which they are transmitting and receiving from each other, but both participate in the communication. For instance, the baby soon develops different qualities in his cry which cue the mother as to the problem he is experiencing. Although the mother probably could not explain to an outsider exactly what is different about the cries, she can identify and respond to their

differences sufficiently to take specific action appropriate to meeting the infant's needs. Similarly, the infant senses the mother's comfort or discomfort in his care and responds in turn with comfort or discomfort himself.

Touch is very important in communicating the mother's comfort or discomfort with her baby.[2, 3] There are several components of touch which seem to be important. One of these is temperature. If the mother feels comfortable with the baby, she will enfold him, holding him close to her body and transmitting to him her body heat, which is reminiscent of the intrauterine environment. This association helps him relax and become quiet, a satisfaction response, which helps her in turn to relax and be more comfortable with him. Conversely, the baby can sense muscle tension in the mother. This muscle tension causes him discomfort to which he responds with fussiness, crying, and tension of his own. The mother then feels more tense, the baby's tension increases, and in this way a disruptive cycle may be initiated.

Montague has suggested rather strongly that rocking chairs are a great adjunct to the care of infants,[4] especially in establishing and maintaining mutuality and, subsequently, trust. He feels that rocking chairs recreate the motion to which the infant was accustomed in utero, and that it gives the infant a sense of relatedness and companionship with the mother because of the pressure of her body on his as they sway back and forth. Mothers are also usually more relaxed in a rocking chair, and the motion is soothing for her as well as for the baby, enhancing their mutual relaxation and comfort. Also, rocking has a hypnotic effect which is soothing to an immature central nervous system, thus further increasing the infant's relaxation. It also seems to improve circulation, respiration, and digestion, all of which contribute to a sense of well-being in the infant and help facilitate a satisfaction response. Many pediatric units in hospitals have adopted the custom of providing rocking chairs for the use of both mothers and personnel who care for infants.

The Feeding Cycle

Probably the most important single event in the infant's life, as far as establishment of trust is concerned, is the feeding cycle. It is important that the nurse understand the behavioral components of this cycle.[5] Initially, the infant arouses from a state of sleep because of awareness of discomfort. He, of course, cannot identify the cause for the discomfort, but his response to it is increased physical activity, agitation, and crying. When he becomes agitated, he may be able to get his hand to his mouth and begin sucking, which is one way of alerting his mother to the nature of his discomfort. The mother responds to his crying by going to him and picking him up. If she recognizes that he is hungry, she will prepare him for feeding and then provide him with either the breast or bottle. The baby responds to objects touching his cheek by rooting, that is, by turning his head toward the object and attempting to grasp it in his mouth. The mother can assist him in locating and grasping the nipple, and then the infant takes the active role in sucking and swallowing as he participates in meeting his own need for food. Finally, as the infant takes in the milk and satisfies his hunger, his activity decreases, and he drifts into a deep, relaxed sleep. The mother sees this satisfaction response and feels increased self-esteem and pleasure in her mothering role (Fig. 24-2).

It is important to note here that the sucking is in itself a pleasurable activity, functioning both to release tension and to provide sensory pleasure for the infant. Infants have both a need for food and a need to suck. Normally, they satisfy their need to suck in the feeding process, although they will usually suck more than is actually needed to meet their need for food. It becomes vitally important whenever food must be delayed or withheld that the infant's

need to suck not be overlooked. The use of a pacifier can make a significant contribution toward decreasing the frustration of an infant who must tolerate prolonged physical discomfort or food deprivation.

The very young infant has no capacity whatsoever to relieve his own tensions without outside assistance.[6, 7] Only as he communicates his need and his mother responds will he begin to trust that his needs will be met, and only as this cycle is repeated numerous times will trust become a part of his life expectations. Mothers, particularly first-time mothers, in their desire to meet their infants' needs are very apt to overfeed them, thinking that anytime they cry they need to be fed. These mothers require assistance in identifying other kinds of needs their infants have, such as relief from pressure caused by lying in one position too long, from being too warm or too cold, from some other kind of physical discomfort besides hunger, or the need for socializing.

Sometimes events occur which interfere with the satisfying completion of the feeding cycle. It is not unusual in a pediatric unit of a hospital, for instance, to observe a mother who is having much difficulty in feeding her infant. Usually, she is very tense and awkward in her handling of him, and he responds with crying, spitting up, and general agitation which increases her discomfort. However, a nurse may take the infant from the mother and feed him successfully. It is very important to understand that the infant is responding to the nurse's comfort and relaxation just as he responded to his mother's tension and anxiety. It is also vital that a nurse who does intervene in such a situation explain to the mother the dynamics of the infant's response so that the mother does not come to the conclusion that she is inadequate because she failed where the nurse succeeded. A mother's self-esteem can easily be damaged by an unsympathetic demonstration of professional competence.

Separation from Mother

The very young infant does not differentiate his own body from objects in his environment.[8] He sees the nipple, for instance, as a part of himself, and his mother is also seen as a part of himself. His awareness is focused totally on his own body sensations. As his mother continues to meet his needs, however, he begins to focus on her, and during this period of infancy, he begins to relate to his mother as an object of interest to him. If the mother and infant are separated at this stage, the infant has a separation reaction, although it is not the same as will occur later. Solnit[9] observed that infants as young as 3 months of age, who were separated from their mothers while hospitalized, seem to recover initially from their illnesses, only to die a few weeks later from an undetermined cause which appeared to be apathy and general weakness. Hypothesizing that these infants were grieving for their mothers, he had the mothers reunited with the infants as soon as the crisis of the illness was over and observed that a much higher recovery rate prevailed. He also noted that as the infants began to recover from their illnesses, they became irritable. This irritability was viewed by him as an encouraging sign indicating a mobilization of energy and an increased responsiveness to the environment. If the infants were given extra stimulation and attention when they became irritable, they tended to become more interested in their surroundings and to reach out toward people and objects. If they were ignored or punished for their irritability, they turned again inward and became apathetic. Katharine Banham found that the development of affection follows a pattern of reaching-out behavior which begins to appear normally at about four months.[10] However, if the baby is either rebuffed or overwhelmed with too much attention, or if he is ignored, he turns his energy inward and ceases to reach out.

Short-term separation from mother prior to the end of the second month of infancy is tolerated very well if the infant is provided with a mothering person who is able to meet his physical needs consistently.[11] However, it is important to remember that a person who does not know the infant intimately will not have established mutuality with him and may have some difficulty sensing and meeting his needs.[12] In any event, the infant will sense empathically the difference in handling which he receives from a person other than his mother, and he may react to that difference with discomfort.

Institutionalization of infants in the period of early infancy has drastic detrimental effects. Rene Spitz was a pioneer in studying responses of very young infants to institutionalization.[13] He found that the infants seemed to progress normally for about the first 2 months of life, after which they began to become increasingly retarded in motor and language development and to become apathetic and unresponsive to their environments. Most of the infants studied were those who were cared for in large nurseries where they received the best hygienic care and good food but little handling and attention from nursery personnel. Approximately one-third of them died before reaching their first birthdays. Many never learned to walk or talk even after becoming toddlers and preschoolers. Most of the infants had

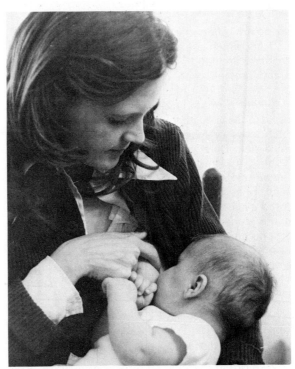

Figure 24-2   As the infant's need for food is met, he develops trust and his mother receives satisfaction in her mothering role. *(Photo courtesy of Penelope Peirce.)*

digestive difficulties, such as vomiting, diarrhea, and rumination. Several of these infants lost weight, became progressively weaker, and finally died. The remainder showed emaciation and a lack of head control and motor vigor normally expected of young infants. Spitz attributed the infants' lack of development and failure to thrive to the absence of mothering. Some investigators since then think that the basic problem may have been a lack of sensory stimulation which the baby would normally have received in the mothering process. Others believe that the critical issue was the lack of a single mother figure with whom to relate. Still others feel that the biggest problem was that the babies did not have an opportunity to practice motor activities which would have brought about their normal development.[14]

Spitz' findings are important because of the nursing implications they suggest. When an infant must be hospitalized for a long period of time, it is important that several things be provided for him. First of all, if possible and if she wishes, his mother should stay with him and care for him. If this is not possible, he should receive frequent handling and attention from as limited a number of personnel as possible. Sensory stimulation and motor development may be encouraged by judicious use of toys.

Toys which are especially helpful in providing sensory stimulation are music boxes or radios, stuffed animals with contrasting textures, rubber bath toys, wooden blocks, and mobiles. Motor development is encouraged by toys which reward active responses from the baby, for example, those which move or make noises when hit by a moving arm or leg. Care must always be taken to provide toys that are safe. They must not have sharp edges or small parts, such as the squeakers in bath toys, which can be removed and swallowed by a baby. Button eyes on stuffed animals should be removed for the same reason. Care must be taken also in suspending toys over a crib to be sure that the baby will not become entangled in the suspension cord. The baby should be encouraged to practice the vocalizations which begin in this early period. The best way to stimulate vocal behavior is to echo to the baby the sounds he is making.

Anxiety in the Parent-Child Relationship

Because of the detrimental effects of anxiety in the parent-child relationship, it is very important to consider sources of anxiety for parents of sick infants.[15] One of the most important sources of anxiety is concern for the child's recovery. The parents, especially the mother, are likely to overreact to their infant's illness. These overreactions are a reflection of the strength of the fusion and affectional bonds which have been established. Severe overreaction may indicate, however, that normal separation has failed to occur in the relationship. A severe overreaction is seen when a mother watches every respiratory movement of the baby and interprets normal variations in respiration as indications of impending death. Other severe reactions may be manifested by the mother's refusal to leave a child in a mist tent, insisting rather on rocking him continuously, or by the mother who frequently complains that her infant is being neglected or mismanaged by medical or nursing personnel. Severe and unreasonable maternal guilt reactions are also manifestations of inadequate separation of mother and child. Reactions severely out of proportion to objective reality may indicate the need for some counseling assistance for the parents.

It is very important in talking with parents that words be chosen carefully so as not to alarm or confuse them. Many parents are inclined to interpret medical jargon incorrectly. For instance, they might confuse inflammation with infection or moniliasis with meningitis. It must be remembered that most medical terms are relatively unfamiliar to the average mother and that any person's ability to comprehend spoken communication may be greatly diminished when under stress. Even mothers who are nurses may be alarmed inappropriately by what is said about their infant's condition. One nurse became very anxious when she was told that her infant's tear duct was infected, probably with "staph," because she assumed "staph" to imply a pathogenic drug-resistant infection, forgetting that nonpathogenic staphylococci are a part of normal skin flora.

It is especially important in working with highly anxious mothers that the same terms be used by all personnel. One mother whose seriously ill child was being treated by a group of staff doctors became very agitated and angry when two doctors in the group used different names for the same drug; she assumed that they either disagreed in their treatment or that one of the doctors was incompetent.

The nurse can help prevent such problems by being present when doctors talk with parents and by recording the substance of the doctor's explanations so that all personnel will know what parents have been told. Misunderstandings which the nurse becomes aware of later should be both clarified to the parents and reported to the doctors as soon as possible.

In addition, special care must be taken to ensure that all nursing approaches are consistent and planned to meet the individual needs of the parents as well as the child. It is especially important in working with highly anxious parents that all nursing personnel do procedures in exactly the same way so that the parents do not come to believe that one nurse is more competent or more caring than another. This is no time for shortcuts, even if they are safe; these parents need the reassurance of consistency. Team conferences and cooperation among personnel are essential. Even such "routine" procedures as the daily bath may need to be outlined in detail and followed consistently in order for parents who are extremely upset to be able to relax and trust the staff. The nurse's ability to remain calm and confident in giving care in such stressful situations will greatly contribute to the parents' eventual ability to recover their emotional equilibrium and to begin to trust that their child will recover.

A second source of anxiety for parents of hospitalized infants is the hospital environment. The presence of strange and frightening equipment and the use of medical jargon may result in a set of very frightened parents. One commonly used piece of pediatric equipment which is especially frightening to parents is the mist tent.[16] Because it resembles an oxygen tent and may be used in conjunction with oxygen administration, its use seems particularly ominous to parents even when it is used for comfort or prophylactically. The purpose for its use should be carefully explained to parents so that they are not unduly frightened by it. With assistance, even a frightened parent may learn to care for an infant in a mist tent. The nurse needs to be alert to other equipment or procedures that parents may find frightening, so that unrealistic fears can be relieved.

3) A third cause for parental anxiety is subordination of the parents, particularly the mother, to the nurse. The nurse who excludes the mother from the care of the child deals a severe blow to her self-esteem. While mothers desire nurses to perform the technical aspects of care, they tend to resent the nurse who performs the mothering activities, such as feeding and bathing the child, when they feel able to do it. It is important for the nurse to be aware of the mother's needs at all times, because a greatly frightened or fatigued mother may desire and need the nurse to perform caretaking activities. The same mother, after a few hours' rest, may wish to perform these activities herself. It is very important when the nurse performs mothering activities that she not imply in her manner or conversation that she feels the mother is incapable of caring for the child; the mother already feels inadequate and has had a decrease in self-esteem simply by the fact of her baby's illness.

4) A fourth source of anxiety for parents is a sense of guilt and self-condemnation for having allowed the child to become ill or for not having recognized the illness earlier. If the infant has suffered an accident, the guilt reaction of the parents is even more severe. These parents are especially sensitive to any real or imagined criticism from medical personnel.

One father whose infant son had sustained a mild concussion from falling off a table where his father had placed him in an infant seat was seen pacing the hall in an agitated manner. The doctor, intending to take the child's history, asked to speak to the father in the conference room. The father immediately began defending his placement of the baby on the table, although nothing had been said by the doctor about the accident. In another instance, a nurse, thinking she was consoling a mother whose infant had been injured in a fall from a high chair, said, "It is hard to watch babies all the time." She was astounded when the mother's reply was, "You needn't get smart with me, young woman!" Such situations must be handled with utmost tact and maturity.

5) A fifth concern of parents when an infant is hospitalized is their worry about other members of the family, particularly toddlers or other young children in the home who also need the mother's attention. Separation of the mother from a toddler may be more detrimental for the overall family welfare than separation of the mother from the very young infant who is hospitalized. Sometimes the nurse may need to help the mother work out a solution to this problem which will consider the needs of all the family members. The needs of the mother and father must be considered, too, in such planning.

The life of one family was greatly disrupted when their young infant was diagnosed with Wilms' tumor. The mother took the baby to a referral hospital 200 miles from home, intending to stay there with him for 3 weeks while his initial treatment was begun. His siblings, 2 and 4 years old, were sent to stay with a grandmother 100 miles from home in a different direction, and the father stayed home to work and commute to the hospital on weekends. After 3 days at the hospital, the mother began getting reports of the older children's unhappiness and discontent, and she herself became very depressed. As the nurses talked with the mother, it became apparent that she felt guilty about being away from her older children and husband. At the same time, she felt it her duty to stay with the infant. Finally, she agreed that it might be better for her to allow the nurses to care for the infant and to go home and care for her other children and husband, with arrangements to visit the baby on weekends. The mother did go home and reunite the other members of the family. She was able to make arrangements for the older children to stay with a well-liked neighbor during her weekend visits to the hospital, and she and her husband were able to have time alone together during the trips to renew and strengthen their relationship. She was able to keep in touch with the nurses during the week by telephone and seemed relaxed in caring for the infant while she was visiting. Because the nurses had followed the mother's usual routines in caring for the infant in her absence, he was not greatly disturbed by the separation.

Not all family disruptions are this dramatic, but if a child is hospitalized for more than a few days, nurses should inquire about the reactions of other members of the family, as mothers may either be so concerned about the sick child that they lose sight of the legitimate needs of other family members, or they may become distressed by reactions of other children or their husbands but not know how to deal with them helpfully.

6) Finally, the parents may be concerned about

costs and the financial drain on an already strained budget. Most families with young infants do not have an excess reserve of financial resources, and they very likely have hospital bills from the infant's delivery which still must be paid.

Coping Behaviors

There are three basic coping behaviors which parents commonly use in working through their anxiety. 1) The most important of these is participation in the care of the infant, which has already been discussed. 2) A second coping behavior is a quest for information and understanding. Characteristically, the parents ask the same questions over and over. It is important to remember that parents are not intentionally being obnoxious in their questioning; they have difficulty grasping and remembering information which is given to them because of their high anxiety levels. As they do assimilate their new information, however, it helps to decrease their anxiety. 3) Finally, many parents are able to become emotionally dependent upon the nurse. These parents may cry and talk with the nurses for long periods of time as they attempt to relieve their tension. It is important that these behaviors be met with genuine understanding and concern.

THE PERIOD OF MIDDLE INFANCY (4 TO 8 MONTHS)

After about the fourth month of infancy, the child begins to become more oriented toward his environment. He becomes interested in toys and their manipulation, and he is able to manipulate them because his motor development has continued to the point where he can purposefully hold on to a toy. New toys are put through a whole repertoire of maneuvers as he tries to learn about his environment. They may be tasted, banged, and looked at right side up and upside down. The physical development of the infant during this middle infancy period includes learning to sit alone and to reach for objects, the ability to crawl, and an increasing interest in self-feeding. It is important in the hospital situation that the infant be encouraged to practice the motor development which he is capable of performing. For instance, if he is used to sitting in an infant seat or chair, it is helpful for him to continue this practice. Some hospitals provide chair tables for infants in the hallway by the nurse's station so that they can not only be stimulated by the activity around them but also practice their motor skills. A careful nursing history taken at the time of the child's admission to the hospital should provide the nurse with information relevant to planning such experiences.

Separation from Mother

The infant in the middle infancy period begins to recognize his mother as a person separate from himself, and sometime between 6 and 8 months he begins to recognize her as a person different from other persons. It is because of this recognition that separation of mother and child during this period of development is especially devastating. During this time, he will usually reject the attention of strangers even if his mother is present, and his reaction to separation from her may range from crying episodes to stark terror. In one study it was found that children between the ages of 6 months and 4 years were the most disturbed by hospitalization and separation from parents.[17] The degree of the disturbance increased when the hospitalization lasted longer than 3 weeks. Infants older than 6 months react first with extreme distress and crying at separation from their mothers. Then they progress to a panic reaction and from there to apathy and depression. This depression is actually a grief reaction such as is seen in older children and adults and should be understood in this way. The infants observed tended to regress in their motor skills when separated from their parents for a long period of time, but unlike the very young infants they did maintain social skills. If they were reunited with their mothers within a 3-month period, a very rapid spontaneous recovery occurred, but after a 5-month separation, they seemed never to recover entirely.[18, 19]

It is important that parents of infants in this age group receive some support and help from the nurse if it is necessary for them to be separated from their infant even for a few hours.[20, 21] Some parents find it helpful to stay with their infants until they fall asleep for the night. If it is necessary for the parents to leave while the baby is awake, a nurse should be available to hold the infant and comfort him during their leaving and to reassure the parents that he will be cared for in their absence.

In approaching infants, it is helpful if nurses make initial contacts with the infant by first chatting with the parents. In this way the infant has time to become familiar with and to begin to view the nurse as a safe person. After the infant becomes somewhat comfortable with the nurse, it is much easier to provide care for him. Again, it is best, to the extent possible, to let the mother keep on with direct care, the nurse doing only those things which the mother cannot or does not want to do. It is also helpful in providing infant care for the schedule in the pediatric unit to be flexible enough to maintain the normal routines which the infant is used to at home. This flexibility helps in maintaining the mutuality and trust which has been established between mother and child and in decreasing the strangeness of the new environment.

Interaction with the Environment

One interesting phenomenon occurs during this age period: the baby begins to teethe. When this event occurs, he takes a much more active approach to his environment, especially in the form of biting behavior. He also begins to sense that he has control over his environment, a magical power. If the persons in his environment are consistent in their response to him, he learns that his behavior causes other people to act in specific predictable ways. He will then attempt actively to control his environment. If an event which he enjoys, such as his mother's singing a song, happens to correspond with his jumping up and down in his crib, then later, when he wants his mother to sing, he will again jump up and down in his crib. Whether his jumping actually will cause his mother to sing is something he will have to learn by watching her responses, but this attempt to control his environment is an important first step in the development of communication skills. Later, he will learn to substitute vocal behavior for physical activity. However, if the responses of others in his environment are not consistent, such as might occur in a hospital unit where his interaction with personnel tends to be more random, his efforts to control his environment and thereby communicate will not be reinforced, and verbal communication may be delayed.[22]

Regression

One common reaction of children to illness is behavioral regression. Usually the last-acquired motor skill is the first to be lost. The younger the child is when he becomes ill, the greater the degree of regression and the sooner it appears.[23] Parents may need help in understanding regression and in coping with it. They tend to see it as a reflection on their parenting skills or as misbehavior in the child. They need to know first of all that regression is an expected, normal response to illness, and that it is in no way a negative reflection of parenting skills. If the nurse is accepting of the child's regression, the parents will find it easier to be accepting also. The

duration of the regression can be minimized by the parents' uncritical acceptance of it, coupled with their awareness and positive reinforcement of each small step toward independence and growth which the child displays as he begins to recover from his illness.[24] Most children, especially infants, have a strong natural drive toward growth and maturation. The nurse can assist the child in continuing his maturation by providing him with opportunities and encouragement to use newly acquired skills such as self-feeding or drinking from a cup. Again, a thorough nursing history taken at the time of admission will provide the nurse with the needed data to plan individualized care appropriately.

THE PERIOD OF LATE INFANCY (8 TO 12 MONTHS)

During the last few months of the infant's first year, he begins to combine simple behaviors which he has learned previously into complex behavior patterns. Since he has not developed any sense of danger, however, his parents must begin to exert some external control over his behavior in order to keep him safe. If the child has been ill during his infancy, the parents will find limit-setting to be rather difficult, and some may not be able to do so at all. This inability to set limits reflects an inability to separate from the child appropriately, and it is very important that some guidance be provided to prevent disturbances from developing in the parent-child relationship.

The child is also likely to be doing some self-feeding at this age, and he may have strong food likes and dislikes. It is important, if he is to be separated from his mother, to find out what his likes and dislikes are and to provide for them as much as possible within nutritionally sound management. One of the common problems of this age is anemia which may result from the parents' not having introduced solid foods sufficiently into the diet and allowing the child to drink too much milk. This practice, which of course must be corrected, is an example of the kind of health teaching to which the nurse needs to be alert when working with parents of older infants.

Separation from Mother

The older infant reacts to separation from his mother much the same as the infant in the middle period of infancy. He tends now to be even more possessive of his mother and more aggressive in his clinging at the time of separation. However, he is able now to keep an object in mind when it is partially hidden,

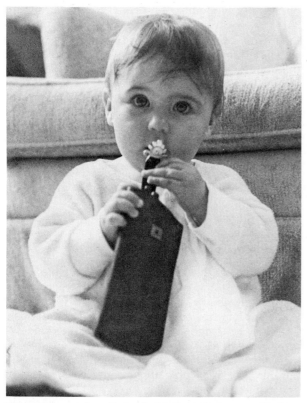

Figure 24-3 A favorite toy helps the infant cope with his mother's absence while they are separated. *(Photo courtesy of Penelope Peirce.)*

and games such as peek-a-boo or partially hiding an object and letting him find it will help him to establish the fact that his mother will return after she leaves him.[25]

Toward the end of the first year, the infant may be able partially to relieve his own tensions and loneliness if he is allowed to keep a favorite blanket or stuffed toy.[26] Care must be taken to ensure that these objects are not lost while the child is in the hospital because he tends to identify with them and their loss will increase his fear of loss or abandonment. The favorite objects, along with thumb-sucking or other comforting behavior will help him cope with his mother's absence when it is necessary (Fig. 24-3). Prolonged separation, however, should be avoided, as the child's tolerance for separation is still very limited, and his anxiety about abandonment is at a very high level.

Intervention during Procedures

Preplanning by the nurse to prepare infants for procedures is a necessity. If possible the child's mother should be with him to comfort him during the procedure. The procedure itself should be explained to the mother in terms of its purpose and what she will see and hear, especially if bleeding is likely or if fluids will be removed from the child's body, as in a spinal tap. If possible the infant should be provided with a pacifier during painful or prolonged procedures. In addition, his mother should be encouraged to talk or sing to him and to maintain physical contact by touching him or holding his hand during the procedure. Persons who restrain him for the procedure should do so with gentle firmness so that he senses security in their care. The baby should be comforted after the procedure is finished by being cuddled or rocked until he is quieted. Mothers usually prefer to provide this care, but if they cannot or do not wish to, the nurse should take the time to do so.

Allowing the child time to become familiar with simple equipment, such as a stethoscope, prior to its use in his care will also decrease his anxiety.

A tremendous amount of development occurs in the first year of life. The infant changes from a neonate whose response to his environment is entirely that of reflex activity to a 1-year-old who can manipulate and direct his environment sufficiently to begin to relieve his own anxieties and fears. Only the infant who has experienced a stable relationship with his parents can progress to this extent in his first year. Nurses who care for infants must keep the importance of the parent-child relationship in mind and strive constantly to strengthen it.

REFERENCES

1 Theodore Lidz, *The Person: His Development Throughout the Life Cycle,* Basic Books Inc., Publishers, New York, 1968, pp. 117–158.
2 Lienne D. Tempesta, "The Importance of Touch in the Care of Newborns," *Journal of Obstetric, Gynecologic, and Neonatal Nursing,* 1(3):27–28, 1972.
3 M. F. Ashley-Montagu, *Touching: The Human Significance of the Skin*, Harper & Row, Publishers, Incorporated, New York, 1971, pp. 92–165.
4 Ibid., pp. 149–157.
5 Roberta A. O'Grady, "Feeding Behavior in Infants," *American Journal of Nursing,* 71(4):736–739, 1971.
6 Erik H. Erikson, *Childhood and Society,* W. W. Norton & Company, Inc., 1963, pp. 247–251.
7 Lidz, loc. cit.
8 Lidz, loc. cit.
9 Albert J. Solnit, "A Study of Object Loss in Infancy," *Psychoanalytic Study of the Child,* 25:257–272, 1970.
10 Katharine Banham, "The Development of Affectionate Behavior in Infancy," in M. L. Haimowitz and Natalie Reader Haimowitz (eds.), *Human Development: Se-*

lected Readings, Thomas Y. Crowell Company, New York, 1960, pp. 166–172.

11 Wayne Dennis and Pergrouhi Najarian, "Infant Development Under Environmental Handicap," in M. L. Haimowitz and N. Reader Haimowitz (eds.), Human Development: Selected Readings, Thomas Y. Crowell Company, New York, 1960, pp. 173–189.

12 Myriam David and Genevieve Appell, "A Study of Nursing Care and Nurse-Infant Interaction," in Leo Kanner, Child Psychiatry, Charles C Thomas Publishers, 1972.

13 Rene Spitz, "Motherless Infants," in M. L. Haimowitz and N. Reader Haimowitz (eds.), Human Development: Selected Readings, Thomas Y. Crowell Company, New York, 1960, pp. 166–172.

14 Dennis, loc. cit.

15 Florence Bright, "The Pediatric Nurse and Parental Anxiety," Nursing Forum, 4(2):30–47, 1965.

16 Florence Bright, "Parental Anxiety—A Barrier to Communication," ANA Clinical Sessions, San Francisco, 1966, Appleton-Century-Crofts, New York, 1967, pp. 13–19.

17 David A. Vernon, Jerome L. Schulman, and Jeanne M. Foley, "Changes in Children's Behavior After Hospitalization," American Journal of Diseases of Children, 3:581–593, 1966.

18 Lidz, loc. cit.

19 Spitz, loc. cit.

20 Madeline Petrillo and Sirgay Sanger, Emotional Care of Hospitalized Children, J. B. Lippincott Company, Philadelphia, 1972, pp. 139–140.

21 David and Appell, loc. cit.

22 Lidz, loc. cit.

23 Vernon, et al., loc. cit.

24 Gerald R. Patterson and M. Elizabeth Gullion, Living With Children, Research Press Company, Champaign, Ill., 1971, pp. 73–79.

25 Lidz, loc. cit.

26 Lidz, loc. cit.

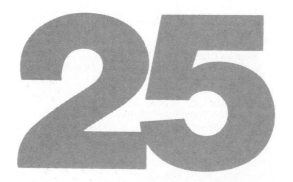

EFFECTS OF ILLNESS ON THE TODDLER

MARGARET SHANDOR MILES and JOYCE OLSON

The toddler period is usually defined as encompassing the years of approximately one to three. During this period, the child moves out of the infancy period and more clearly defines his own independent identity. While still emotionally dependent on his parents, he begins to *actively* move out to explore and investigate other people and new places and things. He is constantly in motion—walking, running, climbing, dumping, turning, pouring, or trying to lift something bigger than himself (see Fig. 25-1). Many of these activities are related to his inquisitive and curious nature; he wants to "discover the world," but with his mother close by. The routines and rituals of his world provide structure, limits, and safety in his new adventures.

Some of the developmental tasks that the toddler is working on include development of a sense of autonomy and independence; increase in language and communication skills; control of bowel and bladder function; increase in neuromuscular coordination, including locomotion and manual dexterity; decrease in egocentrism with an increase in cooperative behavior; and beginning development of a more reality-based sense of time, space, and causality.

Because of the many developments during this period and the uniqueness of each individual toddler as he goes through this stage of development, the generalizations made about the toddler may not fit a specific child or age within the toddler period. A broad range of variations in development can be expected. One child at 15 months may be developing quite differently from another. Peter, at 15 months, was fiercely independent and demanded to feed himself even when the food did not lend itself to his clumsy abilities. Jane at the same age still required much assistance at mealtimes and took a bottle at nap and bedtime.

In addition, the child at 1 year is quite different from the child at 3. At 1 year of age Amy was still holding onto furniture when she walked from place to place. Her gait was wide-based, and she was quite clumsy. By 3, Amy was able to run, climb stairs, and ride her tricycle. Thus, accurate assessment of the individual child is vitally important in planning intervention.

Illness and hospitalization, whether a sudden episode or a chronic illness, represent many unknowns and many threats to the toddler's developing identity and his interactions with the world he is just beginning to know.

The toddler's reactions to illness and hospitalization are affected by many factors including:

1 His family: their past experiences, their relations to

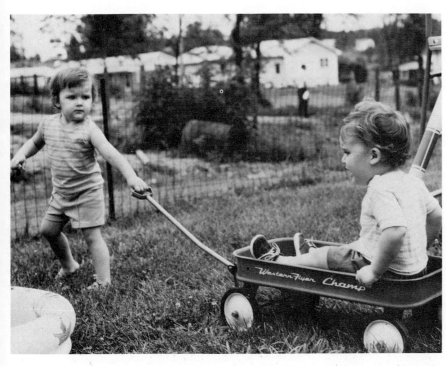

Figure 25-1 The toddler is in constant motion.

each other and to him; their reaction to his illness; and their ability to support him during his illness

2 His personality and developmental struggles as a toddler: the child's unique personality; his developmental level and the stresses it has imposed; and his unique way of coping with stress

3 His past experiences in life: illness or death of significant others, including family members, friends, or pets; a past illness or hospitalization experience; past experiences with strangers

4 His particular illness and experiences in the hospital: the type of illness; the particular treatment needed; the diagnostic tests involved; prior preparation for the hospital experience

Because of the importance of these factors, a nursing history should be prepared at the time of the toddler's admission to the hospital or clinic. Data can be collected by talking with the parents and by observing the child's interaction with them and with the nurse. The history should be used to assess the strengths and weaknesses of the family, to determine their problems and needs related to this hospitalization, and to plan appropriate nursing intervention for the child and his family.

DEVELOPMENTAL TASKS, HOSPITALIZATION, AND NURSING INTERVENTION

The reaction of the toddler to illness and hospitalization is closely related to and influenced by his developmental needs. His reactions may be the result of frustration and interference with attainment of developmental tasks.

Separation Anxiety

The most obvious source of stress for the hospitalized toddler is separation. His relationship with his mother has become very intense and meaningful and he feels secure in her presence. He longs for constant attention from her and is fearful when she is gone for even a short shopping trip. At the same time, he is becoming more socialized. He develops a close relationship with his father; his siblings become important.

In discussing the toddler's separation anxiety during hospitalization, most authors refer only to his acute anxiety reaction to being separated from his mother. The toddler also faces stress in being separated from his father, particularly the toddler who has a very close relationship with his father.

The reactions seen in the toddler experiencing this separation include protest, despair, and denial. During the protest phase, the toddler cries, screams, and uses other overt behavior to let everyone know that he does not want his parents to leave (see Fig. 25-2). When they are gone, he lets the nursing staff know that he wants his parents back immediately. This protesting behavior can easily be misunder-

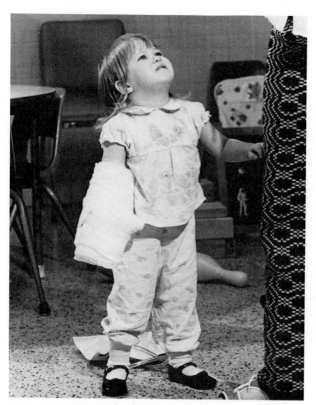

Figure 25-2 The hospitalized toddler experiences separation anxiety when his parents leave.

stood by the nursing staff and his parents as well. Not understanding what he is trying to communicate, they insist that he should be a good little boy. This request tells him that he should not be expressing these deep and significant emotions. Some toddlers have even been punished for their continued crying. Sally, age 2½, was standing near the nurses' station screaming following her mother's departure. Lacking an understanding of her needs, the nurse placed Sally in her crib and shut the door.

Sometimes parents are afraid to return to visit their children because they feel that their visits are upsetting to them. Parents need help in understanding the normalcy of the toddler's protestations. They also need to know how they can best help the child cope with the separation. Leaving a familiar item which belongs to his mother or father with the child, returning as often as possible and staying as much as possible, telling the child truthfully that they are leaving and that they will return are all ways of helping the grieving child cope with the loss.

Nursing intervention with parents and toddler should take place at the time of the parents' depar-

ture. For example, Billy, a 2-year-old, began screaming and kicking when his parents told him they were going to leave to get some supper. His mother then began to cry and was reluctant to leave him. The nurse explained to the parents that Billy's reaction was quite natural, recognized the fact that his behavior was upsetting to them, and offered to help Billy with the separation. As the parents left the room, she picked him up and held him for a while. When Billy later expressed concern about his parents whereabouts, the nurse said, "Mommy and Daddy are eating supper. I know you miss them very much. They will be back to play with you."

If the parents cannot return frequently or cannot stay long because they have other pressures at home or must travel a long distance from the hospital, the toddler will need special help from the nursing staff. He may seek out a certain nurse and follow her around for the entire shift, protesting when she leaves. Ideally the toddler is assigned to one or two nurses who see him consistently and who establish a trusting relationship with him. The nurses assigned to him may need help in knowing how to handle the protesting and grieving toddler. He needs constant reassurance that his mother and father love him, will return to see him, and will take him home eventually so that he does not feel abandoned. A note on his bed or in his nursing care plan indicating when his parents will return is helpful so that everyone says the same thing to him. He also will need love, attention, cuddling, and diversional activities such as play. Jay's mother could visit only in the evenings. He liked to sit in his nurse's lap as she charted, spend time with the playroom lady, and visit with another 8-year-old patient.

When the parent does not visit the child frequently and consistently and when he does not receive attention and consistency from the nursing staff, the child may exhibit the second and third stages of separation anxiety—despair and denial. Despair is characterized by withdrawn, depressed behavior. The child may refuse to eat, to leave his room, or to relate to anyone. When his mother arrives, he may cry intensely or he may react with anger and distrust. Some children may reach for the nurse in preference to their mother. Denial is evident when the child appears not to care when his mother and father returns. He may ignore them, reach for another adult instead, or remain quietly in his crib. Nursing staff often erroneously interpret this phase as positive adjustment to the hospital, since the child cries less and relates more to the staff. Because he forms superficial relationships with many staff members, he may become the ward favorite. He really needs the opportunity to form a trusting relationship with one individual to foster his psychosocial development.

Increasing use of rooming-in facilities, the lengthening of visiting hours, and the shortening of hospital stays for toddlers have minimized the problems which stem from separation anxiety. However, it is important to remind nurses that the toddler still experiences stress from separation—separation from the rest of his family and from the familiar surroundings of his home. All these losses are important to the toddler and create feelings of insecurity and grief. In the midst of separation from familiar family members and familiar surroundings, the toddler is faced with unfamiliar frightening surroundings and interactions with many strangers on a daily basis. The importance of consistency of personnel cannot be overemphasized.

Grandparents or friends should be allowed to visit and also stay overnight so they can relieve the parents from their bedside vigil. If the hospitalization is a long one and if the child's condition becomes stabilized, he should be allowed to visit siblings or talk with them on the telephone. It also helps if photographs of siblings, grandparents, parents, pets, and his home are hung on his walls. Other familiar objects from home, such as favorite toys, blankets, and clothes, are also helpful.

Rituals and Routines

Another source of stress for the toddler during an illness and hospitalization is the major change in his daily routines and rituals which occur in the hospital environment—an environment which imposes a new set of routines and rituals on him. The routines of his daily life are important to the toddler's sense of security; he knows what to expect and when to expect it. Even a vacation can be very upsetting to him. Because of the loss of familiar routines, he may exhibit many different behavioral changes during or after a vacation such as night fears or regression to bedwetting.

In addition to routines, toddlers tend to set up precise and involved rituals around the important activities of eating, sleeping, or bathing. A ritual is a rigid pattern of procedures which the toddler expects his parents or babysitters to follow. These rituals assure him that he can know what to expect and allow him to exert some control over the situation.

It is important in planning nursing care for toddlers to learn about their special rituals and their usual routines so that plans can be made to attempt to follow some of them during his hospitalization. Bedtime for toddlers can include such rituals. Jim, a 15-month-old, had developed a precise repertoire of activities which he expected his parents to perform at bedtime. These activities include rocking him and singing special songs as he commanded them by name, kissing him on both cheeks and ears, closing the door exactly the right amount, and saying, "Good night, I love you" to him and his stuffed dog. During hospitalization, his parents tried to continue the ritual as closely as possible with the result that he slept quite well during his brief hospital experience.

Another area in which loss of rituals and familiar surroundings becomes important is that of eating. Eating patterns in toddlers are easily affected by changes in self, the person who feeds him, and the environment. Since the toddler's appetite is erratic anyway, the effects of change may lead to refusal of food. Certainly hospitalization creates a change in the environment, feeding person, time, and the food which is received. In addition, the toddler's illness or drugs he is taking may cause some anorexia or nausea. Thus, a decrease in appetite can be expected until some adjustments are made by the child and his physical condition improves. It is not uncommon for him to eat only one good meal a day, so it helps to know what he has eaten at previous meals. Attempting to force a toddler to eat will be unsuccessful, as eating is one activity he can control. It will help if the nurse attempts to follow the ritual used at home, to have a familiar person help with the meals, and to let the toddler feed himself as much as possible.

Closely related to the problems created by the changes in routines and rituals is the toddler's poor time sense. They simply do not understand the abstract concepts involved in time. Yet, hospital routines revolve around time schedules—a certain time for eating, a certain time for playroom, a certain time for a bath. Nurses and parents need to realize that telling a toddler something will happen at a certain time means nothing to him. However, if he is told that something will happen after his nap, he will have a little clearer idea of the time. Thus, time schedules for a toddler revolve around his activities and not around a clock.

Independence and Autonomy

One of the outstanding features of this period is the toddler's egocentric view of life. He feels that the world should revolve around his desires and wishes. His egocentrism is closely related to his developing sense of independence and autonomy. He is the focus of his world. When events do not go exactly as he expects and wants them to go, the toddler is prone to react. He usually reacts through the familiar mode of temper tantrums. Through the tantrum, he is trying to express his desire to be respected as an individual and his desire to control the world.

This type of negativistic behavior is quite evident in a hospitalized toddler. Hospitalization and illness, as already discussed, impose many restrictions on his behavior, his activities, and ultimately on his independence. Painful and frightening things are done to him without his having any control over the situation. In many hospital settings, he is consulted about nothing and given no choice in what happens, nor even an explanation. The result is a negativistic, hostile toddler.

The toddler needs help in finding appropriate outlets which allow him to maintain some sense of independence and autonomy, thereby decreasing his negativistic outbursts. He needs to be allowed the privilege of making choices whenever and wherever possible. Making his own decisions will help him to preserve his sense of independence and autonomy. Never offer him a choice which is unacceptable after he has decided upon it. A typical example is the nurse who asks, "Lisa, would you take your medicine?" Lisa's choice of refusing to take the important medication cannot be accepted. She *can* make a choice about whether she wants the red liquid medicine from a paper medicine cup or from a straw. Or she could be offered the choice of taking the crushed tablet mixed in applesauce or grape juice.

Physical settings for toddlers should ideally be planned to encourage their independence by making it easy for them to eat, dress, and use the bathroom by themselves. A potty chair near the bed, feeding tables, and an accessible area for clothes and belongings will help. Another way of helping toddlers increase their sense of autonomy is to let them explore their environment within the limits needed for their safety. They will feel more independent when they know that they can leave their room, go to the playroom themselves, and find their nurse when they want her.

Despite the nurse's efforts to allow some control, there are still many aspects of hospitalization which lead to temper tantrums and negativism. The negative behavior may be expressed directly at the time of the incident or may be generalized to many other areas. They may express this behavior mainly with their parents, who are "safer." They may express negativism at meals, an activity with which they feel a sense of control. Handling of the negativistic toddler is a highly individualistic problem, depending on the child and the situation. Some toddlers respond to being ignored at this time; some need to be held firmly until they gain control. Diversion through play or another activity such as showing the child an interesting toy, directing him to look out the window, or getting him to help another person with something may also be successful.

Communication

A very significant problem for the hospitalized toddler is related to his developing, but still incomplete, comprehension and use of language. Since the toddler is only beginning to use and understand language, verbal communication between him and the rest of the speaking world is limited and incomplete. Thus, the toddler will have a hard time understanding verbal explanations and in communicating concerns, desires, and needs. Even when he attempts to communicate something that is very important to him, it may be misunderstood or not even heard by the adults with whom he is trying to communicate.

The toddler's parents are the nurse's most important resource in attempting to establish communication. It is important to find out from the mother the important words in the child's vocabulary and his unique way of communicating his needs and concerns, both verbally and nonverbally. For the toilet-trained toddler it is vital that words used to communicate toileting needs are understood. He becomes frustrated when the nurse does not respond to his need and then chastises him for wetting the bed.

Nonverbal behavior is a very important avenue of communicating with the toddler. His facial expressions, body movements, and body restrictions can all be clues in helping the nurse understand how he feels about a situation. Nonverbal communication is a two-way exchange; nurses must remember that their feelings and frustrations are communicated to the toddler by facial expression, tone of voice, body movement, and gentleness or roughness of handling. For example, Mike had a cleft palate repair and had refused fluids from his nursing student. The instructor gently picked Mike up and placed him in her lap. In a calm, gentle tone she said, "It's time to have a drink." He responded by reaching for the glass and drank the milk. Using the same approach later, the student was also successful.

Important points to remember in communicating with toddlers are:

1 Give one direction at a time, using simple words that have meaning for them.
2 Be gentle in manner and tone.
3 Approach them on their level—*verbally and physically*.
4 Be positive by suggesting what to do rather than what not to do.

Body Integrity Fears

A lack of understanding about body functions and misconceptions of causality present one of the greatest difficulties for hospitalized toddlers. They are unable to understand what is wrong with their bodies and the reasons for the treatment and diagnostic measures. Their incomplete and inaccurate understanding cause fear, anxiety, frustration, and anger.

The toddler is rapidly becoming more aware of his external body. He has started to name body parts and is becoming aware of and interested in the bodies of others. He delights in learning that he has some of the same body parts as his mother or father. He is puzzled when he finds sexual or other differences. He will notice a mole on his mother's chin or a bruise on another child and become concerned. Because of his new awareness about his body, injury or loss of a body part tends to create concern about his body integrity (wholeness). Thus, the toddler is concerned about the slightest injury. He shows his injured part to everyone he sees and may demand that it be covered up with a bandage to restore his sense of body wholeness.

An additional stress is added by his incomplete knowledge about what is inside his body. He cannot understand explanations which refer to internal body parts or to the cause of illness. Explanations given to him are understood in a very egocentric, limited manner. It is hard to assess just what he is thinking about the situation; he may attach all sorts of fantasies to the experiences and explanations or he may feel that he has done something wrong. He may also blame the illness experience on his parents, who until now have been his protectors. For example, Jane, a 2-year-old, returned from the operating room following a tonsillectomy. Upon being greeted by her parents, she turned her head away in anger.

Nursing and parental support of the toddler are very important in helping him overcome his fears and fantasies. The toddler feels supported if he knows that his parents and nurses understand some of his fears. For the older toddler, simple, basic explanations about his illness and about diagnostic and treatment measures should be given to him by his parents or his nurse. Even if he does not understand exactly what is said, he will be comforted in knowing that the significant adults in his world do understand what is happening. Staying with the toddler when procedures are being done is also a very important means of support for him. He needs someone whom he trusts to hold his hand and allow him to express his fear and anxiety through crying, holding on tight, or talking.

For example, Jim, a 20-month-old, saw the needle and syringe to be used for blood withdrawal and he became hysterical. Holding Jimmy in her lap, the nurse slowly and calmly said, "I know you are afraid of needles because they hurt you. We don't like to hurt you but we need to do this blood test to find out why you are sick. You can help us get finished quickly by holding your arm still. When it hurts you can squeeze my hand or cry. I'll be here to help you." Jim stopped screaming hysterically and cried only when the needle was inserted.

Since explanations are ineffective to comfort the child following a painful procedure, physical and psychologic comfort can be provided instead by holding him for a short period.

If the procedure is one where the parents may be present if desired, two factors need to be considered. One factor is the parents' choice. They may or may not want to be present, and the decision is theirs. The second factor is their capacity to support the child. If the parents understand what is going to happen and can serve as an emotional support to the toddler, parental participation is helpful. If, however, the parents' anxieties and fears inhibit their ability to help the child cope, their presence may be detrimental.

After procedures or injections, the toddler may become very insistent about having a bandage put over the puncture site. Some toddlers refuse to have any of these "security objects" removed for days. This need to preserve body wholeness needs to be understood and respected.

Mobility

Another important development in the toddler period which may be affected by illness and hospitalization is the development of mobility—the ability to move around in the world on one's own two feet. Mobility is such an important task for him that the toddler may fight going to bed or sitting in a chair at mealtimes. He wants to keep moving. Mobility provides him great pleasure, gives him a feeling of independence, helps him learn about the world, and gives him an important avenue for coping with frustration. Running, kicking, rolling, and dancing are all important outlets for feelings which cannot be expressed verbally.

If an illness or hospital experience imposes a restraint on this very important activity, one can expect great frustration. Bedrest, casts, traction, and other types of restraints which limit walking and mobility are indeed a source of stress for the young child. He may react by fighting against the experience: climbing over siderails, tearing off a restraint, or trying to walk with the cast. Some toddlers react verbally by screaming and crying for hours on end. A few toddlers may react by withdrawal and depression. Whatever the reaction, the child needs help from his parents and the nursing staff to find effective ways of coping with the restrictions.

An important rule for the nurse to remember regarding immobilization is to replace the lost activity with another form of motion. Walking can be replaced by other means of motion such as a stroller, swing, wheelchair, or by moving the bed (see Fig. 25-3). Some hospitals even have special carts for young children who need to move around despite the presence of casts or an order for bedrest. Attempting to keep a toddler on bedrest is almost impossible. He will be much quieter and happier if held or put on a moving cart and taken to the playroom where he can be a passive observer of others' activities.

If an arm or leg restraint is necessary because of intravenous therapy, surgery, or equipment, the restraint needs to be removed several times a day under close supervision so the child can exercise the limb (unless movement is contraindicated) and so the nurse can examine and care for the skin. Restraints on a toddler are often overused when simple explanations or other means of protection would be less traumatic and more successful. For example, hand mitts were placed on Roger, a 2-year-old, for the purpose of keeping him from removing his esophageal string. Because of the mitts, he could not use his hands to play or to feed himself. Removal of the mitts under supervision for several days indicated that he never tried to remove the string. Finally the mitts were removed totally after a careful explanation about the importance of leaving the string alone. Use of his hands changed Roger from a depressed, sad boy to a happy, active toddler.

Immobility may decrease the child's opportunity to learn about himself, other people, and his environment through tactile, kinesthetic, and visual means. He needs opportunity to develop through these sensory modalities. Water play, mirrors, body games, and back rubs are helpful replacements. Lack of mobility also decreases the toddler's opportunity to use his abundant energy and to express his aggressive feelings. Activities such as tearing paper, pounding, or throwing balloons should be offered.

Regression

Since the toddler has so recently acquired new abilities and more mature behavior, the stresses of illness and hospitalization can cause a regression in behavior. Regression can be expected in the areas of toileting, self-feeding, verbal communication, thumbsucking, and an increased need for security objects. Regression may be increased by undue anxiety, type of illness, or poor communication between child and staff members. Nursing staff may also encourage regression by not accurately assessing the individual toddler's level of development. Toddlers are often automatically placed in diapers, fed by the nurse, or given a bottle.

Conversely, the toddler's parents or his nurse may expect him to maintain prior behavior at a time when this is very difficult or impossible. They may scold him, thus increasing his feelings of insecurity and inadequacy. Assessing the toddler's individual developmental levels and planning care accordingly may prevent regression. When regression occurs, the best approaches to helping him are accepting his behavior, assuring him that he is understood, and helping him overcome the regression when he is ready. Michael was crying and upset when the nurse approached his bed. When he pointed to his wet pants, the nurse said, "Michael's upset because he didn't make it to the potty on time. That's O.K., we'll get you some dry ones. Let's find a potty chair and put it by your bed, so it will be easier for you the next time."

Play

The toddler spends most of his waking hours in activities which are lumped together under the word *play*. Play encompasses his activities with toys, motion, touch, sound, and exploration. Play, then, is an important process for learning about the world, for communicating feelings, for overcoming boredom, and for developing motor skills and independence.

The need for play does not cease in the hospital, but becomes even more important. Play is helpful in making the hospital a more familiar place—toys are a universal sign of friendliness. Play can help in the establishment of a trusting relation with a toddler, and it can serve as a means of communication with him. Through play he may express many nonverbal feelings. Play can serve as a diversion from pain and fears which he is experiencing. Play can become a replacement for mobility and can be helpful as an outlet for anger and frustration. It can also help the toddler feel more independent by giving him control over something, and a sense of accomplishment. Thus, the toddler needs to have an opportunity for play in the hospital environment: play in a supervised playroom, play in his bed, play with his parents, and play with his nurses (see Fig. 25-4).

Play activities for the toddler must be chosen with regard to safety needs, illness limitations, developmental level, and individual personality. Specific goals such as muscle strengthening, increasing coordination or dexterity skills, or learning about hospital routine and procedures may also be considered in selecting play activity.

The following are examples of play materials which can be used with the hospitalized toddler:

Soft toys such as stuffed animals and rag dolls
Action toys such as push and pull objects, a hobby horse, tricycle, or riding animals
Toys for water play such as bubble pipes and plastic bottles
Toys for building and nesting such as blocks, nests of blocks or other shapes, pyramid rings
Books, especially cloth or heavy cardboard picture books
Musical toys, including record players, music boxes, musical telephones
Throw and catch toys such as balls, beanbags, or balloons
Kitchen items such as pots, pans, dishes, or spoons
Artistic items such as large crayons and paper or finger paints for the older toddler
Empty-and-fill toys such as a bottle and clothes pins, a small plastic container with spools or other items to place in it and dump out (always avoid items small enough to be placed in the child's mouth, as he may choke)
Simple trains, boats, cars, and trucks
Toys which are fun to feel and manipulate such as playdough or clay

PARENTAL RESPONSE, COPING ABILITIES, AND NURSING INTERVENTION

A major overriding factor which affects the child's reaction to illness and hospitalization is the reaction of his parents to the situation and to the illness. Children are very sensitive to the moods and attitudes of their parents. Toddlers can detect the slightest change in attitudes or feelings, even when they are not verbalized, and they react to these changes. Whether the illness is acute, short term, or chronic, all parents need some help in some areas.

Contact with parents of the toddler at the time of admission sets the stage for further intervention.

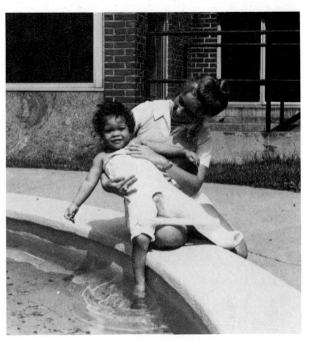

Figure 25-3 Walking can be replaced by another means of motion.

A nursing interview to obtain information about the child and family, to give information about what to expect during the hospitalization, and to indicate who will be caring for their child help in establishing a trust relationship with both parents and child.

Since rooming-in should be encouraged with the toddler, clarification of the roles of mother and nurse need to be established upon admission. Rooming-in parents need to know what they can do for the child, where necessary supplies can be found, who can be asked for assistance, what to expect from the nursing staff, and where to take care of their own personal needs. Continuous open communication between parents and staff is vital to the success of rooming-in.

The nurse working with parents must be sensitive to their feelings and needs. The expression of anxieties and feelings about the child's illness and the hospital experience is often difficult. Yet, parents who are burdened with anxiety and fears about the child's illness and expected outcomes may affect their child's behavior by increasing his anxiety. Parents who are hostile and negative and who lack trust in some or all aspects of the hospital experience will probably have a child who is especially frightened by hospital personnel, experiences, and procedures.

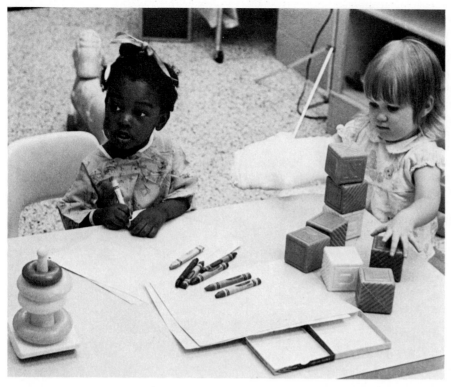

Figure 25-4 The need for play becomes more important to the hospitalized toddler.

Some parents may react to the illness with a deep sense of guilt, particularly when the illness was caused by an accident or when the illness is congenital or chronic. To overcome their feelings of guilt, parents may overprotect the child and set no limits with him. The child, in turn, is never satisfied and becomes quite grouchy, unhappy, and insecure. This behavior tends to increase the guilt feelings of the parents, and the overprotective behavior continues. A vicious circle of behavioral reactions can occur, and intervention is needed to help the parents in limit-setting and dealing with their feelings of guilt and insecurity.

Mr. and Mrs. R. continually brought Janie toys, candy, and other gifts that she had requested, hoping that these items would make her happy. Instead, she became more demanding and cried frequently. The nurse began to see the parents daily and helped them express and face their feelings about Janie's illness and her behavior. At the same time, she helped them begin to gradually set limits with Janie. Janie, in turn, became less demanding and irritable.

Other parents may react to the situation with a deep sense of inadequacy. Rather than face the child's protesting behavior, they may try to avoid these reactions by leaving when a painful procedure is planned or when they can no longer cope. Recognition of their feelings of inadequacy is vitally important to avoid labeling parents as uncaring. Working with them to increase their coping abilities and supporting them during traumatic times is necessary in helping them overcome their feelings of inadequacy and helplessness.

Some parents view the child's behavior as a reflection on themselves and make it very clear to the toddler that he should "be a good boy," or that "good boys don't cry." In essence, these parents are telling children not to express their feelings; they need help in understanding the normal reactions to hospitalization.

All parents need open channels for asking questions and getting information about the illness, treatment, and anticipated responses to the treatment. Some parents communicate their concerns and questions openly, others are afraid and need help to formulate and ask their questions.

Parents also need preparation for discharge, including some information about how to deal with both the physical and emotional needs of the child at home. Anticipatory guidance related to expected behavior changes in the toddler can make the return home easier. Clinging, fear of strangers, separation anxiety, night fears, and bed-wetting are common posthospital reactions which gradually diminish if the parents are sensitive, patient, understanding, and consistent with the child.

Nurses have tended to concern themselves with the mother-child dyad and leave the father out of the picture during hospitalization. With the younger generation of parents, fathers are becoming more actively involved in the care of their children. Many toddlers have a strong relationship with their fathers, and he should be encouraged to visit and be helped in his support of the child and mother. The father may have greater difficulty in defining his role with the sick toddler and therefore may need more assistance and guidance in caring for and helping the child.

Fathers frequently can visit only after work in the evening. Since the toddler may be tired and irritable, the father may need help in understanding the need for his presence and attention when the child's behavior appears to say the opposite.

In one-parent families others may be important in helping the toddler and his parent. Whether these be grandmother, grandfather, aunt, friend, or others, their capabilities and limitations in helping the child cope must be recognized.

SPECIAL PROBLEMS OF INTERVENTION
Surgery

Preparation of the toddler for surgery can best be done by his parents with the help of the nurses. Therefore, it is important to find out what the parents know about the planned procedure, how much they have prepared the child so far for the hospitalization, and if and how they plan to prepare him for surgery.

The authors have noted a variety of parental responses to these questions. Some parents have a good understanding of the procedure and have sensitively prepared their child. Some parents feel that preparation of the child should be done but feel uncertain about how to proceed. A few parents will strenuously object to telling the child anything because they are afraid to frighten him.

In preparing toddlers for any procedure, there is a fine line between over- and underpreparation. A toddler's capacity to understand may be far greater than his capacity to verbalize. His interpretations are literal; words that are used must have meaning to him. To individualize the approach, consideration should be given to the child's age, level of maturity, anxiety level, past experiences, relation to parents, and the surgery planned.

With the young, immature toddler, very little preparation can be done. The presence of his parents, when possible, and of a nurse whom he knows and trusts is his biggest support. The older mature toddler may need to have a *very simple basic* explanation about the operation and about his postoperative status. "The doctor is going to fix your heart so you won't get so tired when you play. After the operation, you will be in this special room in a special little house (tent). Your mommy and daddy will be close by and come to see you very often."

The most traumatic aspect of surgery for the toddler is separation from his parents. Emphasis needs to be placed on where his parents will be waiting and when he will see them again. It is ideal if a nurse whom he trusts can go to the operating room with the child and be in the recovery room when he awakes. Favorite pillows, blankets, or toys should also go with him to help maintain contact with the familiar and secure.

Postoperatively, the nurse may need to help the child understand about the various treatment measures, restraints, tubes, or other equipment. Again, a very simple explanation in a calm, reassuring manner is sufficient.

Most of the toddler's "pain" during the postoperative period is caused by psychologic stress. Separation from parents, lack of physical contact with parents (being held and cuddled), and imposed immobility are all very painful experiences to the toddler. Restriction of fluids can also be difficult for him, since it is hard for him to understand why thirst cannot be immediately alleviated with a drink. Physical pain is minimized if the toddler has the needed psychologic support.

The parent is again the major source of comfort and support to the toddler during the postoperative period. To provide this support, the parents must know what they can do to provide comfort and assistance in recovery. They need to know whether the toddler can be held, what he can drink or eat, how they can help with ambulation, and who will help them if they need assistance.

The Child with a Long-Term Disease

Congenital defects, hereditary disease, and chronic terminal illness present some unique needs for the toddler and his parents.

Parents of a toddler who has just been diagnosed as having a long-term chronic disease may be expected to have an intensified reaction to their child's illness. They need a constant person who can help them over a long period of time as they adjust to the diagnosis and progressing change in their child. They need to learn as much as possible about the disease, cause, and treatment measures. They will also need help in gaining insight about the child's possible reaction to the illness and how they can best help him cope with it adequately.

Parents who react to the diagnosis with intense feelings of guilt, anxiety, and insecurity may excessively protect their child. The overprotection of the child tends to make him feel insecure, frustrated, and manipulative. Unless someone intervenes and helps the parents discuss their feelings and helps them in limit-setting, a vicious circle of behavior reactions can occur, as discussed earlier. The child's manipulation, anger, and insecurity lead the parents to feel more guilty and insecure, which intensifies their overprotective behavior and thus compounds the problem. Consistency on the part of the parents with a toddler who has chronic disease is very important from the start.

The child with any type of long-term illness is greatly affected by his parents' view of his illness and their feelings about him. The toddler's self-concept and self-image are very closely related to his parents' attitudes, reactions, and feelings toward him. Some parents may need help in resolving their grief reaction, in realistically accepting the child and his illness, and in identifying with their child's individual personality and uniqueness.

Although the child with a congenital defect or long-term disease may have experienced many hospitalizations, traumatic and painful procedures, and separations, he should not be expected to adjust more quickly than another toddler. Some parents and nurses feel that he should be "used to" the hospital and should thus be the "ideal, good patient." If the past experiences have been positive and supportive, a few older toddlers may feel trusting and at ease. Most of the time, however, these past experiences serve only to compound the normal anxiety and fears experienced by the hospitalized toddler. Separation anxiety, body integrity fears, regression, and dependency may all be problems for these children. It is very important that they experience a consistent trusting relation with nursing personnel; ideally these relations are consistent from hospitalization to hospitalization. If the nurses can also see the child during his intervening visits to the outpatient department, trust will be more firmly established.

The parents of a hospitalized toddler with a congenital defect or hereditary disease may also have some unique needs. If the child has had many hospitalizations in the past, his parents may have some idea of what to expect during the hospitalization, and some parents may be less anxious and more relaxed. Other parents, however, may be even more anxious, especially if the past hospitalizations were long and difficult. They may be personally exhausted, very tired of hospitals, and financially drained.

For some parents, the toddler's hospitalization may mark the end of a long series of continuing illness, hospitalization, and surgery. The end of their problems seems close at hand, and hope is high. If the outcome is not as expected, these parents may have a great deal of hostility and frustration. For example, Angela was admitted for her third operative procedure for congenital hip. Her parents were told that this would be her last operation as her hip would *finally* be repaired. Before discharge, however, they were informed that another operation was necessary. Understandably they became very hostile and complained about every aspect of the hospitalization. After the parents had vented their feelings and frustrations to the nurse, they were again able to cope with the situation.

Some parents of children with birth defects or hereditary disease may be experiencing an adjustment to their toddler's new developmental level. They have concerns about how his developing maturity will be affected by his illness. Anxieties may revolve around such areas as development of mobility in a child with a motor handicap, development of speech in a child with a cleft palate or hearing loss, development of self-image of a child with a visible difference such as phocomelia, cognitive development in a child with mental retardation, and social acceptance of a child who is experiencing difficulty in toilet training because of a neurogenic bladder. Some of these conflicts may be verbalized during hospitalization. Nurses can assist parents in appraising problems realistically and in finding various approaches to helping their child achieve his greatest potential in development. For example, Jimmy, age 2½ years, was born with kidney problems and phocomelia of the left arm. He was beginning to go out to play with children in the neighborhood and with friends of his 5-year-old sister. His mother was concerned about how to answer other children's questions with respect to his arm. The nurse helped her verbalize her concerns, explore the way the children and Jimmy might be viewing the situation, and discuss the positive coping mechanisms already demonstrated by Jimmy and his sister. After this discussion, Mrs. J. felt more confident about her ability to answer questions as they came.

Illness and hospitalization can create many threats and stresses for the toddler. When consideration is given to the toddler's developmental level and the strengths and limitations of his family, nursing intervention is a critical factor in reducing the trauma produced by illness and hospitalization.

BIBLIOGRAPHY

Blake, F.: "Nursing Intervention To Reduce Suffering from Separation Anxiety," *Conference on Maternal and Child Nursing*, Columbus, Ohio, Ross Laboratories, 1965.
———, Wright, F., and Waechter, E. H.: *Nursing Care of Children*, J. B. Lippincott Company, Philadelphia, 1970.
Erickson, F.: "Therapeutic Relationship of the Nurse to the Parents of a Sick Child," *Conference on Maternal and Child Nursing*, Columbus, Ohio, Ross Laboratories, 1965.
———: "Helping the Sick Child Maintain Behavioral Control," *Nursing Clinics of North America*, 2(4):695–703, 1967.
———: "Nursing Care Based on Nursing Assessment," in B. Bergerson et al. (eds.), *Current Concepts in Clinical Nursing*, vol II, The C. V. Mosby Company, St. Louis, 1969, p. 171–177.
Fraiberg, S.: *The Magic Years*, Charles Scribner's Sons, New York, 1959.
Freiberg, Karen H.: "How Parents React when Their Child Is Hospitalized," *American Journal of Nursing*, 72(7):1270–1273, 1972.
Gyulay, J. E., and Miles, M. S.: "The Family with a Ter-minally Ill Child," in D. Hymovich and M. Barnard (eds.), *Family Health Care,* McGraw-Hill Book Company, New York, 1973.
Hines, J.: "Father—the Forgotten Man," *Nursing Forum*, 10(2):177–199, 1971.
Kunzman, Lucy: "Some Factors Influencing a Young Child's Mastery of Hospitalization," *Nursing Clinics of North America*, 7(1):13–26, 1972.
Lindheim, R., Glaser, H. H., and Coffin, C.: *Changing Hospital Environments for Children*, Harvard University Press, Cambridge, Mass., 1972.
McDermott, J. F., and Akina, E.: "Understanding and Improving the Personality Development of Children with Physical Handicaps," *Clinical Pediatrics*, 2(3):130–134, 1972.
Petrillo, M., and Sanger, S.: *Emotional Care of Hospitalized Children*, J. B. Lippincott Company, Philadelphia, 1972.
Plank, E.: *Working with Children in Hospitals*, The Press of Case Western Reserve University, Cleveland, 1962.
Riddle, Irene: "Nursing Intervention To Promote Body Image Integrity in Children," *Nursing Clinics of North America*, 7(4):651–661, 1972.
Robertson, J.: *Young Children in Hospital*, Tavistock Publications, 1958.
Waechter, E.: "Developmental Correlates of Physical Disability," *Nursing Forum*, 9(1):90–108, 1970.
Wolff, S.: *Children under Stress*, The Penguin Press, London, 1969.
Yancy, W. S.: "Approaches to Emotional Management of the Child with a Chronic Illness," *Clinical Pediatrics*, 11(2):64–67, 1972.

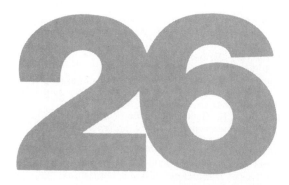

26

EFFECTS OF ILLNESS ON THE PRESCHOOLER

EILEEN GALLAGHER NAHIGIAN

The Child as an Individual within the Family

Now more than at any time previously the child must be recognized as an individual within his family constellation, whatever the nature of his family. This fact requires no memorization by anyone regularly exposed to the preschool child! His presence and needs are communicated actively and boisterously. What must be learned by the professional is the "why" for the preschooler's behavior and "how" the rest of the world might sensibly respond to this erupting new person. The "why" and the "how" bear significant import for the family or professional who further seek to understand the way a child of this age reacts to illness, hospitalization, and intrusive procedures.

Historical Importance of the Child and Family

Observation and study readily reveal that the preschooler's reaction to these experiences, as well as the nurse's correlated care, are very much a function of the child's and family's developmental history. Various assumptions *might* be made effectively, but if a nurse presumes to care for a "textbook" preschooler exclusively, or for any child independent of his family, sad realizations of failure will be encountered. The nurse intercepts and interacts with a given family, for purpose of aid, at one or several needful points along their life continuum. Equally important, the family encounters the *nurse* at a particular moment in its own life experiences—it may be legitimately expected that the character of any ensuing mutual activity will be partially governed by incidental circumstances of each one's life. Acknowledgment of this reality by nurses will substantially contribute to the therapeutic value of their interactions with families.

To appreciate the impact of the preceding statement, briefly ponder what constitutes family life from its inception through the child's third birthday anniversary. As a simple example, consider a family of young parents with their first child; more complex is the situation of a couple in their forties with their eighth child. This historical frame of reference admits a mutual as well as a personal history for each family member, simultaneously recognizing that each new experience will have modified their various perspectives in life.

Effecting this historical/developmental approach in patient care requires a working knowledge of developmental theory, of the child's and family's own development, and of their current need. It further necessitates not only awareness of their education and occupation, but also a familiarity with coping behavior established in response to prior trauma, stress, or crisis. In assessing their patients without such a broad data base, nurses invite failure because they inject none of the person into the assessment and care plan.

Coping

Because so much of a person's response to life is influenced by his ability to cope, and because the preschooler has achieved a level of development which demands a certain degree of self-control, it is appropriate to review here related concepts of coping behavior. The importance of coping resides in its empowering a person to emerge from difficulty unabashed and renewed in self-confidence. Despite attempts to shield people from adversity, neither child nor adult can realistically be protected from every potential stress, nor does it seem desirable to avoid all such experiences. It is preferable, then, to encourage growth by mastery over stressful events.

In considering the preschooler's coping, one should concern oneself with this phenomenon in both the child and his parents. For the child, adult cognizance of limitations on his ability to cope, as well as of his need to cope, is imperative. According to Murphy[1] there are at least four capacities operable in a child faced with stress which, either alone or in combination, may promote a favorable resolution. Knowing this, the wise nurse will elicit relevant information from the earliest observations and interviews with the family.

1   If a child should experience initial frustration in a situation, he might achieve satisfaction from substitute gratifications or sublimated activities. This facility is an expression of the child's warmth and sincerity toward his object world.

2   Some children skillfully mobilize resources toward an alternative route to satisfaction. They possess a fortunate resilience when difficulty threatens, which is fostered by a positive response to all life holds for them. Such a child displays a sense of self-pride and courage to face reality.

3   A child's constructive and flexible implementation of a variety of coping devices and defenses will strengthen his potential to withstand stress. Escaping excessive stimulation or temporarily denying desires may preclude scars otherwise suffered from anxiety-producing situations.

4   While regression has often been considered in negative terms, it is supported in Murphy's theory as a positive measure when employed for a specific and limited purpose. Properly understood, regression permits the child a brief retreat to a less mature period. Protected from the rigid expectations of his oedipal personality, he can then accept, for example, a kind of care more appropriate to a younger child. Recuperation may thus be fostered, since his vulnerability is abated. *adults, too.*

Overall effectiveness of any child's coping attempts is further determined, as earlier suggested, by parental response to his behavior. How do his parents acknowledge his coping maneuvers? Are they able, for example, to accept temporary regression? Are they secure enough to permit their child's utilization of any of the previously mentioned attempts toward a positive resolution of stress; or, contrariwise, do they demand continued "maturity" and attention to reality?

One might better ask, primarily, how the parents themselves cope with problems. What has been the nature of previous events requiring *their* coping? How have they surfaced from stress? How much support need the professional interject for them?

Influence of Nurse on Reaction to Illness

To complete the circle of interrelationships it is necessary to admit that nurses must also cope. Are they sufficiently self-aware to be supportive of, and unthreatened by, the family groups who need them? Can they remove themselves from the immediate scene to assess needs realistically and to arrive at a workable and flexible plan of care, a plan to favorably modify the patients' potential reactions to illness and its accompaniments? This chapter will presuppose a mature nurse, but it would be negligent to ignore the many instances when nurses, encumbered by their own unresolved experiences, have aggravated an already trying situation for a preschooler and his family.

The theory presented in this chapter can come alive in the nurse/client contact only if all features of it are correlated and adapted to specific cases. The preschooler's developmental characteristics strongly determine his reaction to illness, hospitalization, and intrusions. The essence of the present chapter lies in implementation of theory in order to modify the probable reactions discussed. Excerpts from actual contacts are included to substantiate this approach which, it is hoped, will increase the effectiveness of nursing care administered to preschoolers and their families.

REACTION TO ILLNESS, HOSPITALIZATION, AND INTRUSIVE PROCEDURES
Probable Reactions

The ill or hospitalized preschooler qualifies as candidate for innumerable fears and anxieties because of the major characteristics of his struggle toward maturity. The preschooler requires security and stability of his environment, as well as opportunity to understand his environment. Having only recently achieved control over some body functions, he would favor conditions suitable to maintaining the status quo. Protective of his body intactness, he hesitates and worries over imagined or real physical threats.

Threat, in the sense of stress, may occur when any balance in the child's world is challenged by illness, hospitalization, and/or concomitant care and treatments. Such stress experienced by hospitalized children has been dramatically depicted by Erickson[2] via a variety of preoccupations evidenced by children subjected to professional alleviation of their ills. The nurse's capability of producing similar suffering if he is insensitive to the child should be experienced with awe.

Fear of Unfamiliar Environment Among the preschooler's probable reactions are a host of fears. If one were to reflect on his initial adult impressions of a hospital, perhaps a beginning appreciation of the child's plight could be attained. A nurse might also recall a sense of confusion or disorientation temporarily felt in a strange institution after having already achieved some sophistication about hospitals! Sensitivity to such impressions might better prepare the nurse to identify and respond to the child's fears regarding unfamiliar people, places, paraphernalia, and procedures.

People are important to preschoolers, who tend to categorize them in terms of "mother," "father," "boy," or "girl." Some of this interest in roles, especially in parental roles, is evidenced when the child questions the nurse: "Are you a mommy?" Associated misconceptions are frequently demonstrated in conversation or play concerning doctor and nurse as marital partners. Perhaps the child is trying to locate himself in this new "family" to which he has gained entry. He is unlikely to differentiate readily the various professionals and their associates or the nonprofessional hospital personnel to whom he will be exposed. Further misunderstandings are apt to exist as to who can and cannot fulfill his various needs. (After all, at home, Mommy can do everything!) Depending upon their progress through the oedipal or Electra situation, boys may experience difficulties with male personnel, girls with female personnel.

Significant home routines are modified or ignored without adequate explanation to the child. Which child is accustomed to having meals served in bed on a bulky tray? What happens to bedtime rituals—in fact, who is the "Mommy" who puts the youngster to bed? Toileting continues as an obstacle: Where is the toilet? By what name is it known? How does one communicate his need to defecate or urinate? (A listing of the terms to identify these functions would prove a tremendous aid to novice personnel.) Why all the concern over "if" and "when"? Why must a child who has recently achieved independent toileting be observed for the integrity of his urinary stream? Why must he use a small plastic cup, bedpan, or urinal and allow a strange nurse to "save" his stool and urine? It is insufficient that nurses know all the answers; they must anticipate these unverbalized and verbalized queries, and be prepared with legitimate answers *before* anxiety mounts.

Places! There are bedrooms and treatment rooms, medicine rooms and linen closets, nurses' stations and pantries, playrooms and radiology labs, operating rooms and elevators, eye clinics and ear clinics, cast rooms and who-knows-what-else-rooms! While it is true that each room might serve a special and beneficial purpose, the preschooler, nevertheless, experiences some consternation at wondering to which room he will be transported next, and for what reason. These rooms advertise an array of policies governing their use: off limits certain hours, no parents allowed, patients only, danger/keep out (e.g., cobalt or surgical suite). Some are wide-open spaces and brightly lit; others are crowded and dim. More than one child has drawn the hospital as a "jail" with cells in which the patient occupies a restricted corner of the drawing paper.

We also use many frightening objects in the hospital: "shots" that "don't hurt"; tubes that drain bladders, fill stomachs, give oxygen; restraints that immobilize; wheelchairs and carriers that insist on movement, sometimes with squeaky and wobbly wheels to magnify the monstrosity; masks that "put you to sleep"; masks that "don't put you to sleep"; beds with side rails that are not cribs; cribs for "babies"; signal bells or lights "if you need the nurse, but . . ."; stethoscopes to "take" heart beats; something else to "take" blood pressure; enemas; x-ray cameras; tilting tables; urine drainage bags. These are all used threateningly without intended threat, but if the nurse neglects some explanation of them for the child, he deserves, along with the object, to be feared. Who wants to be feared by a youngster?

Also active are the preschooler's auditory and olfactory senses. Sometimes each nurse should close himself in a hospital room for several hours, allowing odors and sounds to filter in, to grasp a minimal appreciation for this experience. The child has no foreknowledge of such sounds as the elevator, a fallen bedpan, an intravenous flow rate alarm, a hungry baby, or professional staff rounds; consequently he gathers ample data for fantasy, fantasy of personal threats. Imagination can create poisonous gases from the smells of strange soaps and cleaners or medications. An immobilized 4-year-old girl, isolated in a private room, heard the clapping of postural drainage from another child's room. She asked: "What's that? Sounds like horsies comin'. Is there horsies here? Sounds like clomping!"

In short, the child might well feel victimized by hospital features whether or not they are directly intended for him. It behooves the nurse to respond accordingly.

Fear of Abandonment and Punishment Especially for the 3-year-old, the threat of separation and abandonment lurks beneath the maturing ego. Adjustment to hospitalization is partially dependent upon the child's ability to retain a mental image of his mother during her absence. Also needed is his realization that mother, with all her "bad" qualities, is also the "good" mother who loves him and wishes him no harm. This ability is achieved normally at about the transition point between toddlerhood and the preschool years.[3]

Threats of abandonment are also contingent upon a fear, wish, or need for punishment. Fantasies created by the preschooler may contain vengeful wishes for the death or maiming of parent or sibling; such evil thoughts, which are related to the oedipal situation, cause the child to expect retribution. Very sad and difficult is the child who interprets his illness or hospitalization as vindication for or by his fantasied victims. Since it is unclear to the preschooler that his fantasies are veiled from the knowledge of others, and since his developing ego (self) and superego (conscience) exert rigid controls with censure, the hospitalized preschooler may yield to any of a number of causes for an unfavorable emotional reaction to the experience.

Fears Related to Body Integrity The entire theme of body intactness, alone, generates ample fear in the preschooler, whether or not other fears exist. In fact, it contributes to some fears already mentioned. Castration, per se, a fear often linked to the oedipal phase, restricts us; preferred is Schilder's[4] broader reference to a wish for body integrity and a fear of being attacked or mutilated. The hospitalized child is provided, simultaneously, a multitude of threats for both *body* mutilation and loss of *identity*.

A sense of vulnerability evolves in the child because of his repeated subjection to various clinical equipment or "gadgets" which interfere with his ability to differentiate himself from his environment.[5] Not only "gadgets" but also surgery and *most* required treatments are seen by the child as hostile invasions, designed to damage or destroy body and being.[6,7]

One dare not assume that the child's conception of skin integrity is nearly so accurate as the adult's. The preschooler does not possess knowledge that he will not exsanguinate via an injection site; neither does he understand the process of wound healing. Rather, he knows that pierced balloons burst, and that clothes hold together only so long as stitching remains intact. Why should his skin differ? With this cognitive base, he doubts the integrity of his body boundaries when he witnesses his tracheostomy, ileal bladder, or blood oozing from a surgical wound. His general cognition is further tested when he is expected to differentiate a needle for injection from a needle for aspiration, or test tube of blood from capillary tube of blood; depending upon which aspect he "centers," he manifests varying success.

Under such circumstances how should a child respond at the hands of a "hypocrite" who mechanically tells him "hold still," "don't worry," "it won't hurt," "just a little blood"? Always before, his parents protected him from strangers; now his parents may be forced to stand idly by or to leave the room while all sorts of inhumane attacks are perpetrated in the name of healing. Surely a parent would not participate in this cruelty except as retaliation for evil wishes!

Communicated Fears Meantime the parents, too, often ignorant of the bases for their child's fears, try to disguise their own fears. For the preschooler to cope, he needs assurance from his parents' conviction that this hospitalization is right and good. Yet how often have mothers with masklike faces been heard to admonish their preschooler: "Boys don't cry! Not another word! No more crying. There's nothing to fear. Hospitals are nice places to make Johnny feel better." Then later, "Go to sleep or I'll call that nurse to give you a shot!" How does Johnny reconcile these incongruities? How does he, as a surgical patient, allow the hospital and its agents to "cut him open," and then surrender himself to these same villains for relief? What protection has he from repeated surgeries at anyone's whim?

If his mother is also afraid of the hospital, who is able to protect him? Furthermore, if his parents are afraid, why should he be brave? Parents often telegraph their nervousness to their child by their incessant and uncharacteristic doting, or by constantly seeking reassurance from the professional staff. The parental behavior is, assuredly, understandable—but to the nurse, not to the confused child. When the parents' fears are communicated to their child, a tragic cycle may ensue as is graphically depicted in the following case excerpt.

Five-year-old **Leo K.** had experienced repeated hospitalizations for evaluation of urinary incontinence. Eventual diagnostic studies revealed need for corrective surgery, and a ureteroneo-cystostomy was performed. The surgeon, known for his satisfactory relations with children, had detailed to the parents the nature of surgery and postoperative course. Preparation was continued during hospitalization by the nurse specialist.

Leo's parents were in their early thirties; Mrs. K. was an elementary school teacher; Mr. K. was a young executive; there were two siblings. Leo had apparently tolerated prior admissions during which he had seldom been left unattended by an adult relative. Superficial preparation for surgery had been given him prior to admission, and minimal instruction was continued the evening prior to surgery. Obvious anxiety in parents and child limited instruction. The nurse specialist visited Leo in the recovery room and oriented him to his various paraphernalia; the parents were also informed of his progress immediately postoperatively.

Leo's convalescence was marked by loss of emotional control and almost continual clutching at his genitals. His oedipal fantasies and fears of mutilation were nurtured by the required dressings and catheters, hematuria, bladder spasms, and his hovering parents who hardly gave him breathing space. Questions were answered for him, and everything he desired was given. Attempts were unsuccessful to alter this "concern" or to have nursing personnel occasionally relieve the parents' vigil. Leo continued to whine, holler, and grasp his penis; this behavior was exacerbated with periodic bladder spasms. Warm or cold compresses, explanations, diversions, attempted projective techniques, and medication failed to soothe him. Whatever were the K.s' initial fears, Leo's reaction

perhaps worsened them. They grew unable to set any limits, and acquiesced to their son's every wish. Finally, Mrs. K. required emergency room care, was diagnosed to have an ulcer, and was instructed to spend a week in bed beginning immediately. Mr. K. was phoned at work and requested to come to the hospital to reassure his wife and to substitute for her with Leo.

When Mr. K. arrived, he was coincidentally met by the nurse specialist. Wide-eyed, flushed, and anxious, he fumbled: "Is he gone?!" Mr. K., convinced his son was dying, had not heard the entire phone message. It had been necessary for his employer to give him a tranquilizer prescribed for himself, before driving him the 8 miles to the hospital. A circuitous route was taken to the hospital, to allow Mr. K. opportunity to regain some composure. In no condition to meet his son, he was accompanied to the nurses' lounge. The surgeon arrived and joined the nurse in summing up Leo's condition and prescribing action to hopefully curb Leo's fears and hasten his recovery.

Mr. K. was helped to recognize the fear cycle which had developed and was receptive to professional insistence that it be interrupted. He calmed sufficiently to visit his son, explain that Mommy was sick, and return to work. (By this time the maternal grandfather had arrived.)

Only gradually was the family able to leave Leo unattended for intervals, but beginning attempts to rectify the situation were noted immediately. Leo continued an uncomfortable course, but began to slowly cooperate with care. Once Mr. K. recognized and admitted his own fears, he was able to support Leo; once his fear was less apparent, his son could hope for recovery.

Most often, communicated fear is more subtle in its effect, and parental self-controls do not shatter so totally. The same potential exists in all instances, however.

Ego Defensiveness Fortunate is the preschooler who can positively employ defense mechanisms to aid his adjustment to hospitalization. Ego defenses, by somehow distorting consciousness, allow the child to sidestep some of life's disturbances. The child's ego defenses are only beginning to emerge, and prolonged need for them hinders their healthy implementation. Nevertheless, if used for limited periods and/or used in combination, they may constitute a positive adjustment. If abused, pathologic dependence may result.

Regression In the past, when a 3-to-6-year-old was observed to cuddle his blanket, suck his thumb, and return to his bottle, the signal was immediately raised in red letters "REGRESSION," and his caretakers industriously plotted to remove the blanket, glove his hand, and cast away the bottle. A dramatic statement perhaps, but such archaic care persists at times, totally ignoring the needs behind the behavior. Regression, appropriately employed, allows the growing child a brief return to a less mature and demanding period, so that need-meeting by adults can be accepted without threat. Requiring help with toileting or feeding may additionally reduce fear by eliciting close attention from protective adults. The incontinent preschooler's infantile crying may say, in effect, "It's okay to dirty my pants; I'm only a baby." In another instance, the boy who had previously been admonished that "Big boys don't do that" (a common adult response to normal masturbation in the oedipal period), may find less superego conflict if he whines during examination of his cryptorchidism.

Repression   Repression has been called the cornerstone of all other defenses because it tends to participate in their manifestations. This defense diverts cathexis (the investment of psychic energy) from the undesirable and unpleasant present, thus inhibiting affect. Repressed content is then manifest only symbolically via the absence of normal characteristic behavior.[8] Other reactions might also be observed as a consequence of the child's *total* energy reserve being required to *maintain* repression of threatening material. If the child should be described as "not curious about the treatment," he is to undergo, one should suspect repression.

Denial and Withdrawal   Two mechanisms likely to accompany repression are denial and withdrawal, which allow the child to ignore interruptions and disavow any thought or feeling that would be painful to experience. When a preschooler *totally* absorbs himself in play, television, or sleep, or when he denies pain from an obviously uncomfortable procedure, his passivity may represent a function of these two ego defenses. (Passivity may also result in response to imposed loss of former self-controls.)

Displacement and Sublimation   Additional defenses may be operative, two of which have been considered by some to be healthier than those already mentioned. Displacement and sublimation alter the aim of impulses so that they find expression in other situations. These mechanisms may be active in the symbolic artwork or play of hospitalized youngsters,

permitting emotions such as anger to be redirected via "creativity."

Projection   If unable to tolerate objectionable elements in his personality, the preschooler may "project" these to others in his environment. Thus, the angry child uses strong language to describe a "witch nurse" or "monster doctor," or he kicks and claws at his mother while screaming "You're awful! You, you, I...*you hate me!*" In this way, he succeeds in accusing the environment of anger toward him. This defense can particularly upset parents and personnel when the hospitalization objectively produces discomfort for the child as an essential part of diagnosis and care (e.g., bone marrow aspirations or chemotherapy for leukemia).

Summary about Defenses   Whichever defenses are used, Anna Freud[9] cautions that distinguishing them on a broad index is better than on the basis of pathologic versus healthy. Defenses should be weighed according to age adequateness, balance among a variety of mechanisms, intensity of usage, and reversibility (the ability to cease defensive behavior once the real danger ceases).

Fantasy   Fantasy, sometimes called a waking dream, may be a part of ego defenses or it may be a phenomenon in itself. Deriving from both objective and subjective experiences, it is a mental activity the value of which centers on reality-adaptation.[10] Hospitalized preschoolers are exposed to almost infinite occasions requiring ready adaptation. It is conceivable that fantasy assists their adaptation via brief excursions into a nonthreatening nonreality to achieve resolution of real threats.

Adults continue to question whether fantasy should be fostered, ignored, or forbidden. How often are heard the warnings: "Stop daydreaming!" "An idle mind is the devil's workshop!" Regardless, fantasy life eludes control from others. As with ego defenses, of course, perverted use of fantasy would be an undesirable aberration; however, the ego support and growth afforded by fantasy recommends it. One must remember that fantasy activity, which determines the seriousness of illness and hospitalization in the child's mind, will occur quite naturally. The adult needs to acknowledge this fact in order to be prepared to help the child cope with his interpretations of what is happening to him.

Fantasy which occurs totally within the child's mind is obviously not available for adult interpretation. Quite frequently, especially if equipment is accessible, the child's activities will manifest his fantasies. In such instances, it is possible to correlate evident fantasy material with other observations to build a data base for planning care.

One 4-year-old girl in traction, on the eighth day of her hospitalization, continued to work through her fears of abandonment and displacement within her family. She had been playing with dolls representative of a family, a nurse, and a doctor. She had already placed most of the dolls in specified spots on her overbed tray. Doing so required frequent shifting of her own position and was accompanied by deep sighing. Finally she reached for the baby doll (who, it was thought, represented herself) and attempted to locate it satisfactorily. She stood the baby doll first to the left near the "mother," then to the right near the "doctor," then between the "doctor" and the "father," then on the opposite side of the "father," finally back near the "mother." When questioned, she could not explain why the baby doll was moving all around. Nevertheless, prior and subsequent observations supported belief that she was working through her displacement from home to hospital and her hoped-for eventual return home.

Oedipal fantasies may also be revealed. Worry that "some boy might climb in my bed" or questions such as "Why are babies here? Are they here for . . . like . . . for when people get married?" hint strongly of latent concerns. Alone, such childhood revelations mean little. In context of the child's history, nature, and duration of hospitalization, they give the alert professional a series of insights into the patient's difficulties with hospital adjustment and into apt responses toward easing that adjustment.

Aggression   For whatever interpretation one might prefer to assign to aggression—whether to consider it destructive, constructive, or neutral in intent—support is available in psychoanalytic literature. Let it suffice here to consider an aggressive act as any behavior which is either threatened or performed against the person of another.

Activity provides a significant outlet for aggressive tendencies. Recall the normal activity of a preschooler as depicted in Chapter 12. How much more intrusive would the child have been in a less formal and regulated environment! Consider how much of this activity would be curtailed if the child were hospitalized, how much more if confined to bed. What supposed responses should be expected from him in such instances? Since activity constitutes the preschooler's most effective natural protection

against threat, intense aggression may be manifest when confinement and immobilization are necessitated. Verbal insults, attacks displaced onto toys, and biting are among his repertoire of aggressive responses displayed especially when his mobility is restricted.

Many potentials for generating behavior are inherent in hospitalization, the most obvious of which may be intrusive procedures which are directly related to hostile attack from the hospital's agents. Another ever-present threat is deprivation, which the child senses as aggression.[11] Actual or potential separation from parents, fasting required for certain diagnostic and therapeutic procedures, and loss of normal routines and developmental opportunities are a few of the deprivations experienced during hospitalization. It has been shown that deprivation may result in inadequate satisfaction of the child's constructive drives which then become disorganized into hostile or destructive aggression.[12]

Often aggression may be energetically controlled or hidden behind certain ego defenses.[13] However, external release is imperative if it is not to be excessively dammed up and internalized.[14] Any pediatric nurse will attest to the frequent external release via kicks, bites, hair-pulling, and punches. Less physical expression takes the form of shouting, screaming, and name-calling; sometimes it is still more subtle as in voiced disapproval of how the nurse or parent has met his need. Unsocial though it may seem, all this behavior is deserved and desirable when viewed from the child's perspective.

Difficulties Related to Mutilation and Body Image
This topic differs somewhat from the discussion earlier in this chapter of "Fears Related to Body Integrity," although it is based on the same considerations. Essentially, the question of this present adjustment problem is "How does the preschooler assimilate body alterations into his body image?" The developing personality is ill-prepared for such an assignment, especially should the libidinal, physiologic, and sociologic spheres of this body image elaboration be disregarded. The nurse might expect too ready an adjustment to experiences of anesthesia, surgery, sutures, scars, bleeding, dressings, restricted mobility, intrusive equipment, and ministrations by strangers if the influence of any of or all these experiences on one's image of oneself is ignored.

Schilder[15] has described body image according to three spheres of life. With the preschooler's personality and cognitive characteristics in mind, Schilder's theory is reviewed here in relation to hospital experiences which might compromise the accuracy of a child's body image.

On the *physiologic* level, body image is influenced by pain, limb motility, definition of body boundaries, and other experiences of an optic, tactile, or kinesthetic nature. Optic messages from a massive bandage might cause the child to sense his bandaged part as much larger than normal. Immobility adds another insult since increasing information about the body depends upon data provided only by movement. Interference with the child's sense of equilibrium, effected by anesthesia or narcotics, is another concern. A 4-year-old girl had been confined to bed for 17 days in an awkward position with skeletal traction to her right arm. Having been medicated with meperidine hydrochloride preparatory to manipulation of her fracture, she later related: "Feels like my eyes are pulling out!" "Feels like I'm standing upside down." Her physiologic reference had been grossly disturbed as she tried to maintain contact with her body.

Positive or negative interests invested in the child's body by others will influence his body image, according to the *libidinal* sphere, second in Schilder's list. The child's intuitive thinking creates a special challenge to nursing personnel in this regard, since it is important to also remain mindful of the preschooler's cognitive egocentricity and centering. Several principles related to the libidinal sphere find particular applicability in this context:

1   The relative value of body parts is partially governed by emotional influences.
2   One part of the body may symbolize another part.
3   The actions and attitudes of others influence a person's body image elaboration.
4   A person modifies his interest in his body according to interests he observes others to have in their bodies.
5   A person loses interest in his body and in the outside world when he experiences depersonalization, a state in which he feels totally changed from his previous self.

The caretaker who evidences repulsion at a child's ileal bladder, or avoids him for any reason, may aggravate his body image distortion. Or when the body is repeatedly intruded upon by insulin injections, the preschooler might interpret the treatment as punishment for his fantasies or transgressions of parental orders.

Depersonalization constitutes a menace especially for children who require frequent observation or manipulation of all or part of their bodies, as though they have become objects in exchange for personalities. Consider the burn-scarred child who, first of all, must face himself as *objectively* changed. Throughout his therapy program he is wrapped, un-

wrapped, prodded, poked, bathed, rubbed, grafted, immobilized, the primary focus always being "the burn" or "the graft." Comparable is the experience of a child who has had an ileal bladder created: interest focuses on "the stoma," "the bag," and "no more wet diapers." Where is the person and his personality?

That the interest others have in their bodies will influence the child's interest in his body is particularly relevant for the preschooler who is in the stage of "identifying." In imitation of her nurse or roommate the preschooler might allow her hair to be combed, wear a "nurse's cap," or change to clean pajamas. On the other hand, this same influence might operate detrimentally. While children admitted to wards might reap many benefits from peer relation, the possibility also exists that they will be threatened by abnormalities or treatments observed.

The *sociologic* sphere, third in Schilder's list, equally relevant to this discussion, is elaborated later in this chapter when modification of the child's reactions to hospitalization, illness, and intrusions is considered.

The preschooler, struggling with his identification process and body image organization, reacts to any bodily defect, temporary or permanent. Because his "stigma" is either evident and known by, or readily visible to, others,[16] his behavior often suggests a preoccupation with catheters, surgical wound, nasogastric tube, diarrhea, or extra toe. To the intrusive-minded child any of these may portend what Goffman[17] has termed a naked exposure to, and invasion of privacy by, nonstigmatized persons. In response, some children try to hide their defects; others make a great display of them.

Probable Reactions to Acute and Chronic Illness

It is virtually impossible to view reactions toward illness separately from those toward hospitalization and intrusions since they are often seen in combination, and since there are so many similarities. Although hospitalization entails all varieties of reactions, illness and intrusions can and regularly do occur outside the hospital. For this reason, acute and chronic illnesses are discussed here without reference to hospitalization.

Acute Illness   Acute illness strikes the child especially harshly because of its suddenness. Even the adult may spend days of irritability, nausea, or headache without realizing he has been caught in the vise of illness. Perhaps the preschooler's first reaction, then, will be one of confusion and fright at the internal turmoil which menaces his body integrity. Possibly anxiety will have developed even before his parents recognize he is sick.

Since his cognition has not yet conquered the process of change, he has difficulty understanding how and why he became ill. At some time during and following the illness he will grapple with this problem of explaining his sickness. Mothers of preschoolers often tell how months later their children spontaneously ask, "Remember last day when I was sick? Why did that doctor come? Why did you give me that awful 'mehacin'?"

The nurse's first premise with an ill child should be that the child's interpretation of his condition in no way correlates to the adult's. All that has already been said about the preschooler's development, for example, his inability to synthesize and analyze, and his limited experiential history, attests to his inability to accept illness without some emotional reaction.

Some of the possible reactions have been studied by Anna Freud[18] as a means of determining the child's inner mental state. Meek submission, which many adults consider "good" behavior, may constitute a manifestation of regression whereby the child takes pleasure in passivity. Sometimes, too, a mother is heard to comment that her young daughter indignantly wanted to care for herself while sick; such a reaction might portend a feeling of dissatisfaction at having been poorly mothered.

Fears, to which the preschooler is especially subject, may approach obsession if he becomes overwhelmed by a combination of fantasies, vulnerable emotions, and disease symptoms.[19] Finally, any reaction is dependent on cumulative factors, including the child's basic personality and parental reaction to the illness.

Chronic Illness Of considerable interest in the child's reaction to chronic illness is a sense of loss which may be communicated to him from parental grief and mourning process. Grief and mourning, in relation to chronic illness, are not limited to the possibility of death since they have been recognized in response to such experiences as body mutilation and the birth of a baby with a congenital defect. Yet, death fears *are* a real component of chronic illness, and the wise nurse remains sensitive to overt and covert evidence of them. Some of the manifestations of death fears include the following: Parents who spend as little or as much time as possible with their child, children who withdraw from peer contact, repeated insistence that "I'm never going to get well!," or refusal to entertain any discussions of future plans. Verbalizations may emphasize the past

tense, as in statements such as "Ralph always rode his bike on Sunday," even though Ralph would still ride his bike if allowed by his parents.

The preschooler's death fears are related to his fantasy life and superego development, along with body integrity concerns. Especially for the youngster who cannot yet conceive of permanent lifelessness, his fears center on experience of separation. Only ignorance can direct the nurse to assume no such fears among preschoolers, when communication media continually intrude their experiences with sounds of death and threats of death, whether by news of war or of the latest ban on some food additive. Pets and plants also provide data about death, although pets are often replaced and plants return alive with each spring. In short, to adequately cope with this aspect of the chronically ill child's needs, one needs to be aware of his prior experiences about death.

In chronic illness, possibly more than in any previously mentioned circumstance, parental reaction and coping determines the preschooler's reaction. Adequate resolution of the identification process requires healthy parent/child interchanges which permit a positive outcome of the oedipal situation. Both of these needs may suffer concurrently, or they may flourish satisfactorily.

On the basis of a diagnosis of a chronic disease or handicap, a child might be totally rejected by a parent. Denial of the diagnosis or manifest insecurities regarding its ramifications may usurp any potential for normal parent/child interaction. Patterns of care have repeatedly resulted in which either the child's development is stifled, or he is allowed to manipulate his parents. When this happens, the preschooler may experience either restraint at an earlier developmental period, or a sense of instability and insecurity under threat of losing control over his parents.

Another variation of reactions is an exaggerated mother/child symbiosis, ignoring the husband/father. A vicious circle of resentment, envy, and aggressiveness may then undermine the family group, eventuating in its actual or effectual dissolution. The preschooler, so needful of normal family relations to develop his identity and sense of self-worth, especially suffers in such an instance.

MODIFYING REACTIONS VIA IMPLEMENTATION OF DEVELOPMENT THEORY
General Needs

Awareness of Environment It seems such a little thing, yet so much is achieved by an orientation tour to specific areas of the hospital environment. Considering the preschooler's attention span, "centering," and anxiety aroused by the experience, wisdom suggests orienting initially and again as opportunities arise. Especially for the oedipal child, orientation may help reduce night terrors and fears of going to bed.

The preschooler may identify with his environment through "helping" his caretakers. This can be accomplished in such activities as cooperating in bed-making, assisting the ward clerk assemble new charts, or showing a new patient to the playroom. One 5-year-old boy enjoyed standing at the doorway and singing while the nurse soothed a crying baby. He was thereby not constrained to fantasy why the infant cried, and was allowed to overpower his environment to relieve stress. Others use doll play toward the same end.

Ongoing instruction regarding his experience is essential to ease adjustment. As will be seen later in the chapter, these explanations must be kept simple and comprehensible at the child's level. Similar guidance for the parents is also necessary, to extend their own adjustment and their ability to continue meaningful parental support of their child. It is painful to witness frightened and dubious parents attempting to put their child at ease. "Ongoing" instruction, meaning "repetitive" in this context, might be the single most difficult of the nurse's tasks, also the single most helpful. Often a nurse might prefer to reprimand an inquiring parent, stating that he has discussed the entire topic previously and has no more to tell the parent. Wisdom and sensitive nursing care preclude such a response to vulnerable people. This does not, however, rule out required limit-setting in discussion, which is at times indicated to help the parent gain control and cope more positively.

Maintenance of Former Object Relationships Security within the family remains a primary need for the preschooler, whether sick at home or in the hospital. Especially for the young preschooler, separation threatens this security. Since the subphase for development of object constancy as described by Mahler[20] may or may not have been achieved yet, it is likely that the youngster cannot retain the internal image of his mother for prolonged periods. Therefore, while his mother may not need to remain constantly at her preschooler's side, she hopefully is readily available to him. In the instance of hospitalization, this need is intensified because of inherent pressure toward regression. Normal object relations should also entail continuation of security via limit-setting and discipline. Parents need help, usually, to

understand that excessive permissiveness granted the "poor sick child" will weaken his sense of security.

Sibling relations and, to an extent, peer relations suffer when illness and/or hospitalization interrupt the child's normal life. Whether by a psychosocial or by a physical separation, normal patterns of interaction are modified and/or temporarily discontinued. Explanations of the separation must be meaningful for each of the people involved. For Johnny to survive his temporary indisposition satisfactorily, his siblings and playmates should understand his irritability and/or absence from home. Johnny needs to know that his playmates continue their normal life and that he will rejoin them when he becomes well. This assurance is especially important if the child's prior experience would cause him to believe otherwise, for example, if his grandfather had recently died while hospitalized.

Maintenance of former relations may be facilitated by interjecting siblings' names into conversation, or by sending messages and drawings home and to the hospital from each other. Direct use of the telephone may also prove valuable. True, the nurse might have a crying child to manage following the phone call, but the crying will be healthier than that caused by a sense of abandonment. Occasionally visits between well and sick children are indicated and arrangements for these should be possible. Of course, it is presupposed that parent contact can be maintained as constantly as desired by the family, and that parents may participate in hospital care of their children if they wish.

Continuation of Growth and Development A rather gloomy outline of possible reactions has been presented, but let it be understood that some children continue positive growth and development throughout their experience. This is certainly to be encouraged so long as it does not exert additional stress on the child. When he can be permitted fairly normal motility and when his intrusive questioning and behavior is respected, the preschooler can learn a tremendous amount about himself, his hospital environment, and new relations, even at his relatively immature level of comprehension. His ability to tolerate separation can be extended, and his coping devices enhanced. Careful planning of an activity program can further broaden his horizons and mollify his adjustment.

Play Activity
Normal Play Preschoolers play. Ill or hospitalized preschoolers can also play; better yet, opportunity can be provided for free and planned activity of an

appropriate nature. Children's minds can almost atrophy in some hospitals where they are left completely to their own devices except for medical/nursing care and protection from bodily injury! A listing of the kinds of diversion enjoyed by this age-group of children is included here more as a challenge than as a suggestion. Can these activities be incorporated into *your* care of the sick child? *Three years*: cooperative play, spontaneous play in groups for short periods, storytelling (especially about own infancy), "dress-up," play "house," coloring, simple books, scissors and paper, "pouring fluids," tricycles, fire engines. *Four years:* longer group activities, "dramatic" play, drawing, stories, "helping" adults, pounding nails, expressive play (e.g., making clothespin dolls, making paper chains, stuffing animals, "sewing" pictures). *Five years:* being read to, simple records, simple letter and number games, scrapbooks and other creative activities as at age 4, costumes, cars and trucks, matching pictures and forms, organized simple group play, rhythmic activities, gross motor activity, opportunity to use substances such as mud, stones, and snow.

Therapeutic Play   Normal play can be employed as therapeutic techniques which allow the child to express his concerns in a nonthreatening manner to an observing adult who then utilizes the data in planning more effective care for the child. Story telling and story completion techniques, when the child cooperates, may help to reveal his internal fears. Drawing has been discussed frequently in the literature regarding its usefulness in depicting body image concerns, for example, as evidenced by absence, exaggeration, or diminution of a body part in a drawing of a man.

Whether play is implemented on a more formal basis as in the play interview[21], or as free play created by the child, it provides a real source of data experienced *and* fantasied by the child.[22,23] This mechanism assists the child in at least three unconscious objectives: (1) Working through his life's experiences to achieve some understanding, resolution, or mastery of them; (2) assuming the role of others in his environment (perhaps the aggressive nurse or doctor!), as if to gain control; (3) notifying the sympathetic adult observer of his innermost concerns and needs.

Implementation of This Theory

Child/Family's Relevant History Myelomeningocele is a congenital defect accompanied by a host of physical problems and potential psychosocial problems to further complicate a child's life. For this reason, and because preschoolers have often been hospitalized for therapy related to the primary and secondary manifestations of myelomeningocele, the care of these children poses a challenging example for implementation of the foregoing theory. Their more obvious symptomatology resides in neurologic, orthopedic, urologic, infection control, plastic revision, cognitive development, physical growth, and psychosocial areas; few additional possibilities could remain!

The prime nursing problem with these children is often to undo what has been done, or to do what has never been attempted in support of parents and child, particularly regarding their adjustment to a chronic situation. (This will have been handled from birth onward, it is hoped, but too little evidence exists to support belief in adequate early care.) Whatever the reason for admission to an acute-care hospital, most parents exhibit a need not only to sit and discuss the present hospitalization with an informed nurse, but also to relive their life with the child—a kind of grief work. Such a session is of tremendous value to parents. Additionally it provides significant information for the nursing history, especially insofar as the nurse gains a perspective on the parents' and child's coping, on their needs, and on the child's developmental history.

Five-year-old **Kenny V.** was admitted for urinary diversion via an ileal conduit. His history was one of myelomeningocele which had been surgically repaired in infancy; he had had lower leg casts and a shunt for hydrocephaly. The nurse specialist visited Kenny and Mrs. V. early on their second day, *introduced herself, and promised to return* to discuss the surgery with Mrs. V. Mrs. V. commented that she knew little of Kenny's problem and anticipated surgery. When the nurse reflected her comment, Mrs. V. immediately poured forth her story. "Nobody has ever explained all this to me. What causes it? I remember when Kenny was born I heard a cracking sound. Could that have been it? I didn't even know how big a problem he had for some time. The nurse told me he had a cut on his back and his feet were turned in. She said he would be transferred to a larger general hospital 50 miles away. I was worried. She told me not to worry, that his back would be bandaged and his feet casted and in a few months I'd never know he had any problem." She continued, hardly breathing between thoughts, to relate her horror at final discovery.

Indeed, Kenny's congenital defect remained not only obvious, but also a deterrent to his functioning.

His legs had failed to grow normally, and he required low leg braces and crutches for mobility. Fortunately he had had no complications from his shunt, and he was appropriately intelligent. Now this! He had never achieved bowel or bladder control and could not be accepted for kindergarten until his elimination problems were remedied. Besides, he had developed a threat of urinary complications. "Why? What causes all these problems? I wish someone could tell me."

The nurse *listened* and waited her turn to reply. *First of all she acknowledged that Mrs. V. was burdened.* She then told her: *"We can talk about Kenny's* problems before we discuss surgery. Right now, I want you to know that the defect did not occur at the time of Kenny's birth. It had to have happened earlier when the bone in his low back didn't close. Also, despite your probable concern that you yourself caused the defect, no one has yet discovered a precise cause. As for his other problems, they are all interrelated. *I'll give you a pamphlet with explanations and diagrams.* After you've had a chance to read it, I'll stop by for our talk." (Simple literature is usually available or the nurse can devise some.)

This kind of approach informs parents of the nurse's concern and readiness to help; it exonerates the nurse of any suspected judgmental attitude; it affords the parents an opportunity to refresh their memories and to formulate more specific questions; and it identifies the nurse and family to each other so that their discussions become humanized and personalized. Explanations such as preoperative preparation can then be achieved without having the parents' attention diverted by basic anxiety precipitated in part by ignorance.

To obtain a history, specific questions must sometimes be asked, but *open-ended interviewing* often provides more, and more meaningful, information than that elicited with a rigid interview schedule. Introducing hospitalization with a relaxed interview often succeeds in comforting the parents who realize that they have helped to prepare the nursing staff to meet their child's essential needs. More at ease, they are better able to assist their child's adjustment. Their guilt feelings acknowledged, and at least temporarily relieved, the parent/child relation is less likely to produce anxiety over oedipal wishes and death fears.

Mrs. V.'s story has been rephrased and repeated frequently by other mothers, even by those whose recorded history indicates that they had been previously instructed about the defect. It is as though each new threat demands the reexploration of painful memories.

Five-year-old **Victor W.** displayed numerous deficiencies. His mother, in her late twenties, reaped verbal punishment from a pediatric intern who had made inaccurate assumptions and presumptions on the basis of physical examination alone. Victor truly was pathetic on admission: he had two enormous ischial decubiti, contractures holding him in a frog-leg position, absence of bowel and bladder control, poorly developed lower extremities with paresthesia, uncoordinated fine motor ability of the upper extremities, nystagmus, a temperamental atrioventricular shunt, scarring from previous closure of his myelomeningocele sac, immature communication patterns, and underdeveloped intelligence.

Having been consulted about how the nursing staff might proceed with this "bad" mother, the nurse specialist planned a visit during the mother's visit with her son. The first several minutes of the visit were spent *observing the maternal/child interaction* in progress on the nurse specialist's arrival. Mrs. W. worked with dexterity and with anticipation of Victor's needs as she cleaned him following bowel incontinence. She spoke softly and tenderly to a boy who responded with the cooperation expected.

Later, in a comfortable lounge setting, apart from Victor, Mrs. W. related some history. She was the second wife of a father of three healthy children. Victor was *her* first child by her husband (and a witness, perhaps, of her incompetence in producing?). She expressed feelings of being helpless and overwhelmed, of having had questions ignored by physicians, of professional indecision about Victor's care, of one neurologist who had referred to Victor by a most derogatory term, and of their own parental inability to determine a course of action for long-term care planning. Her support system was minimal; potential baby-sitters expressed a fear of Victor and refused to assume any responsibility for him because he often convulsed. She had little relief; yet she insisted that the family would not also assume a handicap. She told of group activities with all the children, including a plane trip she had managed unaided because her husband had to work.

Mrs. W. also had questions regarding plans for the current hospitalization which supposedly would include correction of the decubiti, ileal conduit, and orthopedic evaluation and therapy. Three specialized groups of physicians were to manage Victor; of these, she had met only the urologist.

Family responsibility prevented her staying constantly, but she could visit several times a week if she could locate transportation. She smoked during the interview, and half-slumped over the desk as she talked. She was much too heavy for her frame; her carriage and clothing aroused suspicion that she had little interest in her own appearance, yet her well-kept hair and appropriate makeup suggested the opposite. Her confusion and need were apparent; effectual care had been lacking for this family.

In a later conference with the physical therapist and the nurse specialist, Mr. and Mrs. W. further embellished this history. The W.'s verbalized their quandary for almost an hour, during which time the professionals offered a few suggestions as to how they might proceed and offered themselves as contacts for coordinating Victor's care. At termination of the conference, Mrs. W. remarked with exuberance: "Thank you so much! No one has ever been so helpful or told us so much before. For the first time we feel as though we understand." In fact, of course, the parents had done more "telling" and the professionals more listening!

Based on information thus obtained, improved communication was established with the various physicians involved, a more positive approach by the nursing staff was encouraged, and a postdischarge conference with the public health nurses promised a better future for the W.'s. Gradually Mr. and Mrs. W. were able to listen and respond to suggestions for improving their son's care, and Mrs. W. felt comfortable initiating support from involved professionals. Throughout a prolonged hospitalization requiring skin grafting for one decubitus and a later ileal conduit, Mrs. W. responded positively to guidance in her child's care. She quickly learned effective care related to Victor's ileal bladder, and preferred doing it herself if necessitated during her visits.

Awareness of Environment   The value of orientation tours has been explained in Chapter 30; they are indispensable for preschoolers. Orientation also includes awareness of the time, which presents problems to children even in a home setting. A specially constructed calendar which shows admission day and each successive day of hospitalization has proved helpful with some children. These calendars can be made of colorful construction paper and decorated with pictures of flowers, baseball players, or whatever is meaningful to the particular child. A side effect of these has been to stimulate cognitive growth by prompting the child to experiment with numbers and colors.

Alleviation of Fears Related to Body Integrity   Once initial relations have been established with child and parents, the nursing-care plan must provide for needs pertinent to the child's hospitalization. Again,

the child with a myelomeningocele presents a working example, since he is especially vulnerable to the required therapy.

A child scheduled for an ileal conduit is scheduled also for a remarkable insult to his body integrity. A simple explanation "The doctor will fix you so you'll have no more wet diapers" is fine as introductory material prior to hospitalization. It is too simple prior to surgery, however. This fact can be appreciated by a cursory consideration of how the child will see himself following surgery. He will be supine, possibly restrained to avoid self-injury. Nasogastric intubation, which he views from a distorting vantage point, will necessitate a disturbing drainage pump. On his abdomen he will spy a red "stoma" draining into a plastic bag; alongside will be a dressing hiding surgical sutures. He will have awakened thirsty and be refused oral fluids, but he "shouldn't be thirsty" since he will be receiving intravenous fluids. Repair of the myelomeningocele itself, at this age, is equally disturbing. Postoperatively the youngster must maintain a prone position constantly, with mobility limited more than preoperatively.

How does one prepare a child for such horrors? Several factors are important: content, timing, method, and the people involved.

Mrs. V. said she had not been prepared prior to admission, but Kenny knew that the doctor intended to rid him of wet diapers. Mrs. W. had an inkling of proposed therapy, but Victor denied any knowledge. Obviously there is no single technique which would adequately provide preparation for both of these families. Each family requires a unique approach, based on their situation.

Cognitive and psychosocial elements must be considered in any plans preparatory to explaining an intrusive or mutilating procedure to the preschool child. Specifically to be considered are his "concreteness," "centering," "irreversibility," and inability to ponder the activity of transformation from one state to another. Oedipal fantasies and fears of body mutilation must also be respected. The ultimate directive in preparations is to move slowly and specifically, and to choose nonthreatening vocabulary.

Timing, taking into consideration the length of preoperative hospitalization, is best judged on the basis of individual personalities involved. Very early preparation is detrimental since it places too great a demand on the child's coping and defensive behavior. Some preparation is best left to within an hour or so of the anticipated procedure, sometimes immediately before and *during* the procedure. In surgical cases it is sometimes appropriate to give very little information beforehand, and follow this with immediate resumption of support beginning in the recovery room and continuing throughout the postoperative course. Parents can be very helpful in determining appropriate timing by informing the nurse of how the child copes with stress. For example, does he profit from having a period to gain control or from instantaneous treatment followed by a period to work it out?

Too complete an explanation disregards a child's "centering" and inability to appreciate the process of change. The preschooler's anxiety level will partially protect him from too informative a discussion; when he wanders away bodily or mentally from the instruction, it will be obvious that his tolerance has been—or is about to be—overextended.

Several preoperative attempts were made to prepare Victor. He avoided every attempt by turning to toys, requesting the nurse to play with him, asking for his mother, playing with his television control, or saying he would go home "tomorrow." The nurse consequently kept preparation to a minimum, and followed this up postoperatively via several methods including the use of a stuffed animal who had had "surgery."

More thorough preparations, conducted by both nurse and parent, were possible with Kenny. Once his mother had gained control of some of her heightened feelings, she participated in the nurse's instruction of her son by (1) allowing the preparation; (2) interpreting misunderstanding; (3) answering questions in the nurse's absence, and (4) notifying the professionals of how Kenny was responding to the preparation.

Kenny's preparation followed this sequence. First contact: Nurse introduced herself and began a friendly relation; elicited child's understanding of his hospitalization; promised to return later. Second contact: Nurse continued friendly relation; "borrowed" mother for conference aimed at relieving her anxieties. Third contact: While administering physical care, the nurse began preparation more directly. "Dr. C. told me he plans to help you stop wetting your diapers. He'll do that in a special way in a couple of days. Then you'll have a special bag to hold your urine till you can get to the toilet, just like other boys! Won't that be something?! Other boys have a bag inside them; your bag will be outside, but you will keep it under your clothes so no one will see it unless you want them to see it." Kenny responded in terms of what this would mean to him, "Then I can go to kindergarten, too." "Yes, then you can go to kindergarten." Later when the nurse was about to leave the room, she suggested, "Think about that new bag I told

you about, and when I come back I'll answer all the questions you think up for me about it, okay?"

Fourth contact (Some children would have no questions since their ego might be too weak to cope this way. In such cases it might be necessary for the nurse to suggest questions.): Kenny asked, "How is Dr. C. gonna fix me?" (A preschooler does not expect surgical details in answer to such a question, but wants to know when he will have surgery and whether it will hurt.) He was told that in 2 days he would have the operation, and anesthesia was explained to him. Points included about anesthesia were (1) its difference from regular sleep, (2) no pain would be felt, (3) he would sleep for the entire operation, and (4) after the operation he would awaken in the "wake-up" room. The nurse used an ileal bladder doll to demonstrate how the rectal anesthesia would be administered and how Kenny's abdomen would appear after surgery. Kenny was shown the "stoma" on the doll and told that some children think it looks like blood even though it is not blood. "Thast stoma is like the new hole Dr. C. will make for your urine to come from. Your urine will flow into a bag like this. Every time the bag fills up you will go to the bathroom and empty it. It'll sound just like other boys going to the toilet." (This last statement usually is welcomed by boys for obvious reasons.)

Fifth and continuing contacts: Opportunities were provided for Kenny to work through his understanding of the preparation given him, and to offer more essential details. The doll was reintroduced, for example, and a dark thread was added to the nostril to resemble a nasogastric tube. (Prior explanation of the nasogastric tube seems important since it intrudes the body, feels odd, and may cause a sore throat, besides being totally incomprehensible to the child.) Terms such as "stomach pump" were avoided so as not to have Kenny conjure up a fantasy such as of a football pump. "When Dr. C. does the operation, your stomach will need a rest. So Dr. C. will also give you a special tube to keep your stomach empty so it won't have to work till you start feeling better. It will look something like this. As soon as it's time for your stomach to start working again, the nurse will remove the tube and you won't need it anymore."

This, as is true of all explanations, was interrupted several times by the child's or parent's questions, or by the child's need to change the subject temporarily to relieve his anxiety.

Most questions are generated after surgery when denial becomes increasingly difficult. Continued availability of the nurse is therefore mandated postoperatively to help the family cope with the new body alterations and the required "gadgets" being used. The doll may continue to benefit the child, and may therefore be placed in the child's recovery bed and allowed to remain with him for the duration of his convalescence.

The benefit of the doll may reside in the processes of identification and of assimilation of body changes into the body image, as explained by Schilder's theory. His physiologic and libidinal spheres have already been discussed. The sociologic sphere[24] seems, however, to have more particular application in this instance because the preschooler readily animates the doll and relates to it as if to a person. Essentially what happens is that the child can (a) through his various senses, specifically sight and touch, gain an impression of the doll's stoma; (b) assign some meaning to this impression, based on his emotional reaction to it; and (c) make some judgment regarding the doll's stoma. Thereafter he can begin to respond to his own stoma. Beneficially employed, this phenomenon can be directed toward the child's ease of adjustment.

Alleviation of Fears of Abandonment and Punishment

Four-year-old **Patty** expressed her fear of abandonment while playing with her security blanket. She held one corner of the blanket and let the rest of it extend down from the bed. Gradually she began dropping it to the floor, waiting, then asking the nurse to retrieve it for her. Finally, she dropped it with an announcement, "It fell!" The nurse joined in, "The poor blanket, oh, the poor blanket." Patty explained, "The poor blanket, nobody wants it!" The nurse picked up the blanket and and set it back on the bed, saying "Patty wants you, blanket."

Patty perhaps was wondering if, since she had fallen from her tricycle, her mother would no longer want her (she was broken). Or, if the blanket symbolized her mother, perhaps she abandoned it in retaliation for having been abandoned to the hospital.

Five-year-old **Lou Ann** suffered lesions of her feet from running barefoot outside. Since she had a history of paresthesia, she had been frequently reprimanded for similar misbehavior. Finally she had "disobeyed" once too often and had incurred a wound which refused to heal. She was eventually hospitalized for skin grafting. Her mother had been administering most of her personal care, and the nurses consequently spent little time with her.

Lou Ann cried loud and long in anticipation of skin grafting. She had overheard snatches of conversation between her mother and the surgeon. Her pediatrician, sensitive to her probable fears, consulted the nurse specialist. During ensuing puppet play, the child verbalized her fear of amputation—actually a natural fear based on her developmentally appropriate expectation of punishment for transgression, and on her heightened body integrity concerns. Subsequently "play therapy" allowed her to cast her doll's legs in the same position hers would be for immobilization of the skin graft. She was thereby able to inject some reality into her fantasies about what would happen.

In attempting to resolve fears of punishment such as this one, it is sometimes wise and sometimes unwise to use the child's own doll for the play procedure. The nurse really needs to take clues from the child as to whether it would be more or less traumatic to in turn punish her own doll. Sometimes, if the procedure has first been played out with the nurse's doll, the child is then more ready to experiment with her own doll. This technique is applicable to boys as well as to girls, although sometimes the boys, and especially their fathers, are more receptive if an animal or a boy doll is used.

Support for Ego Defensiveness *Regression* Initially it is proper to allow regression, but to recognize it for what it is. Rather than admonishing, "Big boys don't cry," which, after all is a lie, the nurse can offer ego strength. Saying "It's all right to cry; you're scared" while cuddling a frightened child, tells him he is accepted despite his behavior, and profits his self-esteem.

Thumb and blanket perhaps bring the hallucinated mother closer in times of feared abandonment. As the child is assisted to realize he is not being abandoned, he will become able to voluntarily release his regressive tools. A 4-year-old girl, whose mother could visit only a few hours each day, resorted immediately to substitute gratification from her thumb and blanket. Hospitalization included the added and unforgivable trauma of having been taunted by some personnel about being a baby because she was enuretic a few nights. Yet, with these and other supportive measures, she managed to cope. One day, having observed the nurse place a pillowcase on the overhead traction bar, she requested that her security blanket also be placed there—she was ready to move forward.

Repression, Denial, and Withdrawal Since repression, denial, and withdrawal may place a heavy toll on the ill preschooler's energy reserves, they might also interfere with his convalescence. If allowed to persist, development may be interrupted and the ego may be weakened. Nursing care must provide opportunities for healthy resolution of the child's inner stresses which necessitate this kind of defensiveness. Pertinent care might consist of a combination of the following: (1) offering self as a steady and trustworthy adult support; (2) continuing to explain the experience to the child in nonthreatening and understandable terms; (3) encouraging substitute coping devices for the undesirable behavior; (4) fostering continued parental support and contacts with normal aspects of daily life; and (5) providing for reality orientation.

Substitute devices might take the form of "play therapy," or perhaps of "chores" or other contrivances to promote mobility within, and identification with, the environment.

Displacement, Sublimation, Fantasy, and Aggression If angered by personnel, parents, or circumstances, how can the preschooler express his emotion without further jeopardizing himself? If he is frightened, can he lose face by admitting it? If his superego accuses him of having caused his own illness/hospitalization, how can he accept the blame? Displacement and sublimation offer him an "out."

Planned play programs afford opportunity to hammer and slam objects, to hop and run, or to draw the dreariest picture. Unplanned opportunities can also be effective if materials for similar purposes are spontaneously introduced. None of this, however, will optimally benefit the child unless personnel attitudes are in accord. The value of such opportunities is not so much in the professional's observing the behavior expressed and interpreting it as in the child's pure expression of his inner feelings. When the child uses this mechanism to relay his understanding of the experience, the informed nurse can modify her care to allay his anxieties, however.

Drawing One 4-year-old girl drew pictures for her mother and 5-year-old sister Kathy. Her pictures took the form of a "cat" face, ostensibly to represent her pet cat. She always denied any connected story, but said "They're just pictures of kitty cats." The cats at times seemed more human than feline, having hair and expressive mouths. She drew a total of 18 pictures during her hospitalization, all of which were addressed "To Mommy and Kathy"; all but two bore resemblance to cats. On the fourth day of her hospitalization she drew the first three cats; her fourth picture was described as she drew it: "I did it good." Asked what it was, she replied, "I don't know." "It's gonna be

night and they'll have to look outside for it. . . . to find it." "It's not a big lady." "I can't figure it out." (See Fig. 26-1.)

Considering her total response to hospitalization, it was felt that this picture at least partially represented her feeling of loss and abandonment.

The following day she produced five more pictures. She had no story for her drawings, except for one. As she drew with the green crayon, she said: "Now I'm gonna draw a sad one." With the green crayon she outlined a face, then eyes, nose, and whiskers. She started to put some dots by the right eye: "Look what's happening. These are tears." She added "tears" to the left eye; then she drew a downturned mouth (Fig. 26-2). What a graphic representation of her own sadness this seemed to be!

Toys Five-year-old **Freddie** placed a multitude of controls on his aggressiveness. It was essential that he be provided ample materials for external release of this aggression. He played with a truck during one play period. The nurse asked him what the truck contained and he replied: "Soldiers. Soldiers to attack everything." When asked what they would attack, he responded: "Phillipsburg" (his hometown). "Everybody in Phillipsburg. 'Cause I don't like them." Freddie has plenty of reason to despise his parents, siblings, hometown, hospital, and everyone else connected with his 5 years of repeated hospitalizations, surgeries, tracheostomy aspirations, and threatened family disintegration. In this and many other play sequences Freddie displaced socially unacceptable behavior to a safe object via an acceptable channel, fantasy.

Play kits Interestingly, Erikson[25] calls playing a natural *autotherapeutic* measure of childhood which is employed in response to a need to rid oneself of the past and/or to prepare for the future. As such, play therapy ought to be an ever-present resource to the ill and hospitalized child, perhaps more so if his hospitalization is especially marked by traumatic procedures. Since the two avenues open to the intruded child are withdrawal and retaliation, a need exists for children manifesting either of these responses to project their feelings to a play situation.

Erickson's[26] work demonstrates the invaluable use of play interviews with hospitalized preschool children. The child is offered a kit full of both threatening and nonthreatening items with which to play. Threatening objects might be a stethoscope, needle and syringe, thermometer, catheter; nonthreatening are more familiar items such as a doll family and furniture. The nurse's role in implement-

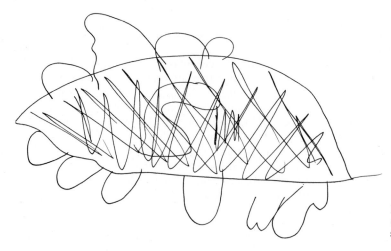

Figure 26-1 Perhaps this drawing expressed Patty's sense of loss and abandonment.

ing the play kit for an "interview" is to provide the materials, then observe and record what transpires. Unless the child should endanger himself, he is allowed to continue without direction until he disrupts his own play.

Items specifically pertinent for a particular child can be added to the play kit, to elicit expression of suspected underlying feelings. Devices for oxygen or anesthesia administration, for example, have been employed effectively. One boy used this medium to express his understanding of what happened during surgery. An anesthesia mask was included in the kit. He restrained a doll on a table top, placed the mask over the doll, directed the doll to count to three, then attacked its neck: "Shot, shot, shot!" This was the same Freddie previously mentioned, a child with a permanent tracheostomy.

Television Wise selection of television programs has proved therapeutic with some children. Caution is paramount, however, that already vulnerable children not be exposed to further stresses from ill-chosen programs. Most "hospital" programs contain anxiety-producing situations that readily contribute to the preschooler's fantasies. "Soap operas" often suggest loss and abandonment, and may multiply fears already being fought by the child.

Fortuitous happenings on children's shows might be incorporated into explanations of the hospital experience. "Misterogers' Neighborhood," a well-known children's program, proved significant for one little girl, Patty, who had unverbalized questions about her bandaged arm: Mr. Rogers removed his sock and slipper to display a bandaged foot. He stated that as a child he sometimes thought that when a bandage covered a foot or a finger, that maybe the foot or finger was no longer there; he had learned that he was wrong. The nurse turned to Patty and suggested, "But you know your arm is under the bandage, huh?" She replied: "Yes, . . . 'cause you washed it." Mr. Rogers then showed a film supposedly taken when the doctor had originally bandaged his foot. Patty said excitedly, "Look, that's just like we're bandage!" and the nurse agreed. Mr. Rogers then asked the doctor to remove his bandage to assure the children his foot was still there. Patty countered, "But you don't wrap it like that." When asked for clarification, she explained that the nurse did not wrap, unwrap, and rewrap her bandage. The nurse answered, "No, because your bandage was already on and you know your arm is there." Patty agreed.

Storytelling Fictitious stories can be created to help preschoolers work through their experiences of sickness, injury, hospitalization, and all the concomitants. It is important to end such a story happily with health and homecoming if the child's prognosis is such. A more difficult variety would be for the chronically ill child who might be helped in another manner. Stories for the chronically ill child could perhaps terminate with a suggestion for compensation or sublimation via an appropriate channel.

The nursery rhyme *Humpty Dumpty* may aggravate fears for an injured child who feels the doctor may be unable to "put him back together again." Animism and other cognitive elements require that the preschooler by some means have the story placed in perspective. A suggested concluding comment is the following: "But little boys and girls are different from eggs. When their bones break, they can be fixed. Besides, mommies and daddies could never find someone to replace their boy or girl. Mommies and daddies tell the doctor to do a good job, and then they take their children home when they're better."

Projection and limit-setting The goal of all nursing care is the eventual return of acute patients and their families to optimum health. This means that the nurse maintain some sense of normalcy and discipline for the child, and that the child gradually be weaned from dependency and defensiveness.

One day a mother reported to the nurse that on a preceding evening her daughter, Patty, had accused her of wanting her to be in the hospital. She had asked her mother, angrily, "Why did you let me stand on that bike? Why did you leave me here?" The mother had let her say these things without redress, knowing that it is common for children to project blame as a means of relieving their consciences. This was the same girl who had the habit of dictating "letters" for the nurse to write for her mother. The letters served as a communication system, and were really quite informative. Patty always instructed the nurse to place the letters in an obvious spot atop the television.

On the thirteenth day of hospitalization, Patty became unhappy that her nurse was leaving earlier than usual. She cried for the letter to be handed to her; when it was given to her, she placed it securely between her knees. Suddenly she grabbed for the letter with such emotion that only after fumbling with it was she able to maintain a grasp on it. She threw it deliberately to the floor during this outburst. It was thought that she may have been displacing her anger to the letter in retaliation for unacceptable emotions which she had safely assigned to both her mother and her nurse.

The nurse, by chance, was prepared to cope with Patty's behavior. She took a ping pong ball from her pocket and held it up: "Balls are for throwing; letters are not for throwing." As she picked the letter from the floor, she tossed the ball into Patty's bed. Patty immediately displaced her anger to a game of throwing and catching the ball. The nurse expanded her limit-setting as she joined the game: "You're a big girl to be crying. When you're angry, you can say that you're angry. It's all right to be angry. I know that you're angry because I'm leaving. But you're a big girl and can say that you're angry instead of crying." (This incident might have been improved had the nurse referred to the throwing of the letter, and emphasized the crying less, since crying certainly provides an acceptable outlet at times. The intention here was specifically to give Patty some way of controlling her

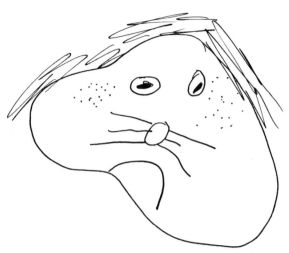

Figure 26-2 The tearful, sad "cat" likely represents Patty's sadness.

feelings, and to inform her that the adults in her environment were in sympathy with her plight.)

Then and for many days afterward, Patty invested her energies in the ball game. She quickly learned to ask for the game when she needed relief. Gradually she was able to admit her feelings and to divest the game of its obvious anger component.

Some examples are more apparent, as when the child says, "You hate me. You don't like me!" or "I didn't wet the bed, that bad boy came in and did it." The adult, in the first instance, might reaffirm his love and concern for the child by verbalizing, "I do love you Nicky, but you are angry at me because you had to come to the hospital. Neither of us wants you to stay here; you will come home with me just as soon as you are well enough." In the second situation, a responsible reaction is also required. One suggestion is, "I know you wet the bed, Anne. That sometimes happens when a little girl is sick. It's okay that you did it. Next time you think you need to use the bedpan, try to call the nurse before you wet the bed."

Summary

The reader very likely knows of additional reactions of the child, and of measures to help modify these reactions. It should furthermore be noted that there is frequent overlap among the reactions manifest and the measures employed to modify them, since probably no behavior could be an example of one exclusive emotion. If the nurse were to direct his care toward alleviation of even one of the child's needs, he could, however, expect the others to benefit. ~~Most beneficial in any situation, remains the offer-ing of self with all that implies.~~

REFERENCES

1 Lois Barclay Murphy, "Preventive Implications of Development in the Preschool Years," in G. Caplan (ed.), *Prevention of Mental Disorders in Children*, Basic Books, Inc., Publishers, New York, 1961.

2 Florence Erickson, "Stress in the Pediatric Ward," *Maternal-Child Nursing Journal*, 1(2):113–116, 1973.

3 Margaret S. Mahler, in collaboration with M. Furer, *On Human Symbiosis and the Vicissitudes of Individuation, vol. I, Infantile Psychosis*, International Universities Press, Inc., New York, 1968, pp. 23–31, 222–225.

4 P. Schilder, *Contributions to Developmental Neuropsychiatry*, Lauretta Bender (ed.), International Universities Press, Inc., New York, 1964, p. 80.

5 Emmy Sylvester, quoted by V. Calef, "Psychological Consequences of Physical Illness in Childhood," report of panel presented at annual meeting, San Francisco, May, 1958, *Journal of the American Psychoanalytic Association*, 7:159, 1959.

6 Anna Freud, "The Role of Bodily Illness in the Mental Life of Children," *Psychoanalytic Study of the Child*, 7:14, 1952.

7 Florence Erickson, op. cit., p. 113.

8 Anna Freud, *Normality and Pathology in Childhood*, International Universities Press, Inc., New York, 1965, p. 15.

9 Ibid., pp. 177–178.

10 Heinz Hartmann, "Ego Psychology and Its Problem of Adaptation," in *Organization and Pathology of Thought*, trans. by David Rapaport, Columbia University Press, New York, 1951, p. 373.

11 P. Schilder, op. cit., p. 277.

12 Lauretta Bender, "Aggression in Children," *American Journal of Orthopsychiatry*, 13:397, 1943.

13 Eileen Gallagher Nahigian, "A Five-Year-Old Child Controls His Aggressive Response to Body Intrusion," *Current Concepts of Clinical Nursing*, 4(15):134–142, 1973.

14 Anna Freud, *The Ego and the Mechanisms of Defense*, in *The Writings of Anna Freud*, based on translation by Cecil Baines, II, International Universities Press, Inc., New York, 1966, p. 56.

15 P. Schilder, *The Image and Appearance of the Human Body*, John Wiley & Sons, Inc., New York, 1950, pp. 170–173, 138–140.

16 E. Goffman, *Stigma*, Prentice-Hall, Inc., Englewood Cliffs, N.J., 1963, p. 4.

17 Ibid., p. 16.

18 Anna Freud, *Normality and Pathology in Childhood*, p. 19.

19 W. S. Langford, "The Child in the Pediatric Hospital: Adaptation to Illness and Hospitalization," *American Journal of Orthopsychiatry*, 31(4):678, 1961.

20 Margaret S. Mahler, op. cit., pp. 222, 275.

21 Florence Erickson, "Play Interviews for Four-Year-Old Hospitalized Children," *Monographs of the Society for Research in Child Development, Inc.*, 23(3), serial no. 69, 1958.

22 Melanie Klein, "The Psycho-Analytic Play Techniques: Its History and Significance," in Melanie Klein, Paula Heimann, and R. E. Money-Kysle (eds.), *New Directions in Pyscho-Analysis*, Basic Books, Inc., Publishers, New York, 1957, p. 8.

23 R. Waelder, "The Psychoanalytic Theory of Play," *Psychoanalytic Quarterly*, 2:208–224, 1933.

24 P. Schilder, *The Image and Appearance of the Human Body*, p. 226.

25 E. H. Erikson, "Studies in the Interpretation of Play," *Genetic Psychology Monographs*, 22:561, 575, 1944.

26 Florence Erickson, "Play Interviews for Four-Year-Old Hospitalized Children," op. cit.

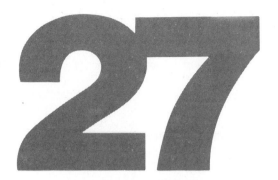

EFFECTS OF ILLNESS ON THE SCHOOL-AGE CHILD

EILEEN GALLAGHER NAHIGIAN

INTRODUCTION
School-Age Child in His Environment

So recently a *preschooler*, the child now joins that mass called *schoolchildren* for his next 6 years. He hopefully arrives at this station in life well prepared for the necessary independence and sense of self which will be tested throughout his school years. Since effective nursing care depends on the nurse's alertness to the child's normally expected behavior and his likely regression secondary to illness and hospitalization, a familiarity with growth and development is required of the nurse in planning and carrying out the school-age child's care. Chapter 13 presents the normal development of middle childhood in detail. Major characteristics are touched upon below.

Family Member Once the child has experienced day-long or even summer-long separations from home and parents, his status as a family member becomes significantly altered. He is influenced in large measure by his outside contacts as he tests the dogmas of his home, establishes his personal code of right and wrong, and formulates his own perspective on the world. In this he may well remain very close to his former beliefs; however, to the family he may seem newly distant, taciturn, and insolent.

As the child's industry remains latent or expresses itself, parents experience a sense of censure or reward, commonly vacillating between the two. Yet, at this time the child especially needs confident parents secure in their own identity and beliefs since he is required to substitute his "identity as group member" for "identity as individual."

Responsibility within the family ought to be evidenced in tasks required and fulfilled. Manifest sibling rivalry, considered undesirable and irresponsible by some adults, is normal at this time and should dissipate with maturity. Especially in early school years while his moral code remains rigid, the child may be expected to admonish parents and siblings for their imperfections, thus making life at times taxing and at times intolerable.

The school-age child is a different patient from what he was in his earlier years. All his experiences and responsibilities influence his interpretations and responses to illness, hospitalization, and intrusions. His responses continue to be highly influenced by parental reactions, particularly if he experiences illness, hospitalization, or both for the first time during these years. Awareness of his role in the family and of the family's coping patterns is required if the nurse expects to facilitate the family's adjustments.

Peer The school-age child lives in a much more expansive world than formerly. He moves into a world of strangers—mostly peers, although teachers, scout leaders, and employers also constitute much of his world.

From his multitude of contacts the child verifies and perhaps alters his views on life, self, and others. His subculture is one of many paradoxes in which he must act with "maturity" alternately with the "immaturity" inherent in prank activities.

Psychosomatic Complaints

Among the new experiences of this age period are many for which the child is ill-equipped. This is particularly true for the less mature child whose earlier years were marked by parental inability to allow the evolution of normal and necessary independence. Newly aware of their bodies and no longer permitted to cry when distressed, many of these children exhibit psychosomatic illnesses. Psychosomatic illness is briefly discussed here because, although it is itself an illness, it may also occur in response to other illnesses or necessary treatments and because it is commonly manifest during the school years.

Psychosomatic is a term misunderstood and dreaded by parents as well as by adult patients so diagnosed. The child merely knows he is sick, does not understand why, and desires relief. Relief will be achieved once the initiating cause has been identified and eradicated. Some frequent causes are new experiences; autocratic or overly permissive parents or teachers; a new neighborhood and/or school; a frightening dog along the route to school; and an inability to reconcile conflicts with peers, siblings, family, or life in general.

An 8-year-old boy had been admitted to the hospital because of several vague allergies, "fainting," "falling down," and "headache." His mother described herself as overprotective; his father had been paralyzed since Joe was 8 weeks old, as a result of meningitis following brain surgery.

Joe was rather uncommunicative especially in his mother's presence, and frequently requested that she reply to questions posed to him. However, when asked why he had so many allergies, his response was, "Human nature." When asked why he spent long periods studying about United States Presidents instead of his regular school work he answered, "No

one else knows the Presidents like I do. I showed it off in second grade and now I want to show it off in third grade." His mother reported that Joe says he doesn't want to grow up because "I don't want to stay in bed like Daddy." (Perhaps this is why he fidgeted constantly whenever he lay in bed.)

His mother revealed numerous personal problems she had in rearing Joe, including anger ("I turn purple!") whenever he sassed her. She punished him for sassing by sending him to bed or depriving him of something he wanted. She had previously spanked him for punishment, but that had resulted in nightmares, bedwetting, and vomiting.

Joe's story becomes increasingly involved, but these few glimpses suggest ample nonphysical cause for his somatic complaints in the absence of any physical findings.

PROBABLE REACTIONS TO ILLNESS, HOSPITALIZATION, AND INTRUSIONS
Response To Trauma In General

Hospitalization is just one of the many potential traumata occurring during childhood (divorce, sexual assault, death of a loved one, handicaps, and disgrace being among the others). Any event of illness or hospitalization might be experienced as a single trauma of mild to severe consequence, or as one aspect of *cumulative* trauma in which relatively minor events gradually amount to a major and possibly pervasive insult. Few events offer a single cause for pain or anxiety; for example, hospitalization—even for the older child—includes elements of separation, strangeness of environment, pain and punishment, and threat to the self. The more experienced child may suffer further trauma as a retroactive interpretation of earlier and less understood events when new data produce a revival of his past.

The school-age child may respond to trauma immediately or not for months after its occurrence. His response will then depend in part on his own interpretation of the event and in part on how it is viewed by his peer group who may either mitigate or exaggerate its effect. Observed manifestations have included a vast number of behaviors such as acute anxiety and panic, physical complaints, tremors, repetitive dreaming, inappropriate laughing or crying, inhibition, anger, excessive talking, or silent "acceptance." These may constitute coping measures or may require recourse to other coping devices.

In coping with his plight, he will surely seek answers as to why the trauma occurred and who is responsible for it. How he copes depends very much on his developmental and experiential history. It is this coping for which the nurse must be vigilant to determine the need for professional assistance (see discussion on coping in Chap. 26).

Some Carry-Overs from Preschool Years

Without discussing broadly the concept of regression, let it simply be stated that regression is to be expected of school-age children as of any other, especially early in the school years. Even in later years the possibility remains, most likely occurring inconsistently and at times of heightened anxiety, sudden acute illness, or both. In these instances the child's reaction is often intensified by anxious parents or obviously concerned personnel. The regressive pull also frightens the child who, though aware of his immature inclinations, cannot control his response or accept it in himself.

Heightened Concerns Related To Privacy, Modesty or Disgrace

Early in the school years and again at about 11 or 12 years of age, children experience intensification of rigid superego controls and of body awareness. The resultant sense of increased self-consciousness may easily interfere with physical examination and/or questions about personal behavior and hygiene. Since each of these requires care, whether the child is ill at home or in the hospital, an already uncomfortable situation is intensified for him.

Frequent occurrences which evidence heightened concern about privacy, modesty, or disgrace include the child's repeated "forgetting" to save a stool or urine specimen, denial of constipation, hesitancy to confide symptoms truthfully, refusal to have a rectal temperature checked, and reticence to ambulate dressed in hospital attire. A more dramatic example occurred in the following situation.

Seven-year-old **Anna** had been admitted to a ward on an adult unit because of overcrowding in the pediatric unit. Her roommates were a 10-year-old girl admitted for cardiac catheterization and a 4-year-old girl readmitted for evaluation of acute leukemia. Both roommates were accompanied by doting and anxious parents. Anna's parents had returned home shortly after her admission, having promised to return later that evening.

The pediatric nurse specialist had been consulted to assist the 10-year-old girl's very worried mother. Anna appeared to listen to the nurse's explanations to her roommate's mother, then requested the nurse to talk with her.

"Tell me what they're going to do to me." The nurse checked Anna's records and returned. She was to have a ureteroneocystotomy the following morning. Since she'd been hospitalized previously for diagnostic roentgenogram and cystoscopy, she had real experience with which to relate. She seemed most concerned about anesthesia, fearful that a needle would hurt and that a mask would frighten her. She was assured that her anesthesia would be administered rectally, and its instillation was simply described. Anna accepted this explanation quietly but did not settle down in bed. She brightened when the nurse promised to be with her during the induction.

About 15 minutes later the mother of the 10-year-old located the nurse and asked her to return to Anna who was then "hysterical." Anna was found screaming with tears flooding her flushed face. When she calmed sufficiently to communicate, she sobbed that she did not want anyone looking at her "bottom." She lost control again as she talked. The nurse held her close, calmed her, and accompanied her to a quiet office where they could talk alone. During their session Anna repeatedly related that it would be "bad" to let a stranger see her "bottom," and that her mother would not allow it. Fortunately she accepted the nurse's repeated explanations that it would be done only with her mother's permission and in such a way that her modesty would be protected. After requiring further confirmation of the nurse's statement that she would be with her during anesthesia induction, she asked to return to her room. With both her mother and the nurse present, induction was markedly facilitated the following morning.

All school-age children are subject to these same worries. The only difference is in their ability or inability to shield themselves and others from obvious manifestations of concern.

Discontinuities of Normal Life Activities

For security the school-age child depends heavily on his well-established place in society—family, peer group, community, and other organizations. Any threat to his position in any of these situations arouses marked discomfiture. Illness, especially when associated with hospitalization, strikes a severe blow since he becomes physically isolated from most daily life; friends avoid him "like the plague" either by choice or by necessity.

Considering the numerous incidental social and cognitive lessons of daily life during childhood, it appears that a sick child sacrifices a tremendous amount of experience when constrained to relative abnormalcy. His peace of mind and his future goals may be compromised, particularly if his "isolation" continues for days, weeks, or months.

Whether by missing (1) the developmental milestones of his infant brother, (2) significant classroom discussion of historical issues, (3) the most strategic little league game of the season, or (4) the experience of seasonal change, the sick child suffers from more than the illness itself. It becomes the responsibility of his caretakers at home or hospital to limit the effect of such discontinuities in his life.

Fear of Being Displaced

A related concern is the fear of being displaced, a fear especially prominent during the early years when the child is less sure of his importance. He may fear, for example, permanent loss of his place as class "math whiz" or usurpation at home by a new sibling. He, therefore, needs evidence of continued importance in his former roles.

Docility Related to Imposed Passivity

Imposed passivity is interpreted as punishment by the latency-age child, who does not yet reliably use causal thinking to determine explanations. With further threat of punishment inherent in the family reaction to his illness or injury, the child's docility becomes more understandable. It is unrealistic to assume that all families immediately rally to support and encourage the ill child. In reality, one child's illness may interfere with a planned vacation, may place too great a burden on the family budget, or may demand too much of the parents' time away from the family or household activities or work. In any such instance normal aggressiveness in response to the imposed passivity of illness may be replaced by docility.

In discussing reactions to physical restraint caused by illness, Bernabeu[1] refers to several defenses utilized by children. One of these, suppression, relates to docility in that the child consciously attempts "mature" behavior and denial of symptoms; suppression produces a guarded and superficial affect which may without warning yield to the aggressive tendencies being held in check.

Few episodes in a nurse's life can be so trying as caring for a docile child: no complaints, no evidence of improving or worsening symptoms, little conversation beyond "yes" and "no," not even a challenge to parenteral medications. While eventual compliance is always hoped for, the normal spirited hesitance to cooperate is expected.

Docility resembles denial in its allowing the child to maintain his former self-image amidst challenges to it. Since "saving face" is most important for continued peer group acceptance and self-acceptance, it is easier to return to the group and truthfully relate: "I let them do anything they wanted without complaining. Nothing hurt. It really wasn't so bad."

Fear Of Disability and/or Death

Since school-age children are actively engaged in life, they depend upon mobility provided chiefly by their own bodies. When illness occurs or threatens, their concerns involve curtailment of activities and of the ability to preserve themselves intact from any insult.

Bernabeu[2] records some rather interesting responses of children to experiences of crippling, including frustration, anxiety, rage, guilt, fixation on the idea of motor activity, and a feeling of threat to self-preservation. Similar responses are occasionally observed in temporarily immobilized children as well.

Enforced inactivity may refer to situations of relatively minimal restraint, for example, restraint for intravenous therapy, or to total paralysis. The child's subjective interpretation of his restriction compounds any objectively real disability. The four examples that follow illustrate how the ill child might respond.

1 A 10-year-old girl, following cystoscopy and insertion of a Foley catheter, claimed an inability to move and maintained a rigid supine position. Further exploration of her claim revealed her reasoning: previously she had shared a room with a paralyzed girl who incidentally had been catheterized. Explanation that the catheter had not produced the paralysis lessened the girl's anxiety and she was encouraged to ambulate.

2 A 10-year-old girl had sustained a fractured pelvis and had been maintained for several weeks on bedrest with a pelvic sling almost constantly in place. She manifested a cheerful exterior most of the time but evidenced her deeper feelings in a nonchalant attitude about most of her experiences: (a) she complained regularly of the placement of the bedpan and preferred only certain nurses to assist her with toileting, even allowing herself to soil the bed during the night; (b) she despised the pelvic sling and complained that it soiled easily from perspiration and

elimination; (c) she expressed security only when certain nurses provided her care.

The nurse specialist tried repeatedly and unsuccessfully to encourage verbalization of her anxieties, but she continued to deny her true emotions. Not until a few weeks postdischarge did her suspected feelings gain release. The girl was visiting the nurse at home. In a casual and unrelated conversation the nurse facetiously remarked: "Ask me anything—I'll tell you!" The girl (still in her wheelchair) immediately countered, "Am I going to die?!" Nurse: "I'll bet you wondered that quite often while hospitalized." Girl: "Yeah. I must say I thought of it many times." From then on an explanation of the normalcy of her concerns and assurance that her fractured pelvis would not cause her death ensued.

3 A 9-year-old boy hospitalized with a severely paralyzing acute illness had progressively lost and eventually regained respiratory, speech, and total motor ability. He had had an emergency tracheostomy after a few days of hospitalization and spent several weeks in the intensive care unit while being maintained on intermittent positive pressure breathing apparatus. He never lost his mask of cheerfulness despite having been exposed to many horrifying sights including his own treatment and that of others. Later attempts by the nurse specialist to verbalize for him some of his probable fears resulted in a flood of tears as he was forced to recall what had happened. Still later when he was able to vocalize, the nurse planned with him that he could make a tape recording describing the intensive care unit—ostensibly to help other children know what to expect.

His volunteered story was peppered with assurances that there was nothing to worry about because the nurses watch the patients closely; he told of the happy experience of having had another boy in the unit with him part of the time. Only with direct questioning did he admit to his real worries: (a) He had feared falling to sleep because the nurse might not hear if he started choking (he knew the tracheostomy would preclude sound). (b) An old and disoriented patient had tried repeatedly to struggle from his restraints. Jack feared the man would come after him and he would be unable to defend himself. (c) He worried that the nurses would drop him whenever they turned him from back to abdomen. (d) His dreams about running scared him lest he might fall out of bed during them.

4 An 11-year-old boy whose growth and mobility were severely hampered as a result of spina bifida and myelomeningocele had been provided crutches, braces, and eventually an ileal diversion to ensure

some self-control over his voiding. While being encouraged that he would soon be able to ambulate to the bathroom to manage his toileting, he denied this possibility, referring to himself and his disability as "a poor helpless little boy like me." This comment is additionally revealing in light of a belief that disabled children assume less self-responsibility and have lower self-esteem than do nondisabled children.[3]

Less obvious immobility may affect children whose eyes are bandaged. A recent study suggests that school-age children who are "blinded" by eye bandages are confronted as well with restricted mobility which interrupts their normal ability for self-care.[4] Their sense of identity is compromised by social deprivation, and they feel estranged from the real world which ordinarily would affirm their identity. Loss of personal identity, it seems, should rank alongside loss of physical identity and the fear of disability in this regard.

Acute or chronic illness of any degree, then, may be accompanied by definite anxieties related to one's own death or disability beyond efforts for self-preservation. The parent and the nurse must accept responsibility to present reality, to allow verbalization and acting-out of fears, and to encourage progress toward normalcy.

Fears Related To Strange Environment

Whether ill at home or in the hospital, the child may still react toward the strangeness of his environment. Home treatment of measles, for example, includes darkening the room (blankets over the window, a dim light, wearing dark glasses); extended home care during illness may require the acquisition of a hospital bed, a bedpan, or other unusual equipment and procedures.

Made anxious by reports from peers and siblings, the school-age child approaches the unfamiliar environment dubious of his safety within it. His fears of separation, abandonment, body mutilation, and death, among others, are all multiplied by his new predicament. A very simple example of his difficulties was demonstrated in the instance of 11-year-old Gary. Gary had just visited his 4-year-old sister who was immobilized in traction. He echoed his sister's question: "How come if they want to put the bones together, they're pulling them apart?"

The school-age child is better able to deal with the hospital environment than the younger child. When exposed to the unfamiliar, the 6-to-12-year-old benefits from advancing cognitive skills which he can implement more purposefully than can a preschooler. The nurse can capitalize on these cognitive skills to help ease the child's adjustment.

Utilization of Defense Mechanisms

The schoolchild's defenses retard the regressive pulls associated with the oedipal conflict and its resolution, as well as negating any sense of inadequacy or inferiority which might threaten his sense of industry, as described by Erikson.[5] Among the many defenses now operating are repression, reaction formation, sublimation, and obsessive-compulsive behavior which becomes a hallmark of late latency. The child's use of defenses stabilizes toward the end of this developmental period as he becomes more self-directed and self-assured, less constrained by conscience, and more realistic.

Reaction formation temporarily resolves conflicts in the child's mind. A curiosity about the body may be concealed by disgust at looking at certain body parts, blood, or another's injury or deformity. Reaction formations are essential to growing up, but, since they are too rigid to be maintained for long, they are mollified with age. In situations of illness or hospitalization the need to watch treatments or the refusal to do so may actually exemplify a reaction formation, as might a rigid expression of "respect" or regard for a feared physician.

Frequently repression conceals fears or guilt related to illness and hospitalization. This defense masks the child's true affects and causes him to gird himself for the onslaught of a threatening environment. At least two ill effects result. First, repression may generalize so that it colors the child's total life situation. Second, when his true feelings are so controlled, they may become displaced against innocent persons and objects.

Depression may be exhibited as boredom, lack of interest, or restlessness. Less prepared personnel may interpret such behavior as simple annoyance or anger at having been restricted to certain areas or placed in a room with younger children—factors which do contribute to the basic depression. Depression, however, is unhealthy, and measures must be instituted to help the child overcome this state.

Isolation of affect is observed in the following case in which the child, having suffered extensive burns, relates the event flatly and admits no fear connected with it. Eddie told the nurse he had noticed his pants had caught fire from a low gas heater. "First I patted it out. No, I wasn't scared. . . . I wasn't scared 'cause we play with fire a lot. . . . We go camping. My Dad sets the fire and uses gas sometimes if it doesn't light right away. . . . He tells us to get back far in the water. . . . Yeah, he don't tell me to get that far back, but he tells my sisters to 'cause they'd just stand around and scream.''

The most common defense of older schoolchildren is obsessive-compulsive behavior. Recurrent thoughts are prime offenders in this defense; when applied to conditions of illness and hospitalization, the content of recurrent thoughts may easily prove threatening by virtue of their hostile or fearsome nature. Also witnessed has been the need to repeatedly wash a specific body part to be certain it is clean, or the need always to wash one's hands before touching any object. It is conceivable that isolation technique and forced awareness of physiologic functions might compound some of these behaviors for ill children.

Sublimation is one defense that can be directed positively during latency for informing the nurse of the child's true reaction to hospitalization and for keeping in touch with one's peers. Letters written back and forth, especially if shared with the nurse, afford valuable assistance to understanding the child. One 9-year-old girl was asked to write a poem about her hospital experience. She found it too difficult to express her own feelings, but she located a get-well card she had received, copied the long and "comical" verse from it, and actively displayed this as her own.

COPING WITH REACTIONS TO ILLNESS, HOSPITALIZATION, AND RELATED FACTORS

How the child copes and how the adult facilitates his coping are keys to his achieving a satisfactory resolution of a disturbing interruption in his life. Theoretical discussion must concern itself with situations from the mildest to the most severe, whether viewed objectively or subjectively.

One of the most traumatizing situations one could expect is reported in Kikuchi's[6] case story of a 12-year-old boy who required tracheostomy, craniotomy, and bilateral guillotine amputation of both forearms following the explosion of a bomb he had been making. Although his conflicts were far from resolved during the initial hospitalization, his nurse had helped him approach cognitive preparation for discharge during that time. Regardless of the nature of his illness, the child profits from the nurse's accepting responsibility to assist his coping.

Eliciting the Child's Thoughts and Feelings

Enhanced Availability School-age children tend to idealize adults, a tendency which transfers to their interactions with nursing personnel. Also operative might be infatuation toward any nursing personnel of the opposite sex. Both facts portend serious responsibility for nurses who not only administer specifically indicated care to their young patients, but also contribute incidentally to the children's continuing personality and character formation.

The ill child needs adult support related to his illness and hospitalization. But just being available is insufficient. Enhanced availability means that parent, nurse, or other competent person provides a sense of openness and constancy to the child. While he may not require constancy of the same degree required by a preschooler, neither does he benefit from superficial contacts with a variety of persons. For therapeutic sharing, he relies on a feeling of confidence and security with his nurse which allows him to seek mature advice regarding his illness or other matters.

Scheduling the same nurse regularly to a child's care and encouraging that nurse to plan for the child's total care, and employing nurses who both *listen* with all senses and *respond* on the proper level are among the administrative measures which foster expression of the ill child's concerns. The staff nurse who is encouraged to work under this kind of philosophy proves the merits of pediatric care.

One 8-year-old girl scheduled for urinary surgery had been judged calm and prepared by several nurses who had intermittently cared for her. Another nurse who had spent time with her and promised to care for her preoperatively *and* postoperatively was with her the morning of surgery when she first expressed her feelings. She began to cry and say she did not want to have the operation. When asked to explain, she confided to the nurse, "I saw a man on *Dr. Casey* who had kidney surgery and he died! I don't want to die." She calmed after being instructed that her operation was to prevent kidney damage so that she would not need kidney surgery later. A sketchy diagram of the urinary system was used to help her understand the relation of bladder to kidney. A few days postoperatively when a mist mask was prescribed to treat her respiratory congestion, she expressed death fear again. The same nurse, aware of the depth of her anxiety, was then prepared to present the therapy nonthreateningly and let her adapt to it gradually.

Projective Techniques When simple conversation fails (although one must not lose sight of the merits of conversation), the prepared nurse employs alternate routes to elicit the child's concerns and facilitate his coping. If one is alert to the environment, projective devices "appear"; for example, television, books, or games frequently afford opportunity to encourage verbalization of thought.

A 9-year-old boy recovering from acute paralysis was prompted by a television advertisement about cerebral palsy to compare his predicament with that of the child in the advertisement. He questioned the differences in their conditions and asked about the brace he would be wearing until he regained full motor ability. A 10-year-old girl who could not openly express her anger toward her parents concocted occasions to play board games with her nurse. In these games she sought to win aggressively without regard to the rules; she also handled the game pieces roughly. At times she attempted to manipulate the nurse to play when it was convenient only to herself. After a few similar occasions, the nurse reflected on the girl's behavior and encouraged her to talk of her anger toward her parents.

A technique employed by Gellert[7] elicits data regarding the child's understanding of his body and his illness. The child is asked to name the parts of his body under his skin, then to state the function of these body parts, and finally to suggest what would happen if each of these parts was missing. The following cases demonstrate how this technique might be employed.

Eleven-year-old **Richie** had been hospitalized with a complaint of recurrent constipation alternating with fecal soiling. He continually changed the subject when the nurse attempted discussion of his condition. When subsequently asked to help the nurse learn how much school-age children know about their bodies, he agreed, and the Gellert questions were posed. He explained his intellectual approach to this test by stating that he had studied about the body in school and in his encyclopedia. His answers to the third question evidenced a concern about paralysis and death, indicating that without a stomach or large or small intestines "you'd die." He was then asked to draw into a human outline each body part he had named (see Fig. 27-1A). His drawing was rather precise and complete (though not entirely accurate), and he requested a second outline so that his picture

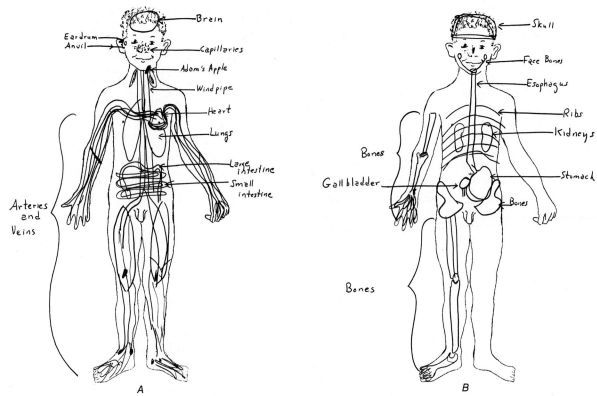

Figure 27-1 Richie's physiologic drawings. *A.* Rather precise completion of outline. *B.* Without a stomach or intestines "you'd die."

would not be cluttered (see Fig. 27-1B). (Cleveland Metropolitan General Hospitals employs this kind of body outline and makes copies of it and of other physiologic drawings accessible to area hospitals. This technique and others have been reported by Plank[8] in a very useful reference.)

By contrast Eddie, who had been confined to a wheelchair to allow healing of a graft on his burned leg, stated no connection between the digestive tract and death, but claimed that muscles were important because ". . . . If you couldn't move you'd probably have a heart attack." (See Fig. 27-2, p. 406.)

Children of this age enjoy creating puppet shows. Sometimes a little initial direction removes any potential threat; the nurse might suggest, for example, that they devise a skit to orient a child to the good and bad parts of being hospitalized. A similar idea was utilized effectively with a passive 10-year-old girl following open-heart surgery. She cooperated in assisting the nurse to write a puppet play about heart surgery. She was the "nurse" and

the nurse was the "inquiring child." In her script she described nurses as "kind and generous," said it was wise to have heart surgery so one wouldn't be "puny," and verbalized distaste for injections. She extolled the virtues of having surgery and of being in the intensive care unit. The nurse, attempting to draw her out more realistically, expressed the "inquiring child's" eagerness to also have surgery. In an almost inaudible mutter, the "nurse" was caused to scoff at such naïveté.

The play interview as employed in the preschool period is also of value. Play settings may be used by preparing a doll for surgery and allowing the child to assume the professional's role. One example of the way a nurse used this technique to elicit the feelings of a child is shown in the case history on the next page. Sean, an 8-year-old foster child, was hospitalized in anticipation of heart surgery. His very anxious manner is evidenced by his behavior and his comments, as listed in the left-hand column. In the right-hand column are the nurse's brief interpretations of what the boy's latent worries seem to be.

The nurse brought a Teddy Bear to help explain to Sean how the doctor would fix his heart. Sean: "Does he have a bad heart too?" So assured, Sean moved his finger across the bear's chest and said: "You gotta cut his heart out!" Nurse: "Is that what you think the doctor will do to you?" Sean denied this, shaking his head negatively. Nurse: "Well, he's not, and we're not going to take the Teddy's heart out either. That stays right where it is."

Sean indicates awareness of reason for own hospitalization.

Sean's fantasy: He needs verbalization that his heart will not be removed. May be concerned with mutilation and death. (Nurse's reply may have been better if less direct, perhaps a simple reflection of his inference.)

Sean was disturbed and distracted by the absence of one of the bear's eyes. He fingered the place of the missing eye without comment. The nurse assured him of that difference between him and the bear and that no one would disturb his eye. He remained distracted. Nurse: "We could pretend one of your own toys needs to get fixed." Sean nodded approval and volunteered his stuffed monkey.

Mutilation fantasy may have extended to possibility that he, too, could lose an eye.

Nurse, laying the monkey beside Sean: "You know the doctor won't fix your heart until you're asleep, don't you?" He nodded. "But not when you're asleep at night; he'll do it when you have a special kind of sleep. We'll give you some medicine to help you sleep."

Child needs to have fear of sleeping allayed.

Sean: "Yeah! A pill!" Nurse: "No, I think it won't be a pill; it'll be medicine into your leg with a needle." She demonstrated by a pinch on each of the monkey's thighs, and explained that the needles would be over with fast and that he wouldn't feel them for too long. He nodded. The nurse further explained that this medicine would make him drowsy but not completely asleep.

Denial of the needle as a defense.

This explanation was intended to allay fear that he would awaken prior to anesthesia induction.

Holding an anesthesia bag, the nurse explained that after he went to the operating room he would be given more medicine to keep him asleep during surgery. He was told the mask would be placed over his face, that he would then be asked to blow into it and breathe normally, and that he might be asked to count to 3.

A tangible ability provided him with a means of temporarily controlling the situation. He diverted the explanation and also actively participated by counting.

Sean responded by counting to three. When the nurse suggested he might count higher before falling asleep, he counted as high as he could (to 78), and smiled when praised for his ability.

Sean then experimented with the bag, smelling its rubber, squeezing it rhythmically and placing it over his own, the nurse's, and his mother's faces. He asked the nurse to anesthetize the monkey. As she complied with his request, he covered the monkey's eyes and asked: "How will I cover my eyes?" The nurse demonstrated by putting the mask to her own face, closing her eyes and feigning sleep.

He was developing a familiarity with the bag and assuring himself of its safety.

(Continued)

His mother remarked, "She's falling asleep. It must be real!" At that the nurse "awakened" and laughed, saying it was only pretend. Sean laughed and the nurse continued anesthetizing the monkey. When it was decided that the monkey was asleep, the mask was removed and the nurse started applying a dressing to the monkey's chest. Sean picked up the monkey: "Ow! He's awake!" The nurse set the dressing down and said: "Oh, no, that'll never do. We can't fix him unless he's asleep. We'll have to put him to sleep again. You know, Sean, this is a special kind of sleep so that you can't even feel anything while you're asleep."

> Success of the instruction might depend on Sean's belief that it was make-believe; therefore, no suggestion of reality could be entertained.
> He is testing whether surgery depends on his being asleep.
> He needs to know he will not feel hurt during surgery.

Anesthesia and dressing were reenacted. Sean watched, then played with the anesthesia bag again, experimenting with squeezing its breeze on his face, nose, and ear. He repeated these actions with the nurse and with his mother, observing their reactions to having the air squeezed into their ears. He then asked where the tube that led from the bag originated and terminated and an explanation of the anesthesia gas was given him. His mother suggested the gas would smell like fingernail polish remover.

> He seems to be reviewing and experimenting to aid assimilation of the lesson.
>
> Specific information sought to aid understanding and therefore control.

The nurse placed a monitor lead on the monkey's chest and Sean commented, "They look like Band-Aids." Mrs. F. offered that they might also look like lollipops. He was told that the leads would be connected to a machine he would not see. A chest tube was placed on the monkey. Sean took the free end and put it into his own mouth. The nurse explained that the tube would connect to a bottle under his bed. He said he would see that because he would look. He took the tube and tied it around his foot, calling the nurse's attention to a scar on his lower leg. The nurse remarked that it appeared healed and he agreed.

> Attempts were made to relate these strange things to something familiar.
> May suggest regressive orality and/or his identification of a known orifice in place of an unknown one.
> He attempts to control at least part of his situation.
> He may be seeking reassurance that a new wound will also heal.

He disrupted the explanation to again play with the anesthesia bag. Then the pediatric urine collector was applied to the monkey and explained to Sean. The nurse indicated that was the end of the surgery and Sean asked her to fix another toy. A discussion ensued in which the nurse encouraged Sean to do the next "surgery." He was hesitant, saying he did not want to be a doctor because he did not want to chop off people's heads. He was assured the doctors did not do this, that they were in the hospital to fix children, not to hurt them. He agreed to instruct the nurse in performing the next "surgery" instead of doing it himself. Nurse: "Okay, what do I do first."

> His fantasy and fears are evidenced.
> He assumes a *passive* role of identifying with the aggressor by indirectly doing the surgery.

Sean: "First you gotta take all that stuff off the monkey. Now put the bandage on." The nurse began to bandage the monkey but was interrupted: "No, you gotta give the needles first." This was done, and his mother prompted him about the anesthesia mask; he instructed the nurse to anesthetize the monkey. The nurse counted for the monkey until it appeared he slept. Sean idled a while with the anesthesia bag, then handed the nurse the monitor leads and instructed her to

> He needs more time to assimilate the sequence. He may also be exercising some denial by forgetting needles and needing prompting.

apply them. He next followed his mother's prompting to have the nurse place the catheter on the monkey's chest.

Value of having parent included in preparation: helps to resolve parents' anxiety and encourages them toward some cognitive mastery over their child's hospitalization.

Sean decided they should practice on him. He took the dressing from the nurse and placed it in his axilla over his pajamas. The nurse repositioned the dressing correctly. He lay down and asked the nurse to put him to sleep. The mask was placed over his face, he was told to breathe and to count until he fell "asleep." He was told to close his eyes and pretend to be asleep. He did so, and the nurse removed the mask. He stirred. Nurse: "Oh no, you have to be asleep." The anesthesia was reenacted and he remained still. His mother helped the nurse apply the monitor leads, chest tube, and dressing. The urine collector was placed at the crotch of his pajamas. He was told he was through with surgery and that he could awaken. He opened his eyes but lay still. Nurse: "You know, Sean, you won't wake up in *this* room. You'll wake up in a bigger room, and probably noisier room where they will have a lot of machines making noise." His mother added that the nurse would be with him when he awakened and the nurse verified this remark. Sean sat up and removed his paraphernalia. Asked if he wanted to do more surgery, he indicated he did not. He changed the subject to a game of riddles.

Assured that his monkey survived, he seems more secure and able to practice on himself.
He continues to test the reality of his fear that he will awaken during surgery. Probably he cannot yet understand all that will happen to him.

He needs assurance that he *will* awaken, but also needs to be oriented about where he will be.
He has benefited all he could with his coping ability.

Observation   Since the child's contacts with staff members often differ from contacts with others, observation of these encounters provide the nurse with more meaningful information regarding the child's true feelings. In Kikuchi's[9] report the injured boy's eager and uninvited display of his amputee stumps perhaps informed his nurse more truthfully of his needs than did his protestations that he resented the curiosity of others. Equally revealing is the situation of a docile girl who "didn't mind" being catheterized but refused to ambulate where the catheter drainage might be viewed by strangers. Another example is presented by an immobilized child who voiced no concern about his roommates but was later overheard questioning, taunting, and bullying them.

Frank Conversation   Mutual respect between the nurse and child is perhaps fostered best by honest conversation between them. Especially is this so in the later school years when the child has achieved some realistic self-appraisal of his significance and is more responsible for himself.

Effective conversation with the family should be at least threefold: (1) with the parents, (2) with the child, and (3) with the child and family together. It is not unusual for the child to relate facts or fears to the nurse and to conceal them from his parents. It is also not unusual to ignore symptoms, assuming that since they were neither mentioned nor noticed they do not exist. Clever interviewing skills are essential to avoid later learning that information was not conveyed because "You never asked me that" or "Oh! I didn't think that was important enough to mention."

Bobby had been admitted for evaluation and treatment of obvious obesity. Repeated interviewing by physicians and nurses revealed little more than that Bobby ate the same foods as his family and friends in the same quantities. Further delving for specifics proved successful: Bobby (1) ate a high intake of eggs and potatoes daily; (2) finished his schoolmates' lunches along with his own meal (the mother had been aware of this but did not mention it because she blamed the lunchroom supervisor for allowing it);

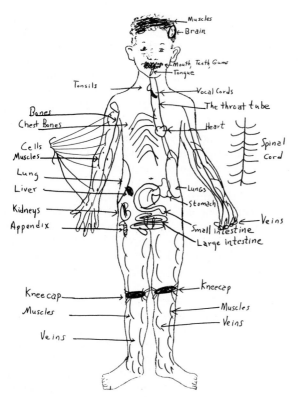

Muscles
Brain
Mouth, Teeth, Gums
Tongue
Tonsils
Vocal Cords
The throat tube
Bones
Chest Bones
Heart
Spinal Cord
Cells
Muscles
Lung
Liver
Lungs
Stomach
Kidneys
Appendix
Veins
Small intestine
Large intestine
Kneecap
Kneecap
Muscles
Muscles
Veins
Veins

Figure 27-2 Eddie's physiologic drawing. Muscles are important because "If you couldn't move you'd probably have a heart attack."

(3) stated that his only incentive to lose weight was a promise from his father that he could then sit in the front seat of the car with him. Very interestingly, Bobby's father was very thin and his mother was grossly overweight.

Hess and Shipman[10] describe two systems of communication between adults and children which are applicable to this discussion. In the "restricted code" there is no specificity or exactness in instruction so that the child has no standard by which to measure his response. Restricted statements are short and simple. In contrast, "elaborated codes" are more complex and individualized, giving reasons and examples as a part of directions. When seeking information from patients and their families, the nurse succeeds most often if he elaborates on his communications with them.

Similarly, directions or policies require explanation for understanding, and treatments need to be explained meaningfully so that the child has an opportunity for cognitive and emotional adjustment to

the requirements. Rigid codes in these instances are very seldom rational and can be justified only on the basis of personal expediency. Impersonalized explanations which require compliance because "I say so" or "That's the rule" deny the child or his family their dignity. Rigid codes are efficient for emergencies where vital time must be saved and where lengthy explanations flirt with the ridiculous as well as with danger.

Another aspect of frank conversation requires verbalization of both points of view in certain patient-nurse relations, as this case study illustrates. Eddie, driven by anger and depression, repeatedly ignored the doctor's order for immobility of his leg. The nurse verbalized for him since he seemed unable to admit his feelings: "I'm sure that wheelchair isn't too pleasant for you. You're accustomed to being up and running around and that's what you like to do. But the fact of the matter is that for your leg to heal you have to follow these rules. . . . I'm sure you're angry and I don't blame you. If I were you I'd want to have a pair of boxing gloves and a punching bag and really bang it up. . . . But in the meantime I think you can understand what the facts are." Later he did work out some of his anger in the playroom.

Rules versus Reality One of the greatest truths is that children need discipline and rules to help govern their behavior and contribute to their sense of security and feeling of being loved. When ill or hospitalized, this is no less true; were the child permitted free access to his former way of life, disaster might well threaten. Being in a weakened state of both self-control and physical stability, and having his concerns introverted, the child most certainly would be less likely than at other times to make wise judgments in his own behalf. Consequently, policies must be established as a means of protection.

As is equally true in health, however, the policies may lose their perspective in application. (Rather, those who apply the policies may lose their perspective). A common failing among parents of ill children and among hospital personnel is that the rule becomes the end rather than the means to an end. Illness and hospitalization are themselves experiences of severe isolation and personal threat, and the cause of many discontinuities in the child's life. Occasional relaxation of rules is therefore indicated to lessen the impact of the experience. Application of Piaget's[11] theory regarding children's consciousness of rules eases their relaxation.

Usually prior to age 10, the child learns to modify his rigid adherence to rules. He wants some participation in their codification and can cooperate in a democratic alteration of rules acceptable to the group. It is on this basis that certain department policies might effectively be relaxed occasionally (such as "Lights out" or "No visitors under 16") to express faith in the children as *persons* and to lessen the threat inherent in loss of normalcy. Permission to accompany a nurse or parent to the coffee shop or to have food brought from home might encourage fluid intake more easily than a mandate to drink 4 oz of juice every hour. An informative tour of the laboratory might spark later cooperation with specimen collection. Accordingly, cooperation can be attained to respect one another's varying needs, for example, the quiet required by a fresh postoperative patient or the help appreciated by a bedfast patient in retrieving dropped articles.

Familiarity with the Hospital

Familiarity with the hospital beyond the incidental department tour conducted on admission is helpful to the school-age child.

Eddie, who felt punished by his relative immobility and several weeks of confinement in one unit, responded with excitement at the offer to tour the hospital with a nurse. His need was apparent in his verbalized fantasy to spend 24 hours away from his unit. He outlined the tour which was to begin in the basement and continue upward through the entire building. He and a friend visited the carpenter shop, the kitchen, central supply room, and record room. In the record room they showed great interest in the nature of information recorded. Eddie had previously stated he would like to visit the operating room where he had had skin grafts; when restriction was placed on this request, he did not object. He challenged the nurse about all other restrictions, however. When he passed a laboratory display of test tubes and venapuncture equipment, he said it reminded him of "dope." Along with relieving his anxiety of being isolated (the tour required 2 days for completion), it also informed the nurse of some of his previously unverbalized needs.

Tours of the cardiac catheterization laboratory have been widely used in one hospital to acclimate children who remain awake for the procedure. With no immediate threat from the environment, the tour has successfully elicited questions and comments from children and parents regarding the procedure. When accomplished the day prior to catheterization, the schoolchild has time to allay his anxiety and prepare for the unavoidable test. Such a tour should be conducted only if the nurse later follows it up with personal attention of a supportive nature.

An explanatory picture book of hospital areas serves a similar purpose for those reluctant to participate in a tour.

Providing Outlets

Organized Activities Anxieties associated with illness, hospitalization, and their accompaniments are eased somewhat when the child is not left to flounder aimlessly in his strange environment. Organized activity, whether related to recreation or schooling (preferably both), structures an otherwise whimsical world of strange events. A recreation director, a school program, a library cart, planned events such as weekly movies or visits from celebrities, and a selected time in the playroom just for school-age children are some of the many successful attempts toward facilitating adjustment.

Social and benevolent organizations usually want to entertain sick children on special holidays or provide them with gifts. Since too much of this kind of activity in a short span of time proves too stimulating and disorganizing for the children, it would seem wiser for institutions to encourage interested persons to space their generosity throughout the year so that more of the children would benefit.

Normal "Problem" Behavior Legitimate opportunities for self-expression of a rowdy nature are required; preferably these opportunities occur via playroom activities of punching, throwing, pounding, and general noisemaking. However, any nurse caring for school-age children should anticipate occasional subjection to ridicule, disobedience, ignorance of policy, and mimicking. This is not to suggest that child-rule is desirable or that limits are not to be set and maintained; it merely calls for common sense and mature judgment, based on awareness of the reasons behind the child's antagonistic behavior. A nurse with a firm self-concept can maintain his equanimity and avoid involvement in petty quarrels with the children by applying his theory of development and of the effects of hospitalization on behavior. The normal industriousness of the schoolchild can be cleverly redirected to constructive activities which actually will satisfy the child more than does his misbehavior.

Providing for Mobility Mobility provides a sense of self-sufficiency and control as well as a most desirable and socially acceptable outlet for aggression. The ability to acquire, employ, and rid oneself of the services of his environment ranks high in a person's appraisal of his self-sufficiency. When loss of this ability is threatened or effected, one's identity and self-esteem are undermined.

Children who are immobilized or anticipate immobility seek assurances of their competence for employing the services of others. Seeley[12] distinguishes three types of coping behavior instituted by an 8-year-old girl whose postoperative period included immobility imposed by a hip spica cast. Even prior to surgery she insisted on being wheeled in the wheelchair and having objects handed to her, as if testing her ability to profit from vicarious mobility. She adapted to her early postoperative concern with loss of control by allowing herself to regress, by evaluating what was happening to her, and by requesting and demanding changes in her environment. Progress was evident during her final 3 days in the hospital when she displayed cognitive curiosity about her cast, participated in her own care, and completely rotated herself without assistance. So great was her need to be active that she refused to be hampered by circumstances.

Similar response might be encouraged in other instances of immobility. The nurse who understands the dynamics inherent in a child's incessant requests for company and for retrieval of objects out of his reach will probably plan for reducing the associated stresses. Providing for appropriate placement of articles reduces stress on patient and personnel alike; the patient realizes some self-sufficiency, and personnel are freed for other responsibilities. To occasionally move the patient in his bed to another area such as the playroom or outside patio helps relieve much anxiety associated with accumulated energies. These and other nursing interventions are essential for immobilized children.

Formal Instruction

The school-age child's coping is facilitated by intellectual control of his own progress; the nurse's coping with the child's adjustment problems is also enhanced by a definite and ongoing plan to inform him of his status and of how he can limit his symptoms.

An illustrative situation is that of a diabetic child, either newly diagnosed or found uninformed about his diabetes. To teach him effectively—in a way which will assist him to accept his condition and to appropriately alter his daily habits—requires that the nurse know (1) the child's and the family's responses to the diabetes, based on developmental and other factors; (2) the physical facilities available to the child; (3) the child's and parents' ability and willingness to learn; (4) theory of diabetes and its management. Furthermore, it demands the nurse's ability to cooperate with allied professionals inside and outside the hospital for optimum care.

The schoolchild hopefully has become accustomed to the classroom atmosphere which includes the need for study, review, and testing sessions. All these elements can be incorporated into an effective teaching plan, even though it be an individualized and one-to-one lesson. Concentration on essentials, repetition for mastery, and provision for continuing education are also prime considerations in the instruction.

Hopefully while awaiting confirmation of the diagnosis, the nurse-family relation will have been effected; upon diagnosis simple instruction can then be begun immediately, and developed according to patient-family need and ability. It is criminal to waste valuable time, only to attempt a "crash" program belatedly, since such a program serves to exaggerate anxiety.

A teaching plan should be established *for the child* since he must begin immediately to adapt at *his* cognitive and emotional level, but it must also involve parents and/or other significant persons who will help further the child's health needs. Special parental needs include relief of their guilt, knowledge of the condition, and understanding of the child's problems of adjustment to it.

Similar strategy is possible on other levels related to acute illness, avoidance of hazards, or preparation for procedures or operations. In any case, certain basic realizations will assist the nurse. In most instances that the nurse encounters, learning is related to a heightened emotional state which might influence the outcome by having either a disorganizing or an intensifying effect on the child's and family's motivation. At best such learning is narrow and deep and needs to be extended by repetition. A great degree of literalness is indicated for effectiveness, particularly with the school-age child whose cognitive skills do not yet encompass abstraction.

Continuation of Normal Life

Certain basic elements make up the school-age child's normal life, viz., peer contact, self-responsibility, recreation, and schooling. It is a simple matter to continue these, if only vicariously, by encouraging contact with the "news" from his world. Welcome is the person who informs the child of the latest athletic scores, the storm center moving in, the highlights of the national scene, the new dress a friend is wearing, or any topic which interests him, the depth of discussion being adapted to the child.

Letters or phone calls to and from family and peers are very useful measures toward continuing normality. When separation is prolonged, photographs or tape recordings provide another worthwhile dimension. Unless specifically contraindicated, visits from peers and siblings might be encouraged.

One 9-year-old hospitalized for several months enjoyed the antics of his 11-month-old brother when the physician finally permitted sibling visitation. Between visits he eagerly shared his brother's developmental progress with the nurses. This same patient had previously spent several weeks in the intensive care unit and had had a friendly relationship with one of the nurses who entertained him with stories and pictures of her dog. She continued to visit him when he was transferred to the pediatric unit, and one evening arranged to have boy and dog "meet" in his hospital room. This kind of activated awareness of childhood needs and pleasures relieves the "sick" atmosphere for a child and enhances his response to overwhelming circumstances.

The child also needs to know that his normal status in the family remains intact during his temporary indisposition. If someone has assumed his chores, he should be informed that he will resume them on his return to health. A little confession that "No one does it so well as you do" will go far to restore his waning sense of self-worth. At the same time, one must be cautious not to convey a dire need for his immediate return to health, lest a particularly serious youngster anguish over having caused so much upheaval for everyone.

If siblings are allowed to visit, the nurse might casually suggest to the mother that visitors should not be dressed in the sick child's clothing even though they might ordinarily interchange wardrobes. Verbalizing that the child is missed by siblings and peers as well as by parents and that he will return home when well frequently answers unmentioned worries.

One other very important—though often most dreaded—aspect of continuing reality in the sick room is completion of school assignments, including provision for tutoring if necessitated. Few children are so ill for extended periods as to preclude their fulfilling responsibilities for daily assignments. One commercially available device allows for telephone connection between sickroom and classroom so that the child can actively participate in learning with his peers. On another level, parents or siblings often carry assignments between teacher and child or monitor tests in the home. Few school systems have no means for continuing the child's education while ill.

In anticipation of discharge or return to normal daily life, the child profits from opportunities to prepare for the big event. Calendars help him plan ahead for *the day*; newspapers or other media keep him informed of what is important to others; an ingenious parent can help by having him plan his homecoming wardrobe and party.

Fatal Illness

To hide a fatal diagnosis from a school-age child is probably one of the least possible achievements any parent ever attempts. Whether fatality is related to an acute or chronic illness, a natural defense-like mechanism establishes itself—a mechanism which dictates "appropriate" behavior and nonbehavior toward the child. Avoidance is exercised on a physical, emotional, and/or social plane. The immediate change in the parent-child relationship confuses the child whose data sources conflict with each other: on the one hand he is told there is no problem, while on the other his nonverbal messages shout of threat. As a result he is without significant relationships at a time when he needs them most. Essentially, then, attempts to shield the child from the nature of his illness are futile.

For further discussion, see Chap. 29, "The Terminally Ill Child."

REFERENCES

1 Ednita P. Bernabeu, "The Effects of Severe Crippling on the Development of a Group of Children," *Psychiatry*, 21:169–194, 1958.
2 Ibid.
3 S. A. Richardson, A. H. Hastorf, and S. M. Dornbusch, "Effects of Physical Disability on a Child's Description of Himself," *Child Development*, 35:894, 1964.

4 Irene D. Riddle, "Communicative Behaviors of Hospitalized School Age Children with Binocular Bandages," monograph I, *Maternal-Child Nursing Journal*, 1(4):348–350, Winter 1972.

5 E. H. Erikson, *Childhood and Society*, 2d ed., W. W. Norton & Company, Inc., New York, 1963, pp. 258–261.

6 June Kikuchi, "A Preadolescent Boy's Adaptation to Traumatic Loss of Both Hands," *Maternal-Child Nursing Journal*, 1(1):19–31, Spring 1972.

7 Elizabeth Gellert, "Children's Conception of the Content and Function of the Human Body," *Genetic Psychology Monographs*, 64:293–405, May 1962.

8 Emma N. Plank, *Working with Children in Hospitals*, 2d ed., The Press of Case Western Reserve University, Cleveland, 1971.

9 Kikuchi, op. cit.

10 R. D. Hess and Virginia C. Shipman, "Early Experiences and the Socialization of Cognitive Modes in Children," *Child Development*, 36:869–886, 1965.

11 J. Piaget, *The Moral Judgment of the Child*, trans. by Marjorie Gabain, The Free Press, New York, 1965, pp. 50–84.

12 Esther F. Seeley, "Coping Behaviors of an Immobilized Eight Year Old," *Maternal-Child Nursing Journal*, 2(1):15–21, Spring 1973.

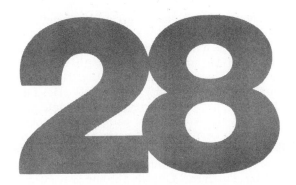

28

EFFECTS
OF ILLNESS
ON THE
ADOLESCENT

MARY JEAN DENYES and ANNE ALTSHULER

Illness may cause disruption in a child's life situation at any stage of his development. To the adolescent caught up in the task of forging his dreams into concrete plans for the future as he makes the transition from childhood to maturity, illness may be perceived as an especially difficult experience. Even when illness seems overwhelming to the adolescent, it may provide opportunities for growth that strengthen his inner resources and thus prepare him to cope more effectively with future crises of human existence.

The effects that illness may have upon adolescents are dependent upon a variety of factors. The major ones to be considered in this chapter include: (1) the strengths that adolescents have available to them to deal with illness and treatment programs; (2) the nature of imposed illnesses and treatment regimens; and (3) the character of the environment, which includes the quality of the support systems available. Knowledge of these factors provides a base for identifying how nurses can intervene to assist adolescents in adapting to their health states and the health care system in ways that promote achievement of their potential for optimal physical and psychosocial growth.

ADOLESCENT STRENGTHS

The basic question of adolescence is "Who am I?" In seeking an answer to this question, young people work at mastering a variety of developmental tasks. They strive to adapt to the physical changes occurring in their bodies, to develop satisfying heterosexual adjustments, to realign their roles within the family and community, to identify and define meaningful personal value systems, to select and prepare for vocations, and to develop their intellectual skills more fully. These developmental issues markedly influence adolescents' adaptation to health and illness states and need to be considered when providing nursing care.

Knowledge of adolescent development and understanding of the goals toward which these young people are striving enables the nurse to view as strengths many behaviors that might otherwise be perceived as limitations.

For example, while **Steve**, age 16, was being evaluated as a possible candidate for a kidney transplant, it was determined that his father was a potential donor. When Steve learned this fact, he flared with this response: "I don't want *his* kidney! . . . We never got along anyway. . . . I won't live off his kidney!"

411

The staff's immediate interpretation of Steve's behavior was one of concern about the obviously poor relationship Steve had with his father, and Steve's inability to understand the positive significance of having a kidney available for transplant. Their plan was to reteach him about the severity of his renal disease and the value of the kidney transplant and to "do something" about the family relationships. The nurse specialist reviewed with the staff the need of the adolescent to strive for independence from his parents. Immediately one of the nurses exclaimed, "Of course! How much more dependent could you feel upon your father than to know you were alive because his kidney was inside of you!" It was then possible to view Steve's response not as evidence of a limitation in ability to deal with his health state but as evidence of a strength. He had begun to express openly his feelings of conflict related to sacrificing independence in order to achieve wellness. By recognizing his response as an assertion of independence and by identifying it as a strength, it was possible to design nursing care that facilitated physical wellness and also supported his drive for independence. The above example and those that follow are included to illustrate some ways in which nurses can provide knowledgeable care by focusing on the strengths adolescents possess in dealing with illness and treatment regimens.

Adaptation to Physical Changes

Major physical changes that occur during adolescence were described in Chapter 14. These changes have great impact on the course of adolescents' physical illness states and on their psychosocial adaptation to them. In the following example the nurse responded to the developing awareness and concern related to bodily changes expressed by a hospitalized young adolescent girl.

Cindy, age 13, called the nurse into her room one day. She had had an operation to correct the curvature of her spine and was at that time lying on her abdomen sobbing hysterically. "The pain is just terrible! I can't stand it; I just can't stand it!" The nurse knew that Cindy had received medication earlier for back pain and was uncertain as to the meaning of the present outburst. To learn more, the nurse looked toward Cindy's back. Then she said to her, "What do you think might be the problem?" "No, no, not in my back! I have pain right here!" Cindy cried as she reached down toward her iliac crest. Recalling the kind of operation Cindy had had, the nurse said, "Yes, you know you had the bone chips from your

hip removed and placed in your back and . . ." "No! No! Not on that side; it's on the other side, and it's just terrible, and that's what's so scarey because there shouldn't be anything wrong with that hip." The nurse realized what was happening; Cindy was lying on the firm mattress in a position that placed pressure on her unoperated iliac crest, and she could not figure out why she would have pain there. Thinking that she might be unaware of parts of her anatomy, the nurse said, "Cindy, do you know why you have pain there?" "No," Cindy interrupted. "There is something wrong, I'm sure." Quickly the nurse went on to relieve her tension, "Cindy, you can't feel your own bone, so reach over here and put your hand on this bone on me." Cindy placed her hand on the nurse's prominant iliac crest. Her eyes lighted up and her expression seemed to say, "What is this? Is that part of me too?" To the casual observer it might seem strange that Cindy was not aware that she had that particular bone, but the excitement of self-discovery was clear. Once Cindy understood what was happening to her, she relaxed, ceased her fearful crying, and was able to help the nurse decide what could be done to alleviate the pressure and thus the pain.

The next day the nurse was walking by the room and Cindy called out to her again. "Mary, come here, I've got something else!" She was having trouble because her back hurt, and once again the pain was not at the surgical site. This time she had discovered her scapula! Cindy's concerns were viewed as strengths in that she was growing in awareness of her body and learning to adapt to its form and functions. By responding to her awakening awareness of her own body and providing information to Cindy, the nurse was able to free the energy Cindy was expending in fear and distress for use in learning and growing.

Adolescent Behavior Pattern*

In order to interpret the behavior of young people such as Steve and Cindy, it is helpful to have knowledge of a pattern of response frequently seen in adolescence. Often we become disturbed by the behavior we observe and move in impulsively to counter the actions of adolescents. In so doing, we fail to recognize that if we are patient enough to wait even a few minutes, adolescents are likely to alter their behavior to a tolerable, more balanced, mature level without our assistance.

* Material in this section is based on clinical experience of the authors, study with Florence G. Blake, and the writing of Irene M. Josselyn.

A frequent pattern of adolescent behavioral response is one characterized by an exuberant and undaunted approach to life situations often resulting in overextension of self, sufficient to provoke anxiety and fear. Then suddenly the assertive, enthusiastic youngsters may retreat in fear and regress while reassessing what is happening to them. When their dependent behavior is accepted by others, the adolescents may be protected, in part, from loss of self-esteem. However, once they recognize that they have regressed, a sense of guilt is experienced because they acted like babies and gave up the drive for independence. That recognition of what has happened spurs them on to strike out again toward adulthood. When both dependent and independent drives are expressed and accepted, adolescents have energy to assert themselves again and restart the cycle of behavior. Figure 28-1 and the following description of Coreen illustrate this pattern of adolescent behavior.

The nurse specialist received a telephone call from Mrs. R., the mother of a 14-year-old girl, who related her problem this way: "We're really having troubles. You know Coreen said we never really understood her. Well, the other night she really put us right out of our minds. She'd been lying around saying, 'You don't understand ... I've got too many restrictions from you and I can't do anything I want to! I'm going out with my friends!' She went out with her friends. During the evening they decided that this was the night they would experiment with drinking. Everyone had themselves a time and Coreen got 'woozy' from drinking beer. Then she got scared of what would happen when she got home and so she stayed out all night."

The nurse specialist reviewed in her mind the events that probably had transpired. Coreen must have realized what had happened, that she had gone out to show her parents that she really could manage herself, was grown up, and could do what everybody else was doing. She found out that she was into more than she knew how to handle, then became anxious and so afraid of possible repercussions from her parents that she did not go home.

Mrs. R. continued, "She went to school the next day and phoned me from school and asked me to pick her up. I went after her, and when she got home she stayed in her room by herself at first unwilling to talk with us." The nurse specialist knew that Coreen usually got herself to and from school easily, but on that day she pulled back and became dependent on her mother, became nonverbal, and retreated to her room. Coreen's regressive, dependent

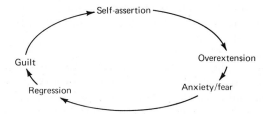

Figure 28-1   Pattern of adolescent behavior.

behavior and her withdrawal to reassess what was happening to her were accepted though not clearly understood by her mother.

"Later, when she came out of her room," Mrs. R. reported, "Coreen said she felt really lousy about what happened, but she wanted to go out again tonight!"

Coreen moved from self-assertion through overextension, anxiety and fear, regression, guilt, and back to self-assertion. These apparently conflicting messages and rapid changes in behavior were troublesome to her mother, as they often are to those living and working with adolescents.

Having knowledge of the above pattern of behavior that adolescents often evidence makes it possible for the nurse to recognize it, bear it, and respond in helpful ways. If adolescents are being assertive, the nurse can support this behavior by encouraging the self-assertion but protecting them from overextending to a degree they are totally unable to manage themselves. In the face of regression, time must be allowed for the self-reassessment and problem solving that can take place if adolescents are protected from feelings of loss of self-esteem and guilt related to regression. The supported self-reassessment and problem solving strengthen the adolescents' inner resources which help them deal more effectively with new situations. Eventually, the adolescents gain energy to reassert themselves and thus more effectively to learn and grow.

Viewing the above behavior pattern as one common in adolescence increases the nurse's ability to predict behavioral responses and determine when it is helpful to move in with support or limits and when to take a "hands-off" approach. It also helps nurses learn to trust that this pattern of behavior will contribute, in time, to the more stable behavior patterns associated with adulthood.

Achievement of Heterosexual Adjustments

The following example describes the behavior of an adolescent who was dealing with his adjustment to heterosexual relationships and the responses observed in the adults who were confronted with his behavior.

One day when the nurse specialist arrived on the hospital unit, the security guard was present and clearly distraught. He explained that the nursing staff had lost one of the patients (a 16-year-old boy), and that it was only after an extensive search of the hospital that he was finally found with his girl in the Meditation Room! General staff reaction was one of annoyance and distress: "What did Bob think he was doing anyway? He's so busy being a big shot and acting out and trying to get on people's nerves . . . as teenagers always do! There's only one thing to do, and that's not to allow him to leave the unit again!"

In interpreting Bob's behavior and determining how to assist him, the nurse specialist viewed the situation as one in which Bob was working hard at figuring out who he was with respect to himself and his girl, and that they needed a place to go where they could have privacy. Throughout their lives young people are aware of and relate with others of the same and opposite sex. However, during adolescence these relationships become crucially important to them in identifying for themselves and for others who they are. Bob had asserted and overextended himself in his striving for increased understanding of heterosexual relationships. The nurse specialist saw it to be especially important that Bob be allowed to continue to gain understanding in this area as he was paraplegic, was immobilized in a body cast, and had been hospitalized for nearly a year. These factors markedly limited the opportunity Bob had to progress with normal developmental experiences, and the nurse specialist wished to protect him from the regression that might occur as a result of punitive staff approaches. She made her office (adjacent to the unit) available to Bob so that he and his girl could sit and talk in the evening as they said they wished to do. This arrangement provided them with privacy and avoided the need for them to sneak away in search of a place where they could be alone. With this understanding, Bob began telling the staff where he was going when he left the unit and appeared to feel less secretive and guilty about his activities.

Although heterosexual behavior is not the same in all phases of adolescence, the need to support each developmental stage remains constant. Russ, age 13, was busy giggling with several young teenage girls he had recently met on the adolescent unit. When the supper trays arrived, he announced that he wanted to "eat in the girls' room." In this situation all the nurses did was grant Russ his request. He then followed through with his supper plan. During the meal Russ received a school picture from his "special girl" that he displayed on his bedside stand for 3 days until she went home and a new girl who interested him was admitted.

While it was easy to give Russ and the girls an opportunity to learn about each other, illness and hospitalization very often interrupt such contacts with peers of the opposite sex. It might have been simpler for the nurse to have Russ follow the usual routine of eating supper in his own room. The nurse might also have viewed Russ's request as a teenager's attempt to manipulate the system and have responded as if it was disruptive adolescent behavior that should be ignored, erased, or punished. Basing nursing intervention for adolescents on system efficiency or assumed behavioral limitations is to fail to promote achievement of adolescents' optimal growth potentials.

Realignment of Roles within Family and Community

The realignment of roles within family and community that normally occurs during adolescence is an important consideration when caring for ill teenagers. In the presence of chronic illness in particular, we often expect that the move from dependence on parents toward interdependence is not realistic or is, at best, slow and difficult.

The need for several months of immobilization at home in a body cast following a spinal fusion for idiopathic scoliosis was especially threatening to 14-year-old Emily, who was fighting hard to become less dependent upon her mother. The same situation was a less difficult problem for Susan, an adolescent comfortable enough with her own identity to allow her to temporarily accept help from her mother without threat or loss of self-esteem.

Strengths in the adolescent that reflect striving toward independence can be identified and used to help him grow, as can strengths in the parents.

Dan, age 18, had cystic fibrosis. He had been dependent upon his mother for an extensive treatment regimen for many years. Unlike the child with diabetes, who can usually learn to test his urine and give his own insulin injections, Dan had to rely upon a person other than himself to do his percussion and postural drainage treatments twice daily. He also experienced frequent acute episodes of his illness that required hospitalization. Through the years his mother had assumed much of the responsibility for his care at home and had stayed with him during hospitalizations. During Dan's early adolescence the nursing staff noted frequent signs of readiness for increasing independence. He asked to have his mother present when he was very ill, but sought peer companionship when he began to feel better. The nurses recognized the importance of supporting adolescent moves toward dependence on self and peers rather than on parents. They shared with Dan's mother their perception of his gains and encouraged her to maintain contact with him by visits and telephone calls during his convalescent periods. Over time, the trust she had developed in the medical and nursing staff's ability to care for Dan also helped her to separate from him. Dan began to rely increasingly upon himself and professional staff for care, calling upon his mother for help predominantly when he regressed during acute illness episodes.

In late adolescence independence can be facilitated for youngsters with chronic illnesses such as cystic fibrosis by providing alternatives for parental care, such as outpatient physical therapy or assistance by the school nurse. In Dan's situation, however, by late adolescence both he and his mother appeared comfortable and pleased with his increased reliance on himself and his peers. She readily relinquished her role in treatments to the young woman whom Dan selected as a marriage partner.

Dan moved from dependence upon his mother to interdependence with his wife. By identifying his readiness to grow and his mother's ability to free him for growth, it was possible to assist Dan in his transition from adolescence to young adulthood and to do so without threat to his health care.

Establishment of Personal Value Systems

Another necessary component of the task of adolescence is selection of a meaningful personal value system. This choice is made after much consideration and weighing of values held by parents, peers, and other persons of significance to the adolescent. The meaning of health and illness and its relative importance in life is one value examined by youth. Previously accepted treatment measures may be rejected and reconsidered by ill adolescents; they must evaluate for themselves during adolescence the possible consequences of deviation from treatment plans determined by others.

Sandi had a birth defect that caused bowel impactions; she had learned to regulate her bowel by daily enemas. At age 15, she decided she could skip some of the enemas because they were "a pain to do every day!" Unfortunately, she had not considered the possible consequences of her decision; a bowel accident at school resulted, and Sandi decided that daily enemas were worth "the pain." As a consequence, independently she resumed her daily enema regimen. The nurse who has contact with adolescents whose behavior is similar to Sandi's can try to protect them from overextending and asserting their independence in ways that may be harmful to them, and help them sort values by discussing the consequences of altering their treatment programs. If they do experiment, however, responding to their exploratory behavior in a nonpunitive fashion can help in reestablishing their equilibrium and in learning. For Sandi, it was primarily a social discomfort that resulted. The nurse needed only to indicate to Sandi that she was pleased she had learned from her experience and had made the decision to continue with her program.

For others, the consequences of deviating from the treatment programs are more life-threatening than those cited above, and there is less opportunity to learn from testing. Steve, as noted earlier in this chapter, had severe renal disease and was awaiting a kidney transplant. His threats to "skip" dialysis treatments represented, in part, a need to test out the meaning of health, illness, and treatment as it related to himself. It also probably related to his need to become increasingly more independent of his parents. Throughout childhood, parents are usually identified as primary care providers. Therefore, rejection of care by the adolescent may represent rejection of childhood dependency states.

The nurse accepted Steve's verbal rejection of treatment and dependence and indicated to him that it made sense to be angry and rejecting. Also, the nurse clarified that, although these feelings were reasonable and were similar to feelings of others, Steve needed to find ways to deal with the reality of illness in his life. In response, Steve "sounded off." Then he settled down and began reconsidering what he understood and valued in relation to his health and to life in general. "Isn't it strange," he said "that in your head you can want to be well so badly, and yet your body, which is part of you too, can make you sick?" The nursing interventions used with Steve assisted him in asserting himself verbally and protected him from overextending and harming himself physically. They helped him in continuing to learn and to work toward finding meaningful values relevant to his life.

Preparation for the Future

Adolescents expend great amounts of time and energy identifying goals and preparing for the future. As adults we often become impatient or consider it strange when a teenager focuses his concern on a goal that does not seem realistic, crucial, or relevant to us. The young adolescent's goals may be ones that are relatively close at hand, and they often relate to school or community activities. With the older adolescent, preparation for a specific career goal may assume major importance. When nurses are clear about the direction in which the adolescent is headed, they can provide care that facilitates rather than retards his progress toward attainment of his goals.

Russ, the 13-year-old boy described earlier as wanting to have supper with "the girls," had a specific concern about his future. The nurses caring for him in the hospital had concerns, too—ones that often clouded their ability to focus on Russ's needs instead of on their own. He had cancer, was going to have his leg amputated, and might not live more than 6 months. The goal that Russ had worked toward and had attained before cancer was diagnosed was to become captain of his basketball team. He knew he had cancer, but his energy was tied up in dealing with the amputation of his leg and the resultant loss of his chance to play on and lead his school team. At first the nurses' energy was expended in dealing with their own feelings about the eventual death of this delightful young adolescent.

To help Russ deal constructively with the discrepancy between *his* goal and the reality imposed by illness, a nurse asked Russ what he thought about his situation, listened to what he said, and talked with him about his feelings and about ways to make things more tolerable. She was able to focus on his concerns rather than on her own. This kind of intervention was repeated many times with Russ, and gradually over time he was able to say with sadness and with pride, "I wish I could be playing myself 'cause the team is really good, but they did ask me to be manager and that's something I can do well with one leg."

Russ's family and the nursing staff perceived his continuing interest in sports to be a strength and encouraged exploration of his abilities in athletics. In the following year he not only saw his basketball team in the championship playoff games, but he also delighted many people with his developing skill in golf, swimming, and baseball. He did explain, however, that "the Little League uses a pinch runner for me when I bat!"

If Russ's concerns and goals had not been identified and thoughtfully considered, the focus of nursing care might have been placed on helping Russ deal with death and dying when he was focused on living. Later when Russ's condition worsened, he had the strengths and ability to adjust his goals and voice his new concerns. Each time his previously made plans seemed out of reach, he actively sought help from the nurses to assist him in dealing with the difficult readjustment of his goals.

Development of Intellectual Skills

In each of the areas discussed, it has been implied that adolescents possess an ability to problem solve. Too often intellectual skills are not identified on the list of strengths that this age group has available for dealing with illness and hospitalization. The adolescent, having developed to the highest cognitive level, can use thought processes to manipulate pieces of information and achieve solutions of problems. Once he finds a solution to a problem, he can consider the consequences without actually having to act it out. Frequently the adolescent lacks the pieces of information that he needs for problem solving and the extensive experience that would assist him in deciding whether his solution will achieve his goals.

Illness and hospitalization may interfere with intellectual growth by restricting the usual learning opportunities available to adolescents. Nurses can offset this problem by providing care that assists adolescents in identifying their problem-solving abilities, in using these abilities, and in gaining confidence in use of their intellectual skills (Fig. 28-2). Adolescent intellectual capacities can be stimulated by the multiple and varied problems encountered while ill in the hospital environment.

Ken was a young adolescent, age 12, who had been hospitalized for 2 months for a psychiatric illness. When planning for discharge to his home, Ken expressed concern about returning to his bedroom where the event triggering his overt illness had occurred. His parents and several staff members immediately offered elaborate suggestions about how he could handle the bedroom problem. Then the nurse intervened by asking Ken if he had any ideas about what he could do. Immediately he beamed and said, "Yes, I've been thinking a lot about it and I think that when I'm ready to go to bed I could run up the stairs,

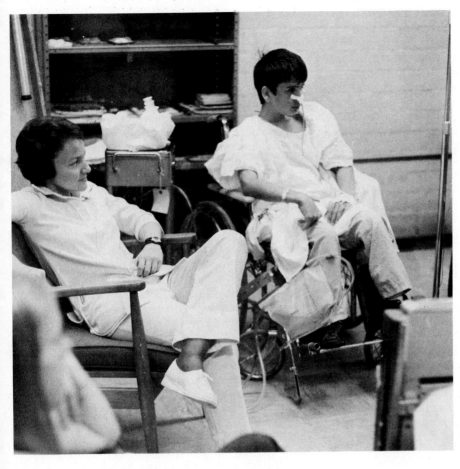

Figure 28-2 In peer discussion groups, nurses can assist adolescents with problem solving.

get into bed, and go to sleep as fast as I can so I don't have much time to think about being afraid." The solution was far simpler than those anyone else had considered, and it was one Ken thought would work for him.

The adolescent is often best equipped to know which actions will fit most comfortably into his own life-style. He knows his home routines and his school day better than anyone else, and he needs to help determine what actions are reasonable and workable for him in his own life and setting.

Fifteen-year-old **Helen** was extremely shy and modest and was upset about going home in a body cast following a spinal fusion. In talking with her nurse over a period of several weeks, she was gradually able to begin working out methods to preserve her need for privacy even while spending 3 months in a hospital bed in the family living room. She decided to ask her father to let her wear some of his shirts (something

she viewed as a special privilege), which she felt would cover her cast well. She also helped her mother design and sew some attractive clothes that would fit over the bulky cast. She thought of a way to set up a screen for privacy and decided that she would plan to use the bedpan before any company was expected to arrive. Because she was able to anticipate situations that she felt would present special difficulties and work out her own solutions, she was not overwhelmed by problems when they actually arose. These were her ideas, and she felt proud and pleased to be able to figure them out herself. She made a constructive adjustment to life at home in a body cast.

It is obvious that adolescents need to be included in plans for their treatment, to be accepted as vital members of the health care team, and to be given the kind of information they desire and need to enable them to participate in their care. They can be helped to decide what kinds and amount of information and supports are most appropriate in helping them prepare for and deal with potentially traumatic procedures. As they learn to recognize the actions that have been most helpful to them, they can begin to think them up by themselves, and thus to expand their repertoire of methods to help themselves. By recognizing adolescents' ability to work with ideas and to problem solve skillfully, and by encouraging them to practice these skills, the nurse enables them to resolve perplexing problems independently. In so doing, they are also helped to heighten their self-esteem, to reduce their dependence upon others, to become increasingly explicit in problem solving, and thus to grow toward maturity.

NATURE OF IMPOSED ILLNESS AND TREATMENT

The nature of the imposed illness and treatment regimen is a second major factor that influences the way in which an adolescent deals with stress. It is one that must be considered in designing the nursing care plan and the way in which the plan is implemented. As was noted earlier, the major physical changes that occur during adolescence clearly affect both physiologic and psychologic responses to illness.

When the illness is clearly a temporary discomfort, it may be much easier to bear than one which has an uncertain outcome or a course with no definite end in sight. This is a distinction that is not possible for the young child to make.

Ellen, age 16, was hospitalized for a rhinoplasty. She had decided to pursue a career as a ballet dancer. She felt that the rhinoplasty was important in reaching her long-term goals. She had participated in planning the time of and place for the operation. She was knowledgeable about and willing to undergo the temporary discomfort and changes in appearance that were involved. She was able to seek and use guidance from the hospital staff, her roommates, and her mother. As a consequence she was able to bear discomforts during the fairly brief hospital stay.

Cindy, who was mentioned previously, was also able to deal constructively with the discomforts of a spinal fusion once she understood the specific causes of them.

Adolescence is a time for the person to come to grips with himself and to accept his body as it is, with all its strengths and imperfections. A child born with a congenital defect will have to struggle anew in adolescence to accept the fact that he is different from his peers and unlike the way he would like to be

(Fig. 28-3). Only then can he plan goals which are realistic and consistent with his actual abilities. This takes time. He knows his body and his limitations well. His challenge is to accept the ways in which he differs from his peers, to identify his strengths and limitations, to establish realistic goals, and to discover ways to develop himself to his fullest potential. His problems may be quite different from those of the adolescent who has always taken good health for granted and then suddenly must make large-scale and unexpected changes in his self-image and goals for the future because of a sudden illness or an accident with incapacitating or disfiguring complications. The need to give up dreams and plans that were counted upon, and to reassess and reestablish relationships and roles on the basis of new and threatening changes, require considerable time and support. Yet there is some evidence to suggest that children who acquire handicaps after a period of optimal physical fitness have more self-esteem and are able to deal with anxiety better than those children who were born with congenital defects.[1]

The same illness, seen in several adolescents, may evoke strikingly different emotional responses, behaviors, and coping patterns. How an adolescent perceives and responds to an illness and hospitalization is influenced by his own particular strengths and limitations and by all his past experiences. Where he is in the course of his adolescent growth and development is of great importance. Is he in early, middle, or late adolescence? How far has he progressed in mastering the tasks and concerns that are commonly encountered during adolescence? How clear is he about his goals and his sense of himself? How does he relate to himself, to others, and to the experiences he is meeting? What kinds of accidental crises has he faced in the past, and how has he dealt with them?

Specific questions that may be raised in determining the impact of the illness on the adolescent might include the following:

1 Timing
   At what age did the illness, incapacity, or development of significant new symptoms occur?
   How much time has the adolescent had to adjust to his illness or incapacity?
   Did they appear at a time when he was using his energy and resources to deal with other changes or problems, so that the onset of illness posed an unusually potent threat?
   If so, what were the problems he was faced with when he first became ill?
2 Nature of illness
   Is the illness common and familiar, or is it one that is relatively unknown?

Is the illness socially acceptable, or is it one that tends to cause embarrassment, shame, or guilt?

Is the illness one whose very name tends to arouse unusual fears (e.g., cancer, leukemia)?

Does the illness threaten fulfillment of the adolescent's appropriate sex role or bear genetic or other implications for his children?

3   New experiences imposed

In the course of diagnosis and treatment, how much will the adolescent be asked to adjust to or cope with in the way of new experiences, people, places, treatments, and equipment?

4   Changes in body and self

What major changes in the body and self will the adolescent be forced to adjust to?

How will the illness or treatment affect his *appearance*? To what extent will his appearance differ from what it was prior to the onset of the illness? From what he desires it to be like? From the way in which he perceives the appearance of his peers?

What new *bodily sensations* must he deal with? How much physical discomfort or pain will be involved?

What illness or treatment-related changes in emotional state or response may occur (e.g., drugs that cause depression or illnesses that cause personality changes)?

How will the illness and treatment affect his *abilities and skills*, the things he enjoys and can do independently for himself?

5   Expectations for the future

To what extent will the illness cause a *change in lifestyle*? Will it necessitate separation from home, school, friends, normal activities, and interests? What major goals and dreams will have to be modified or relinquished?

Does the illness or treatment have a limited course, or is the length of the course unknown?

Is the outcome clear or uncertain?

Will the treatment of his health problem result in improved health and functioning? Eventual return to full health? Limited ongoing disability? Severe incapacity and change? Death?

How closely is the course of his illness following or deviating from set expectations?

By collecting data relating to the impact of the disease on the adolescent, the nurse will gain invaluable insights. These insights can be used to help the youngster master natural developmental tasks and also to design and implement plans of care which will support adaptations to his altered state of health in a growth-producing manner.

CHARACTER OF THE ENVIRONMENT

The character of the environment in which the adolescent must come to terms with his illness and treatment is the third major factor in determining how effectively he will cope with his problems. The concern of the persons around him and the support they are able to provide are important influences on

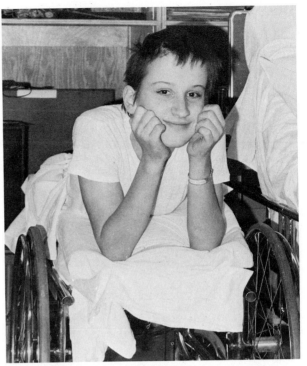

Figure 28-3   The adolescent with a congenital defect struggles anew with his body image.

the formation of adaptive responses to both long- and short-term experiences with illness. A group of peers who support the ill adolescent assist him in maintaining a sense of self-esteem and a meaningful place in his world. A family who understands and cares about him provides him with strength and stability to cope with illness. Knowledgeable and concerned school, clinic, and hospital staff members can help him gain new skills to deal with change and crisis.

When treatment necessitates hospitalization, great strain may also be put on the teenager's ability to cope with the demands of a concurrent natural, developmental crisis. This is further reason why it is so necessary that the hospital setting be designed to provide a growth-enhancing environment for adolescents. When groups of adolescents are cared for in one location, staff members can be recruited who are knowledgeable about their care and who find working with this age group an exciting, enjoyable, and challenging experience. A staff with both male and female members can give the adolescent some opportunity to have experiences with those persons he can relate to most comfortably. A staff composed of persons with a variety

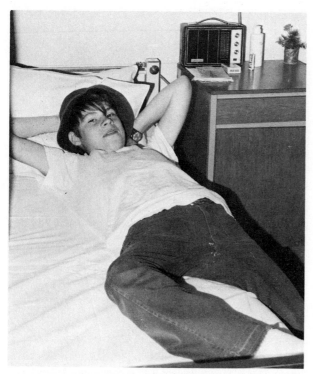

Figure 28-4 Whenever possible, adolescents should wear their own clothes during hospitalization.

of interests and talents can also help to develop each others' skills in such areas as purposeful listening, teaching, and use of humor (not teasing or ridicule, however). They can also share those methods of guidance which they have found most helpful in working with an adolescent population.

Hospital school programs can challenge adolescents to keep up with their classmates and to make progress in achieving their educational goals. This also helps to provide some semblance of normality in their disrupted life-style. Recreational programs are also of help in overcoming boredom, in releasing tension through activity, in obtaining pleasure from sharing with others, and in producing something of special value to them. Nurses can play an important role in collecting data to substantiate a need for or to point out to both lay and professional people the benefits of such programs to adolescents.

When possible, an area of the hospital should be set aside where teenagers can enjoy without disturbing others the kind of music, games, and socializing which is especially meaningful to them. For example, a lounge equipped with Ping Pong or pool table, record player, television, books and magazines, and soft-drink machine is very helpful to teen-

agers. If an outdoor area is available, a basketball and a place to shoot for baskets will be widely used, even by those adolescents who are confined to wheelchairs.

When units for adolescents do not exist, a conscious and deliberate effort will need to be made to provide individualized school and recreational programs which interest and stimulate teenager involvement. It is helpful for a nursing staff to compile a list of resource people who can be brought in to provide such services to adolescents in general hospital units. Such a list might include high school teachers or tutors, nurse specialists, recreation workers, and volunteers who have expertise in working with teenagers.

The adolescent may want to participate in making the decision of whether to be admitted to a pediatric or to an adult unit when no adolescent unit exists. Many teenagers find real satisfaction in being able to share their experiences as a means of helping to prepare other patients for special procedures, tests, or experiences in the hospital or clinic. They may enjoy and benefit from recognition of any contributions they can make in the hospital setting. They may want to help feed or entertain an elderly or a young patient in the same area of the hospital. They may want to deliver the mail or help with some of the clerical work at the nurses' station. One student in an art school proudly donated several of his paintings to decorate the unit on which he had been hospitalized.

Flexibility of institutional rules, made with respect for the growing sense of independence and responsibility on the part of adolescents, can also be of help. For example, 17-year-old Jim, hospitalized far from his home for several weeks of radiation therapy for Hodgkin's disease, left the hospital "on pass" with friends, family, staff members, or alone, whenever he felt well enough to go out after his treatment. He assumed complete responsibility for signing out and returning according to plan. Hospitalized adolescents enjoy sending out for a pizza together, or watching a late television program and having their need to "sleep in" the next morning respected. All these activities respect the worth of teenagers, convey a sense of caring about them as individuals, and demonstrate the staff's ability to bend institutional tradition to provide for the satisfaction of personal needs.

Adolescents have to maintain their sense of identity in the face of a changed body, an unfamiliar setting, new expectations, and difficult problems. Making it possible for them to wear their own clothes if they so desire and to decorate their bed

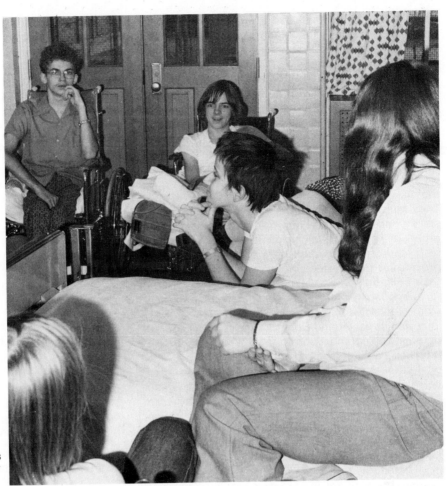

Figure 28-5 Adolescents frequently derive support from discussions with peers who are coping with similar problems.

and room to express themselves and to make them uniquely theirs also manifests respect for their personal likes and dislikes (Fig. 28-4). Bulletin boards at each bedside can allow for hanging of favorite posters or cards. When possible, provision of a space for privacy where an adolescent can be alone if he feels a need to be is also of importance. A quiet conference room for private conversations, as well as provision for privacy while bathing, dressing, being examined, and treated, are essential to meet the needs of teenagers. Access to mirrors in rooms and bathrooms is also needed and especially valued by both sexes.

Most teenagers are dependent on their peer group for support. When they are ill and hospitalized, access to friends is important. Whenever the teenagers' conditions permit, their friends should be welcomed in the hospital and space provided where they can meet without disturbing others. Adolescents are usually quick to make new friends in the

hospital and frequently derive much support from peers who are coping with similar problems. This characteristic can be supported by appropriate selection of roommates, by provision for regular meetings of teenagers in the hospital, and also by setting up group meeting hours in clinics for adolescents with similar health problems (Fig. 28-5). School nurses can play a vital role in helping adolescents meet and support each other in dealing with health-related issues. Bedside telephones are invaluable to hospitalized teenagers. With them they can maintain contact with their friends at home and continue to derive support from them. Telephones also serve to preserve interest in an activity which was probably an important part of their life-style at home.

Many parents of adolescents are at a stage in their lives when they are nearing the end of their childbearing and perhaps of their child rearing years as well. Even though they welcome this period in their lives, they may feel shut out while their adolescent sons or daughters are struggling to establish their own identities. More and more, personnel in health care facilities are dealing directly with adolescents rather than indirectly through their parents. The recent growth of birth control information centers, venereal disease treatment units, and abortion clinics has contributed to this trend. While this may serve to help the adolescent feel responsible and respected on his own right, many parents feel excluded while their offspring are being treated in clinics or in the hospital. They love and have concern for their children regardless of their age. Parents, too, have questions and fears when children are ill. They want to know about the course of their youngster's illness and the rationale of the treatment regimen. They need to feel that hospital and clinic staff members care about them as parents and will provide for their needs and concerns as well as for their children's.

Each family must be studied and evaluated individually to determine the most helpful plan of guidance for its members. Some adolescents and their parents will feel most comfortable when the nurse's interviews are held with them separately during hospital admission or clinic visits. Others will prefer to be interviewed together. Some benefit most by an opportunity to talk together as a family and also separately with the nurse. In some instances a nurse can be instrumental in helping a family discuss their problems more openly together than they have before and thus take steps toward their resolution. In all instances, both the adolescent and his parents will need to feel that the nursing staff respects and understands their problems, concerns, and particular needs for help.

SUMMARY

Three major factors to be considered in providing nursing care for adolescents who are ill have been identified. They have been discussed and illustrated with examples of behavior, nursing care, and adolescents' responses to it. The factors are: (1) the strengths that adolescents have available to them to deal with illness and treatment programs, (2) the nature of imposed illnesses and treatment regimens, and (3) the character of the environment, which includes the quality of the support systems available. Nurses' abilities to make sensitive and careful observations and analyses of what they see, hear, feel, and think, and to use the information gathered to plan

and provide nursing care in a thoughtful, purposeful manner, will be a decisive factor in determining the outcomes of their nursing interventions.

The nursing care of adolescents has special characteristics. It cannot be called easy, nor is it always difficult. It is energy-consuming, but it is also stimulating, thought-provoking, and challenging. Special rewards will await those nurses who persist in working through the ofttimes painful problems that present during initial experiences with ill adolescents. Understanding adolescents' strengths and needs makes it possible for nurses to use their creativity fully and as a consequence also get the joy that comes from observing growth and realizing that they have had a hand in making it possible.

REFERENCES

1 Beverly A. Myers, S. B. Friedman, and I. B. Weiner, "Coping with a Chronic Disability: Psychosocial Observations of Girls with Scoliosis Treated with the Milwaukee Brace," *American Journal of Diseases of Children*, 120(3):181, September 1970.

BIBLIOGRAPHY

Blake, Florence: "Immobilized Youth: A Rationale for Supportive Nursing Intervention," *American Journal of Nursing*, 69(11):236–2369, November 1969.

Brunswick, Ann F.: "Health Needs of Adolescents: How the Adolescent Sees Them," *American Journal of Public Health*, 59(9):1730–1745, September 1969.

Dempsey, Mary O.: "The Development of Body Image in the Adolescent," *Nursing Clinics of North America*, 7(4):609–615, December 1972.

Fine, L. L.: "What's a Normal Adolescent? A Guide for the Assessment of Adolescent Behavior," *Clinical Pediatrics*, 12(1):1–5, January 1973.

Josselyn, Irene M.: *The Adolescent and His World*, Family Service Association of America, New York, 1952.

Lindheim, Roslyn, Glaser, Hellen G., and Coffin, Christie: *Changing Hospital Environments for Children*, Harvard University Press, Cambridge, Mass. 1972.

Lowenberg, June S.: "The Coping Behaviors of Fatally Ill Adolescents and Their Parents," *Nursing Forum*, 9(3):269–287, 1970.

Reif, Laura: "Managing a Life with Chronic Disease," *American Journal of Nursing*, 73(2):261–264, February 1973.

Robischon, Paulette: "The Challenge of Crisis Theory for Nursing," *Nursing Outlook*, 15(7):28–32, July 1967.

Schowalter, J. E., and Lord, Ruth D.: "The Hospitalized Adolescent," *Children*, 18(4):127–132, July-August 1971.

Scofield, Cheryl: "Adolescents in the Hospital," *Maternal Child Nursing Conference*, Department of Pediatric and Obstetric Nursing, University of Pittsburgh, 1966, pp. 1–4.

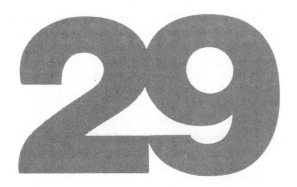

THE TERMINALLY ILL CHILD

JEANNE QUINT BENOLIEL

There is no more difficult problem in nursing practice than providing care for the terminally ill child and his family. The purpose of this chapter is four-fold: to provide some general information about the cultural, social, and psychologic dimensions of death and dying as critical problems in nursing practice; to clarify the special meanings associated with the death of a child and the high-stress nature of nursing work with children who have terminal illnesses; to provide some guidelines to assist nurses in their ongoing interactions with children who are facing death, with members of their families, and with other members of the health care team; and to identify some specific ways by which nurses can function to help dying children and their families during the final period of time they have together.

UNDERSTANDING THE CONTEXT OF DYING
Influence of Cultural and Social Values

Since the beginning of human life, birth and death have existed as moments of significance in the ongoing life of social groups. These important events serve as markers of transition and change, and social rituals and special practices are used by groups to identify the rites of passage associated with the gain or loss of a member. Customarily, special functionaries such as priests or healers are designated to officiate at these ceremonies and assist the other members of the group through the period of transition. In the case of death, all human societies have developed one or more cultural systems—combinations of words and actions—which serve to help the members come to terms with and adapt to the personal and the social meanings of death.

Human beings learn to interpret death on the basis of the cultural and social values of the society in which they live. The values which dominate in the society determine to a great extent the settings in which people die, the events which take place when a person is defined to be dying, and the behaviors which are expected of the various people who are involved. In a real sense, the orientations toward death in any society are expressions of the general character of the culture of that society.

In the United States death expectations and attitudes have been greatly influenced by the dominant values of the white, Anglo-Saxon, middle-class culture which stresses mastery over nature, emphasis on future-time orientation instead of past or present, individualism, and an activity-orientation of *doing* instead of simply being or becoming.[1] As far as each individual is concerned, the personal meanings of death are also influenced by other cultural and social conditions: the amount of direct exposure a person has to death and dying; his membership in an ethnic subgroup with values and beliefs at variance with the dominant system; and membership in a particular religious denomination. Concerning the latter point, there are wide variations in beliefs about death and afterlife among the many religions of the world, and in many cases these religious beliefs play a part of considerable importance when someone is about to die.

Today the death expectations and attitudes of people in the United States have been affected by four important conditions. First, with the increase in longevity has come a tendency for people to transpose death from an immediate and always present menace to a distant and remote prospect. It is no longer natural to die at an early age, and death has come to be equated with being old. Second, Americans in general are insulated from perceptions of death and direct experience with persons who are dying because the ill and the elderly tend to be removed to special institutions and communities. Third, the growth in scientific knowledge and applied technology in the twentieth century has created the expectation that death, too, can be defeated if enough time, energy, and money are invested to solve the problem. Finally, people no longer participate in a society which is dominated by tradition, by lineage and kinship ties, or by accepted dogma. The old systems of social control once clearly provided by church, state, and family have given way to the concept of individual freedom, accompanied by a sense of personal responsibility and increased levels of anxiety.

As these changes took place in the United States, a sociocultural system evolved which has led to a depersonalization and fragmentation of the experience of human death.[2] From the perspective of sociology, such a system serves to protect society from the disruptive influences of death by separating the dying from the living and by developing bureaucratic procedures for managing death and dying as routine social matters.[3] Psychologically, however, persons who are facing death—whether as patients with incurable illness, as members of families, or as caretakers—are not provided with easy answers for the problems they encounter nor have they been prepared for effective performance in the new roles and role-relationships which the event of death brings into being.

Influence of Technology on Caretaking

One important feature of the modern death system is a division of labor among various specialists, some of whom offer services to the dying, some to the dead, and still others to the survivors. Heavily influenced by the high value attached to science and technology in Western society, the education of these many specialists (funeral directors, clergymen, physicians, nurses, social workers, and others) has emphasized the technical aspects of their work. Relatively less attention has been given to preparing these many specialists for the task of providing psychosocial care to patients and families faced with life-threatening illness or with the emergency of sudden and unexpected death.

In the case of health-care workers, education for terminal care has by and large stressed the application of medical technology to prevention of death and has encouraged the development of attitudes of "life-saving at all costs." Thus, the importance attached to science and technology has led to educational practices which emphasize the *cure goal* of practice somewhat at the expense of the *care goal*.

The influence of technology on caretaking in the twentieth century is epitomized in the development of life-prolonging machinery and techniques. Since the Second World War new surgical techniques, antibiotics and chemotherapy, advances in parenteral medication and treatment, and life-assisting mechanical devices all make possible the prolongation of living—and the prolongation of dying. Useful as these discoveries may be, the new technologies have added to the complexity of medical decisions when the threat of death is present.[4]

Social Structure and Social Relationships

Medical specialization and applied technology have also contributed to the development of a variety of special-purpose hospital wards, a number of which are designed specifically to offer intensive treatment through application of highly specialized techniques and life-saving procedures. At the same time there has been an increase in specialization among physicians and a tremendous growth both in numbers and types of paramedical workers. These two outcomes of medical specialization have combined to create problems in the delivery of *personalized services*—not only to patients who are facing death, but to patients in general.

These two changes—the great increase in numbers of different types of health-care workers and the development of special-purpose wards in hospitals—have had important consequences for both patients and staff. The organizational structures of hospitals have become extremely complex, resulting in barriers to effective patient care. For example, communication between and among the many different health-care workers employed in the hospital is difficult to achieve. More than that, the heavy focus on life-saving at all costs and the development of intensive-care wards in which large numbers of patients are facing the threat of death have increased the psychologic stresses and strains of hospital work when patients are thought to be dying. These problems are exceptionally acute in settings where nurses are faced with life-and-death choices at frequent intervals; recent reports have described in some detail the situational and psychologic stresses and strains experienced by nurses on intensive-care wards.[5, 6]

Clearly, the problems associated with death in the hospital have increased in intensity. At the same time, more and more people are being sent to hospitals to die. Reflecting the primary values of society, the hospital system places a high priority on the delivery of life-prolonging services. Such a system serves to perpetuate the general societal pattern of denying the reality of forthcoming death and facilitates a depersonalization of experience during the final period of living.

A major characteristic in modern society is the social isolation of the person who is dying. This isolation takes two forms: placement in special settings remote from home and family, and limitations in opportunity to talk about the reality of forthcoming death. The removal of those who are dying into hospitals and other special institutions means that increasingly nurses and other health-care personnel are involved in social affairs that once belonged primarily to the family, to the extended kinship group, or both. In addition, nurses are faced with many situations in which the goals of care and cure come into conflict.

The Goals of Care and Cure

Nurses and doctors have always been caught between the two somewhat conflicting goals of practice: to do everything possible to keep the patient alive, *but* to do nothing to prolong pain and suffering uselessly. The availability of life-prolonging machines, organ transplants, and other extreme treatments has contributed to the development of hospital environments in which *care of the person* has become secondary to prevention of death. For nurses, there are two matters that are of serious concern today: the difficult choices and decisions faced by them when the conflicting goals of recovery care and comfort-until-death care converge, and the management of the social and psychologic aspects of care when patients are dying.

The basic dilemma for nurses centers around the problem of delivering personalized care in a context which attaches prime value to cure. Whereas the cure goal deals with the objective aspects of the case, the care goal deals with the subjective meaning of the disease experience. In essence, personalized care requires practitioners to be concerned with the subjective elements of the situation and to behave toward the patient as a human being, not as a "case." In addition, personalized care means facing the reality that patient care today is provided by groups of practitioners who together provide services to patients. I think of personalized care for each patient as having three components: *continuity of contact* with at least one person who is interested in him as a human being; *opportunity for active involvement* in social living to the extent that he is able—including participation in decisions affecting how he will die; and *confidence and trust* in those who are providing his care.[7]

The delivery of care for patients facing death requires the combined efforts of many disciplines. The provision of personalized services needs a systems-oriented approach to planning based on the assumption that *continuity* as well as *care* must be built into the system when multiple numbers of people are involved. More than that, persons holding key positions in the system must be willing to assume leadership in the direction and management of the social and psychologic components of care.

Within the organized system of health-care services, nurses hold key positions in the communication networks which influence what happens to dying children and their families. Not just nurses in hospitals are influenced in these matters. Nurses in doctors' offices, in clinics, and in schools can often play vital parts in the ongoing daily experiences of children faced with shortened life spans. To assist these children, however, nurses must be willing to accept responsibility for the difficult task of helping people cope with the changes associated with forthcoming death.

Teamwork is especially critical in matters of psychosocial care where the "expert" who is needed by the patient and/or family may or may not be a physician. As later sections of the chapter indicate, children with fatal illnesses as well as their families need different kinds of assistance at different points in time, and they face many problems that are nonmedical in nature. Furthermore, the child's need for help may be quite different from that required by the members of his family, and often more than one helping person is needed if effective family-centered care is to be implemented. Thus, the goal of personalized, family-centered services can be achieved only when communication, collaboration, and cooperation among the different health-care professional and nonprofessional workers is valued and encouraged.

In today's complex health-care system, the goal of personalized care cannot be achieved by any one discipline alone. In fact, achievement of the goal requires that teamwork be recognized as a necessary commodity by *all* members of the health-care team. In addition, practice at teamwork needs to take place if persons in different disciplines are to learn how to solve difficult problems of patient care together. Furthermore, each member of the team must be willing to accept responsibility for his contribution to the overall plan and program of care and to be held accountable for the outcomes. I submit that nurses must be willing to accept responsibility for their choices and actions in the provision of terminal care if the human needs of patients are to receive attention comparable with that presently given to life-saving activities and procedures.

The Meaning of Death in Childhood

Difficult as is the provision of psychosocial care in general, the problem increases in complexity when the person who is dying happens to be a child. In any country which places a high value on youth and childhood, the death of a child assumes uncommon proportions. In the United States, to die as a child is to die out of phase, and such deaths are conceived as carrying a high social loss.[8] The public expectations for "miracles" in the application of curative measures add to the stresses for families and health-care workers whenever a child is threatened with death. Thus, for everyone concerned, the appearance of life-threatening disease in childhood means difficult problems of adaptation to a critical change with many psychologic and social dimensions.

Each member of the family responds to the change in terms of its special meanings for him. In the case of the child with the terminal illness, psychologic and social stresses come not only from the threat to his life per se but also from the attitudes and actions of those around him. Sources of stress for the siblings (as with the fatally ill child) rest as much with the effects of the terminal illness on the behaviors of others (especially the parents) as with their own personal responses to the child who is ill. For parents there is probably no more devastating experience than the fatal illness and loss of a child. In fact, the child's final experience of living depends on how his parents and other signifi-

cant persons come to terms with his forthcoming death.

In addition to these personal reactions, the family as a functioning unit is faced with a major crisis of adaptation. Life-threatening illness introduces many different kinds of stress and strain into the social system of family relationships. In the case of sudden death, the family faces adjustment to an unexpected and unforeseen loss, and young families in particular have had little or no experience to prepare them for coping with such events. When the crisis extends over long periods of time, as is true with certain chronic diseases, the adjustments required of the family vary and change depending on the stage of illness. That is to say, the stresses and strains for families will be different at the time of diagnosis, during periods of exacerbation of illness, at the point when death occurs, and during the postdeath period of bereavement.[9]

There are also serious stresses and strains for health-care practitioners when the threat of death in childhood is present. Nurses, for example, encounter many difficulties in the provision of psychosocial care for patients and families simply because they *feel* themselves *caught* between the conflicting goals of cure and care. When there is very little that they can do to prevent death, nurses often find themselves caught up in feelings of helplessness, hopelessness, and sometimes despair. At times they experience anger and frustration; on other occasions they can feel guilt. Not uncommonly, they find themselves experiencing a deep sense of personal identification with the patient or his family because of reminders of their own situation.

Reactions of this nature are to be expected in anyone who must face the frustrations of a life-threatening situation. In addition, the daily contact with dying children and their families during periods of hospitalization makes nurses especially vulnerable to feelings of loss when the patient finally dies. Those who are beginning as practitioners need to be aware that dying in childhood is a high-stress situation for all concerned. The ability to provide personalized services under these difficult circumstances means learning to cope constructively with many difficult feelings and decisions and to develop the capacity to remain compassionate in the face of multiple stresses and strains.

UNDERSTANDING THE EXPERIENCE OF DYING
The Child's Concept of Death

Nurses who work with dying children and their families can be most effective if they understand the complex circumstances that influence the meaning of death to children (and to the significant others in their lives). A child's behavior in response to a death or a perceived threat to life, either his own or another's, is determined by several factors in combination. Among these factors are three that have been found to be extremely influential: ideas about the meaning of life and death as a function of concept development; socialization into particular cultural patterns of bereavement; and amount of direct exposure to death, dying, and life-threatening situations.

Stages of Concept Development The development of a concept of death takes place by stages that are directly related to the normal developmental sequence of biological and psychologic growth. That is, the age of the child influences his ideas about death, and these ideas in turn influence the way he responds when he is faced with death as part of his personal situation. Movement toward comprehension of death from an adult perspective is a steplike process through which a child passes as he comes to understand death both as an abstract entity and as a universal human experience. How the process takes place is determined in great measure by the adults who are responsible for socializing the child. Whether adult comprehension is eventually attainable does, of course, depend on the child's having an intact and functioning neuroendocrine system.

The child who is 3 years of age or younger does not distinguish between death and absence, and for this reason, the departure of mother (or other significant person) is experienced as abandonment. When these young children must be hospitalized, they generally respond to the departure of parents with expressions of anger and loud protest. In his studies of young children's reactions to the experience of hospitalization, Bowlby described three phases of response to separation: protest, followed by despair, and then detachment—during which phase the parents may be completely ignored by the child.[10] These and other studies have shown clearly that children under the age of 5 years respond with *separation anxiety* long before they are able to consider the possibility of their own deaths.

Because the child under 3 years has not yet learned to separate life and death, he thinks of death as a reversible fact. Not surprisingly when he is informed that someone has died, he continues to talk about the dead person from his own frame of reference—as a living being. The young child's pattern of thinking is not the same as that used by an adult, and fantasy and reality are not sharply separated from one another.

Between 3 and 6 years the majority of children begin to understand death as something that happens to others. Children at this age are better able to tolerate short separations than are younger children, but their ideas about death are strongly affected by their feelings in response to relations with their parents. For example, the child's aggressive impulses and actions as he strives for autonomy are often thwarted by his parents, and he in turn develops hostile death wishes toward them. During this period of developmental conflict, the child tends to personify death, and often the concept becomes confused in his mind with magical thoughts, mystery, and punishment. The diagnosis of serious illness in the child at this time in his development can easily be experienced as a retribution for "bad thoughts" or actions.

The child of 6 to 11 years moves closer to identifying death as a personal event. According to several studies, children in this age group conceive of death as caused by an external agent. Also during these years, children are prone to associate injury and mutilation with death itself. As many psychoanalytic writers have noted, children are unable to differentiate in the mind between the *wish* and the *deed*; hence they easily feel remorse and guilt even though those reactions are not at all logical to the realities of the situation. It is useful to be aware that children in preadolescence are vulnerable to intense feelings of guilt in association with death because of patterns of thinking and reacting that are characteristic of development during these years.

By the time of early adolescence, most children intellectually understand the universality and permanency of death. Although in a general and abstract sense these young people conceptualize death as an inevitable process, in the personal sense they may not truly comprehend death as an event occurring to persons close to them.[11] Applying the concept of death to themselves is a devastating experience for young people in adolescence. Physical illness in and of itself is hard to bear during this time when physical beauty and physical activity are important standards of personal esteem and social worth. To know that life is being cut short by fatal illness means *death before fulfillment*—a fate which few if any can face with equanimity.

Cultural Patterns of Bereavement Although the conceptual understanding of death can be shown to follow a definite developmental sequence roughly the same in children in all societies, attitudes and expectations associated with death are not necessarily the same and are learned out of experiences in particular cultures. Through a combination of direct and indirect practices by adults, children are socialized to behave toward death in patterned ways that are typical for the society in which they live. Not only do children learn particular sets of ideas about death, they also learn particular ways of acting and reacting when someone dies. Bereavement behaviors derive from patterned systems of family and kinship relationships; and these relationships influence the range, frequency, intimacy, and quality of interaction among the persons who compose the system.

Patterns of emotional attachment are not the same in all societies, and typically different bereavement behaviors are observed in societies with different kinship structures and customs.[12] In Western societies of the Northern European traditions, for example, the open expression of grief is not encouraged, and controlled behavior in public is expected during the period immediately following a death. By comparison, in traditional Arab communities the open expression of grief is anticipated, and mourning among family and friends is demonstrated loudly and obviously immediately following a death.[13] Knowledge about cultural and ethnic differences such as these is essential information if effective services for psychosocial care are to be made available.

The development of emotional responses to death is critically influenced by the attitudes and actions of the family members who socialize the child into the customs of his society. Not only do they introduce him to the roles he will be expected to play, they also provide him with ways of conceptualizing the meaning of life—the latter generally taking place through a form of religious training. In particular, religious upbringing influences what a child will learn about death and afterlife, and religions differ in what they teach about life, death, and the existence of an afterlife. Schowalter is of the opinion that children exposed to death in a nonfrightening way tend to be less fearful than those without such exposure, and belief in a benevolent God and reunion after death may be more hopeful than belief to the contrary.[14] By comparison, religions that espouse severe punishment after death do not provide much consolation, and children socialized into such systems of belief may respond to serious illness with intense fear—even terror. The point is that religion per se cannot be viewed as a safeguard against fears about death, and the nurse, to be effective in interaction, needs to understand the patient's responses in terms of his religious beliefs rather than her own.

Direct Exposure to Death   The amount of direct exposure a child has to death has also been found to influence the way he conceptualizes its meanings and its causes. A study of death conceptualization in Midwestern children and youth revealed that death due to violence was found more frequently among children of lower socioeconomic status than in those of a higher socioeconomic level.[15] Black children who grow up in the inner cities, unlike their counterparts in the white suburbs, are exposed to the fact of death early—sometimes in brutal ways.[16] So, too, are the children who are born and reared in countries ravaged by war and constant internal strife.

Children are very vulnerable to the loss of persons important in their lives. Recent evidence suggests that loss of a significant person during childhood not only influences ideas about death but may also seriously interfere with personality development and may even contribute to behavior disorders in later life.[17] In a very real sense, the defense mechanisms developed by a child for coping with death are dependent on the child-rearing practices used by the adults who socialize him in combination with direct experiences that are perceived by the child as threatening to his existence.

Psychologic Impact of Life-Threatening Disease

To think about death in the abstract is one thing. Direct experience with the psychologic impact of death as a personal threat is quite another. For both the child and his family, the process of living with life-threatening disease requires psychologic adjustments that take place by stages. In general, the process begins with the announcement of the diagnosis.

Crisis of Discovery   For parents, the crisis of discovery begins when they are told the diagnosis of fatal illness, although often they are aware that "something is wrong" prior to this event. Typically, parents respond to the announcement with feelings of "shock," sometimes disbelief. During this critical period of initiation, emotional reactions of guilt and self-blame are frequent. So also is a persistent effort to seek information about the disease by asking questions, by reading newspapers and magazines, and by actively seeking data that will refute the negative prognosis.[18]

The child's reaction at the time of diagnosis depends on a combination of circumstances. His age, what he is told about what is happening, whether he is hospitalized—all influence the child's behavior in response to his illness. If the crisis begins with an acute episode of physical illness, the child may display little psychologic response or open expression of emotions, simply because his energies are taken up in combating the disease process. For example, fever and dehydration are physically depleting experiences; under these conditions the child is prone to be both lethargic and apathetic.

Because children tend to be sensitive to the covert as well as the overt reactions of their parents, children will respond to the tensions they sense in their parents even though the name of the disease and the prognosis are not understood by them. They undoubtedly know that something is wrong, but the extent to which they associate what is happening at this point with their own death at some time in the future varies a good deal.

Course of Illness The process of discovery marks the beginning of a social experience which has been termed the *dying trajectory*.[19] There are several types of dying trajectories, and the social characteristics of each are directly tied to the course of the physical illness. In some cases, the crisis of discovery is followed rapidly by the child's death, as can happen after an accident or an acute fulminating illness. Under such circumstances, the family has little opportunity for *anticipatory grief* and must abruptly find ways of adapting to the sudden loss of a child.

Death may not always take place immediately, however, and the time interval prior to the end may extend for a few days to several weeks. This relatively short-term pattern of dying can be precipitated by accidents and other injuries, serious burns, acute communicable diseases, and infections that do not respond to treatment. When the course of illness is extended and death is delayed, the persons involved have time to begin the adjustment to forthcoming death by anticipatory grieving. The extent to which they can do so, however, depends on whether they are able to face the reality that the child is dying and are allowed or encouraged by others to enter into mourning.

Facing the prospect of loss of a child may be especially difficult when the anticipated death is due to an accident, and markedly so if the parents see themselves as having been causative agents for the injuries sustained by the child. Severe reactions of guilt can be expected under these conditions, often effectively interfering with initiation of the process of grieving. (Similar reactions can also appear in siblings, though the hospital staff is not always aware that other children in the family are caught up in these feelings of guilt and blame.)

A somewhat different situation occurs when a child is born with a life-threatening disability such as congenital defect of the heart. A child so born essentially begins the dying trajectory at the moment of his birth, and families find themselves living with a "dying" child from the very beginning. In situations of this type, the change in the child's status may come about only through surgical intervention which, if successful, can result in "cure" for the life-threatening situation. Sometimes, of course, such intervention brings an end to the trajectory—with the child's death occurring either in the operating room or during the early postoperative period.

Another type of pattern of dying is one in which the course of disease spreads across a number of years. Leukemia, for example, is a disorder which is marked by exacerbations and remissions of physical illness and which persists for something like 3 to 5 years in children before death finally comes. Under these conditions, the child and his family find themselves having to learn to live with the ambiguities of an uncertain future. The adaptational tasks required of these families have been described as follows: The parents must maintain an investment in the welfare and future of the sick child while at the same time preparing for his death through anticipatory mourning. The parents face the dilemma of maintaining a sense of mastery while at the same time coming to terms with the terminal nature of the child's illness. The child himself faces the equally problematic dilemma of integrating the losses and changes produced by his illness while still fulfilling his personal potential for life to the extent that he is able.[20]

A similar pattern of living with uncertainty, but one that often exists for long periods of time, follows when a child is diagnosed as having cystic fibrosis. Although generally labeled as chronic rather than fatal, cystic fibrosis (especially when the respiratory system is involved) introduces families to a cyclic pattern of acute exacerbations of respiratory infection and a progressive tendency for multiple complications to develop. Because of its genetic origins, cystic fibrosis is also likely to appear in more than one child in a family. Needless to say, the psychosocial difficulties of daily living can be compounded tremendously when a family finds itself having to cope continuously with the special needs of several children with chronic disease.

Not only do parents of children with cystic fibrosis undergo the same intrapsychic reactions that have been reported in parents of leukemic children, they are faced with a time-consuming set of treatment procedures that openly impinge on other types of family activities. The life-threatening nature of cystic fibrosis produces another set of stresses reported by parents to include the following: extreme stress when the diagnosed child asks questions about the prognosis of his illness; the presence of siblings who are aware of the prognosis; and a feeling of anticipatory anxiety about a living cystic fibrotic child when there has been a prior death of a child from cystic fibrosis.[21] The extent to which the "death concerns" associated with cystic fibrosis produce a social context of chronic stress has perhaps not been fully appreciated.

Stages of Psychologic Adjustment The process of learning to live with life-threatening illness takes place by stages. Everyone involved—family members, health-care personnel, the child himself—goes through a series of psychologic steps through which he assimilates the change in status into his own concept of reality. The process of psychologic adaptation to forthcoming death takes place through five stages: shock and disbelief during which denial is a commonly observed pattern of behavior; gradual awareness of the reality of the change in condition accompanied generally by expressions of anger and guilt; reorganization of relationships with other people; resolution of the loss through active grieving; and a reorganization of identity incorporating the changes that take place.[22]

Concerning preparation for death, the third stage may include efforts to strike a bargain (usually with God, but sometimes with the doctor) to have death postponed. Once the person begins to assimilate the reality of what is happening, he moves into depression and active grief. If enough time and energy can be given to mourning and preparation for death, the point of acceptance can finally be reached.[23]

These psychologic stages of dying—the means of coming to terms with death—do not necessarily take place in a straightforward and easy manner. Rather, people generally have to repeat the stages each time they go through a serious episode of physical regression and/or hospitalization. Those who work with dying children and their families need to recognize that the stages can repeat themselves over and over again.

People also vary a good deal in their capacities to experience the full impact of anger, frustration, guilt, sadness, and grief and to display these emotions openly. Persons who have been taught from early childhood that the open expression of feelings is legitimate will by and large move through the stages of psychologic adaptation with greater ease than will those who identify overt expression of emotion as a sign of weakness or loss of control. Indeed, Lindemann's well-known study of the processes of grief showed that resolution of grief required some capacity to come to grips with guilt and mourning and that unresolved grief led to pathologic outcomes.[24] Respect for individual differences in background and life experience is a necessary characteristic for nurses who seek to help dying children and their families come to terms with forthcoming death.

During the course of fatal illness in childhood, the child will commonly be in and out of the hospital several times before he dies. Each episode of acute illness can serve as the triggering mechanism for renewed concerns about death, but hospitalization per se can in and of itself contribute to difficulties. As noted before, very young children respond to separation from their parents as a form of abandonment, and repeated hospitalizations can lead to high levels of anxiety and a tendency to cling fearfully to mother. The child who is somewhat older can come to associate hospitalization with active rejection by his family, and his concerns about separation are generally compounded by his fears about shots and other painful procedures. Caught up in emotions of fear and anger, a child can easily respond to reentry into the hospital by openly rejecting his parents through direct verbal attacks or by complete withdrawal from interaction with them. Either of these reactions is difficult for the majority of parents to bear, and either reaction adds to the problems faced by nurses when the disease is known to be a fatal one.

Because hospitalization often means painful procedures and difficult treatments for the child, readmission to the hospital is a difficult experience for the parents as well as for him. Very much in contrast, during periods of remission of the disease the parents and the child can easily deny the reality of the life-threatening situation. When hospitalization is again required, both are reminded once more of the terminal disease which affects their daily lives.

Psychosocial Problems and Adaptations

Psychologic Reactions and Role Relationships The onset of a life-threatening illness in a child marks the beginning of a time interval during which major psychologic and emotional adaptations are required of all persons involved. For the young person himself, the diagnosis serves as the marker initiating a major change in identity. Facing the prospect of a shortened life is especially difficult for adolescents who understand, more so than do younger children, that their lives are being cut short. Not uncommonly, young people of this age feel bitter and resentful, often expressing these reactions quite freely and openly to those around them. Other young people can turn these reactions inward, and respond by withdrawing from social contacts and social relationships.

A number of important changes are initiated by the diagnosis of fatal disease. In the first place, the child finds himself faced with "being different," and this phenomenon contributes to changes in self-perception and role-performance. If the physical changes produced by the illness are severe, these visible signs of "being different" add further to alterations in self-concept, in performance of roles, and in role-relationships with significant persons.

The young person finds himself having to cope with and adapt to the changed reactions of other people toward him. Withdrawal by his friends may be extremely difficult to endure, and these actions by other people can add to the feelings of anger and futility produced in response to the illness. The process of disease is bound to interfere with the normal sequence of events associated with growing up and to alter the new roles and role-relationships which are important to the social development of the child becoming an adult.

The loss of peer relationships can be notably traumatic for young people who already feel isolated by the disease itself. The experience of being cut off from such important peer activities as dating, competitive sports, overnight slumber parties, and other social events is a cogent reminder that fate has dealt an unfair hand in the game of life.

The members of the family are also faced with the emotional impingement of this new experience on their roles and activities. The parents may react by becoming overly protective of the child with the illness, and the "favorite child" syndrome can result in all manner of difficulties among the siblings in the family. Overprotection by the parents can also prevent the child from leading a normal existence, even when physically he is quite capable of doing so.

Like the child himself, the members of the families find themselves caught up in complex emotional reactions that include sorrow, anger, and guilt. Feelings of sadness may cause them to feel physically tired much of the time and unable to function effectively in their ordinary tasks. Anger and irritation may lead to family arguments, or, not uncommonly, the members of the health-care team become targets for the expression of irritation. Evidence from a number of studies shows that the presence of a child with fatal or chronic illness serves as a stressor on the marriage relationship. In a very real sense, the marital ties are put to the test when parents are faced with the problem of fatal illness in one of their children. Not all families are able to survive the strain.

Changes in the child's physical appearance can be extremely upsetting and especially difficult for the parents to see. Sometimes one or more members of the family cannot cope with the tensions produced by the situation and withdraw from active involvement in the ongoing social affairs of the family. This withdrawal by a family member adds yet another dimension of strain to the already burdened social system of human relationships.

The introduction of life-threatening disease into a family clearly adds to whatever stresses and strains already exist within that family circle—and often the extended kinship group as well. In a profound sense, the fatal illness can never be completely forgotten. The experience of living with fatal illness can serve as a mechanism for drawing people closely together, or where strain already exists among the members, it can add to their problems in daily living. The adaptational task of living with uncertainty over a period of years is an energy-depleting experience. People may reach the point of "wishing the child were dead," an emotional response that often triggers secondary reactions of guilt and self-blame. If the child takes a long time to die once he has reached the terminal stage, the parents and other relatives may have completed most of the mourning process long before he reaches the point of biological death. When circumstances of this nature arise, the child is treated as though he were dead already. The family members withdraw from their emotional attachments to him, and the delivery of personalized care often becomes a difficult nursing problem.

Social Adaptations to Treatment Regimen   The psychologic reactions precipitated by terminal illness are difficult indeed. They are not the only outcomes of fatal illness, however, and often the treatment regimen can be such as to require major adaptations by the family in its style of living. Two examples are used to illustrate these problems of adaptation.

Although diabetes mellitus is not generally considered a fatal disease (at least in the same sense as leukemia), nonetheless it is life-threatening when a proper treatment plan is not followed. In the case of juvenile-onset diabetes, insulin must be taken at the proper times and food eaten at proper intervals to avoid hypoglycemia and to prevent the onset of ketoacidosis. The implementation of an effective diabetic regimen in insulin-dependent diabetes requires a time-bound kind of existence, and the diagnosis of diabetes in childhood has been found to require major adaptations in living by all members of the family. The parental style of behavior as the agent of delegated treatment is a factor of great importance in family adaptations to diabetes. Empirical evidence obtained in a study of young diabetics and their families showed that the patterns of adaptation varied depending on whether the parental style was protective, adaptive, manipulative, or abdicative.[25]

In the situation of cystic fibrosis, prevention of pulmonary complications requires several time-consuming and arduous activities: use of a mist tent at night, postural drainage at specified intervals each day, and regular exercise to facilitate respiration and proper ventilation. Implementation of this rigorous regimen is an enterprise which impinges heavily on the parents' time and energy. In a sense, cystic fibrosis can make the parents—especially the mothers—captives in their own homes. Guided by the middle-class norms of the health-care system, the parents of these children are expected to modify their personal activities to accommodate to the demands and requirements of the medical treatment. Families, however, may not be able to survive as intact social systems under these arrangements, and parental separations are not uncommon occurrences following the appearance of chronic illness in childhood.

The Awareness Dilemma A problem of singular concern for the parents of a child with fatal disease centers around the question of how much the child knows, or should know, about the diagnosis and prognosis. In the case of diabetes mellitus, talk about the disease, its treatment, and its prognosis tends to be open. In the case of leukemia and cystic fibrosis, conversations about prognosis tend often to be marked by ambiguity and evasiveness. The difficulty of talking directly with a child about his life-threatening situation has a direct relation to the perceived "lack of cure" for the disease. Health-care personnel as well as the public are prone to avoid conversation about the future outcomes of these conditions and to focus attention on medical treatments and other cure-related matters.

In general, there are two viewpoints about what the child with fatal illness should be told. Those who take the protective approach suggest that the ill child's (and often his siblings') emotional well-being is dependent upon shielding him from the meaning of his illness and upon maintaining a "normal" family life. The protective viewpoint includes a belief that the ill child be shielded from knowledge about the disease, diagnosis, and prognosis. In contrast, those who advocate the open approach argue that the child with fatal illness and his siblings need an environment in which they can ask questions and can know what is happening. The open approach advocates giving the child information about his illness and his future.[26]

The general tendency for parents to shield their children from hearing the diagnosis and prognosis may well be tied to a general parental tendency to protect their children. There is also reason to think, however, that parental inability to deal openly with the reality of fatal illness is tied more to their own concerns about the loss of a child than to concerns about helping him to cope with it.

Research to ascertain children's reactions to fatal illness suggests that despite parental efforts to protect them from knowledge about the prognosis, children with fatal disease are aware of more than other people seem to recognize. Very young children, although they do not directly verbalize a fear about death, do demonstrate in their behavior a high degree of concern about separation, disfigurement, or pain. A number of reports provide evidence that children of 4 years and older, even when not told directly about the prognosis, show in other ways that they are aware of the seriousness of their condition. In a study of children 6 to 10 years of age, Waechter found that those with fatal illnesses do indicate considerable preoccupation with death in fantasy, along with feelings of loneliness and isolation, and a sense of lack of control over the forces impinging on them.[27]

The extent to which other people (notably adults) are unaware of how much the child with fatal illness knows about his condition rests with the fact that they are for the most part unwilling to talk with him about it. A second reason, however, derives from the fact that children, especially very young ones, speak in symbolic language—a sort of language all their own in which words and phrases have cryptic and personal meanings, with messages often conveyed by action rather than through talk.[28] Becoming aware of how much a child knows and understands about his life-threatening situation means learning to listen carefully to children at play and to observe with an open mind what they say and do. Observation of the child as he is drawing or is playing with his toys can provide useful clues to the thoughtful observer about the child's state of

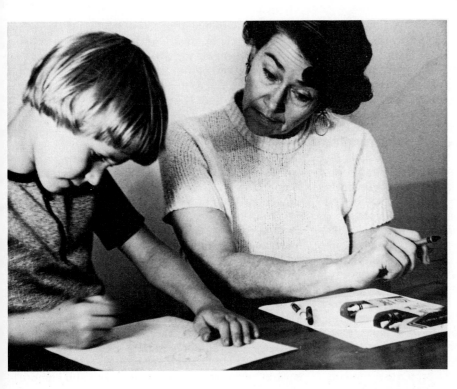

Figure 29-1 The nurse observes as a child draws a self-portrait and talks about it. *(Courtesy of Betty E. Hunt and Douglas Benoliel.)*

mind and state of feeling. The nurse in Fig. 29-1 has asked the child who is waiting to see the doctor to describe his drawing, and she anticipates learning something about his underlying concerns from the story that he tells.

Recent evidence suggests that the efforts used by adults to protect children with fatal illness from knowledge about the disease may, in fact, do just the opposite by causing them to worry about that which is unknown. A 2-year demonstration project in which 51 children with leukemia were provided honest answers to their questions about their illness produced no major adjustment problems among these children but instead relieved them of many worries and serious concerns.[29] The findings from the study are persuasive that children can cope with far more than adults will allow and that children appreciate the opportunity to know and to understand what is happening to them.

Differences in Families

Nurses need to recognize that families are social systems with different capabilities and capacities for adapting to the impact of life-threatening illness, sudden death, and bereavement. Families that can be defined as low in risk are those with plentiful resources to assist them in living through the experience of losing a child through death. At the other extreme are high-risk families, those with few resources for coping with the multiple stresses produced by life-threatening disease.

In studies about the effects of sudden and unexpected death, several different familial responses have been observed and described. Families that were amenable to crisis intervention activities were found to be atomized, nuclear families accustomed to the idea of professionals and experts to assist them and with the financial resources to do so. A second group of families were part of a cohesive cultural subgroup and had their own resources and ways of coping with bereavement without assistance in the form of crisis intervention. A third group consisted of atomized, nuclear families that had minimal social ties with the society at large, were resistant to crisis intervention, and were also highly vulnerable to physical and mental depletion in response to the crisis of death.[30]

Nurses should be aware that family systems have differential abilities to adapt constructively to the stresses and strains of living with fatal illness of a member. These strains are particularly acute when the member happens to be a child. Any family or other social group that is deprived in social, psychologic, or economic resources can be defined as "high-risk" in vulnerability to the consequences of life-threatening situations.

The study of diabetic families mentioned before suggested that several family-types appear at greater risk than others in adapting to the requirements of a chronic, progressive disease. The family with only one parent was seriously handicapped in taking over the adaptive responsibilities of chronic illness. By comparison, the child's adaptation to the diabetes was facilitated when both parents participated actively as socializing agents—a pattern observed in the middle-class families. In contrast, within the working-class families, child-rearing practices were such that the burden of care fell mainly on the mothers. In these families the lack of paternal involvement was an element of some importance affecting the child's adaptation to the stresses and strains of diabetes. To judge from these findings, the life-style of working class families makes them a high-risk group for coping with the stresses and strains of life-threatening illness in ways that protect the child from social isolation and scapegoating.[31] On the other hand, availability of extended kinship groups may sometimes provide resources for support among working-class groups not available or utilized by middle-class families.

Some years age City of Hope Medical Center in California initiated a Parent Participation Program to help families of children with leukemia or cancer to deal in a constructive way with the catastrophic consequences of fatal illness. Despite the overall success of the program, some families did not benefit from the service, and efforts were made to identify the reasons. The conditions found to be associated with diminished capacity of families to cope adequately with the fatal illness included the following: low capacity for coping with life's tasks in general; a history of prior marriages in one or both parents; a diagnosis (such as nonoperable sarcoma) with few if any remissions; and a child 10 years of age or older.[32] Judging from these findings, families with one or more of these characteristics can be expected to encounter serious difficulties in adapting to the multiple strains imposed by terminal illness. If help is to be made available to such families, the services offered to them—including that provided by nurses— may need special modifications and additions in order for a usable support system to evolve.

Nursing interventions with a family faced with a life-threatening situation can be most effective when the nurses are knowledgeable about the social and cultural features of the particular family system. Nursing activities need also to take account of the stage in which the family finds itself, the family's previous experience with death and dying, the resources available to them, and any other circumstances that critically influence the meaning of the death of this child.[33]

COMMON SITUATIONS IN NURSING PRACTICE
Sudden and Unexpected Death

One of the most difficult situations likely to be encountered in nursing practice occurs when a family is confronted with the sudden and unexpected death of a child. Accidents are probably the most frequent cause of these psychologically traumatic events. In recent years, SIDS (sudden infant death syndrome) has also assumed importance as an identified cause of sudden and unanticipated death during the first year of life.[34]

Nurses who work in emergency wards are often in contact with families faced with sudden death. These persons are usually in an active state of psychologic shock in reaction to an unexpected and generally unwanted incident. The behavior which can be expected from persons in this state can be of several types. Some people are dazed and immobile. Others respond with hysterical laughter, crying and wailing, or with overt expressions of frustration and rage. Still others may respond by taking charge of the situation and telling others what to do.

No matter what the behavior pattern displayed, the chances are high that the person will remember very little of what he is told during this period of acute psychologic crisis. Health-care personnel who are assisting these persons should not expect them to remember information clearly and should be prepared to repeat information several times. At this time nurses can assist the recovery process by open acknowledgement of the psychologic crisis. That is, by simple words or touch, a nurse can express concern for the persons who are caught up in their own personal tragedy. They may or may not be able to respond to this overture. The nurse needs to be aware that their preoccupation with themselves limits their ability to communicate in response.

As the shock begins to wear off, the survivors may want to talk about the situation—often in rambling and disconnected ways. This need to talk is a way of sorting out what has happened, and a good listener can often serve as a sounding board for the grieving ones to work out their thoughts and feelings about what has happened. The need to talk about what has taken place does not always occur while the persons are still in contact with the health-care facility. In fact, one of the major obstacles to "working through" the psychologic process of recovery comes from a lack of helping services in the community to assist people in adjusting to the aftermath of sudden death.

The Child Who Attempts Suicide

If the sudden and unexpected death of a child is due to suicide, the family is highly vulnerable to psychologic problems and emotional disturbances. Because suicide is unacceptable in the Judeo-Christian tradition, people in Western societies generally respond with feelings of shame to suicide by a member of their family. The usual reactions of psychologic shock are generally compounded by strong feelings of guilt. Feelings of anger against the person for "doing this to me" are likely to be present, but they are not usually expressed openly because of the cultural norms against such behavior. Often family members are found to have difficulty in experiencing grief following death by suicide, and these difficulties in coming to terms with the death increase if they blame themselves intensely for what has happened.

The child who attempts suicide but does not succeed poses another set of problems. Because suicide is viewed as unacceptable behavior, the staff tends to attach moral meanings to the event and to behave toward the child as though he carries a stigma. Family members, too, can react negatively to the child for bringing shame upon them, but they also experience ambivalence because of their other feelings of concern for the child. It is important to be aware that unsuccessful suicide is a situation which precipitates strong feelings in staff and family alike.

To assist the child and his family, the most important step for any helping person means coming to terms with his own feelings about suicide. It is not uncommon for health-care personnel to have strong reactions of anger against patients who have attempted suicide and to resent them for taking a nurse's time away from other patients. Anger can easily breed a tendency to treat these patients as objects, and treatment as an object is precisely not what the suicidal person needs.

The young person who attempts suicide is not a happy person. The difficulties that led to the attempt to end his life are not easily resolved. Anyone who has made such an attempt is extremely sensitive to the actions of others toward him, especially any actions which add to his devaluation of himself. Effective treatment for this problem generally requires psychologic treatment for all members of the family over a somewhat extended period of time. On a short-term basis, genuine interest and concern for the young person can do much to help him through a traumatic period of transition.

Terminal Stages of Illness

A third and very common problem in nursing is that of providing care during the terminal stages of illness. Although the child who has cancer or other fatal illness often has several hospitalizations, there comes a time when the "nothing-more-to-do phase" appears. At this point, curative treatment of the disease is no longer effective, and only palliation is left to be used.[35] The nothing-more-to-do phase represents the end point of the dying trajectory; several serious nursing problems are likely to be present during the final period of the child's life.

Nursing Problems in Care Delivery A nursing problem that is markedly difficult to manage takes place when the family and physician decide that the child is not to be told what is happening. For the nursing staff, the psychologic difficulties can be intensified when curative life-prolonging treatments are continued and the child clearly does not want them. The difficulties can also be exacerbated if the child indicates that he no longer has trust in them or in anyone else. The youngster may respond to the context of closed awareness which others impose by withdrawing into himself. When a child turns his face to the wall, both the family and the staff are likely to be very upset because they feel that the child has rejected them.

When parents are unable to face the reality of the child's forthcoming death, it is the child who suffers—in the pain of social isolation and in the lack of opportunity to make his wishes known. Sometimes this suffering includes the indignity of dying in the intensive care unit (ICU) surrounded by strangers and with no chance to say goodbye and to share the final moments of separation with those who are dear to him. Prevention of this latter form of suffering requires that the parents be helped to recognize the reality of their situation and to allow the child to be moved into a quiet, caring environment as his life draws to a close. In a very profound way, the major task that nurses face during the final phase of the child's illness may be the provision of support and care to the parents so that they in turn can support and care for the child.

A second type of difficult problem is that of the child in a coma. If the unconscious child dies in only a matter of hours or days, the problem for the nurses soon resolves itself. When the child exists for weeks or months in such a state, the problems for the family and for the staff are multiplied. Sometimes the family can precipitate this difficult situation by not being able to "let go" of the patient and by insisting on continuation of heroic treatments. Sometimes it is the staff who cannot let the patient go, and they may perpetuate the use of intensive treatments even though the treatments have little to offer except additional expense.

The setting into which the child is placed has a definite influence on the services that are provided. The continuation of heroic life-saving interventions is bound to continue if the child is hospitalized and placed in an intensive care unit. They are least likely to be used if the child is permitted to remain at home to die.

Another difficult situation for staff and family occurs when the child's terminal illness is marked by extensive pain and discomfort. Under these circumstances, the other feelings of distress precipitated by the child's forthcoming death are compounded by a disquieting sense of helplessness associated with the inability to offer him comfort and relief from suffering. A related problem, and equally difficult, occurs when the child is clearly frightened by what is happening to him. Once again, the staff can experience strong feelings of helplessness, but they can also be forcefully and uncomfortably reminded of their own unresolved fears about the prospect of death.

Teamwork and the Caretaking Process Finding solutions for these difficult problems requires a willingness to recognize that they exist and depends on teamwork and open communication among the many disciplines involved.

Facing up to the reality that death is about to happen is not an easy matter, and there are many difficulties to be overcome in obtaining open and effective communication. Without effective communication, however, the child is likely to end his days in social isolation, and decisions are likely to be made without consensus among the persons involved.

This terminal period of illness is a time when choices are available and decisions must be made. This is a time when the family must decide whether to leave the child in the hospital or to take him home to spend his final days. This is a time when members of the medical staff must decide about the continuation or cessation of heroic life-sustaining interventions. This is a time when decisions about what to tell the child are again brought to the fore.

The final period of living for the child is a time when the staff who are providing care have their own needs for support. It is a period when there is need for regular meetings at which problems can be discussed and decisions made about steps to be taken. The achievement of death with dignity for the child is a process which takes place by helping the parents and key members of the family (and the staff) come to terms with what is happening. Only as they can face the reality of the child's death can they be willing to permit the cessation of life-saving measures.

Often at this time, the family and the staff are so caught up in their own problems that they forget about the child's need to talk about what is happening to him. There is a tendency for both parents and health-care personnel to be overly protective toward the child. One of the ways by which overprotection is manifest is avoidance of conversation about what is happening. Avoidance of talk can also be accompanied by avoidance of contact. Because the child is sensitive to the behavior of others, these patterns of withdrawal by others can add to his deep-seated fear of abandonment.

Nurses are often in a position to offer the child outlets for talking about his concerns. The extent to which he will have realized his forthcoming death and be able to talk about it, of course, depends on how much his parents have permitted him to do so in the past. If the parents have been open and able to talk with the child about the reality of his death, it is unlikely that there will be need for another person to be his listener. It is when the parents themselves have been unable to face the situation that the child is most in need of someone to serve as his confidant.

Nurses who wish to assume the caretaking role need to be aware that children frequently use symbolic language to talk about their own deaths. Learning the individual's symbolic language means paying special attention to the words that he uses and observing carefully what he does. Nurses who assume this special caretaking role with children need especially to learn how to handle their own anxieties about death. There is, perhaps, no greater tragedy in human experience than that of losing one's life before it has scarcely begun. The meaning of the time available to the child or adolescent whose life has been cut short by a life-threatening disease is determined in great measure by the other people around him. He can be placed in social isolation; at the other extreme, he can be involved in finding meaning out of each day that he has—until he is ready to let go.

NURSING FUNCTIONS IN TERMINAL ILLNESS

Because illness with fatal outcome is psychologically and socially depleting to a child who bears the disease, he and his family need several kinds of assistance as they move from the point of diagnosis to the point of death—and even beyond, for the family. Nurses are often in contact with these children and their families at critical points along the way; therefore, they are in position to play a singularly important part in providing assistance to them, and can do so through supporting, teaching, coordinating, and caring functions.

The Supporting Function

As this chapter has outlined, the child with fatal illness and his family undergo a series of critical experiences including the final interval which ends in death. These critical experiences include the point of diagnosis, periods of hospitalization, and family crises which overlap with the many problems posed by the illness. Because nurses frequently are with the child and the family at points of psychologic stress, they are clearly in position to offer emotional support and other kinds of assistance during these critical moments.

The supporting function begins with the ability to listen with sensitivity and genuine concern. This ability is facilitated when the nurse understands the stages of psychologic adaptation to terminal illness, and at the same time can recognize when the person shows readiness to move to another stage. The most difficult periods for any listener are those during which the other person (whether child, parent, or staff) is expressing anger or is experiencing depression. Yet often it is at these times that people most clearly need to be able to express how they truly feel in order to move psychologically toward the point of acceptance.

Although listening is clearly important, the supporting function also includes helping the child and his family to find other resources as needed. The types of assistance can vary a good deal. The family may need help in financial matters. They may need day-care services or help in finding someone to assist them at home. When the illness worsens, they may need referral to a visiting-nurse association. Not infrequently, families may be unaware of the many services available through voluntary agencies until these matters are brought to their attention. Families may also find support through contacts with parents' groups, such as the Candlelighters, composed of families who have themselves lost a child through death and who want to help other families faced with the same experience.

A third way by which the supporting function is implemented is through competent performance of the technical tasks of nursing care. There is a special kind of support provided by physical ministrations which are deftly given. The nurse who can relieve the child's pain by the skillful administration of an injection provides an additional element of support to his care. As the child becomes weak and dependent on others for his physical well-being, the supporting function demonstrated in good physical care looms high in importance to him (and to his family).

Whenever children are seriously ill or psychologically disturbed, they tend to regress to earlier patterns of behavior. To the consternation of parents, for example, old habits such as thumb-sucking or bed-wetting may reappear in an 8- or 9-year-old child as the disease process continues. The physical regression so commonly observed as the illness progresses probably reflects a need for attention and care at a very primitive level of existence.

When the illness reaches the point of producing a state of complete physical dependency, the child's needs for care are much the same as they were during his infancy, and communication by means of touch becomes extremely important. No matter what his chronological age may be, the child who is approaching death wants to be held in his mother's arms. In fact, physical contact with someone who cares may be the primary source of comfort at this time, yet hospitals are often effectively organized to prevent this kind of care from being offered. For the child, nothing can replace the comfort of being held in his mother's arms. As Fig. 29-2 suggests, a special kind of relaxation takes place in the child who is permitted to experience communion of touch with the person who gave him birth.

Caught up in her own needs, however, the child's mother may not be able to recognize his wishes, or she may be afraid to touch him for fear of causing pain or other discomfort. Sometimes mothers (and fathers, too) need help in being able to share this important experience with their children. Nurses can do a great deal to provide support for children facing death by allowing this kind of paren-

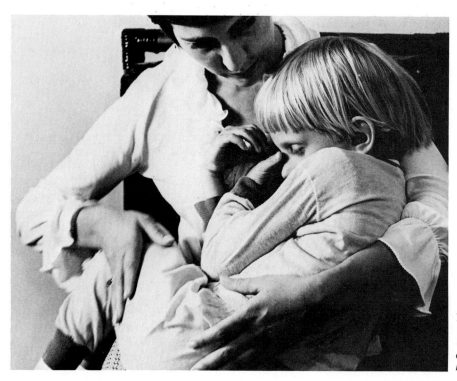

Figure 29-2 A special kind of relaxation occurs when a child is held by his mother. *(Courtesy of Betty E. Hunt and Douglas Benoliel.)*

tal caretaking activity to take place in the hospital and by encouraging parents to participate actively in the provision of physical care.

The Teaching Function

A second important way by which nurses can contribute in their ongoing contacts with terminally ill children and their families is through the teaching function. This function is implemented through the provision of information and guidance to assist them directly in learning to live with the life-threatening disease and the treatment regimen that has been recommended.

A major segment of instructional assistance is the teaching of self-care activities and medical treatment procedures to be done at home, and effective teaching includes periodic follow-up sessions by the nurse to ascertain whether the child and his parents have a clear understanding of what they are doing. One key to the success of this component of teaching is the provision of information necessary to clarify their knowledge and understanding of the treatment, procedures, and routines to be done. The nurse also needs to be aware that a certain amount of repetition and reexplanation may be necessary along the way. Reexplanations may be

particularly essential during the early stages of illness when the parents are caught up in the immobilizing effects of psychologic shock.

The teaching function also means answering questions about the disease, its treatment, and related matters at the time that these loom as important to the child and his parents. One explanation is often not sufficient for true understanding to take place, and sensitivity to the instructional needs of the patient and family is an important attribute for nurses to develop.

An important component of the teaching function is that of interpretation of the physician's orders and explanations. This component of the teaching function may be especially important when the family has had contact with a variety of different medical specialists who use technical language and perform intricate procedures as they engage in consultation at the request of the primary physician. It can also be important, however, after any kind of contact with medical authority. To assist families in understanding special tests and unusual therapies, the nurse can identify misunderstandings and misinterpretations only by taking the time to talk with the families. Opportunity for discussion with the nurse *directly after* contacts with the doctor must be built into the plan of care or, as otherwise can happen, the parents' needs for explanation are lost along the way.

A final point about nurse-physician communication seems in order here. To be highly effective in helping the child and his parents to understand the physician's orders and explanations, the nurse needs an effective, mutually respectful working relation with physicians. Only by having a clear understanding of the physician's plan of treatment can the nurse provide explanations which the child and the parent will find most useful. When nurses are not informed about the physician's approach to therapy, they can easily add to a family's confusions instead of helping them to achieve understanding.

The Coordinating Function

Because patient care today is offered by multiple numbers of health-care workers, the child and his family often find themselves involved with many different caretakers without clear direction as to the management of their situation. One of the important contributions that nurses can offer is the facilitating and coordinating function, i.e., the team concept in action. Activities central to implementing this function are the arrangement of regular conferences as needed to plan the care for and with the patient and his family, and referrals to other facilities and services as needed, with adequate follow-up to ensure that the services desired were in fact given.

The facilitating and coordinating function is centrally concerned with the goal of *continuity of care*. In this regard, the facilitating and coordinating function often breaks down unless there is clear designation as to which nurse is to be the primary caretaker for the child and his family. Very often the nurse who works in a cancer clinic or physician's office occupies a key position for serving as leader in the task of coordination, but the nurse to be effective must be willing to assume responsibility for these activities and not to expect the physician to do so. If a goal of nursing is to help children with fatal illness and their families to cope with the *situationally derived* needs which result from the terminal situation and their reactions to it, the coordinating function may be a singularly important contribution that nurses can make to the ongoing services available for children faced with terminal illness.[36]

The Caring Function

The caring function consists of activities that assist the child in coping with the subjective experience of his terminal illness *on his own terms*. This function has the goal of personalizing care for the child by providing continuity of contact with someone who is concerned about him and encouraging his participation in social living for as long as he is able.

The caring function allows the child opportunity to direct activities and to let his wishes be known (the principle of control over his own dying). The caring function is implemented by setting realistic limits for the child when in an authority relationship with him and by adhering to these limits with regularity (the principle of consistency) while providing nursing services. Another way by which the nurse can implement the caring function is to intervene on behalf of the child with members of his family, physicians, and others who are involved when his (the child's) wishes and desires are not being heard (the principle of advocacy).

In addition to helping the child maintain some measure of control over his life, the nurse can also help to find simple enjoyments—for example, by having fun together to the extent that his physical condition permits and he so desires. Perhaps most of all, the caring function means a willingness to hear the child when he indicates that he wants to talk about something important to him. When the child mentions death, either directly or indirectly, he is letting the nurse know that he is concerned about himself and is reaching out for human contact.

When he begins to cry, to ask questions about death, or to review his past, the child is indicating a desire to cope with his forthcoming death by approaching it directly instead of using avoidance behaviors.[37] He is reaching out for relationship now. The nurse who postpones the opportunity to share these moments with him will probably not have another chance. People who are dying initiate conversations about death when they are ready to do so. The caring function depends on nurses who have flexibility in their approaches to the planning of nursing care and ability to make rapid shifts in priorities when the human needs of the terminally ill child are in jeopardy.

REFERENCES

1 Florence Rockwood Kluckholn, "Family Diagnosis: Variations in the Basic Values of Family Systems," *Social Casework*, 39:63–72, 1959.

2 R. Kastenbaum and R. Aisenberg, *The Psychology of Death*, Springer Publishing Co., Inc., New York, 1972, pp. 205–208.

3 R. Blauner, "Death and Social Structure," *Psychiatry*, 29:378–394, 1966.

4 R. J. Glaser, "Innovations and Heroic Acts in Prolonging Life," in O. Brim et al. (eds.), *The Dying Patient*, Russell Sage Foundation, New York, 1970, pp. 102–128.

5 D. Hay and D. Oken, "The Psychological Stresses of Intensive Care Unit Nursing," *Psychosomatic Medicine*, 34(2):109–118, 1972.

6 Davida R. Michaels, "Too Much in Need of Support to Give Any?" *American Journal of Nursing*, 71(10):1932–1935, 1971.

7 Jeanne Benoliel, "Nursing Care for the Terminal Patient: A Psychosocial Approach," in B. Schoenberg et al. (eds.), *Psychosocial Aspects of Terminal Care*, Columbia University Press, New York, 1972, pp. 145–161.

8 B. Glaser, "The Social Loss of Dying Patients," *American Journal of Nursing*, 64(6):119–121, 1964.

9 J. Wiener, "Reactions of the Family to the Fatal Illness of a Child," in B. Schoenberg et al. (eds.), *Loss and Grief: Psychological Management in Medical Practice*, Columbia University Press, New York, 1970, pp. 87–101.

10 J. Bowlby, "Grief and Mourning in Infancy and Early Childhood," *Psychoanalytic Study of the Child*, 15:9, 1960.

11 A. Portz, "The Child's Sense of Death," in A. Godin (ed.), *Death and Presence*, Lumen Vitae Press, Brussels, 1972, pp. 139–154.

12 E. Volkart, "Bereavement and Mental Health," in R. Fulton (ed.), *Death and Identity*, John Wiley & Sons, Inc., New York, 1965, pp. 272–293.

13 J. Racy, "Death in an Arab Culture," *Annals of the New York Academy of Sciences*, 164(3):871–880, 1969.

14 J. E. Schowalter, "The Child's Reaction to His Own Terminal Illness," in B. Schoenberg et al. (eds.), *Psychosocial Aspects of Terminal Care*, Columbia University Press, New York, 1972, p. 60.

15 Matilda McIntire et al., "The Concept of Death in Midwestern Children and Youth," *American Journal of Diseases of Children*, 123:529, 1972.

16 B. Rose, "Death Is Alive and Well in the Ghetto," in E. Shneidman (ed.), *Death and the College Student*, Behavioral Publications, Inc., New York, 1972, pp. 3–11.

17 E. Markusen and R. Fulton, "Childhood Bereavement and Behavior Disorders: A Critical Review," *Omega*, 2(2):107–117, 1971.

18 S. Friedman et al., "Behavioral Observations on Parents Anticipating the Death of a Child," *Pediatrics*, 32(4):610–625, 1963.

19 B. Glaser and A. Strauss, *Time for Dying*, Aldine Publishing Company, Chicago, 1968.

20 I. Hoffman and E. H. Futterman, "Coping with Waiting: Psychiatric Intervention and Study in the Waiting Room of a Pediatric Oncology Clinic," *Comprehensive Psychiatry*, 12(1):68–69, 1971.

21 J. H. Meyerowitz and H. V. Kaplan, "Family Responses to Stress: The Case of Cystic Fibrosis," *Social Science and Medicine*, 1:249–266, 1967.

22 Marjorie Crate, "Nursing Functions in Adaptation to Chronic Illness," *American Journal of Nursing*, 65(10): 72–76, 1965.

23 Elisabeth Kübler-Ross, *On Death and Dying*, The Macmillan Company, New York, 1969.

24 E. Lindemann, "Symptomatology and Management of Acute Grief," *American Journal of Psychiatry*, 72:141–148, 1944.

25 Jeanne Benoliel, "The Developing Diabetic Identity: A Study of Family Influence," *Communicating Nursing Research: Methodological Issues*, Western Interstate Commission for Higher Education, Boulder, Colo., 1970, pp. 14–32.

26 Lynda Share, "Family Communication in the Crisis of a Child's Fatal Illness," *Omega*, 3(3):187–201, 1972.

27 Eugenia Waechter, "Children's Reactions to Fatal Illness," in A. Godin (ed.), *Death and Presence*, Lumen Vitae Press, Brussels, 1972, pp. 155–168.

28 B. Bird, *Talking with Patients*, 2d ed., J. P. Lippincott Company, Philadelphia, 1973, pp. 290–293.

29 M. Karon and J. Vernick, "An Approach to the Emotional Support of Fatally Ill Children," *Clinical Pediatrics*, 7(5):278, 1968.

30 Rita Vollman et al., "The Reactions of Family Systems to Sudden and Unexpected Death," *Omega*, 2(2):101–106, 1971.

31 Jeanne Benoliel, "Assessments of Loss and Grief," *Journal of Thanatology*, 1:190–191, 1971.

32 M. B. Hamovitch, *The Parent and the Fatally Ill Child*, City of Hope Medical Center, Duarte, Calif., 1964, pp. 111–116.

33 J. F. Scott, "Brief Comments on Situational and Social Structure Implications for the Loss of a Loved One," in D. Moriarty (ed.), *The Loss of Loved Ones*, Charles C Thomas, Publisher, Springfield, Ill., 1967, pp. 167–176.

34 A. B. Bergman, "Sudden Infant Death," *Nursing Outlook*, 20(12):775, 1972.

35 B. G. Glaser and A. L. Strauss, *Awareness of Dying*, Aldine Publishing Company, Chicago, 1965, pp. 177–225.

36 P. J. Wooldridge et al., *Behavioral Science, Social Practice and the Nursing Profession*, The Press of Case Western Reserve University, Cleveland, 1968, pp. 74–88.

37 June Lowenberg, "The Coping Behaviors of Fatally Ill Adolescents and Their Parents," *Nursing Forum*, 9(3):285, 1970.

BIBLIOGRAPHY

Benoliel, Jeanne Quint: "Talking to Patients about Death," *Nursing Forum*, 9(3):254–268, 1970.

———: "The Concept of Care for the Child with Leukemia," *Nursing Forum*, 11(2):194–204, 1972.

Brim, O. G., Jr., et al. (eds.): *The Dying Patient*, Russell Sage Foundation, New York, 1970.

Browning, Mary H., et al. (eds.): *The Dying Patient: A Nursing Perspective*, Contemporary Nursing Series, The American Journal of Nursing Company, New York, 1972.

Easson, W. M.: *The Dying Child: The Management of the Child or Adolescent Who is Dying*, Charles C Thomas, Publisher, Springfield, Ill., 1970.

Fulton, R. (ed.): *Death and Identity*, John Wiley & Sons, Inc., New York, 1965.

Grollman, E. A. (ed.): *Explaining Death to Children*, Beacon Press, Boston, 1967.

Lasagna, Louis: *Life, Death, and the Doctor*, Alfred A. Knopf, Inc., New York, 1968.

Quint, Jeanne C.: *The Nurse and the Dying Patient*, The Macmillan Company, New York, 1967.

Switzer, D. K.: *The Dynamics of Grief*, Abingdon Press, Nashville, Tenn., 1970.

Weisman, A. D.: *On Dying and Denying: A Psychiatric Study of Terminality*, Behavioral Publications, Inc., New York, 1972.

30

HOSPITAL ADMISSION AND ENVIRONMENT

JUDITH A. TRUFANT

Hospitalization is an interruption of the child's active cycle of growth and development and of his and his family's life-styles. The child is removed from the daily routines of homelife, and his contact with siblings, relatives, and peers may be limited. He may be required to experience strange and painful events and to communicate with strangers.

Preparation for such dramatic change is essential for both the child and his parents. The first contact with the hospital can set the tone for the rest of the hospital stay, so the admission procedure should be carefully planned and carried out. The hospital environment should be planned to provide comfort for the ill child and his family as well as to meet their emotional and developmental needs.

PREPARATION FOR HOSPITALIZATION*

Preparation prior to hospitalization is essential to make the transition from home to hospital as nondisruptive as possible. The well-prepared family should know what to expect before their child is admitted to the hospital. The child's developmental level as well as his relation with his parents determine when preparation should begin and in how much detail it should be carried out.

The Role of Parents

Parents who know the strengths and weaknesses of their child and who can communicate with him are essential for helping prepare him for admission and for interpreting to him the events that will take place in the hospital. The parent may not always be the best person to give the child support, however. Parents may be too emotionally "shocked" to be supportive, or an accident may have left one or both parents physically unable to be with their child upon admission. Parents may rightfully express and feel inadequacy in accompanying their child upon admission and may delegate this responsibility to a friend or relative. Whatever the circumstances, the child needs a familiar and understanding person to help prepare him for and support him during admission to the hospital.

Preadmission Preparation

Preadmission preparation is most effective when the admission is planned and there is enough time for the nurse to provide necessary information to the

*The author gratefully acknowledges the assistance of Jean Carol Wilson, R.N., M.N., in the preparation of this chapter.

family and to make sure that they understand it. The child's parent should be the main interpreter and facilitator of information for the child. Through direct participation in learning about what hospitalization will be like, the parent's anxiety may be somewhat alleviated. As the parent helps communicate to the child, he gains information which may answer many of his own questions, therefore allowing him to more constructively support his child.

Admission Information The physician is the primary source for facts concerning the purpose, therapeutic plan, and expected outcome of hospitalization. The information he offers should include a description of physiologic and/or psychologic aspects of treatment which will be carried out as well as an estimated length of stay in the hospital.

After the physician's explanation the office or clinic nurse may provide immediate follow-up by eliciting from the family their understanding of the admission plans, and may add and clarify information for them. Families are often emotionally upset over the initial revelation that hospitalization is needed, and they may not be able to comprehend all the information that is given. Therefore repetition and clarification at a later time is very important and should take place some time between the first knowledge that hospitalization is necessary and the actual admission.

Many hospitals provide a booklet which describes the routines of their pediatric unit. Such information may be given to the family by the nurse or sent directly from the hospital. In any event the family should receive such materials before admission to help them in planning for hospitalization. The information in preadmission booklets should be written for the parents and the child. Simply written, factual information that can be easily read by people with elementary reading skills and pictures of the pediatric unit can communicate a story by themselves. Families need to know what they should bring with them to the hospital and what the physical accommodations will be. They also need to know who will be taking care of their child and some of the routines and procedures to expect. Part of an admission booklet should be for the child. It might be written with simple words in large print and have pictures to color or a puzzle related to the hospital.

The nurse should assume an active role in helping parents prepare their children for hospitalization. Depending upon the age of the child, the nurse may prepare the parents, who in turn can communicate the information to their young child. Parents of older children may be given information by the nurse. The child may also be prepared by the nurse in a separate meeting or with the parents present. Parents are then prepared to reinforce information which their child has received.

Printed materials, movies, slides, and a variety of playthings can be used to help prepare the child for hospitalization. There are many books about going to the hospital written especially for children which the nurse can provide or recommend for parents. Some of these are listed in the Bibliography at the end of this chapter under "Hospital Books for Children." The nurse may also instruct the parents in simple play techniques which they can use to help them help their child understand what will happen in the hospital. For example, if a child is to have a tonsillectomy, the nurse can demonstrate for the mother what will happen before and after the operation using dolls that represent the child (patient), nurse, doctor, and others involved in the hospital care. Then the child's mother can enact this drama with her child at home to help him learn what to expect in the hospital.

Going to the Hospital Children should be told openly that they are going to the hospital. Preparation depends upon when and how the child's parents usually prepare him for a new experience. The child's ability to conceptualize time may be used as a guide for determining when to tell him about going to the hospital. In general, children over 7 years may be told as much as 2 weeks in advance of admission as they are able to comprehend how far in the future "2 weeks" will be. The younger the child under the age of 7, the shorter should be the interval between the time he is told he is going to the hospital and the day he is admitted.

The child needs to participate as much as possible in planning his hospital visit. Depending upon his age, he may want to take part by choosing which toy he will take with him, explaining to his friends why he will be gone from school for a few days, or picking out new pajamas to wear. He may also participate by packing his own bag to take to the hospital.

The Emergency Admission Instances of sudden illness or injury pose added problems for a child admitted to the hospital when the first impressions may be those of the sights, sounds, and smells of the emergency room. An accident may leave one or both parents unable to be with their child. The child's own injuries or illness may make his perceptions of the strange surroundings inaccurate and frightening.

A sudden injury or illness may precipitate feelings of guilt in both the child and parents. The child may have disobeyed his parents, or the parents may feel that they did not provide adequate supervision.

The perceptions and feelings of families must be dealt with as an emergency just as is the physical disruption. If the child is able to communicate, he should be oriented as soon as possible to his surroundings and to the events taking place. Information should be obtained from the parents, and they should be given support in expressing their feelings about what has happened in any way that is appropriate.

ADMISSION PROCEDURE

From the time that the child and his family enter the hospital doors, the admission procedure should be carried out in a friendly and efficient manner. From the admitting area to settling in their room, the child and family should receive the utmost courtesy and attentiveness during this initial phase of transition from home to hospital.

Admission to the pediatric unit and helping the family learn about their new surroundings are nursing responsibilities. The nurse is the best person for answering the family's questions about all aspects of hospital life and he can, during the admission procedure, detect possible problem areas in the family and assess ways of dealing with them.

There are two objectives which should be carried out during admission. They are (1) to acquaint the family with the physical facilities and services of the hospital, and (2) to exchange information with the family about their child's care.

Physical Facilities and Services

In order to accomplish the first objective, a definite plan for activities must be carried out at admission which will ensure that the family will be informed about all aspects of their new environment. Many pediatric units develop a system for orienting families to their surroundings which is constructed on the basis of identified family needs. A list of all activities and information needs which should be carried out is a helpful tool. Each nursing staff should plan an admission procedure which is specific to their own unit facilities and to the needs of the families using it.

Orientation to the Pediatric Unit   When the family arrives at the pediatric unit, they should be shown the room where their child will stay and the toilet facilities he will use. If the bathroom is "down the

hall," a landmark pointed out may be helpful in remembering which way to go. It is important to demonstrate exactly how the faucets turn on and off and how the toilet is flushed, as they may work differently from the ones the family uses at home.

The approximate times when meals are served to children should be provided for the family. This information may be particularly important for parents who plan their visiting time to coincide with the time their child eats. For the child, knowing when his meals will be served provides the beginnings of a routine for his day, and mealtime can become a way for him to judge the passage of time. Children need to know that "snack food" is available, and they can be shown the kitchen and snack supply on the unit.

If meals cannot be made available to them in their child's room, parents need to know where they can eat their meals. They should have directions about how to get to the cafeteria or coffee shop and the hours these facilities are open. It may also be important to give an estimate of food cost to some families.

Showing the child the playroom soon after he comes to the pediatric unit will let him know that there is a place in his new environment which may seem somewhat familiar. The playroom and the play equipment offer nonthreatening activities for the child who may feel threatened by real or imagined events in the hospital. Many children want to explore the playroom immediately and will relax noticeably amidst toy trucks, dolls, books, and blocks. It is comforting for parents to know that there is a play facility to help them entertain their child.

Soon after admission it is important to explain to parents and children where and how they can call a nurse if they need help. The nurses' desk or charting station should be identified to parents as a place where they can come to get help. The call button or intercommunication system in their own room should be demonstrated, and it is a good idea to have the family participate in using this equipment as it is explained. If there is no phone in their room, the family should be shown the closest phone they may use. Having a phone available is particularly important for families who must be separated during hospitalization.

Providing for Parents   Parents need to know how their daily living needs will be met while their child is hospitalized and they are staying with him. Facilities may allow them to "live in" with their child, or they may spend varying amounts of time with their child. If a living-in arrangement is not available to the parents, the nurse should explore with them how much time they will spend with their child and how they will manage this time away from the rest of the family. They may need to know about available housing close to the hospital and about convenient transportation. If the family must drive in and out of a large city, they may want to know the easiest route to and from the hospital. A small map of the hospital and how to get to their child's room may also be helpful.

When living-in is possible, the parents should be given a clear understanding of the particular facilities available to them such as those for eating, sleeping, and bathing. Knowing which parts of the pediatric unit and hospital are "out of bounds" as well as those which they may utilize will make the family feel more comfortable and secure.

Facilities where parents can relax or socialize with other parents should be pointed out. It is important that parents who spend a lot of time with their sick child have an opportunity to engage in some type of recreation or diversion. A list of churches and synagogues in the immediate area of the hospital may be given to families, and they should be shown the hospital chapel.

One of the first questions that parents often ask upon arrival at the unit is, "When are visiting hours?" The family needs time schedules as well as suggestions of who may visit and how often. This is also a good moment to explain anticipated reactions of their child to having them leave and return for visits.

The Nursing Interview

The second objective of admission, exchanging information, is accomplished by conducting a nursing interview with the parents and their child. At this time the nurse can learn why the child has come to the hospital and the concerns and expectations he and his parents have about this event. During this interview the nurse can communicate to the parents what they can expect of him and what he will expect of them. Through this informational exchange the nurse begins to communicate his professional role, and the nurse-patient relationship is begun.

Conducting the Interview It is important to have a quiet place for the interview where parents, child, and nurse will feel comfortable and at ease. As much as possible the interview should be conducted in one session with no interruptions.

When appropriate (usually according to the age and developmental level of the child) the interview should be carried out in three phases: (1) nurse, parent, and child; (2) nurse and parents; and (3)

nurse and child. This sequence allows each individual the confidentiality of exchanging and receiving personal information. During the interview between nurse, parent, and child, which should be conducted first, the nurse explains to the family members the sequence of interviews. There may be instances in which the nurse assesses that the two parents should be interviewed separately, or the parents may initiate this request.

While the parents and nurse are talking and the child is present, he may be provided with a quiet activity such as books or drawing materials. The child should be included in the interview whenever he wants to contribute or when the nurse detects that he wants to say something. During this part of the interview the nurse can assess to some extent how the parents interact with their child, how he reacts to discipline, and how independent he is in expressing himself.

The nurse-parent interview is necessary for providing information about the child's illness or proposed treatment which might be upsetting for the child to hear. During this time the parents have an opportunity to express their own fears.

The child in his interview with the nurse has an opportunity to express the fears about his illness and hospitalization that he might be unable to show in his parents' presence. At this time the nurse has an opportunity to further establish an individual relationship with the child.

It is a good idea to explain to the family at the beginning of the interview the purpose of the informational exchange and to give a brief description of what will be discussed. As the interview progresses, the family's facial expressions, gestures, and body movements, not just their verbal responses, should be carefully noted. These mannerisms may indicate sensitive areas which should be explored in greater depth or which should be discussed at another time (providing the information is not vital to immediate care).

Exchange Information A variety of interview guides have been developed to help in the informational exchange process. Some are quite detailed in enumerating in checklist fashion characteristics of the patient and details pertinent to his nursing care. Others are more open-ended and require that information be written in a narrative form similar to the traditional medical history. Regardless of form, some type of guideline is necessary for organizing and recording data obtained during the informational exchange process. The interview guide should be a workable, usable tool for the nursing staff who use it, and it should help them to assess, plan, and evaluate nursing care more accurately.

There are specific types of information which should be acquired in an interview; they are described below. As these topics are discussed with the family, the nurse needs to keep in mind that although information about the child's illness and his deviations from the established "normal" are important, it is equally important to establish the "normal" patterns of growth, development, and behavior for the individual child. The focus of the informational exchange should be on determining what the child and his parents can do for themselves and what the nurse can do for them while they are in the hospital.

The giving of information is just as important as acquiring information in the nursing interview. As information is obtained in each area of the history, the nurse should explain to the family how he will use that information to meet their individual needs during hospitalization.

GUIDELINES FOR THE NURSING INTERVIEW

Identification
    Hospital identification stamp
    Child's nickname
    Chronologic age and birthdate
Health and physical development
    Length, symptoms, and nature of present illness
    Past illnesses and health care
    Allergies to medications, food, or other substances
    Immunizations
    Names of medications child has taken
    Form in which medication was given and how child accepted
    Gross motor development, i.e., sitting, walking, jumping
    Fine motor development, i.e., eye movements, grasping, writing
    Sensory development, i.e., vision, hearing, smell, taste, touch
    General physical appearance
Hospitalization
    When and where previous hospitalizations occurred
    Helpful or harmful incidents during previous hospitalizations
    Treatments and procedures performed
    Preparation for present admission
    Expectations for hospitalization
    Experiences with hospitalization and illness of family members
Social-Cultural
    Geographic and neighborhood setting
    Type of dwelling
    Ethnic background
    Religious preferences
    Parental and family relations
    Friends and other people important to child
    Recent changes in environment and family relations
    Present level of social development
    Educational level of parents
    Economic status
    Hospitalization financing
Nutrition
    Types of food, fluid, and formula
    Current food and fluid likes and dislikes
    Special diets
    Mealtime patterns
    Ability to feed self
Elimination
    Frequency of bowel movement and urination
    Constipation problems and remedies
    Present level of bowel and bladder control
Sleep
    Sleeping arrangements, i.e., type of bed and with whom child sleeps
    Hours for day and nighttime sleeping
    Wakeful or sound sleeper
Communication
    Present level of language development
    Special words: i.e., words for bowel movement, urination, hunger
Behavior
    Habits or rituals
    Reaction to stress and comforting measures
    Methods of discipline and reaction to discipline
    Behaviors for which punished
    Types of punishment
    Interaction with others
Play
    Playmates and pets
    Special games and hobbies
    Favorite playthings
    Playthings brought to the hospital from home

Reinforcing Information   Although a great deal of information is exchanged between nurse and family during the orientation and the interview, the nurse cannot assume that all this information will be retained by the family. It is therefore important to provide reinforcement of information, particularly throughout the first days of hospitalization. Whenever appropriate, all members of the nursing staff can reinforce information which they know is a part of the admission procedure.

HOSPITAL ENVIRONMENT

Hospitalization and the possibility of living in the hospital environment provide conditions which are stressful to most families. Separation, decreased mobility, enforced dependence, unfamiliar routines, and fears and misunderstandings can all cause the child and his family varying degrees of anxiety. The nurse can help the hospitalized child and his family maintain normalcy by sustaining an environment which will meet the physical needs of parents who stay with their child and contribute to the child's developmental progress while he is in the hospital surroundings.

The Infant

Parent Participation The infant's immediate surroundings are usually limited to the world of his crib and to the closeness of his mother's arms. The sensations he receives are mainly visual, tactile, auditory, and oral, and through these modes he learns in the first few months of life to identify his mother. It is therefore important for the basic development of trust that the infant's needs for food, warmth, and love be met by his mother or a constant mother figure throughout the period of infancy.

Providing for infant-mother interaction is particularly important when the infant must be hospitalized, not only for the infant, but also for his mother as well, since most mothers need the satisfaction of mothering and caring for their infants. For some mothers, demands at home may rightfully take precedence over staying at the hospital with their infant. In this instance nursing care should be planned to allow the same person to care for the infant each day, so that his needs are met by a consistent mother figure.

A rooming-in or living-in arrangement which allows at least one parent to stay with their infant 24 hours a day is the best way to continue the close relationship necessary during this period of development. There are also other advantages in this type of arrangement. Having parents present gives the nursing staff an opportunity to assess more closely family strengths and weaknesses and to teach parents to give care that will be necessary after discharge. Parents are available to participate in the child's care, making them feel as though they are providing a real contribution to helping the child get well.

Living-in also allows for more informal contact with the nursing staff and contributes to a freer exchange of information. Families can give each other support as daily contacts bring them closer together. A lounge or small corner with table, comfortable chairs, and coffeepot can provide an informal environment to help stimulate interaction among parents, families, and staff.

In order for living-in to be beneficial to the family and the nursing staff, it must be well planned, supervised, and evaluated. Policies concerning rights and privileges of families should be carefully planned and explained. A brochure which describes appropriate ways parents can participate in their infant's care can help them feel more comfortable and secure in their hospital role. Some considerations for living-in policies should include hygiene facilities, eating and sleeping arrangements, and recreation and relaxation privileges.

Environmental Stimulation for the Infant The infant's environment—his crib world—should be kept well supplied with a variety of objects for auditory, tactile, and oral stimulation. Very often crib playthings of varying colors, shapes, and textures can be hung over the top and on the sides of the crib. The infant's ability to grasp and move about should be assessed so that the playthings can be placed where he will receive the most benefit from them and where they will be safely secured. For example, the infant under 6 weeks keeps his head turned toward one side or the other when he lies on his back. Objects for his visual stimulation should therefore be attached to the sides of his crib rather than strung over the top.

Special seats designed to help the infant maintain an upright position are very useful in helping provide a change of scene. He can be safely placed in his seat inside his crib and be in a new position to reach for dangling playthings, thereby encouraging the development of his eye-hand coordination (see Fig. 30-1). In his special seat the infant can comfortably be placed in a variety of places throughout the pediatric unit where he can be stimulated by a change of scene and still be carefully observed by the nursing staff.

An important part of the infant's development is learning about himself through the discovery of his own body. The placement of a mirror on the side of his crib or on the wall near his crib can aid this aspect of his development. Tactile stimulation by those who dress, bathe, and change his diapers will also help him become aware of his body.

As the infant's gross motor development progresses, he needs to be provided with more space where he can creep, crawl, and scoot about. An area of the playroom can be set aside for the supervised infant to play on a carpeted or padded floor. Small walking and scooting toys can be used to further stimulate development of gross motor skills.

Providing a change of scene other than the crib surroundings or one room is particularly important for the infant over 6 months of age. Regular trips to the playroom, rides up and down the hallway in a stroller, and merely sitting in an infant seat at the desk while the nurse works nearby can all provide this type of necessary stimulation.

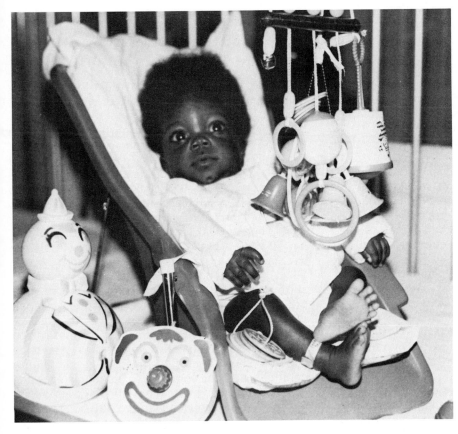

Figure 30-1 The hospital environment can encourage infant development. *(Courtesy of Lynn Brown.)*

The Toddler

Need for Parental Support The toddler is beginning to develop the ability to separate from his mother, but if his mother must leave him in the hospital, it is usually a distressing experience for all concerned. As the toddler actively explores his environment by using his newly developed motor skills, he practices separating from his mother. It is necessary for him to return to her frequently, however, to assure himself that she is there. When he must be separated from his mother, he feels concern for her whereabouts, and he cannot tolerate long periods of separation without expressing his feelings of being abandoned.

Most toddlers are in the process of learning bowel and bladder control: hospitalization can be a real disruption to this process. His limited vocabulary makes it difficult for him to express his needs or to be understood, and he may even have his own personal words or meanings. Consequently it is important to provide living-in or unrestricted visiting privileges for the toddler's mother, so that she can help interpret his needs and tell him what is happening and so that she can help provide continuity in his personal care.

Toddler Safety The toddler has developed increased skills in walking and in the manipulation of objects. These new abilities plus an inability to judge situations and objects which may be harmful to him make the toddler particularly vulnerable to the many safety hazards which can be found in the hospital environment. These factors make it necessary to continually assess the environment and the individual child's needs for care and supervision within it.

Floors and walls in all areas of the pediatric unit which are accessible to the toddler must be kept as clean as possible. The floor is one of the toddler's favorite play areas, and vinyl or similarly surfaced hard floors should not be too highly waxed and polished or they may lead to falls. An easily cleaned indoor-outdoor carpeting is ideal for the pediatric area as it provides protection against tumbles and softness and warmth for play with trucks, blocks, and pull toys.

The use of child-size furniture in children's rooms and the play area will minimize risks that the toddler will fall or be injured. Furniture such as high chairs, toddler-size tables, and strollers should be periodically inspected for safety.

Electricity is an integral part of the hospital environment and offers a variety of hazards to the toddler's safety. Light switches should be in good working order and when possible should be located out of the toddler's reach, as the curious child may injure himself or others by turning a power source on or off. Electrical outlets should be securely covered at all times when not in use to prevent the curious toddler from poking his fingers or conductive toys into a dangerous opening. Numerous pieces of electrical equipment such as mist machines, heating pads, and suction machines must be considered as potential hazards to the toddler and must be regularly checked by the nursing staff.

Particular attention should be given to the storage and disposal of drugs and small pieces of expendable equipment. Many storage areas can easily be closed off from the toddler who might wander in. The control of disposable equipment is more complex, and the nursing staff should be alert for dangerous objects discarded in trash cans accessible to children. Toddlers at eye level with waste cans may discover tempting playthings in discarded equipment.

Play materials, a controllable part of the child's environment, must be continually assessed. Parents may provide toys which are not suitable for their child, particularly if his illness has interfered with his usual ability to play. By discussing the child's play habits with his parents, the nurse can help them choose safe toys for him to use in the hospital. All playthings that the child uses should be appropriate for his level of development and suitable for the activity allowed by his illness.

Environment for the Toddler Although the toddler is in the process of developing fine motor skills, the development of gross motor skills predominates. Locomotion and the movement of the large muscles of his body are particularly important in his everyday activity. In planning the environment suitable for the toddler, his need for development of large muscles should be a primary purpose for providing equipment and activities.

In many hospital environments the playroom is the most appropriate place for the toddler to engage in play, and he should spend some time there every day. The playroom should be supplied with a variety of push-and-pull toys, and large push-apart and put-together toys. Rocking horses, small wagons, and pounding toys are all appropriate for the playroom, and their use can encourage large-muscle development.

If his illness does not permit him to leave his own room or his bed, appropriate gross motor activities should be provided to suit the toddler's condition. Even quiet activities such as play with large boxes, nesting toys, light-weight sponge balls, and blocks can stimulate gross motor development.

In addition to gross motor development the toddler's language skills are developing during this period as he learns the names of things in his environment. Picture books can provide endless possibilities for introducing new words to the toddler. His surroundings in the hospital can also be planned to provide more experiences. This can be accomplished by placing colorful pictures on the walls or by having bulletin boards where new pictures can be displayed. Other decorative devices such as printed curtains, sheets, and bedspreads can also supply colorful scenes or figures. Hospital equipment and any object in the toddler's surroundings are potential sources of language learning for him, and it remains only for his nurse or his parents to stimulate him by telling him the names of things, repeating them, and helping him learn new words.

The toddler is also learning new social skills such as how to feed himself and how to control his bowel and bladder functions. Equipment should be provided which is as much like what he uses at home as possible. The toddler table is lower in height, provides more space for eating, and serves the same function as the standard high chair which many toddlers use at home. Portable toddler-size toilet seats are necessary equipment to help provide as much continuity as possible in toilet training, which is usually in progress during the toddler period.

The Preschooler

Parent Participation The preschooler has a beginning understanding of past and future and an increased ability to retain a mental image of his mother when she is not present. He may therefore be capable of spending periods of time in the hospital without a parent staying with him.

The preschooler may regress when ill and hospitalized, and the presence of a parent can minimize regression. His daily routines and patterns of toileting and feeding can also be better carried out with a parent present. It is important to provide facilities for parents of preschoolers to live-in or spend as much time with their child as they think and as the nurse assesses is necessary.

The preschooler's language interpretation and understanding of words are more highly developed than the toddler's, but he may have his own private meanings for words, and these need to be interpreted by his parent and recorded on the nursing interview form. During this period of development the preschooler's emerging self-concept is influenced by the approval of significant people; this is another reason for having his parents with him most of the time.

During this period of development the young child is beginning to enjoy play with children his own age, and he can cooperate with his peers. Having a roommate near his age or the same age can provide opportunity for group play which is important at this time. Together, preschoolers may begin to act out some of their feelings through group play. Sharing a room may bring disadvantages, depending upon the complexity of illness of the children. Careful consideration should be given to the types and severity of illness of preschoolers who are allowed to share a room. Privacy is necessary when procedures such as a bandage change may be viewed by a roommate, and painful treatments should be carried out in the treatment room.

Environment for Preschool Play The preschooler needs to work through the problems which may be presented by his illness, hospitalization, or normal growth and development. He is able to explore and solve many of his problems through group play and expressive play. As much as possible, his environment should allow and contribute to these types of experiences.

Either a child's own room or a corner of the playroom may become an area for several preschoolers to express themselves with puppets, a play house, miniature store, or other types of dramatic play. Dress-up clothing may be made available to allow the child to assume roles of family members or people he sees in the hospital. Although this type of play should be well-supervised, an element of privacy is needed to allow the child the feeling of complete freedom in acting out his feelings.

Activities such as simple crafts and imitating adult tasks can serve as expressive play (see Fig. 30-2). Supplies for drawing, painting, and other creative efforts can also be provided. Bulletin boards in

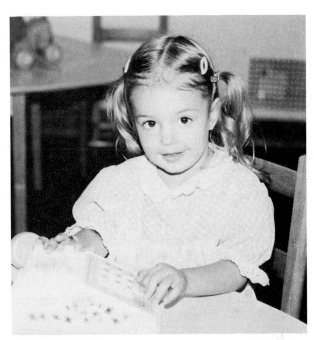

Figure 30-2 The preschool child needs to engage in expressive play. *(Courtesy of Lynn Brown.)*

the child's room or in the hallways should be provided for displaying the child's handiwork as most preschoolers take pride in their efforts and their creations.

Most preschoolers are able to take care of many of their simple hygiene needs by themselves, and their environment should be structured to allow them to do this. Child-size toilets and other furnishings can aid in self-care and minimize frustration. The child can also help to maintain his environment by assuming simple responsibilities for keeping his room in order and his toys in their proper place. By participating in all these self-care activities, the preschooler can be encouraged in his ability to be independent.

The School-Age Child

School Activities To the school-age child illness and hospitalization lead to a discontinuity in formal and informal learning. Most school-age children thrive on and have a genuine interest in learning about everything both in and out of the formal educational setting. In appropriate cases when the child's illness can allow him to continue his studies and when he is to be hospitalized for a considerable length of time, he should participate in some type of formal learning experience. Many hospitals have a regular school program with a teacher who can meet the child's individual educational needs. If this service is not available, a special tutor or a visiting teacher may be obtained. When possible, continuity with the child's own school program should be provided so that he can continue with his regular schoolwork.

An adequate environment and supplies for learning should be provided for the school-age child. He needs a place to keep his books and other materials and a place and specific time to do his work. An over-bed table may serve the purpose, or he may use a desk or table in the schoolroom or playroom. For the child who must be immobilized, lap boards can be used to aid him in accomplishing written work.

Regardless of whether it is appropriate to continue formal learning, the child's desire to learn can continue to be stimulated in the hospital environment. Seeing hospital equipment such as stethoscopes, intravenous bottles and tubings, syringes, and wheelchairs provides new ground for questioning and learning. His own experiences with the use of equipment and traveling to other parts of the hospital, such as x-ray and physical therapy sections, give him valuable learning experiences. The nurse can contribute to the child's learning and development by answering his questions openly and honestly and by offering information about his surroundings. She may also take an active part in helping other health care workers throughout the hospital understand that learning is an important part of the school-age child's development.

Clubs and fads are important to the school-age child, and the nurse may expect the child to want a poster of his favorite sports star or singing idol pinned up in his room. Collections and hobbies are also important, and the child may bring a collection to the hospital with him (see Fig. 30-3). When possible, shelves, bulletin boards, or a special table may be used to display these items. The child may also need a work table for his hobby, and this table should be left undisturbed if it cannot be in his own room.

The school-age child is beginning to take an interest in assuming tasks and responsibilities in the real world. This phase of his development can be furthered if he is allowed to help with simple tasks on the pediatric unit. He may assist in serving snacks, delivering mail, or keeping the playroom in order.

Maintaining Peer Relationships Peer relationships are an important part of the school-age child's development. He should be encouraged to maintain contact with his friends at home and at school through writing letters, making telephone calls, and visiting when possible. He may quickly form new friendships in the hospital, and these types of peer relationships may be enhanced by roommate selection and placement.

As much as possible, school-age children of the same sex, age, and level of development should be placed in the same room. At times it may also be advisable to place children with similar diagnoses together. By this type of roommate grouping, the important peer relationship may be promoted, and the children may lend each other support during times of stress. For example, 10-year-old Carla, who had had her blood specimen taken the day before, watched as her roommate, 9-year-old Beth, had her blood specimen drawn. As the needle was inserted, Beth wrinkled her face in pain and yelled "Ouch." Carla, from her bed next to Beth's, said "Don't worry, Beth, I had my blood taken yesterday and it hurt, but only for a few minutes." Beth was able to turn toward her roommate, smile, and relax.

Sharing secrets and playing together in small groups are characteristic of the school-age child. Privacy is important to these activities and should be allowed by the nursing staff, yet play needs to be discreetly supervised. A small meeting place or "clubhouse" in a corner of the playroom or a special area of the pediatric unit may become the gathering place for a small group of children to meet and share secrets or work on a special project.

The Adolescent

Adolescent's Own Environment The adolescent is in a transition period from childhood to adulthood and is actively striving for independence. He may seem moody at times as he seeks to master his emotions and his physical body changes. He is capable of more abstract thinking and is beginning to develop his own standards and values. He may rebel against restraints, yet he still needs protection and may ask for it in very indirect ways. He is interested in spending a great deal of his time with other adolescents and may take special interest in a member of the opposite sex. For all these reasons he should have a special environment in the hospital.

Many large hospitals can provide a separate

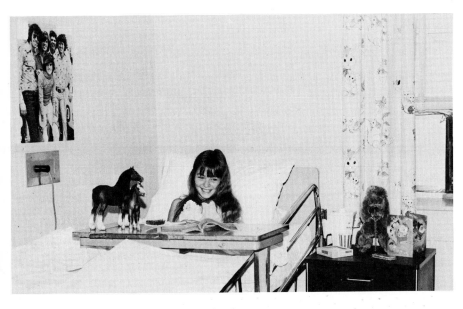

Figure 30-3 School-age patients enjoy decorating their rooms with favorite posters and collections. *(Courtesy of Lynn Brown.)*

adolescent unit just for this age group. If this unit is not possible, a separate wing of the hospital or even a few rooms in one area may be designated for adolescents. The atmosphere of this area should be as unrestricted as possible to help give the adolescent a feeling of independence. Adolescents may even be included in helping set rules and restrictions for living in their area of the hospital.

Physical surroundings should be casual and geared to the interests of adolescents. They need space for their personal belongings, books, hobbies, and mementos which are important to them. An area where groups of young people can get together for meals, parties, or other activities should be available. A supply of snacks for between-meal hunger is a welcome feature.

Responsibility for Care Because independence is important to the adolescent, he and his parents may decide that he can spend most of his time at the hospital without them. Unless the adolescent's illness demands a great deal of support from his parents, he may be quite secure in staying at the hospital, particularly when he has young people with whom he can share this experience. Roommate selection is important for the adolescent; when possible, adolescents with similar interests should be placed in the same room or ward.

The adolescent can assume responsibility for all his personal care if provided with supplies for his

hygienic needs. When able to be out of bed much of the day, adolescents may want to wear their own clothing rather than a hospital gown as their appearance is very important to them. With proper assessment and teaching, the adolescent may assume responsibility for performing simple treatments related to his illness.

BIBLIOGRAPHY

Care of Children in Hospitals, 2d ed., American Academy of Pediatrics, Evanston, Ill., 1971.

Dodson, F.: *How to Parent*, New American Library, Inc., New York, 1971.

Freiberg, K. H.: "How Parents React When Their Child Is Hospitalized," *American Journal of Nursing*, 72:1270–1, 1972.

Godfrey, A. E.: "A Study of Nursing Care Designed to Assist Hospitalized Children and Their Parents in Their Separation," *Nursing Research*, 4:52, 1955.

Hardgrove, Carol, and Dawson, Rosemary: *Parents and Children in the Hospital*, Little, Brown and Company, New York, 1972.

Heiting, K. H.: "Involving Parents in the Residential Treatment of Children," *Children*, 18:162–167, 1971.

Hymovich, D. P.: "ABC's of Pediatric Safety," *American Journal of Nursing*, August 1966.

Issner, N.: "The Family of the Hospitalized Child," *Nursing Clinics of North America*, 7(1):5–12, March 1972.

Kunzman, L.: "Some Factors Influencing a Young Child's Mastery of Hospitalization," *Nursing Clinics of North America*, 7:13–26, March 1972.

Oremland, E. K. and Oremland, J. D.: *The Effects of Hospitalization on Children*, Charles C Thomas, Publisher, Springfield, Ill., 1973.

Petrillo, Madeline: *Emotional Care of Hospitalized Children*, J. B. Lippincott Company, Philadelphia, 1972.

Plank, Emma N.: *Working with Children in Hospitals*, 2d ed., The Press of Case Western Reserve University, Cleveland, 1971.

"Preparing the Child for the Hospital Experience," *Trainex Corporation*, Garden Grove, Calif., 1972.

Wilkins, Gladys N.: "The Role of the Nurse in the Admission of Preschool Children to Hospitals," *Nursing Research*, (1):36–40, 1952.

Hospital Books for Children

Clark, Bettina, and Coleman, L. L.: *Pop-Up Going to the Hospital*, Random House, Inc., New York, 1971 (5–9 yr).

Deegan, P. J., and Larson, B.: *A Hospital: Life in a Medical Center*, Amecus Street Books, Inc., Mankato, Minn., 1971 (8–15 yr).

Falk, Ann Mari: *The Ambulance*, Burke Publishing, Ltd., Toronto, 1966 (4–10 yr).

Froman, R.: *Let's Find Out about the Clinic*, Franklin Watts, Inc., New York, 1968 (5–9 yr).

Haas, Barbara S.: *The Hospital Book*, The John Street Press, Baltimore, 1970 (4–11 yr).

Hallqvist, Britt G.: *Bettina's Secret*, Harcourt Brace & World, Inc., New York, 1967 (8–13 yr).

Kay, Eleanor: *The Clinic*, Franklin Watts, Inc., New York, 1971 (8–12 yr).

————: *First Book of the Emergency Room*, Franklin Watts, Inc., New York, 1970 (9–13 yr).

————: *First Book of the Operating Room*, Franklin Watts, Inc., New York, 1970 (8–13 yr).

Margaret's Heart Operation, Children's Hospital of Philadelphia, Public Relations Department, 1740 Bainbridge Street, Philadelphia, 1969 (3–12 yr).

Michael's Heart Test, Children's Hospital of Philadelphia, Public Relations Department, 1740 Bainbridge St., Philadelphia, 1967 (3–12 yr).

Rey, Margaret, and Rey, H. A.: *Curious George Goes to the Hospital*, Houghton Mifflin Company, Boston, 1966 (4–9 yr).

Schima, Marilyn, and Bolian, Polly: *I Know a Nurse*, G. P. Putnam's Sons, New York, 1969 (6–9 yr).

Shay, A.: *What Happens When You Go to the Hospital*, Reilly & Lee Company, Chicago, 1969 (4–11 yr).

Tamburine, Jean: *I Think I Will Go to the Hospital*, Abingdon Press, Nashville, Tenn., 1965 (4–11 yr).

Watson, Jane Werner, Switzer, R. E., and Hirschberg, J. C.: *My Friend the Doctor*, Golden Press, New York, 1972 (4–6 yr).

Weber, A.: *Elizabeth Get Well*, Thomas Y. Crowell Company, New York, 1970 (5–10 yr).

Welzenbach, J., and Cline, Nancy: *Hello Hospital!*, Med-Educators Inc., Chicago, 1970 (4–12 yr).

———— and ————: *The Hospital See-Through Machine*, Med-Educators Inc., Chicago, 1970 (4–12 yr).

———— and ————: *The Hospital Sandman*, Med-Educators Inc., Chicago, 1970 (4–12 yr).

———— and ————: *A "Mill-Yun" Hospital Questions*, Med-Educators Inc., Chicago, 1970 (4–12 yr).

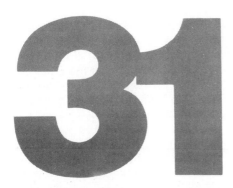

PREPARATION FOR DISCHARGE FROM THE HOSPITAL

JOYCE M. OLSON

NEED FOR DISCHARGE PLANNING

In the effort to provide comprehensive nursing care for the hospitalized pediatric patient and his family, nursing intervention will involve several interrelated functions. The nurse is concerned with providing (1) direct physical care pertinent to the disease or illness process; (2) psychologic support for the child and his family; and (3) appropriate activities to promote the continued growth and development of the child and utilize his capabilities fully. These activities are necessary whether the illness is of an acute or chronic nature.

The long-range goals in the care of the child hospitalized with an acute illness episode are (1) returning the child to the highest possible level of physical and emotional health; and (2) maintaining the family integrity. With the chronically ill child, the long-range goal is the maintenance of the highest possible level of physical and emotional health for both child and family. In the event that the child and family are faced with a terminal illness, the long-range goal is keeping the child at home for as long as possible while providing support for the child and family to maximize coping abilities and family function. With any hospitalization, one of the goals is also to minimize the psychologic trauma to the child.

When these long-range goals are a part of the care plan during hospitalization, the integration of the components of the nursing process (assessment, planning, intervention, and evaluation) will include planning for discharge. The pediatric nurse will be concerned with what happens to the child and family upon discharge and return home. Continuity of care has become a frequently used phrase in nursing practice, but it has also been said that discharge planning is often done poorly and seldom evaluated for effectiveness.[1]

Extending nursing intervention beyond the spatial and temporal setting of the current hospitalization to provide for the ongoing physical, psychosocial, and cognitive needs of the child and family is necessary if we are to provide continuity of care. The nurse assumes a leadership role in assessing the need for ongoing care after discharge. He is also instrumental in the planning for, implementation of, and evaluation of the plan for discharge and post-discharge care.

FACTORS WHICH INFLUENCE DISCHARGE PLANNING

The degree of continuity or effectiveness of discharge planning will depend upon the abilities of the health care disciplines involved to communicate and work cooperatively toward common goals established with and for the child and family.

The general objectives of discharge planning are (1) to ensure that there will be no interruption in the care required by the child and his family; (2) to provide the family with adequate information and instruction to allow them to care for the child; and, (3) to involve appropriate other agencies as needed and provide them with the necessary information to ensure continuity.[2]

Planning for discharge begins with the admission of the child. During the admission interview, the nurse will obtain information that will be useful in this planning. The reason for admission, the initial patient and family understanding of the illness process, and data about the family constellation, patterns of daily living, geographic location, and financial status provide the basis for beginning to plan for discharge.

Throughout the child's hospital stay, additional information is gathered which will help the nurse identify learning needs and determine capabilities of the child and family. Several variables will influence the specifics of the discharge planning as it evolves. Consideration must be given to the physical needs related to the illness, to growth, and to developmental, emotional, social, and environmental needs. The delineation of need priority will be further influenced by (1) the age of the patient, (2) the severity of the health problem, (3) the patient and family response to medical and nursing intervention, (4) the strengths and resources of the family in providing for the child's continuing care needs, and (5) the involvement of the child and family in the planning for discharge.

Readers can refer to other sections of this book for discussions of normal growth and development, factors which influence or impair growth and development, reactions to hospitalization by children of various ages, and health problems common to the age groups.

COMPONENTS OF DISCHARGE PLANNING

Identification of learning needs and assessment of the family's ability to provide care and cope with the illness ramifications provide the core of the discharge plan.

How does the nurse identify the learning needs of the child and family? Some needs will be easily identified. If the child is a newly diagnosed cardiac or diabetic, the need to understand medication and diet management is obvious. The ability of the child

and/or family to understand the disease process, deal with acceptance of the illness or injury, and provide long-term care at home is less easily determined. Observation of the child and family, and involvement of them in care during the hospitalization, are necessary if needs are to be adequately identified.

Other needs will be identified as the child or family ask direct questions of the nurse. Will Johnny's activity be limited when he gets home? How am I going to keep a 4-year-old quiet for a month? Where can I buy the special formula my baby needs? What should I do if the tube comes out?

Learning needs related to direct physical care are more easily identified by both the nurse and the family. However, the nurse must remember that many families are hesitant to ask questions. Careful listening to the parents as they talk to the nurse or to the parent and child as they interact will help the nurse further identify needs to be met in preparation for discharge. For example, Billy, age 4, has had a temporary colostomy performed because of Hirschsprung's disease. As the nurse enters the room, Billy's mother is saying, "I wonder what your sister is going to think about this bag you have to wear." Is she concerned about explaining it to siblings? Is she concerned about Billy being "different"? Only by talking with Billy's mother will the nurse determine the real concerns and intervene to meet the need.

Observation of the behavior of the child and family may provide the nurse with additional information. Comprehensive nursing care involves the assessment of the parent-child relationship. Anticipatory guidance and teaching may be needed in the areas of discipline management, realistic behavior expectations, management of fears and anxieties, or in helping the parent cope with normal developmental tasks.

Communication between the physician, nurse, and other health-team members is vital in the preparation for discharge. The disciplines involved will vary with the particular child and family. All must cooperatively determine the goals and identify needs relevant to preparing the child and family for discharge. The contributions of each toward meeting the goals must be clearly understood. It is the nurse's responsibility to initiate communication and coordinate planning. This can be most easily accomplished if the primary-nurse concept is utilized. One nurse then has the responsibility for planning care of the child throughout the hospitalization, and can effectively coordinate the planning for discharge. In this age of specialization, we often find several physicians and multiple disciplines involved with one child and family. Involved in the care of the child with a meningomyelocele will be a neurosurgeon, urologist, orthopedist, physical therapist, bracemaker, nurse, and perhaps the social worker and schoolteacher. The nurse has the greatest opportunity to integrate plans and reinforce teaching with the child and family. The nurse is also best able to assess readiness for discharge and must assume a major responsibility for communicating this status of the child and family to other members of the team.

In addition to effective verbal communication and cooperative planning, a *written* plan for discharge is essential. It should include the goals for the individual child and family and specific instructions necessary to carry out the plan. Movement toward the goals and completion of specific parts of the plan are also indicated in writing. This written plan allows for consistency between disciplines and between the three shifts of nursing personnel providing care to the child and family.

Another important aspect of the preparation for discharge is the identification of need for and appropriate use of persons, agencies, or facilities to assist in providing follow-up care. Again, it is the nurse's responsibility to know the community resources that are available or to communicate with someone in the hospital setting who has this knowledge. In metropolitan areas, resources are usually available; in rural areas, necessary follow-up may be more difficult to arrange. When preparation for discharge is initiated early, appropriate plans can be made.

In some settings, the hospital nurse will move into the community to provide follow-up care and continuity. In the future, we may find this occurring more frequently. In many hospitals, a nurse is employed as a community health coordinator to facilitate discharge planning, communication, and continuity.

Early involvement of the person or agency who will assist the family postdischarge is important. It is ideal if the community health nurse, social worker, mental health worker, or other appropriate person sees the child and family in the hospital and is included in the team planning for discharge.

In the event that the geographic location does not have necessary follow-up services, a longer hospitalization may be required, or arrangements made which place a greater burden on the family in terms of time, travel, or expense. The family needs sufficient time to make whatever arrangements are necessary.

Verbal communication via the telephone can be utilized during the planning for discharge and at the time of discharge. A complete written referral form or discharge summary which includes family data, goals for the child and family, known or anticipated assistance needed, teaching carried out in the hospital, and current status of the child and family should be immediately available to those providing follow-up care. It is also important that the family and person or agency providing care know whom to contact, should they have questions. Many questions related to the day-to-day care of the child at home can best be answered by the nurse who has cared for the child during hospitalization. Parents need to know that they may call in and seek assistance at any time.

The family needs clearly written instructions and information regarding medications, dressing changes, exercise, activity, and any similar procedures they are expected to carry out.

TEACHING THE CHILD AND FAMILY

Since teaching is a primary tool utilized by the nurse in preparing the child and family for discharge, a brief review of some of the basic principles of teaching as discussed by Redman is appropriate.[3]

Learning goals can be classified into three domains. The cognitive domain focuses on understanding; the affective domain, on attitudes; and the psychomotor domain, on motor skills. Teaching necessary in preparation for discharge most commonly involves all three domains. The nurse is concerned with the child's and family's understanding of the illness process or injury effect, the acceptance of the illness or injury by the child and family, and the development of the motor skills necessary to management. Specific learning goals will vary with the individual child's or family's abilities and situation. Goals for the child and the teaching methods used must take into consideration his intellectual level, motor skill ability, and psychosocial development.

Motivation is required if the individual is to learn. Telling the child or family about the illness process or treatment method does not ensure learning. Learning is most effective when the individual is ready to learn. Motivation and learning readiness must be continually assessed by the nurse while planning for and implementing the teaching for discharge.

In the hospital situation, several factors can interfere with or delay the readiness of the child or family to learn. The process of adaptation will vary with the severity of illness and its implications for the child and family. Early in the adaptation process, denial or disbelief is often present. Even though the nurse must begin planning for discharge upon admission, it may take several days of support and reinterpretation of information before acceptance begins to occur and the child and family are ready to begin learning. Helping the child and family to reach this point is a part of preparation for discharge. The child or family faced with birth defects, diabetes, leukemia, or serious trauma such as burns, head injuries, or multiple system injuries may have a prolonged adaptation period.

The nurse will also need to consider the hierarchy of human needs when assessing readiness to learn. Maslow lists physiologic needs as most basic, followed by safety, love and belonging, self-esteem, and self-actualization. The child who is in pain or who is frightened of all that is happening to him will not be receptive to teaching. The family that is extremely insecure and anxious cannot be attentive to teaching. A mild level of anxiety is helpful in learning, but increasing levels are detrimental.

Closely intertwined with the emotional readiness to learn is the experiential readiness. Learning most easily moves from the known to the unknown. Does the child or family possess the knowledge needed as a basis for learning a new skill? Are attitudes present that will interfere with learning? Assessment of prerequisite knowledge and behaviors is necessary if the nurse is to carry out teaching in a manner meaningful to the learner.

The material to be learned needs to be presented in a form that can be understood by the child and family. A variety of teaching methods are available to the nurse. One-to-one or group discussion can be used and supplemented with audiovisual materials such as booklets or filmstrips. Often, the nurse will have to use ingenuity in adapting materials to fit the situation. When the requirement is the learning of physical skills necessary to care, demonstration, return demonstration, and practice are the most effective. This teaching should utilize the materials the family will be using at home. As a part of discharge preparation, the nurse will plan with the family to allow time for practice. The child and family must be able to "get into the act" if changes in behavior, development of understanding, and competency in motor skills are to occur. Perhaps the best way to accomplish this is to have the mother room with the child and assume responsibility for care while someone is available for support and assistance.

It is also important for the nurse to remember that materials to be learned should be presented in small parts and sequential order. It is easy for the family to be overwhelmed by what seems to be "so much to learn." An overview of what needs to be accomplished before discharge is helpful, but this must be coupled with the assurance that the objective will be to accomplish "one step at a time." The learner needs to receive feedback as to his accomplishments and progress toward the goals. Positive feedback and successes will provide motivation to continue the learning process.

Teaching also requires that some method of evaluation be used to determine its effectiveness. Again, the nurse may want to use a variety of methods such as oral questions and answers, written quizzes, or return demonstrations. This is done during the hospitalization to determine effectiveness of teaching at that point in time. It is continued after discharge to determine the persistance of the change in behavior and evaluate the ability of the child and family to continue care in the home setting. Feedback from the community health nurse, evaluation at later clinic visits and physician visits, or other communication with agencies providing follow-up is necessary if improvement in preparation for discharge is to occur.

CASE STUDIES
Adolescent with Chronic Illness

Jean, a 13-year-old girl with myelodysplasia, was admitted for evaluation of her total health status, but with a chief complaint of an open wound on her thigh and burns on both feet.

Past Medical History Jean's meningomyelocele had been closed soon after birth and hydrocephalus had not developed. Initial treatment had been carried out in another state. She had been followed at another health care facility for 8 to 9 years and then "lost to follow-up." Past records were not available.

Social History Jean lives with her parents, both in their forties, and two brothers, age 16 and 18. Her father is a minister and her mother is also employed full-time. They reside in a community of 11,000, approximately 150 miles from the center where Jean is hospitalized. Some financial assistance is available through the Crippled Children's Commission, and the family also has insurance. Jean had at one time attended regular school, but because of problems with urinary and bowel incontinence had not gone for 3 years. Tutoring in the home had been sporadic with none for the past year. Jean appears to be of average intelligence.

Physical Findings on Admission

Sensory level at L3

Large decubitus on right posterior thigh

Probable neurogenic bladder with urinary incontinence

Bowel incontinence

Obesity—weight 145 pounds

Flaccid lower extremities

Chronic hip subluxation

Rotatory scoliosis

Healing second-degree burns on both feet

Consultations included urology, orthopedics, nursing, physical medicine, plastic surgery, social service, dietetics, and child psychiatry. In addition to the multiple physical problems, it was felt that Jean was also socially and intellectually deprived. She was at home alone most of the day, and seldom taken out of the home.

After the initial assessment and evaluation was completed, a conference involving the patient, family, urologist, orthopedist, and nurse was arranged. At this time goals and priorities were discussed with the family, and additional information obtained from them. As the various goals were discussed, comments and questions from the family helped the health care team to determine their understanding of and attitudes toward Jean's problems and probable methods of treatment.

Goal: Control of Urinary Incontinence

Summary of interaction   Control of urinary incontinence by indwelling catheter had been tried before without success. Urine had leaked around the catheter necessitating mother leaving work to take Jean home from school and resulting in her eventual withdrawal from school. The family had previously heard about an ileal conduit and asked if this would be more feasible. The urologist agreed that this might be necessary, but pointed out that Jean's obesity would make the surgery technically difficult and that it would also create problems with appliance management. The family agreed to having a cystoscopy and cystourethrogram performed to determine whether a mechanical problem such as bladder stones or partial innervation might be causing the leakage problems. If not, they were willing to try catheter drainage again.

Goal: Control of Bowel Incontinence

Summary of interaction   A training program had not been tried before. The technique was explained to the family. Since regularity is a requirement of the training program, an evening time was decided upon to better fit into the family's activity schedule. The possibility of Jean managing this function independently was discussed. The parents had been told several years earlier that Jean would need a colostomy, and they asked if this would be easier to manage and have better results. The reasons for not doing a colostomy seemed to be understood by the family.

Goal: Closure of the Decubitus by Skin Grafting

Summary of interaction   Skin grafting was necessary to provide coverage that would not easily break down again as Jean returned to using a wheelchair. This procedure was readily accepted by the family. Both parents and Jean asked that grafts be taken from an area other than the lower thigh if possible so that scars would not be visible when Jean wore short dresses.

Goal: Weight Loss

Summary of interaction   Both parents were pessimistic as to achieving weight loss, commenting that they and relatives on both sides of the family tended to be heavy. Jean's father had read about "bypass surgery" and asked about the possibility of doing this at the same time the ileoconduit, if necessary, was performed. The family seemed to accept the reasons for this not being a realistic method of treatment for Jean. The 1200-cal diet which had already been started, was mentioned, as was Jean's 1-lb weight loss to date.

Goal: Return to School

Summary of interaction   Both parents indicated a desire to get Jean back in school. However, they were concerned about transportation and about there being no school nurse to assist Jean. Jean's 16-year-old brother had in the past pushed her the eight blocks to school when weather permitted.

Goal: Ambulation (delayed but eventual goal)

Summary of interaction   Jean's father expressed disappointment that ambulation was not given high priority and again questioned the goal of weight loss prior to attempting ambulation.

The family also asked questions about the effect of myelodysplasia on Jean's menstrual function and sexual development. Goals relevant to planning for discharge at this time were stated in the care plan.

1 Patient and family will understand the process of bowel training and demonstrate ability to carry out the program.

   a Assist Jean in assuming responsibility for

bowel management program—regularity, use of suppository, Valsalva maneuver

b Plan with family for time to include them in teaching

2 Patient and family will be able to select foods appropriate to weight reduction diet and plan meals.

a Dietitian to instruct patient and family in 1200-cal diet

b Jean to assume responsibility for selecting menu

c Continue to assess motivation and ability to adhere to diet

3 Patient will be using wheelchair for mobility.

a Contact Crippled Children's Commission for financing and make necessary arrangements for family to obtain.

b Obtain flotation pad for use in wheelchair and on bed.

4 Patient and family will understand the need for physical therapy program and demonstrate ability to perform exercise routine.

a Physical therapist to instruct patient and family in exercises for strengthening upper extremities, preventing further contractures of lower extremities, and maximizing hip and knee flexor potential.

b The nurse caring for Jean will reinforce teaching.

5 Jean will increase socialization and intellectual activities.

a Involve hospital schoolteacher

b Obtain books from local school

c Contact local school system to plan for homebound teaching after discharge until physical status permits return to school.

d Involve Jean in occupational therapy program and ward activities.

6 Jean will assume responsibility for activities of daily living.

a Continue to assess Jean's motivation and ability to function independently

b Jean is to care for personal hygiene needs and manage bowel and exercise programs. (Planned surgery will temporarily alter this goal.)

7 Staff will help Jean to verbalize her feelings, concerns, and aspirations about the future and in relation to the developmental tasks of adolescence.

a Provide continuity in the caring person and develop a milieu of trust and confidentiality that will allow Jean to verbalize

b Attempt to ascertain the family's view of Jean's potential

8 Begin planning with follow-up services.

Contact the Community Health Nurse to determine resources available in the local community for physical care and psychologic and developmental support.

During the next week of hospitalization, indwelling catheter drainage proved effective in maintaining bladder continence. An additional goal could then be added.

9 Jean and her family will understand the care and management of the indwelling catheter and demonstrate ability to perform the necessary skills.

a Jean and her mother will do perineal care twice daily and after each bowel movement

b Jean and her mother will irrigate the catheter twice daily using aseptic technique.

c The Community Health Nurse will change the catheter every other week and as needed

d Jean and her mother will demonstrate knowledge of the need for adequate fluid intake and of the signs or symptoms indicating the need for catheter change or a beginning urinary-tract infection.

The decubitus was grafted and closed during the third week of hospitalization. Both the wound and donor sites healed well. Jean continued to improve in her ability to manage daily activities but required much encouragement to carry them out. Verbalization of her feelings and concerns was limited throughout the hospitalization. Behavior at times was manipulative and demanding with staff and family. As the family could visit only once a week, teaching sessions were planned for that time. Discussion of the need to encourage independence and discourage manipulative behavior was also included.

As wounds healed, limited sitting was allowed, and transfer from bed to wheelchair was included in the teaching. As the time for discharge neared, both Jean and her family demonstrated understanding of the treatment plan and the ability to perform the techniques required. The motivation of the patient and family to maintain the program over a long period of time was still questionable.

Jean was discharged at the end of 6 weeks with arrangements made for:

Tutoring on a daily basis

Assistance in the home when family not present

Community Health Nurse to visit twice weekly to assess Jean's physical and psychologic status and promote continuation of the bowel, bladder, and exercise programs

Return to paraplegic clinic on a regular basis where she would be seen by the urologist, orthopedist, dietitian, nurse, and physical therapist

Both telephone and written summaries of care during hospitalization and current status of the patient and family were provided to the Community Health Nurse.

As of 6 weeks postdischarge, the treatment program was progressing well at home. Jean was able to be up in the wheelchair for several hours at a time and plans were made to return her to school. Weight loss totaled 6 pounds at this time.

This abbreviated case study is far from inclusive of all that occurred during the hospitalization but is meant to point out the need for beginning discharge preparation early, communication between health team members, involvement of the child and family in realistic goal setting, and utilization of appropriate and available resources to provide continuity of care.

School-Age Child with Acute Illness

Paul, a 7-year-old, was admitted following an accident. He had been hit by a car while riding his bicycle. His presenting problems were a fracture of the left femur, multiple abrasions, and a mild cerebral concussion.

Past Medical History Paul has had measles, chickenpox, and the usual colds and gastrointestinal upsets. No illnesses requiring hospitalization. Immunizations were up to date.

Social History Paul lives with his mother, father, and a sister age 4. All family members are in good health. Father is employed as a maintenance man for the local telephone company, and mother is a housewife. They have insurance which will cover most of the hospital costs.

Treatment Paul's condition was relatively stable on admission. Physical and developmental assessment revealed no abnormal findings other than the fracture, abrasions, and concussion. He was responsive but frightened unless mother was close by. The abrasions were cleansed and the left leg was placed in Russell's traction to maintain immobilization and alignment. The physician explained to the parents that Paul would be in traction for 2 to 3 weeks and then placed in a spica cast for several weeks. He would probably be discharged a day or two after the cast was applied.

With the overall goals of returning the child to the highest possible level of physical and emotional health and maintenance of the family integrity, much of the care in the hospital was carried out with preparation for discharge in mind.

Problem: Paul's parents were both anxious and verbalized, "We shouldn't have let him ride his bike in the street."
In-hospital intervention and application to postdischarge care Listened, empathized with normal concerns for Paul's safety. Reinterpreted normal activity levels of 7-year-old, need for independence, and impossibility of their watching him constantly. Reassured them that the accident was not their fault. Allowed parents to verbalize feelings about the accident. Prevented overprotection and limitation of activity and independence after recovery.

Problem: Paul expressed worry about missing schoolwork and not being able to ride his bike again.
In-hospital intervention and application to postdischarge care Assured Paul that he would be able to ride his bike again. Explained in simple terms the need for the leg to rest and get better. Used appropriate pictures of bones and casts. Arranged for Paul's family to bring in his books and assignments from school so that the hospital schoolteacher, family, and nursing staff could continue his lessons. (If hospital teacher is not available, contact local school system for tutoring.) Allowed for clarification of the temporary nature of the immobility and helped Paul understand the reason for the traction and cast. Maintained intellectual stimulation and developmental level making return to school easier.

Problem: Paul's mother felt she needed to bathe him and help him with every meal.
In-hospital intervention and application to postdischarge care Permitted early in the hospitalization, with discussion of the need for Paul to help himself as much as possible. Fostered independence and self-care as much as possible during hospitalization and postdischarge.

Problem: Immobility interfered with need for activity and industry, occasionally leading to anger and frustration.
In-hospital intervention and application to postdischarge care Provided activities for release of aggressive or angry feelings—punching bag suspended from traction bar. Provided activities to foster creativity within the confines of the traction—construction projects, painting, drawing, scrapbook. Met needs for activity and industry in the hospital and showed mother ways of meeting these needs at home.

Problem: Immobility and hospitalization interfered with sibling and peer contact.

In-hospital intervention and application to postdischarge care Used telephone and parents to maintain home and sibling contact. Encouraged mother to have classmates and friends send cards and letters. Fostered reintegration of the family and peer group relations after discharge and recovery. Maintained contact with the outside world.

Problem: Home assessment in preparation for discharge.

In-hospital intervention and application to postdischarge care Explored the living situation at home. Paul's bedroom was upstairs. A daybed was available downstairs, and Paul's father felt he could carry him up and down. A bed board was to be obtained by the family. The family car was a station wagon, and so transportation to and from the hospital and inclusion of Paul in some family outings would not be a problem. A bedpan and urinal were also obtained by the family. Because discharge needs were anticipated, the family was prepared to leave the hospital ahead of schedule.

Problem: Need for family to feel comfortable and competent in caring for Paul in his cast.

In-hospital intervention and application to postdischarge care The mother was involved with his care after the hip spica was applied. Teaching included the care of the cast, observation of toes for circulation, observations of the cast which might indicate an infection underneath, inspection of skin for irritation from cast edges, checking for small objects which might become lodged underneath the edges of the cast, and the proper method of turning and positioning. Instructions titled "Going Home in a Cast" were also given to the family.

As Paul's parents felt they would be able to manage well at home, a referral was not deemed necessary. They were given the unit number to call should problems arise.

Preparation for the discharge of Paul focused primarily on assisting the mother in meeting the physical and psychosocial needs of a 7-year-old who was to be immobilized for several weeks.

REFERENCES

1 Sister Anne Ambrose, "Discharge Plans—The Weakest Link," *Hospital Progress*, 54:58–60, March 1973.
2 Lynne Power Deakers, "Continuity of Family-Centered Nursing Care between the Hospital and the Home," *Nursing Clinics of North America*, 7(1):83–93, March 1972.
3 Barbara Klug Redman, *The Process of Patient Teaching in Nursing*, The C. V. Mosby Company, St. Louis, 1968.

4

THE DEVELOPMENT, FUNCTION, AND PATHO-PHYSIOLOGY OF BODY SYSTEMS

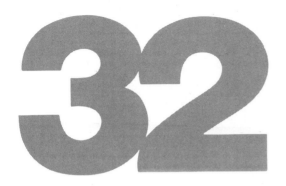

THE NERVOUS SYSTEM

REBECCA SISSON, STEPHANIE CLATWORTHY,
and JOYCE ZADROGA

EMBRYOLOGY

Fetal development consists of three periods of growth. The first period of development is the *pre-embryonic* period, which includes the first 3 weeks of gestation and is concerned with fertilization of the ova and the formation of the embryonic disk. This disk contains three layers, the entoderm, mesoderm, and ectoderm, from which the central nervous system (CNS) develops. The second period of development is termed the *embryonic* period and includes the fourth to eighth weeks of gestation. During this period there is rapid growth, differentiation, and organization of cells which form all the major organs. The third period of development, the *fetal* period, includes the ninth to fortieth weeks of gestation and consists of the completion of fetal growth and development.

Preembryonic Period

The nervous system develops from the ectoderm, which has been established by the third week. The protoplasm of ectodermal tissue is conductive in nature and supports the conduction process found in the nervous tissue.

Embryonic Period

A neural plate is formed by the twenty-first day on the cephalic end of the embryo and rapidly develops a neural groove. On the twenty-second or twenty-third day, fusion of the neural groove begins to form the neural tube, which eventually becomes the CNS. The fusion process takes 5 to 6 days, beginning in the middle of the neural groove and extending simultaneously toward the cephalic and caudal ends of the embryo. The fusing process is a crucial period of development for the nervous system, for it is during this time that CNS malformations may occur because of improper closure of the neural tube. With the closure of the neural tube, three vesicles are formed at the cephalic end; they become the forebrain, midbrain, and hindbrain. The remainder of the neural tube becomes the spinal cord, and the mesenchymal tissue surrounding the neural tube becomes the meninges (see Fig. 32-1 and Table 32-1).

The cells within the neural tube form the neuroglial and nerve cells. The neuroglial cells migrate and take up positions as supporting tissue within the CNS. Some of the cells within the neural tube migrate to the periphery and form the mantle layer, which becomes the gray matter, and some cells from the wall of the neural tube form the marginal

463

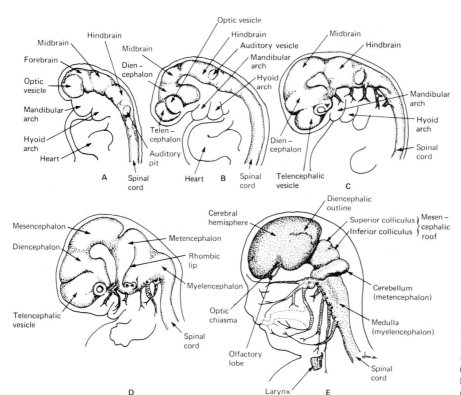

Figure 32-1 Embryology of the central nervous system. Development at (*A*) about 3½ weeks; (*B*) about 4 weeks; (*C*) about 5⅓ weeks; (*D*) about 7 weeks; (*E*) about 11 weeks.

layer, which becomes the myelinated white matter of the CNS. In the fifth week of gestation the cerebral hemisphere begins to develop as evaginations of the forebrain. In addition, the pons and the cerebellum begin to develop in the hindbrain vesicle. From the floor of the future third ventricle a diverticulum erupts, creating the infundibulum; by 8 weeks this contacts Rathke's pouch, which becomes the anterior pituitary.

Fetal Period

The cerebral cortex becomes very cellular in the twelfth week as a result of the migration of nerve and neuroglial cells. The cerebellar hemispheres are evident in the twelfth week, and by the sixteenth week fissures have developed on these surfaces. The ventricles, choroid plexus, medulla, and midbrain complete their development during this period. By the sixteenth week the spinal cord lies at the level of the third lumbar vertebra. At the sixteenth week the spinal cord is beginning to show cervical and lumbar enlargement which corresponds to the development of the extremities, and myelination of the sensory fibers begins. By the twenty-fourth week myelination

begins in the brain. The vestibular nerve is the first sensory fiber that is myelinated; therefore, hearing is well developed at birth. Myelination of the cerebellum begins in the thirty-fourth week.

Late in fetal life the endocrine system begins to influence the function of the CNS. By the fortieth week neurocytes are differentiated in the cerebral cortex. At the time of birth the optic nerve is myelinated, and the descending motor fibers are beginning the process of myelination which continues into the second year of life. Most of the brain is still nonmyelinated at birth; therefore there is little cerebral function, and the motor reactions of respiration, sucking, and swallowing are essential reflexes during the newborn period.

PHYSIOLOGY OF THE NERVOUS SYSTEM

The nervous system is the most highly organized system in the body and controls it in its adjustment to the environment. The system consists of two primary components, the central nervous system and the peripheral nervous system. The central nervous system is the brain and the spinal cord (Figs. 32-2 to 32-4), and the peripheral nervous system is the cere-

Table 32-1 PROGRESSION OF EMBRYOLOGIC DEVELOPMENT OF THE CENTRAL NERVOUS SYSTEM (CNS)

Names in embryonic period	Names at fifth week	Divisions at fifth week	CNS structures	Cranial nerves	Ventricles
Forebrain vesicle	Forebrain (prosencephalon)	Telencephalon	Cerebral hemispheres	I	Lateral ventricles or first, second, and part of third
		Diencephalon	Thalamus, hypothalamus, posterior lobe of hypophysis, optic chiasma, eyes, optic nerves	II	Third
Midbrain vesicle	Midbrain (mesencephalon)	Remains the mesencephalon		III, IV	Cerebral aqueduct (aqueduct of Sylvius)
Hindbrain vesicle	Hindbrain (rhombencephalon)	Metencephalon	Pons varolii, cerebellum	V, VI, VII, VIII	Fourth
		Myelencephalon	Medulla oblongata	IX, X, XI, XII	Fourth

brospinal nerves and the autonomic nervous system which carry impulses to and from the central nervous system (Figs. 32-5 and 32-6). The purpose of the nervous system is accomplished by an intricate conduction of impulses to and from specialized areas of control by electrical and metabolic means.

Properties of the Nervous System

Structure The structural unit of the nervous system is the neuron, or nerve cell, which is composed of a cell body and one or more processes. All but one of the cell processes of the neuron are dendrites which conduct impulses toward the cell body. Neurons have only one axon, which conducts impulses away from the cell body. A neuron is designated as afferent, efferent, or internuncial, according to its function. The afferent neurons are sensory, the efferent are motor, and the internuncial transmit impulses from one neuron to another within the spinal cord or the brain. The connections between axons and dendrites in a chain of neurons are called *synapses*.

Nervous tissue has two basic characteristics known as *excitability*, the ability to be affected by stimuli, and *conductivity*, the ability to transmit impulses from one area of the nervous system to another. A nerve impulse is self-propagating and travels at its own speed, depending on the thickness of the myelin sheath and the size of the nerve fibers, with larger fibers being the most rapid in conduction. Appropriate levels of oxygen, glucose, sodium,

and potassium are necessary to support the property of conduction.

Regeneration Healing of nervous tissue is dependent upon the presence of centrosomes, or neurilemma, which are found in only two component parts of the nervous system. Neuroglial cells, the connective supportive tissue of the CNS, contain centrosomes and therefore can be replicated. The axons and dendrites of the peripheral nervous system (PNS) contain neurilemma which regenerate and allow for the continuation of nervous function. Regeneration within the PNS is slow and may take up to 1 year for completion. Damage to the CNS creates permanent disability as the components of regeneration are not present.

Protective Mechanisms Because the nervous system is so vital to the total body function, it is afforded much protection. The bony structure, meninges, cerebrospinal fluid, and blood-brain barrier all contribute to the maintenance of its integrity.

The blood-brain barrier is a poorly understood phenomenon which protects the central nervous system by preventing specific substances from entering the brain tissue and the cerebrospinal fluid.

Vulnerability The more specialized a tissue is within the body, the less it is able to adapt to deficits; thus the nervous system is highly vulnerable to alterations in its metabolism. Of prime concern are the oxygen and glucose levels. The CNS requires 20 percent more oxygen than the rest of the body,

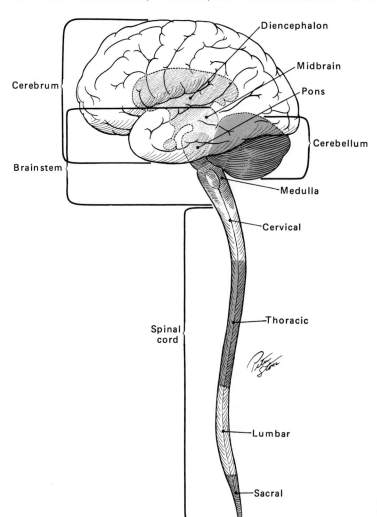

Figure 32-2 Lateral view of the central nervous system. *(From L. L. Langley et al., Dynamic Anatomy and Physiology, 4th ed., McGraw-Hill Book Company, New York, 1974.)*

and its need for oxygen remains constant regardless of the stress or activity of the rest of the body. Insufficient oxygen to the CNS results in permanent brain damage in 4 to 5 minutes. Decreased glucose to the nervous tissue creates a buildup of acid substances within the CNS that interferes with the metabolic process. When appropriate glucose is not supplied, nervous tissue is destroyed.

NEEDS OF CHILDREN WITH SPECIFIC NEUROLOGIC SYMPTOMS

Children manifest neurologic disorders in a number of ways. Alterations in sensation, seizures, signs of increased intracranial pressure, and alteration in level of consciousness are frequently seen as the presenting symptoms. Although these symptoms

vary with disease process and age of the child, all require specific and knowledgeable nursing care.

Alterations in Sensation

Touch Alterations in tactile sensation are manifested as paresthesia (the sensation of burning, crawling, tingling, or prickling); hyperesthesia (exaggerated sensitivity of the skin to touch); hypoesthesia (diminished sensation to touch); or anesthesia (absence of sensation to touch). Two forms of touch sensibility are recognized; (1) simple touch which includes light touch, light pressure, and some tactile localization; (2) tactile discrimination or proprioception which includes the sense of deep pressure, spatial localization, and the perception of the size and shape of objects.

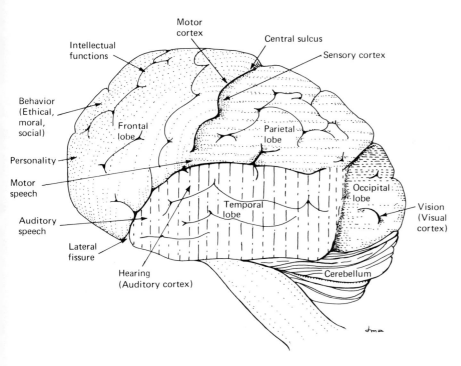

Figure 32-3   Lateral view of the cerebrum.

The cause of altered sensations of touch may be specific pathology, such as infection, trauma, tumors, toxins, and degenerative diseases, or medications which invade the nervous system. Diagnosis is based on the findings of a complete neurologic assessment and specific diagnostic studies to identify any pathologic condition (see Table 32-2).

Nursing management   The nursing goals for children with altered sensations to touch include prevention of atrophy and injury to the affected part and the maintenance of physical and psychologic comfort. Frequent assessments are needed to evaluate the progress of the child and the effects of nursing interventions.

Altered sensations to touch create immobility in the affected area. Nursing intervention should be established to prevent muscular atrophy, contracture of joints, and pressure areas. The decrease in circulation that accompanies immobility enhances the potential for tissue breakdown; therefore active and passive range of motion exercises, proper positioning, frequent turning, and skin care are necessary to prevent further destruction of the affected area.

Children with altered sensations of touch are endangered because they cannot use their sense of touch to accurately evaluate their environment.

These children are not aware of pain, pressure areas, or extreme temperatures, all of which may be harmful. The nurse must teach the child and parents how to maintain a safe environment in the absence of a sense of touch in the affected parts, e.g., how to judge the temperature of bath water, inspect the body area for lacerations or pressure at frequent intervals, and maintain appropriate body positions during sleep. It may be necessary to avoid excess handling of the affected area, use a bed cradle to reduce sensory stimuli, prevent injury by padding, alter environmental temperature, or provide medication. Much of the care will involve spending time in teaching and reassuring the parents. It is frightening and distressing to the child when touch sensations are abnormal. Realistic support must be given to the child and the parents as changes occur and as plans for treatment are established.

Pain   Pain is a disagreeable, uncomfortable sensation caused by the stimulation of specialized nerve endings in the body. It is created by nerve impulses which travel to the posterior horn cells of the spinal column where they decussate to the anterolateral pathways, then to the brainstem, and on to the thalamus, where they are relayed to the somesthetic area of the parietal lobe. Awareness of crude pain occurs when the impulse reaches the thalamus.

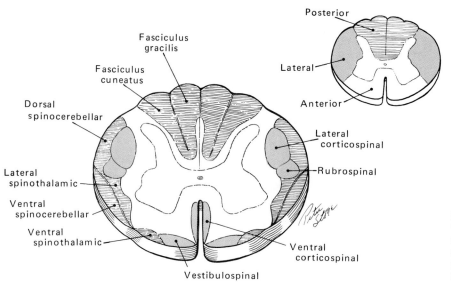

Figure 32-4 Cross section of the spinal cord. *(From L. L. Langley et al., Dynamic Anatomy and Physiology, 4th ed., McGraw-Hill Book Company, New York, 1974.)*

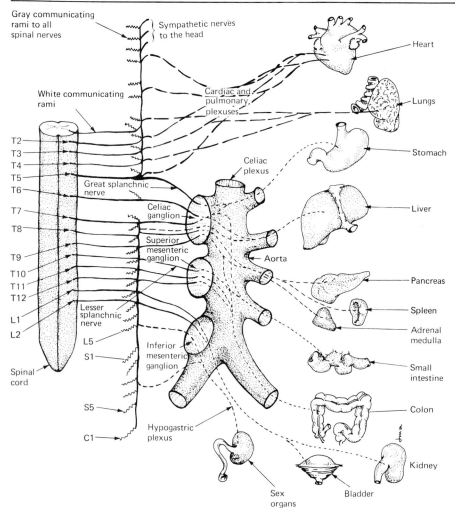

Figure 32-5 Sympathetic fibers of the autonomic nervous system.

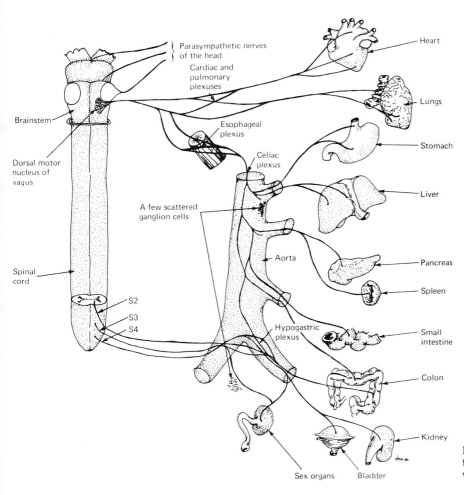

Figure 32-6 Parasympathetic fibers of the autonomic nervous system.

Other qualities of pain are perceived when the impulses reach the parietal lobe of the cerebral cortex and are integrated with other sensory stimuli.

There are special nerve endings which receive specific stimuli from pressure, distention, inflammation, friction, contraction, or cell destruction and create the perception of pain. These special nerve endings respond to selected stimuli. Certain areas of the body respond only to selected stimuli according to the composition of their nerve endings. Thus pain is *elicited* by cell destruction in the skin and external mucous membranes; pain is *caused* by friction, stretching, and inflammation of the arterial walls, dura mater, pleural, and peritoneal surfaces; and pain is *perceived* with contractions and distention in the hollow viscera. Pain may be described as severe, throbbing, dull, hot, searing, crushing, burning, or aching, depending on the location and degree of involvement to the nerve endings. *Referred pain* may be evident when pain is perceived in one area while the actual pain stimulus is located in another

area. Pain may be experienced with emotional disorders in the absence of organic pathology; this type must be treated by health care personnel in the same manner as other pain.

Pain is diagnosed by communication with the child. The communication may be a verbal description of the type and location of pain or nonverbal communication, such as crying, restlessness, irritability, anorexia, insomnia, perspiration, pallor, shallow respirations, splinting, or rigidity of body movement. Pain is a significant symptom of the specific pathology and must be assessed as to its severity, location, type, and pattern to aid in revealing the pathology. Characteristic body language in children may indicate pathology, e.g., pulling at the ears to indicate earache, exaggerated or frequent swallowing to indicate sore throat, or pulling of knees up to the abdomen to indicate abdominal pain.

Nursing management   Each child has his own threshold for pain, and this will also vary according to his

Table 32-2 NEUROLOGIC DIAGNOSTIC TESTS

Name	Purpose	Procedure	Nursing care (before test)	Nursing care (after test)
Electroenceph-alogram (EEG)	To examine brain waves and electrical activity to: Identify damaged or nonfunctioning areas Identify seizure disorders Follow progress of child after encephalitis, encephalopathy, or head injury	Multiple electrodes are placed on various areas of head with adhesive Readings are taken sleeping, awake, and hyperventilating May be done on outpatient basis	Explain purpose to parents and child Explain placements of electrodes and that EEG is not painful May shampoo hair to remove oils that would interfere with electrode readings Do not give coffee, tea, Coca Cola, or alcohol on the day of the examination (contain stimulants or depressants) Do not give medications unless specifically ordered Sleep-deprive 8–10 hr prior to study if ordered	Wash electrode paste from hair Allow patient to rest Provide means of resolving feelings, e.g., therapeutic play
Skull series	To study bony configuration of skull to identify: Skull fractures Developmental disorders of bony growth, i.e., premature or post-mature closing of fontanels Tumors or hemorrhage Presence of old fractures to rule out child battering	X-ray taken of head May be done on outpatient basis	Explain to parents and child x-ray equipment which may be frightening, that there is no pain, and describe procedure Remove glasses, hearing aides, dentures, barrets, hairpins, etc., from mouth or head	Allow child to express feelings created by this procedure
Pneumoenceph-alogram	To demonstrate shape, size, symmetry, and position of ventricular system and subarachnoid spaces to identify: Space-filling abnormality of brain and meninges (except hydrocephalus) Tumors or masses	Air is injected into subarachnoid space from lumbar or cisternal site X-rays of head General anesthetic given Hospitalization required	Explain to parents and child the procedure, NPO for 6–8 hr prior to study, preoperative and postoperative occurrences	Keep flat, rest, check neurologic signs q.½°x4, then q.1–2° as appropriate Observe and care for headache, vomiting, irritability, fever, meningeal irritation, intracranial pressure Encourage fluids if not contraindicated to assist in repletion of CSF Provide for means of resolving feelings when condition is satisfactory
Brain scan	To identify brain tumors, some vascular lesions, and masses	Iodinated human serum (I^{131} HSA) or Hg^{203} Neohydrin is given I.V. 2 hr prior to scan X-rays taken of head May be done on outpatient basis	Explain to parents and child the procedure, its purpose, that I.V. medication is given; describe x-ray equipment	Allow child to express feelings, e.g., therapeutic play

Study	Purpose	Description	Nursing Intervention (Preparation)	Nursing Intervention (Care)
Ventriculogram	To visualize ventricles of brain to identify: Hydrocephalus Masses, lesions	Air injected into ventricles X-rays taken during and after General anesthetic given Hospitalization required	Explain to parents and child NPO 6–8 hr prior to study, medication, preoperative and postoperative occurrences	Keep flat, at rest, check neurologic signs q.½°×4, then as appropriate Severe headache likely for 12–48 hr—provide comfort Encourage fluids to replenish CSF Observe for alteration in intracranial pressure Provide for therapeutic play when condition is improved
Myelogram	To visualize subarachnoid space of spinal cord to identify: Tumors, masses Interference in flow of CSF Fractures, dislocations, foreign bodies	Air or iodinized contrast medium injected into subarachnoid space via lumbar or cisternal puncture X-rays taken Iodinized medium is removed Hospitalization preferred	Explain to parents and child procedure, purpose, NPO for 6–8 hr prior to study, sedative p.r.n.	Keep flat, at rest Observe for headache, alterations in intracranial pressure, temperature for 24–48 hr Comfort Encourage taking fluids Provide for therapeutic play to resolve feelings
Angiogram	To identify: Vascular anomalies, lesions Hemorrhage Tumors, masses	Radiopaque substance is injected into carotid, brachial, vertebral, or femoral artery or vein or a dural sinus General anesthetic given Surgical exposure of vessel to be injected may be necessary Hospitalization required X-rays taken	Explain to parents and child NPO for 6–8 hr prior to procedure, sedative, preoperative and postoperative procedures	Observe for complications of: transient hemiplegia, seizures, petechiae, transient loss of vision, thrombus at injected site, hemorrhage or hematoma at injected site (emergency tracheostomy may be needed if jugular was used), alterations in intracranial pressure and level of consciousness Provide for complications if they occur Comfort Help to resolve feelings with therapeutic play
Lumbar puncture	To identify: Intracranial pressure Culture, sensitivity, cell count, sugar, protein of CSF Hemorrhage in CNS To reduce intracranial pressure	Needle is inserted into lumbar area of subarachnoid space Manometer attached to determine pressure Queckenstedt test performed CSF is collected in tubes which have to be numbered and labeled accurately May be on outpatient or inpatient basis	Explain to parents and child procedure, purpose, need for sedation, and that some pain is encountered During procedure: Position child on side with knees flexed on abdomen and head flexed on chest to open lumbar space Hold child firmly Provide constant verbal support Observe child for tolerance of procedure Label and number tubes of CSF in order of their collection	Keep flat, at rest Observe and care for headache Encourage taking fluids Provide for therapeutic play

(Continued)

Table 32-2 NEUROLOGIC DIAGNOSTIC TESTS (Continued)

Name	Purpose	Procedure	Nursing care (before test)	Nursing care (after test)
Subdural tap	To identify: Subdural effusions Subdural or ventricular hemorrhage Bacteria in subdural or ventricular spaces To obtain fluid for laboratory analysis To relieve intracranial pressure To instill medication	Needle is inserted into subdural space or ventricle through open anterior fontanel or during craniotomy Hospitalization usually required	Explain to parents and child procedure and need for consent concerning shaving area on head Shave the hair over open anterior fontanel During procedure: Position child on back with head facing forward Hold head securely Observe child for tolerance of procedure Label tubes in order they were collected Tape tubes of fluid to the child's bedside unit, label tubes according to day and time of collection	Keep flat, at rest Observe for alterations of intracranial pressure, leakage of fluid from tap site
Ventricular tap (procedure is the same as for a subdural tap)				

age and to his fatigue, anxiety, and stress, and the degree of pain stimuli. The way the child communicates his degree of pain is governed in part by his age, culture, family expectations, and by previous experiences with pain.

Pain may be reduced by the application of heat or cold. Heat dilates vessels, increases circulation, and thus promotes healing. Moist heat conducts to the deep underlying tissue; dry heat conducts primarily to the surface areas. Cold constricts the vessels, decreases metabolism to the cells, and reduces edema; therefore, cold is best applied soon after injury, and heat is best applied once edema and inflammation have developed. Splinting or immobilizing the affected area decreases pain. Often the child will do this on his own, or the nurse can provide means to help immobilize the affected part. There are hazards inherent in the application of heat or cold or in immobilization; therefore, collaboration with the physician is necessary prior to instituting these forms of therapy.

Analgesics, sedatives, narcotics, tranquilizers, and antispasmodics are types of drugs used to control pain in children. Once the nurse has assessed the severity and cause of the child's pain, other variables concerning the use of medication should be considered, such as the child's physical stability. Narcotics, which are CNS depressants, are contraindicated whenever there is shock or CNS disorders because they may further inhibit respirations and mask important symptoms.

Seizures

An insult to the central nervous system can result in a seizure, which is described as any abnormal, involuntary neuromuscular activity which encompasses a specific part or the total body and may create loss of consciousness and of bowel and bladder control. The neuromuscular activity of a seizure is described as *tonic* (rigid) or *clonic* (alternately rigid and relaxed). The cause of insult to the CNS and the maturity of the child govern the specific seizure activity. Seizures are most frequently encountered as sequelae to immaturity of the nervous system, brain damage, metabolic disorders, elevated temperatures, alterations in fluids and electrolytes, and invasions of the nervous system by infections, toxins, and drugs. Seizure activity may be temporary or permanent, on the basis of the cause and treatment.

Seizure activity is diagnosed by the history and the observation of abnormal neuromuscular activity. An electroencephalogram (EEG) confirms the diagnosis in the majority of children. Anoxia from seizures creates additional brain damage; therefore, seizures must be identified and treated rapidly. The primary means of treating seizures is to remove the causative factor or prevent it from occurring; but when the causative factor cannot be controlled, medications help prevent and regulate seizure activity. Barbiturates are the most frequently used drugs to control acute seizure activity. Because of its rapid action, amobarbital is the drug of choice when a child is demonstrating seizure activity. Phenobarbital, alone or in conjunction with Valium, Benadryl, or Mysoline, is used prophylactically to prevent seizures.

Nursing Management Nursing care is primarily directed toward providing safety and making astute observations of any seizure activity. Measures should be taken to prevent seizures, but if they occur, the nurse must care for the child during the seizure.

Seizure precautions, designed to prevent injury to the child, consist of the following:

1 Place the child in a quiet room to prevent additional stimuli, which may trigger seizure activity, and in a nursing unit where he can be easily observed.
2 Provide a bed with side rails that are padded.
3 Tape a padded tongue blade or rubber airway to the head of the bed.
4 Provide suction equipment, endotracheal tubes, oxygen, and emergency drugs at the bedside.
5 Place a seizure chart in the child's room.

When a child demonstrates seizure activity, the first steps are to protect him from additional injury and to notify the physician. Toys and other objects should be removed from his immediate environment. Once a seizure has started, the child should not be moved, but the head should be turned to the side to prevent aspiration of pooling secretions. A small, folded blanket placed under the head prevents head trauma if the seizure takes place when the child is on the floor. No attempt should be made to restrain the child because the force of the tonic-clonic activity can cause fractures and dislocations if there is resistance to movement of the extremities. If the tonic-clonic activity is noted in the face and jaw, the padded tongue blade or airway may be placed between the teeth to prevent damage to the tongue and cheeks. The tonic-clonic muscular activity of the thoracic muscles may inhibit respirations, causing anoxia, and oxygen may be administered by mask. If adequate oxygen levels are not maintained, apnea may develop, and intubation will be required following the seizure. When the seizure activity has ceased, the child may appear very lethargic and sleepy, and may have no recollection of the seizure activity. The nurse should return him to bed, assess the level of consciousness, motor response, pupil reaction, and vital signs, and allow him to sleep.

Necessary observations during and immediately after a seizure include noting the time of onset, the location of the neuromuscular activity, the type of activity (tonic, clonic, or both), the length and pattern of the seizure, the child's activity immediately preceding the seizure, the incidence of incontinence, and the child's level of consciousness. This information must be recorded on the seizure chart and in nursing notes to help those caring for him recognize his unique seizure pattern.

When the child awakens after his seizure, vital signs should be checked and the neurologic status should be evaluated frequently. The child may need readjustment to reality as he will have difficulty remembering the episode. Older children may feel guilt and embarrassment secondary to the incontinence and the loss of body control. Transient personality disorders which have been seen in some children following seizure activity require specific nursing care.

Increased Intracranial Pressure

An increase in intracranial pressure (ICP) occurs whenever the amount of tissue, cerebrospinal fluid (CSF), or blood increases within the cranium. Increased ICP causes irritation to the nervous tissue and, if allowed to proceed, leads to brain damage and ultimately permanent disability or death.

The rapidity and severity of symptoms of increased ICP are determined by the maturity of the CNS and the stability of the cranium. The infant with open fontanels and an immature system does not develop evidence of increased ICP as rapidly as the older child who has a closed skull.

The symptoms of increased ICP may occur in a matter of hours or months, depending upon the cause of the increasing pressure (see Table 32-3). As death and permanent brain damage may occur at any time, early diagnosis and institution of treatment are vital. X-ray studies are done to diagnose underlying pathologic conditions; EEGs are used to diagnose and monitor the progression of brain damage; lumbar puncture is performed to measure the ICP and obtain CSF for laboratory analysis. If lumbar punctures are done, the child must be carefully observed for signs of shock. The sudden release of

pressure through the opening can create herniation of the brainstem, resulting in a medical emergency.

Treating ICP may involve removing masses or tumors by surgery and radiation, controlling hemorrhage and edema, and removing pooled secretions by tapping (subdural or lumbar puncture) or shunting. When the cause of the increased pressure cannot be alleviated, palliative measures such as removal of skull plates, creation of burr holes, or decompression of masses are instituted to reduce the effects of pressure.

Barbiturates and tranquilizers are frequently ordered to control seizures and promote rest. Cerebral edema may be controlled with diuretics, corticosteroids, or hypertonic solutions, such as 50 percent glucose, 10 percent sodium chloride, or salt-poor serum albumin, which alter the osmotic effect of the cerebral tissue fluid. Antipyretics, analgesics, antiemetics, and stool softeners are instituted as necessary.

Evaluation of blood gases is necessary at frequent intervals when there is respiratory depression or the child is being maintained on respiratory equipment. Increased carbon dioxide levels cause dilation of blood vessels and thus increase cerebral volume and pressure. Conversely, if the carbon dioxide level is low, the blood vessels constrict, resulting in decreased oxygen in the cells.

Administration of intravenous fluid is necessary for the child with altered levels of consciousness. The fluid volume and electrolyte levels, particularly of potassium, sodium, and calcium, must be monitored carefully, because an imbalance creates increased ICP, edema, and nervous tissue irritability. Therefore, blood is drawn for electrolytes every 4 to 8 hours.

Nursing Management The care of a child who has increased intracranial pressure requires a perceptive nurse who can quickly detect any change in status and institute proper nursing care. Frequent assessment is required to evaluate the degree of pressure and to prevent unnecessary complications. Life or death depends on the quality of nursing care.

A neurologic check is a systematic nursing assessment that allows for rapid evaluation of the child's neurologic status. The four major components of the evaluation are (1) level of consciousness, (2) pupillary response, (3) vital signs, and (4) motor activity.

The level of consciousness indicates the highest level of cerebral activity and is evaluated by deter-

Table 32-3 SYMPTOMS OF INCREASED INTRACRANIAL PRESSURE

Early symptoms	Intermediate symptoms	Late symptoms
Irritability	Projectile vomiting	Decreased level of consciousness
Restlessness	Tense, bulging fontanel in child under 18 months of age	Decreased reflexes
Anorexia	Severe headache	Decreased respirations
Headache	Sluggish, unequal response of pupils to light	Elevated temperature
	Papilledema	Herniation of optic disk (creates blindness)
	Blurred vision	Absent doll's eye maneuver
	Diplopia	Sunset eyes
	Decrease in pulse and increase in blood pressure	Decerebrate rigidity
	Seizures	Death

mining degree of alertness and orientation to person, place, and time. Ability to awaken, degree of lethargy, knowledge of being in the hospital, and recognition of parents and staff are but a few of the signs by which the level of consciousness is assessed.

The pupillary response includes reaction to light. The normal pupil has an equal, rapid constriction in response to light. When observing the pupils, the nurse should assess the movement and position of the eyes because an abnormality could indicate cranial nerve involvement. Strabismus, nystagmus, absent doll's eye movement, sunset eyes, and inability to move the eyes in all four quadrants are examples of abnormality.

The effect of increased intracranial pressure on the vital signs should be evaluated. A decrease in pulse and respiration accompanied by increased blood pressure is evidence of increasing intracranial pressure. Any change in neurologic status is cause for close and frequent observation because even the slightest change is significant.

The quality and strength of motor activity are evaluated by having the child move all four extremities, grasp or squeeze the examiner's hand with both hands at once, and push against the examiner's hand with both feet. The facial muscles are also observed by having the child smile, bare his teeth, and squeeze his eyes tightly shut. Any inequality is noted in motor strength. Generalized weakness, tremors, ataxia, or altered sensation of position are significant indications of nervous system pathology.

It is also important to prevent or reduce the occurrence of increased pressure of a normal, transient nature in a child who already has ICP. The Valsalva maneuver and pressure on the jugular veins are two common causes of transient pressure increases. Whenever the child cries, sneezes, coughs, vomits, strains at stool, or resists restraints, the Valsalva maneuver is elicited. Pressure on the jugular veins occurs when an infant is held in the upright sitting position on the lap for bubbling or when he is held for lumbar puncture.

To help control cerebral edema, fluid intake must be monitored. Children whose oral fluids are restricted should have their quota of oral fluids distributed over the 24-hour period. Intravenous (I.V.) fluids are carefully monitored to prevent overhydration, which increases the production of CSF. Infusion pumps may be used to control the rate of flow of I.V. fluids. Elevating the child's head may decrease cerebral edema. Shock blocks at the head of the bed will both elevate the child's head and maintain straight body alignment, promoting comfort and adequate respiratory exchange.

The child with increased ICP may demonstrate an elevated temperature because of an inflammatory process, a systemic infection, or irritation or damage to the temperature-regulating mechanism in the brainstem. When a child's temperature is 37.7 to 38.9°C (100 to 102°F), the nursing treatment consists of cooling the environment by removing excess bed linen and clothing, opening the window, or turning on the air conditioner. Children with temperatures of 38.9 to 40°C (102 to 104°F) require more direct nursing interventions. Antipyretics, such as Tylenol, may be administered orally or rectally. (Aspirin should be avoided as it interferes with the clotting time and creates gastric distress.) Tepid baths are effective cooling measures, but during the tepid bath, care must be taken that the child does not become chilled.

Shivering, the normal compensatory mechanism of the body to warm itself, counteracts the effects of this cooling measure. During the bath the child's temperature should be taken at 15-minute intervals, and the temperature should not be allowed to drop more than 0.5°C (1°F) per hour. Once the temperature has been reduced, it should be monitored at 1-hour intervals. If it rises again, the bath must be reinstituted. Ice baths, alcohol sponges, and ice enemas should be avoided with all children because the rapid reduction of temperature may lead to shock and possibly death. Children who have temperatures of 40 to 41.6°C (104 to 107°F) or who cannot maintain an appropriate temperature require the use of a hypothermia mattress; this must be set at 1°C below the body temperature for safe cooling. Because the mattress may increase skin breakdown from pressure and burning with the cold temperature, lanolin or appropriate lotion must be applied to the skin.

Safety and comfort measures such as seizure precautions must be instituted. The child who is vomiting should be refed because vomiting is caused by neurologic difficulties, not gastric irritation; however, if vomiting persists, feeding should be withheld to prevent the transient increased ICP encountered with vomiting. Headache may be reduced by maintaining the elevation of the head, applying ice bags to the head and neck, and administering appropriate analgesics. The child with blurred or distorted vision requires additional communication with the nurse to alleviate anxiety and promote orientation to reality. Appropriate play and diversionary activities should be provided.

Alterations in Levels of Consciousness

The level of consciousness is the most important single indicator of cerebral function. Alterations in the level of consciousness may be slight or severe enough to render the child unable to respond to his environment. General anesthesia, intracranial pathology, trauma, toxins, and metabolic disorders are the primary causes.

Alterations in levels of consciousness generally follow a sequential pattern. Initially the child is alert and knows who and where he is. He can readily engage in purposeful play and responds to his parents and surroundings as any child according to the norms for his age. The progression of disorientation is usually time, place, and lastly person, which may be evaluated even in young children. With continued alterations in his level of consciousness, he becomes restless and irritable. His thrashing, restless behavior is not alleviated even with comfort from his parents.

He becomes drowsy and may not be awakened from sleep, and if previously toilet trained, he may become incontinent. Although he is not able to awaken totally, he can respond to direct commands, and painful stimuli elicit withdrawal of a part or facial grimaces.

As the level of consciousness decreases, there are specific levels which can be described:

1 Unconscious, purposeful response to pain
2 Unconscious, nonpurposeful response to pain
3 Unconscious, flexes to painful stimuli
4 Unconscious, extends to painful stimuli
5 Unconscious, decorticate posture-position of adducted, rigid flexion of arms and fingers with internal rotation of the hands.
6 Unconscious, decerebrate posture—all extremities in rigid extension and adduction, back arched, and toes pointed inward
7 No response

Observation of altered levels of consciousness should be based on a description of behavior rather than on nebulous terminology such as *confused, stuporous, delirious, semicomatose,* or *comatose.* The nurse should report, for example, the child's ability to turn his head and produce facial grimaces in response to a loud noise or deep pain stimulus.

Nursing Management Observation at frequent intervals and maintenance of bodily functions are major nursing responsibilities. The nursing assessment must include a neurologic check and appraisal of reflexes (e.g., gag, swallow, corneal) and neuromuscular abilities, including asymmetry of face and extremities.

Ineffectual gag and swallow reflexes require specific nursing interventions to provide for respiration and nutrition. Absence of these reflexes creates pooling of secretions; thus the child must be positioned on his side, and his mouth and nose must be suctioned at frequent intervals to prevent aspiration pneumonia and asphyxiation. Frequent turning, postural drainage, and mechanical respiratory assistance are necessary to prevent hypostatic pneumonia. Good oral hygiene is necessary to maintain the integrity of the oral cavity.

The corneal reflex must be checked frequently. When the eye does not close completely, the cornea becomes dry and ulcerated, and these ulcerations can result in permanent blindness. Saline eye drops, or artificial tears, and lubricating agents such as methylcellulose can be used to keep the eye moist. If applied with caution, eye patches may be used; however, they must be checked frequently to make sure the eye is not open under the patch. Some physicians recommend the use of clear tape to hold the eye closed so that it will be quite obvious if the eye opens.

Children with decreased levels of consciousness are subjected to the hazards of immobility, and specific nursing care to maintain the integrity of the muscles, bones, skin, circulatory system, bowel, and bladder are required. Nursing interventions include frequent range of motion exercises to decrease atrophy and frequent turning and positioning to prevent contractures. A child who is able to do active range of motion exercises must be encouraged and helped to perform these exercises at least three times each day. Range of motion exercises incorporated into play activities increase their frequency and provide diversional activities. Passive range of motion is done three to four times a day for the child who is unable to perform active range of motion. The immobilized child should be turned and positioned every 1 to 2 hours to help prevent pressure on specific skin breakdown and contractures. The use of sheepskins, alternating pressure mattresses, rubber pads, pillows, and splints can help maintain the proper body alignment and the integrity of his skin.

Atrophy of the bones is seen as decalcification and is termed *osteoporosis*. It is reduced with application of stress to the bones, for example, by having the child sit or stand by means of a Circo-electric bed, rocking bed, or standing board. Upright positions also assist in the drainage of the urinary system, promote circulation, and maintain equilibrium.

Maintenance of bowel and bladder function is essential for the child who is immobile and is best fostered by providing a diet that is well balanced with adequate amounts of fluids, fruit juices, and stool-softening medications. Rectal suppositories or small enemas may be given to assist in the evacuation of feces in accordance with the bowel schedule.

These children are particularly susceptible to cystitis secondary to urinary retention and stasis. Incontinence and increased calculi development are additional problems. Medications, increased fluids, and cranberry juice maintain the urine in an acid state, which decreases the possibilities of infection and calculi formation. The specific gravity and pH of the urine should be measured at 8-hour intervals to determine concentration and acidity. A Foley catheter may be inserted to promote adequate drainage. The catheter should be clamped at all times and released every 3 to 4 hours for drainage to maintain the tone of the bladder.

Circulatory stasis in the immobilized patient may lead to phlebitis and thrombosis formation, and elastic stockings may be ordered by the physician. Postural hypotension occurs when the child's position is rapidly changed from horizontal to vertical and is evidenced by low blood pressure, pallor, circumoral cyanosis, weakness, syncope, thready pulse, diaphoresis, or cool and clammy skin.

Sensory distortion due to sensory overload or deprivation easily occurs in children who have decreased levels of consciousness. People assume that these children are unable to comprehend or hear what is being said, although hearing is the last sense to be lost in an unconscious patient. Parents may sit by the bedside for hours without speaking to the child, and the nurse quietly hovers over him and does not say a word. The background noise of machines beeping and humming and of people working is not meaningful to the child, and he sinks further into a world of oblivion. When hearing is the only touch with the real world available to the child, much can be done with the voice to bring about comfort, companionship, pleasure, knowledge of what is happening, trust, and understanding.

The child should be called by name, read stories, and given explanations of procedures at an appropriate level for his understanding. Television programs and music that are familiar to the child bring comfort to him, provided they are supplied for specific amounts of time and are not allowed to drone on and to become monotonous.

NEUROLOGIC DISORDERS IN THE NEWBORN
Hydrocephaly

A neurologic abnormality which may be present at birth or may become evident soon after is *hydrocephaly*, the abnormal increase in cerebrospinal fluid volume within the intracranial cavity. Unless otherwise stipulated, hydrocephaly refers to internal hydrocephalus, a condition in which the fluid accumulates under pressure within the ventricles.

Two forms of hydrocephaly should be noted for clinical clarity. *Noncommunicating*, or *obstructive*, internal hydrocephaly is caused by a blockage within the ventricles which prevents cerebrospinal fluid from entering the subarachnoid space. (See Figure 32-7.) *Communicating* hydrocephaly occurs when the obstruction is located in the subarachnoid cistern at the base of the brain and/or within the subarachnoid space.

As the fluid begins to accumulate, the intracranial pressure increases, the cerebral cortex becomes thinner, the scalp veins dilate, and the cranial suture lines begin to separate. When the infant demonstrates a tense or bulging anterior fontanel and

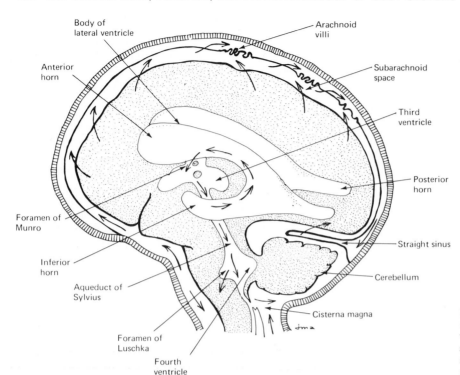

Body of
lateral ventricle

Arachnoid
villi

Anterior
horn

Subarachnoid
space

Third
ventricle

Posterior
horn

Foramen of
Munro

Straight sinus

Inferior
horn

Cerebellum

Aqueduct of
Sylvius

Cisterna magna

Foramen of
Luschka

Fourth
ventricle

Figure 32-7 Normal circulation of cerebrospinal fluid from the ventricles to the subarachnoid spaces around the brain and spinal cord and through the central canal.

when cranial suture separation is apparent, hydrocephaly is suspected. Other clinical symptoms include vomiting, a wide bridge between the eyes, and bulging eyes in the classic "sunset" sign showing the upper scleras. In the severe form, head size increases rapidly, the infant's cry is shrill and high-pitched, and hyperirritability and restlessness are noted.

Subsequent neurosurgical intervention offers the best prognosis for survival and intellectual functioning. The degree of neurologic impairment cannot be predicted: some children grow up to function normally, while others may be minimally or profoundly retarded. Their ultimate potential is difficult to forecast.

Shunting procedures have become popular with the development of inert plastics which are well tolerated by the body. Although no shunt is invariably successful, satisfactory results are frequently obtained. A wide variety of bypass methods may be implemented. One type of silicone valve permitting cerebrospinal fluid flow in one direction only has resulted in the development of a bypass from the ventricle into the right atrium via the jugular vein. Another type involves sacrificing a kidney so that cerebrospinal fluid is drained through the ureter. The

pleural and peritoneal cavities have also been used as sites into which cerebrospinal fluid is drained.

Of the many types of shunting procedures available in treating hydrocephaly, the preferred method depends on the site of the obstruction and the neurosurgeon who is directing the team's activities. Success depends on the careful, individualized treatment of each hydrocephalic infant.

Nursing Management Observation is essential, as is conscientious collection of data, including measurement of the head circumference and a check of the size and fullness of the anterior fontanel. Noting any change in the infant's behavior is also important.

Nurses have a direct responsibility for the nutritional requirements of these newborns, but feeding may be a particularly time-consuming activity for the staff. When the infant is irritable or vomiting, various techniques should be attempted to provide adequate nutrients and fluids. Techniques that are successful for a particular infant should be shared with all persons involved in feeding him, including the parents. Feeding times should be flexible, and small feedings at frequent intervals may prove more successful than rigid nursing routines.

The increased head size makes positioning a

potential problem, especially when the head circumference is increasing rapidly. Hydrocephalic neonates may develop decubiti if not turned often. Frequent linen changes and the use of lamb's wool also help deter skin breakdown. The infant should be turned cautiously for the increased head size places an additional strain on its neck.

These neonates also have emotional needs which should not be dismissed. They enjoy being held or cuddled. Although some nurses may be hesitant about handling the baby, it is important to remember that dexterity comes through experience. Such an endeavor on the part of one health team member may support and encourage others to do likewise.

Microcephaly

The presence of a head which is smaller than chest circumference is diagnosed as *microcephaly*, a condition secondary to micrencephaly, or a small brain. It may be caused by maternal infections such as toxoplasmosis, irradiation, or any one of a number of factors genetically or environmentally induced. Although the sutures close prematurely in microcephaly, they may be open at birth or in early infancy. With the arrest of brain growth, there is generally profound retardation which may be complicated by cerebral palsy or seizure activity. Therefore, a craniotomy is to no avail. In contrast, a condition known as *craniosynostosis*, in which brain size is normal but the fontanels and suture lines have closed at birth or in early infancy, necessitates surgical intervention which will allow the brain to continue to grow.

Nursing Management   Since microcephaly cannot be surgically corrected and mental retardation is a consequence, the problem of giving birth to a deformed infant is further complicated by knowledge of the infant's limited intellectual ability. Specific nursing interventions for these infants are not enumerated because the care given is routine from the standpoint of meeting their physical, emotional, and nutritional needs. The nurse should, however, offer a great deal of support to parents, for they are frequently faced with making difficult decisions which may include institutionalization. If these infants are cared for by parents, the community resources available should be identified for them.

Neural Tube Malformations

Occasionally at delivery a neural tube malformation is identified. Although *spina bifida* refers to a congenital problem in which there is a defective closure of the vertebral column, whether this problem will be one of minimal involvement or whether the defect will have devastating consequences for the neonate depends entirely on the site and the extent of the anomaly. Considering the variety of internal and external forces with genetic and/or environmental interactions affecting embryonic development, it is no wonder that such defects occur. (See Chap. 19.) While the cause of these malformations is unknown, since closure of the neural tube occurs by the fourth week, it appears that these midline neurologic deviations must occur by that time. The two major categories of spina bifida are occulta and cystica.

Spina bifida occulta is a condition commonly seen and found in about 10 percent of the routine spinal x-rays of children and adults. Usually the 5th lumbar and 1st sacral vertebrae are affected with no protrusion of intraspinal contents. Many times it is discovered accidently when other radiologic studies are being performed. The skin over the defect may reveal a dimple, a small fatty mass, or a tuft of hair.

Spina bifida cystica is a more serious defect in which a cystic lesion develops in the midline of the vertebral column. Two common types of lesions are meningoceles and meningomyeloceles (myelomeningoceles). A *meningocele* is a protrusion through the spina bifida which forms a soft, saclike appearance along the spinal axis and contains spinal fluid and meninges within the sac. A more severe malformation is the *meningomyelocele*, which is also an external protrusion along the midline, but the contents of this mass include spinal fluid, meninges, spinal cord, and/or nerve roots.

Meningoceles and meningomyeloceles are covered by a thin, transparent membrane, a thicker, irregular epithelium, or normal skin. The neurologic manifestations of a meningocele may be minimal; however, the symptoms manifested by the presence of a meningomyelocele vary and depend on the extent of the defect and the site of the protrusion.

Parents' rights in the decision-making process regarding surgery for a neonate born with a major defect such as meningomyelocele are a highly controversial issue.[1, 2] A discussion of the moral, ethical, and legal aspects of the dilemma of "informed consent" extends beyond the scope of this text. However, if parents withhold permission for surgical intervention, nurses working with these infants and their parents must be aware of the differences in a family's abilities to deal with deformed babies, of the anguish experienced in arriving at a decision, and of the needs of families to verbalize their feelings. While offering support to parents, these nurses must also identify and offer support to colleagues who grapple with their own reactions to denial of surgery.

When permission for surgery is granted, the protrusion is excised, the nervous tissue is placed into the spinal canal, and fascia and skin are sutured over the defect. With larger, more difficult repairs a neurosurgeon and a plastic surgeon may collaborate to close the neural tube malformation.

Nursing Management These serious types of defects are usually identified at birth. In the special-care nursery, before surgery, the neonate must be handled carefully. Rupture, infection, irritation, or leakage from the protruding mass may occur, placing the neonate's life in great jeopardy. Avoiding pressure over the meningocele, meticulous skin care, and positioning become important nursing measures. In observing the newborn, attention is also directed to the anterior fontanel, noting its tense, full, bulging, or normal status.

If the question of whether the patient presents a meningocele or a meningomyelocele has not been answered, astute nursing observations and assessments may contribute to the final diagnosis. In consideration of a neonate with a meningomyelocele, the dribble of urine, the absence of anal sphincter control, and characteristic deformities of the feet emphasize the extensive neurologic involvement. The location of the lesion determines the extent of lower-extremity involvement. There may be paralysis, flaccidity, spasticity, or no impairment whatsoever.

Methods of protecting the meningocele or meningomyelocele vary and depend on the physician, the skin covering the protruding mass, and the time interval before surgery. Sterile dressings should always be utilized, but the decision to apply topical ointments or antiseptic solutions depends entirely on the treatment selected by the physician responsible. Generally, if surgery is not performed immediately, some method of protecting the mass must be devised. Abdominal combines rolled, covered with gauze, and made into a doughnut shape to fit around the defect may be the basis for one type of protective dressing. Sponge rubber may also be used in a similar manner. After careful cleansing of the skin over the defect, sterile gauze is draped over the area, and a plastic square, previously cleaned with alcohol, is placed over the gauze covering. The doughnut-shaped appliance is then positioned around the spinal defect, protecting and supporting it. Finally, some type of wide gauze bandage, functioning as an abdominal binder, is cautiously wrapped around the dressing to secure it in place.

Postoperatively, the baby is placed in a prone position in an incubator or on a Bradford frame, and the head is lowered 8 to 10° to decrease the likelihood of spinal fluid leakage from the site of the operation. Since positioning on a frame lessens the possibility of contaminating the dressing with urine or feces, a disposable plastic bag partially split at the sides for attachment to both the head and foot canvas portions of the frame facilitates the collection of urine and feces. Such receptacles should be changed every 3 or 4 hours. Because of poor anal sphincter control, the anal area must be cleaned often.

Since the neonate will remain in a prone position for 7 to 10 days, bedding must be kept wrinkle free and dry to prevent skin breakdown. Whether the young patient can be held for feedings during the immediate postoperative period is determined by the neurosurgeon; however, if permitted, the patient should be kept prone, lying across the nurse's lap, in a reasonably comfortable position for the patient and the nurse. Like all infants, these newborns enjoy being held.

After a repair, nursing observations should focus on assessing the baby's neurologic status, sphincter control, and movement of the lower extremities. Dressings are kept dry and clean. Many neurosurgeons utilize an elastic type of adhesive covering which facilitates keeping the wound clean and dry. Daily head circumference measurements are taken routinely because of the high incidence of hydrocephaly (70 percent) following neural tube closures. A bulging anterior fontanel, hyperirritability, a shrill, high-pitched cry, and vomiting indicate increased intracranial pressure. Passive range of motion exercises should be done with impaired lower extremities. (See Chap. 40.)

While these newborns face repeated hospitalizations, innumerable surgical procedures, and multiple, chronic problems, eventual rehabilitation depends on many factors. An interdisciplinary team approach, early parental involvement in the baby's care, a thorough knowledge of community resources, and parental understanding of the long-range implications greatly influence and affect this newborn's early years.

NEUROLOGIC DISORDERS IN THE INFANT
Narcosis

A severe depression of the central nervous system due to an overdose of narcotics is termed *narcosis*. A newborn may show evidence of narcosis when the mother has received large doses of narcotics within 3 hours of delivery. The incidence in the new-born has been greatly diminished by the acceptance of "childbirth with participation" because the use of narcotics during the second stage of labor is reduced. Narcosis is still present when mothers require narcotics secondary to complications of their labor.

The narcotized newborn is nonresponsive at birth (low Apgar score, depressed respirations, and bradycardia). When respiratory function is depressed to a level which creates anoxia, permanent brain damage occurs.

Nalline is administered to counteract the effects of the narcotic, and respiratory assistance is instituted to prevent anoxia. The newborn is placed in an incubator to conserve his body temperature and thus reduce the depletion of his energy stores. Unless anoxia has occurred, the newborn recuperates from the effects of the narcosis within the first 12 to 18 hours of life and has no sequelae.

Nursing Management   The narcotized newborn is admitted to the high-risk nursery where appropriate nursing care utilizing incubators and respirators is available. (Refer to Chapter 33 for specific care of the newborn in an incubator and in respiratory distress.)

Seizures of the Newborn and Infant

The immaturity of the infant's nervous system renders him very susceptible to neurologic responses resulting from alterations in his physiologic state. Skilled assessment is needed to differentiate seizure activity of fine twitching or jerking of the extremities from the normal random, uncontrolled movement of the infant. Generally the infant having a seizure demonstrates other clinical signs such as rigidity of the tremulous extremities, fixed staring of his eyes which may be accompanied by nystagmus, and an abnormal Moro reflex. Rarely does the infant lose consciousness with seizure activity. The most frequent causes of seizures in the infant are elevated temperature, hypoglycemia, and hypocalcemia (see Chap. 39).

The incidence of hypoglycemia is increased in premature infants, low-for-birth-weight infants, and those born to diabetic mothers. Hypoglycemia is also encountered in infants who are in stress situations as with respiratory distress syndrome, sepsis, and cardiac distress because these infants rapidly deplete their glucose storage reserves. For this reason the premature and other high-risk infants are provided with additional glucose. Hypoglycemia has

also been noted in infants who have been on parenteral fluids which were suddenly discontinued. It is believed that while a patient receives glucose intravenously, insulin production increases. When the glucose is suddenly removed, the insulin is still being rapidly produced, and the infant develops hypoglycemia. The hypoglycemic infant appears to be having seizure activity because he is jittery, listless, hyperirritable, and restless. The diagnosis is made by determining the blood glucose level.

Persistent hypoglycemia will lead to seizure activity; permanent brain damage and mental retardation may ultimately result.

Nursing Management   The nurse's knowledgeable assessment of the behavior of all infants is necessary if abnormal activity is to be identified. Specific nursing care for the child with seizure activity is discussed earlier in this chapter.

Subdural Effusion

A collection of fluid in the subdural space usually of 2 cc or more in volume is termed a subdural effusion. The cause has not been clearly identified; however, head trauma and meningitis are known to increase the incidence. Subdural effusions are primarily found in infants, with an increased incidence at 7 months of age.

The first sign of *acute* effusion is rapidly increasing ICP. The most frequent symptoms of *chronic* effusions are convulsions, irritability, stupor, and projectile vomiting. In addition, head enlargement, failure to thrive, and developmental lags have been reported to occur with chronic subdural effusions. Transillumination, subdural tap, and in some cases angiography are used in diagnosis. The fluid in the subdural space is characteristically found to have increased protein levels and may be accompanied by red blood cells.

If the infant has no evidence of neurologic changes, he should be observed closely. No treatment is instituted because some children have had resolving effusions with no sequelae. Subdural taps are done with all those who evidence clinical signs of neurologic dysfunction. Generally no more than 30 cc is removed at one time. Taps are usually done as needed every 1 to 4 days until fluid production in the subdural spaces has ceased. If fluid production continues more than 14 days, a craniotomy to remove the fluid-producing membrane may be performed. Repeated taps may still be necessary following surgery; if continuation of fluid development persists, shunting may be instituted.

Nursing Management The nurse must be alert to any signs of increased intracranial pressure. A neurologic check done at frequent intervals is particularly important after a subdural tap as signs of increased pressure could develop suddenly following a period of decreased pressure. Close observation of the fontanels for signs of bulging and daily measurement of the head circumference are important nursing measures.

Since the infant may be subjected to repeated, painful subdural taps, the nurse should take time to hold and fondle him to help develop a trust relation. Allowing the parents to be with the infant as much as possible will decrease their anxiety and help overcome feelings of separation. The parents of these infants are very distressed because it may be many weeks or months before the full potential of their child can be identified.

NEUROLOGIC DISORDERS IN THE TODDLER
Cerebral Palsy

The term *cerebral palsy* is used to describe disorders created by damage to the motor centers of the brain. This damage may occur before, during, or shortly after birth and may result from anoxia in the perinatal period, trauma at birth, or infections or kernicterus during the postnatal period. One infant in 1,000 live births are born with this condition every year. Of the 6 out of 7 who survive, some will be profoundly retarded and may be institutionalized; others will be so mildly affected that little or no treatment is necessary. The remaining children will have moderate to severe handicaps.

Cerebral palsy is characterized by various neuromuscular abnormalities such as weakness, paralysis, or incoordination of voluntary movements. Other disorders include seizures, visual and hearing difficulties, emotional disorders, speech problems, and mental retardation.

The clinical manifestations of cerebral palsy are categorized by the type of motor disturbance. These are spasticity, athetosis, ataxia, rigidity, tremors, and atonia. Athetosis refers to constant, irregular, and involuntary slow movements. Spasticity refers to exaggerated reflexes and jerky, uncertain movements. Cerebral palsy is suspected in the infant who fails to respond normally to a neurologic examination and who demonstrates flaccidity; rigidity; prolonged tonic neck, Moro, or fisting reflexes; and fixed positioning, or scissoring of legs when picked up.

Nursing Management Early diagnosis helps the parents accept their child as an individual with basic needs for love and care. The parents who have accepted the child initially as a "normal" child, with "normal" potential, encounter greater difficulties in accepting their child with his handicaps at a later time. Denhoff describes three emotional phases a parent of a handicapped child exhibits. The first phase is hostility to the doctor who has confirmed their fears that something is wrong with their child. The second phase is the search for a doctor who will reverse the first diagnosis. The last phase is acceptance. Until the period of acceptance has been reached, therapeutic interventions are not helpful.

A major nursing goal is to foster in the child with cerebral palsy a positive self-image—his motivation to learn, his development of independence, and his need to socialize and be accepted by his "normal" peers. This goal is difficult for the child to achieve because he is so often frustrated by his inability to coordinate the muscular activity required for speech, mobility, posture, and facial expression. The level of the acceptance and support offered to the child with cerebral palsy from people significant to him and his degree of neuromuscular involvement determine his ability to function within society. Meeting this nursing goal provides support which prevents the family from raising a child with a "handicapped" personality. It must be stressed that children with cerebral palsy are like normal children in their need for love, independence, success, and acceptance by others; the only difference is that they cannot control their body with ease.

Once the parents have accepted their child, the remainder of the medical treatment is related to preventing deformities and promoting "normal" growth and development. (See Chap. 40.) Training of the child who has cerebral palsy is ideally managed by an interdisciplinary team and carried out in a relaxed setting. The sequence of training and the goals established are in accordance with the abilities and handicaps of the individual and should help him reach the highest level of functioning.

Head Trauma

Most head trauma is accidental. The most common types are concussions and fractures (linear, depressed, basilar), both of which may be accompanied by intracranial hemmorrhage. A *concussion* is the jarring of the skull contents which may create a loss of consciousness. A *contracoup concussion* is created when the skull contents strike against the skull wall on the side opposite the blow. A *simple fracture*, in which there is no displacement of bone, is called a *linear fracture*. A fracture creating a displacement of the skull is called a *depressed skull fracture*. A *basilar fracture* refers to one found in the base of the skull.

Concussion is the most frequent type of head trauma in children. The shifting of skull contents during a blow to the head may result in a brief loss of consciousness. The child regains consciousness rapidly, may complain of pain, but quickly returns to his play. Trauma to the brain may cause bleeding or edema which develops slowly, allowing the child to be asymptomatic for 6 to 18 hours following the injury. As the hemorrhage or edema increases, the child demonstrates symptoms of increased ICP, usually lethargy, irritability, nausea, and vomiting.

The diagnosis of skull fracture is confirmed by x-ray. Depressed fractures may be found by palpating and observing the contour of the head. The diagnosis of basilar skull fractures is further supported with evidence of drainage of CSF or serosanguineous fluid from the nose, mouth, or auditory canal. Incidence of brain laceration and invasion of foreign bodies is greatly increased with severely depressed or compound fractures to the skull.

Children with head trauma may display minor symptoms or may demonstrate severe neurologic deficits. The symptoms of head trauma are not specific but appear with the development of cerebral irritation or increased pressure due to edema or hemorrhage. Hemorrhage is classified according to its location and may be found in the subdural, epidural, or subarachnoid spaces and within the cerebral tissues.

Subarachnoid hemorrhage occurs within the subarachnoid space from bleeding of damaged vessels on the surface of the brain. The onset of symptoms is gradual, within 24 to 48 hours after injury. Increased ICP and meningeal irritation are manifested by elevated temperature and alterations in level of consciousness. Laboratory findings demonstrate blood in the CSF. The treatment consists of rest and reduction of pressure. The prognosis depends on the degree of hemorrhage, with massive brain damage evident in the severe cases.

Subdural hematoma is a unilateral or bilateral collection of blood between the dura and the arachnoid mater. The symptoms may not develop until 2 to 4 weeks after head trauma. Infants demonstrate tight or bulging fontanels, enlargement of the head, ano-rexia, irritability, vomiting, low-grade fever, hyperactive reflexes, retinal hemorrhage, and increased transillumination. Older children demonstrate signs of increasing ICP. The diagnosis is based on EEGs, carotid angiography, and subdural taps. Treatment consists of daily subdural taps to decrease the intracranial pressure.

Extradural hematoma is bleeding into the space between the dura and the cranium. The onset of symptoms may be rapid, constituting a surgical emergency. The child shows evidence of concussion with lateralizing neurologic signs, hyperactive deep tendon reflexes, positive Babinski sign, and increasing ICP. The lumbar puncture shows clear fluid and slightly increased pressure. Immediate surgery is imperative.

Treatment of head injuries is primarily supportive until the degree and location of the injury are identified. Children with no immediate evidence of CNS involvement may not require formal medical attention. Parents, however, should be instructed to observe their child for lethargy, vomiting, irritability, and muscular weakness. If these signs of increasing pressure occur, the child is hospitalized. Frequent, complete neurologic assessments are necessary to rapidly identify the site of cerebral trauma and the correct treatment to prevent further brain damage.

Surgery is performed when there is massive hemorrhage and rapidly developing intracranial pressure. The primary purpose of surgery is to decompress (reduce pressure), control bleeding, or to remove bone fragments and foreign bodies. Slow bleeding or edema formation may be best controlled by allowing the pressure developing within the skull to act as local pressure on the bleeding sites.

The child who has incurred severe head trauma may have permanent brain damage which cannot be evaluated fully until all cerebral edema has subsided. This process may take weeks or months. Approximately 3 percent of children with closed head trauma have seizure activity as a sequela to the trauma. Seizure activity is found in 50 percent of the children with open head injury. For this reason children with moderate to severe head injuries are placed on seizure medications prophylactically for a minimum of 1 year. Psychosis and neurosis are sometimes encountered in the convalescent period but rarely persist.

Nursing Management The primary goal in the care of the child with head trauma is to prevent further brain damage. This means that the nurse must be alert at all times for the slightest change in the child's condition. Frequent assessment of the neurologic status is important, especially the level of consciousness. Any complication, such as respiratory distress, dehydration, skin breakdown, or persistent hyperthermia could be life-threatening.

The child with a head injury and the family need reassurance and support in a possible life-threatening situation. Allowing a family member to stay with the child is helpful. The nurse should explain all procedures to the family to allay fears; his presence at frequent intervals is also reassuring.

In contrast to the child with brain surgery, who has a clean surgical incision draining small amounts of serosanguineous fluid, children with head trauma have increased drainage onto their dressings because of the deep traumatic nature of their injuries. The amount of fluid loss must be carefully measured by weighing the head dressing before its application and after removal and by circling the drainage area with a nonabsorbable pen. The chance of a child's developing an infection is compounded in the traumatic open injury; therefore it becomes vital to reinforce or change moist dressings to prevent capillary induction of pathogens into the wound. A child with a basilar skull fracture may have serosanguineous drainage from the nose, mouth, or ears which could be cerebrospinal fluid. Because the presence of such drainage increases the chance of admitting pathogens directly to the CNS, sterile dressings may be applied loosely to the child's ears or nose to prevent contamination.

Since the majority of head traumas are the result of accidents, the nurse should stress to the family the safety measures that might prevent a similar accident in the future.

Lead Poisoning

With the passage of federal laws prohibiting the use of lead paint, the incidence of lead poisoning has greatly decreased. Children living in old buildings, where peeling exposes the old lead paint, are more likely to develop lead poisoning. This condition is often seen in a child with pica, an appetite for unusual foreign materials.

Ingestion or inhalation of toxic levels of lead causes encephalopathy. Lead poisoning may be acute or chronic, but in either case residual damage to the nervous system occurs. Acute lead poisoning is usually caused by ingestion of lead salts. The onset of symptoms is rapid, and the child presents in a critical condition with nausea, vomiting, abdominal pain, seizures, and eventually coma. Renal failure leading to death can occur in 1 to 2 days.

Chronic lead poisoning is more common, and the symptoms are insidious in onset, proceeding from mild to severe. Early diagnosis and treatment are important to prevent serious sequelae. On admission to the hospital, the child could have symptoms such as weakness, irritability, vomiting, abdominal pain, loss of appetite, and anemia.

Diagnosis is made following blood studies and urinalysis. X-ray of long bones shows an increased density at the ends. The blood shows low hemoglobin and red cell count; lead is present in the urine. Other findings could be a blue lead line along the gums, presence of lead in the blood, a lowered cell count, increased protein, and traces of lead in the CSF. Treatment of acute lead poisoning begins with gastric lavage, which must be done immediately. Magnesium sulfate is administered after the lavage to aid in the catharsis of all lead particles. Milk is given to counteract the storage of lead in the bones. Once the acute stage has been resolved, the child develops the more typical appearance of chronic lead poisoning.

Medications are given to prevent lead absorption and promote lead excretion. Such drugs as calcium disodium edetate (EDTA) and dimercaprol (BAL) aid excretion of lead. These drugs aid in the absorption of lead by the bloodstream, which carries lead to the kidneys for excretion.

EDTA, a frequently used chelating agent, is given intramuscularly, in daily divided doses, usually over a 5-day period. In the presence of very high lead levels, BAL may also be used concurrently with EDTA. Urine and blood lead levels are usually obtained daily to determine drug effectiveness. A repeat drug regimen may be necessary. Rotating intramuscular sites is an imperative nursing action.

Nursing Management Implications for nursing the child with lead poisoning are many. Neurologically, the child can manifest seizures, muscular incoordination, or loss of consciousness. The child must be observed closely for any change in neurologic status.

The family members need understanding and support for they may feel guilt concerning the child's condition. Referrals to social service and the community nurse could be helpful. Detection of toxic levels of lead is the major goal in preventing lead poisoning.

NEUROLOGIC DISORDERS IN THE PRESCHOOLER

Meningitis

Meningitis is an inflammation of the meninges. It can be caused by a number of organisms, both bacterial and viral. Table 32-4 describes the most common organisms and symptoms and the age group generally affected.

The diagnosis of meningitis is based on symptoms and the culture of spinal fluid and nasopharyngeal material. A lumbar puncture reveals an increased CSF pressure and, in bacterial meningitis, a cloudy color. In meningococcal meningitis the organism is found in the purpural rash exudate.

If meningitis is treated early, the prognosis is good, but there may be complications and long-term effects. Subdural effusion is frequently a result of H-flu meningitis. Other sequelae may be hydrocephalus, impaired intelligence, seizure disorders, visual and hearing defects, and personality changes.

Nursing Management Whenever there is elevated temperature, nausea and vomiting, restlessness, or the possibility of seizures, the nurse must provide rest and quiet, prevent dehydration, and institute safety measures. Medications, generally phenobarbital and Valium, are given to control restlessness and prevent convulsions. General comfort measures are important, and frequently the nurse must use ingenuity to provide comfort and adequate rest to the irritable, restless child.

Since the child is initially quite ill, observations of any signs of a change in condition are critical. Any indication of increased intracranial pressure requires immediate attention and should be reported at once. Vital signs and neurologic evaluation are done hourly at first, or more frequently if necessary. When I.V. fluids are administered, the danger of increasing intracranial pressure is very real, and the fluid volume must be monitored closely.

A position flat in bed is generally more comfortable for the child with meningitis, especially when there is opisthotonic nuchal rigidity. Because sitting and movement of the head cause increased pain, care is taken to have as little movement as possible. If opisthotonos is present, the child is positioned on his side. Adequate hydration is important, and fluids

Table 32-4 TYPES OF MENINGITIS

Causative organism	Symptoms	Age group affected	Need for isolation
Bacterial			
Hemophilus influenzae, type B (H-flu)	Chills, fever, vomiting, headache, stupor, convulsions, nuchal rigidity; positive Kernig's and Brudzinski's signs	Infant to school age	None
Meningococcus	Same as above with sore throat, purpuric rash	Preschool age	Respiratory isolation
Pneumococcus	Same as H-flu (following respiratory infection)	Preschool age	None
Streptococcus	Same as H-flu	Preschool age	None
Staphylococcus	Vomiting, irritability, high-pitched cry, convulsions, bulging fontanel	Infant	None
Enteric bacteria (*Escherichia coli*)	Same as *Staphylococcus*	Infant	None
Viral			
Coxsackie B	Fever, headache, vomiting, lethargy, stupor, stiff neck	Preschool age	Excretory precautions
Echo	Same as above	Preschool age	Excretory precautions
Rubella virus	Same as above	Preschool through school age	Excretory precautions
Mumps virus	Same as above	Preschool through school age	Excretory precautions
Herpesvirus	Rapid onset, severe and rapid deterioration; severe brain damage Death usually results	Infant	

should be encouraged, preferably in ways that do not require sitting. Straws should be used, and gelatin desserts or popsicles may be offered.

Medications are administered intravenously for 2 to 3 weeks. These medications, toxic and irritating to the vein, tend to create phlebitis during prolonged administration. Medication sites should be observed for evidence of infiltration or development of tissue irritation. If the nurse administers the medication slowly in a dilute form, irritation can be prevented. The nurse must know the characteristics of the specific medication he is administering, including the proper dilution and the side effects. The child should be restrained in a functional position which safeguards the integrity of the I.V. infusion and still allows for mobility. When able, the child should be allowed to ambulate and play.

Encephalitis

The term *encephalitis* describes an inflammatory process of the brain. The encephalitic process is usually created by the invasion of a virus or as an allergic reaction to a virus. Chickenpox, measles, mumps, and herpes simplex may cause encephalitis as a complication of the disease process, and encephalitis may occur as a complication following routine vaccinations for smallpox, poliomyelitis, diphtheria, pertussis, and influenza.

The clinical features of encephalitis vary according to the invading organism and its prime location within the brain. Characteristically there is a sudden or insidious onset of headache and elevated temperature which may be followed by drowsiness, then can progress to a deep coma. Sometimes the onset is marked by changes in behavior and hyperactivity. Seizures are more likely to occur in the infant, whereas paresis of one or more of the cranial nerves, disorders of speech, ataxia, weakness of muscle groups, diplopia, alterations of reflexes, and disturbances of the autonomic nervous system may occur as single entities or in combinations in the preschool child with encephalitis.

Diagnosis is based on the history of the onset of symptoms and the result of laboratory studies. The CSF is often within normal limits initially, but a moderate increase in leukocytes may be evidenced after 48 hours. The sugar content of the CSF is usually normal but may be low, and the protein count is either normal or slightly elevated.

The prognosis is guarded. Recovery may be dramatically sudden within a few hours or may not occur for days, weeks, or months. Death may be the result. Infants are more likely to have permanent residual effects than are older children. Residual effects may be in the form of seizure disorders, hemiplegia or monoplegia, bizarre behavior patterns, and mental retardation. Evidence of residual damage may not be apparent until the child fails to meet developmental levels or has difficulty with learning.

Nursing Management   The symptoms dictate plans for nursing care. The child is placed in an area where he can be observed closely for evidence of seizures and increased intracranial pressure. The child with encephalitis may demonstrate signs of respiratory distress from paralysis of the respiratory muscles or involvement of the respiratory center of the brain. If the child has difficulty swallowing, pooled secretions may contribute to his respiratory difficulty. To maintain adequate respiratory function, the child may require intubation or a tracheostomy.

If the child is comatose, he may emerge rapidly or somewhat slowly from this state, often with some immediate residual affects such as ataxia, behavior changes, and general confusion. The child must be oriented to time and place and told what has happened. Play should be incorporated into the care according to age and physical abilities to foster return of neuromuscular function. Working with clay, stringing beads, and throwing balls are possible, enjoyable, and beneficial activities. Living with and accepting the unknown create anxieties for both the parents and the child during his convalescence, but the full potential for residual effects may not be known for many months. The nurse should assist the parents in their acceptance of their child with his current disabilities and project hope for the future that is based on reality. The family that must eventually accept the child with permanent disabilities needs additional support from the health team.

A schedule for routine evaluation of the development level should be established as part of the discharge plan. A referral to the public health agency provides necessary follow-up.

NEUROLOGIC DISORDERS IN THE SCHOOL-AGE CHILD
Brain Tumor

Brain tumors occur most commonly in the 5- to 7-year age group. Because approximately two-thirds of the tumors occur in the posterior fossa, signs of increased intracranial pressure develop early. Seventy-five percent of brain tumors in children are gliomas. It is uncommon for children to have metastatic tumors.

Five major forms of brain tumors are most frequently seen in children. *Astrocytoma* can occur at any age, but usually has a peak incidence at 8 years of age. This tumor is usually located in the cerebellum. Astrocytoma is divided into four grades, depending on its malignancy—grade 1 is the least malignant and grade 4 the most malignant. The tumor has an insidious onset and a slow course. The child usually presents with signs of focal disturbances, increased ICP, hypotonia, diminished reflexes, and papilledema, which may lead to optic atrophy, blindness, and nystagmus. Without surgery the prognosis is poor, but surgical removal of the tumor with complete cure is possible.

Medulloblastoma is a highly malignant, rapidly growing tumor usually found in the cerebellum. The peak incidence is in the 6- to 7-year age group. The manifestations of this tumor are usually an unsteady walk, anorexia, vomiting, and an early morning headache. As the tumor progresses, the child develops ataxia, papilledema, drowsiness, and nystagmus. Death usually occurs in 1 year.

Brainstem *gliomas* have a peak incidence in children of 7 years. The clinical manifestations are multiple cranial nerve palsies and ataxia. The child demonstrates little sensory loss; increased intracranial pressure slowly develops. The course of the glioma is slow. The tumors are inoperable, but radiation has increased the survival time.

Ependymoma is a tumor which is located in the first, second, or fourth ventricle. There is no sex or age predilection. The clinical manifestations are increased ICP, nausea, vomiting, unsteady gait, and headache. Children with open sutures may demonstrate enlargement of the head, and hydrocephalus may occur. The primary treatment consists of incomplete internal decompression of the tumor followed by x-ray therapy.

Craniopharyngioma occurs late in childhood; the tumor is usually located near the pituitary gland. The clinical features are pituitary or hypothalamic dysfunctions, with diabetes insipidus being the most common hormonal symptom. Pitressin is given on a long-term basis to control the diabetes insipidus. The child may have stimulated growth, myxedema, delayed puberty, visual defects, alterations of personality and memory, and increased ICP. Complete surgical removal is usually impossible, but radiation therapy may control the growth of the tumor for years.

Diagnosis of brain tumors in the early phase is very important but often difficult because of the insidious onset. Vomiting in the morning may be the initial symptom. Because of the age of the child, vomiting is often attributed to school phobias. Headache should prove valuable in diagnosis as this is not a common complaint of children. Changes in vision are difficult to evaluate and may not be recognized until the child begins to stumble into furniture or fall over objects. Late-developing strabismus should give warning of tumor activity, but other disease entities could cause this. Unilateral weakness may develop very slowly, allowing the child to compensate, and thus fail to evidence the difficulty until it has progressed.

The diagnosis is confirmed after specific diagnostic procedures such as EEGs, pneumoencephalograms, skull series, ventriculograms, arteriograms, brain scans, and lumbar punctures to measure pressure as well as chemical analysis of the CSF. Depending on the type and location of the suspected lesion, a complete diagnosis requires a biopsy, which is usually done by craniotomy. These procedures have obvious inherent risks and discomforts and should be done only when there is sufficient evidence to warrant their use. The child and family require much support and care during the diagnostic phase.

Nursing Management The nursing care of the child with a brain tumor may be divided into basic phases: diagnostic, preoperative, postoperative (maintenance), radiation, and discharge. Throughout each of these phases the nurse must assess the child for evidence of alteration in neurologic status and for response to the diagnostic or therapeutic measures.

Diagnostic phase When a brain tumor is suspected, the child and his family approach hospitalization and the diagnostic studies with great anxiety. Many parents feel guilty for not seeking help earlier because they thought the child had flu or did not want to go to school. A slow change in personality may be one of the symptoms indicating serious disorder. Many parents express the fear that their feelings will be confirmed, yet they also want an explanation for the changed behavior. The child also is concerned about what will happen to him. A trusting, therapeutic relation with the parents and child must be established at the time of admission. The best way to accomplish this is to take a nursing history during the admission interview. A therapeutic relation is very important since the nurse will provide primary care not only during hospitalization but possibly for the life-span of the child. A nursing assessment of the family unit and its coping mechanisms should be made at this time.

Following diagnosis, a decision is made regarding the most appropriate medical treatment for the child. If no treatment is appropriate, the child is discharged with only supportive measures, and the family must be taught to care for the child at home. A liaison within the community to provide continuous support for the family would be helpful.

Preoperative phase   If surgery is a part of the treatment of the child with a brain tumor, the nurse must understand the purpose of the surgery and prepare the child and his parents for the craniotomy procedure. (See Chap. 27.)

The child and the parents need careful explanation and preparation for the change in appearance postoperatively. They need to know that the child's head is shaved and that massive head dressings will be in place. Some physicians advise that the entire head be shaved; others advocate cutting the hair short and shaving only the incision area; still other surgeons shave only the operative site and leave the rest of the hair intact. Regardless of the technique, the loss of hair can be very traumatic to the child and his parents. It may be possible for the child to pick out a wig prior to surgery, but specific preparation of the head should be planned in collaboration with the neurosurgeon and the child.

The parents must also be prepared for the appearance of facial edema and the possibility that their child will be in a comatose state immediately following surgery. The nurse must understand that parents have difficulty comprehending such possibilities as they watch their child preoperatively.

Postoperative phase   During surgery and postoperatively, the nurse who has assumed responsibility for continuity of care must be available to the parents for continued support. When the child has regained consciousness, the nurse who is providing primary care should visit with him several times a day in the intensive care unit. At this time of increased stress the total family benefits much from the therapeutic relation established by the primary care nurse in the preoperative period.

Postoperative care of the child who has undergone brain surgery is critical. The nurse must assess this child frequently for evidence of increased ICP, caused by edema or hemorrhage, and for alterations in level of consciousness.

The nurse must assess the child for edema, frequently located in the neck, face, and intracranial spaces. Edema may inhibit respirations and ability to close the eyes, thus increasing the child's discomfort. Positioning, with the child's head elevated and the body turned on the unoperated side, reduces the edema and decreases the ICP. Methylcellulose applied to his eyes prevents corneal damage, and cool compresses applied to his head, face, and neck reduce the edema and promote comfort. Severe edema in the neck may necessitate use of respiratory apparatus. To control cerebral edema, the child may be receiving medications such as Medrol; hypothermia may be instituted to further control edema and reduce the metabolic needs. Astute monitoring of the I.V. infusions is necessary to prevent increased cerebral edema secondary to overhydration.

The child must be carefully watched for signs of nervous tissue irritation resulting from damage secondary to the surgical procedure or from the edema. Areas of the brain which control respirations may be affected, creating the need for mechanical respiratory assistance. If the temperature control area of the brain has been irritated, the child will have a high fever which is best controlled with a hypothermia mattress. An elevated temperature secondary to CNS disturbance rarely responds satisfactorily to the conservative treatment of aspirin, Tylenol, or tepid baths.

Infections in the postoperative period may prove fatal to these children. Immediately after surgery the child should be isolated from anyone with an infection, and antibiotics may be given prophylactically.

The nurse should observe the head dressing carefully for signs of drainage. Should drainage occur, the color, amount, and odor should be reported immediately. The area of drainage should be circled with a pen or pencil and timed. Do *not* use felt tip pens as this ink is rapidly absorbed to the incision level. With a simple craniotomy, drainage should be slight and consist primarily of serosanguineous fluid from the skin. If burr holes have been used or skull plates removed for decompression, the drainage is likely to be greater. If large amounts of drainage are noted, the nurse may reinforce the dressing with additional material and report the situation to the physician immediately.

When the child's condition is stabilized, he is returned to his previous unit. During the recovery period, he is allowed and encouraged to return to independence, although this may be complicated for the child who has residual affects from his surgery. The child and parents need to be told that these residual effects are due in part to edema and the surgical trauma and thus may disappear as the healing process is completed. The nurse may also help return parent-child relations to the presurgery level. Many parents are so relieved that the surgery is over and have such concern for the child who experienced surgery that they tend to be overprotective and indulgent. Both the parents and the child must return to the "well role."

Play should be encouraged for fun as well as its therapeutic results. Care must be taken, however, that the child does not hit his head or fall until he is completely healed. Stocking-knit and head dressings may provide enough protection, depending on the type of surgery and the child's age. For some children a football helmet or wig is necessary to prevent trauma should they fall.

Postoperatively, children do not usually have difficulties adjusting to their altered appearance from loss of hair as long as the dressing is in place. When the dressing is no longer needed, many children exhibit extreme difficulties in accepting their baldness and adjusting to their body self-image. Stocking-knit caps, head scarves, or hats may be enough to allow the child to cope with his baldness and once again interact with other children and resume active participation in his recovery phase. Some children do better if a wig is supplied until the hair has grown in. If the head has not been totally shaved, the creative nurse may be able to comb the child's hair so that the area of loss is not so evident.

Radiation phase   Radiation therapy may be used as the singular mode of treatment or in conjunction with surgery. As with all procedures, the child requires preparation prior to radiation therapy. The radiologist outlines in ink the areas to receive the radiation, and these marks must not be washed off. Since radiation therapy destroys or inhibits the growth of cells, it is given in small doses for a prescribed length of time, usually three times a week for 5 to 6 weeks. Depending on the location of the tumor and the amount of radiation received, the child may not demonstrate untoward effects from the therapy until the second to fourth day. General malaise and headache may occur as early side effects. The most severe side effects are due to the destruction of normal cells; skin breakdown, loss of hair, leukopenia, and decrease in platelets occur most often. Supportive and comfort measures must be instituted by the nurse when the child demonstrates these untoward effects of radiation.

Discharge phase   Although hospital staffing patterns and policies do not usually allow the primary nurse to maintain contact with the family in the community, the nurse may be able to see the child in the clinic and maintain contact by telephone. Whether or not this is done, a referral should be made to a community health nurse to reinforce teaching and maintain therapeutic support for the family. There should be contact with the child's teacher and school nurse so that they are able to support the child on his return. They can prepare the child's classmates for his return and help them with their feelings of concern for the change in appearance and behavior. These explanations should include some information about the child's inability to engage in contact sports. Rest periods may need to be provided at school, and attendance should be on a part-time basis initially. Although school is fatiguing, it is a normal part of a child's life, and the satisfaction of learning and socializing with friends is important.

Minimal Brain Dysfunction

The term *minimal brain dysfunction* (MBD) is used interchangeably with minimal brain damage, minimal cerebral dysfunction, and learning disabilities. Children with MBD have impairments in perception, conceptualization, language, memory, control of attention, impulses, or motor functions. They are differentiated from the mentally retarded in that they have an IQ that is normal, and yet they have difficulty in learning. The terminology is somewhat confusing because these children rarely demonstrate intellectual impairment; however, a majority have a history of prenatal or perinatal traumata which might result in brain damage. About 50 percent of these children have abnormal EEGs, despite the absence of seizure activity. There are no accurate data concerning incidence.

Most children with MBD are males and are diagnosed at 7 to 12 years of age. They are seldom identified before school age because their behavior does not impair intellectual or social development until confronted with the structured classroom experience.

The clinical manifestations vary. A typical child is brought to the pediatrician by his mother, who complains of the child's disorderly and unmanageable behavior in school and home. Failing grades (including reading abilities) are her greatest concern. His restlessness, hyperactivity, short attention spans, and aggressive behavior toward siblings are typically described. When scolded or reprimanded, the child with MBD is likely to scream, throw himself on the floor, or noisily retreat to another room, only to return shortly and continue with the unacceptable behavior. When shopping, the child touches and handles everything, including other shoppers. In restaurants he is likely to leave the table, walk around, or constantly look over the back of the booth, interfering with other diners. Again, when reprimanded, he screams and throws temper tantrums. The mother says, "He makes me tired just watching him."

The teacher's description is similar. He shuffles his feet, stands up, sits down, or squirms in his chair. He is constantly poking the children around him, and does not follow simple classroom rules. If the teacher is reading he is likely to get up, walk down the aisle, or go to a window. When the rest of the class is quietly working, he is rattling paper or crying out in nonsense phrases. Although capable, he does not read, and the teacher states that he just does not try.

Both the mother and teacher describe him as having characteristic behavior of emotional liability. Peers refuse to play with him because he does not follow the rules, and he responds to their rebuke by screaming or retreating and crying. All who have contact with him report their frustration and inability to control him.

The diagnosis of MBD must be made carefully. Of particular importance is a history of delayed developmental milestones, small or large muscle incoordination, confusion in laterality, general irritability, insatiable demands for attention, compulsive activities, unexpected phobias such as fear of animals or loud noises, and persistent automatisms such as head-rocking, head-banging, or staring at objects.

In addition, a complete physical assessment of the child and referral to a pediatric neurologist for a complete neurologic assessment should be done. A neurologic assessment often reveals abnormalities, so-called "soft" neurologic signs. These symptoms include unsustained ankle clonus, hyperactive tendon reflexes, asymmetric deep tendon reflexes, pupillary inequality, inconsistent Babinski reflex, motor awkwardness, choreiform movements of fingers, difficulty differentiating left from right, strabismus, nystagmus, articulation disorders in speech, hyperactivity, tic, auditory impairment, intention tremors, and inability to stand and hop on one foot. Hearing and vision testing may identify specific sensory dysfunction.

A psychologic assessment is included because these children often have overriding emotional difficulties. The psychologic examination should include intelligence testing. The WISC or Stanford-Binet test is most frequently used as either eliminates some of the socioeconomic barriers in intelligence tests. The expert must carefully evaluate the child's score and his responses to inquiries. Often the child with MBD has a discrepancy in his verbal and performance scores. The draw-a-man test and the Ammon's-Quick test identify intelligence as well as perceptual difficulties often found in MBD. The child

may have "mirror vision" or difficulty in spatial relations, either with distances or foreground (ability to identify figures on a plain background but not on a textured or marbled background). He transfers numbers and letters, for example, *b* versus *d* and 3 versus *e*. The child may hear and understand what he is told, but when asked to read or write the same, he cannot complete the task. He adds sounds or transposes sounds in his vocabulary, e.g., bat versus cat or at. Speech, visual, and neuromuscular difficulties of this type obviously create learning difficulties, frustrations, and feelings of failure.

Treatment includes patient counseling, psychotherapy, educational management, and drug therapy. Parents need to develop a thorough knowledge of their child's disorder. Usually they have been aware that a problem exists and are relieved to know the cause of the disturbing behavior. They are especially relieved to know that the child cannot control his activities.

Once the parents understand the disorder, they must learn what they can do to alleviate or control behavior. Discipline in MBD is vital, for the child cannot discipline himself, but it must be appropriate and consistent. When necessary, discipline may consist of placing the child in a calmer, more controlled environment, a room, in which he may regain his own self-control.

Parents of the child with MBD have success when they avoid exposing the child to situations in which he is apt to lose control. Large social gatherings within the home, shopping, or dining out should be avoided. Life-style adjustments are necessary, but they should not be detrimental to the needs of the family unit.

Frustrations and frequent failures in learning and establishing relationships with peers and adults may lead to secondary emotional difficulties. Low self-esteem, school phobias, or even truancy are frequently encountered behaviors. Psychotherapy may be necessary and might include the total family because the parents and siblings may need assistance in alleviating angry or hostile feelings toward the affected child.

Educational management is a major concern. Parents and teachers need to assume major roles in helping this child acquire an education. The average classroom is a very poor environment for this child, and the majority of educators agree that the child should be placed in a special classroom with fewer students. Stimulation from the environment should be eliminated so that he can concentrate on learning. Some classrooms have been built without windows, with carpeting, and equipped with special study carrels to decrease stimulation. Teachers should have the knowledge and ability to develop highly individualized learning plans and to help the child develop a more positive self-image so that he can function more effectively in society.

Drug therapy has a definite but limited place in treatment and is directed toward controlling hyperactivity. These children are usually placed on amphetamines or methylphenidate (Ritalin). Barbiturates are avoided as they tend to accentuate the hyperactivity. Other drugs which have been effective include Benadryl, Thorazine, and other tranquilizers. The dosage must be in accordance with the child's needs, thereby avoiding side effects such as lethargy or loss of appetite. The parents and teacher should work closely with the pediatrician in establishing an appropriate drug regime for the individual child.

The prognosis is fair. Limited longitudinal studies are available which indicate that the majority of children appear to outgrow their difficulties in adolescence. Other studies reveal that some children continue to have difficulty establishing and maintaining relationships. A small percentage have been institutionalized for personality disorders or emotional difficulties.

Nursing Management The nursing role in working with children with MBD has three aspects. Providing support to the family and educating the community is the first. The parents can be helped if they have someone with whom they can share their concerns.

A second aspect is acting as a case finder. The nurse is frequently in a position to observe children in schools, doctors' offices, or hospital settings. In assessing the child's behavior and in history-taking, the nurse may identify behavior that is significant of the MBD child. Collaboration with the physician and family may lead to an early diagnosis, treatment, and more effective management.

The third area of concern for nursing is providing care to the child when he is hospitalized. He is usually described as a behavior problem in the hospital. Unable to tolerate being in bed, he roams the halls, gets into bed with other children, or commits other mischievous acts. The hospital setting creates exacerbations of inappropriate behavior because of increased stimulation. Separation from home is very difficult, and although the hospital stimulates his behavior, it does not allow for expending additional energy. One successful nursing intervention is assigning a nurse to maintain a continuity of care therapy, decreasing the number of people with whom the child has contact. This nurse must be patient, consistent, and supportive to the child and his parents. While caring for the MBD child can be very taxing, it is rewarding for those who approach with knowledge and understanding.

Epilepsy

The term *epilepsy* is used to describe recurring seizures of some type. A symptom such as loss or impairment of consciousness, accompanied by tonic-clonic muscular spasms and/or alterations in behavior, is indicative of the disorder. The terms *epilepsy* and *recurrent convulsive disorders* are used interchangeably. The diagnosis is *idiopathic* or *cryptogenic epilepsy* if no cause for the child's seizures can be identified. When a cause for the seizure can be identified, the diagnosis is *organic* or *symptomatic epilepsy*.

Epilepsy is diagnosed primarily from a history of seizure episodes, and it is confirmed by abnormal EEG readings. The diagnostic work-up includes an extensive neurologic assessment to rule out an organic basis.

There are several forms of epilepsy. *Grand mal seizures* are generalized convulsions and are indicative of disturbance in brain function. The onset is abrupt, although many will have a warning known as an *aura*. The aura is described as peculiar feelings, sights, sounds, tastes, smells, or twitching or spasm of small muscle groups. The tonic contraction may occur simultaneously with loss of consciousness. The child falls to the ground, his color becomes pale, the pupils dilate, the conjuctivae are insensitive to touch, the eyes roll upward or to one side, the head is thrown backward or to one side, the abdominal and chest muscles are held rigidly, and the limbs are contracted irregularly or they are rigid. As the air is forced out by the sudden contraction of the diaphragm against a closed glottis, a short startling cry may be heard. The tongue may be bitten by the contracting jaw. Involuntary urination and sometimes defecation occur with the contractions of the abdominal muscles. The pallor may change to cyanosis depending on the length and severity of this phase, for respiration is inhibited. The tonic phase may last 20 to 40 seconds or longer. It is followed by clonic activity which involves the entire body.

The child sleeps after the seizure has stopped. On awakening, he appears drowsy, stuporous, and accomplishes routine tasks in an automatic fashion. This behavior is believed to be caused by malfunction of the neurons which have not yet recovered from the seizure. Occasionally a child has a seizure during sleep, evidenced by bitten areas in the mouth, blood on the pillow, or a wet bed. He awakens with no recollection or memory of the seizure. When seizures are so frequent that they appear to be constant, the child is said to have *staticus epilepticus*, a medical emergency which may result in brain damage because of a decreased oxygen supply to the cerebrum.

Petit mal seizures are transient losses of consciousness. The patient may exhibit eye-rolling movements, drooping or fluttering of the eyelids, drooping of the head or slight quivering of the limb and trunk muscles. These seizures develop after 3 years of age, frequently disappear with adolescence, and are more common among females. The child who has petit mal seizures is frequently described by parents and teachers as having "dizzy spells," "absences," "lapses," or "daydreaming episodes." If he is in the middle of a task, he drops whatever is in his hand; on completion of the seizure, he immediately resumes the activity without knowledge of ever having stopped. Exposure to blinking lights or hyperventilation may initiate a petit mal seizure.

Psychomotor seizures represent the most difficult form of epilepsy to recognize and control. Behavioral abnormalities and purposeful but inappropriate repetitive motor acts are characteristic of this disorder. Frequently an aura of a shrill cry or running to an adult is noted in young children. The child may sleep following the seizure. Sometimes the child exhibits a gradual loss of postural tone and softly falls to the floor, losing consciousness. There are usually no associated clonic or tonic movements. The EEG is normal unless taken during a seizure, and therefore a diagnosis is difficult.

Focal or *Jacksonian seizures* are sensory or motor, depending on the location of disturbed neural discharges. The sensory type is relatively rare in children. Occasionally Jacksonian seizures have been identified in the absence of organic lesions, but they are primarily indicative of a CNS lesion. Focal seizures are preceded by a brief tonic phase; however, they are clonic in nature. They begin in one muscle group and proceed to other muscle groups in a fixed manner, i.e., finger to wrist to hand to arm to face and then to the leg of the same side. When the attacks are brief, there is no loss of consciousness, but if the spread is rapid and extensive, consciousness is lost, and it is followed by a generalized convulsion, indistinguishable from a grand mal seizure.

The treatment of epilepsy is based on controlling seizure activity, accomplished primarily through the use of drugs. Phenobarbital is most frequently used in treating grand mal seizures. It has few side effects and is relatively inexpensive. Dilantin is also used to treat grand mal seizures either alone or in combination with phenobarbital. Dilantin has some side effects, especially stomatitis and hypertrophy of the gums. It has also contributed to deformed teeth when given to children in the predentulous ages. Zarontin, used in treating petit mal seizures, has fewer side effects and is more effective than Tridione or Parodyne. However, Zarontin has been known to cause blood dyscrasias, and routine white blood cell counts should be done on children who are receiving it. Mysoline is given for grand mal and psychomotor seizures. It is relatively nontoxic and may be given in conjunction with phenobarbital.

Whatever drug is used, the appropriate dose is determined by the child's reactions to it and its effectiveness in controlling the seizure activity. As he grows, the dosage must be altered. Drug therapy is a long-term process, as epilepsy is a chronic disease. The condition is usually considered under control when the child has been without a seizure for 1 year or longer. Once seizures are controlled, the medication should be withdrawn gradually, because rapid withdrawal of drugs may result in seizure activity. If seizure activity recurs, medication is reinstituted. Other supportive measures include reducing stress, avoiding loud noises or blinking lights, and developing good family relations.

Nursing Management The attitude of society as a whole is not supportive to a family with an epileptic child. The term *epilepsy* has a stigma attached to it. Throughout history people with epilepsy have been branded as "outcasts," "feebleminded," "beseeched with evil spirits," "witches," or "insane." Even today, some of these attitudes prevail. Many children with epilepsy have been considered mentally retarded, although mental retardation is not found with this disease unless there are organic lesions or it results from status epilepticus. Because of these attitudes and the ignorance of society, the activities of many epileptics are restricted.

The nurse must be cognizant of the fact that initially the parents have the same misconceptions about their child's diagnosis as most of society. The nurse can help by teaching the family about epilepsy and about the specific needs of their child.

The parents must understand the purpose of the child's medication and be taught to observe for signs of toxicity and evidence that the dosage may need alteration. They should be instructed to always have the drug available, including on trips and vacations. The medication should be stored in a safe place, away from children who may accidentally ingest it. If the child must take the medication at school, an extra supply is often maintained by the school nurse.

or teacher who supervises its administration. If the school cannot support the child in this manner, only the exact dose of medication should be sent to school with him. An epileptic child must be taught that his medication is important to him, but dangerous to other children.

A young epileptic and his family must be aware of safety factors. If he has frequent grand mal seizures, it may be necessary for him to wear a football helmet at all times to prevent injury to his head. Wearing a helmet can and usually does create social difficulties, and it should be utilized only when absolutely necessary. He should not be allowed to participate in activities that would be hazardous, such as swimming or horseback riding, unless he is accompanied by a responsible person. Children with epilepsy should wear Medic-Alert bracelets with all necessary information, such as diagnosis and drug regime, so appropriate assistance may be offered should they have seizures when they are not with their families or close friends.

The nurse can assist the child to develop a healthy self-concept. Children with epilepsy are frequently described as having personality disorders such as egocentricity, shallowness, religiosity, and chronic negativism. These personality disorders can be prevented if the parents accept the child with his disease. Care must be taken to discipline, to set limits, and to love. Some children may use their seizures to "control" their parents, and thus a circular effect of manipulation between the child and his parents develops.

As adolescence approaches, the epileptic child may act out or test his disease, much like the diabetic adolescent. He may stop taking his medication, engage in activities that have been forbidden, and subject himself to undue stress. This type of behavior causes his parents great concern, but the understanding parent recognizes this behavior as essentially normal, allows for the testing, and supports the adolescent in the final resolution of acceptance.

NEUROLOGIC DISORDERS IN THE ADOLESCENT
Spinal Cord Injury

Spinal cord injury occurs when there is compression or destruction of the cord. Accidents are the most common cause of spinal cord injury among children, and diving, boating, snowmobiling, skiing, surfing, and automobile accidents are frequent causes of trauma. Bullet wounds are also responsible for many cord injuries.

Compression is the most common cause of cord damage. Subluxation, crushed laminas, or dislocated fractures are most frequently responsible for pressure on the spinal cord. Since the spinal cord is housed in a relatively small bony area, minimal edema or hemorrhage can compress the cord. Complete or partial severance of the cord is less frequently seen than compression. Initial assessment of the injury is important. Was paralysis immediate or did it slowly progress? The prognosis in gradual paralysis is far better than in immediate and total paralysis. The degree of return depends on the severity of damage from compression as well as the rapidity with which the pressure was removed. When the cord is partially or completely severed, the hope for return of function is lost.

The clinical manifestations of spinal cord injury depend upon the location of the insult. The degree of paralysis is determined by the level of the injury. At high levels (the 3d and 4th cervical vertebrae, C_3 and C_4) there is paralysis of the intercostal muscles and diaphragm, and so respiration is difficult. At lower levels (C_5 and C_6) there is primarily paralysis of all extremities and the abdominal muscles. In either case there is loss of voluntary motor function and bowel and bladder control.

Injury to the thoracic area results in paralysis of the lower extremities, abdominal muscles, bladder, and rectum. The paralysis at first is flaccid but later becomes spastic.

In the lumbar region, injury affects the cauda equina, conus medullaris, and possibly segments of the lower cord. As a result there are flaccid paralyses of the lower extremities and atonic bladder and rectal muscles.

Systemic shock is demonstrated soon after the injury. The suddenness of the loss of function requires the body to initiate massive compensatory actions, and the lack of movement and muscle support to the vascular system create circulatory difficulties. Increased pulse and respirations with a decrease in blood pressure are encountered. The shock response is intensified if the respiratory area has been affected by the insult.

Spinal shock, resulting from sudden insult to the cord, causes a disturbance to the reflex arc which leads to flaccid paralysis. As the reflex arc becomes adjusted to its current state or pressure is removed, the paralysis becomes spastic. The reflex arc, once active again, has a tendency to be overactive, and subsequent spasticity becomes a real problem for the adolescent.

Following a diagnosis of spinal cord injury, x-rays are necessary to evaluate fracture or displacement of the vertebrae, and a thorough neurologic assessment should be done to evaluate loss of function or sensation. Lumbar puncture may be performed to rule out blockage in the flow of CSF or hemorrhage.

Nursing Management   Upon arrival in the emergency room, the adolescent must be evaluated immediately for degree of shock and neurologic function. Intravenous fluids are started to provide a route for emergency medication, and vital signs and neurologic status are monitored every 15 to 30 minutes. Since cervical involvement inhibits respiratory function, respiratory assistance may be needed in the form of an endotracheal tube, tracheostomy, or mechanical respirator. Pain must be alleviated to help reduce shock. A Foley catheter is inserted to prevent bladder distention as well as to monitor kidney function. Once shock and respiratory needs have been treated, a more definitive diagnosis can be made and treatment planned accordingly. The danger of complications secondary to immobility, such as bedsores, contractures, bladder infection, impaction, and circulatory stasis, are of primary concern to the nurse.

Drug Abuse

There is no single definition for drug abuse, but the term includes addiction to narcotics, experimentation with many drugs, and self-medication. The incidence varies with the reporting authority, but general trends have been identifed. Drug abuse is found at all social levels and includes all age groups, but the greatest incidence of drug abuse is among adolescents and young adults. Drug abuse contributes to social, vocational, and educational difficulties, and there is frequently an increased incidence of degenerative disorders and communicable disease within the population of heavy drug abusers. It is said to be the leading cause of death in the 15- to 35-year-old age group.

Many drugs are taken by adolescents to promote physical and psychic changes, often in an experimental way. Generally the type and amount of drug ingested are endemic to certain areas. Once the novelty is removed, new drugs move in to replace the old. Thus the drugs taken by adolescents in different communities change according to the feelings of the adolescent members. They may be taken singularly or in combination, which increases the need for astute assessment when caring for an adolescent with evidence of drug toxicity. Drug abuse is not limited to adolescents but is found in increasingly higher numbers among preadolescent children.

An additional aspect of drug abuse is the increased incidence of drug-addicted newborns. The child of a heroin-addicted mother will also be addicted to the drug. These infants demonstrate all the symptoms of addiction and of withdrawal when the supply of the drug is cut off at birth.

Diagnosis of drug abuse is based on the history of drug ingestion, but relying on the adolescent to supply this information is questionable. Therefore, health care practitioners must utilize observation and selected laboratory studies of blood and urine levels to diagnose drug abuse. Adolescents who appear to have altered levels of consciousness, increased activity, inappropriate affect, or altered perceptions and those who appear malnourished or who have hepatitis should be examined carefully for evidence of drug abuse. The presence of needle tracks on the arms or legs or between the toes or abscesses on the skin are evidence of "mainlining" or "skin popping."

The most frequently used stimulant, depressant, and hallucinogenic drugs [amphetamines, heroin, barbiturates, marijuana, hashish, and lysergic acid diethylamide (LSD)] are listed in Table 32-5 with short- and long-term effects.

Nursing Management   An adolescent suffering from acute drug overdose of stimulants, depressants, or hallucinogenics represents a medical emergency secondary to the alterations in the central nervous system.

Adolescents who have ingested toxic levels of stimulants require seizure precautions, temperature control, and appropriate bland, high-carbohydrate diets. Thorazine or other tranquilizers may be used to better control the central nervous system symptoms. Adolescents who have had prolonged, chronic use of amphetamines experience emotional depression and overwhelming fatigue when the drug is withdrawn. Therapeutic communication with the adolescent who is experiencing acute restlessness and irritability or who is depressed provides a reduction of anxiety and a better understanding of his behavior.

Synthetic narcotics such as Lorfan and Nalline are administered to adolescents with toxicities of depressant drugs (heroin overdose). Barbiturate toxicity is treated symptomatically with infusions, diuresis, hemodialysis, and oxygen (administered via endotracheal tube in severe cases).

Nursing care of adolescents "tripping" on LSD is concerned with preventing injury and restoring reality. The same principles of communicating with any person in a panic, crisis, or aggressive state

Table 32-5 DRUGS MISUSED BY ADOLESCENTS

Name of drug	Slang name	Duration of action, hours	Method of taking	Short-term effects	Long-term effects
Hallucinogens:					
DMT (*N,N*-di-methyltryptamine)	AMT, businessman's high	Less than 1	Injected	Nausea, visual imagery, altered and increased sensory awareness, anxiety, incoordination, exhilaration, increased awareness or consciousness-expansion	May intensify or precipitate an already existing psychosis; panic reactions; may not have any long-term effects
Mescaline (peyote)	Cactus, mesc	12–14	Swallowed		
Psilocybin	Mushrooms	6–8	Swallowed		
STP*			Smoked		
LSD (lysergic acid diethyl-amide)	Acid, sugar, cubes, trip, big D	10–12	Swallowed		
Cannabis (marijuana)	Pot, grass, hashish, hash, tea, weed, stuff, joint, reefer, gage, smoke	4	Sniffed, smoked, or swallowed	Some alteration of time perception, impaired judgment and coordination; relaxation, euphoria, increased appetite, signs of CNS stimulation and depression	Usually none. May become habit forming. May have acute panic reaction.
Narcotics:					
Percodan			Swallowed	CNS depressant, impaired coordination and intellectual functioning, euphoria, relief of pain, and sedation	Addicting with resultant painful and unpleasant withdrawal syndrome. Loss of weight, constipation, anorexia, temporary impotency
Demerol					
Cough syrups	Schoolboy	4	Swallowed		
Codeine					
Heroin	Horse, H, smack, shit, junk, scat, stuff, harry	4	Injected (vein, muscle) sniffed		
Methadone	Dolly	4–6	Swallowed Injected		
Morphine	White stuff, M	6	Swallowed or injected		
Opium	Op	4	Inhaled (smoked)		
Sedatives:					
Barbiturates (Amytal, Nembutal, Seconal, phenobarbital)	Barbs, blue devils, candy, yellow jackets, phennies, peanuts, blue heavens, dolls, red devils, goofballs, sleepers	4	Swallowed or injected	CNS depressants; sleep-inducing relaxation; drowsiness; impaired judgment, reaction time, emotional control and muscle coordination; euphoria	Addicting with severe withdrawal syndrome, irritability, weight loss, possible convulsions, toxic psychosis
Chloral hydrate					
Doriden					
Miltown, Equanil					

* According to Hells Angels and Timothy Leary, serenity, tranquillity, and peace. (From R. R. Lingeman, *Drugs from A to Z: A Dictionary*, McGraw-Hill Book Co., New York, 1969.)

(Continued)

Table 32-5 DRUGS MISUSED BY ADOLESCENTS *(Continued)*

Name of drug	Slang name	Duration of action, hours	Method of taking	Short-term effects	Long-term effects
Stimulants: Amphetamines (Benzedrine, Methedrine, Dexedrine)	Bennies, dexies, speed, wakeups, lid proppers, pep pills, hearts, cartwheels, crystal, meth, x-mas trees, sweets, blues, black bombers	4	Swallowed or injected (vein)	CNS stimulant, anorexia, euphoria, insomnia, alertness, decreased fatigue	May be habit-forming. Restlessness, irritability, weight loss, delusions), hallucinations, toxic psychosis
Cocaine	Coke, carrine, gold dust, Bernice, flake, stardust, snow	Short and variable	Sniffed, injected, or swallowed		
Tranquilizers: Librium Thorazine Compazine Stelazine Reserpine		4–6	Swallowed	CNS depressant (selected); decreased anxiety, tension, hallucinations or delusions; relaxation and generally improved function	May cause blood dyscrasia and death. Usually causes blurred vision, dry mouth, drowsiness, skin rash, and tremors
Miscellaneous: Glue, gasoline, and solvents Antihistamines Nutmeg Compoz Catnip Nitrous oxide		2	Inhaled or swallowed	Euphoria, impaired judgment and coordination	Some may cause hallucinations or liver or kidney damage

must be employed. This "talking down" therapy must continue for the total length of the drug's effect.

Thorazine may be given to control adverse reactions to LSD, but it must not be used when atropine-like fillers have been added to the acid because cardiac and respiratory failure may occur. Diazepam is the drug of choice when Thorazine cannot be used.

The treatment of adolescent drug abusers must be directed toward prevention and to long-term efforts to help meet psychosocial needs. Adolescents who currently abuse drugs require skilled professional help to reestablish a life-style that does not include the use of drugs. Many inpatient and outpatient clinics are being established to assist the adolescent to develop a more positive self-image and life-style.

REFERENCES

1 R. S. Duff and A. G. M. Campbell, "Moral and Ethical Dilemmas in the Special Care Nursery," *New England Journal of Medicine*, pp. 890–894, Oct. 25, 1973.
2 A. Shaw, "Dilemmas of 'Informed Consent' in Children," *New England Journal of Medicine*, pp. 885–890, Oct. 25, 1973.

BIBLIOGRAPHY

Blake, Florence G., et al.: *Nursing Care of Children*, J. B. Lippincott Company, Philadelphia, 1970.

Bray, P. F.: *Neurology in Pediatrics*, Year Book Medical Publishers, Inc., Chicago, 1969.

Carini, Esta, and Owens G.: *Neurological and Neurosurgical Nursing*, 5th ed., The C. V. Mosby Company, St. Louis, 1970.

Charalampous, K. D.: "Drug Culture In the Seventies," *American Journal of Public Health*, 61(6):1225–1228, 1971.

Chusid, J. G., and McDonald, J. J.: *Correlative Neuroanatomy and Functional Neurology*, Lange Medical Publications, Los Altos, Calif., 1967.

Clausen, J., et al.: *Maternity Nursing Today*, McGraw-Hill Book Company, New York, 1973.

Conners, K.: "The Syndrome of Minimal Brain Dysfunction: Psychological Aspects," *Pediatric Clinics of North America*, 14(4):749–766, 1967.

Crowther, D.: "Psychosocial Aspects of Epilepsy," *Pediatric Clinics of North America*, 14(4):921–932, 1967.

Culp, P.: "Nursing Care of the Patient with Spinal Cord Injury," *Nursing Clinics of North America*, 2(3):447–458, 1967.

Ellis, R. W. B.: *Disease in Infancy and Childhood*, E. & S. Livingstone, Ltd., Edinburgh, 1968.

Farmer, T. W. (ed.): *Pediatric Neurology*, Hoeber Medical Division, Harper & Row, Publishers, Incorporated, New York, 1969.

Ford, F. R.: *Diseases of the Nervous System in Infancy, Childhood, and Adolescence,* Charles C Thomas, Publisher, Springfield, Ill., 1952.

Foreman, N., and Zerwekh, J.: "Drug Crisis Intervention," *American Journal of Nursing*, 71(9):1736–1739, 1971.

Gatz, A. J.: *Manter's Essentials of Clinical Neuroanatomy and Neurophysiology*, F. A. Davis Company, Philadelphia, 1970.

Gustafson, S., and Coursin, D.: *The Pediatric Patient*, J. B. Lippincott Company, Philadelphia, 1968.

Guyton, A.: *Structure and Function of the Nervous System*, W. B. Saunders Company, Philadelphia, 1972.

Haywood, C., and Gordon, J.: "Neuropsychology and Learning Disorders," *Pediatric Clinics of North America*, 17(2):337–346, 1970.

Kaulitz, S., et al.: "Bacterial Infections of the Central Nervous System," *Pediatric Clinics of North America, 7(3):* 605–626, 1960.

Kennedy, C., and Wangler, P.: "Encephalitis: A Variable Syndrome in Response to Viral Infections," *Pediatric Clinics of North America*, 14(4):809–818, 1967.

Latham, Helen C.: *Pediatric Nursing*, The C. V. Mosby Company, St. Louis, 1972.

Marlow, D.: *Textbook of Pediatric Nursing*, 4th ed., W. B. Saunders Company, Philadelphia, 1973.

Meachum, W., and McPherson, W.: "The Diagnosis and Treatment of Subdural Fluid Collection In Infants," *Pediatric Clinics of North America*, 17(2):363–372, 1970.

Millichap, G.: "Diagnosis and Management of Convulsive Disorders: With Special Emphasis of Seizures Amenable to Specific Therapies," *Pediatric Clinics of North America*, 7(3):583–604, 1960.

———, and Fernando, A.: "Treatment and Prognosis of Petit Mal Epilepsy," *Pediatric Clinics of North America*, 14(4):905–920, 1967.

———, and Fowler, G.: "Treatment of 'Minimal Brain Dysfunction' Syndrome," *Pediatric Clinics of North America*, 14(4):767–777, 1967.

Moidel, H., et al.: *Nursing Care of the Patient With Medical Surgical Disorders*, McGraw Hill Book Company, New York, 1971.

Paine, R.: "Minimal Cerebral Damage," *Pediatric Clinics of North America*, 15(3):779–801, 1967.

Snell, R.: *Clinical Embryology For Medical Students*, Little, Brown and Company, Boston, 1972.

Robbins, S.: *Pathology*, 3d ed., W. B. Saunders Company, Philadelphia, 1967.

Robe, E.: "Subdural Effusions in Infants," *Pediatric Clinics of North America*, 14(4):831–850, 1967.

Werry, J.: "Development Hyperactivity," *Pediatric Clinics of North America*, 15(3):581–600, 1968.

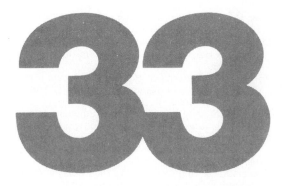

33

THE RESPIRATORY SYSTEM

MARILYN A. CHARD and GLADYS M. SCIPIEN*

EMBRYOLOGY OF THE RESPIRATORY SYSTEM

At about the fourth week of development of the embryo, a median, longitudinal groove evolves in the pharyngeal floor. The entodermal lining of this groove gives rise to the epithelial lining and the glands of the larynx, trachea, and bronchi, as well as to the epithelium of the alveoli.

The margins of this laryngotracheal groove fuse caudally, and as the process extends toward the head, a tube is formed, and the lumen of the laryngotracheal tube becomes separated from the foregut of the embryo. Simultaneously, as the now-separate foregut lengthens, its lumen becomes narrower and the esophagus begins to develop.

This primordial growth, the laryngotracheal tube, extends caudally into splanchnic mesoderm, ventral to and parallel with the esophagus. The distal outgrowth exhibits a pair of knoblike enlargements which are the primary bronchial buds, sometimes called *lung buds*. The elongation process continues in its progressive downward direction until they reach their eventual position in the thorax. Cartilage development begins in the upper portion of the tube which gives rise to the larynx, while the lower segment will develop as the trachea.

Each of the primary bronchial buds grows laterally, and it is interesting to note that, from its beginnings, the right primary bronchus is larger than the left, and it tends to be directed less sharply to the side. This difference in lateral angle development is significant when one stops to consider that more foreign bodies make their way into the right bronchus than the left. With the right primary bronchus dividing into three lobes, and left into two lobular sections, it is apparent that during the beginning of the second month structures comparable to those found in a fully developed lung are present.

The caudal growth of the primary bronchus continues bilaterally, and as it occurs, branching begins; for example, a branch forms on one side of the bronchus while the main portion continues to grow without any change in direction. This tissue division continues, branching and rebranching, until the bronchial tree of the adult lung is formed. The process extends to the sixth month of development, when approximately seventeen orders of branching have occurred. After birth some branching continues until the full complement of twenty-four orders of branches is established.

* The authors wish to acknowledge the assistance in the preparation of this chapter of James Robotham, M.D., Chief Resident, Pediatrics, Boston City Hospital; Instructor in Pediatrics, Boston University School of Medicine.

As the lungs continue to grow, the intraembryonic coelom is evaginated, and the splanchnic mesoderm is pushed out as a covering over the mesenchyme-packed bronchial trees. These regions of the coelom are expanded and walled off to form the pleural cavities. The splanchnic mesoderm becomes thinner, eventually forming the mesothelial layer of the pleura, while the immediate underlying mesenchyme forms the stroma of the pulmonary lobules, the cartilage, smooth muscle, and connective tissue which reinforces the epithelial lining of the bronchi.

Once the branching process of the bronchi has been completed for the most part, the established terminal buds are divided into from three to six passages called *alveolar ducts*, which by the sixth month develop additional outpouchings called *alveolar sacs*, or *alveoli*. Once formed, the alveoli undergo radical change—the columnar epithelium thins to squamous epithelium, and capillaries of the pulmonary system form a rich mesh network. The tissue which separates the blood of the pulmonary circuit becomes thin enough to permit the oxygen and carbon dioxide exchange.

The fetal lung, on microscopic examination, looks like a gland since its alveolar sacs are not distended. At birth, however, with the beginning of respiration, the lungs expand, and most of the alveoli become filled with air. The fluid frequently found in the bronchial tree before birth is a combination of amniotic fluid and the glandular secretions of the lining mucous membranes. It is rapidly removed at birth, probably through pulmonary capillaries as well as the lymphatic system.

PHYSIOLOGY OF THE RESPIRATORY SYSTEM

The main function of the respiratory system is to maintain adequate oxygen and carbon dioxide exchange between the body and the environment. Respiration consists of two phases, external and internal. *External respiration* occurs in the alveoli where inspired oxygen is exchanged for carbon dioxide which is expired. *Internal respiration* occurs as oxygen from the alveoli is carried by the arterial circulatory system to the capillaries, through the capillary wall into the tissue fluid surrounding the cells, and across the plasma membrane. Carbon dioxide passes in the opposite direction by the same route until it reaches the capillaries, where it enters the venous blood to be transported to the lungs for exhalation.

External Respiration

Several muscles are involved in respiration. Normally, only the inspiratory muscles (those that elevate the chest cage) are used. Expiration is the result of elastic recoil of the lungs when the inspiratory muscles relax. The diaphragm is the most important inspiratory muscle. Diaphragmatic movements account for 80 percent of inspired air volume, while rib movements are responsible for the other 20 percent. If inspiratory effort is great, the scalene and pectoralis minor muscles assist in raising the rib cage.

Two pleural membrane layers are found in the thoracic cavity, one covering the lungs and one lining the thoracic cavity. Since the pleural layers are in intimate contact, the pleural space is potential rather than actual. Both layers are moist, causing surface tension which, in turn, causes the lung wall to follow the thoracic wall. Surface tension is present in the alveoli and respiratory passages because of the fluids lining them. The alveoli secrete a lipoprotein called *surfactant* which tends to decrease this surface tension. If surfactant were absent, lung expansion would be difficult. As the lung decreased in size during expiration, surface tension would increase, causing a possible atelectasis.

Surface tension is not the only reason that the pleural space remains potential. Intrapleural pressure is below atmospheric pressure. Thus, the lungs maintain their elasticity. Intrapulmonic pressure (pressure within the lungs) is exactly atmospheric at the conclusion of expiration, no air is flowing, and there is free communication between the atmosphere and the alveoli via the airways. During inspiration, intrapulmonic pressure decreases as the lungs and chest expand, and air enters the lungs. If the chest wall were pierced, the lungs would collapse.

During expiration both intrapleural and intrapulmonic pressures increase. However, intrapleural pressure never reaches atmospheric pressure. Intrapulmonic pressure becomes greater than atmospheric pressure, and air moves out of the lungs. Normal expiration is due to relaxation of the muscles of inspiration. During a forced expiration the internal intercostal muscles and abdominal muscles are utilized.

Internal Respiration

Most of the oxygen transported to the tissues is in the form of oxyhemoglobin. The extent to which oxygen combines with hemoglobin depends upon the partial pressure of oxygen in the blood, the pH of the blood, and tissue temperature. Alveolar oxygen partial pressure is greater than blood oxygen partial pressure. Therefore, oxygen from the alveoli diffuses into the arterial blood. Most of this oxygen combines with hemoglobin, while the remaining 3 percent is carried in physical solution. A blood oxygen partial pressure (Po_2) of 100 mm Hg ensures 90 percent saturation. With partial pressures from 10 to 60 mm Hg, the degree to which oxygen combines with hemoglobin rapidly increases. Since pulmonary disease moderately reduces the Po_2 in the alveoli and the arteries, this plateau from 60 to 100 is important in oxygen supply to the tissues (see Fig. 33-1).

The Po_2 of the blood depends upon the amount of oxygen molecules which are free in solution (only gas molecules which are free in solution can create gas pressure). The oxyhemoglobin does not contribute to this pressure. As blood enters the capillaries, tissue Po_2 is less than blood Po_2. Therefore, the free plasma oxygen diffuses into the tissues. Since plasma Po_2 is now lower than that of the erythrocytes, oxygen is released from oxyhemoglobin and diffuses into the plasma.

The pH of the blood is determined by hydrogen ion concentration. An increase in hydrogen ion causes a decrease in pH. The more acid the blood is (decrease in pH), the less affinity hemoglobin has for oxygen. Tissue temperature affects the formation of oxyhemoglobin in a manner similar to that of pH. Tissue temperature is elevated when tissue is engaged in active metabolism. The release of oxygen from hemoglobin is facilitated as blood flows through these tissue capillaries during active metabolism and by an increase in the chemical 2,3-DPG (2,3-diphosphoglycerate) in the red blood cell.

Once arterial blood has supplied oxygen to the tissues via diffusion through the capillary walls, carbon dioxide diffuses out of the tissue into the venous blood where 8 percent remains in physical solution and 25 percent combines with hemoglobin. The remaining 67 percent is converted into bicarbonate and hydrogen ions primarily in the red blood cells. The hydrogen ions in excess of the amount needed to maintain normal pH of the blood are eliminated by the kidneys (assuming normal renal function). As venous blood flows through the lung capillaries, hydrogen and bicarbonate combine to give carbonic acid which breaks down to carbon dioxide and water. Now that blood Pco_2 is greater than alveolar Pco_2, carbon dioxide diffuses through the capillary walls into the alveoli from which it is expired into the atmosphere. Carbon dioxide moves much more easily across the alveoli than oxygen does. Hence, with disease, the Po_2 changes first.

Ventilation

Ventilation is regulated in several ways. Within the medulla oblongata and pons in the brainstem is a group of neurons known as the *respiratory center*. There seems to be general agreement that there are inspiratory and expiratory neurons which fire alternately back and forth indefinitely, causing the act of respiration.

Increased carbon dioxide in inspired air and an increase of the hydrogen ions in the blood which diffuses into the cerebrospinal fluid increase ventilation. Chemoreceptors, located in the carotid and aortic bodies which transmit signals to the respiratory center, are stimulated by hypoxia, and ventilation increases. When hypoxia and hypercapnia (increased CO_2) are prolonged and severe, the respiratory center is depressed.

The Hering-Breuer reflex limits lung inflation and deflation, thereby preventing overdistention and overcompression. The Hering-Breuer receptors in the bronchioles and, possibly, in the walls of the alveoli stimulate the respiratory center, by way of the vagus nerve, to inhibit inspiration as the lungs fill and allow expiration to occur. As the lungs deflate, the receptors work to stimulate inhibition of expiration. If these reflexes are not intact, respiratory arrest can occur much more quickly than if they are intact.

If the respiratory rate is *increased* for a prolonged period, too much carbon dioxide is expired, and a condition known as *respiratory alkalosis* may occur due to *decreased* hydrogen ions in the blood. This decrease stimulates the respiratory center to decrease alveolar ventilation in order to raise the hydrogen-ion concentration (pH) to normal. If the respiratory rate is *decreased* for a prolonged period, too much carbon dioxide is retained, and *respiratory acidosis* may occur owing to increased hydrogen ions. This increase stimulates the respiratory center to increase alveolar ventilation in order to lower the hydrogen-ion concentration to normal.

PULMONARY FUNCTION TESTS

Pulmonary functional abnormalities may explain the mechanisms of some symptoms, but the results of pulmonary function tests do not provide a specific diagnosis. Their value lies in assessment of the severity of a specific disease, evaluation of treatment, and determination of prognosis. Most tests are accomplished through spirometry, although plethysmography may be utilized to obtain functional residual capacity and total lung capacity results, while a flowmeter is sometimes used to determine the peak expiratory flow rate.

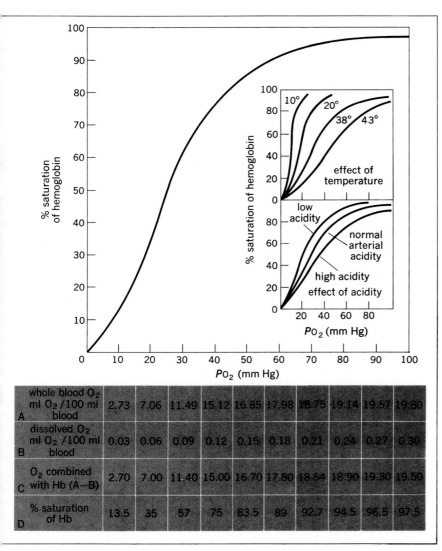

	whole blood O₂ ml O₂/100 ml blood	2.73	7.06	11.49	15.12	16.85	17.98	18.75	19.14	19.57	19.80
A											
B	dissolved O₂ ml O₂/100 ml blood	0.03	0.06	0.09	0.12	0.15	0.18	0.21	0.24	0.27	0.30
C	O₂ combined with Hb (A—B)	2.70	7.00	11.40	15.00	16.70	17.80	18.54	18.90	19.30	19.50
D	% saturation of Hb	13.5	35	57	75	83.5	89	92.7	94.5	96.5	97.5

Figure 33-1 Hemoglobin-oxygen dissociation curve. The large curve applies to blood at 38°C and the normal arterial hydrogen-ion concentration (acidity). The inset curves illustrate the effects of altering temperature and acidity on the relation between P_{O_2} and hemoglobin saturation with oxygen. *(From A. J. Vander, J. H. Sherman, and D. S. Luciano, Human Physiology, McGraw-Hill Book Company, New York, 1970, p. 318. Modified from J. H. Comroe, Jr., Physiology of Respiration, by Year Book Medical Publishers, Inc., Chicago, 1965. Used by permission.)*

Commonly Used Tests

Tests most commonly used to determine pulmonary functional abnormalities provide information about airway resistance regarding trapped air, airway obstruction, and ventilation in relation to blood flow. The results of functional residual capacity, total lung capacity, vital capacity, tidal volume, residual volume, and forced expiratory volume in 1 second yield information in regard to air trapping.

The test for *functional residual capacity* (FRC) is accomplished through spirometry or plethysmography and measures the total amount of gas in the lungs at the end of respiration while the child is at rest. The *tidal volume* (TV), or amount inhaled or exhaled with each respiration, may be determined at the same time. FRC is recorded in milliliters or liters, while TV is recorded in milliliters. Since TV determines ventilation, it does not represent true lung volume. The *total lung capacity* (TLC) is a measurement of the total amount of gas in the lungs at the end of a full inspiration while the child is at rest. Whether a spirometer or plethysmograph is used, results are recorded in milliliters or liters. The *vital capacity* (VC) represents the greatest amount of gas the child can exhale after a full inspiration and is the sum of inspiratory capacity (IC) and expiratory reserve volume (ERV). Results via spirometry are noted in milliliters or liters. The amount of air in the lungs after a full expiration is termed *residual volume* (RV); spirometry is the method utilized to measure it and yields data in milliliters or liters. RV is normally 25 percent of TLC. *Forced expiratory volume in 1 second* (FEV 1) represents the amount of air exhaled in 1 second with a forced expiration and is expressed in milliliters on a spirometer. FEV 1/FVC is the ratio of forced expiratory volume in 1 second to forced vital capacity and is expressed as a percentage. Thus, if FEV 1 is 1,100 ml and FVC is 1,250 ml, then FEV 1/FVC is 8.8 percent. When air is trapped in the lungs, FRC and RV are increased, VC and FEV 1/FVC are decreased, and TLC is either normal or decreased.

The *peak expiratory flow rate* (PEFR) is determined by spirometer or flowmeter as the result of the forced expiratory flow of gas. This test provides an approximate indication of airway obstruction and is recorded in liters per minute. A decrease in PEFR is indicative of obstruction.

Alveolar ventilation (AV) denotes the amount of air circulating in the alveoli and is expressed in liters per minute. The symbol for blood flow is Q and is recorded in milliliters per minute. VA/Q is the ratio between alveolar ventilation and blood flow and is determined by spirometry. The average is 0.8; an increased ratio is indicative of decreased ventilation.

The figures in Table 33-1 are not standardized. Pulmonary function tests can vary between individuals, groups, and sexes. Variations also exist between the results of different investigators. This table has been devised as a guide to readers of this text.

There is little information relative to the course of pulmonary function in the first 4 years of life. Because of the rapid growth rates of infants, testing presents technical difficulties. Only FRC can be measured accurately, and plethysmography is the more practical method, since the infant is enclosed in a chamber similar to an incubator and is disturbed as little as possible during the testing. Use of the face mask may stimulate the rooting reflex. Thus, several trial runs may be necessary to condition the infant to this sensation.

Preparing the Child

Children need to become familiar with the methods used for mouth breathing with the nostrils closed during spirometry. Closure of nostrils is accomplished through the use of a nose clip or by an adult's closing the child's nostrils between two fingers. When tested with a spirometer or a flowmeter, children are usually more cooperative if they are allowed to familiarize themselves with the mouthpiece. A child who is to be tested by plethysmography must be willing to enter the chamber. His imagination may be brought into play by calling this chamber a "space ship," "boxcar," "atomic submarine," and so forth.

Nursing Management

The nurse is in a position to work with the tester and the parents in preparing the child to cooperate when undergoing pulmonary function tests. The nurse may be the one who "conditions" the infant to the use of the face mask, or he may enlist the aid of the parents in performing this task. Whether or not parents display an inclination to become involved in the care of their infant, the nurse should invite their participation. Then the nurse is provided with an opportunity to share information with, and listen to,

Table 33-1 PULMONARY FUNCTION TEST AVERAGES ACCORDING TO HEIGHT AND SEX

Test	Sex	Height, cm/in.						
		110/43	120/47	130/51	140/55	150/59	160/63	170/67
TLC (ml)	M	1,600	2,000	2,500	3,050	3,650	4,300	5,100
	F	1,550	1,950	2,400	2,950	3,500	4,100	5,000
VC (ml)	M	1,250	1,600	1,950	2,400	2,900	3,400	4,050
	F	1,200	1,500	1,750	2,200	2,750	3,300	3,900
FEV1 (ml)	M & F	1,100	1,400	1,700	2,100	2,600	3,100	3,700
FRC (ml)	M	700	850	1,100	1,350	1,650	2,000	2,380
	F	700	900	1,100	1,350	1,650	1,950	2,300
RV (ml)	M & F	380	450	550	650	750	900	1,050
PEFR (liter/min)	M & F	152	200	254	300	350	400	460

Source: Compiled from G. Polgar and V. Promadhat, *Pulmonary Function Testing in Children*, W. B. Saunders Company, Philadelphia, 1971, pp. 209–211.

parents. Another possible outcome is that parents will be invited to accompany the infant when he is tested.

Cooperation between tester, nurse, and parents may also be utilized for children. Demonstrations of mouth breathing with nostrils closed and the use of the mouthpiece by any of these adults may be well accepted by a child who then returns the demonstration. Parents can provide valuable information about the child's interests in preparing him for plethysmography.

METHODS OF IMPROVING OXYGENATION
Oxygen Therapy

When the nurse is administering oxygen to a child, certain facts need to be remembered, for this commonly used gas may have its harmful effects on some structures in the body, particularly in the case of a newborn. The amount of oxygen given should be determined by monitoring the Po_2 level, and it should be commensurate with the cellular needs of the body at that time.

It is important to prevent oxygen toxicity. Increasing amounts of oxygen may create an inability on the part of a newborn to assimilate the gas, consequently increasing his oxygenation needs. High concentrations of oxygen (70 to 80 percent) for a short time, or extended use of oxygen over a long period, may result in a loss of pliancy and a thickening of the alveolar and vascular structures, thereby interfering in the gaseous exchange. These conditions may result in atelectasis and an increased cellularity of the lungs. Cilia may become paralyzed, making the removal of secretions far more difficult for the young patient. Blood gas determinations identify toxic levels which cannot be detected by observation or with the use of an oxygen analyzer.

Although the physiologic effects of hypoxia may occur at an arterial Po_2 level of 50 mm Hg, cyanosis does not become evident, usually, until the arterial Po_2 level falls below 32 to 40 mm Hg. Many medical centers monitor the Pco_2 levels simultaneously. Conversely, it is important to know that Po_2 levels above 100 mm Hg in the neonate may cause retrolental fibroplasia, a type of blindness which can be prevented. As a result, the American Academy of Pediatrics has recommended that arterial Po_2 determinations be available in any hospital which administers continuous oxygen to very young patients over a period of time.

Certain safety principles are vigorously adhered to when oxygen therapy is in effect, for oxygen supports combustion. Electrical equipment must not be used while oxygen is being administered. The clothing or linen used should not be made of wool or synthetic fibers which may produce static electricity. Alcohol or oil should not be used on an infant or child receiving oxygen within a confined environment.

As the patient's condition improves, termination of therapy should be gradual in order to allow him to adjust to the normal atmospheric oxygen concentrations. In an incubator the rate of oxygen flow can be decreased, or the air vents may be opened. In a mist tent zippers may be opened, or a section of the plastic canopy may be flipped over the top of the tent. In either instance, it is important to observe the patient and to note his responses to the decreased oxygen concentrations. Any distress, increase in respiratory rate, retractions, or cyanosis should be reported to a physician immediately, and methods of increasing oxygen intake should be considered.

Administration by Incubator or Hood Closed incubators can deliver 40 to 100 percent levels of oxygen to newborns or infants. It is imperative that oxygen analyzers be used every 2 hours to identify appropriate concentrations, in addition to monitoring blood gases. Oxygen levels greater than 40 percent should not be administered, unless there is cyanosis, or unless it has been specifically ordered by a physician. It is important to remember that the menace lies in the bloodstream concentration, not in the atmospheric oxygen.

Oxygen should always be moisturized before it is delivered to an incubator, and this process is facilitated by the passage of the gas through a type of water vessel or nebulizer. (See Fig. 33-2.) Likewise, sterile water should always be used, unless medications or other agents which liquefy secretions are to be utilized.

Since inhalation equipment is a source of contamination, daily cleaning is imperative. All equipment should be changed every 7 days. Cultures of oxygen tubing, water, and nebulizers as well as the interior of incubators should be taken at least every 3 days.

Closed incubators have a significant loss of heat and oxygen because of imperfectly fitted plastic lids, uncovered vents, and the frequent opening of portholes, thereby contributing to a depletion of the desired heat and oxygen concentrations. If the patient's condition necessitates oxygen levels above 40 percent, plastic circular hoods should be used to maintain that concentration. Maintenance of heat will then be the problem with which nursing must contend, for while 34°C (93.2°F) may be necessary

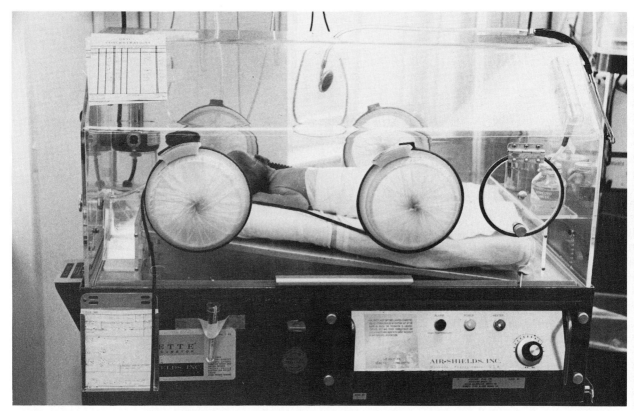

Figure 33-2 A neonate in a closed incubator receiving oxygen and humidity. *(Courtesy of Children's Hospital Medical Center, Boston. Photograph by Boston University School of Nursing, Media Services Department.)*

for small infants, others may need only a supplemental temperature of 30°C (86°F). Fluctuations in a young patient's environment result in a lowering of body temperature and the immediate, rapid metabolism of still larger amounts of oxygen. Simultaneous recordings of the infant's body temperature and the temperature of his environment are essential notations for a nurse to make when working with premature or newborn babies. Members of the health team should coordinate their individual activities in an effort to prevent fluctuations of heat and oxygen which may contribute further to the debilitating status of the young patient. Open incubators deliver radiant heat while procedures are being done or nursing care is being given, and with the utilization of a circular hood the desired humidified oxygen concentration can be maintained without exposing the patient to stressful variations.

Whenever oxygen is being administered, it should be warmed to 31 to 34°C, depending on the baby, and it should always be humidified. Thermal sensors are present in a baby's face, and a blast of cold oxygen produces a typical neonatal response

to cold stress, including oxygen deprivation, metabolic acidosis, rapid depletion of glycogen stores, and a reduction of blood glucose levels.

Administration by Mist Tent Mist tents are usually utilized to increase oxygen levels in young children. Obviously, the size of the patient determines the most appropriate equipment. The mist tent which is frequently used with older infants, toddlers, and preschoolers functions on the basic principle of thermal circulation. The oxygen is cooled over ice and becomes heavier than air, thereby settling in the lower part of the tent, surrounding the patient with a higher concentration of oxygen. Conversely, the warmer carbon dioxide which is being exhaled rises and escapes through the designated exit porthole.

The mist tent is portable and easy to assemble, and facilitates observation of a young patient. Another distinct advantage is that all working parts of a tent are outside the canopy, away from a curious young child's reach. One disadvantage for nursing personnel is that the tent needs to be opened frequently for treatments, procedures, or the monitoring of vital signs, and entry results in the lowering of both oxygen and humidity concentrations. Thought should be given to the organization of nursing functions and the coordination of procedures which will be done by other health team members, too. Consideration should be given to maintaining the desired humidity and oxygen concentrations, as well as providing the patient with substantial periods of rest.

Occasionally a face mask is used simultaneously to supplement oxygen intake. The young child may resist it, initially, and a nurse should offer support to the patient by staying with him until he becomes accustomed to it. Since it is placed over his nose and mouth, caution should be exercised whenever its use is contemplated. In objecting to its utilization, a toddler could cause it to slip above the nose and possibly cause injury to the eyes. Frequent adjustments are imperative. It is essential for the nurse to evaluate the youngster's response to this additional therapeutic measure.

When oxygen therapy is instituted, a nurse should check the tent for tears or malfunctioning zippers which would make it difficult to achieve the desired humid, oxygenated environment. He should also smell the mist being released to be positive that the tubing is not carrying a noxious chemical or the remains of a solution which was not adequately rinsed out after use by a previous patient. The mist tent should be flooded with condensation before the patient is placed inside and covered with a cotton blanket. While a cooled, supersaturated aerated mist provides the desired relief, the anticipated condensation necessitates frequent changes of clothing and linen to prevent chilling of the patient.

As the child improves, he takes a more active interest in his surroundings and demonstrates a desire to play with toys. While he is in the supersaturated environment, it is important to carefully select the kind of toys he will play with, and the material they are made of. For example, stuffed animals and other cloth toys tend to absorb the moisture (becoming excellent media for the growth of microorganisms), and therefore they should not be used within this humidified canopy. A very favorite Teddy bear may not be able to tolerate the mist tent as well as his young friend can. Those toys which retard absorption, are washable, or easily cleaned appear to be the most suitable.

Whenever oxygen therapy is begun, a nurse must know how to use the equipment involved in its delivery to a patient. He must be knowledgeable in its mechanical aspects, in the different models available, in the use of various regulatory devices;

he must be informed regarding the means by which humidity and oxygen determinations are ascertained; he must know how to clean and where to store the innumerable parts. It is he who must maintain the desired concentrations, evaluate the functionability of the equipment, and determine the effectiveness of the treatment in relation to the young patient's respiratory status.

Postural Drainage

Postural drainage is an important, yet simple, procedure to perform on the child who is having difficulty in removing mucus from the tracheobronchial tree. It is frequently utilized when caring for patients who are demonstrating obstructions in aeration due to the secretions present. Changing a patient's position and clapping and vibrating the chest wall dislodge the plugs and facilitate drainage of the bronchi.

Positioning the patient properly is essential because gravity enhances drainage, and, by placing the patient in a series of positions, each segment of the bronchial tree may be emptied. In order to determine the best position for the child, a nurse must be cognizant of the specific lobe involved. Basically, the area to be drained should be uppermost, with the bronchus then in a vertical position. Remember that the lobe to be drained must be higher than the passages through which the secretions move.

The cupping, clapping, or tapping technique percusses the chest wall lying over the affected lobe or segment, loosening the secretions by vibrating the lungs. Trapping air between the cupped hand and the patient produces a hollow sound. In the course of treatment, should a reddened area be observed over the percussion site, treatment must be discontinued immediately. Either an inadequate amount of air is being trapped within the cupped hand or the patient is being slapped instead of being tapped. In either case the treatment is ineffective and useless to the patient (see Fig. 33-3).

In patients with chronic conditions such as cystic fibrosis, postural drainage should be done early each morning to remove secretions accumulated during the night. Likewise, it should be performed just before bedtime to ensure a more restful sleep. Patients who may be receiving intermittent aerosol treatment to open bronchial passages and promote removal of secretions should utilize this additional therapeutic measure before postural drainage is done.

Infants and very young children may be held in one's lap during the procedure, with the patient on

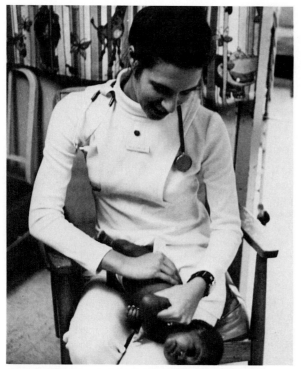

Figure 33-3 A registered nurse assisting an infant with postural drainage. *(Courtesy of Boston City Hospital. Photograph by Boston University School of Nursing, Media Services Department.)*

his stomach and his head down to drain the posterior lower lobes. When the patient is placed on his back with his head down, the anterior portions of both lower lobes can be drained. When initially placed in this position, a baby usually cries, but as the procedure continues, coughing is stimulated. As the mucus is mobilized and moves from the periphery of the lungs toward the larger bronchi, infants and young children may be unable to expel it by coughing. In that case sterile aspirating equipment may be necessary to facilitate removal. Coughing up mucus cannot be accomplished until the child is about 4 years of age.

Older children assume the same basic positions as an adult. Remember that the area to be drained is elevated with the bronchus vertical to assist in removal. These youngsters are usually encouraged to cough and breathe deeply after each positional change.

How long should the treatment be done? The answer lies in the tolerance level of each young patient. Initially it may be done for 5 to 10 minutes, every 4 hours for the first day; however, it is important to understand this arbitrary schedule is totally dependent on the patient's physical status. The time interval should be increased to 20 minutes every 4 hours. In assessing and evaluating a patient's progress, a nurse may elect to do it oftener for shorter periods of time. For localized involvement, treatment may be longer and more intensive for the segment affected.

It is important to remember that chest physical therapy should not be done before or after feedings or meals. If done before mealtime, the child may lose his appetite, and, if done after he has just eaten, he may become nauseated and vomit.

At many medical centers, a physical therapist is consulted regarding the positions to be used in the therapy. He frequently demonstrates all steps to the nursing staff before they assume this responsibility. Generally, the therapist also teaches parents the method they should utilize after the child is discharged. Frequently all positions are taught, regardless of the extent of the involvement. This method is especially true in the case of a child with cystic fibrosis where postural drainage is an integral part of long-range care. These parents must do these procedures often, and they should be comfortable and knowledgeable in all aspects of the procedure.

RESPIRATORY DISEASES AND DEVIATIONS IN THE NEWBORN
Respiratory Distress Syndrome

The most common cause of death in premature infants is respiratory distress syndrome (RDS, hyalin membrane disease). Predisposing factors other than prematurity include a diabetic mother and birth by cesarean section. In full-term infants whose mothers are routinely delivered by cesarean section due to cephalopelvic disproportion, there is no increased incidence. The basic defect in RDS is inadequate pulmonary exchange of oxygen and carbon dioxide due to lack of sufficient surfactant to maintain alveolar stability. The characteristic hyalin membrane found in the alveoli and bronchioles on autopsy is rarely seen in infants who die earlier than 6 to 8 hours after birth. The membrane may be due to intrauterine hypoxia and increased capillary permeability which would cause effusion from the pulmonary capillaries into the alveoli and terminal bronchioles. The resultant formation of a hyalin-like material mainly composed of fibrin reduces alveolar ventilation, and atelectatic areas, therefore, are present. Surfactant is deficient in RDS. Surface tension in the affected alveoli is increased; the alveolar walls will not separate; lack of expansion of affected alveoli reduces alveolar ventilation.

According to Gluck, *surfactant* is composed of phospholipids, for example, lecithin (Le), sphingomyelin (Sph), and their precursors. Lecithin, the principal surfactant component, is decreased in RDS infants. In fetal lung development the amount of sphingomyelin in the alveoli is greater than lecithin until the thirtieth week of gestation. At this time, lecithin increases slowly until the thirty-fifth week, when a sharp rise in lecithin and a decline in sphingomyelin ensue. An Le/Sph ratio of 2.0 signifies the advent of pulmonary maturation to the point where extrauterine life can proceed normally. Lecithin and sphingomyelin are present in amniotic fluid. Through amniocentesis, the Le/Sph ratio may be determined and lung development accurately assessed before birth.

Surface-active lecithin is synthesized in utero by two major pathways: the methylation pathway, primarily from the eighteenth through the thirty-fifth week of gestation, and the choline pathway, primarily from the thirty-sixth week on (although both pathways continue to operate). When the Le/Sph ratio has reached 2.0, the choline incorporation pathway of synthesis, the more stable of the two, is in operation.

PDME, a lecithin precursor, is deficient or absent in the premature whose methylation pathway is incapable of establishing marginal alveolar stability and whose temperature indicates hypothermia. Once the hypothermic premature infant with RDS is warmed, PDME appears in tracheal aspirates. As RDS infants improve clinically, PDME also reappears, and surface-active lecithin increases. Full-term infants who become hypothermic do not develop RDS because the more stable choline pathway is in operation.[1]

Usually the infant breathes normally for 1 or 2 hours after birth, but in severe cases he may be symptomatic from the first minutes of life. Respirations become rapid and shallow, increasing to 60 or more per minute. Prominent symptoms are intercostal retractions and expiratory grunt. Other symptoms include nasal flaring, chest lag, xyphoid retractions, chin tug, frothing at the lips, and cyanosis (see Fig. 33-4).

On auscultation, air exchange may seem normal or diminished. On deep inspiration fine rales can be heard over the posterior lung bases. Excessive respiratory effort produces increasing evidence of air hunger and fatigue. Death occurs within a few hours. In mild cases, a peak is reached in 3 days. Improvement is gradual and the prognosis is good.

Prevention would aim toward elimination of prematurity and unnecessary cesarean sections plus careful management of diabetic mothers. Since the basic defect in RDS is inadequate pulmonary exchange of oxygen and carbon dioxide with resultant metabolic acidosis, the infant tries to compensate by increasing the rate and depth of respirations and by *grunting*, thereby increasing alveolar ventilation. Grunting, with closure of the glottis, is nature's positive-end expiratory pressure, thus increasing oxygen transfer and making ventilation perfusion increase evenly. Inserting an endotracheal tube would prevent grunting, allow alveoli to collapse, and, thus, decrease alveolar ventilation. Therefore, the use of an endotracheal tube should be avoided. Chilling causes pulmonary vasoconstriction and increases the metabolic need for oxygen and production of carbon dioxide. The premature infant has little sub-

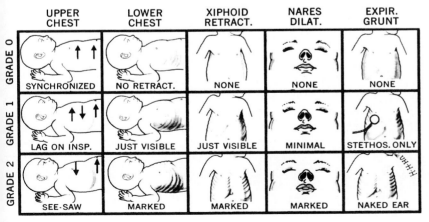

Figure 33-4 Observation of respiratory difficulty. *(Courtesy of Mead Johnson and Co., Evansville, Ind.)*

cutaneous fat for insulation. If the abdominal skin temperature can be kept at 36 to 37°C (96.8 to 98.6°F), as indicated by thermoregulating equipment, and humidity at 30 to 60 percent, chilling is avoided, and metabolic oxygen need is minimal. In the absence of this special equipment, an incubator temperature of 32 to 34°C (89.6 to 93.2°F) and 80 to 90 percent humidity will maintain the infant's thermal stability.

Hypoxia and acidemia can not only result from but also cause pulmonary vasoconstriction. Therefore, oxygen and buffers are given in the treatment of respiratory distress syndrome (RDS). The best method for maintaining a constant oxygen environment for the infant is the use of a plastic circular hood which is just large enough to house the infant's head (see Fig. 33-5). This hood permits a constant flow even when direct care is being given by nursing and/or medical personnel. Oxygen and carbon dioxide values and blood pH are monitored periodically to determine the degree of hypoxia, hypercapnia, and acidosis. If acidosis is untreated, hyperkalemia results. The effects on the heart of excessive potassium in the blood are manifest by electrocardiogram. Rarely must hyperkalemia be treated in the newborn. Blood pH is regulated with 10 percent glucose and water and sodium bicarbonate and by controlling the respiratory function of an infant who is on a respirator or positive-end expiratory pressure. An intravenous infusion for the infant with RDS would contain varying concentra-

tions of glucose and sodium bicarbonate relative to blood pH and carbon dioxide content. Recent data suggest that sodium bicarbonate may not be indicated and that perhaps only plasma is needed.[2] In treatment, the administration of glucose has the highest priority while calcium is next in importance.

There are two schools of thought on the administration of prophylactic antibacterial agents. Some physicians give them routinely because pneumonia is a frequent complication of RDS. The risk of infection also accompanies the use of assisted ventilation and indwelling vascular catheters (for monitoring blood values). Other physicians believe that prophylactic antibacterial agents are unnecessary and will only select out organisms which are resistant to them for infection.

Nursing Management   Although the respiratory system functions well by 27 weeks of fetal life, the premature infant's rib cage is unstable, his chest muscles are weak, and the alveoli and capillary blood supplies are incompletely developed. These factors, in themselves, predispose to respiratory failure. If a premature infant seems to be breathing normally for the first 1 or 2 hours following birth and then suddenly develops rapid, shallow respirations, the nurse should consider the possibility of RDS and notify the physician immediately. The advent of intercostal retractions and expiratory grunt indicate that the infant is attempting to compensate for inade-

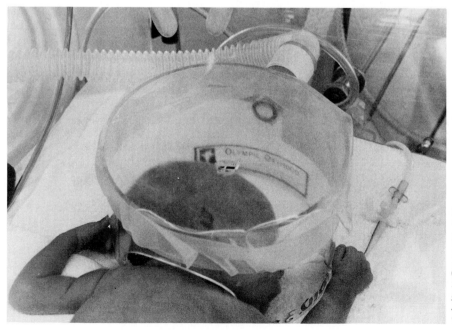

Figure 33-5   A premature infant whose head is enclosed with a plastic circular hood that maintains a constant humidified and oxygenated environment. *(Courtesy of Children's Hospital Medical Center, Boston. Photograph by Boston University School of Nursing, Media Services Department.)*

quate exchange of oxygen and carbon dioxide. Immediate responsibilities will involve initiating life-saving measures by gathering the necessary equipment, working with the physician in carrying out these measures, and monitoring machines, such as the thermoregulating equipment, oxygen apparatus, and an intravenous pump. The nurse is responsible for maintaining the necessary skin temperature, humidity, oxygen flow, intake and output, and intravenous rate. If antibacterial agents are ordered intramuscularly, he must calculate the dosage and administer it in the vastus lateralis muscle. He may also work with laboratory personnel who are monitoring the infant's blood values.

As the hours advance, the nurse observes the infant for signs of increasing air hunger. He notes and carefully records the skin color, rate and depth of respirations, severity and type of retractions, and the presence of flaring of the nostrils, chin tug, chest lag, expiratory grunt, restlessness, and frothing at the lips. The physician is kept informed of the infant's progress. If the infant survives the first 18 hours of life, his symptoms probably will reach a peak in 3 days. Improvement follows, and the prognosis is good. The nurse's evaluation of the infant's response to interventions is important to the physician's evaluation of the infant's progress, and it should be shared with him.

Parents are now allowed to enter some intensive care and/or premature nurseries after carefully washing their hands and donning cap, gown, and possibly mask. Whether they observe only or observe and participate in the infant's care depends on the infant's condition and the parents' feelings about involvement in his care. With so many machines in evidence, the parents may have difficulty (along with the nurse and doctor) in realizing that an infant is present. As time progresses, the nurse and physician prepare the parents to care for the infant at home.

More often than not, though, the nurse will be helping parents work through their grief. Should the infant die, parents may wish to see him, and their desire should be granted. This experience may be the only way the infant's death can become a reality for them. At this time, their questions should be answered openly, and the way paved for more parent counseling and teaching.

Asphyxia Neonatorum

A newborn is expected to begin breathing within 30 seconds of delivery; however, if apnea is present, or if there is total respiratory failure, asphyxia neonatorum may be the diagnosis. The failure of a neonate to breathe spontaneously is usually attributed to any of or all the three most common causes: cerebral injury, anoxia, or narcosis. A cerebral injury, such as a brain hemorrhage, may damage the respiratory center, but the use of forceps in a difficult vaginal delivery may also harm the infant.

Since the fetus is dependent upon the placenta for its oxygenation needs, any interference with that system may have devastating results, and so an abruptio placenta and, in some instances, a placenta previa cause concern and anxiety. A prolonged labor with an excessive compression of the cord, while the baby is confined to the birth canal, in addition to the beginning separation of the placenta after the uterus becomes partially emptied is directly responsible. A prolapsed cord which interrupts the fetus's blood supply may also contribute to the anoxia. An asphyxiating episode in utero may cause the fetus to gasp, and in so doing amniotic fluid including meconium particles or vernix caseosa may initiate the aspiration syndrome.

In the United States the commonest cause of respiratory depression in the neonate is maternal analgesia or anesthesia, since both sets of agents are capable of depressing the respiratory center.[3] An infant already experiencing compromised placental circulation is placed in even greater jeopardy by his inability to discard the inhalatory anesthetic, or conjugate drugs, properly within the liver.

Rapid physicochemical alterations occur as a result of the hypoxic state of the neonate. Acidosis develops quickly, with a lowered blood pH, elevated P_{CO_2} and diminution of buffer base content. The mild to moderately asphyxiated neonate manifests signs of *asphyxia livida*, with cyanosis, a delay in the first cry, a delay in establishing spontaneous respirations, tachycardia (more than 160 beats per minute) or bradycardia (less than 120 beats per minute), and hypotonus or hypertonus, as well as a mildly exaggerated or diminished response to stimuli.

The severely asphyxiated newborn demonstrates symptoms of *asphyxia pallida*, with shock present, in addition to pallor, a prolonged delay in crying and breathing, flaccidity, bradycardia (less than 100 beats per minute), and no response to sensory stimuli.

In describing the status of infants, the scoring method suggested by Apgar is reproducible with prognostic significance. Utilizing that particular scoring device, a slightly depressed baby could have an Apgar of 7 or 8, a moderately to severely depressed neonate's Apgar score could be 4 to 6, while a severely depressed (flaccid-pallid) baby would be in the 0 to 3 range.

Some resuscitative maneuvers which could be anticipated by a nurse when the diagnosis of asphyxia is made follow.[4]

Clinical Manifestations	Resuscitation Measures
Fetal heart present just before delivery, but absent at birth.	Immediate intubation and external cardiac massage.
Profound depression, heart rate less than 100 beats per minute and falling, no respiratory effort, or strenuous efforts without air entry into the lungs.	Attempt bagging initially, if response is unsatisfactory, intubation is done, followed by aspiration and mouth-to-tube respiration.
Moderate depression	Mask oxygen with intermittent positive pressure to 35 cm H_2O.
Mild depression, heart rate greater than 100 beats per minute, occasional gasps.	Mask oxygen only.

When laboratory studies have been done and the results indicate acidosis, $NaHCO_3$ and glucose are usually started, being administered through a scalp vein infusion. If the depression is severe, medications may be given directly into the umbilical vein by blunt-edged needle or catheter either in the delivery room or on arrival in the newborn nursery.

Nursing Management The asphyxiated neonate transferred to a special care nursery or a pediatric intensive care unit needs constant, diligent observation, and nurses are called upon to deliver skillful care, utilizing their knowledge of the neonate, their familiarity with the complex equipment sometimes essential for sustaining his life, and, in addition, their understanding of the plight of the helpless father and the very concerned but absent mother.

Of primary importance is the infant and its survival. It is important to remember that a neonate has a large surface area for heat loss and hypothermia is common; therefore, thoroughly drying the infant and applying an external source of heat are immediate essential nursing interventions. It is imperative that the neonate's body heat be conserved, for cooling of the infant contributes to the fall in his pH. Infrared lights facilitate its maintenance, but if none is available, the nurse needs to be cognizant of repeated entries into a closed incubator, which tend to decrease the temperature within that controlled environment. It is also important to remember that these infants are frequently without clothing for better observation, for placement of monitoring leads, and for other purposes, and because of this the authors support the use of open incubators which maintain the desired body temperature, permit accessibility to the critically ill infant without disturbing the heat and oxygen concentrations essential in his new environment, and also allow much closer observation.

Oxygen and suction equipment should be in constant readiness, for a patent airway is of prime importance. Should a nurse assess a patient and select suctioning as the appropriate intervention, then the obstructive substance can be removed from the mouth, nasopharynx, or trachea, reestablishing respirations swiftly. All these anatomic structures are small, and the slightest amount of secretions may obstruct them. Caution must be exercised, for excessive suctioning without intermittent oxygen or positive pressure may result in further deterioration. In selecting a suction tip, the size of the infant must be considered; therefore, a no. 8 or no. 10, soft, French tip should be selected. Remember to be gentle when suctioning a neonate to prevent injury to his mucous membranes. After the procedure has been completed, the suction tip is discarded. Aseptic technique should always be carried out when suctioning an infant, for this neonate is already in jeopardy without introducing an additional contaminant and a possible complication.

Monitoring vital signs, as ordered by the physician, is important; however, should a question arise or an irregularity or a radical change occur, repeat the process. Never hesitate to increase frequency of the readings with the aim of early detection of an impending problem. When observing the neonate, include the status of muscle tone, reflexes, and hypo- or hyperirritability. Every sign being demonstrated by the neonate indicates his status.

Intake and output records should be meticulously updated and kept at the bedside. Intravenous intake should be recorded at least every hour, running at the appropriate rate of flow. The infant's intravenous site should be closely observed for signs of infiltration or the development of phlebitis. It is also important when immobilizing the heads of these infants for infusions to check the ears frequently to ensure that no pressure areas are developing. When the urinary output is recorded, writing "one wet diaper" is adequate, unless the physician has requested a more accurate output, which would necessitate "bagging" the infant, or weighing his saturated, disposable diaper. Specific gravity readings should be done on all urine obtained.

Positioning looms as a major nursing problem. These neonates should be turned about every hour, and all efforts should be directed toward maintaining the intravenous therapy, being careful not to disturb monitoring devices or dislodge the endotracheal tube if one has been inserted. The entire body should be examined closely to prevent pressure points from developing. Most nurses consider this period the ideal time to remove restraints from the upper extremities in order to exercise the arms.

Generally an abundance of equipment is used in the care of an infant with asphyxia neonatorum, and all of it should be handled meticulously, particularly that which is involved in the ventilatory system. All tubing, suctioning equipment, nebulizers, and other similar pieces of equipment should be changed every 24 hours. If there is a department within the hospital which assumes this responsibility, those members of the team will carry out this procedure, but for the most part, nurses will find that they themselves must do it, and they must remember that this tedious task is most important to the infant's health status. Gas sterilization and proper degassing before replacement are imperative in avoiding a saprophytic contaminant such as *Pseudomonas aeruginosa*.

When oxygen is used, the nurse may find himself faced with increasing the concentration temporarily to relieve respiratory embarassment. If it is not being administered, then the oxygen may be given through a tube held in front of the baby's mouth and nose, or it may be attached to a funnel in the same position. The inspired concentrations should be held to a minimum for acceptable blood levels. Remember the toxic effects of oxygen on the neonatal lung with prolonged usage.

Typically, should an apneic spell occur, sensory stimulation is adequate in initiating a respiratory response. When the apnea monitor alarm sounds, simply changing the baby's position or snapping the soles of his feet should serve as instigators. As he changes an infant's position, the nurse must observe the extent of a neonate's response to the process.

The prognosis depends upon the severity of asphyxia. Newborns, fortunately, tolerate oxygen deficits better than older individuals, and most recover completely. However, some will die, and others, as they grow, will evidence some neurologic impairment.

Atelectasis

Primary Atelectasis Normally, at the time of delivery, negative intraplural pressure causes air to be drawn into the alveoli, and lung expansion occurs. However, when this process is not demonstrated, *primary (congenital) atelectasis* or a failure of the lungs to expand may result. It is commonly seen in premature infants and in neonates with central nervous system damage. Some explanations are needed in order to understand what causes the plight of these newborn babies who experience respiratory embarrassment.

The failure of alveoli to expand may occur as the result of a poor quality of respirations, immature lung tissue, poorly developed respiratory and accessory muscles in addition to the soft thoracic cavity which collapses on the lungs as a result of negative pressure being exerted by the contracting diaphragm. Other causes which deserve consideration include the oversedated baby, central nervous system damage, a mucous plug, and aspiration.

On delivery, in severe primary atelectasis, the neonate is hypotonic, respirations are irregular, rapid, and shallow, and an expiratory grunt is often present. Mottling of skin, nasal flaring, apnea, and cyanosis are common. In mild cases, shallow respirations and minimal cyanosis relieved on crying or with the administration of oxygen may be the primary clinical findings. The prognosis is dependent upon the severity of involvement.

Secondary Atelectasis When the lungs have been aerated for a period of time and suddenly collapse as a result of an occlusion, *secondary atelectasis* occurs. This condition is also known as acquired atelectasis and is relatively common in infancy and childhood.

Some intrabronchial obstructions which may result in secondary atelectasis are the aspiration of a foreign object, mucous plug, or the mucoid secretions common to cystic fibrosis or asthma. Extrabronchial obstructions may result from a compression of the bronchi by hilar or mediastinal lymph nodes due to infections, bronchiectasis, cardiac enlargement, or some neoplastic tissue. Congenital anomalies of the diaphragm, such as eventration or diaphragmatic hernia, may also exert pressure on the pulmonary parenchyma preventing expansion. Osseous deformities such as lordosis and scoliosis, in addition to some neuromuscular conditions such as poliomyelitis or amyotonia congenita, have also been contributing causes of acquired atelectasis.

When a bronchus is obstructed, air is trapped in the parenchyma of the involved pulmonic area, and as it is absorbed into the blood, a perfusion of that part of the lung occurs. After the collapse of a segment or lobe, ventilation is minimal, and although perfusion of the area is only slightly decreased, the ventilation-perfusion relationship is disturbed with a resultant circulatory adjustment. Concomitantly, there is an accumulation and stasis of secretions in the involved section of the lung, which is an excellent microorganism media. Responsible for the initial distention of the affected area, as the secretions are absorbed, there is a contraction of the obstructed lung tissue.[5] The signs and symptoms of secondary atelectasis, as expected, vary. The causes reiterate an ill child with a myriad of organic problems, where a cough and a fever already may be present. Although one observes decreased chest expansion, diminished breath sounds and a wheeze may be evident, suggesting an atelectatic process. In many instances the diagnosis is confirmed by chest roentgenogram.

When a previously well child demonstrates respiratory distress, an aspirated foreign object may be suspected. But if a patient experiences increasing respiratory distress after surgery, then aspiration, subsequent bronchial obstruction, and resultant secondary atelectasis should be suspected.

An acute, acquired atelectatic episode resolves itself in a short period of time with efforts being directed toward treating the infection. The chronically ill and children with recurrent pulmonary infections are much less fortunate. There may be bronchial damage, and resolution may take a long time because of the delay in expelling accumulated secretions which would facilitate ventilation. The causative agent of repeated pulmonary infections needs to be identified and treated. Bronchoscopy is performed only after the child has not responded to medical treatment. Conversely, if a child has had a sudden coughing episode, or choking spell with a unilateral wheeze, bronchoscopy is done immediately, for any delay in removing the aspirated object alters the prognosis.

Nursing Responsibilities Neonates with total atelectasis may not live long, but those with partial involvement can survive, provided nursing measures are directed toward assisting the expansion process. Positioning becomes an extremely important responsibility for nurses. Changes in position should be done conscientiously, every 2 hours. Raising the head of the platform within the incubator relieves pressures of visceral organs upon the diaphragm, thereby increasing the area of rib cage expansion. The infant's upper extremities should be placed on either side of his trunk or chest, for their placement on his rib cage increases the weight of the thoracic cavity upon the lungs.

Observing the neonate, monitoring his vital signs, noting his skin color, and evaluating his respiratory status should be done hourly, and in some instances more frequently. Changes will occur rapidly in these babies, with little warning.

Generally these infants are placed in incubators open or closed, dependent upon the institution where temperature and humidity can be more easily controlled. Since some of these babies have subnormal temperatures, maintaining body warmth may be a problem that needs to be resolved quickly, for it may contribute to his deterioration. Oxygen levels should be determined with the use of an analyzer every 3 hours, and the data appropriately recorded. The humid environment facilitates liquefaction of secretions, and permits their removal, but suctioning may be necessary to assist the infant. Postural drainage should be initiated as soon as the patient's condition warrants the procedure.

Since these infants have an oxygenation deficit, a nursing care plan which best utilizes the time a nurse spends with the baby needs to be devised. In doing so, one should consider the baby's physical status, the necessary medical and nursing procedures which must be performed, in addition to daily radiologic studies, and innumerable, unexpected interruptions. Effective use of time may extend the sleep and rest periods which are important to recovery.

When oral feedings are instituted, caution must be used. These babies should be fed slowly and burped frequently to decrease the possibility of abdominal distention. Although these neonates should be allowed to cry for short periods of time, for this activity aids in lung expansion, nursing interventions geared toward preventing a baby from crying after feedings should be implemented. By such actions the possibility of vomiting and aspirating, which lead to additional complications, can be avoided.

Pneumothorax and Pneumomediastinum

When air escapes from the lungs into the pleural space because of ruptured alveoli on the pleural surface, *pneumothorax* results. If the ruptured alveoli are not on the pleural surface, *pneumomediastinum* occurs due to pulmonary interstitial emphysema which results in mediastinal emphysema. A pneumothorax follows a pneumomediastinum if the mediastinal wall ruptures. Pneumomediastinum and/or pneumothorax may occur in any ball-valve bronchial or bronchiolar obstruction due to aspiration which causes severe alveolar overdistention with resultant alveolar rupture. Pneumothoraxes may also occur from trauma, such as puncture wounds; from a ruptured lung abscess in association with staphylococcal pneumonia; and as a result of atelectasis.

Asymptomatic pneumothorax is diagnosed through x-ray, percussion, and auscultation. X-ray reveals emphysema. On percussion, the affected lung is hyperresonant. Diminished breath sounds are heard on auscultation.

The onset of symptomatic pneumothorax may be sudden or gradual. The degree of respiratory distress may vary from tachypnea to severe dyspnea with grunting and cyanosis. Since bilateral involvement may occur, symmetry of the chest *does not* rule out pneumothorax. If asymmetric involvement is present, an increased anteroposterior chest circumference and bulging intercostal spaces occur on the affected side. A mediastinal shift is present, with the heart displaced toward the affected side and the diaphragm displaced downward. With a right-sided pneumothorax, the liver is also displaced downward. Because of the mediastinal shift, heart sounds and impulses are not heard in their usual sites. An x-ray depicts the collapsed lung and mediastinal displacement.

In pneumomediastinum, respiratory distress varies in accordance with the amount of trapped air. When this amount is great, bulging of the midthoracic area, distended neck veins, and low blood pressure occur. On auscultation, heart sounds are distant and may be barely audible, while breath sounds are normal.

Asymptomatic pneumothorax requires no treatment. With symptomatic pneumothorax, 100 percent oxygen is administered periodically. Needle aspiration is utilized followed by thoracotomy and water-seal drainage. Aspiration is ineffective in the treatment of pneumomediastinum. The only treatment to date is administration of 100 percent oxygen. Any acid-base imbalance and blood gas abnormalities which occur in either condition are treated in the same manner as that described for respiratory distress syndrome.

Nursing Management A shift in the location of the apical pulse in the newborn in respiratory distress should alert the nurse to the need for needle aspiration. Prior to thoracentesis the nurse administers 100 percent oxygen via hood or tight-fitting mask to hasten the resolution of accumulated air and retard further accumulation. (Nursing care of the pediatric patient with water-seal drainage is covered in Chapter 34.) Difficulty in finding the heartbeat of the newborn and/or swelling and crepitus in the mid-thoracic region and subcutaneous tissues of the neck should alert the nurse to the possibility of pneumomediastinum. Mediastinal shift is absent.

RESPIRATORY DISEASES AND DEVIATIONS IN THE INFANT
Congenital Laryngeal Stridor

A noisy, harsh, crowing sound on inspiration is termed *stridor*. When stridor persists or appears after the first few days of extrauterine life, the epiglottis and supraglottic aperture are the most commonly involved structures. *Laryngomalacia* refers to congenital laryngeal stridor caused by a flabbiness of the epiglottis and supraglottic aperture. It is the most common cause of congenital laryngeal stridor, and symptoms usually disappear by 1 year of age.

The diagnosis is made by laryngoscopy, by which abnormalities of the epiglottis, vocal cords, and other laryngeal structures may be visualized directly. Causes of laryngeal stridor other than laryngomalacia include chondromalacia of the larynx and trachea, malformations of laryngeal cartilages, intraluminal webs, anomalies of the vocal cords, cysts, tumors, and birth trauma.

Symptoms in addition to noisy, crowing sounds may include dyspnea and supraclavicular, intercostal, and subcostal retractions on inspiration. Cyanosis is rare. With respiratory infections, symptoms become exaggerated.

Laryngomalacia rarely requires treatment. Symptoms gradually disappear by 1 year of age. The greatest problem may be feeding the infant. If respiratory efforts are great, normal sucking and swallowing are inhibited. Therefore, slow, careful feeding is required. In more severe cases, lavage or gastrostomy feedings may be indicated. Since respiratory infections exaggerate all symptoms of stridor, infants with laryngeal stridor must be protected from these infections.

Nursing Management Sometimes a flabby epiglottis will occlude the larynx and shut off air flow to the trachea when the young infant is in a recumbant position. Until the epiglottis is more stable, a prone or semi-Flower's position is preferable.

The crowing noise produced on inspiration due to laryngomalacia can be frightening. It is especially apparent during feedings. Since sucking interferes with breathing, the nurse feeds the infant slowly, stopping frequently. The respiratory process is more important to the infant than his desire for food. When the infant stops sucking to breathe, the nurse waits for a few moments and offers the nipple again. If the infant has difficulty in swallowing, the nurse is alerted to the possibility of aspiration and removes the nipple at once. The infant is *never propped* for feedings. Slow, careful feeding may be accomplished by using a small, hard nipple, or "premie nipple," on the nursing bottle, a dropper, or a glass. With a "premie nipple" the infant not only can suck but also obtain satisfaction from sucking.

Difficulty in respiration is indicative of infection and/or aspiration. In order to prevent respiratory infection, the infant should not come into contact with affected persons. He is also kept warm and dry, away from drafts, and in an environment of high humidity.

Parents need to be reassured that the increase in stridor during feedings is normal and will decrease in severity as the child becomes older. The nurse instructs the parents in methods of feeding and affords them support during the process of feeding their infant. Parents may indicate fear of the unknown verbally and nonverbally. A look of anxiety when holding the infant and questions about noisy respirations, feeding, and ability to breathe alert the nurse to teaching needs. Parents are allowed to experiment with the different feeding methods while the infant is still in the hospital. In this way, the feeding method that seems easiest for both mother and infant is discovered before the infant goes home. The nurse discusses with the parents why the infant stops sucking and what to do. Parents are also encouraged to become familiar with the sound of the infant's crowing when he is feeding, crying, and resting so that they can judge if and when stridor becomes worse and notify the physician if necessary.

Sudden Infant Death Syndrome

The most common cause of death during the first year of life (excluding the first week of life) is the sudden infant death syndrome (SIDS). It strikes 1 out of every 300 live-born infants each year. SIDS is seen more frequently in prematurely born infants and those who live in overcrowded settings, is more prevalent during the winter months, and occurs almost exclusively while the infant is asleep. Its peak incidence is at 2 to 3 months of age, but it is rarely seen before 3 weeks or after 8 months of age.[6]

When an apparently healthy, symptomless infant is put to bed and found lifeless sometime later, SIDS should be considered. A positive diagnosis is made on autopsy. The findings include a minor inflammation of the upper respiratory tract, petechiae over the pleura, and often some lung congestion caused by common cold viruses. Many theories have been postulated to account for a sudden, unexplained death with minimal postmortem findings. The latest theory, offered by Bergman and his associates, is that a viral infection affects the nerves controlling the vocal cords in such a way that spasm causes a sudden closure of the vocal cords during sleep, occluding the airway.[7] Judy F. Rosenblith and Rebecca B. Anderson-Huntington of Brown University's Institute of Life Sciences theorize that some unknown neurologic problem exists which interferes with the infant's respirations. The infant who is prone to SIDS fails to open his mouth and, instead, clamps his mouth shut, dying quietly in his sleep. Most recent studies seem to point to some type of neurologic involvement in impaired respiratory function. Research in England with newborn lambs, calves, and monkeys points to laryngeal sensory receptors. When fluid or regurgitated gastric contents come in contact with these receptors, respiratory arrest occurs overriding the stimulation normally supplied by central and peripheral chemoreceptors. A theory proposed in the United States is related to decreased CO_2 sensitivity and lack of hypoxic drive with resultant prolonged periods of apnea. Another possible cause of apnea being investigated regards normal, prolonged apneic periods which occur during rapid eye movement (REM) sleep and their relation to postnatal age.[8]

As yet, no known way of treating SIDS exists. The treatment lies in supporting parents and siblings who not only grieve over the death of the infant but also wonder if they could have prevented the death. People who may come in contact with the family after the infant's death—policemen, firemen, coroners, doctors, nurses—need to understand the nature of SIDS so that they can guard against thoughtless remarks. Someone who is knowledgeable about SIDS and skilled in helping families deal with grief (whether nurse, doctor, or other health professional) should provide information and counseling as early as possible.

Nursing Management The three most common *parental concepts* of the cause of sudden infant death are suffocation, choking, and unsuspected illness. If the infant was seen by a physician (a routine visit) before death, both parents and physician wonder what signs and symptoms were missed. During the acute phase of grief which may last for several weeks, parents at first express disbelief that the infant is dead. They speak of the infant in both past and present tenses. They may also express anger, helplessness, loss of meaning of life, fear of going insane, and guilt regarding the death. Physical symptoms may include "whirling around," "pressure in the head," "heartache," and "stomach pain." A sad expression, sighing, insomnia, and restlessness are associated with these strange visceral sensations.[9]

Following the acute phase of grieving, parents often have mood fluctuations. Their hostility may be directed toward friends and relatives, and they have difficulty concentrating. Denial of the infant's death may be expressed in behavior, such as preparing the infant's food and bath. Many parents dream about the infant and are afraid of being left at home alone. Those parents who have no close ties are apt to move from the area after the infant's death.[10] The preceding description of the grief reaction is normal and follows Lindemann's classic description.

If nurses are to help families with their grieving, they must be able to discuss the symptoms of grief with the parents and assure them that they are not going insane. Some physicians make referrals to a skilled public health nurse who realizes that parents will be upset and unable, perhaps, to utilize factual information immediately. Therefore, the nurse may have to make several home visits in order to repeat the factual information and assist the parents with the grieving process. Many parents decide to have another child and may need support, factual information, and counseling during the decision-making process, pregnancy, and first year of the subsequent child's life.[11]

Members of the National Foundation for Sudden Infant Death propose a compassionate and medically sound procedure in every community for handling SIDS. The procedure includes mandatory autopsies in all cases of sudden infant death. Results of the autopsy would be relayed promptly to parents by a physician, nurse, or other health professional who is knowledgeable about SIDS and skilled in helping parents deal with their grief. Coroners and medical examiners would be informed of criteria for diagnosing SIDS on autopsy, and the term *sudden infant death syndrome* would be utilized on the death certificate.

Strategy to accomplish these proposals would include provision for dissemination of information to instruct the public, including those most apt to come in contact with the family; alliance with professional medical and health organizations; and involvement with the government on local, state, and national levels to ensure the necessary legislation for compassionate and medically sound handling of all cases of sudden infant death. Nurses can be prime movers of appropriate legislation by contacting their legislators, disseminating information to them, and helping to instruct the public who, in turn, can contact legislators.

Bronchiolitis

In *acute bronchiolitis* a blockage of the egress of air from the alveoli results in overdistention of the lungs, dyspnea, cyanosis, and exhaustion. It occurs during the first 2 years of life, with its peak incidence at 6 months of age. It is most often seen in the winter and early spring. Viral invasion causes widespread inflammation of the bronchial mucosa, and tenacious exudate within the lumens of the bronchioles acts like a ball valve. Air may be permitted to enter the alveoli during inspiration, but the orifice closes and traps air during expiration. The lungs become progressively distended, and many alveoli lose their normal function of aerating blood (atelectasis). If a critical portion of alveoli is affected, adjacent alveoli cannot compensate for the inadequate ventilation. As a result, hypoxia occurs, carbon dioxide is elevated, pH decreases, and the infant is in respiratory acidosis. Small amounts of pneumonia may be present in the lungs.

In making the diagnosis, any condition associated with generalized obstructive emphysema must be ruled out. Of these conditions, asthma is the one most commonly confused with acute bronchiolitis. Since asthma rarely occurs in infancy, acute bronchiolitis should be the first diagnostic consideration during the first year of life.

Symptoms of acute bronchiolitis include flaring of the alae nasi and an overdistended chest which collapses poorly on expiration and retracts intercostally and subcostally on inspiration. Respirations range from 60 to 80 per minute and are labored but shallow due to lung distention. Varying degrees of cyanosis may be present. The infant is restless, has a hacking cough, and eats and sleeps poorly. Fever may be absent, intermediate, or high, or the infant may be hypothermic. The acute phase lasts for 2 to 3 days following the onset of cough and dyspnea. When this critical period is over, recovery is dramatic and rapid. About 1 percent of affected infants die from exhaustion and the inability to oxygenate blood or a complicating pneumothorax.

Since the causative agent is viral, there are no antimicrobial agents which will be therapeutic. Tracheostomy is not indicated because the obstruction is at the bronchial level. The value of corticosteroids is questionable. One dose of epinephrine may be given to see if there is an element of response. Otherwise, since bronchodilating drugs increase restlessness and oxygen requirements, they are usually contraindicated. Therefore, treatment is symptomatic. High humidity via cold vapor to help liquefy secretions and decrease edema and oxygen for dyspnea are readily supplied through the utilization of a mist tent or oxygen tent (see Fig. 33-6). Since anxiety and restlessness accompany dyspnea, they will be allayed through an adequate supply of oxygen.

Positioning is important. Placing the infant on his abdomen fosters better drainage, and the weight of the back assists in compressing distended lungs during expiration. Putting the infant in semi-Fowler's position, with slight extension of his neck, allows for fuller chest expansion and a clearer airway.

If the infant tires easily when sucking and because of tachypnea, he is placed on "nothing by mouth," and intravenous fluids are started. Tachypnea in itself may have a dehydrating effect, and supplemental intravenous fluids may be given along with oral fluids. Respiratory acidosis is helped through the administration of appropriate parental fluids, with better perfusion of the lungs and V/Q ratio.

Nursing Management Observation of the infant's vital signs, skin color, skin turgor, and anterior fontanel and accurate recording and reporting of these observations are extremely important during the critical 48 to 72 hours following the onset of cough and dyspnea. These data, in conjunction with findings on auscultation and palpation and laboratory findings, provide important clues to the infant's status. They also alert the nurse to impending respiratory acidosis and secondary dehydration.

The nurse checks the oxygen tent frequently to ensure its proper functioning in providing high humidity and oxygen at a comfortable temperature. Higher oxygen content aids in breathing, and the mist helps to liquefy secretions, thus making coughing less distressing to the infant. The infant's response to oxygen therapy is ascertained through observation of his color, nature of his respirations, the degree of restlessness, and determination of arterial blood gases. If the infant's nares are blocked, he will breathe through his mouth. Nasal secretions should be removed with cotton-tipped applicators or with cotton cones. Positions as described in the treatment should be maintained to aid in oxygenation.

If fluids are tolerated, the infant is offered water between feedings. In the event that he cannot be removed from the mist tent due to his respiratory status, the nurse supports his head and back with one hand while holding the bottle with the other. If the infant's breathing is labored, medications and feedings are given very slowly. The nurse notes the infant's behavior during feeding to ascertain the need for stopping oral feedings. The rate and flow of any intravenous fluids are observed frequently to prevent over- or underhydration and/or electrolyte imbalance.

Croup

Croup is a term applied to several conditions characterized by cough, inspiratory stridor, hoarseness, and signs of respiratory distress. Bacterial croup is seen more commonly in the 3- to 7-year age group, while viral croup is seen more frequently from 3 months to 3 years of age. Males, for no known reason, have a higher incidence of croup. The disease seems to occur more often in cold weather. Parainfluenza viruses account for the majority of infectious croup cases. Epiglottitis and diphtheria, the bacterial forms, are discussed later in this chapter. Clinical varieties of viral croup include laryngitis, laryngotracheobronchitis (the most common form), and acute spasmodic croup.

Laryngitis is usually mild except in the young infant. The high obstruction causing respiratory distress in the infant is due to edema of the vocal cords and subglottic area. With laryngotracheobronchitis (LTB), as the name suggests, the infection extends downward from the larynx to the bronchi. Children with acute spasmodic croup, for little or no apparent reason, develop episodes of severe laryngospasm at night.

Laryngitis begins with an upper respiratory infection followed by sore throat, cough, and croup. When the clinical course is severe, obstruction occurs in the subglottic area. Marked hoarseness, deep suprasternal and substernal retractions, severe inspiratory stridor, dyspnea, and restlessness occur. As the course progresses, air hunger and fatigue appear, at which time the infant alternates between periods of agitation and exhaustion secondary to decreased P_{O_2} and increased P_{CO_2}.

The onset of LTB is characterized by an upper respiratory infection which lasts for several days before cough and inspiratory stridor indicate the advent of respiratory distress. As the bronchi and bronchioles become involved, expirations become labored and prolonged, and the infant appears restless and frightened. Fever may be slight, or the temperature may reach 39.4 to 40°C (103 to 104°F). The illness lasts for several days, a week, or longer. It is initially distinguished from epiglottitis by its slower

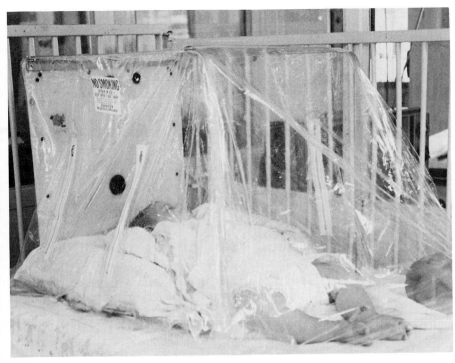

Figure 33-6 An infant in a mist tent receiving oxygen and humidity to relieve his respiratory difficulty. *(Courtesy of Children's Hospital Medical Center, Boston. Photograph by Boston University School of Nursing, Media Services Department.)*

onset as opposed to the explosive onset and more rapid course of epiglottitis.

Acute spasmodic laryngitis occurs most commonly between 1 to 3 years of age. Since anxious and excitable children seem more prone to this condition and a familial predisposition may be present, allergy and psychologic factors may be implicated along with viruses. Following a mild to moderate coryza and hoarseness, the child awakens at night because of respiratory distress. He exhibits a barking, metallic cough, noisy inspiration, anxiety, and fright. The child is afebrile. His respirations are slow and labored with supraclavicular, suprasternal, substernal, and intercostal retractions. His pulse is rapid, and his skin is cool and moist. If the child becomes excited, dyspnea increases and intermittent cyanosis may occur. Severe symptoms usually last several hours and then decrease. Increasingly milder attacks may occur on one or two subsequent nights. Eventual recovery is complete.

The aim of treatment is to ensure adequate exchange of oxygen and carbon dioxide at the alveolar level. High humidity with cold mist aids in preventing the drying of secretions and in reducing mucosal edema. If an infant is in severe respiratory distress, oral feedings may be discontinued and parenteral fluids given. Thus, physical exertion is lessened, and the probability of aspiration of vomitus is decreased.

Cyanosis may be an indication for tracheotomy. Therefore, when oxygen is administered to alleviate anoxia and apprehension, the infant must be observed carefully for other signs of impending need for a tracheotomy. Indications for a tracheotomy include advancing cyanosis, restlessness, and tachycardia. In lieu of tracheotomy, some physicians elect to intubate their young patients for 24 hours. Others believe that inhalation of racemic epinephrine is helpful.

Sedatives are *contraindicated*, since restlessness is one of the criteria for ascertaining the need for tracheotomy. In those rare instances where sedation might be essential due to the infant's extreme agitation and fright, chloral hydrate or paraldehyde (never I.V.) may be given, since neither dries secretions nor depresses the respiratory center. No medications are of value in treating viral croup with the exception of subemetic doses of syrup of ipecac to relieve laryngeal spasm in spasmodic croup. Emetic doses of ipecac result in vomiting due to probable vagal stimulation.

Nursing Management Frequent reassurance by the nurse will aid in keeping the infant calm and quiet. This reassurance may be accomplished through the nurse's tone of voice, touch, and physical presence. The nurse must observe the infant frequently. Careful noting, recording, and reporting of the degree of hoarseness; type of cough; type and severity of retractions; degree of stridor, cyanosis, and restlessness; presence of labored and prolonged expirations; pyrexia; and tachycardia are essential in determining the infant's progress. The pattern of increased heart rate, decreased respiratory rate, and decreased stridor spell emergency. Stridor decreases as the infant moves less air. Heart rate increases in response and respiratory rate decreases as P_{CO_2} rises above 60 or 70.

The nurse should note the infant's behavior during feedings. If he becomes tired, oral feedings may be discontinued and parenteral fluids started. Rate of flow, amount, and type of intravenous fluid must be recorded at least every hour. Signs of infiltration of parenteral fluids should be reported immediately and recorded.

If an infant suffers an attack of croup at home, instant steam may be provided by fully turning on all hot water taps in a closed bathroom. The infant may then be placed in an atmosphere of high humidity. This procedure may be done in lieu of cold mist, but cold mist vaporizers for home use are commercially available. Families on welfare may obtain them at no cost if a doctor writes a prescription for one. In the hospital, the infant may be in a "croup" room or a mist tent with oxygen and mist.

If a high fever is present, sponge baths with tepid water may be given. These sponge baths last for approximately 15 minutes. If at any moment during that time cyanosis; weak, irregular pulse; slow, shallow respirations; or chills occur, the sponge bath should be discontinued, because of impending circulatory collapse.

Increased restlessness, pulse rate, and fever and the presence of dyspnea and retractions *before cyanosis occurs* are indications for a tracheotomy. The infant may have an anxious expression on his face because of his inability to aerate his lungs adequately. The alert nurse reports the advent of these manifestations to the physician.

After a tracheotomy has been performed the nurse observes the infant for and reports restlessness, extreme fatigue, dyspnea, cyanosis or pallor, fever, rapid pulse, retractions, noisy respirations, bleeding, crepitance, and infection around the incision. Symptoms of obstruction in the tracheotomy tube include blue or ashy color, especially of the infant's ears, face, and lips; noisy, moist respirations; substernal retractions; restlessness or apprehension; and increased pulse rate. Adequate suctioning, changing, and cleaning of the inner cannula should prevent obstruction in the tracheotomy tube.

The infant's arms are restrained to prevent his removing the tube with random arm movements. The nurse may assure the infant through tone of voice, touch, and physical presence. The infant is provided with oxygen and mist, usually by way of mist tent. Immediately following a tracheotomy, the infant is suctioned frequently and then every hour. As he improves, his need for suctioning decreases. A mediastinal shift or decreased breath sounds on one side are indicative of tension pneumothorax, a rare complication following tracheotomy.

Since the infant cannot cry, he needs a sense of trust in himself and others. Trust is provided through the love of his mother and the nurse caring for him. His vital signs are taken as ordered or more frequently, according to the nurse's assessment. Changing the infant's position frequently prevents pooling of secretions. The infant is offered small amounts of water at frequent intervals unless oral feedings are contraindicated. At this time, arm restraints may be removed under the nurse's supervision to provide range of motion exercises.

Parents need factual information and constant reassurance during the acute phase of the illness. Following an explanation of the child's condition and the reasons for treatment and nursing measures, parents can determine, with the nurse's help, the degree of their involvement in the care of the child. This involvement can pave the way for parents and infant for the return home.

Sometimes the infant with LTB is discharged with the tracheotomy tube in situ. Parents who have been involved in the care of their infant know how to carry out procedures and are aware of danger signals. They are also cautioned to be careful when bathing the infant to prevent water from entering the tube. If parents need help in caring for the infant at home, a referral is made to a community health nurse.

Retropharyngeal Abscess

Behind the posterior pharyngeal wall are several small lymph nodes which drain portions of the nasopharynx and posterior nasal passages. The nodes normally disappear by 3 to 4 years of age. They sometimes become infected when an infant has an acute nasopharyngitis or pharyngitis. An infection of these small lymph nodes behind the posterior pharyngeal wall results in *retropharyngeal abscess*. The usual causative organism is a group A hemolytic streptococcus.

Following an upper respiratory infection, the infant abruptly develops a high fever accompanied by difficulty in swallowing and refusal to eat. His respirations are noisy and often gurgling. He lies with his head hyperextended. With dysphasia, secretions accumulate in the mouth, and dyspnea increases. Presented with these clinical features, the physician will examine the infant for a retropharyngeal mass by placing him in Trendelenburg's position. The danger is rupture of the abscess under nonoperating room conditions with massive aspiration. Therefore, the infant is placed on his abdomen. Suction apparatus should be available to prevent aspiration if the abscess ruptures. Regional cervical lymph nodes are markedly enlarged. Leukocytosis, with polymorphonuclear cells predominating, is present. The mass may not be visible or palpable when it is in the lower pharynx, but may be revealed by a lateral view of the neck on x-ray.

Once retropharyngeal abscess is the suspected diagnosis, penicillin G is started parenterally. When the abscess is fluctuant, it is drained. The mass is first aspirated. If blood is obtained from erosion of blood vessels, the incision into the abscess is not made. With serious bleeding involving the carotid vessels, ligation of the carotid artery is necessary prior to incision to prevent exsanguination. Penicillin therapy is continued for several days following surgery.

Nursing Management The nurse who is assisting the physician in examining the infant's throat ensures that this examination is done quickly and gently without damage to the wall of the pharynx and with minimal pain to the infant by applying a mummy restraint. The infant is placed in Trendelenburg's position. The nurse immobilizes the infant's head by placing his hands gently but firmly on either side of it. This same technique is utilized when the physician incises and drains the abscess to prevent aspiration of purulent material into the larynx.

Preoperatively, when the infant's fever is 39.4°C (103°F) or above, the nurse carries out those nursing measures which will prevent febrile convulsions. Observations of the infant's respirations, his ability to swallow, and his assumed position are important points to record and report. With an accumulation of secretions due to dysphagia, the nurse provides gentle oral suction, being careful to stay away from the infant's pharyngeal area. Suction should be of the *mouth only* for the purpose of removing secretions which have collected there.

Postoperatively, in order to facilitate drainage, the foot of the bed is elevated and the infant is placed in a semiprone position. If the infant becomes restless and attempts to change his position, restraints are applied. When the swallowing reflex returns, he is given fluids by mouth. Frequent swallowing may be an indication of bleeding, and the physician should be notified. The infant is observed for signs of respiratory distress which would be reported to the physician immediately. The nurse should observe the infant pre- and postoperatively for any allergic reactions to penicillin. Scrupulous mouth care will help in keeping the infant's mouth and lips moist and in dispelling halitosis.

Parents probably need the most support when the infant is first brought to the hospital. An infant who has gurgling respirations and accumulated oral secretions appears mortally ill to his parents. Thus, they need factual information and a nurse with a listening ear.

Pertussis

The infant has no temporary immunity to pertussis (whooping cough) in the first few months of life and is highly susceptible to this communicable disease. The highest mortality from pertussis occurs in the first year of life.

Pertussis, an acute infection of the respiratory tract, is caused by a bacterium known either as *Bordatella pertussis* or *Hemophilus pertussis* and is spread by droplet infection or direct contact. It is characterized by a paroxysmal cough which ends in a prolonged inspiration or "whoop" and, frequently, vomiting. The structures most affected are the bronchi and bronchioles. Some inflammation may be seen in the trachea, larynx, and nasopharyngeal mucosa. Lymphocytes and some neutrophils infiltrate the respiratory passages causing an interstitial pneumonitis. Sometimes, small mucous plugs in the bronchioles cause obstructive emphysema and atelectasis.

Symptoms may occur anywhere from 7 to 14 days after exposure. The disease proceeds in three stages: catarrhal, spasmodic or paroxysmal, and convalescent stages. The entire course lasts about six weeks.

The *catarrhal stage* has an insidious onset with a mild cough, usually at night. For the following 10 days to 2 weeks the cough becomes progressively more severe and occurs during the day. Coryza, sneezing, and, sometimes, hoarseness occur. The infant may be anoxic. Recovery of the causative organism from a cough plate or nasopharyngeal swab culture during this phase is helpful in making the diagnosis.

At the end of 10 days or 2 weeks of the catarrhal

stage, the infant enters the *spasmodic or paroxysmal stage*. During a severe paroxysm, a series of explosive efforts occurs. The infant's face becomes red from this exertion and may even turn cyanotic. This cyanosis may become severe enough to require artificial respiration and administration of oxygen. As the paroxysm ends, a sudden inspiratory whoop occurs. This episode may be followed by vomiting or by coughing up or swallowing large amounts of thick, tenacious, mucoid sputum. In small infants, choking spells may occur in place of the characteristic whoop. Following the coughing spasm, sweating, congestion of neck and scalp veins, mental confusion, convulsions (especially in infants), and exhaustion may occur. Paroxysms are aggravated by excitement, sudden changes in temperature, activity, and inhalation of irritating fumes, like smoke. The white blood cell count averages from 15,000 to 45,000/cu mm with a progressive lymphocytosis.

The *convalescent stage* begins about the fourth week of the clinical course. The number and severity of paroxysms decrease, vomiting subsides, and appetite returns. An intercurrent respiratory infection may cause a recurrence of all major symptoms of the disease process.

Pertussis is readily recognized during the paroxysmal stage. Sequellae include hemorrhages (epistaxis, hemoptysis, conjunctival extravasations, and intracranial hemorrhage), respiratory tract infections (otitis media, bronchopneumonia, atelectasis), nervous system complications (encephalitis), and digestive tract complications (emaciation due to prolonged vomiting and hernias due to straining on coughing and vomiting). Residual conditions include bronchiectasis and pulmonary fibrosis due to severe respiratory complications and epilepsy, mental retardation, and personality changes due to cerebral edema and intracranial hemorrhage.

The infant with suspected pertussis is isolated to prevent spread of the disease. During the early stages, hyperimmune gamma globulin, given intramuscularly once a day for 3 days, may lessen the severity of the clinical course. The infant must be observed continually to provide oxygen and suction as needed. He is offered small, frequent feedings to maintain his nutritional status. If he vomits a feeding during a paroxysm, he is refed in 15 to 20 minutes. An oxygen tent is used when the infant has convulsions or persistent dyspnea to provide adequate oxygen to the tissues. Excessive mucus is removed by gentle suctioning and placing the infant on his abdomen with his head lower than his body to facilitate drainage. Drugs effective against *Bordatella pertussis* include the tetracyclines, α-amino-benzyl penicillin, and chloramphenicol, but the latter is not used routinely because of its toxic effects.

Nursing Management Since pertussis is highly contagious, the infant is placed in isolation. Spread of the disease must be prevented, and the affected infant must be protected against secondary infection. Though paroxysms of coughing are inevitable, they can be decreased if the nurse enters the room quietly and talks to the infant before touching him or lowering the cribside. All sudden noises and sudden changes in temperature should be avoided. By maintaining a quiet environment, the nurse minimizes excitement (laughter, fright, crying) in the infant.

During paroxysmal coughing spells, the nurse reassures the infant by talking to him in a quiet voice. He supports the infant's muscles to prevent any weakening of abdominal musculature during these severe paroxysms. The infant is kept in a humidified environment to liquefy secretions. Oxygen is given if he becomes cyanotic, and chilling is avoided. Sometimes, an infant's respirations cease following a paroxysm, and the nurse provides artificial respiration. If he vomits or has excessive mucus, he is suctioned in order to maintain a patent airway. Meticulous nose and mouth care is given to prevent excoriation of the skin around the nose and lips due to nasal secretions. If the infant convulses following a coughing spasm, he is protected from hurting himself and from occluding his airway.

In order to assess the infant's progress, the nurse must observe, report, and record the severity and frequency of paroxysms; the amount, type, and frequency of vomiting; the infant's color before, during, and after coughing episodes; the type and amount of mucus; and the condition of the infant following a paroxysm. The nurse should also observe, report, and record any signs and symptoms of complications and/or sequellae.

Surely whooping cough must be frightening to parents. They need constant reassurance and factual information during the course of the disease. They are taught isolation technique in order to spend time with their hospitalized infant and, if they desire, become involved in his care. Parents may also need information about immunization schedules and booster "shots" for any eligible sibling.

Pneumonia

Bacterial pneumonia may be caused by several organisms. Clinically they may be difficult to distinguish. Pneumococcal pneumonia is presented here. Staphylococcal, streptococcal, and pneumonia caused by *Hemophilus influenzae* are presented briefly in Table 33-2.

The highest incidence of pneumococcal pneumonia is during late winter and early spring. In childhood, it occurs most frequently in the first 4 years of life. In infants, bronchopneumonia is more common, whereas in older children and adults one or more lobes are involved in the disease process without affecting the remainder of the bronchopulmonary system. The clinical course in older children is similar to that in adults. In bronchopneumonia, there is a consolidation of scattered lobules and the mucosa is inflamed.

The infant usually has a mild upper respiratory tract infection of several days' duration consisting of a stuffy nose, fretfulness, and decrease in appetite. This initial phase is followed by an abrupt onset of fever from 39.4 to 40.6°C (103 to 105°F), restlessness, apprehension, and respiratory distress. The infant may have a generalized convulsion due to high fever. Observation of the infant may reveal flushed cheeks; circumoral cyanosis; flaring of the alae nasi; supraclavicular, suprasternal, intercostal, and subcostal retractions; tachypnea; and tachycardia. A cough appears as the clinical course progresses. Abdominal distention may be due to swallowed air or paralytic ileus. Meningism may be present. The white blood cell count ranges from 15,000 to 40,000/cu mm. Polymorphonuclear leukocytes predominate. On x-ray, a patchy infiltration of one or several lobes is found, indicating bronchopneumonia. The causative organism is recovered in secretions from the trachea or from pleural fluid obtained by thoracentesis. The most common complication is empyema. The prognosis is favorable.

Penicillin G is the most effective antimicrobial agent in the treatment of pneumococcal pneumonia. If the infant is allergic to penicillin, erythromycin or cephalothin is an effective agent. The remainder of the treatment is symptomatic and supportive: bed rest, an abundance of oral fluids, and antipyretics for fever. Oxygen and mist are administered to alleviate respiratory distress and anxiety. If empyema occurs, a thoracentesis is done. Intravenous fluids are given to combat dehydration and electrolyte imbalance.

Nursing Management The infant who has pneumonia needs rest and is disturbed as little as possible. His respiratory status is assessed frequently and appropriate measures instituted. Fluids are necessary to maintain electrolytes and a normal specific gravity of the urine, but the infant should not be forced to eat since he is anorexic. Intravenous therapy may be necessary. The infant may tend to lie on his affected side to relieve pain. Frequent position change will prevent the pooling of secretions and maintain adequate circulation. Postural drainage and clapping may be necessary to assist the infant in relieving congestion.

Taking an accurate temperature is important in preventing febrile convulsions. If the infant's temperature is 38.9°C (102°F), the nurse administers the prescribed antipyretic. A fever of 39.4°C (103°F) or above necessitates a sponge bath with tepid water. A distended abdomen may be indicative of constipation, paralytic ileus, or swallowed air due to mouth breathing. A rectal tube may provide some relief for constipation and swallowed air, or the physician may order an enema. Excoriation due to copious nasal discharge may be prevented through effective skin care.

The nurse observes the child for signs of tension pneumothorax due to empyema, particularly if the pneumonia is staphylococcal in origin. An abrupt onset of pain, dyspnea, cyanosis, and absent or diminished chest movements on one side indicates the need for a thoracentesis.

The spread of a staphylococcal infection is a nightmare in a pediatric unit. The infant with staphylococcal pneumonia is placed on strict isolation, and meticulous precautions are observed by all who care for him. The nurse may have to intervene with allied hospital personnel by teaching them the importance of carrying out strict isolation technique. The infant needs oxygen therapy and blood determinations for electrolytes, hemoglobin, hematocrit, white blood cell count and differential, and so forth. Therefore, the nurse aids in the prevention of spread of a staphylococcal infection by ensuring the observance of strict isolation technique by hospital personnel.

RESPIRATORY DISEASES AND DEVIATIONS IN THE TODDLER
Aspiration of Foreign Objects

Toddlers who are up and about, investigating their environments, are particularly prone to the aspiration of a variety of objects and foods. The severity of the problem depends on what has been aspirated and the degree of obstruction. Although there is choking, gagging, wheezing, or coughing initially, there may be a symptom-free period of days or weeks when the original precipitating episode is forgotten. The time interval produces little pathologic change or a total respiratory response. What occurs depends upon the object aspirated.

Table 33-2 BACTERIAL PNEUMONIAS

Organism	Age	Signs and symptoms	Laboratory reports	Treatment
Staphylococcus	Under 1 year	History of furunculosis, recent hospitalization, or maternal breast abscess. Respiratory infection, upper or lower, for several days to 1 week followed by abrupt change—fever, cough, respiratory distress, tachypnea, grunting respirations, sternal and subcostal retractions, cyanosis, anxiety. Lethargic if undisturbed, irritable if roused. Pyopneumothorax, pneumatoceles, and empyema as clinical course progresses.	WBC: normal range in young infant, 20,000/cu mm with predominant polymorphonuclear leukocytes in older infants. Tracheal aspiration and/or pleural tap culture positive. X-ray: patchy infiltration or dense (bronchopneumonia or lobar).	Symptomatic and supportive. Oxygen. Semi-Fowler's position. Parenteral fluids during acute phase. Methicillin or penicillin G for 3 weeks I.V. or I.M. Thoracentesis. Closed chest drainage with extensive involvement for 5–7 days. Hospitalized 6–10 weeks.
Streptococcus group A	3–5 years	Mild prodromal symptoms followed by sudden onset of high fever, chills, respiratory distress. Clinical course similar to staphylococcal. Complications: empyema and bacterial foci in bones and joints.	WBC elevated with polymorphonuclear leukocytes predominating. ASO titer elevated. Positive culture. X-ray: disseminated infiltration.	Symptomatic and supportive. Penicillin G. Thoracentesis. Closed drainage.
Hemophilus influenzae	Infants and young children	Mild or severe. Insidious onset. Clinical course subacute and prolonged, of several weeks' duration. Signs and symptoms similar to pneumococcal. Signs and symptoms in young infants associated with bacteremia and emphysema. Complications: bacteremia, pericarditis, cellulitis, empyema, meningitis, pyarthrosis.	Bacteremia. Positive cultures. Moderate leukocytosis with lymphopenia. X-ray: lobar consolidation.	Symptomatic and supportive. Ampicillin.

Laryngeal-Tracheal Aspiration A foreign body located in the larynx or trachea causes hoarseness, a croupy cough, aphonia with hemoptysis, and dyspnea with wheezing; cyanosis may also occur. If the object is opaque, it can be detected on roentgenographic examination; however, if it is nonopaque, it can be identified by the physiologic effects produced. A direct laryngoscopy confirms the diagnosis and provides access to the foreign body.

Bronchial Aspiration Symptoms related to aspirated objects which lodge in the bronchi are affected by the degree of obstruction and the local pathologic changes which have occurred. A nonobstructive foreign body may produce few symptoms even after a prolonged period, while an obstructive object may produce signs and symptoms and pathologic changes quickly. If there is a slight obstruction, wheezing will be present, but in a more severe form, emphysema or atelectasis may be produced with subsequent chronic pulmonary disease. Metallic or plastic aspirants may produce obstructions because of their size and injury to tissue because of their shape. If the foreign body is of a vegetal source, such as a peanut, bean, pea, or watermelon seed, it has a tendency to swell many times its size and is serious because a bronchitis may develop with a resultant cough, fever, and dyspnea.[12]

Again, the diagnosis is made with x-rays and a physician's physical findings. Only 2 to 4 percent of the aspirated objects are spontaneously coughed up, but about 99 percent can be safely removed by bronchoscopy. A rare complication of a vegetal aspirant is the formation of a lung abscess.

Nursing Management These toddlers are usually frightened, coughing, wheezing, and cyanotic. Relieving the child's distress, gaining his confidence, and establishing a meaningful relationship with his parents promotes trust between the child and the nurse. Although he may not fully comprehend, procedures should be explained to him. Since these admissions are usually of an emergency nature, initial preparation of the patient is limited to bare essentials.

After a laryngoscopy or bronchoscopy has been performed, the youngster is usually placed in some type of oxygen/humidification device. Transfer to this confined environment might be made less frightening for the child if the nurse refers to the device as a tent or plastic house. The desired oxygen and humidification levels must be maintained. Occasionally the physician prefers liquefying agents. An important nursing observation after a bronchoscopy or laryn-

goscopy is the patient's ability to reestablish his swallowing reflex. Clear fluids initially offered should be given slowly and cautiously. When the child has reacted fully and has no difficulty in swallowing, fluids should be urged, for they tend to decrease the amount of soreness experienced. The patient should also be observed for laryngeal edema which causes an airway block and increases respiratory distress. Monitoring respirations and identifying any breathing difficulty (increased respiratory rate or retractions) are important.

Since he has been hurt, the toddler usually rebels by crying and screaming, which tend to increase the irritation of the respiratory tract. An effort should be made to calm him. His parents may be of tremendous assistance.

Chemical Pneumonia

The severity or intensity of the manifestations of chemical pneumonia depends on three factors which should be considered in every case of aspiration or ingestion: the material ingested, the individual child's response to that substance, and the amount involved. Most chemical pneumonias seen in clinical pediatrics fall into one of two categories, hydrocarbon and lipoid pneumonias. Some authorities believe the aspiration of lipids and hydrocarbons during swallowing, vomiting, or gastric lavage is the cause of lung involvement, while others state those results occur after absorption from the gastrointestinal tract and "excretion" into the lung fields.[13] Perhaps both should be considered important in producing the pulmonary response.

Hydrocarbon Pneumonia Kerosene, gasoline, and turpentine are potentially harmful substances which are often accidentally ingested by children, particularly curious toddlers. Other substances include furniture polish, certain insect sprays (where the propellant is usually kerosene), and lighter and cleaning fluids. If the amount swallowed is in excess of 10 cc, the toxicity increases greatly.[14] Within an hour after ingestion nausea, vomiting, and coughing may occur, with evidence of central nervous system involvement, such as drowsiness, evident as a result of the inhaled vapors. Gastroenteritis will be present in those youngsters who have ingested kerosene, but it does not occur in those children who have swallowed gasoline. These patients are frequently febrile with temperatures from 38 to 40°C (100 to 104°F). Methemoglobin formation may also be demonstrated. About 40 percent of these children develop pulmonary complications. Cyanosis and dyspnea may also be manifested. On physical examination, there may be suppressed breath sounds, rales and diminished resonance on percussion; however, roentgenographic studies most frequently depict the extent of pulmonic involvement.

Although complications such as pneumothorax, subcutaneous emphysema of the chest wall, and pleural effusion including empyema may occur, in most instances recovery is in 3 to 7 days. The differences in subsequent recovery depend upon the patient and, in the case of a kerosene ingestion, the constitution of the kerosene, for it varies according to the temperature at which the cracking process was carried out.[15]

Generally if a small amount of the hydrocarbon has been ingested, a gastric lavage is not advised; however, when large amounts are involved, a gastric lavage is done with great care to prevent aspiration. Saline cathartics are usually ordered. An oil preparation is usually administered to decrease the absorption rate within the gastrointestinal tract. Gerarde's investigation indicates that olive oil is more effective than mineral oil in diminishing the amount of the hydrocarbon absorbed in the gastrointestinal tract,[16] but conflicting data exist.

Nursing Management These young children need very careful respiratory monitoring, for deterioration of their status can be determined by an increase in respiration rate, increasingly labored respirations, or dyspnea. Frequently these patients are febrile, and antipyretic administration as well as other cooling measures should be carried out as ordered by the physician. Observations of vital signs, done hourly initially, can be decreased appropriately as the patient's condition stabilizes or improves.

In the case of kerosene ingestions, gastroenteritis may be a problem; therefore the patient's output should be recorded at the bedside after each stool. His skin turgor should be assessed carefully, as should his state of hydration.

The institution of oxygen therapy with humidity is common, and all the equipment should be checked frequently, including a measurement of oxygen levels at 3-hour intervals with a Beckman analyzer or some other device.

Observing the patient and evaluating his comfort are essential components of nursing care. Cyanosis and dyspnea may occur, and hence observation is imperative. In addition, the child's position should be changed every 3 hours to prevent additional pulmonary complications. Postural drainage should be done conscientiously.

Since drowsiness may be a clinical manifestation, the patient's level of consciousness should be monitored. Although twitching, convulsions, and coma are rare, the nurse may be responsible for preventing these sequelae through the use of observational skills.

Should methemoglobin formation occur, a blood transfusion may be considered by the medical staff. If such a procedure is necessary, the nurse is expected to prepare the child, observe him for a blood reaction, and assume those nursing responsibilities associated with transfusions described in Chapter 35.

Parents of children who have accidentally ingested a harmful substance are usually overwhelmed by the sudden onset of symptoms, the emergency measures, and the equipment used. They may verbalize feelings of negligence or guilt, and it is important to listen to them and to understand the emotions they are experiencing.

Lipid Pneumonia Lipid pneumonia, caused by the aspiration or accumulation of oil in the alveoli, is a chronic condition which may occur in children with cleft palates; in debilitated infants with improper swallowing or depressed cough reflexes; in children who are force-fed or maintained in a horizontal position. The aspiration of milk is a common cause of lipid bronchopneumonia in the first year of life. Administering substances with oily bases such as mineral oil, castor oil, and cod-liver oil to crying toddlers may result in lipid pneumonia.

As a rule, vegetable oils such as olive oil, cottonseed oil, and sesame oil are the least toxic and the least irritating lipids. They are not hydrolyzed by lung lipases, cause little damage, and are removed, mainly, by expectoration. The exception in the case of vegetable oils is chaulmoogra oil which results in extensive pulmonic damage. Furthermore, animal oils, such as cod-liver oil, are very dangerous because they have a very high fatty acid content, and when hydrolyzed by lung lipases, the liberated fatty acids combine with those present in the originally aspirated substance and produce severe inflammatory responses.

After aspiration an initial interstitial, proliferative inflammatory response occurs. The second phase involves the development of diffuse, proliferative fibrosis, which is followed by the formation of multiple, localized nodules.[17]

A cough is present, and dyspnea may be evident in severe cases; however, there may be no other manifestations, unless there is a superimposed infection. As expected, secondary bronchopneumonic infections are common. Roentgenographic chest films reveal patchy to nodular infiltrations or densities, especially in the right lung.

The prognosis is dependent upon the extent of involvement, whether administered oil preparations are continued, and the overall physical status of the young child. Treatment is symptomatic, and the prevention of secondary infections is essential. Surgical resection may be considered later, should pulmonic involvement be localized to one segment or lobe.

Nursing Management It is imperative for nurses to remember the causes of lipid pneumonia. Although feeding a child slowly is time-consuming, particularly if he objects to eating or is debilitated, the nurse must do so if the likelihood of aspiration is to be decreased. Cradling the child or holding him upright while he is being fed may enhance his oral intake. If the child is bottle-fed, the hole in the nipple must not be too large or the flow of fluid may be too much for the child. If the hole is too small, his oral intake will not be adequate. There should be an ongoing evaluation of his sucking and swallowing reflexes. It is also important that such information be placed on the young patient's Cardex or in his nursing care plan to assist personnel in identifying nursing problems and successful interventions.

Realistically, toddlers may resist certain oily base medications which the nurse is attempting to administer. Thus, several methods of gaining the child's cooperation are explored and evaluated. When parents are expected to continue the medication at home, sharing what has been learned by the staff is most helpful information for them.

Proper positioning of the young patient is another nursing function, for if changes are not considered, hypostatic pneumonia may be an additional complication. Placing a child on his side or abdomen will lessen the possibility of aspiration and is essential if he has a tendency to regurgitate or vomit after feedings. Parents may need some instruction about administering feedings, vitamins, and other medications. Including them in the care of their child, where feasible, decreases their anxiety and apprehension.

RESPIRATORY DISEASES AND DEVIATIONS IN THE PRESCHOOLER AND SCHOOL-AGE CHILD
Epiglottitis

Epiglottitis, an infectious form of croup, is seen more commonly in children from 3 to 7 years of age, whereas croup of viral origin is seen more in infants and younger children. The onset of illness, often abrupt, is preceded by a minor upper respiratory infection in approximately one-fourth of affected children. Epiglottitis is a severe, rapidly progressive infection of the epiglottis and surrounding area and is most commonly caused by *Hemophilus influenzae* type b. The identical disease may also be produced by pneumococci and group A streptococci. Children may progress from an asymptomatic state to one of complete airway obstruction in *2 to 5 hours*.

In younger children, the presenting symptom is sudden onset of high fever, while in older children the initial complaints are severe sore throat and dysphagia. The rapid progression of the disease is exhibited within minutes or hours of onset when the child displays severe respiratory distress with inspiratory stridor, cough, dysphagia, hoarseness, irritability, and restlessness. The child's temperature can range anywhere from 37.8 to 40.6°C (100 to 105°F) with an average of 39.4°C (103°F). With dysphagia, drooling may occur.

The younger child may assume a position of neck extension, but other meningeal signs are absent. The older child seems to prefer leaning forward in a sitting position, mouth open with tongue protruding. The severity of disease in some children is displayed in a rapid progression to a shocklike state characterized by pallor, cyanosis, and seeming loss of consciousness.

Observation of the child reveals severe respiratory distress and inspiratory stridor with flaring of the alae nasi and suprasternal, supraclavicular, intercostal, and subcostal inspiratory retractions. On examination of the child's oral cavity, pharyngitis and excessive mucus in the faucial regions are usually visualized. When the child's tongue is depressed with a blade, a large, edematous, cherry red epiglottis is seen. This finding is pathognomonic of epiglottitis. The use of a tongue depressor to visualize the child's epiglottis may lead to sudden and complete obstruction in the child who is seriously ill. Therefore, a tracheotomy set must be immediately available when this procedure is performed on a seriously ill child with the suspected diagnosis of epiglottitis. On palpation of the neck, a mild to moderate cervical adenitis may be found. Use of auscultation may reveal diminished bilateral breath sounds indicative of poor air exchange. If mucus is present in the upper respiratory tract, ronchi will be heard. Laboratory tests reveal a white blood cell count of 15,000 to 25,000/cu mm with a predominance of polymorphonuclear cells, and a bacteremia caused by *H. influenzae* or pneumococci.

Because of the high mortality rate without routine tracheotomy, most centers advocate immediate tracheotomy once the diagnosis of acute upper airway obstruction secondary to epiglottitis is made, whether or not the child is having severe respiratory problems at the time.[18] Following tracheotomy, the child is placed in the intensive care unit (if one is available). Antimicrobial therapy is instituted. Parenteral ampicillin 150 mg/kg/day is the drug of choice. Supportive measures include high humidity with cold mist, parenteral fluids, and reduction of fever. The tracheotomy tube is usually removed in 4 days without complications. Most children can be discharged in less than 1 week.

Nursing Management The place in a hospital—emergency room, operating room, or elsewhere—where the child undergoes a tracheotomy depends on his condition and the protocol of the particular hospital. The nurse's first contact with the child and his parents may be in a hectic emergency room. The physician will most likely be the one who first talks with parents and explains procedures. The nurse can later reinforce what the physician has said. If an intensive care unit is not available, a nurse should be in constant attendance. The nursing care for the child with epiglottitis is essentially the same as that described for the infant with laryngotracheobronchitis following tracheotomy, taking into consideration the age of the child. Since the preschooler's great fear is bodily harm, the child needs much reassurance once a patent airway has been restored.

Diphtheria

Another form of infectious croup is a specific infectious disease known as *diphtheria*. Unlike pertussis, the immune mother provides a temporary passive immunity to diphtheria for her infant. This immunity is absolute for the first 3 months of the infant's life and partial until he is 6 months of age.

Diphtheria, caused by *Corynebacterium diphtheriae*, is characterized by a local pseudomembranous lesion on the tonsils, pharynx, and adjacent tissues. This pseudomembrane absorbs a powerful toxin which is produced by the causative organism and causes constitutional symptoms. Symptoms appear from 2 to 7 days after exposure. In the United States, the majority of affected children are under 5 years of age. As a result of immunization, sanitation, and other preventive health measures, the incidence of diphtheria has declined greatly, although a slight rise in morbidity and age incidence has occurred since 1965. This rise supports the need for continued "boosters" throughout the school years. Infection is spread through contact with a person who has active disease or is a carrier of virulent organisms.

The three main forms of diphtheria are faucial, nasal, and laryngotracheal. *Faucial* diphtheria, especially in partially immune persons, may cause catarrhal inflammation without membrane formation. Therefore, the diagnosis may be overlooked in the absence of bacteriologic examination. Sore throat may or may not be present, and fever is usually low grade. Congestion and slight swelling of tonsillar and pharyngeal tissues occur during the first day, followed by small yellowish white spots on the tonsillar surfaces. These spots coalesce and extend to the pillars, uvula, soft palate, and postpharyngeal wall. This membrane may continue upward into the nares, causing a bloody, serous nasal discharge with an offensive odor. Swelling of soft tissues and cervical lymph nodes occurs. The pulse becomes rapid and of less volume, the blood pressure decreases, and prostration becomes more evident. Constitutional symptoms include difficulty in swallowing, noisy breathing, nasal voice, regurgitation of liquids through the nares when attempting to swallow due to palatal paralysis, and diminished or absent patellar reflexes. Laboratory tests reveal polymorphonuclear leukocytosis and albuminuria.

Laryngotracheal diphtheria is more common in the infant. The mortality rate is high. Initial symptoms include hoarseness, brassy cough, and noisy breathing. Inspiratory stridor is indicative of progressive laryngeal involvement. An increase in suprasternal and subcostal retractions is accompanied by increased anxiety. Examination by laryngoscopy reveals edema, congestion, and pseudomembrane. Unless the obstruction is relieved, cyanosis will develop, and death may occur from suffocation or cardiac failure.

Nasal diphtheria occurs primarily in the nose, although it may extend to the nasopharynx, throat, and larynx. If the infection remains localized, constitutional symptoms are absent or slight. A foul-smelling, sanguineous nasal discharge may be the only pathologic sign. Nasal diphtheria tends to be chronic if not treated, and is, therefore, a continuous source of contagion.

Part of treatment involves prevention of spread of the disease. All those who have had close contact with the child are subjected to Schick tests, nose and throat cultures, and daily inspection. They also receive penicillin either intramuscularly or orally. Previously immunized contacts are given booster injections. Anyone with a negative Schick reaction and positive cultures is treated as a carrier and receives penicillin or erythromycin. Contacts who have positive Schick reactions and positive cultures receive 2,000 units of antitoxin and either penicillin or erythromycin.

The affected child is isolated until two negative nose and throat cultures on consecutive days have been obtained. A week after the onset of the disease, the first culture is taken. If the second culture is positive, the doctor waits 5 days before ordering the next culture series. Three weeks following the onset of illness, the child may return to school.

General treatment consists of complete bed rest for 2 weeks. Daily physical examinations are essential in determining the course of the disease. Since there is a tendency toward hypoglycemia due to the toxemia produced by the causative organism, intravenous injections of 10 percent glucose solution are given. A fluid or soft diet containing ample vitamins is provided. Symptomatic treatment includes saline throat irrigations, an ice collar for cervical lymphadenitis, and codeine and aspirin for relief of headache and sore throat.

Since the affected child has active diphtheria, he is given both penicillin and antitoxin. Before antitoxin is administered to either contacts or patients, sensitivity to horse serum is determined through the intracutaneous injection of 0.05 ml antitoxin or horse serum in a 1:20 dilution. With either a local or general reaction to the preliminary test, careful desensitization of the child or contact is accomplished through serial injections of antitoxin at 15-minute intervals, provided no reaction occurs. Because of the possibility of anaphylactic shock, a syringe containing epinephrine chloride solution should be available whenever antitoxin is being administered.

Complications of diphtheria include bronchopneumonia, atelectasis, circulatory and cardiac failure, albuminuria, nephritis, and paralyses of the palate, ocular muscles, and phrenic nerve. Treatment is provided according to existing complications.

In *laryngeal diphtheria*, tracheotomy may be required to relieve the obstruction. Therefore, the child is observed carefully for increasing restlessness, anxiety, increasing suprasternal and substernal retractions, and cyanosis. When cyanosis occurs, tracheotomy is urgent. Since sedatives can conceal the preceding symptoms of inadequate air exchange due to obstruction, they should be withheld. During the cannulation period of 7 to 10 days, antibiotic therapy is maintained.

Nursing Management Since diphtheria is contagious, the child with this suspected diagnosis is placed in isolation. He is usually kept flat in bed for 2 weeks or longer to prevent acute toxic myocarditis and toxic peripheral neuritis. Intravenous therapy is often necessary. The nurse observes the child for respiratory obstruction. If he displays increased restlessness, anxiety, increasing suprasternal and substernal retractions, and cyanosis, the nurse notifies the physician and prepares for a tracheotomy, which is *urgent*. The child is suctioned as needed and is usually in a mist tent with oxygen.

If the child has cervical lymphadenitis, an ice collar usually eases his pain. Headache and sore throat are relieved by the administration of prescribed analgesics. A bloody serous nasal discharge with an offensive odor, an increased pulse with decreased volume, and decreased blood pressure are indicative of spread of the pseudomembrane into the nares and should be reported to the physician. If the nurse observes that the child regurgitates liquids through his nares when attempting to swallow, palatal paralysis is considered, and the physician is notified.

In the care of the child, chilling should be avoided, and he should be kept as warm as possible. If he has difficulty in swallowing, small frequent meals will minimize vomiting. The skin of the child's lips and nose can be protected from excoriation by the use of a soothing ointment, such as zinc oxide or petroleum jelly. A moist humid atmosphere prevents or decreases irritation to the nose and throat. The child who has a tracheostomy may need to be fed by nasal gavage, unless the pseudomembrane has extended into the nares. Otherwise, his only nourishment may be from intravenous fluids until the membrane has been aspirated via laryngoscopy. The child should be observed for any sensitivity to penicillin so that another drug may be substituted, if necessary.

Complications which may occur after discharge from the hospital include paralysis of the ocular muscles and paralysis of the phrenic nerve. The nurse should discuss these complications with the parents. Ocular paralysis usually does not occur until the third week or later. If the parents notice that the child has difficulty in reading, crossing of the eyes, or a drooping eyelid, they should inform the physician. Phrenic nerve paralysis usually does not occur until the fourth to eighth week. Cough, difficult breathing, and cyanosis should be reported to the physician, and the child should be readmitted to the hospital. Parents should be assured that recovery from paralyses following diphtheria is usually complete. The child should not return to school until at least 3 weeks after the onset of diphtheria.

Cystic Fibrosis

Cystic fibrosis is a hereditary disease of the exocrine glands. Although the basic genetic defect is unknown, investigators agree that it is transmitted as an autosomal recessive trait. Cystic fibrosis occurs most often in Caucasians and is one of the most common of the serious and chronic childhood diseases in this country. Thick, tenacious excretions of some mucus-producing glands cause obstructions mainly in the pancreatic ducts and bronchi. The secretory acini and ducts are dilated, and the exocrine parenchyma suffers secondary degeneration. The pancreas, and often the salivary glands, are firmer, smaller, and thicker than normal. With pulmonary involvement, the bronchioles are the structures first occluded, followed by the main bronchi. Eventually, chronic lung disease results, followed by emphysema due to obstructive overinflation. The heart, in trying to adapt to bronchial obstruction and pulmonary hypertension, develops a right ventricular hypertrophy. The secretions from sweat and parotid glands demonstrate an abnormal chemical composition. Children with cystic fibrosis are extremely susceptible to respiratory infections, although the immune response is normal.

Clinical manifestations include meconium ileus, chronic pulmonary disease, pancreatic insufficiency, and cirrhosis of the liver. Meconium ileus occurs in only 5 to 10 percent of children. Since cirrhosis is focal, hepatic manifestations are usually absent. Most affected children have chronic pulmonary disease. Its onset may occur weeks, months, or years after birth. It begins with a dry, nonproductive cough followed by signs of generalized bronchiolar obstruction with secondary infection. Some degree of respiratory distress is evident and may be severe. With subsequent respiratory infections the manifestations are repeated and eventually may result in death. As the thick, tenacious secretions accumulate in one or more bronchi, obstructions and dilatation result. The disease state progresses through irreversible bronchial damage to pulmonary insufficiency followed by death in 1 to 3 years. Without bronchial damage, antibiotics may hold the disease process in check. As the pulmonary disease progresses, the functioning alveoli are overaerated causing chest distention (compensatory emphysema). The child then displays a barrel-shaped chest.

Clubbing of the fingers and toes may also be noted. Hemolytic *Staphylococcus aureus* is the organism most commonly recovered from the child's nasopharynx, sputum, and lungs. Complications of severe pulmonary involvement include lobar atelectasis, lung abscesses, asphyxia, hemoptysis, spontaneous pneumothorax, emphysema, and cor pulmonale. Sinusitis may be demonstrable via x-ray, and the child may have a nasal voice, postnasal drip, and polyps.

Over 80 percent of children with cystic fibrosis have pancreatic involvement. Pancreatic insufficiency manifests itself through symptoms of intestinal malabsorption. Although the child has a voracious appetite, he may appear strikingly undernourished. His abdomen is distended, and his stools are frequent, bulky, fatty, and foul. Since most children are given prepared vitamins orally, vitamin deficiencies, with the exception of vitamin E, are usually absent. Diagnosis is made through family history, increase in sweat electrolyte concentration, absence of pancreatic enzymes, and chronic pulmonary disease. Although all four criteria may not be present, (1) a combination of increased sweat electrolytes and either pulmonary disease or pancreatic insufficiency or (2) a combination of pulmonary and pancreatic manifestations suggests cystic fibrosis.

The iontophoresis sweat test is simple and reliable in diagnosing this condition. A sweat chloride above 60 mEq/liter is diagnostic, and levels from 50 to 60 mEq/liter are suggestive. Sweat sodium values are approximately 10 mEq/liter higher than chloride. Chronic lung disease with emphysema is demonstrable by x-ray. Pulmonary function tests reveal increased residual lung volume, decreased ventilatory flow rates, increased airway resistance, and uneven gas distribution throughout the lungs. Pancreatic deficiency may be determined through examination of duodenal contents for pancreatic enzyme activity and a stool for trypsin content. Trypsin is absent in over 80 percent of affected children. Stools are also examined for fat content, and various other fat absorption tests may be ordered. Steatorrhea is present if the amount of fat in the feces is excessive. Serum electrolytes are normal unless the child has severe pulmonary disease.

About 50 percent of children with cystic fibrosis will survive to the age of 10 years. Thirty percent may reach the age of 20, and 20 percent may live to be 30 years of age.

The treatment of these children requires an interdisciplinary approach by the physician, nurse, physical therapist, and medical social worker. The child is allowed as nearly normal a life as possible, and care is taken to prevent his domination of the family. Children with severe pulmonary involvement need repeated intensive antibiotic therapy in the hospital, as do those with moderate pulmonary involvement when they have acute pulmonary exacerbations. The choice of drug is based upon results of culture and sensitivity of the offending pathogens. Physicians are not in agreement on continuous antibiotic therapy. Physical therapy is provided to promote bronchial drainage. A mist tent with aerosol solutions by nebulizer is also utilized to increase hydration of secretions, thereby facilitating expectoration. If oxygen therapy is needed, blood gas levels are monitored frequently to prevent carbon dioxide narcosis.

When the child returns home, physical therapy to the chest and aerosol by nebulizer at night are continued indefinitely. Some believe there is too great a risk for increasing resistance of bacteria to antibiotics, but others believe that severely ill patients cannot be adequately controlled without this therapy. At times, expectorants and bronchodilators may be helpful. During the winter months especially, a dry atmosphere may be combatted with nebulization of aerosol via tent. In the summer, temperatures within the tent may be uncomfortable. A room air conditioner will help to decrease the heat.

The pancreatic deficiency is treated through a high calorie, high protein, moderate fat diet in addition to pancreatic enzymes. A double dose of liposoluble vitamins prepared in a water-miscible liquid is given daily. Pancreatic extract is given with each meal.

Excessive perspiration in hot weather results in a great loss of sodium and chloride. An intravenous saline infusion to prevent cardiovascular collapse may be necessary. Thus, during hot weather supplemental sodium chloride should be given orally.

Nursing Management Observation, recording, and reporting of the character of feces will aid in assessment of pancreatic activity, while observation, recording, and reporting of the child's respiratory status will aid in assessment of pulmonary problems. Adequate preparation of the child, if he is old enough to understand, for sweat iontophoresis, chest x-ray, pulmonary function tests, nasopharyngeal cultures, duodenal aspiration, and stool collection will ensure better cooperation.

The nursing care for children receiving oxygen therapy is the same as that previously described. Although a physical therapist may be providing the chest therapy to promote bronchial drainage, it behooves the nurse to know these techniques in the event that the therapist cannot always come at specified times.

As the child nears discharge, the nurse should stress the importance of treating him as nearly normal as possible. For example, the child should be allowed to exercise and play according to his individual tolerance. The school-age child should attend regular classes when physically able. Parents should be included in the child's care whenever possible. Before he returns home, they must learn how to perform physical therapy to the chest, how to set up a mist tent with aerosol solution by nebulizer, and methods of giving pancreatic enzymes with meals. Parents are also instructed in ways of trying to prevent respiratory infection and are encouraged to ask questions and discuss fears.

Asthma

Asthma is an allergic manifestation characterized by smooth muscle spasm of bronchi and bronchioles in conjunction with edema and an overabundance of mucus. The lumens of the bronchi and bronchioles are narrowed because of spasm, resulting in the advent of signs and symptoms of lower respiratory tract obstruction. House dust can be the offender in children of any age, foods can be the allergen in younger children, and pollen and molds can be the incitant in older children.

In the child an asthmatic attack may occur after vigorous exercise or at night after he has fallen asleep. A poor parent-child relationship may also be responsible for the child's asthmatic episode. For example, severe attacks may reflect a child's struggle against an overprotective mother or his fear of being separated from her.

During an acute attack, a ball-valve type obstruction occurs (as explained in the discussion on bronchiolitis earlier in the chapter) in the smaller bronchi and the bronchioles owing to spasm and excessive mucus. The lungs become emphysematous. With frequent asthmatic episodes over a long period of time, chronic emphysema may develop because of the thickening of the bronchiolar walls and the child's persistent effort to aerate his lungs. Physical characteristics of this chronic condition include prominent sternum, rounded back, and increased anteroposterior chest circumference which produces the "barrel chest" so typically found in asthmatic children.

A diagnosis of asthma is more likely in the presence of the following data: a family history of asthma, repeated attacks of bronchiolitis in the same infant, eosinophilia, immediate positive response to epinephrine, sudden onset without preceding respiratory infection, or extremely prolonged expiration. Eczema in infancy may be a precursor of asthma in childhood. Bakwin and Bakwin suggest that children who have eczema associated with bronchial asthma have personalities similar to asthmatic children. They exhibit irritability, aggression, overanxiety, and insecurity.[19]

Diagnosis is based mainly on clinical findings. The onset may be abrupt or insidious. When a febrile incident precedes an attack, wheezing may occur for a day or two after the appearance of rhinorrhea. Resolution may take place in a few hours or a few days. An abrupt onset may be accompanied by a coughing paroxysm. Sometimes coughing is associated with itchiness of the chin, anterior part of the neck, or chest. As the attack progresses, increasing dyspnea, prolonged expiration, and expiratory rales occur. If the attack is severe, pulmonary ventilation is decreased. Flaring of the alae nasi, retractions, cyanosis, and hypercapnia indicate the air hunger which results. The child becomes restless and tired, his heart and respiratory rates increase, his sputum becomes tenacious, and he may perspire.

Eosinophils may be found in the peripheral blood, nasal secretions, and sputum. If the child has an accompanying infection, a polymorphonuclear leukocytosis may be present. Early in an acute attack, the P_{CO_2} may be normal. When it exceeds 50 or 60 mm Hg, the pH is apt to fall rapidly, and respiratory acidosis increases. At this time, assisted ventilation is necessary. Pulmonary function tests reveal diminished maximal breathing capacity, tidal volume, and timed vital capacity.

Confirmation of the diagnosis of bronchial asthma is made through chest x-ray, examinations of the sputum and peripheral blood, tests for hypersensitivity, and pulmonary function tests. Chest x-ray *may* indicate hyperventilation during an asthmatic attack through elevation of the rib cage, depression of the diaphragm, and increased translucency of the lung fields. Bronchial obstruction and infection may result in pneumonic consolidation, revealed in segmental or lobar collapse or patchy shadows.

In asthma, sputum is mucoid or mucopurulent. Bronchial casts and eosinophilia are present. With superimposed infection, bacteria and pus cells may be found.

Although the best evidence of an allergic causation for asthma is obtained through careful history-taking, skin testing for allergens may support an allergic basis for the disease process. Skin testing is accomplished through pricking or scratching especially prepared antigens into the skin of the forearm or through intradermal injection. Intradermal injection causes a more severe wheal and erythematous flare than pricking or scratching the skin.

Increased air resistance may be discovered through several pulmonary function tests. The forced expiratory volume in 1 second (FEV 1), FEV 1/FVC (forced vital capacity) ratio, and peak expiratory flow rate (PEFR) are decreased during an asthmatic attack. Total lung capacity (TLC) may be normal or increased in association with increased residual volume (RV) and functional residual capacity (FRC). Nevertheless, vital capacity is diminished. Following an asthmatic attack, these findings may return to normal with the exception of some persistence of increased RV. Uneven distribution of ventilation and decreased alveolar ventilation is confirmed with high VA/Q ratios (alveolar ventilation perfusion ratios). Serial recordings of FEV 1 or PEFR are valuable in determining progress and assessing the value of various therapeutic agents in long-term management of bronchial asthma. In the majority of children, asthma may be brought under control with adequate treatment.

Treatment consists of preventive measures, management of the acute attack, and long-term management. Preventive measures include hyposensitization, removal of incitants, and the use of bronchodilators. Treatment by hyposensitization seems to be most effective in seasonal asthma. The child who has gross pollen sensitivity is given a preseasonal course of pollen antigen injections which vary in number according to the preparation used. Although hyposensitization of children who are allergic to house dust, animal danders, molds, and various insects has been less effective in treatment than has hyposensitization to pollens, it is utilized in those children who cannot avoid contact with such antigens. Removal, as far as possible, of offending antigens is a more effective step in the general management of the asthmatic child, and the child may have to forego some household pets. Foam rubber pillows may be substituted for those containing feathers, and regular bed clothes may be replaced with bedding made entirely of man-made fibers. Additional precautions include plastic curtains, no rugs, no pets, and the destroying of moldy old dolls.

Bronchodilators used in the general management of asthma are described in Table 33-3. Ephedrine may be prescribed three or four times daily for the child who has mild asthma or at the beginning of an attack. Rapid, though sometimes short-lived, relief of symptoms may be derived from isoprenaline aerosol (isopropylnorepinephrine). Aminophylline,

Table 33-3 BRONCHODILATORS FOR ASTHMATIC CHILDREN

Drug	Rationale	Action	Method	Dosage	Side effects
Ephedrine	Prophylactic relief of nocturnal paroxysms and wheezing with exercise	Slow; prolonged duration; bronchodilation	Oral	Varies from 8 mg for preschooler to 25 mg for older children	Tachycardia. Central nervous system stimulant. Vomiting.
Pseudoephedrine	Same as ephedrine	Same as ephedrine	Oral	About twice the dose of ephedrine	Relatively free of side effects.
Epinephrine	Severe asthma; relief of paroxysm	Rapid; short duration; bronchodilation	1:1000 solution s.c. 1:100 solution by inhalation *(never used for injection)*	Small doses at 20–30 min intervals; 0.05 ml for infant; 0.2 to 0.3 ml for older child	Pallor, tachycardia, and palpitation
Epinephrine aqueous suspension	Relief of paroxysm, especially frequent ones	Rapid, sustained (8–10 hours)	1:200 aqueous suspension s.c.	Maximum single dose 0.15 ml, 0.005 ml/kg	Anxiety, restlessness, tremor, headache, dizziness, pallor, respiratory weakness, and palpitation
Ethylnorepinephrine	Same as epinephrine	Same as epinephrine	s.c. or I.V.	Same as epinephrine	Relatively free of side effects
Isopropylnorepinephrine	Relief of paroxysm	Same as epinephrine	Aerosol: *Use must be supervised by an adult.*	1 to 2 "puffs" or sprays at ½ to 1 hr intervals—*total daily "puffs"* 4 to 6	Status asthmaticus with prolonged use. Overdose with daily use: hypotension and cardiac arrest.
Aminophylline	Relief of paroxysm when ephedrine has failed	Slow; prolonged; bronchodilation	Suppository: only whole suppository given as drug unevenly distributed. Orally in chlorine preparation or as elixir. I.V. in a 2.5% sol. *slowly* to avoid cardiac arrythmias or hypertension.	3–4 mg/kg q. 8 h. Total daily dose by all routes should not exceed 12 mg/kg.	Initial signs of toxicity, increasing restlessness, irritability, and vomiting. Life-threatening signs of toxicity, increasing excitement or delirium, vomiting of blood and convulsions. N.B. *Never* given in conjunction with epinephrine or ephedrine *unless aminophylline dosage reduced.* Otherwise, toxic effects potentiated.

Note: s.c. = subcutaneous.

531

by suppository at night, may provide relief from nocturnal wheezing. Chromolyn sodium, a recent drug for *chronic use only* may be prescribed for children 5 years of age and older. This drug is supplied in 20-mg capsules. The powder of one capsule is emptied into a special turboinhaler. The medication is readily absorbed by the lungs. Since it is short-acting, it is inhaled every 6 hours. Chromolyn sodium is prescribed as an adjunct to existing treatment, as a seasonal additive, and for steroid-dependent children. Since it inhibits the release of histamine and slow-reacting substance of anaphylaxis (SRS-A), chromolyn sodium has a prophylactic action and, therefore, has *no role in the treatment of an acute asthmatic attack, particularly status asthmaticus.*

During the early stages of an *acute asthmatic attack*, if the preceding general measures have failed to provide relief, two alternative bronchodilators that may be given are epinephrine and aminophylline (see Table 33-3). The most useful agents for the relief of dyspnea are epinephrine and its analogues. Epinephrine given subcutaneously provides rapid relief. If the child becomes unresponsive to epinephrine, diphenhydramine intravenously *may* reestablish responsiveness. When epinephrine has failed to provide relief, aminophylline (theophylline ethylenediamine) or other preparations in which theophylline is the active principle may afford relief of a paroxysm. These drugs are used cautiously because of the severe reactions which may occur (see Table 33-3).

Expectorants may be utilized in conjunction with epinephrine and its analogues. Some physicians advocate a mixture of equal parts of syrup of hydroidic acid and syrup of ephedrine or pseudoephedrine according to the child's need for ephedrine. Other physicians may prefer potassium iodide and potassium quaiacholate in combination with syrup of ephedrine or pseudoephedrine. Cold or warm vaporized water inhalations may add to the child's comfort.

If sedatives are prescribed, they are used sparingly because of their unpredictable effects, and opiates are contraindicated. Adequate hydration is provided. If acidosis occurs due to inadequate gas exchange, sodium bicarbonate is given intravenously. This correction of acidosis may reestablish responsiveness to the epinephrine-fast child. With the advent of cyanosis, oxygen is administered.

If the child does not receive adequate relief within several hours from the drugs and supportive measures mentioned, a corticosteroid may be prescribed. The use of corticosteroids in the management of the asthmatic child is limited. Growth retardation and steroid dependency may result from prolonged use. Therefore, most physicians will prescribe one or two doses of 25 mg cortisone orally, the second dose being administered 8 to 12 hours after the first.

When a child with severe asthma fails to respond to epinephrine or aminophylline, he is in *status asthmaticus*. During a prolonged or unusually severe attack, the child may be unable to move tenacious secretions from the bronchioles. Fatigue and diminishing pulmonary function result, breath sounds become diminished or absent, and cyanosis appears. With the resultant rise of the arterial P_{CO_2}, a mixed acidosis occurs: respiratory acidosis due to retention of carbon dioxide and metabolic acidosis due to anoxia. If the P_{CO_2} rises above 60 mm, assisted ventilation is usually prescribed. Positive pressure breathing by mask may be intermittent or continuous (see Figs. 33-7 and 33-8). If the child is unable to help in this method, for any reason, assisted ventilation is provided via an endotracheal or a nasotracheal tube. When an endotracheal tube is in place, aspiration of secretions from the bronchial tree is facilitated, and bronchial lavage with warm physiologic saline solution may be accomplished. Sometimes a tracheostomy is necessary to provide adequate assisted ventilation and bronchial lavage. Cupped-hand percussion to the chest and postural drainage may facilitate bronchial aspiration (see Fig. 33-3).

The child who is receiving such heroic measures of care requires the cooperation of physician, anesthesiologist, nurse, inhalation therapist, and physical therapist. Also, continuous monitoring of body temperature, electrocardiograms, central venous pressure, and peripheral arterial pressure require an intensive-care setting. Arterial blood must be examined frequently for pH, P_{CO_2}, and O_2 in order to provide adequate control of ventilation. The child's electrolyte balance is identified through determination of serum sodium, potassium, and chloride values. The heroic measures taken to save the child in status asthmaticus may result in complications such as pneumomediastinum, pneumothorax, subcutaneous emphysema, cardiac arrest, and tracheal or glottic stenosis.

Long-term management of the asthmatic child consists of adequate drug therapy, avoidance of precipitating factors, physical therapy, and psychotherapy as necessary. With asthma of mild or moderate severity, ephedrine preparations and isopropylnorepinephrine are used intermittently to suppress attacks. Precipitating factors include known allergens, respiratory infections, and respiratory obstruction due to enlarged tonsils and adenoids. Known allergens are avoided, if possible. Respiratory

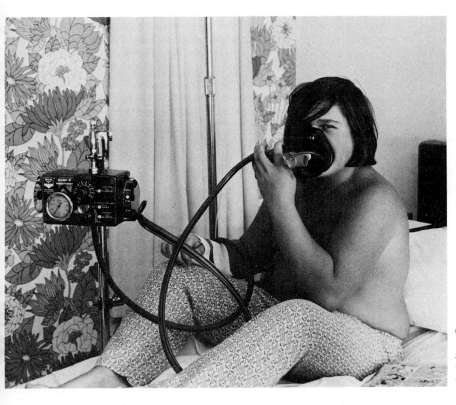

Figure 33-7   An adolescent administering his own IPPB. *(Courtesy of Children's Hospital Medical Center, Boston. Photograph by Boston University School of Nursing, Media Services Department.)*

infections caused by bacteria are treated with specific antibiotics. Since tonsillar and adenoid tissues diminish following adequate allergic management, their removal is not undertaken unless the child fails to respond to an adequate program of allergic management, including hyposensitization. The physical therapist can teach the child how to improve ventilation by controlling his breathing pattern. The need for psychotherapy will depend on the degree of warmth and insight parents exhibit in responding to the child and the child's response to the parents. Educating the parents about the child's real needs may be all that is indicated. If conflicts and anxieties within the family seem to initiate or perpetuate severe attacks, psychiatric consultation may be necessary. In most instances, tensions and adverse family situations are amenable to psychotherapy.

Nursing Management   During the early stages of an asthmatic attack, the nurse cooperates with the physician in providing therapy. The nurse observes the child for and reports side effects of prescribed drugs (see Table 33-3) and provides cold or warm vaporized inhalations as ordered. If acidosis occurs and sodium bicarbonate is to be given intravenously, the rate and flow of the fluid are monitored carefully to prevent overloading the heart. When the nurse observes that the child eats slowly in the presence of increased respiratory difficulty, the child is allowed sufficient time to eat and is provided with small, frequent meals. This regimen is less tiring than large meals at longer intervals.

If the nurse observes cyanosis, oxygen is administered, usually by way of a mist tent. In this way vapor and oxygen are supplied. A sitting position with the child's arms on arm rests provides greater chest expansion than a reclining position. The child needs adequate rest and seems more comfortable in a sitting position.

The nurse, by sharing with the physician and psychiatrist his observations of the child's behavior with other hospitalized children and hospital personnel, can help identify the emotional factors involved in the child's asthmatic attacks. Information about mother/child interactions during hospitalization will also be helpful. If emotional factors contribute to asthmatic attacks, the child should be kept as calm as possible through simple amusements and quiet play with other children. Although the nurse is patient with the child, limits are set. Inconsistency tends to create emotional conflicts which increase respiratory difficulty.

The child in status asthmaticus is too ill to com-

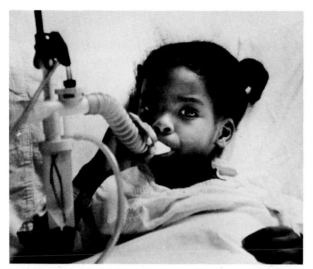

Figure 33-8 A preschooler administering her own IPPB. *(Courtesy of Boston City Hospital. Photograph by Boston University School of Nursing, Media Services Department.)*

prehend explanations of the heroic measures being carried out. The nurse can provide some reassurance for the child through a running commentary on what is happening and the use of touch. Parental anxiety may be relieved somewhat with an explanation of what is happening and what these measures can accomplish.

When the child no longer requires intensive care, the nurse can teach his parents about home treatment by involving them in the child's care in the hospital. The nurse explains to the parents how to avoid known allergens, including respiratory infections. The physical therapist can teach the parents chest percussion and postural drainage. Both mother and child are taught how to use the nebulizer or aerosol equipment and the importance of avoiding overuse of aerosol medications. If the child is to attend nursery school, the nurse may be involved in calling a team conference with the teacher, the school nurse, and the mother to ensure that nursery school personnel understand the problem.

Acute Pharyngitis

In most upper respiratory infections, pharyngeal involvement is present. In its strictest sense, acute pharyngitis refers to all infectious conditions in which the principal site of involvement is the throat. Since the presence or absence of the tonsils does not affect the frequency, course, or complications of or susceptibility to the illness, the term "pharyn-

gitis" includes tonsillitis and pharyngotonsillitis. The peak incidence of the disease occurs between the fourth and seventh years of life. Though generally caused by viruses, group A β-hemolytic streptococci are found in approximately 15 percent of affected children.

Clinically, it is difficult to distinguish viral from streptococcal pharyngitis because of overlapping signs and symptoms. In *viral* pharyngitis, the onset is gradual with early signs of fever, malaise, and anorexia. Within a day or so, the child complains of a sore throat. This discomfort reaches its peak in a day or two. Rhinitis, hoarseness, and cough are commonly noted. Usually, pharyngeal inflammation is slight. Moderately enlarged and firm lymph nodes are generally discovered. The white blood cell count may be normal or as high as 30,000/cu mm with a predominance of polymorphonuclear leukocytes in the early stages of the infection. The duration ranges from 24 hours to 5 days.

In *streptococcal* pharyngitis, the child's initial complaints consist of headache, abdominal pain, and vomiting. Although fever occasionally does not occur for several hours, initial symptoms may be accompanied by a fever of 40°C (104°F). In several hours, the child may complain of a sore throat, which may be mild or severe enough to make swallowing difficult. Approximately one-third of affected children have tonsillar enlargement, exudation, and pharyngeal erythema. The other two-thirds may have only mild erythema, with slight tonsillar enlargement, and no exudate. Tender anterior cervical lymphadenopathy occurs early, and fever may last from 1 to 4 days. If the child is severely ill, he may be incapacitated for as long as 2 weeks.

Since 10 to 15 percent of normal children carry group A streptococci in their throats, a positive throat culture is not necessarily conclusive evidence of streptococcal pharyngitis. Complications with viral pharyngitis are rare, although purulent otitis media may occur. The complications which may be manifested following streptococcal pharyngitis include peritonsillar abscess, sinusitis, otitis media, and, rarely, meningitis. Acute glomerulonephritis and rheumatic fever are generally allergic manifestations of the toxins emitted by group A β-hemolytic streptococci. Therefore, children with proved streptococcal pharyngitis are reexamined 2 to 3 weeks following thier illness.

No known specific therapy is available for viral pharyngitis. Streptococcal infections respond well to penicillin. The present recommendation is LA Bicillin to eliminate the compliance problem. If a clinical response is not noted within 24 hours following an appropriate dose of penicillin, streptococcal infection is ruled out unless complications are present. In proved streptococcal infections, oral penicillin therapy, if prescribed, is continued for 10 days. If the child is allergic to penicillin, erythromycin is a satisfactory substitute.

Although peritonsillar and retrotonsillar abscesses are usually found after 5 years of age, they may accompany a pharyngotonsillitis. A *peritonsillar abscess* displaces the tonsil backward and pushes the uvula to the opposite side, whereas a *retrotonsillar abscess* displaces the tonsil forward. The child complains of severe throat pain, has progressive difficulty in opening the mouth due to spasms of the pterygoid muscles, and may refuse to swallow or speak. Fever may reach 40.5°C (105°F). Without treatment, either type of abscess becomes fluctuant and will point in a few days. Unless the abscess is incised, spontaneous rupture occurs. An intensive regime of penicillin G may prevent suppuration. Analgesics are prescribed for the relief of pain. As soon as the abscess becomes fluctuant, it is incised, and antibiotics are continued. After the inflammation has subsided, tonsillectomy is scheduled in 3 to 4 weeks.

Nursing Management The child with acute pharyngitis may or may not be hospitalized. If the course of the illness is only 1 to 2 days, he most likely will be treated at home. If the child is hospitalized, nursing care is symptomatic. The child needs rest, and quiet play activities are provided. When a child's fever is 38.9°C (102°F), the prescribed antipyretic is given. If his temperature is 39.5°C (103°F), a sponge bath with tepid water is given. Excoriation around the nostrils due to rhinitis can be prevented by gently swabbing with cotton-tipped applicators and using a soothing skin ointment. The child should be observed for allergic reactions to penicillin.

If the child has a sore throat, either hot or cold compresses to the neck will provide relief; the child can decide which method he prefers. If the child knows how to gargle, warm saline gargles are effective in relieving the pain of a severely sore throat. Aspirin may also be prescribed. If the child experiences pain on swallowing, cool bland liquids are tolerated well. No attempt should be made to force the child to eat. Dyspnea and symptoms of respiratory obstruction are indicative of peritonsillar or retrotonsillar abscess. The nursing care is similar to that described for the infant with retropharyngeal abscess.

Tonsillitis

Tonsils and adenoids are lymphoid tissues circling the pharynx and are part of *Waldeyer's ring*. Adenoids are, in reality, the *pharyngeal tonsil*. Those lymphoid structures commonly referred to as tonsils are found on either side of the pharynx and are called *faucial* tonsils. Waldeyer's ring is thought to filter and protect against invasion of the respiratory and alimentary tracts by pathogenic microorganisms. It is also believed to have a role in antibody formation.

Up to the age of 5 years, the child's susceptibility to respiratory infection is greater than in later childhood. Tonsils are normally relatively larger at this time than in later years. As a child's immunity increases through immunizations and exposure to respiratory infections, the protective function of Waldeyer's ring decreases. Therefore, tonsillectomy is usually delayed until 4 to 5 years of age.

Acute tonsillitis has been considered in the section on acute pharyngitis. Principal tonsillar disturbances are infection and hypertrophy which is usually secondary to infection. When tonsils are chronically hypertrophic and infected, the child is said to have *chronic tonsillitis*.

Clinical manifestations of chronic tonsillitis include a persistent sore throat or repeated attacks of sore throats. Complaints of obstruction to swallowing or breathing are usually the result of hypertrophied adenoids. Although some children complain of dryness and irritation in the throat and may have an offensive breath odor, these symptoms are not diagnostic. Chronically infected tonsils may be large or small. Enlargement of cervical lymph nodes provides supportive evidence of infection.

Clinical manifestations of chronic *adenoiditis* include mouth breathing and persistent rhinitis. If mouth breathing is constant, rather than only during sleep, the mucous membranes of the mouth and lips are dry. Frequent or constant chronic nasopharyngitis may be present. Other manifestations include a nasal, muffled voice; a harassing cough; offensive breath; and impairment of taste, smell, and hearing. Confirmation of the diagnosis is made by palpation, visual examination with a pharyngeal mirror, or x-ray. Chronic otitis media may be associated with chronic adenoiditis.

Indications for removal of faucial tonsils include chronic infection, hypertrophy, and peritonsillar and retrotonsillar abscesses. Tonsillectomy and adenoidectomy may be recommended for persistent diphtheria carriers. When the clinical manifestations of chronic adenoiditis are present, adenoidectomy is recommended.

Although surgical removal of both tonsils and adenoids may be accomplished at the same time, during infancy adenoidectomy alone may be indicated. Faucial tonsils are rarely removed in a child under 3 years of age. Often, when the operation is postponed beyond 3 years of age, the need disappears within a year. The need for adenoidectomy, though infrequent, is more common in these first few years of life than is tonsillectomy. Generally, tonsillectomy is postponed until 2 to 3 weeks after an infection has subsided.

Preoperatively, a complete history, including bleeding tendencies, is taken; a thorough physical examination is conducted, including observation for loose teeth; bleeding and clotting times are determined. Preoperative medications include a barbiturate and atropine. Food is withheld for several hours before surgery.

Postoperatively, the child is kept in bed for the remainder of the day. Eating and drinking are encouraged as soon as nausea from the anesthetic has disappeared. Allowing the child to rinse his mouth with an alkaline solution will help remove the disagreeable taste he is experiencing. Aspirin may relieve discomfort. Discharge instructions include rest at home for several days and avoidance of contact with infection.

The efficacy of tonsillectomy lies in the decrease of persistent throat infections, removal of diphtheria bacilli from carriers, and a decreased incidence of cervical lymphadenitis. Following adenoidectomy, the function of affected senses should improve.

Nursing Management The treatment for chronic tonsillitis and adenoiditis is surgical removal. Preoperatively, the nurse working in the clinic or the doctor's office may observe that both mother and child have questions about the operation. The nurse should talk with the mother about the nature of the operation and preparation for admission. Information the mother can then impart to the child includes the facts that his tonsils are causing his sore throats and he will be better off without them. The mother can help prepare the child for what will happen by reading a book to him about a child who undergoes a tonsillectomy.

Some hospitals provide tours of pediatric tonsillectomy care units for parents and children under the direction of a pediatric nurse. At this time, children may familiarize themselves with the surroundings and ask questions about hospitalization and tonsillectomy.

When the child is admitted to the hospital, he is given a complete physical examination, and his bleeding and clotting times are checked. Before the child goes to surgery early in the morning, the nurse checks his mouth for loose teeth and administers his preoperative medications.

Postoperatively, the child is brought to the recovery room where all necessary equipment is available. In order to facilitate drainage, the child is placed partly on his side and partly on his chest with his uppermost knee flexed (semiprone) until he is alert and can handle his own secretions. During this time, he is observed for adequate drainage, bleeding, and aspiration.

Quality and rate of pulse, degree of restlessness, and frequency of swallowing and vomiting are noted. A persistent pulse rate of 120 per minute while the child is quiet, pallor, and continuous swallowing are indicative of hemorrhage. Normally, with a combination of preoperative atropine and dehydration, the child's face is flushed. Involuntary continuous swallowing (five to six times per minute) may be due to a small trickle of blood within the mouth. If this swallowing persists, the stomach will fill with blood and emesis result. The surgeon should be notified of rising pulse rate, pallor, and continuous swallowing; he may have the child returned to surgery to prevent hemorrhage.

Once the child is alert, he may be more comfortable if he is allowed to sit upright. In an hour or two, he may have chipped ice or flavored popsicles, small amounts of clear liquids, and gelatin desserts. Aspirin chewing gum and an ice collar are helpful in relieving a sore throat. The act of eating provides a better blood supply to the throat, inducing more rapid healing. The nurse encourages the child to eat small servings of soft food. A small breakfast should be served as though the nurse expects the child to eat.

The night of the operative day, the nurse should observe the child for and report blood trickling from the nose and mouth, the presence of fresh blood in vomitus, and pallor. Cyanosis indicates obstruction—the surgeon is notified. Raising the child by his hips and slapping him between the shoulder blades usually clears the airway. Another method is to pull the child's head and shoulders over the side of the bed and slap him between the shoulder blades. If the nurse cannot keep the tongue forward by supporting the jaw, the jaw muscles are probably in spasm. The nurse should then open the child's mouth and apply a tongue depressor. Tongue forceps may be needed to pull the tongue forward. The child is then suctioned to remove accumulated secretions.

The child is discharged the day after surgery if his temperature is normal and there are no complications. Parents are instructed that the child should eat only soft, easily swallowed foods for several days. His activities are restricted for about one week. Instructions should include other suggestions for the mother to follow in caring for the child and information about any prescribed medications. If the child does not have a private physician, the mother should be given the name and telephone number of a physician to call for advice or emergency care and the location and place where the child will receive follow-up care. Specific instructions vary with physicians and institutions. Printed instruction sheets are usually available, and the nurse may review this printed material with the child and parent.

Mumps (Infectious Parotitis)

The child with *mumps*, an acute contagious generalized viral disease caused by one of the myxoviruses, usually presents with painful enlargement of the salivary glands, primarily the parotids. The immune mother provides the infant a temporary immunity for the first 6 to 8 months of life. Any clinical or subclinical infection produces life-long immunity. Mumps is spread by direct contact, airborne droplet nuclei, and fomites contaminated by infectious saliva. The disease may be transmitted person-to-person from 24 hours before to 3 days following the appearance of parotid swelling.

Initially, the virus is believed to multiply in the cells of the respiratory tract, from where it enters the bloodstream and travels to many tissues, causing swelling. The majority of affected children are under 15 years of age. Although epidemics may occur at any time during a given year, they are slightly more frequent in late winter and spring. The incubation period lasts from 14 to 24 days, reaching a peak at 17 to 18 days. Prodromal symptoms, though rare, include fever, muscular pain, headache, and malaise.

The usual presenting clinical manifestation is pain and swelling in one or both parotid glands. If bilateral, one gland is generally affected 1 to 2 days prior to the other. Since edema of the skin and surrounding tissues extends beyond the glandular swelling, the condition is readily seen. Maximum size is reached within a few hours, with a peak in 1 to 3 days. The taste of sour liquids and highly seasoned foods produce pain. The tonsil on the affected side may be displaced medially because of edema of the pharynx and soft palate. The child may complain of pain when opening his mouth. Fever rarely reaches 40°C (104°F) or greater. The causative virus may be recovered from saliva, urine, spinal fluid, or blood. Complications include meningoencephalitis, orchitis, epididymitis, oophoritis, pancreatitis, nephritis, myocarditis, mastitis, deafness, dacryoadenitis, optic neuritis, arthritis, and thrombocytopenic purpura. Meningoencephalitis is the most common complication in childhood. Orchitis and epididymitis are common after 14 years of age and rarely result in *complete* infertility. Other complications are rare, although mumps is considered to be a leading cause of unilateral nerve deafness.

Treatment is symptomatic. Bed rest does not prevent complications. Diet is governed by the child's ability to chew. Lumbar puncture relieves the headache which accompanies meningoencephalitis. Local support and bed rest is the treatment for orchitis, and corticosteroids relieve the pain accompanying this condition but do not prevent atrophy.

Mumps vaccine may be given as part of the child's immunization schedule at the physician's discretion but may have to be repeated at a later date. This vaccine does have a protective effect against exposure and may, therefore, be given to exposed adults and adolescents. Immunity may be detected by the presence of CF antibodies to the V (viral) antigen of mumps and by a positive skin reaction similar to the tuberculin skin test.

Nursing Management Since mumps is contagious, the hospitalized child with this suspected diagnosis is placed in isolation for several days. If at home, he is separated from other children and susceptible adults for several days. An ice collar may relieve local pain, or a sedative may be ordered. The nurse develops the child's diet in accordance with an assessment of his ability to chew. Citrus and tomato juices, pickles, and highly seasoned foods are avoided. If the child has a fever, nose and mouth care as well as sponge baths may afford comfort.

The advent of sudden fever, headache, vomiting, moderate stiffness of the neck, and possibly convulsions 3 to 10 days following the onset of the disease should alert the nurse to the possibility of meningoencephalitis. Within 8 days of parotitis, an abrupt onset of fever, chills, headache, nausea, and lower abdominal pain in the adolescent male could spell the presence of orchitis. The nurse should report symptoms of meningoencephalitis and orchitis to the physician.

While the child is isolated, the nurse instructs the parents in precautionary measures. If parents and other family members are susceptible to mumps, they need to know that mumps vaccine is available.

The child may return to school after the swelling has subsided.

RESPIRATORY DISEASES AND DEVIATIONS IN THE ADOLESCENT
Viral Respiratory Infections

About one-half of all respiratory infections in children and adolescents are caused by viruses which can be identified in the laboratory. A majority of these infections are not influenced by antibiotics, and the treatment is symptomatic. It is important to understand the great variation in the frequency of viral infection which changes from season to season and area to area.

To compound the problem further, one virus may result in the presentation of multiple symptoms, and several viruses may also be involved in one clinical syndrome. While it is true that the respiratory tract is limited in its responses to an infection, it is also true that the clinical manifestations presented by a patient depend on the resistance of that person.

Many viruses change their antigenic properties over a period of years; therefore vaccines and natural infections fail to provide protection to the host. Although some vaccines are available for immunization against respiratory diseases due to influenza, parainfluenza, adenovirus, and rhinovirus, they are of limited value. In the case of the influenza virus, the vaccine is usually prepared from the most recent, current antigenic variant, and good immunity can be induced for a short period of time.

Influenza pneumonia can be very serious in some children and adolescents. This viral infection leads to a decrease in lung compliance, an increase in alveolar fluid, and an increase in pulmonary venous pressure; therefore, patients with heart disease, cystic fibrosis, and asthma are prone to pulmonary decompensation.

Three large categories of viral agents are responsible for many respiratory infections seen in pediatrics; they are the myxovirus, the adenovirus, and the picornavirus groups. Table 33-4 includes the most common viruses within each category.

Nursing Management   Viral upper respiratory infections are common in children and adolescents. Often hospitalization is not necessary. A proper diet and an adequate amount of sleep strengthen a person's resistance to these infections. The nurse should teach the concepts of good health whenever the opportunity arises.

In almost all instances treatment is symptomatic. Should a child be febrile, fluids should be encouraged and antipyretics should be given as ordered. Complaints of "aches and pains" may require confinement to bed. Isolation decreases exposure and hence communicability. Adenoviruses may cause a conjunctivitis which a youngster finds bothersome, and compresses may be helpful. Ulcerations, found in herpangina, and located in the oropharynx, are uncomfortable. Mouth washes will bring relief.

Patients with asthma, cystic fibrosis, and heart disease may become more seriously ill as a result of pulmonary complications. In those instances, assessing their respiratory status and administering humidified oxygen may be necessary. Viral infections render any patient more susceptible to secondary bacterial infections such as pneumococcus, staphylococcus, and streptococcus.

Primary Atypical Pneumonia
(Mycoplasma pneumoniae)

Pleuropneumonia-like organisms (PPLO) are the smallest known microorganisms of the genus *Mycoplasma*. Within this group, *M. pneumoniae* is the cause of a respiratory problem identified as primary atypical pneumonia. Commonly affecting adolescents, it may result in pneumonia; however, it has also been responsible for the development of bronchitis and upper respiratory disease. While the prevalence varies from year to year, the lowest incidence is usually found during the summer months. The disease spreads readily among college students, military recruits, and families.

Adenoviruses, influenza viruses A and B, parainfluenza viruses, and RS virus have also been the cause of atypical pneumonia. After an incubation period of 10 to 20 days, there is a rapid onset of fever, malaise, and persistent cough. Chills, headache, and conjunctivitis occasionally develop. A rhinitis will be evident, enlarged cervical nodes are present, and decreased breath sounds are heard.

The microorganism is usually isolated from the nasopharynx, and x-ray findings show an infiltration from the hilum to the periphery. Usually this disease lasts 1 to 2 weeks with otitis media occasionally developing. Since *M. pneumoniae* is resistant to penicillin, tetracycline and erythromycin are frequently prescribed.

Nursing Management   Symptomatic treatment is important. Humid aerosol therapy is important in loosening tenacious mucus. Postural drainage also should facilitate its removal. These adolescents must have more than an adequate amount of fluids, and they should be allowed to assume this responsibility.

Table 33-4 COMMON VIRAL INFECTIONS

	Virology/epidemiology	Clinical manifestations	Laboratory results	Treatment
1 Myxoviruses				
a Influenza virus	Influenza virus type A has a tendency to develop many variant strains. It is recognized in swine, horses, ducks, and fowl as well as man. This type is commonly encountered in epidemic form, rising abruptly and spreading rapidly, especially from early autumn to late spring. Types B and C are found only in man, and the latter appears infrequently. Effective immunity is type-specific and strain-specific, and its duration is short. Although it has a low mortality rate, the morbidity rate can be 10–30% of the population. Entry is gained through respiratory mucus-producing epithelial cells.	Incubation period is 1–2 days, followed by chills, aches, pains, and temperature of 38.3–40°C (101–104°F). Some diseases such as croup, bronchitis, bronchiolitis, and upper respiratory infections (URI) can occur in the presence of this virus.	Blood counts are usually within normal limits; however, leukocytosis may be present. Nasal and throat washings identify causative agent.	Primarily symptomatic. Secondary infections by staphylococci are common in children, and antibiotics may be ordered until the results of the bacterial cultures are obtained.
b Parainfluenza virus	Types 1, 2, 3, and 4 are found in monkeys, mice, pigs, cows, and man. These infections are endemic, and although there are seasonal peaks, they are more commonly found in the colder months.	Mild rhinitis, pharyngitis, and a fever which lasts 1–2 days. Type 1 is commonly associated with croup. Type 3 is responsible for some cases of bronchitis and bronchiolitis found in children. All 4 types are found in adolescents and adults suffering from upper respiratory infections.	Nasopharyngeal cultures identifying the virus.	Supportive in all instances.
c Respiratory syncytial virus (RS virus)	There appears to be one type of RS virus which is found in chimpanzees and man. It is widely distributed, appearing in the colder months, in thickly populated areas, spreading from person to person. Reinfections are frequent and may result in severe lower respiratory tract infections.	Low-grade fever, coryza, sore throat, and cough. Infection in infants may result in bronchiolitis and pneumonia; adolescents and adults may develop URIs. Pneumonias which evolve can be severe.	Leukocyte count is 5,000–20,000/cu mm. Diagnosis made on identifying the agent through culturing and a rise in titer during convalescence.	Symptomatic except in those instances where respiratory complications are evident.

(Continued)

539

Table 33-4 COMMON VIRAL INFECTIONS *(Continued)*

	Virology/epidemiology	Clinical manifestations	Laboratory results	Treatment
2 Adenoviruses	About 28 different types of adenovirus are known to man. More common in the summer months but there are peaks in the winter and spring. Frequently seen in summer camps and military barracks. Although primarily endemic types 3, 4, and 7 have been involved in epidemics. Antibodies for types 1 and 2 are usually found in children, while antibodies for types 3, 4, 5, 6, and 7 are found in adolescents and adults. Entry may be through conjunctiva as well as respiratory tract.	Temperatures up to 39.4–40°C (103–104°F) lasting 1–10 days, sore throat, conjunctivitis, headache, and listlessness. Acute respiratory disease (ARD) is associated with this virus. Its onset is gradual, the temperature is 37.8–40°C (100–104°F); chills headache, and malaise are characteristic. Coryza, cough, and sore throat appear less commonly. Types 4 and 7 are associated with ARD.	Pharyngeal, ocular, and lower respiratory tract secretions are used in the identification. Antibody titer rises during convalescence which aids in diagnosing cause; however, it identifies an adenoviral infection but gives no clue regarding the specific type.	Symptomatic. Secondary bacterial infections are rare.
3 Picornaviruses *a* Rhinovirus (formerly called "common cold viruses" or coryzaviruses)	There are two large subgroups, H and M. The M strains occur in winter and spring months, while H strains are more common in the summer and fall. Rhinoviral infections are transferred from one person to another. Viruses are recovered from nasal secretions and throats prior to the onset of the illness and 1 to 6 days after. The incubation period is 2 days.	Symptoms of cold including a slight sore throat, nasal stuffiness, sneezing, mild headache, and fever.	Identification of virus from nasopharyngeal secretions.	Symptomatic. Antibiotics are contraindicated unless a secondary bacterial infection occurs.
b Enteroviruses (1) Coxsackie viruses A, B	There are 23 types of Coxsackie group A, and 6 types of Coxsackie group B. It is encountered in populated areas throughout the world. Transferred from person to person by direct contact, flies, and dogs. Communicability seems to be highest in the home environment. It has been recovered from nasopharyngeal secretions and feces.	All signs indicate acute respiratory illness. A9 is sometimes found in patients with pneumonia. A21 is frequently cultured out in adolescents and young adults with respiratory problems, while B3 and 5 have been found in patients with croup, bronchiolitis, pneumonia, and pleurisy.	Isolation of virus in laboratory confirms diagnosis. There is an increase in antibodies.	Complete recovery after symptomatic treatment, except in newborn infants, in whom infection with a group B virus may be very, very serious.

The incubation period ranges from 1–14 days with a mean of 3–5 days. Coxsackie B viruses are found in outbreaks of febrile respiratory illnesses in families, camps, and institutions, especially in the summer and fall. Coxsackie A, types 1–6, 8, 10, and 22 have been associated with herpangina, a febrile, acute, self-limiting disease. It is seen in the summer months; onset is rapid; incubation period 2–4 days.	Temperature to 40.6°C (105°F) for 1–4 days with anorexia, dysphagia, sore throat, headaches, abdominal pain, red pharynx, ulcers of the soft palate, uvula, and other areas of oropharynx.	White blood cell count is normal or just slightly elevated.	Recovery is usually uncomplicated after symptomatic treatment.
(2) Echo viruses About 30 types of echo virus are known. Infection with this virus is much more common in warm seasons, in lower socioeconomic conditions, and among children. More frequently found in feces than in the oropharynx. Occasionally an exanthum has been associated with echo infections.	Echo type 11 is found in adults and children with acute respiratory infections. Pharyngitis and conjunctivitis are also seen in these patients.	Causative agent is identified after culturing oropharyngeal secretions. The antibody titre rise is significant.	Symptomatic.

Intravenous therapy may be instituted in the young child who is hospitalized and dyspneic.

Again, since adolescents and college students may develop this disease more than any other age group, health teaching should be done routinely. The need for a balanced diet and adequate sleep should be emphasized.

Tuberculosis

Childhood tuberculosis (TB) and its many manifestations are usually considered a single disease entity with the initial infection demonstrated in the lungs and complications seen in all parts of the body. Although the tubercle bacillus, *Mycobacterium tuberculosis*, is usually inhaled through droplets from an adult with active pulmonary tuberculosis, it may be ingested or enter through an abrasion in the skin or mucous membranes.

There is no evidence of a genetic predisposition to tuberculous infection, but the following factors should be considered: the resistance of the person, the defenses of the host, the virulence of the invading organisms, the size of the infecting dose, and the number of bacilli present.

In the United States, nonwhites, particularly the American Indians, have a higher mortality rate from TB, a fact that may be attributed to poor hygiene and environmental conditions, such as inadequate housing. Both factors present opportunities for frequent reinfections. The fatality rate is highest in infancy and adolescence, with the mortality and morbidity greatest in females in late childhood and adolescence. Chronic fatigue, chronic illness, and malnutrition may also reduce resistance to TB.

Once the invasion into the parenchyma of the lung has occurred, the bacilli create a small inflammatory area, the primary focus. Simultaneously bacilli begin to migrate through the lymphatics to the nearest lymph nodes which drain the area. The combination of the primary focus and the regional lymph node involvement is known as the *primary complex*.

In the affected area of the lung polymorphonuclear leukocytes accumulate, followed by the formation of epithelioid cells. In the process of proliferating, they surround the bacilli and create the typical, walled-off tubercle formation. Eventually, the lesion becomes calcified in children.

The incubation period for tuberculosis varies, with 2 weeks the minimum and 10 weeks the maximum; however, the average range appears to be 3 to 5 weeks. At the end of that time hypersensitivity is evident in the positive tuberculin reaction which occurs if the causative organisms are present in the body of the host. There may be no other symptoms present in the child except the positive skin test. Although an early diagnosis is imperative, no obvious clinical manifestations can be identified.

Tuberculin skin testing appears to be the most effective method of determining the infectious process in children. A positive skin test signifies only that the child has been infected with the tuberculosis bacilli at one time or another. It does not signify an active or inactive infection, nor does it define acuteness or chronicity. The size or intensity of the reaction is not related to the severity of the disease. If the procedure was done routinely on all children, in addition to those identified as coming in contact with an active adult tuberculous patient, chemotherapy could be instituted more quickly, thereby decreasing the possibility of its innumerable complications.

The tuberculin solution used in testing is available in two forms, old tuberculin (O.T.) and purified protein derivative (P.P.D.). The three most common methods of testing can be found in Table 33-5. All

Table 33-5 COMMON METHODS OF TUBERCULIN SKIN-TESTING

Test	Method of administration	Reading time interval	Results
Mantoux	0.1 cc of O.T. or P.P.D. is injected intradermally under skin. A wheal *must* be produced.	48–72 hours	Area of induration is measured at greatest transverse diameter. <5 mm, negative 5–9 mm, questionable 10 mm, positive.
Heaf gun	Heaf gun injects concentrated P.P.D. with six punctures simultaneously 1 mm in depth.	3–7 days	Presence of four or more papules is positive.
Tine test	Four tines predipped in O.T. are pressed into the skin.	48–72 hours	One or more papules 2 mm or larger, positive.

tests are conducted on the volar surface of the fore-arm. Any one of these tests should be performed on all infants at 6 to 8 months of age and annually thereafter. However, in a study of 2,500 pediatricians, 55 percent did tuberculin testing routinely, and 21 percent used the test only after the age of 3 years.[20] In view of the high mortality rate in children under 3 years, it would appear that a valuable case finding method is not being utilized to the fullest.

In addition to a positive tuberculin reaction, the bacillus itself must be found in order to confirm the diagnosis, and a gastric washing is performed for this purpose. Children tend to swallow organisms which reach the pharynx from the lungs. A gastric lavage done on three successive mornings, after an overnight fasting period, aids in identification.

There are no known antimicrobial agents which eradicate the causative organism, and the aim of treatment is to arrest the existing condition and prevent complications. The three drugs of greatest efficacy in treating TB in children are given in Table 33-6. They have largely been responsible for the drastic reduction in deaths from TB. Para-amino-salicylic acid (PAS) and isoniazid (INH) are frequently used in combination; triple therapy which would include streptomycin has little advantage except in severe forms of the disease, such as tuberculous meningitis or miliary TB.[21] The incidence of toxic hepatitis in some patients receiving INH has prompted the use of cycloserine (Oxamycin) recently.

Several attempts have been made to introduce artificial immunity against TB, the most successful of which is bacillus Calmette-Guérin (BCG) vaccine. According to the World Health Organization (WHO) the vaccination produces an immunity lasting at least 10 years. It is used on those children who are living in a home in which there is an adult with a tuberculous infection, or one in which there is a potential danger, as in the case of a mother discharged from a sanitorium as arrested. To be eligible the child must have a negative tuberculin test and a negative chest roentgenogram within the previous 2 weeks. Eight to twelve weeks after vaccination these diagnostic measures are repeated, and the skin test should be positive at that time.

Common Complications Clinical evidence of the complications of TB may appear within 1 month after the onset of the primary infection; however, for the most part they are evident within 6 months to a year. The most serious, meningeal and miliary TB, may be evident within 3 months. As the bacilli are disseminated and migrate to other parts of the body (before hypersensitivity), some of the infecting organisms may die, or their subsequent development may be arrested by the host. In the latter, these tubercle bacilli lie dormant, and at a point in time when the host's resistance is lowered by injury, disease, or malnutrition, they may become active again.

Progressive Primary Pulmonary Tuberculosis In the progressive type of TB, there is an enlargement of the primary pulmonary complex, and the area of caseation liquefies. As the latter process occurs there is a dissemination of its contents into the bronchi, thereby setting up new focal points of infection. The symptoms of fever, anorexia, and loss of weight, typically associated with TB, are present. It is a severe form of the disease in young children, and the mortality rate is just above 50 percent. Treatment

Table 33-6 DRUGS COMMONLY USED IN TREATING TUBERCULOSIS

Agent	Action	Dose	Route	Side effects
Isoniazid (INH)	Penetrates cell membrane; moves freely into CSF and into caseous tissue; prevents complications.	20 mg/kg; 500 mg maximum daily dose	Oral; I.M.; intrathecal	Neurotoxic, with seizures or peripheral neuritis; allergic reactions or gastrointestinal dysfunction.
Streptomycin (SM)	Inhibits growth of tubercle bacillus.	20–40 mg/kg/day; 1 Gm maximum daily dose	I.M.	Toxicity involves eighth cranial nerve. Loss of vestibular function may be permanent.
Para-aminosalicylic acid (PAS)	Bacteriostatic effect on bacilli; also acts to delay resistance to SM.	200 mg/kg 3–4 divided doses/day	Oral	Gastrointestinal disturbances; hypokalemia; severe allergic reactions.

of primary pulmonary TB would prevent the development of this progressive form of the disease.

Obstructive Lesions of the Bronchus When lymph nodes become tuberculous as a result of the initial infection, an edematous process occurs. The subsequent pressure is applied to the walls of a bronchus causing an occlusion, and possibly atelectasis. In addition to the antimicrobials described previously, some authorities have also used steroids in successfully treating this particular complication.

Acute Miliary Tuberculosis Although acute miliary TB is a generalized disease, the pulmonary manifestations are most common and appear within 6 months after the onset of the disease. The multiple tubercles develop as a result of bacilli migrating to and lodging in capillaries, where necrosis occurs. These patients frequently have elevated temperatures, but no other symptoms of respiratory disease. Within 2 weeks after the acute onset, the mottled lesions are evident on roentgenograms. In untreated cases, there is almost 100 percent mortality; however, with the initiation of triple therapy, the figure may be lowered.

Pleurisy with Effusion Pleurisy with effusion is a common complication in primary pulmonary TB, especially in the school-age child. Some of the clinical signs are high fever, chest pain especially on inspiration, and dyspnea. Tachycardia may be evident when a massive effusion is present. A thoracentesis is done to relieve some of the patient's discomfort. Since pleural fibrosis and pleural adhesions may result, thereby restricting the patient's ventilatory capacity, antimicrobial treatment is imperative.

Superficial Lymph Node Involvement Although lymph nodes may be infected as a result of the primary complex, generally their involvement occurs as a result of metastasis at that point in time before hypersensitivity has been realized. When tubercular bacilli begin their migration to nearby nodes, they reach a certain location where they remain quiescent until an infection or an injury activates them. The cervical nodes are commonly affected, and a tonsillitis may be severe enough to activate the bacilli. After the initial infection has been treated, lymphatic involvement persists and enlargement continues. Aspiration or drainage of the affected lymph nodes may be required.

Tubercular Meningitis The discharge of tubercle bacilli into the subarachnoid space is responsible for one of the most serious forms of TB. Before streptomycin, mortality was 100 percent; now, however, the survival rate has improved substantially with the advent of triple chemotherapy. A convulsion is usually the first indication of this neurologically involving infectious process, which may extend to unresponsiveness and decerebrate rigidity. The amount of residual neurologic damage depends on the speed with which the diagnosis is made, and this identification is usually made by isolating the bacilli in cerebrospinal fluid.

Tuberculosis of the Bones and Joints When the bacilli migrate from the primary focus and lodge in bones, the bodies of the vertebras, the head of the femur, and the carpal bones and phalanges are usually affected. Since the initial symptoms are mild, intermittent, and relatively painless, treatment may be postponed, and some permanent disability may result. In older children when the vertebras are attacked, there may be a kyphotic deformity (Pott's disease). Some theorize that the dormant bacilli become activated as a result of trauma or bodily injury. When osseous structures are involved, tuberculous abscesses may develop, and surgical intervention may be necessary. Early diagnosis can avert incapacitation as well as a permanent deformity.

Genitourinary Tuberculosis Tuberculosis bacilli within the kidneys are frequently not demonstrated before puberty. The signs of a urinary tract infection, including hematuria and frequency, are common. When persistent manifestations do not respond to treatment, TB should be suspected.

In females, tuberculous salpingitis may be seen in puberty or adolescence. Symptoms may include pain, fever, nausea, and vomiting, on occasion, but ammenorrhea may be the primary sign. If a laparotomy is performed on a pubescent female, with no evidence of inflammation, an examination of the fallopian tubes frequently reveals the source of the symptoms. Sterility is a common sequela.

Nursing Management Nurses in schools, public health agencies, outpatient departments, and inpatient settings all have a role to play in identifying tuberculous children. Follow-up of a known contact is imperative, for an early diagnosis decreases the likelihood of some of the aforementioned complications.

Skin testing, initial isolation, and long-term chemotherapy are essential preventive measures. The use of BCG vaccine, particularly where contacts have been established, will produce the immunity desired. In view of the severity of the disease in adolescents, special attention should be devoted to case finding. Systematic testing of these persons in schools and camps may facilitate the process.

Since TB is difficult to diagnose in its early stages when a diagnosis is important, routine skin testing should be incorporated in all existing pediatric admitting policies, unless testing has been done within the previous year. A positive tuberculin reading should precipitate a most conscientious search for the contact. The public health or community nurse may be the initiator of the investigation, which could involve roentgenograms on all adults who have had contact with the child.

Although bed rest at home or in the hospital may be necessary for a short period, the nurse may be involved in devising play activities whereby the child's interest may be nurtured and maintained. Acknowledgment of the stage of development is imperative in this selection process.

The adolescent is the most difficult person to involve in other activities for he is missing peer group interactions essential to his developmental age. Fortunately, bed rest and isolation are being kept to a minimum with current chemotherapeutic programs. However, concerted efforts should be made to maintain group contact. A phone by his bed or active correspondence with his friends may decrease the possibility of boredom or despair. Active participation in the health team's planning for his care and rehabilitation will permit him to enjoy some control over his environment.

Arrangements for a tutor or "home to classroom" intercommunication device permit children with TB to participate in classroom activities. Fortunately, children on chemotherapy who are afebrile are allowed to resume normal activity, including attendance at school. The only exception is participation in vigorous contact sports.

Long-term antimicrobial therapy is imperative for arresting the tuberculous infection and preventing complications. Administering medications to small children may be a nursing problem. Flavored syrups such as isonicotinic acid hydrazide (INH) may be used to disguise the taste of the medication. Tablets may be pulverized and mixed in applesauce, jam, or jelly. If the patient is hospitalized, recording successful interventions to nursing problems on the chart is helpful to all members of the staff.

A poor appetite initially is typical of the tuberculous child; thus selecting proper foods and those which he will eat is not an easy task. In the acute, early phase of the disease the child's diet should be high in calories and protein. Allowing him to select his menu will usually increase the likelihood of his consuming it, although some children eat better when they are not consulted, for they enjoy the element of surprise. If the child is reluctant to drink milk, adding chocolate syrup or fruit flavors may increase his intake. If the hospitalized child is not eating well because unfamiliar foods are being offered, his parents are usually pleased to prepare familiar foods at home and bring them into the hospital for their child.

Since many children with TB are from low-income families, the parents may need some guidance in budgeting their food money so as to be able to purchase essential foods. In collecting data during history taking, the nurse may identify a potential problem and need to approach other disciplines and appropriate agencies for additional financial allowances. Arranging a consultation between the family and a nutritionist may result in improved nutritional intake of all family members.

The amount of teaching to be done by a nurse caring for a patient with TB is great. Parents have many questions about this infectious disease, particularly the mode of transmission and its communicability to adults and other children in the family. If their fears and anxieties are to be relieved, discussions should focus on the needs which they verbalize. The importance of maintaining chemotherapy, in spite of the absence of symptoms; the need for a diet rich in protein, calcium, and phosphorus; and the need for adequate rest should be integrated in discussions with parents or the teaching plan developed by the nurse. Long-term follow-up should be stressed. The patient and his parents should also be advised that once the patient has reached puberty, return visits will be more frequent, even though there are no signs of the reactivation of this disease.

REFERENCES

1 L. Gluck, "Pulmonary Surfactant and Neonatal Respiratory Distress," *Hospital Practice*, 11:45–56, 1971.
2 Enrique M. Ostrea and G. B. Odell, "The Influence of Bicarbonate Administration on Blood pH in a 'Closed System': Clinical Implications," *The Journal of Pediatrics*, 80:671–680, 1972.
3 Mildred T. Stahlman, "Respiratory Disorders in the Newborn," in E. L. Kendig, Jr. (ed.), *Pulmonary Disorders,* vol. I, W. B. Saunders Company, Philadelphia, 1972, p. 168.
4 Modified from "Indications for Resuscitation" in R. E. Cooke, *The Biologic Basis for Pediatric Practice*, McGraw-Hill Book Company, 1968, p. 1451.
5 Rosa Lee Nemir, "Atelectasis," in E. L. Kendig, Jr. (ed.),

Pulmonary Disorders, vol. I, W. B. Saunders Company, Philadelphia, 1972, p. 351.

6 A. B. Bergman et al, "Studies of the Sudden Infant Death Syndrome in King County, Washington, pt. 3, "Epidemiology," *Pediatrics,* 49:860, 1972.

7 ———, "Sudden Infant Death," *Nursing Outlook,* 20:755–757, 1972.

8 "Case Records of the Massachusetts General Hospital," *The New England Journal of Medicine,* 289:261–265, 1973.

9 A. B. Bergman, Margaret A. Pomeroy, and J. Bruce Beckwith, "The Psychiatric Toll of the Sudden Infant Death Syndrome," *GP,* 40:101–102, 1969.

10 Ibid.

11 Carolyn Szybist, *The Subsequent Child,* National Foundation for Sudden Infant Death, Inc., New York, 1972.

12 Nemir, op. cit., p. 357.

13 W. C. Adams, "Aspiration Pneumonia," in E. L. Kendig, Jr. (ed.), *Pulmonary Disorders,* vol. I, W. B. Saunders Company, Philadelphia, 1972, p. 312.

14 W. E. Nelson, V. Vaughn, and J. McKay, *Textbook of Pediatrics,* 9th ed., W. B. Saunders Company, Philadelphia, 1969, p. 1498.

15 Adams, op. cit., p. 314.

16 Nelson, Vaughn, McKay, op. cit., p. 927.

17 Ibid., p. 927.

18 Carmi L. Marogolis, D. L. Ingram, and J. H. Meyer, "Routine Tracheotomy in Hemophilus Influenzae Type B Epiglottis," *The Journal of Pediatrics,* 81:1150–1152, 1972.

19 H. Bakwin and Ruth Morris Bakwin, *Behavior Disorders in Children,* 4th ed., W. B. Saunders Company, Philadelphia, 1972, p. 563.

20 E. L. Kendig, Jr., "Tuberculosis," in E. L. Kendig, Jr. (ed.), *Pulmonary Disorders,* W. B. Saunders Company, Philadelphia, 1972, p. 656.

21 Ibid., p. 663.

BIBLIOGRAPHY

Abramson, H. (ed.): *Resuscitation of the Newborn Infant,* 3d ed., The C. V. Mosby Company, St. Louis, 1973.

Barnett, H. L. (ed.): *Pediatrics,* 15th ed., Appleton-Century-Crofts, New York, 1972.

Cole, R. B.: *Essentials of Respiratory Disease,* J. B. Lippincott Company, Philadelphia, 1971.

Gellis, S. S., and Kagan, B. M.: *Current Pediatric Therapy,* W. B. Saunders Company, Philadelphia, 1971.

Guyton, A. C.: *Basic Human Physiology: Normal Function and Mechanisms of Disease,* W. B. Saunders Company, Philadelphia, 1971.

Langley, L. L., Telford, I. R., and Christensen, J. B.: *Dynamic Anatomy and Physiology,* 3d ed., McGraw-Hill Book Company, New York, 1969.

Patten, B. M.: *Human Embryology,* 3d ed., McGraw-Hill Book Company, New York, 1968.

Raffensperger, J. G. and Primrose, Rosellen Bohlen (eds.): *Pediatric Surgery for Nurses,* Little, Brown and Company, Boston, 1968.

Slobody, L. B., and Wasserman, E.: *Survey of Clinical Pediatrics,* 5th ed., McGraw-Hill Book Company, New York, 1968.

Vander, A. J., Sherman, J. H., and Luciano, Dorothy S.: *Human Physiology: The Mechanisms of Body Function,* McGraw-Hill Book Company, New York, 1970.

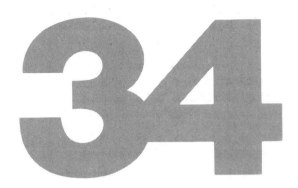

34

THE CARDIO-VASCULAR SYSTEM

SARAH B. PASTERNACK,
GAYLENE BOUSKA ALTMAN,
and GLADYS M. SCIPIEN

EMBRYOLOGY OF THE HEART

Although the heart is not the first organ to make its appearance in the embryo, it reaches a functional state long before any of the other organs and is functional while still in a relatively primitive stage of development. An understanding of the changes that take place during the embryological development of this system is necessary in caring for infants and children with congenital and acquired cardiac disease.

Beginning as a very simple tube through which blood flows to supply the developing embryo, the heart undergoes a most complex period of growth during which it is converted into an intricate, elaborate four-chambered organ. At the end of the second week of development, clusters of mesenchymal cells start to proliferate, forming blood islands and a most primitive vascular system. Scattered clusters of these cells congregate at the cephalic end of the embryonic plate, cephalic to the neural plate. Gradually, these isolated groups of cells fuse to form the *right* and *left endocardial heart tubes*. As the foregut continues to close at the level of the heart, these tubes are brought closer together and fuse into a single, thick-walled blood vessel. (See Fig. 34-1.)

During the fifth week, the endocardial tube begins to grow much more rapidly than the pericardial cavity within which it finds itself. Both the pericardial cavity and endocardial tube rotate on a transverse axis about 180 degrees, and the endocardial tube begins to bulge into the dorsal surface of the cavity, becoming suspended from its dorsal wall by a mesentary, the *dorsal mesocardium*. Simultaneously, the endocardial tube becomes surrounded by a thick layer of mesenchymal cells forming the *myoepicardial* mantle. These cells will differentiate into myocardium and epicardium.

The dorsal mesocardium disappears, leaving the heart tube attached to the pericardium at its cephalic and caudal ends. The cephalic end of the endocardial tube is its arterial end, giving rise to the pulmonary artery and aorta, while the caudal portion is the venous end, from which will emerge the great veins. A primitive heart has developed.

Early, rapid differentiation occurs in the middle of this cardiac tube within that portion which is not anchored down. As it undergoes expansion, several dilatations appear, including the *bulbus cordis*, the *atrium*, the *ventricle*, and the *left* and *right horns of the sinus venosus*. The bulbus cordis and ventricular section elongate swiftly, causing the heart to assume a variety of shapes and resulting in the atrium lying posterior to the ventricle, and the passage between

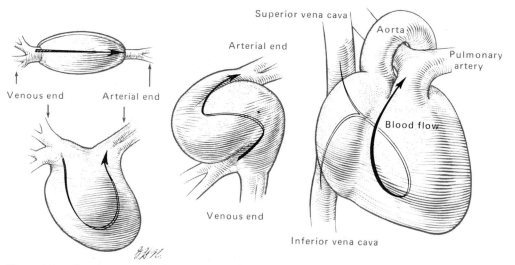

Figure 34-1   Development of the fetal heart. The arrow indicates the direction of blood flow. *(From L. L. Langley, Ira R. Telford, and John B. Christensen, Dynamic Anatomy and Physiology, 4th ed., McGraw-Hill Book Company, New York, 1974, p. 399.)*

the atrium and ventricle narrows to form the *atrioventricular* canal. The atrium, ventricle, and bulbus cordis expand and undergo additional positional changes.

Cellular proliferations within the dorsal and ventral walls of the atrioventricular canal fuse so that the canal is divided by the *septum intermedium*. Simultaneously, the septum primum emerges from the roof of the single atrium, growing downward and fusing with the septum intermedium and dividing this single chamber into the left and right atria. Before fusion is complete, the opening between the lower edge of the septum primum and septum intermedium is called the *foramen primum*. Through a degenerative process which affects the central portion of the septum primum, the *foramen secundum* appears, thereby establishing communication between the left and right atria.

A second, thicker septum, the septum secundum grows down from the atrial roof to the right of the septum primum. While the lower edge of the septum overlaps the foramen secundum in the septum primum, it does not reach the floor of the atrium, and it does not fuse with the septum intermedium. The foramen secundum now becomes known as the *foramen ovale*.

By the end of the third week the heart is beating, and by the fourth week principal divisions of the heart are recognizable, although the heart is still essentially a large blood vessel. The left and right horns of the sinus venosus which emerge as dila-

tations during that period of rapid cellular proliferation become distinct projections into the cavity of the primitive atrium. Eventually the right horn becomes part of the right atrium, while the left horn becomes the coronary sinus.

During the fourth week the ventricular septum begins to project upward from the floor of the single ventricle dividing it into left and right sides; however, communication is maintained through the *interventricular foramen*. Ultimately the interventricular foramen closes as a result of proliferation, fusing with the muscular ventricular septum and forming the *membraneous part of the septum*, thereby shutting off communication between the ventricles.

The distal part of the bulbus cordis, the *truncus arteriosus*, divides to form roots and proximal portions of the pulmonary trunk and the aorta. The two coronary arteries arise as outgrowths of the latter. The *ductus arteriosus* also arises from aortic tissue and provides a shunt for most of the blood entering the pulmonary artery into the aorta and systemic fetal circulation. With the left and right ventricles established, the proximal portion is incorporated into the right ventricle as *infundibulum* and into the left ventricle as the *aortic vestibule*. At about eight weeks three swellings appear at the orifices of the aorta and pulmonary artery, and they become excavated to form the *semilunar valves*.

After the septum intermedium is formed, the atrioventricular canal divides into left and right openings. Raised areas of endocardium appear at the margins of these openings, giving rise to the tricuspid valve at the right atrioventricular orifice and the bicuspid or mitral valve at the left atrioventricular opening. The cusps remain attached to the ventricular wall by muscular strands which become further differentiated into *papillary muscles* and *chordae tendinae*.

Early in development the myoepicardial mantle surrounds the heart. It differentiates and forms cardiac muscle and fibrous tissue of the heart and the visceral layer of the serous pericardium, the *epicardium*. Initially the myocardium of the atria is continuous with that of the ventricles but later it becomes separated by fibrous tissue in the area of the atrioventricular canal.

Undergoing additional differentiation, the connecting muscle strand forms the atrioventricular bundle, part of the conduction system of the heart. The sino-atrial node, the atrioventricular node, and the Purkinje fibers emerge as a result of additional changes within the cardiac muscle. The conduction system of the heart is seen early in fetal life; however, the myocardium is believed to start contracting at the third week of life. Initially these contractions are muscular in origin, but the rhythm is modified after an invasion by afferent and efferent nerve fibers from the sympathetic and parasympathetic segments of the autonomic nervous system.

Once the dorsal mesocardium disappears, the endocardial tube is connected to the pericardial cavity by its arterial and venous ends only. The pericardial cavity is lined by parietal serous pericardium derived from somatic mesoderm, and the heart as well as the roots of its great vessels are covered with visceral serous pericardium or epicardium. The transverse sinus is that area between the arterial and venous sections of the heart tube. As the superior and inferior venae cavae become established, through changes in their relative positions, the oblique sinus emerges. Initially there is communication between the peritoneal and pericardial cavities which is eventually obliterated; in the process, a fibrous pericardium is formed.

PHYSIOLOGY OF THE FETAL HEART

The unique features of the fetal circulation and the changes involved in the transition from fetal to adult circulation, which normally occur at birth, may result in cardiopulmonary abnormalities in newborn infants. For every 1,000 live births, seven to eight neonates have a congenital heart defect, and the incidence is two to three times greater in premature infants.

The circulatory pattern of the fetus depends upon three distinctive anatomical structures: the placenta, a patent foramen ovale, and the patent ductus arteriosus. The placenta serves as the organ of exchange for gases and metabolic wastes. Oxygenated blood returning to the fetal heart from the placenta enters the right atrium through the superior and inferior vena cavae. Some of this blood flows from the right to the left atrium through the patent foramen ovale. This stream then passes to the left ventricle and to the aorta and is distributed to the head via the carotid artery and to the tributaries of the descending aorta including the placental vessels. About one-third of the total flow returning to the right atrium crosses the foramen ovale, and the remaining two-thirds enters the right ventricle. From there about 75 percent of the blood is diverted through the patent ductus arteriosus into the aorta, while only 25 percent flows through the pulmonary artery to the unexpanded lungs.

The major factor influencing the pattern and distribution of fetal blood flow is the relative vascular resistance of the pulmonary and systemic circuits. In the fetus, as contrasted with the adult, pulmonary vascular resistance is very high, and systemic vascular resistance is low. The elevated pulmonary vascular resistance is accentuated by the relatively hypoxic environment of the fetus, hypoxia being a potent stimulus of pulmonary vasoconstriction. The systemic vascular resistance in the fetus is unusually low, primarily because of the large blood flow through the placenta, whose vessels offer little resistance. In the fetus the pulmonary vascular resistance is five times greater than the systemic vascular resistance, and the reverse of that is true in the adult. The result of these factors is that a relatively small volume of blood flows through the lungs, and a large volume passes through the ductus from right to left into the aorta. A considerable portion of the combined ventricular output flows through the placenta.

At birth two major circulatory adjustments occur: closure of both the ductus arteriosus and foramen ovale. Pulmonary expansion occurring at birth leads to a rapid decrease in pulmonary vascular resistance. Therefore, pulmonary flow increases markedly both from the right ventricle and from a left-to-right shunt through the patent ductus arteriosus before its final closure. As a consequence of these pressure changes, the shunting through the ductus arteriosus disappears approximately 24 hours after birth, although permanent anatomical closure may not occur for the first week of life. Left atrial pressure rises (as a result of increased pulmonary flow), and the valve-like foramen ovale closes. The foramen ovale may close as late as the second month of life, but it ultimately closes in 75 percent of children. With the completion of these changes, development of the normal extrauterine pulmonary and systemic circulations is accomplished.

PHYSIOLOGY OF THE ADULT HEART

The basic function of the heart is to pump oxygen (carried by the red blood cells) and essential metabolites to the tissues of the body and remove metabolic waste products such as carbon dioxide from the peripheral tissues. The heart may be viewed as a muscular pump that propels blood into the arterial (delivery) system and collects blood from the venous (return) system (see Fig. 34-2). Blood moves through the heart by both passive filling and muscular contraction of the atria and ventricles. Valves within the heart open and allow blood flow because of differences in pressure within the chambers of the heart. Venous blood returns from the general systemic

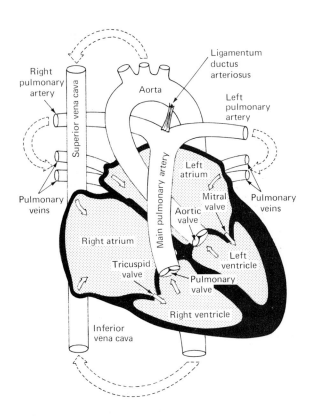

Figure 34-2 Blood flow through the normal heart. *(From Ross Clinical Education Aid #7, Ross Laboratories, Columbus, Ohio.)*

circulation through the inferior and superior vena cava to the right atrium of the heart. The inferior vena cava drains blood from the lower half of the body; the superior vena cava drains blood from the upper half of the body. Blood supplying the myocardium returns to the right atrium via the coronary sinus. The blood returning in the venous system has released oxygen to peripheral tissues and therefore is characteristically dark red in color. The oxygen saturation of venous blood returning to the heart is approximately 40 percent, whereas the oxygen saturation of arterial blood is close to 100 percent. Returning venous blood flows from the right atrium through the tricuspid valve to the right ventricle. The normal tricuspid valve, which separates the right atrium and the right ventricle, prevents the regurgitant flow of blood during ventricular contraction (systole). This oxygen-poor venous blood is then ejected by the right ventricle through the semilunar pulmonary valve into the pulmonary artery and to the lungs. As blood passes through the pulmonary capillaries, its red blood cells lose carbon dioxide and bind oxygen from the inspired air in preparation for reentry into the systemic circulation. Oxygenated blood, which is characteristically bright red in color, returns to the left atrium via the pulmonary veins. After passing through the mitral (bicuspid) valve to the left ventricle, the blood is pumped through the semilunar aortic valve into the systemic circulation. As the blood passes through the systemic capillary bed joining the peripheral arterial and venous circulations, its red blood cells surrender the oxygen to metabolizing tissues and accumulate carbon dioxide and other metabolic waste products.

ASSESSMENT OF CARDIOPULMONARY FUNCTION IN CHILDREN

Of primary importance in evaluating a child with suspected cardiac disease is a thorough medical history and nursing assessment. The *symptoms* of cardiac problems and the *degree of severity* of the symptoms are equally significant and should be elicited early in the history from the parents or the child. It is also possible for children with cardiac disease to be asymptomatic because the condition has not yet created hemodynamic alterations or because the heart has compensated for the defect with only slight hemodynamic changes. In general, however, the nurse caring for children with cardiac problems will observe such obvious effects of alterations in cardiopulmonary function as improper oxygenation and inadequate cardiac output.

Skin Color and Respiration

Without proper oxygenation of its vital organs the body cannot thrive. Oxygenation is the primary responsibility of the heart and lungs; therefore, chief criteria which the nurse can use during daily observation are the color of the skin and the character of respiration. Normal skin color varies from a delicate pink to a ruddy red, and the color is most constant on the trunk and face. *Acrocyanosis* (cyanosis of the extremities) is common in the newborn because the blood does not circulate freely to the extremities. Since skin color is not always a reliable indicator of the degree of oxygenation, it is important to examine the oral mucosa for central cyanosis. Acrocyanosis may tend to clear with increased warmth or activity, whereas cyanosis related to difficulty in tissue oxygenation is made worse by crying or increased activity. If the child is deeply pigmented, reliance must be placed on the appearance of the mucous membranes and the nailbeds. It is important to remember that not all cardiac lesions cause cyanosis. Although generalized pallor may indicate poor cardiovascular function, it is more commonly seen in anemic children.

A continuous problem of poor oxygenation eventually leads to clubbing of the fingernails (Fig. 34-3). Normally, the nail makes an angle of 20 degrees or more with a projected line of the digit. Clubbing causes diminution in this 20 degree angle. While this angle may be entirely obliterated so the digit and plate lie in a straight line, with severe decreased oxygenation the nail may turn downward. A floating nail root may be observed in very early stages with severe cyanosis. This change has been reported as early as 10 days after a tonsillectomy which induced a lung abscess and impaired oxygenation.

It is important to note the character of a child's respirations. The newborn breathes with shallow, irregular, rapid respiration. The rate should be about 40 to 60 per minute during sleep, and ideally, sleeping respiration should be observed to separate normal from abnormal patterns. If a newborn is awake, his respirations may be around 60 to 80 respirations per minute. When recording respirations, the nurse should indicate whether the infant or child was asleep or awake.

The abdomen of an infant usually moves with respiration. Retraction of the chest, grunting, and rapid or labored respiration indicate poor aeration of the lungs. The infant with respiratory difficulty may take a long time to feed and may stop frequently because of shortness of breath.

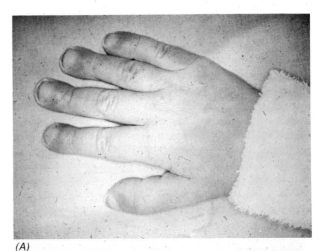

(A)

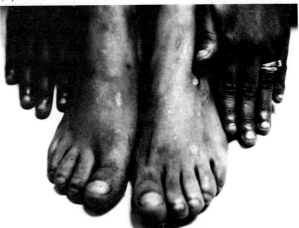

(B)

Figure 34-3 Clubbing in an infant *(A)*. Clubbing and cyanosis in an older child *(B)*. *(Courtesy of Col. James E. Shira, M.D., Chief, Department of Pediatrics, Walter Reed Army Medical Center, Washington, D.C.)*

With the older child, respirations tend to slow to about 20 to 30 per minute. A respiratory rate persistently above 40 per minute is abnormal. Not only is the rate important, but the depth of inspiration and shortness of breath should be recorded. This problem may be observed in a child's having to take a breath before being able to complete a sentence. He may stop to catch his breath while other children his age continue with their activity. The child may also sit up at night or prop his head up on a pillow to facilitate breathing.

Pulse

Cardiac output is the basis of circulatory function. (Stroke volume multiplied by heart rate per minute equals cardiac output per minute.) The apical pulse rate can be difficult to determine in the newborn and should be obtained by auscultation when the infant is asleep, if possible. The infant's rate is 100 to 130 while asleep, 140 to 160 while awake, and 160 to 200 while crying. If he is asleep, the pulse rate should not exceed 160 beats per minute. In the child the pulse rate will steadily decrease until adolescence when the pulse rate is approximately 60 to 75 beats per minute.

It is essential to assess other pulses. The dorsalis pedis and posterior tibial pulses may be abnormally strong on the infant or child with a patent ductus arteriosus or in the older child with aortic insufficiency. This strong pulsation is due to the run-off of blood into the pulmonary artery in a child with a patent ductus or into the left ventricle if the patient has aortic insufficiency.

These pulses in the foot or those in the femoral artery may be absent in coarctation of the aorta. Either defect may also be suspected merely by an inequality of contralateral pulses.

Blood Pressure

Because age and hence size are important variables to consider in obtaining blood pressure readings, selection of a proper cuff is essential. It should not be less than one-half the length of the upper extremity nor greater than two-thirds of its length. With the arm at heart level, a reading can then be obtained. The first audible sound is recorded as the systolic pressure, according to the American Heart Association, and the second or muffled sound heard in children is considered to be the diastolic pressure. Both should be recorded in the appropriate place. Because blood pressures are frequently difficult to obtain in infants by the standard method, the flush method (see Chap. 3) is recommended.

Blood pressure readings of the lower extremities should also be obtained because thigh pressures can be an important indicator of cardiovascular problems. Normally arm and leg systolic pressures are equal in children under 1 year of age. Beyond that age, however, the systolic readings may be up to 40 mmHg higher. Diastolic readings remain the same in all extremities throughout childhood. Identification of a low diastolic figure in the legs may indicate the presence of an anomalous condition such as coarctation of the aorta.

An additional determination that should be made when obtaining the blood pressure is the *pulse pressure*, the difference between the systolic and diastolic values in millimeters of mercury. Generally there is a 20 to 50 mmHg spread. A widened pulse pressure may occur in hypertension, aortic regurgitation, thyrotoxicosis, patent ductus arteriosus, arteriovenous fistulas, and coarctation of the aorta. A narrowed pulse pressure may occur with tachycardia, severe aortic stenosis, constrictive pericarditis, or pericardial effusions. Atrial fibrillation may also cause a decrease in pulse pressure due to the absence of the atria's synchronous contractions and increased blood flow into the ventricles. A weak pulse is felt when there is a narrowed pulse pressure due to the decrease in stroke volume.

Normally, the pulse pressure decreases slightly with inspiration. This phenomenon results from an increase in negative intrathoracic pressure which allows blood to return more freely to the right side of the heart. Blood also freely enters the pulmonary circulation; therefore, less blood returns to the left side of the heart. During respirations of normal depth, no *palpable* variation in pulse volume is demonstrated, although an inspiratory diminution of 2 to 3 mmHg may be noted with the sphygmomanometer. This situation can be accentuated in abnormal states.

A *paradoxical pulse* is defined as a significant drop in arterial pressure during normal inspiration, with a rise or little fall in the venous pressure. Diminution of the pulse volume may be palpated or demonstrated with the manometer. This reduction can occur in the child after cardiac surgery when pericardial tamponade or paramediastinal effusion is present. The cause is attributed to inspiratory traction of the diaphragm on a tense pericardial sac. Less blood is being pumped out of the heart with the decreased pulse.

Another change in pulse pressure that should be evaluated is *pulsus alternans*. There is a normal rhythm and a normal interval between beats, but the pulse waves alternate between those of greater and lesser volume. This symptom indicates myocardial weakness. In less severe situations the difference may not be palpable, but it can be detected by measuring the blood pressure by the auscultatory method. As the cuff is deflated from high pressure, the sounds from the alternate beats are first audible; as the pressure declines, the number of sounds is suddenly double. This phenomenon may be distinguished from *bigeminal rhythm* (coupled rhythm) in which the intervals between members of a couplet are shorter than between pairs. Pulsus bigemini is the result of an electrical mechanism and not a mechanical failure as with pulsus alternans.

Arrhythmias

When a nurse takes an apical pulse, particular attention should be given to the rate and rhythm of the beats heard. If an irregularity is detected, one must then determine whether it is a disordered arrhythmia or whether the irregularity follows a particular pattern. All forms of arrhythmias occur spontaneously in infants and children; therefore, one cannot conclude its presence is abnormal.

A *sinus tachycardia* is not considered abnormal without considering the age of the child or his behavior. A fretful, fussy, hungry infant may have a pulse of 160 beats per minute. It is a characteristic arrhythmia which speeds up with inspiration and slows down with expiration. Asking an older child to hold his breath provides an opportunity to make the differentiation. While the heart rate may exceed 160, the nurse notes that the rate is regular and that there are audible variations. It is a phenomenon which may be present with a fever, exercise, or periods of excitement. Obtaining a sleeping pulse is most helpful, for the apical rate in infants is about 120, decreasing gradually to less than 100 at age 6 years, and less than 80 at puberty. In the presence of a sinus tachycardia, digitalis preparations are never used.

One of the most important rate disturbances seen in pediatrics is *paroxysmal atrial tachycardia* (PAT) when there is a sudden onset of a pulse rate exceeding 200 with no variations in that pulse rate. It is not unusual for the heart rate to be 260 or 300. Since blood flow into the heart is diminished and cardiac output is grossly inadequate, such an occurrence in a small infant is a medical emergency because the symptoms of congestive heart failure may appear in 24 to 48 hours. When obtaining the nursing history, the nurse may note the mother's complaint of the baby's rapid heart beat, the "pounding" left chest, emerging feeding problems, or vomiting. Tachypnea and dyspnea are also obvious.

These paroxysmal episodes may subside spontaneously with a return to normal rate. They also may be terminated by eyeball pressure, unilateral carotid sinus massage, deep breathing (if the patient is old enough to comply) or the Valsalva maneuver, and gagging (physically induced) or vomiting with syrup of ipecac. A digitalis preparation is usually ordered for a period of time after such an episode, especially if it is a recurrence.

Sinus bradycardia is rare in children, especially if the bradycardia is defined as 60 beats per minute or less. This slow, regular rhythm can be demonstrated as a result of a third degree atrioventricular heart block transiently during a cardiac catheterization or in the process of cardiac surgery.

Extrasystoles are occasionally heard; however, most children who demonstrate these premature beats do not have heart disease. When identified, a complete physical, chest x-ray, and electrocardiograms are done to rule out the possibility of disease.

Regular arrhythmias are common in infants and children. The only two causes of *irregular arrhythmias* in pediatrics are atrial flutter with a varying atrioventricular block and atrial fibrillation. Both are extremely rare in children.

Heart Sounds and Murmurs*

Variations in normal heart sounds and/or the presence of heart murmurs are noted in children with cardiac problems. Normally the first sound heard on auscultation (S_1) is the "lub" of the "lub-dub" which indicates the systolic part of the cardiac cycle. The sound is synchronous with the apical or carotid pulse and represents the closing of the mitral and tricuspid valves. The second sound (S_2) is the "dub" of the "lub-dub" and is the sound of the closing of the aortic and pulmonary semilunar valves at the diastolic phase of the cycle. Defects within the heart are reflected in abnormal or unusual sounds or characteristic alterations in the rate, intensity, or rhythm of the heart sounds.

Functional (Innocent) Murmurs A functional murmur is that sound made by the turbulence of blood flowing through a normal heart. Since this type of murmur is caused by the normal "function" of the heart and great vessels, it is not significant and disappears as the child reaches adulthood. It is also important for nurses to be cognizant of the fact that these sounds are usually loud in anxious or febrile patients and generally widely transmitted in thin-chested children.

Venous hum A venous hum is a continuous murmur heard both in systole and diastole under the right and/or left clavicles in young children. It is usually heard during auscultation of the neck vessels and reflects the flow viscosity in the great vessels. Obliteration or change in these sounds can be accomplished by applying pressure at the point of

* The authors wish to acknowledge the assistance of Mary Jane Jesse, M.D., Berenson Professor, Pediatric Cardiology, School of Medicine, University of Miami, in preparing this material.

maximum intensity or by lifting or turning the child's head. The venous hum may increase with exercise and is more evident when a child is in an upright position.

Vibratory or "twanging string" murmur A grade 1 to 3 musical murmur may be heard in early systole in the third or fourth left intercostal space along the left sternal border. The murmurs are frequently heard at the midpoint between the sternum and nipple. Most commonly heard in young children between the ages of 2 and 7 years, these murmurs may persist into adolescence and young adulthood. Characteristically, these murmurs change in sound with a change in position, i.e., the quality of the sound differs when heard while the child is in a sitting position as compared to a lying position. The mechanism is uncertain; however, it is thought that the twanging sound results from the turbulent blood flow across the chordae tendinae. These murmurs will disappear and, therefore, have no significance.

Pulmonic ejection Another common functional murmur is a grade 2 to 3 systolic murmur heard best in the second and third intercostal space at the sternal border. This murmur does not transmit widely. It is short in duration, and its intensity is increased by exercise, fever, and assuming the supine position. It is thought to be caused by the rapid flow of blood across normal pulmonary valves and has no significance.

It is important for nurses to know that these three murmurs account for about 90 percent of the innocent murmurs found in children.

Bruits A bruit is a murmur, or other sound, related to circulation and heard over a specific part of the body. A bruit in the neck may originate in the carotid artery (carotid bruit) at its point of origin from the innominate artery. It is an early to midsystolic murmur. Bruits may be heard in the neck vessels if aortic stenosis or pulmonic stenosis are present. In the absence of these lesions, bruits heard in the carotid vessels of young children are rarely significant.

Almost all neonates have audible bruits in their heads, but they are not significant. A significant cranial bruit is continuous, usually very loud, and seen in the presence of other signs of an emerging problem. For example, a significant cranial bruit is usually accompanied by an increase in the head size of an infant.

Third heart sound This heart sound is best heard at the apex of the heart while the child is in a supine position. It is caused by a rapid diastolic filling which follows opening of the mitral and tricuspid valves. While it may be accentuated with ventricular dilatation, it is frequently noted in children with normal hearts.

Fourth heart sound This sound results from atrial contraction and blood ejection into already distended ventricles. It is very similar to the third heart sound and may be heard on occasion at the apex in the normal hearts of children.

Gallop rhythm A gallop rhythm consists of the first and second sounds accompanied by either a third or a fourth sound. Children with fevers or other systemic illnesses may develop a gallop rhythm which must be accompanied by tachycardia; however, this does not imply that cardiac decompensation has occurred. If the child presents with the signs and symptoms of congestive heart failure and tachycardia with a gallop rhythm is heard, the implication may be that myocardial function is severely depressed. Gallop rhythm in adults has a grave prognosis primarily because the most common gallop rhythms are heard in the presence of severe myocardial damage, usually myocardial infarction.

Rheumatic Murmurs Systolic murmurs arising primarily at the apex of the heart are considered rheumatic in origin until proven otherwise. The systolic murmur heard is caused by mitral valve insufficiency. Middiastolic apical murmurs associated with cardiac enlargement attributed to mitral valve involvement diminish as the carditis diminishes. An accentuated first sound, an indication of mitral stenosis, is uncommon in children. Aortic regurgitation is most frequently heard along the left sternal border, usually in the third or fourth interspace.

Congenital Heart Murmurs
Patent ductus arteriosus (PDA) There are characteristic murmurs found in children with congenital heart disease. The most common murmur heard in neonates and infants is the murmur of a patent ductus arteriosus. Initially, it appears as a systolic murmur in the newborn; however, if the ductus remains open, this murmur will become continuous, i.e., heard in systole and diastole. It occurs because the initial flow through the ductus is from the aorta to the pulmonary artery during systole alone. As the characteristics of the pulmonary vascular bed change and pulmonary vascular resistance drops, blood begins to flow through the ductus during diastole as well as systole. When the blood flow becomes

turbulent enough to hear, the machinery-like murmur of a patent ductus is noted. While heard best under the left clavicle, this murmur may transmit to the second and third intercostal space along the left sternal border.

Ventricular septal defect (VSD) Another common congenital heart murmur heard in newborns and infants is that associated with a ventricular septal defect. It is caused by blood flow from the left ventricle through the VSD (usually in the membranous septum) and directly out into the pulmonary artery. It is loud, harsh, and holosystolic. Generally, it is most audible in the third and fourth intercostal spaces along the left sternal border. At times a palpable thrill may be felt at the site of the murmur. If the flow of blood across the VSD and into the pulmonary vascular bed is very large, a middiastolic, low-pitched rumble may be heard at the apex. This sound is caused by blood flowing across a normal mitral valve during diastole.

Atrial septal defect (ASD) The murmur heard in the presence of an atrial septal defect is caused by the large blood flow across the pulmonic valve. Fully oxygenated blood returning to the left atrium moves across the ASD, into the right atrium, down across the tricuspid valve during diastole, and with systole, across the pulmonic valve. If the shunt is a very large one, a diastolic rumble may be heard at the fourth right intercostal space as the large volume of blood crosses the tricuspid valve. The murmur which is heard in the second left intercostal space is less harsh than that of pulmonic stenosis; however, it may mimic a mild pulmonic stenosis. Characteristically, the second sound in the second left intercostal space is widely split and consists of aortic valve closure followed by pulmonic valve closure. There is a delay in the closing of the pulmonic valve because of the large volume of blood crossing it. The cardiologist's diagnosis is made by hearing the splitting of the second sound and the lack of closure during respiration.

Stenotic murmurs Murmurs associated with aortic valve or pulmonary valve stenosis may be heard at any age. The murmur occurs when blood is ejected across a valve which does not open fully. These murmurs begin after the first heard sound and reach a degree of loudness and then decrescendo before the second sound is heard.

The systolic murmur of aortic stenosis is heard loudest in the second right intercostal space and is transmitted upward into the neck vessels. In children

this murmur may also be noted along the left sternal border. As the stenosis becomes more severe, the murmur may persist to the second heard sound, and, in fact, the second sound may be obliterated by the presence of this murmur. In aortic stenosis the aortic valve is frequently bicuspid. Therefore, the murmur of aortic valve insufficiency, i.e., a decrescendo, blowing diastolic murmur, may be present.

In the presence of pulmonic stenosis, an ejection murmur caused by blood flowing across the narrow pulmonic valve has the characteristics of an aortic stenosis except for the fact that it is heard loudest in the second left intercostal space. A thrill may also be palpable.

The murmur heard in the infant or child with coarctation of the aorta results from turbulent blood flow across the narrowed aortic segment, usually located below the aortic arch in its descending portion. While the murmur is heard best under the left clavicle, it is also always heard posteriorly at the tip of the scapula on the left side. Since hypertension is present in the blood vessels above the coarctation, the murmur is transmitted to the neck. It is also heard at the upper left sternal border.

Other murmurs The murmurs heard in other types of congenital heart lesions are frequently caused by a combination of murmurs. For example, in the child with tetralogy of Fallot, the murmur heard is that of the pulmonic stenosis. Although blood flows across the VSD from the right to the left ventricle, the turbulence is not sufficient to cause a murmur. In the case of a child with severe tetralogy, there is no outlet from the right ventricle to the pulmonary artery; with no blood crossing the pulmonic valve, there will be no murmur. If an infant has transposition of the great vessels without a VSD, there will be no murmur; however, if a VSD is present, that is the murmur that will be heard.

This discussion has concerned the majority of heart murmurs heard in children with normal hearts and in those with congenital heart lesions. It should be clear to the reader that a murmur is insignificant unless congenital heart disease is present. When the diagnosis of a functional murmur has been made, parents will have many questions which need to be answered with honest reassurance. Appropriate, necessary explanations can avoid needless worry and concern on the part of the family.

Additional Physical Assessments

Another major symptom the nurse must evaluate is limitation of activity for the child's age. Exercise intolerance may indicate a failing heart and inability of the heart to meet the metabolic demands for oxygen on exercise. This intolerance could indicate inadequate oxygenation of the myocardium. Poor oxygen delivery occurs in three situations: cyanotic congenital heart disease (arterial oxygen desaturation), congestive cardiac failure (inadequate myocardial function), and severe outflow obstructive conditions (inadequate cardiac output).

Children with cardiac conditions tend to develop infections readily. The parents may complain of the child's constantly having symptoms of upper respiratory infections. Pneumonia may frequently be present in children with a large pulmonary blood flow (as in left-to-right shunts) or in those with greatly enlarged hearts. Poor weight gain and small body size may be found in children with cardiac failure or with cyanotic forms of congenital heart disease.

Congestive heart failure leads to the most frequently described symptom complex occurring in children with cardiac disease. Because of its significance in the nursing care and medical treatment of these children, congestive heart failure is covered in a separate section in this chapter (see "Congestive Heart Failure").

Diagnostic Tests

In addition to a thorough history and physical examination with special emphasis on cardiac auscultation and measurement of arterial blood pressure, there are several procedures which are employed in diagnosis of abnormal heart conditions in children. These include telemetric, radiologic, and certain hematologic tests.

Telemetric Tests Telemetric methods measure and transmit data by electrical transmission to a receiver for recording and analysis. Common diagnostic procedures in pediatric cardiology are electrocardiography, phonocardiography, and echocardiography.

The *electrocardiogram* (ECG) is a recording of heart contractions and relaxation in response to the electrical impulses which originate in the heart. In the normal heart, contraction of the atria results in a first wave, the P wave. The Q, R, S, and T waves are related to the contraction of the ventricles. The shape of the normal P, Q, R, S, and T waves is shown in the diagram of the cardiac cycle (see Fig. 34-4). When used in conjunction with the history, physical examination, and radiographic studies, the ECG is acknowledged to be an important anatomic and functional aid to diagnosis of heart abnormalities. The limits of the normal ECG pattern, which vary widely with respect to the age of the child, have been determined by studying large groups of children. In children, the ECG is of distinct value in the identification of enlargement of specific cardiac chambers because certain anomalies impose hemodynamic burdens on the heart which result in increased muscle mass.

The *vectorcardiogram* is a form of ECG which is particularly helpful in the diagnosis of the severity of congenital heart defects. It is more useful than the standard ECG (which records leads at different times in the cardiac cycle) because it records three leads simultaneously and identifies more precisely the true time relationship between electrical impulses and myocardial responses. There is a distinctive shape and direction of the vectorcardiogram line in normal children, but the line is frequently deformed when various cardiac lesions are present.

A *phonocardiogram* is a graphic representation of the sounds which originate in the heart and great vessels. This measurement offers the advantage of accurate timing of intracardiac sounds and events which are too rapid or too subtle to be detected by auscultation. A phonocardiogram may be obtained externally by placing the sound-sensitive apparatus on the surface of the body over the heart and great vessels. This test may also be incorporated into the cardiac catheterization procedure by placing a special apparatus within the heart or vascular structure where sound originates. When this is performed simultaneously with the recording of intracardiac and intravascular pressures and external tracings, intracardiac phonocardiography provides a permanent tracing which can localize a murmur to the specific cardiac chamber or vessel of its origin.

Echocardiography, a relatively new cardiac diagnostic technique, is a noninvasive procedure which employs ultrasound to reproduce an image of echoes produced by opening and closing of heart valves, blood flow through stenotic valves and vessels, valvular regurgitation of blood, and the presence of anomalous vessels and cyanotic congenital heart defects. Echocardiography provides an indirect method for localizing the origin of cardiac murmurs and may eliminate the need for further diagnostic tests for some patients.

Radiologic Tests Certain roentgenographic and fluoroscopic tests are performed to aid in the diagnosis of heart defects. Alone, x-ray and fluoroscopy do not provide conclusive diagnosis. However, the findings are usually correlated with other tests and

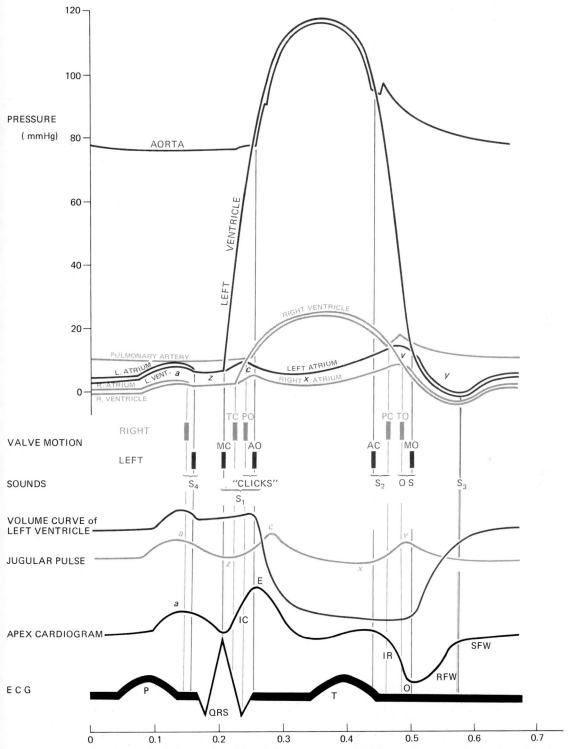

Figure 34-4   The cardiac cycle. Valve motion abbreviations: MC and MO, mitral component and opening; TC and TO, tricuspid component and opening; AC and AO, aortic component and opening; PC and PO, pulmonic component and opening; OS, opening snap of atrioventricular valves. *(From J. Willis Hurst, R. Bruce Logue, Robert C. Schlant, and Nanette Kass Wenger, The Heart, 3d ed., McGraw-Hill Book Company, New York, 1974.)*

physical manifestations to yield a specific diagnosis because they can identify specific anatomic abnormalities as well as other physiologic alterations which have developed as a consequence of the abnormality.

Often the child's tolerance of the procedures and the quality of the films made during the tests depends on the nurse's preparation of the child and family for the x-rays and the nurse's participation in the procedures. In accompanying the child to the radiology department, the nurse is responsible for insuring the child's safety from injury or falling during transportation and during the procedure. The nurse with whom the child is familiar is usually more successful in eliciting the child's cooperation during the test. It may be beneficial for the child and for the parents if parents are allowed to accompany the child to the x-ray department for some of the tests. They are frequently most effective in promoting the child's security and relaxation in the presence of a strange, busy, and somewhat threatening environment.

For most studies performed in the diagnosis of cardiac conditions, the child must swallow a barium preparation. Although the barium is frequently flavored (in an effort to make it more palatable), the child may be more willing to drink the liquid if it is given to him by the nurse or a parent. The nurse's participation is especially important when barium must be given to an infant because the nurse will be alert for dyspnea during administration of the liquid.

The radiologist may ask the nurse or parent to help the child maintain the required position while the films are being made. The amount of radiation used for these is modified for children and is not considered harmful to them. Nevertheless, it is very important that the child and others present or participating be protected from undue exposure to radiation. The American Academy of Pediatrics recommends that adequate shielding of the child's gonads by lead shields and adjustable cones be a routine precaution.[1] The nurse and parents present should be protected by lead rubber aprons and gloves during all radiographic procedures. To prevent overexposure to radiation, it is advisable for nursing personnel who are frequently present during radiologic tests to wear badges which measure the amount of radiation exposure.

Roentgenography, or x-ray photography, can reveal alteration in the size and position of the pulmonary artery and aorta, the size of the heart, and enlargement of any of the heart chambers when the esophagus containing barium provides a contrast area. The four basic views of the child's up-right chest which are most helpful in evaluation of the heart are posteroanterior (PA), lateral, right anterior oblique (RAO), and left anterior oblique (LAO).

In a *fluoroscopic* examination, the child is positioned in front of an x-ray tube, and a movable screen is placed in front of the chest. The room is darkened, and an x-ray beam is passed through the area of the heart, producing light and shadowed areas on the screen. This allows the radiologist to see shadows which represent the dynamic relationship of the heart, pulmonary artery and branches, and the aorta. Areas of abnormal pulsation can also be identified. Some experts now believe that other new and more accurate diagnostic tools eliminate the need for routine use of fluoroscopy in cardiac diagnosis. Whenever fluoroscopy is employed, the radiation dosage must be calculated carefully and the length of exposure limited. Repeated fluoroscopic evaluations are avoided.

Cardiac Catheterization and Angiocardiography
Cardiac catherization is an extremely valuable diagnostic tool which consists of passing a small, soft radiopaque catheter into the cardiac chambers and vessels for the purpose of establishing a complete diagnosis of cardiovascular defects, identifying the severity of the defects, and evaluating their effects on overall cardiovascular function. This procedure is often performed approximately 1 year after cardiac surgery to evaluate the repair and the resulting cardiovascular function of the child.

The objective is to enter as many of the chambers of the heart and the great vessels as possible to: (1) determine the intracardiac and intravascular pressure pulses for each site; (2) determine whether an intracardiac or extracardiac shunt is present and ascertain its location, magnitude, and direction of blood flow by measuring the oxygen concentration of the blood in several sites; (3) measure cardiac output as an indication of myocardial functional adequacy; (4) evaluate the function of the aortic, mitral, pulmonary, and tricuspid valves; (5) visualize major abnormalities by injection of contrast media; and (6) evaluate hemodynamics resulting from existing defects.

Catheterization may be approached through either the right or left side of the heart although both sides of the heart will usually be studied. In infants and young children, the catheter is usually inserted through a femoral venous or arterial cutdown. Umbilical artery catheterization may be preferred to femoral arteriotomy in the neonate.[2] A cutdown in the antecubital vein or a brachial arteriotomy is often the route used for children over 3 years of age.

In older children, a cutdown may be avoided by percutaneous entry, usually to the femoral artery.

Angiocardiography, the injection of a radiopaque contrast medium, usually into the left ventricle, is frequently performed with cardiac catheterization. This part of the procedure provides valuable information concerning hemodynamics when there is a ventricular septal defect, valvular insufficiency, stenosis, obstruction, or a combination of these. Although the injection of radiopaque media may increase the risk of an adverse reaction,[3, 4] its diagnostic potential is so valuable that its use is strongly urged for children with definite cyanotic congenital heart disease, regardless of the immaturity of the child or the severity of the symptoms.[5-8] Angiocardiography is definitely indicated when the premature infant does not respond to treatment for congestive heart failure within 12 hours.[9]

Nursing Management

Preparing the child and the parent prior to these tests is a fundamental nursing responsibility. Information regarding the preparatory measures that are anticipated, the procedures, what the child can expect to see and do during the tests, and what the child may expect following the completion of the procedures should be presented in logical sequence and in language appropriate to the child's age and cognitive development.

Preparation of the child is usually done one day prior to the procedure. However, the older child and adolescent who is hospitalized more than 1 day prior to the tests may be ready earlier for information about the procedures planned. Questions of both older and younger children should be answered succinctly and honestly. Visual aids, such as photographs or drawings of the cardiac lab or a miniature facsimile of the lab and equipment, are effective in helping the child understand the nurse's explanation. If the nurse will accompany the child to the lab and/or remain with him during the procedure, it is important to include this information in the preparatory session. For a more detailed discussion of appropriate explanations and teaching methods for ill children of various ages, the reader is referred to Part 3.

Whenever possible, the parents should be present during the nurse's initial explanation to the child. After the procedures have been explained to the child, it is essential that the nurse provide the parents with an opportunity for private discussion of the anticipated tests. Often, parents will not verbalize their questions and concerns about their child's suspected or known illness and the related diagnostic procedures until the nurse directs attention to their needs.

Although the nurse does not ordinarily participate in the actual procedures, nursing management of the child prior to and following cardiac catheterization and angiocardiography is of paramount importance. The goals in the nursing management of a child undergoing these procedures are (1) promotion of the child's optimal condition prior to, during, and after the tests, (2) detection of adverse reactions to the procedures, and (3) prevention of complications following the procedures.

Frequently, the nurse will accompany the child to the cardiac lab. If a familiar nurse remains with the child during the procedure, this may provide additional comfort and relaxation for the child. Since the procedure usually lasts from 1 to 3 hours (but may be as long as 5 hours), the nurse should be sure that the child is carefully positioned to avoid muscle strain and pressure on blood vessels and peripheral nerves. All extremities should be carefully cushioned prior to the procedure.

In spite of the fact that performance of cardiac catheterization and angiocardiography are encouraged for early diagnosis of severe heart defects during the first hours and days of life, the incidence of complications and mortality following these tests has been found to be highest in the neonate and infant under 6 months of age.[10-13] Although some deaths and adverse reactions may be related to the severity of the defect, vigilant nursing observation and supportive care of the neonate undergoing cardiac catheterization is imperative in the prevention of complications.

Frequent measurement of the vital signs is of critical importance during the first 48 hours following the procedures. The blood pressure, pulse, and respirations should be recorded every 15 minutes for several hours. Because cardiac conditions in children may result in simultaneous changes in more than one clinical sign, the nurse must constantly and astutely observe for subtle changes in clinical signs which may precede cardiopulmonary arrest of the infant. *Bradycardia* is an important sign which occurs in severe heart defects, heart failure, and in infants who have been sedated or anesthetized during the procedure. This sign is significant in that it may be accompanied by hypotension and hypoxia following cardiac catheterization, and either tachycardia or bradycardia may precede cardiac arrest.

In addition to careful detection of the heart rate, the nurse should palpate the *pulses* in the extremity used for entry of the catheter during the procedure.

Weakness of the arterial pulses, unusual coolness, cyanosis, blanching of the extremity, or mottling of the skin in the extremity are signs of arterial thrombosis, the most frequent complication of cardiac catheterization and angiocardiography. Although arterial thrombosis can occur after percutaneous entry of the catheter, the nurse should be particularly alert for these changes when entry was accomplished via a cutdown.

Hypotension is a potential problem following cardiac catheterization of the infant. Inadvertent cardiac perforation during the procedure with resultant tamponade will be manifested by hypotension immediately after the procedure. It is important for the nurse to check the dressing for evidence of bleeding at the catheterization site every 15 minutes. This is particularly essential when the femoral percutaneous route of entry has been used. In this instance, there should be an intact pressure dressing over the site. The nurse should check for evidence of bleeding under the child's hip and thigh, as gravity may pool oozing blood under the extremity. If a femoral percutaneous site develops internal bleeding, the blood will collect in the child's pelvis rather than on the dressing, and the nurse will need to recognize alterations in the vital signs which suggest hemorrhage. Later in the immediate recovery period, cardiac arrythmias and cyanotic periods are likely to result in hypotension in young infants. Hypotension should always be suspected when the nurse notes bradycardia.

Because of the intricate interrelationship of cardiac and plumonary functions in congenital heart defects, adverse reactions to cardiac catheterization in the neonate may be manifested by respiratory difficulties such as apneic periods, dyspnea, sternal retraction upon inspiration, and restlessness. Pulmonary edema and/or hypoxia frequently underlie these signs. Since respiratory acidosis is a frequent complication in neonates during cardiac catheterizations, oxygen in 100 percent concentration is often administered during the procedure to maintain the Po_2 at the highest possible level.[14] The nurse can anticipate that the infant will receive oxygen therapy upon his return to the unit. The concentration should not exceed the generally accepted safe levels of 40 percent, except perhaps for limited periods. (See Chapter 33 for a full discussion of oxygen therapy in the newborn.)

Maintenance of adequate body temperature of the high-risk infant is essential both during and after these tests. Children with heart defects are especially vulnerable to excessive losses of body heat during and following these procedures. When sedation and/or anesthesia is used, the risk of hypothermia is increased. When the neonate's body temperature is decreased, he must compensate by increasing the amount of oxygen normally used to generate heat through metabolism. The survival of an infant who may already be hypoxic due to his cardiac condition will be seriously compromised if his body temperature is not carefully monitored. To counteract conductive heat loss during the cardiac catheterization, the infant should be placed on a UL-approved (approved by Underwriters' Laboratories, Inc.) warming pad. Following the procedure, the neonate should be placed in an open incubator which will maintain the desired body temperature.

Fluid balance of the neonate is essential in the prevention of complications after cardiac catheterization and angiocardiography. Meticulous attention to every detail of the infant's fluid intake and output is a most important nursing responsibility. Because cyanotic infants are polycythemic, they are usually given intravenous fluids during and following the procedure to prevent dehydration and to offset the formation of a thrombus in the artery of entry.

Renal shutdown, in response to the quantity of dye used in the procedure,[15] has been known to occur following angiocardiography. Hematuria is believed to be the most significant clinical sign which precedes renal failure in this situation. Therefore, the nurse should pay particular attention to the characteristics of the urine from the child's voiding, especially the first voiding, after the angiocardiography. Hematuria of renal origin is usually well mixed with the urine and may range from a smoky appearance to a bright red color. Urine which appears cloudy or smoky should be promptly tested for red blood cells and the presence of hemoglobin, and the results should be reported to the physician.

Aside from an infection resulting from inadvertent contamination during the procedures, which is rare, the responsibility for preventing postcardiac catheterization infection at the entry site belongs to the nurse. Strict asepsis is observed in changing the dressing, and it should be protected from moisture at all times. Special care should be taken to avoid contamination of a femoral catheterization site by the child's excreta.

The rate of adverse effects from cardiac catheterization and angiocardiography decreases significantly when these tests are performed after 2 or 3 years of age. In addition, the resulting complications are less severely manifested in older children than in the young infant. However, the older child and the adolescent remain vulnerable to the problems which have been discussed in relation to the infant. Likewise, the goals and principles underlying the nursing management remain the same. Although the child and adolescent have the ability to communicate distressing and untoward reactions, critical and frequent observation of the child by the nurse is nevertheless essential to successful nursing management of the child.

Hematologic Tests The extent to which a child's congenital heart condition is manifested by altered values of blood tests is highly variable. Blood studies are used only as an adjunct to diagnosis of congenital cardiac conditions because the appearance of abnormal test results depends on the severity of the condition, the age of the child, other physiologic effects of the condition, and the existence of other abnormal conditions. Although there is no specific blood test performed to diagnose heart defects in children, the results of certain blood tests are significant.

A review of blood studies done on children with abnormal heart conditions is essential to the nursing assessment. Abnormal results of blood tests are usually a sign of other underlying physiologic effects of the child's heart condition that the nurse must consider in order to plan care which is effective in meeting his special needs.

Infants and children with congenital heart disease, especially those with defects which produce cyanosis, are likely to have an abnormally increased hemoglobin and hematocrit values. Such increases are manifestations of interacting physiological responses to low oxygen content of the child's blood. Because insufficient oxygen in the circulating blood causes hypoxia, the rate of production of erythrocytes is increased. In some children, this results in *secondary polycythemia,* a condition characterized by an increased number of red blood cells. Polycythemia secondary to cardiac defects is usually accompanied by an increase in the blood volume and blood viscosity.

In newborns, polycythemia secondary to congenital heart defects results in a hemoglobin level exceeding 23 Gm per 100 ml of blood and a hematocrit which may rise above 70 percent.[16] In the older infant and in children, a hemoglobin above 16 Gm per 100 ml of blood and a hematocrit above 55 percent is suggestive of secondary polycythemia.[17]

It is, however, quite possible that a child with a cyanotic heart condition may also have anemia. If the child has anemia, the hemoglobin may be near or within normal limits, and the cyanosis will be deceptively less severe. The hemoglobin determination is an important index in the evaluation of a child who is in heart failure. It can detect even a mild anemia (10 Gm per 100 ml blood), which is enough to overwork an already failing heart.

A platelet count and platelet function studies are usually done. Children with cyanotic congenital heart disease and secondary polycythemia are likely to have *thrombocytopenia,* which is associated with a defect in platelet function. Although the reason for this alteration is unclear at this time, the defect in platelet function is more severe in children with a high packed-cell volume and in those with severe polycythemia. It has been observed that platelet function becomes normal following corrective surgery.[18]

The ratio of oxygen content in the blood to the oxygen capacity is measured in order to determine whether a child has a cyanotic congenital heart defect. The test for *oxygen saturation* is performed on a sample of arterial blood. In the newborn, the umbilical artery may be used to draw the blood during the first few days of life. A sample of blood from a heel stick may also be adequate in some instances. The child's foot should then be warmed with towels prior to the withdrawal of blood in order to obtain an accurate arterial sample rather than venous blood which may have pooled in the capillaries of the extremity. In older infants and children, arterial blood is usually obtained via the radial artery. An arterial *oxygen saturation* below 92 percent, or 19 volumes percent, is indicative of cyanotic heart disease. The oxygen saturation of blood in each of the heart chambers and great vessels may be determined during cardiac catheterization.

SPECIAL NURSING PROBLEMS IN CARDIAC CARE OF CHILDREN
Cardiopulmonary Resuscitation

The nurse must be thoroughly familiar with the signs of cardiac and respiratory arrest and always prepared to administer resuscitative measures whenever they are indicated. *Cardiopulmonary arrest* may be defined as cessation of effective respiratory ventilation or circulation of blood. Cardiopulmonary arrest can occur without prior warning in any individual, well or ill, regardless of age.

The *signs of cardiac arrest* are an absence of the heartbeat and an absence of carotid and femoral pulses. Arrest of the heart and circulation may be due to asystole, ventricular fibrillation, and cardiovascular collapse related to arterial hypotension. *Respiratory arrest,* identified by apnea and cyanosis, may be caused by an obstructed airway, depression of the central nervous system, or neuromuscular paralysis.

Cardiopulmonary resuscitation consists of a rapid sequence of activities which are directed toward counteracting cardiopulmonary arrest by ventilation of the lungs and by compression of the heart. Time is of the utmost concern; resuscitation must be initiated as soon as possible. Authorities believe that cardiopulmonary resuscitation should be initiated even if the rescuer is uncertain that arrest exists.[19]

The *first priority* in resuscitation is the *airway*. Vomitus or secretions must be cleared away or all resuscitative measures are likely to be ineffective. The airway may be cleared with mechanical aspiration or manually in the absence of special equipment. The head and neck must be hyperextended and the jaw pulled forward and up. This measure straightens the airway from the mouth to the lungs and prevents the tongue from falling back into the pharynx and obstructing the airway.

The next priority is ventilation. The nurse should place his mouth over the child's mouth and nose, forming a seal, and deliver one breath after every three to four compressions of the heart. If the child is older, the nurse may place his mouth over the child's mouth only and pinch the nostrils to prevent escape of the air. Insufflation should be very gentle for the young infant and stronger for a child. Insufflation can be considered effective if the rescuer notes the rise and fall of the thorax. If the rescuer notes a rise in the abdominal area without a rise of the thorax, this may mean that the stomach has been inflated instead of the lungs. In this case, the nurse can place his hand on the child's abdomen and use light pressure while delivering a breath. This should be sufficient to divert the air through the trachea to the lungs.

If there is a commercially manufactured pediatric resuscitation bag with an attached mask available, it should be used because it is much more effective than the mouth-to-mouth method. The bag is gently squeezed once for every three to four heart compressions.

The technique for *compression of the heart* in children varies for different age groups. In the neonate, the vertebral column is firmly supported while two fingers are used to compress the heart. The fingers should be placed just to the left of the lower sternal border. The chest wall is then depressed one-half to three-fourths of an inch. This should be done 100 to 120 times a minute.[20] In large infants and small children, pressure should be delivered by pressing the heel of the right hand over the sternum, just opposite the fourth interspace.[21] The rate should be

100 per minute. In the large child, the nurse should apply the left hand *over* the right hand to provide the strength of both arms and shoulders during the compression. The rate should be 80 per minute.[22]

The compression and insufflation should be stopped every thirty seconds to determine the presence of spontaneous heart beat and palpable pulses. Resuscitation is discontinued as soon as rhythmic heart beat and respirations begin.

Medical management of cardiopulmonary resuscitation usually includes administration of intravenous sodium bicarbonate to counteract acidosis. Epinephrine may be administered directly into the cardiac muscle when resuscitation and the sodium bicarbonate do not take effect within 3 minutes. The child should be observed closely following recovery from arrest. He will usually be monitored and regulated by electrocardiogram, arterial pressure measurements, and arterial blood pH and gas tensions.

Congestive Heart Failure

Congestive heart failure usually occurs as a result of (1) diminished cardiac output in which oxygenation and nutritional requirements of vital organs are not being met; (2) the pulmonary vascular bed not being emptied efficiently with the result that the pulmonic system is engorged, with subsequent pulmonary hypertension and edema; or (3) diminished blood return to the heart, with venous congestion and a rise in venous pressure. In pediatrics this phenomenon is primarily caused by a wide variety of congenital heart lesions; however, it may occur secondary to systemic disease involvement affecting the renal or pulmonary systems. Regardless of cause, the pathophysiology is the same, and the methods of treatment, while complicated by the presence of another health problem, are those measures frequently employed in treating patients with congestive failure.

As the heart attempts to compensate, the stroke volume increases and cardiomegaly develops. When the cardiac enlargement is severe, the stroke volume decreases. Tachycardia occurs in an effort to maintain an adequate stroke volume for a period of time, but eventually the tachycardia is not sufficient. In a further effort to compensate, catecholamines are released by the sympathetic nervous system thereby increasing systemic vascular resistance and venous tone and decreasing cutaneous, splanchnic, and renal blood flow. The urinary output diminishes. Diaphoresis occurs. As all of these compensatory measures fail, cardiac output decreases further. The young patient is pale and easily fatigued. The newborn or infant, although hungry, has a great deal of difficulty feeding, for as he sucks, he becomes tired and falls asleep exhausted. After a short nap he wakes up screaming, hungry, and anxious to eat, only to have the vicious cycle repeated. This situation is particularly challenging to the pediatric nurse faced with supplying an adequate nutritional and fluid intake to the infant.

In *left-sided failure* dyspnea is a common clinical symptom, and it occurs in part because of the decreased lung compliance due to pulmonary venous congestion and edema. Stimulation of stretch receptors in the left atrium and pulmonary veins may also play a part. Tachypnea is often an early sign, and a constant evaluation of the patient's respiratory status is essential.

A dyspneic episode may be relieved by placing the patient in an orthopneic position because it facilitates a decrease in venous return to the heart and a reduction in pulmonary blood flow. Pulmonary congestion is caused by the increased pulmonary venous congestion resulting in excessive filtration of fluid through the capillaries and giving rise to alveolar fluid accumulation. Hence there is an impaired gaseous exchange. Rales, bloody frothy sputum, wheezing, and cyanosis may be present. These infants also demonstrate a chronic hacking cough because of congested bronchial mucosa caused by the increase in pulmonary venous pressure.

Pulmonary function tests of patients with left-sided failure demonstrate reduced lung compliance, which increases the work involved in breathing. Vital capacity and total lung capacity are diminished. While it is true that tachypnea does increase energy demands, the rapid, shallow respiratory patterns of these infants are most economical in the presence of heart failure.

The above observations may be made in children with coarctation of the aorta or aortic stenosis. It is important to remember that the clinical manifestations of left- and right-sided failure often appear concomitantly in children.

Right-sided failure occurs from systemic venous hypertension. Hepatomegaly is present because of the distention, and it is a reliable clinical sign of this type of failure. Anorexia and abdominal pain are usually also present. Dilated neck veins may be evident in an older child, but this symptom is difficult to evaluate in a neonate or infant because of their short necks. Edema which is present is probably caused by the rising venous pressure exceeding the increased pressure of plasma proteins. The flow of lymph is impaired by the high venous pressure, and

hence there is an increased production but a slower removal of interstitial fluid.

Blood supply to the kidneys is reduced; the glomerular filtration decreases, and tubular reabsorption increases, with the result that sodium and water are retained. The abnormal tendency to retain water is further exaggerated by the action of aldosterone, which enhances tubular reabsorption and promotes the formation of edema.

Diaphoresis is a common sign of failure in children, especially the neonates or infants. A mother often complains that the child's head is "sweaty" or that the sheets at the head of the bed are damp after the infant has taken a nap. These infants also usually have a persistant heat rash.

The clinical manifestations of right-sided failure may be seen in patients who have tricuspid valvular disease, pulmonic stenosis, or large atrial septal defects.

Nursing Management In caring for a child in congestive heart failure the goals are to (1) improve myocardial efficiency, (2) reduce energy requirements, (3) remove accumulated fluid and sodium, and (4) improve tissue oxygenation. Measures implemented include digitalization, bed rest, diuretics and a low-sodium diet, and the administration of oxygen.

The primary action of digitalis on the heart is to improve the force of the systolic contraction, and it is helpful in most cases of congestive heart failure. Digoxin is the most frequently used preparation in pediatrics because it is well tolerated, rapidly absorbed, and quickly excreted. It should always be cautiously administered and only after the apical pulse has been obtained. Checking and rechecking the calculation, the dose, and the route are essential nursing components when administering digitalis.

An initial digitalization dose given by mouth to an infant 1 year is .07 mg/kg; in the 1 to 2 year-old it is .06 mg/kg; and over 2 years it is usually .04 to .05 mg/kg. The first dose is 50 to 70 percent of the calculated amount and it is given immediately; the remainder is given in two divided doses at 6 to 8-hour intervals. The maintenance dose is 30 percent of the digitalizing dose. If the digoxin is given parenterally, the patient receives 75 percent of the dosage calculated for oral administration, with 50 to 70 percent of that amount given immediately and the remainder administered in two doses at 6- to 8-hour intervals.[23] The maintenance dose is also 30 percent of the initial digitalizing dose.

Digoxin is administered to relieve the congestive failure without toxic symptoms. While the above guidelines provide the reader with information related to initial digitalization and maintenance dosage information, it is important to remember that patients and tolerance levels vary. These patients need to be observed closely while they are being digitalized. Vital signs are monitored hourly, and a nurse can evaluate the progress of therapy by careful assessment of the patient and his behavior. Digoxin toxicity is a serious complication; therefore, observing the patient for decreased appetite, bradycardia, nausea, vomiting, and the appearance of arrythmias becomes an important nursing function.

As the child responds to therapy, the dyspnea subsides and the pulse and respiratory rates decrease. There is a reduction in the cardiomegaly and hepatomegaly, in addition to a weight loss.

Electrocardiograms are usually obtained before digitalization is begun in order to complete baseline data. Frequent tracings are done thereafter to help detect impending toxicity.

Rest is essential if the tissue demands are to be met and the energy requirements are to be reduced. Bed rest, while essential, may present a difficult nursing problem. Sedation, as in the case of a hypoxic infant with tetralogy of Fallot, may be necessary. Minimal handling is important; if health team members collaborate in performing their activities at specific intervals, thereby minimizing the number of times a child would need to be disturbed, the infant's rest periods could be lengthened. Small frequent feedings (at least every 3 hours) are essential in order to assure that the infant's nutritional and fluid needs will be met.

It is desirable to place an infant in a cardiac chair, for in this orthopneic position the liver impinges minimally on the diaphragm, venous return to the heart and lungs is diminished, and pulmonary congestion is relieved. The older child can be propped up in bed with his head elevated to produce similar results. Skin care is most important, as is regular, frequent positional change, especially in the case of a cyanotic infant.

Diuretics are employed to facilitate the removal of accumulated fluid and sodium when there is considerable pulmonary or peripheral edema. Since these agents may cause electrolyte imbalance, serum electrolytes are monitored closely.

Mercurial diuretics are effective and have a low toxicity. However, an obvious disadvantage is that they must be given parenterally, and these injection sites may break down. Meralluride and Mercaptomerin are used frequently, but chlorothiazide, hydrochlorothiazide, spironolactone, and aminophylline are other useful diuretic drugs. The drug of choice depends on the preference of the cardiologist directing the team's activities.

The use of diuretics can lead to a potassium depletion. A complication of hypokalemia is weakening contractions and the precipitation of digoxin toxicity, which increases the likelihood of arrhythmias. Therefore, oral preparations of potassium salts may be instituted.

Once the therapy has begun, the patient's weight should be monitored about every 8 hours to identify the fluid loss and evaluate the effectiveness of the diuretic. Weight sheets should be located at the bedside, readily accessible to all concerned.

Since sodium is being retained, restricted sodium intake may be indicated. Low sodium milk is available for infants. In an older child whose salt intake may be limited to less than 1 Gm per day, the diet is low in protein and generally unpalatable. These children may become problem eaters. An astute nurse who identifies the problem and contacts a nutritionist who is skilled and knowledgeable in appropriate substitutions may alleviate a potentially serious problem.

Oxygen therapy may be utilized when caring for a patient with heart failure, especially if he is in an oxygen deprived state. With no apparent cyanosis but the presence of labored respirations, a physician could elect to use a croupette since this cool, humidified tent may ease the patient's respiratory status. (See Chapter 33 for a review of methods used in meeting a child's oxygenation needs.)

CONGENITAL CARDIAC MALFORMATIONS*

There are 35 recognized types of congenital heart malformations, of which 9 common lesions represent 90 percent of these anomalies. Congenital cardiac malformations may be categorized in various ways. A useful classification is based on two clinical features: the presence or absence of cyanosis and the degree of pulmonary vascularity (increased, normal, or decreased). The term *cyanosis* refers to incomplete oxygen saturation of the systemic arterial blood, whether or not visible bluing of the skin and

---

* Because the problem of congenital heart lesions in the nursing of children with cardiovascular defects is so extensive and serious, the format of the following section of this chapter differs from that of other chapters within Part 4. Rather than grouping cardiac diseases and defects according to the age groups in which they occur most frequently, they are divided here into congenital and acquired problems. The intrauterine growth deviations basically responsible for congenital defects are discussed, and ages are specified where appropriate. Congenital defects present serious problems for neonates, infants, and toddlers, while acquired heart diseases are more commonly seen in older children.

mucous membranes occurs. In discussing cardiac deviations, it should be understood that the signs and symptoms presented by a patient may be altered by the degree of severity and/or the presence of coexisting defects. However, basic physiologic principles govern the symptoms of each disease; that is, symptoms are a reflection of hemodynamic alterations.

Acyanotic lesions as a group are the most commonly detected cardiac anomalies, but opinions vary regarding the most frequently identified acyanotic lesion. Some state that ventricular septal defects lead this category, while other longitudinal studies reveal that atrial septal defects or patent ductus arteriosus are the deviations most frequently encountered.

ACYANOTIC HEART DEFECTS WITH INCREASED PULMONARY VASCULARITY

The combination of increased pulmonary vascular markings and acyanosis indicates the presence of a cardiac defect that permits the passage of blood from a high-pressure, left-sided cardiac chamber to a lower-pressure, right-sided cardiac chamber, or the shunting of oxygenated blood to the right side of the heart. Although only oxygenated blood enters the systemic circulation, this is at the expense of an overworked left atrium and ventricle and the exposure of the right side of the heart to higher than normal pressures. Since many of the physical and laboratory findings depend on the volume of blood shunted, a nurse can anticipate a wide variety of symptoms. The direction and magnitude of the shunt is dependent upon either the relative resistance in the systemic and pulmonary circulations and/or the relative compliance of the right and left ventricles. Generally the resistance and compliance of the right side of the heart and in the pulmonary arterial system are less than on the left side of the heart and in systemic circulation. Thus the left-to-right shunt occurs. Patients with left-to-right shunts are subject to the pathophysiologic consequences of volume overload of the specific cardiac chambers involved and to increased pulmonary blood flow. Many of these patients are asymptomatic. However, the larger the volume of blood shunted, the more commonly symptoms appear. In general, the clinical manifestations include congestive heart failure, tachypnea, and poor growth. As in all conditions with an increased pulmonary blood flow, there is a tendency toward frequent respiratory infections and episodes of pneumonia.

Ventricular Septal Defect

A ventricular septal defect (VSD) is an abnormal opening in the membranous portion of the septum that separates the right and left ventricles (Fig. 34-5). Small septal defects may produce no symptoms and may, therefore, require no treatment. Such defects seldom become larger as the child grows older, and about 50 percent have been observed to close spontaneously. However, if the defect is large and the shunt correspondingly great, the systemic circulation may be robbed of a considerable portion of the blood destined for the organs and tissues of the body. In more serious situations, a large shunt may overload the pulmonary circulation and place a heavy strain on the right ventricle. Constriction of the pulmonary vasculature further increases pressure within the pulmonary circuit. The magnitude and direction of the shunted blood are determined by the size of the abnormal communication and the relative resistance to flow into the pulmonary and systemic vascular circuits. Pulmonary vascular resistance may become so high that the shunt becomes bidirectional during different phases of the heart's pumping cycle. Any condition that increases resistance to left ventricular outflow, such as aortic

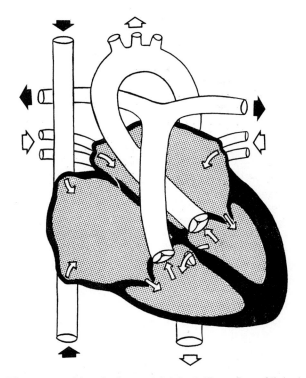

Figure 34-5 Ventricular septal defect. *(From Ross Clinical Education Aid #7, Ross Laboratories, Columbus, Ohio.)*

stenosis or coarctation of the aorta, increases the magnitude of the left-to-right shunt. If the shunt reverses and becomes right-to-left, cyanosis may develop. It is important to remember that the flow of blood through a defect is governed by the same factors regardless of the abnormality present so that basic principles can be applied to an understanding of other conditions in which blood is shunted at either the ventricular, atrial, or great vessel level.

There are two principal hemodynamic abnormalities in patients with an isolated ventricular septal defect: (1) increased right ventricular and pulmonary arterial pressure and (2) increased blood flow to the right ventricle, pulmonary arteries, left atrium, and left ventricle. When the ventricles contract, the flow from the left ventricle through the VSD is almost directly into the pulmonary artery since the defect is usually just below the great vessels. Therefore, the right ventricle is not subjected to the bulk of the volume overload. The augmented pulmonary blood flow returns to the left side of the heart and accumulates in the left ventricle. The left ventricle ejects the blood into the aorta as well as returning it through the VSD. Because of this increased work and eventual left ventricular hypertrophy, left-sided congestive heart failure may occur.

Right ventricular hypertrophy may develop in a situation where pulmonary hypertension exists. In such cases the right ventricle must work against high pressures. Work of the right ventricle is proportional to the level of pulmonary arterial pressure. The cause of pulmonary hypertension is unclear, although increased pulmonary flow may be a contributing factor.

Since cyanosis is not present and usually no symptoms are evident, this abnormality is frequently overlooked at birth. In many patients with a VSD the murmur is not heard until 6 weeks of age because it is not until that age that sufficient blood flows through the defect to cause a murmur. Many children with this defect are asymptomatic throughout childhood; their small- to moderate-sized defects are associated with neither greatly increased blood flow nor increased resistance. Their main risk is the development of bacterial endocarditis. Children with larger defects, however, may develop congestive heart failure and dyspnea. These symptoms usually do not occur until after the third month of life, at which time the lungs have matured sufficiently to permit a large volume of blood flow.

A harsh pansystolic murmur, heard best in the third and fourth left intercostal space, is the classic auscultatory finding in patients with a VSD. X-ray findings in these patients vary with the magnitude of the shunt and the level of pulmonary arterial pressure. Increased pulmonary vascularity, some degree of pulmonary artery dilatation, and, in some instances, left ventricular hypertrophy may be present. The heart size may be normal in patients with small left-to-right shunts and normal pulmonary resistance, while cardiomegaly may be present in moderate-sized and large ventricular septal defects.

Catheterization of the heart demonstrates a higher oxygen content in the blood in the right ventricle and the pulmonary artery than in the right atrium. This increase in oxygen is proportional to the volume of shunted blood. In very small defects no increase is found. Pulmonary arterial pressure in these patients varies from a normal of 25/10 mmHg to levels equal to that in the aorta, depending on the volume of pulmonary blood flow and the pulmonary vascular resistance.

Electrocardiograms show no abnormalities, although occasionally one sees left ventricular hypertrophy or incomplete right bundle branch block if the ventricular septal defect is situated so as to affect the bundle branches. Furthermore, the electrocardiogram findings may vary, reflecting the two potential types of hemodynamic load placed upon the ventricles: left ventricle overload related to increased pulmonary blood flow and right ventricular pressure overload related to pulmonary hypertension. Biventricular hypertrophy may be present if both a large volume of pulmonary blood flow and pulmonary hypertension are present.

Prognosis The prognosis for these children is good in most instances, depending on the hemodynamic alterations and the postoperative course should surgery be performed to repair a large defect. Children with small defects are considered a risk for bacterial endocarditis, and prevention of infection with antibiotics is essential. This treatment should include prophylactic antibiotics when dental work and other forms of medical instrumentation are performed.

Patients who experience dyspnea and congestive heart failure will need treatment. A limitation of activity may be essential for patients with large volumes of shunting. When operative closure of the ventricular septal defect is required, the smaller defects may be simply sutured closed, while larger defects are closed with the insertion of a variety of synthetic materials. If pulmonary hypertension is an early complication, a palliative procedure called a pulmonary artery banding may be performed in order to reduce blood flow and pressure within the pulmonary circulation until a corrective operation can be done. If severe pulmonary hypertension is present, the sudden surgical closure of the septal defect is often dangerous. The pulmonary blood vessels may remain constricted for some time after the operation. This persistent constriction may place such a heavy burden on the right ventricle that heart failure develops on the right side of the heart during the postoperative period. A promising approach that gives the right ventricle and pulmonary circulation time to adjust gradually to the new circulatory conditions imposed by surgery is the use of perforated patches to correct septal defects. The patches contain one or more small openings that eventually close completely, but closure is gradual enough to allow the heart to adjust. The risk of correcting large septal defects accompanied by pulmonary hypertension should thereby be reduced.

Atrial Septal Defect

At birth the foramen ovale is open. It gradually closes during the first few months of life, although in some children closure may be delayed beyond the first year of life. The opening, however, may remain as a small hole or gap or as a possible latent hole between two overlapping flaps of the septum. If no blood is shunting from one atrium to the other, the child will be asymptomatic.

In contrast to a patent foramen ovale, a true septal defect (ASD) is usually large (Fig. 34-6). Because of their size, atrial septal defects readily permit the shunting of blood. Since the atrial pressures are equalized, the shunt results from factors other than the pressure difference between the atria. Later, when cardiac abnormalities develop, the pressure in the left atrium is higher than the pressure in the right atrium, and the defect allows oxygenated blood to flow from the left atrium to the right. This action results in the recirculation of oxygenated blood through the lungs. The shunted blood mixed with unoxygenated blood flows from the right atrium through the tricuspid valve to the right ventricle and thence through the pulmonary artery to the lungs.

The history is important in diagnosing and caring for children with atrial septal defects. The defect is more common in females. Affected children rarely develop congestive heart failure during infancy and childhood. The major hemodynamic abnormality is volume overload of the right ventricle, in contrast to ventricular septal defects where left ventricular hypertrophy is seen more often. As previously mentioned, this is due to the augmented pulmonary blood flow return to the left side of the heart. The right ventricle in a child with a VSD is not as readily

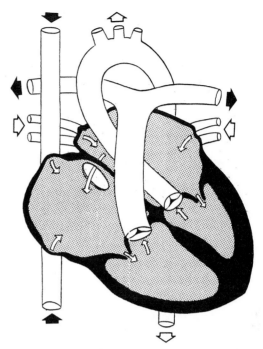

Figure 34-6 Atrial septal defect. *(From Ross Clinical Education Aid #7, Ross Laboratories, Columbus, Ohio.)*

subjected to volume overload since the blood flowing through the defect enters the pulmonary artery almost directly. Because the right ventricle can accommodate larger volumes of blood than the left ventricle, congestive heart failure in infancy is not usually caused by an atrial septal defect.

In caring for the child with an ASD, it is important to note the presence of cyanosis. Increased pressure on the right side of the heart can cause reverse shunting. On occasion, in the first week of life these children may manifest transient neonatal cyanosis. Right-to-left shunting results from decreased compliance of the right ventricle. As pulmonary resistance falls and systemic resistance ensues, changes in ventricular compliance occur and the shunt becomes left to right.

The electrocardiogram may be normal or may show a right-axis deviation or an incomplete right bundle branch block. The chest x-ray may show cardiomegaly and increased pulmonary blood flow. Cardiac catheterization reveals an increase in oxygen saturation at the right atrial level; in children with pulmonary hypertension, however, oxygen saturation may be normal.

Prognosis The prognosis for these children is difficult to determine. Retarded growth may accompany atrial septal defects because of poor tissue oxygenation. Symptoms can occur in infancy or may be delayed as late as the third or fourth decade of life. Normally, cyanosis is not present, but it may develop with congestive heart failure or with pulmonary hypertension. The child may experience exhaustion with activity, which can lead to congestive heart failure and sudden death from paradoxical emboli. Pneumonia and bronchitis are common complications; upper respiratory infections are common and may be the cause of death in the first few years of life. Therefore, prevention of infection and vigorous treatment with antibiotics when infections develop become essential.

Open-heart surgery (with the aid of hypothermia) is employed. The defect may be sutured directly or a patch may be placed in the opening. The operative risk in either procedure is low. The optimal age for surgical treatment is between 4 and 10 years.

Patent Ductus Arteriosus

A patent ductus arteriosus (Fig. 34-7) is probably the most common congenital anomaly in children born to mothers exposed to rubella during pregnancy. It is often present in conjunction with coarctation of the aorta.

During infancy, approximately one in eight affected patients develops serious symptoms such as failure to thrive, breathing difficulty, or respiratory infection. Within this group approximately 15 percent may develop heart failure.

The *ductus arteriosus* is a blood channel that links the aorta to the pulmonary artery during fetal life. It is thought that blood stops flowing through this channel shortly after respirations begin and that it permanently closes within the first 3 months of life. If the ductus remains open, however, the higher blood pressure prevailing in the aorta drives blood through the ductus into the pulmonary circulation. This blood is then recirculated to the lungs. The work load of the left ventricle is thereby increased; the systemic circulation is deprived of a portion of its blood supply; and blood pressure in the pulmonary circulation may rise. The direction of blood flow in a patent ductus is usually from left to right; however, the direction and magnitude of flow depend upon the size of the ductus and the resistance. Since resistance in the pulmonary vascular circuit is usually less than that in the systemic vascular circuit, left-to-right shunting occurs. After birth, pulmonary vascular resistance falls and the magnitude of the shunt increases if the ductus fails to close. The hemodynamics and clinical findings in children

with this malformation are very similar to those in children with ventricular septal defects.

Symptoms result when the ductus is large enough to allow blood to flow from the aorta back into the pulmonary circulation (left-to-right shunt). No cyanosis results, but the volume of blood that the heart must pump in order to meet the requirements of the peripheral tissues is increased. A small opening has no effect on a child's growth or physical activity since the heart can compensate to meet the slightly increased burden. When the volume of blood flowing through the ductus is large, however, both physical activity and growth may be limited.

Examination of the peripheral pulses in a patient with a patent ductus may disclose a wide pulse pressure, as is the case in all other conditions in which abnormal runoff of blood occurs during diastole (such as aortic insufficiency and arteriovenous fistula). Determination of the blood pressure or examination of the peripheral arterial pulses will demonstrate this abnormality. Radial pulses are usually difficult to palpate in newborns or small infants. Therefore, prominent radial arterial pulses in this age group suggest either ductus arteriosus or coarctation of the aorta. If the femoral pulses are bounding, a coarctation is not present.

The classic physical finding in patients with patent ductus arteriosus is a continuous, machinery-like murmur at the left intraclavicular area. When the shunt is small, a systolic murmur may be the only finding. Large shunts produce a diastolic flow murmur across the mitral valve. The pulmonary closure is accentuated in the presence of pulmonary hypertension, whether it is due to increased flow or to increased resistance. Most patients with patent ductus arteriosus are asymptomatic, the murmur being the only evidence of disease.

Congestive heart failure caused by a large left-to-right shunt may occur in early infancy. If it does, such associated lesions as ventricular septal defect, atrial septal defect, or coarctation of the aorta are usually suspected. The electrocardiogram in uncomplicated patent ductus arteriosus may be normal or may demonstrate left ventricular enlargement. A large ductus can produce right ventricular enlargement with the development of pulmonary hypertension. In patent ductus arteriosus the major hemodynamic burden is volume overload of the left atrium and left ventricle.

Cardiac catheterization is usually not necessary to document a patent ductus arteriosus when the clinical picture is typical. Catheterization is recommended in infants with congestive heart failure to exclude associated lesions. The ductus may also be demonstrated by aortogram, either through a brachial artery retrograde injection or direct aortic catheterization.

Chest x-ray findings typically exhibit increased pulmonary vascularity and left atrial and left ventricular enlargement. Usually both the aorta and the pulmonary trunk are enlarged. Patent ductus arteriosus is the major cardiac malformation with a left-to-right shunt in which there is enlargement of the aorta. This enlargement occurs because the aorta carries not only the systemic output but also the blood to be shunted through the lungs. The heart and aorta, of course, will vary from normal to greatly enlarged in size depending on the size of the opening and the pulmonary vascular resistance.

Prognosis Spontaneous closure after infancy is extremely rare. Without surgical intervention the life expectancy is shortened, on the average, by 23 years in men and 28 years in women. Occasionally infants die due to congestive heart failure. Bacterial endocarditis, a complication of late childhood, may result in the development of pulmonary and systemic emboli. Surgical intervention is necessary and should be accomplished 3 months after the infection has subsided.

As previously mentioned, pulmonary vascular changes that lead to increased resistance may occur. Surgery should be performed well in advance of such changes. Surgical correction entails closing the abnormal blood channel with sutures or dividing it and suturing the ductus. Ordinarily the procedure is simple and involves little risk. The operation is usually performed between 3 and 10 years of age.

Endocardial Cushion Defects

The mitral and tricuspid valves emerge from the atrioventricular septum, from growth centers known as endocardial cushions. Intrauterine growth deviations may affect the atrial septum (ostium primum defect) or the ventricular septum (atrioventricular communis), resulting in endocardial cushion defects. The defect consists of a cleft of the septal leaflet of the mitral and/or tricuspid valves making them less competent.

Symptoms manifested by a patient vary and depend on the size of the defect as well as the degree of mitral insufficiency. Some patients may be critically ill and in congestive heart failure. Pneumonia is common. Endocardial cushion defects are found frequently in children with Down's syndrome.

The physical findings are more similar to those of a ventricular septal defect than a simple atrial

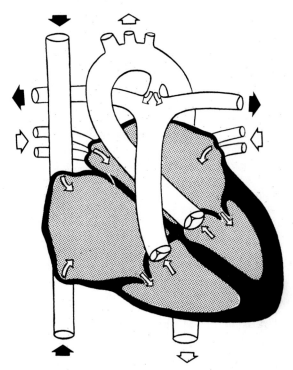

Figure 34-7 Patent ductus arteriosus. *(From Ross Clinical Education Aid #7, Ross Laboratories, Columbus, Ohio.)*

septal defect. There is a well-split second heart sound and a rumbling apical diastolic murmur, signifying left-to-right shunting. The apical systolic murmur is indicative of mitral insufficiency.

An ECG tracing demonstrates a right ventricular hypertrophy and an incomplete right bundle branch block. Vectorcardiograms, fluoroscopy, x-rays, angiocardiography, and a cardiac catheterization are essential in diagnosis.

Prognosis Open-heart surgery is usually done at 5 to 8 years of age, and it is aimed at reducing the left-to-right shunting and repairing the mitral valve. There are technical difficulties associated with the repair, and residual mitral insufficiency is not uncommon.

ACYANOTIC HEART DEFECTS WITH NORMAL PULMONARY VASCULARITY

Coarctation of the aorta, aortic stenosis, and pulmonic stenosis are termed obstructive lesions because they obstruct the flow of blood from the heart. The usual response to this obstruction is myocardial hypertrophy as the ventricles and atria must push against the obstruction to create an adequate cardiac output. The degree of hypertrophy is proportional to the amount of obstruction. Eventually ventricular fibrosis develops as a result of sustained elevated pressures. This fibrosis alters the contractile properties of the myocardium so that ventricular dilation and eventually cardiac enlargement occurs.

The degree of obstruction and, therefore, the degree of hypertrophy varies. The smaller the size of the narrowed orifice, the greater the level of pressure that the ventricle must develop to deliver adequate cardiac output. Mild obstruction may be associated with no symptoms, while severe forms may lead to cardiac failure early in life. Dilatation of the vessel beyond the site of obstruction usually occurs as a result of turbulence produced as the flow crosses the restricted orifice.

Coarctation of the Aorta

Coarctation of the aorta (Fig. 34-8) is a relatively common anomaly, comprising 5.6 percent of congenital heart disease in one series.[24] A *coarctation of the aorta* may be defined as a constriction of the lumen of the vessel at any point. Most commonly the constriction is limited to the aortic arch. Frequently the coarctation occurs just below the ductus arteriosus at about the level of origin of the left subclavian artery. This is the so-called adult type, or postductal coarctation. The infantile type of coarctation is preductal, which means that the constriction occurs above the entry of the ductus arteriosus. The development of collateral circulation, which is necessary for survival and therefore present in the adult type of coarctation of the aorta, is established by the interior mammary artery, the first three intercostal arteries, the thyroid arteries, and the thoracic and subscapular arteries. These collateral vessels join the intercostal branches of the descending aorta and branches of the femoral artery, allowing the passage of arterial circulation around the aortic constriction. All vessels involved in this auxiliary circulation become extremely enlarged.

Patients with coarctation are usually healthy males, the lesion having been discovered on routine examination. Heart failure is rare with the isolated lesion. The patient may complain of leg pains with exertion or may have symptoms secondary to hypertension. Blood pressure is high in the vessels arising above the constriction, while impaired circulation is found in the lower extremities. Absence of the left brachial pulse may occur if the coarctation is proximal to the left subclavian artery.

Myocardial weakness can appear at any time in these patients. Headache, epistaxis, and left ventricular failure may occur as a result of the hypertension. Cerebral vascular accidents can also occur. Cold feet and muscle spasm in the extremities may be present as a result of the impaired circulation.

In adult type of coarctation of the aorta it is important to note that there is a difference in the blood pressure and arterial pulsations between lower and upper extremities. The pulse in the upper extremities is bounding, but is weak and delayed or absent in the lower extremities. Normally, the systolic blood pressure in the legs should be 20 to 40 mmHg higher than in the arms as a result of peripheral resistance. However, in coaractation the systolic pressure in the legs is lower than in the arms. During the first few years of life, hypertension of the upper extremities is mild if it occurs at all. In older patients the pressure may become extremely elevated and is accentuated by exercise. Patients with infantile (preductal) coarctation may have a bidirectional shunt at the ductal level causing cyanosis. These patients may develop heart failure.

Children with coarctation usually have a normal-sized heart, although there may be moderate enlargement accompanied by a prominent left ventricular apical impulse. A nonspecific systolic murmur is heard along the left sternal border and over the left back. In addition, patients with coarctation of the aorta may develop murmurs due to collateral flow that may mimic the murmurs of mitral or aortic valve disease. The pathognomonic physical finding is the absence of femoral pulses. When present, femoral pulses are delayed.

The electrocardiogram demonstrates right ventricular hypertrophy during the first 6 months of life; later, a pattern of left ventricular hypertrophy develops. The patterns may vary, of course, in the presence of associated lesions.

Chest x-rays demonstrate a normal cardiac silhouette or ventricular enlargement and some prominence of the ascending aorta. As these children grow older, pulsating collaterals will erode the ribs and can be detected on x-ray as rib notching.

Prognosis The prognosis varies generally with respect to the position of the coarctation—pre- or postductal—and the development of adequate collateral circulation. While treatment is aimed at relieving the heart failure, surgery is indicated in all children with coarctation of the aorta. Such surgery should be performed on an urgent basis only when the lesion causes heart failure. If the child is not symptomatic and not hypertensive, surgery is deferred until he is 8 to 10 years of age. Elective surgery in childhood avoids the late complication of cerebral vascular accident and aortic rupture.

Infants with coarctation of the aorta who develop congestive cardiac failure and respond fully to medical management should be carefully followed and operated on at a later time. Since the anastomotic site of coarctation repair does not grow proportionally with the growth of the aorta, "recoarctation" develops, often necessitating a second operation at a later date. This occurs more frequently among children operated on in infancy, but it is a small price to pay for a life-saving procedure.

Pulmonic (Pulmonary) Stenosis

Pulmonic stenosis refers to any lesion that obstructs the flow of blood from the right ventricle. There are various types of obstruction, but generally the pulmonary valve cusps are altered or distorted in their development so that they fuse and form a membrane with a small opening in the center. Anatomically, the stenotic pulmonary valve is dome-shaped and has a narrowed central orifice. Because of the restricted pulmonary valve orifice, the level of right ventricular pressure must increase to maintain normal cardiac output. With elevation of the right ventricular pressure, right ventricular hypertrophy and, occasionally, right atrial enlargement occur. Pulmonic stenosis can be associated with various other congenital heart defects, or it can occur alone. In about one-third of the cases there is an associated atrial septal defect.

Patients with pulmonary stenosis are generally asymptomatic, although decreased exercise tolerance may be present. In severe valvular obstruction, dyspnea is present, and generalized cyanosis may occur when right ventricular end-distolic pressure increases, thus elevating the right atrial pressure and fostering a right-to-left atrial shunt. Congenital pulmonic stenosis, if severe, can cause extreme hypertrophy of the right ventricle and produce a clockwise rotation of the heart. This changes the caliber of the apical impulse; and pulsations in the third and fourth left parasternal spaces are seen. Occasionally, some patients complain of precordial pain.

Patients with valvular pulmonary stenosis have an ejection murmur over the pulmonic area. This systolic murmur associated with a thrill is maximal at the upper left sternal border with radiation to the suprasternal notch. Pulmonary closure is delayed in severe stenosis, therefore, causing a widely split second heart sound which is usually diminished in intensity.

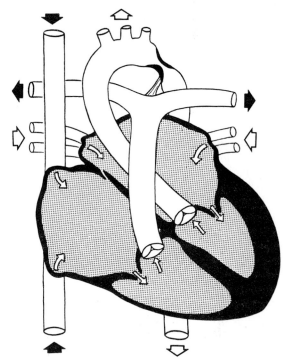

Figure 34-8 Coarctation of the aorta. *(From Ross Clinical Education Aid #7, Ross Laboratories, Columbus, Ohio.)*

The electrocardiogram may be normal in the mildest forms of pulmonary stenosis, but some degree of right ventricular hypertrophy is usually present. The presence of a Q wave in the right precordial leads indicates severe right ventricular hypertrophy and is seen with severe stenosis. The finding of T-wave inversion in association with right ventricular hypertrophy indicates right ventricular strain. This is a sign of the most severe degree of stenosis.

The chest x-ray demonstrates varying degrees of right ventricular enlargement. A prominent, dilated (poststenotic) main pulmonary artery is seen after the first 2 years of life. The peripheral pulmonary vascular markings are normal or decreased.

Cardiac catheterization and angiocardiography document the degree and location of stenosis. Catheterization shows right ventricular hypertension with reduced or normal pulmonary artery pressure. Cardiac output is decreased in severe stenosis. Right atrial pressure may be elevated in the presence of moderate or severe stenosis.

Prognosis The life-span of patients suffering from pulmonic stenosis with a normal aortic root depends upon the severity of the stenosis. Patients with mild stenosis have normal longevity if they can avoid contracting bacterial endocarditis. Infants with severe lesions may experience acute right-sided heart failure.

In general, mild pulmonic stenosis is well tolerated and does not require surgery. Severe stenosis, with right ventricular pressure of systemic range, is an indication for surgery. The presence of a strain pattern on the electrocardiogram would make surgery urgent. With moderate stenosis, the child should be followed with repeat of cardiac catheterization in an effort to define the course of the particular disease. Peripheral pulmonic stenosis is not at present amenable to surgery. Surgical correction of valvular or infundibular pulmonic stenosis results in normal to near normal cardiac function. An induced pulmonary valve insufficiency is usually well tolerated.

Aortic Valvular Stenosis

Various types of aortic stenosis have been identified according to the anatomic site. (See Fig. 34-9). The most common form is related to a stenotic congenital unicuspid or bicuspid valve. Other causes of stenosis involve supravalvular or subvalvular lesions. Regardless of the site of obstruction, the left ventricular pressure rises in order to maintain a normal cardiac output to meet the demand of the body tissues for nutrients and oxygen. As a result, left ventricular hypertrophy develops. Although rare, sudden death may occur in children on exertion as a result of an imbalance between the increased oxygen requirements of the hypertrophied left ventricle and the amount of oxygen that can be supplied to the myocardium. This myocardial ischemia is followed by fatal cardiac arrhythmias, causing sudden death. Myocardial infarctions have also been observed in these situations.

Children with aortic valvular stenosis are rarely symptomatic during childhood. Congestive heart failure is seen in about 5 percent of the children with aortic stenosis in the first year of life. It is a disease found predominately in boys. As some of the asymptomatic children approach adolescence, they may develop chest pain that has the characteristics of angina. This complaint may signify myocardial ischemia and the possibility of sudden death. Therefore, children with aortic stenosis and chest pain should be catheterized to determine the severity of stenosis and the need for surgical treatment.

Children with aortic stenosis and pulmonic stenosis display the two cardiac defects with an associated significant murmur at birth in contrast to other cardiac conditions in which the murmur is not recognized until later in infancy or childhood. Physical examination reveals a thrill and a harsh systolic ejection murmur that are maximal at the upper right sternal border with radiation to the neck and left lower sternal border. The early decrescendo diastolic murmur of aortic insufficiency may be present. A constant ejection click is frequently present, and the second sound is usually normal. This click is a reflection of the poststenotic dilatation of the aorta.

Another significant finding is a narrow pulse pressure and weak peripheral pulses. If aortic insufficiency develops, a water-hammer or collapsing pulse becomes apparent. Infants with moderate to severe stenosis may fail to thrive and may be dyspneic, suggesting degrees of heart failure. Older children with moderate or severe stenosis complain of dyspnea and fatigue with exertion. An alarming symptom that may develop in the adolescent or adult is syncope, especially with exertion, and angina pectoris with exertion. Patients with aortic stenosis generally appear normal although the small group of patients with supravalvular aortic stenosis demonstrate a peculiar and characteristic facies.

The precordial impulse suggests left ventricular hypertrophy. The chest x-ray usually shows a normal-size heart in patients with aortic stenosis who have not developed heart failure. Variable degrees of left ventricular hypertrophy may occur. A common finding in all degrees of stenosis is the prominence of the ascending aorta due to poststenotic dilatation. With severe obstruction the left ventricular diastolic pressure will increase, causing secondary pulmonary venous engorgement and increased pulmonary artery pressure. There may, therefore, be secondary right ventricular hypertrophy. With mild degrees of aortic stenosis the electrocardiogram is usually normal, but with increasing obstruction left ventricular hypertrophy becomes apparent. Left precordial T-wave inversion (strain pattern) is considered evidence of severe stenosis.

The type and severity of aortic stenosis are best determined by cardiac catheterization and angiocardiography. Congestive heart failure, angina, syncope, or a left ventricular strain pattern on electrocardiogram indicates severe disease and the need for early cardiac catheterization. The active child with symptoms of aortic stenosis presents a special problem. It is advisable to study such a patient at about 1 year of age to document the degree and nature of stenosis and to make firm recommendations regarding physical activity.

Prognosis   The prognosis is good; however, surgery for aortic valvular stenosis carries the risk that aortic insufficiency may result. There is also the probability that restenosis will occur following an adequate valvulotomy. If a valvulotomy is not possible, prosthetic replacement of the valve is necessary, but few pediatric patients require a prosthesis. In children, growth is not complete; therefore, patients with aortic valvulotomy may require a valvular prosthesis in adulthood if the valve becomes calcified. It is important for the child and the family to realize that the surgery is not a cure and that symptoms may recur. With these factors in mind, aortic valvular surgery is attempted only on those children in whom the risk of sudden death is great. This would include the group in which moderate gradients plus syncope, angina, congestive heart failure, or evidence of left ventricular strain have been documented by electrocardiogram.

CYANOTIC HEART DISEASE (RIGHT-TO-LEFT SHUNTS)

In most children with cyanosis related to congenital heart disease an abnormality is present that permits some of the systemic venous return to bypass the lungs and enter the systemic circulation directly. Right-to-left shunting results from two types of cardiac malformation: conditions that permit admixture of the systemic and pulmonary venous returns and conditions that result in obstruction to pulmonary blood flow.

The common defects resulting in cyanosis may be divided between those with increased pulmonary vascularity (such as transposition of the great vessels, total anomalous pulmonary venous connection, and truncus arteriosus) and those with decreased pulmonary vascularity (such as tetralogy of Fallot, tricuspid artresia, and Ebstein's malformation). Cyanosis in the newborn and young infant presents a problem somewhat different from cyanosis in the older child. The older child may have symptoms and not be in acute distress, but the cyanotic newborn presents an emergency situation. Tetralogy of Fallot is the most common lesion causing cyanosis in the older child. Hypoplastic left-heart syndrome is the most common cause of heart failure and cyanosis in the newborn. The cyanotic newborn may also suffer from lung disease, eventration of the

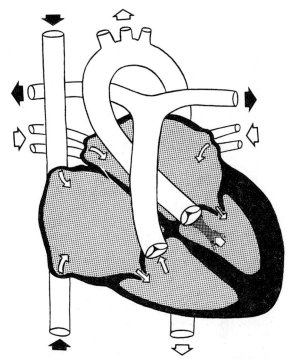

Figure 34-9   Subaortic stenosis. *(From Ross Clinical Education Aid #7, Ross Laboratories, Columbus, Ohio.)*

diaphragm, or methemoglobinemia and should be carefully evaluated for the cause of cyanosis.

Regardless of the type of defect, cyanosis is associated with polycythemia, clubbing, slow growth (the result of hypoxia in the tissues), and a tendency to develop cerebral abscess. Cerebral abscess is believed to result from the bacteria's having direct access to the systemic circuit because of the shunt. A need exists for adequate iron stores to keep pace with hemoglobin needs in polycythemia. In response to the hypoxia associated with cyanosis, the bone marrow is stimulated to produce an increased red cell mass for additional oxygen-carrying capacity. The hematocrit reflects the volume of red cells, and the hemoglobin reflects iron stores. In a person with cyanosis and normal iron stores, hemoglobin and hematocrit values will be elevated and appropriately related. In infancy, however, iron deficiency is common, and the cyanotic infant may show an elevated hematocrit value but have an improper hemoglobin value. Such an infant would have an iron deficiency anemia. Normally the numerical value for hematocrit should be three times that of the hemoglobin; if it is not, the patient is probably anemic and needs an iron supplement.

CYANOTIC HEART DEFECTS WITH INCREASED PULMONARY VASCULARITY

In most cardiac malformations in this group, a single chamber receives both the systemic and pulmonary venous returns. The hemodynamics of admixture lesions are similar to those of left-to-right shunts occurring at the same level. The systemic arterial oxygen saturation or the hemoglobin and hematocrit values are valuable indicators of the volume of pulmonary blood flow, in that the larger the volume of pulmonary blood flow, the lower the hemoglobin and hematocrit values. With the development of pulmonary vascular disease, the volume of pulmonary blood flow decreases. Thus the amount of fully oxygenated blood mixing with the systemic venous return decreases. The patient becomes more cyanotic, and the hemoglobin and hematocrit values rise.

Complete Transposition of the Great Vessels

Transposition of the great vessels refers to a change in the anatomic relationship of the pulmonary artery and the aorta (Fig. 34-10). In this condition, the aorta arises from the right ventricle and the pulmonary artery from the left. However, the great veins are not similarly transposed. Thus, the pulmonary veins still empty oxygenated blood into the left side of the heart, which pumps it back to the lungs. Unoxygenated blood from the body returns to the right side of the heart which pumps this blood back into the systemic circulation. Therefore, two independent but ineffective circulations, the systemic and pulmonic, exist. Only if a sizeable defect exists in the atrial or ventricular septum or if a patent ductus arteriosus or patent foramen ovale exist can enough oxygenated blood reach the systemic circulation to sustain life.

This defect is seen more commonly in males. Those neonates with an intact septum often die in the first month of life (50 percent), while 90 percent of those untreated die by the age of 1 year. Those who survive usually have a large atrial septal defect. A natural, developing subvalvular pulmonic stenosis, decreased pulmonary blood flow, hypoxia, and increasing polycythemia contribute to the death of the remaining children, usually by the age of 2 years.

Cyanosis becomes evident after birth. The communication between the two sides of the circulation is often narrow, such as through a patent ductus arteriosus, and this communication may follow a normal neonatal course of closure. When that occurs, many infants demonstrate profound cyanosis. The degree of cyanosis and physical findings are dependent upon the type of associated malformation. A greater degree of mixing occurs between the two circulations in patients with a large communication.

Almost all these newborns exhibit dyspnea and other signs of cardiac failure in the first month of life. Neonates with an intact ventricular septum develop symptoms earlier and are more intensely cyanotic than those with a coexistent ventricular septal defect which allows some oxygenated blood to be distributed systemically.

On examination these infants may have no murmur or may have varying murmurs caused by flow through the ductus arteriosus or foramen ovale. Signs of heart failure may not be present early; however, once identified they progress rapidly. Associated ventricular septal defects or outlet obstructions cause their characteristic murmurs.

The electrocardiogram at birth may be normal in an uncomplicated transposition. In other children, signs of right ventricular hypertrophy may be evident. Since the aorta arises from the right ventricle, the pressure in that ventricle is elevated, leading to right ventricular hypertrophy. The electrocardiogram reflects this pressure elevation and shows a pattern of right-axis deviation. Patients with a large volume of pulmonary blood flow, as with a coexistent VSD, may also exhibit left ventricular hypertrophy because of the volume load on the left ventricle.

A chest x-ray reveals increased pulmonary vasculature. Cardiomegaly is almost always present.

In conjunction with cardiac catheterization, oximetry data help establish the diagnosis by showing little increase in oxygen saturation values within the right side of the heart and little decrease in oxygen saturation within the left side of the heart. As a result, oxygen saturation values from the pulmonary artery are higher than from the aorta, a finding virtually diagnostic of transposition of the great vessels. In an uncomplicated transposition, right atrial saturation is low and left atrial saturation is normal. The presence of a significant atrial communication causes an averaging of these saturations. In the newborn without a ventricular septal defect or pulmonary stenosis, left ventricular pressure is only mildly elevated.

Prognosis Most infants with transposition of the great vessels will die in infancy unless a palliative procedure is performed. The immediate difficulty in neonates is severe hypoxia resulting from an extremely low effective pulmonary blood flow. Hypoxia leads to death from metabolic acidosis. Infants with large ventricular communications may not have marked cyanosis, but they suffer with congestive heart failure caused by marked pulmonary over-circulation. As with any patient with a right-to-left shunt, decreased oxygen saturation leads to polycythemia and increased blood viscosity; therefore the possibility of vascular thrombosis exists. Cerebral thrombosis is a constant concern and may be avoided by adequate hydration. Paradoxic bacterial embolism, with venous blood carrying bacteria to the arterial circuit, may occur causing such infections as cerebral abscess. Although an uncommon occurrence in infancy, it should always be considered in the differentiation of fever in any patient with right-to-left shunt.

Management of transposition of the great vessels involves establishing intracardiac mixing compensation to prevent congestive heart failure, protecting the pulmonary vascular bed, and eventual total correction. At this time complete correction can seldom be performed without great risk. However, to keep the infant alive until corrective surgery is possible, palliative efforts are made to divert oxygenated blood into the systemic circulation and to decrease pulmonary congestion. At the time of diagnostic cardiac catheterization, an atrial septostomy is usually done, using Rashkind's balloon catheter.[25] If adequate mixing is established, documented by a decrease in left atrial saturation, an increase in systemic saturation, and a decrease in left atrial pressure, the patient may then be medically managed. Should severe hypoxia persist, an atrial septectomy may be done. In this Blalock-Hanlon procedure a large opening or defect is created (or an existing one enlarged) in the septum between the right and left atria, allowing blood in the pulmonary and systemic circulations to intermix.

Because children with associated large ventricular septal defects are prone to congestive heart failure, banding of the pulmonary artery may be done to improve compensation and protect the pulmonary vascular bed.

A promising new procedure (Mustard procedure) for the complete correction of transposition of the great vessels involves, first, removal of the atrial septum to create a single receiving chamber. In the next step of this procedure, an intracardiac baffle is created, using Dacron or tissue obtained from the pericardium. When sewn into place, the baffle forms a tunnel-like structure running across the receiving chamber. It is positioned so as to divert pulmonary venous return to the tricuspid valve and systemic venous return to the mitral valve. This total

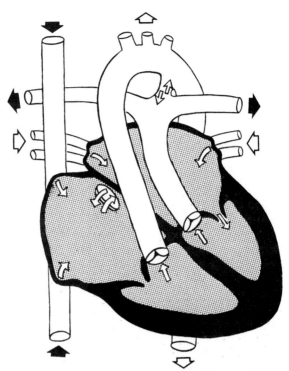

Figure 34-10 Complete transposition of the great vessels. *(From Ross Clinical Education Aid #7, Ross Laboratories, Columbus, Ohio.)*

correction should be carried out when the patient can be maintained on cardiopulmonary bypass.[26]

Total Anomalous Pulmonary Venous Return

In this cardiac defect, the pulmonary veins drain into the systemic venous circulation (Fig. 34-11). The defects are classified as those which enter either the venous circulation above the diaphragm or those entering below the diaphragm. Vessels of entry above the diaphragm enter the left innominate vein, the superior vena cava, the azygous veins, right atrium, or coronary sinus. While the pulmonary veins often have a single trunk, left and right common pulmonary venous trunks may enter combinations of the above sites. Those entering the venous system below the diaphragm involve a single pulmonary venous trunk entering the portal vein, ductus venosus, hepatic veins, or inferior vena cava. In these anomalies the common trunk is usually obstructive to the flow of blood at some point with an associated pulmonary hypertension. In both types there is a complete mixing of pulmonary venous and systemic venous blood at the right atrium. Survival occurs because the systemic blood is shunted through a

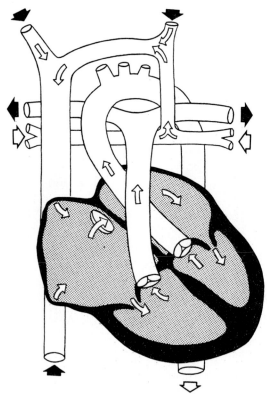

Figure 34-11 Anomalous venous return. *(From Ross Clinical Education Aid #7, Ross Laboratories, Columbus, Ohio.)*

patent foramen ovale or an atrial septal defect to the left side of the heart.

Children who do not have pulmonary vascular disease have enormous pulmonary blood flows, with mixtures in the right atrium composed of four to five times as much pulmonary venous blood as systemic blood. With the blood volume greatest within the right side of the heart, the right side dilates and hypertrophies while the left side remains relatively small. In the presence of these hemodynamics, these infants are minimally cyanotic.

When pulmonary vascular disease is present, resistance to blood flow increases, with pulmonary and systemic venous compartments contributing equal volumes of blood to the right atrium. These children demonstrate noticeable cyanosis. This particular anomaly exemplifies bidirectional shunting: right-to-left at the atrial level and left-to-right with the pulmonary venous blood returning to the right side of the heart.

When pulmonary hypertension is absent, there is a mild pulmonic systolic murmur, three heart sounds, and a middiastolic or prediastolic rumbling murmur at the apex. The second heart sound is well split. While congestive heart failure is common, cyanosis is very mild, and it may be nonexistent in infancy.

With pulmonary hypertension present, there may be a loud second heart sound and little or no systolic murmur. Congestive heart failure is common, dyspnea may be severe, the cyanosis may be marked, and death may occur early in infancy.

The ECG demonstrates a right ventricular hypertrophy, except in the case of shunting below the diaphragm when the heart is within normal limits. A cardiac catheterization and angiography identify the anatomical deviations, which is essential in planning surgery.

Prognosis The prognosis for surgical correction of anomalous vessels entering below the diaphragm is very poor. With entry above the diaphragm, there is a poor prognosis for infants; however, surgical repairs are more successful in children older than 2 years of age. Unfortunately, many infants are in serious difficulty before 6 months of age, when surgical intervention is mandatory for survival.

Truncus Arteriosus

The *truncus arteriosus,* a single large vessel, arises from both ventricles astride a large ventricular septal defect (Fig. 34-12). A single, malformed semilunar valve is also present. When the ventricles contract, the output of both is ejected into the truncus where systemic venous and pulmonary venous blood mix completely.

Clinically, infants with this defect have mottled skin and an almost constant ashen color. As the pulmonary vascular disease increases in severity, cyanosis also increases. Congestive heart failure is severe, and growth retardation is typical. Hepatomegaly and cardiomegaly are common findings. Death frequently occurs before the first year of life.

A systolic murmur is usually heard, and the single semilunar valve produces a loud second heart sound which is not split. The ECG reveals a right-axis deviation and right ventricular hypertrophy. X-rays confirm an enlarged heart and a prominent aorta. While additional diagnostic tests are essential, there is an associated high-risk factor.

Prognosis If a larger percentage of these infants are to survive, surgery is imperative. This intervention involves separating the pulmonary arteries from the aorta, repairing the associated defect, and then closing the ventricular septal defect. Although this type of corrective surgery is new and the mortality rate is high, repairs performed on children between the ages of 5 and 12 years have been the most successful.

CYANOTIC HEART DISEASE WITH DECREASED PULMONARY VASCULARITY
Tetralogy of Fallot

This anomaly is the most common cause of cyanotic congenital heart disease beyond infancy. The malformation called tetralogy of Fallot includes a defect in the interventricular septum, dextroposition of the aorta so that it overrides the VSD, hypertrophy of the right ventricle, and stenosis of the pulmonary artery (Fig. 34-13). Blood leaving the right ventricle encounters an abnormally narrow opening into the pulmonary artery. As a result, much of this blood flows through the opening in the interventricular septum and into the aorta and left ventricle. Unoxygenated blood therefore enters the aorta and flows into the systemic circulation, and cyanosis develops because of this abnormal mixture. The right-to-left flow through the interventricular defect is determined in part by the position of the aortic opening and in part by the hypertrophied right ventricle.

The clinical status of the patient with tetralogy of Fallot is related to the size of the ventricular septal defect and the severity of pulmonary stenosis. These two factors determine the degree of right-to-left shunting. Most children have large ventricular septal defects which present no obstruction of blood flow and permit equalization of ventricular pressures. When the resistance to flow into the pulmonary bed is less than systemic vascular resistance, there may be little or no right-to-left shunt. When pulmonic stenosis is severe enough to cause a greater than systemic resistance, right-to-left shunting will occur. The right-to-left ventricular shunt with decreased pulmonary blood flow is the major physiologic abnormality in tetralogy of Fallot.

Most patients with tetralogy of Fallot do not appear cyanotic at birth; however, this symptom is present in 75 percent of the cases by 1 year of age. The time of appearance and the severity of the cyanosis depend on the severity of the pulmonic stenosis. Exercise, sleep, crying, fever, and other factors also affect the degree of cyanosis. Physical growth is poor.

A characteristic of this defect is the "tetrad spell," or hypoxic episode. On vigorous and persistent crying, cyanosis becomes intense, severe dyspnea develops, and the infant faints because of cerebral hypoxia. (This occurs especially if the fall

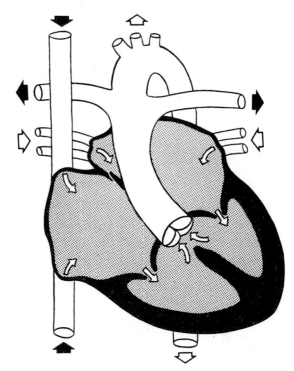

Figure 34-12 Truncus arteriosus. *(From Ross Clinical Education Aid #7, Ross Laboratories, Columbus, Ohio.)*

in the arterial oxygen saturation of the blood is rapid and marked.) Seizure activity can occur during these episodes. The attacks may occur several times a day and last from several minutes to several hours.

On physical examination a harsh systolic murmur is heard, and the second heart sound is not split. Murmurs of bronchial collateral circulation can be heard over the chest. Polycythemia and clubbing of fingers and toes are present. An ECG reveals right ventricular hypertrophy, while chest x-rays show a heart of normal size with a "boot-shaped" configuration. As part of the diagnostic work-up, cardiac catheterization and angiocardiography are done. These procedures are important in identifying the precise anatomic problem.

These children *never* develop congestive heart failure because there is no volume overload of the left ventricle and the blood in the right ventricle has free egress through the VSD, regardless of the severity of the pulmonic stenosis. The major symptoms the nurse will observe are cyanosis, rapid pulse, dyspnea, tachypnea, and exertional fatigue. Exercise tolerance levels in these children vary greatly. As they begin to walk, these toddlers discover the relief they obtain from the dyspneic episodes by assuming a characteristic squatting position, resting on their

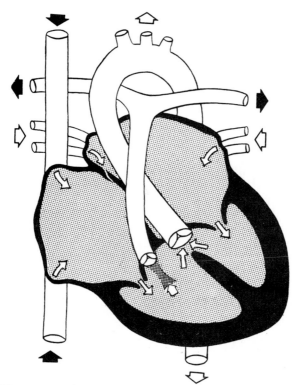

Figure 34-13 Tetralogy of Fallot. *(From Ross Clinical Education Aid #7, Ross Laboratories, Columbus, Ohio.)*

haunches. The precise mechanism by which this position offers such relief is unknown; however, it is known that squatting returns the arterial saturation more rapidly to its normal resting value. There is evidence which suggests that squatting increases the venous return from the legs to the heart and lungs.

These children, as in the case of all children with cyanotic heart disease, are prone to cerebral thromboses and brain abscesses. Assuring adequate hydration is absolutely essential.

Medical treatment involves decreasing hypoxic episodes. This action should include not allowing the infant to cry for any length of time and placing him in a knee-chest position. At times, morphine may be necessary to relieve the symptoms. Oxygen may or may not be helpful.

Should the cyanotic episodes increase or the infant fail to thrive, surgical intervention may be necessary. The Blalock-Taussig procedure involves a subclavian artery–pulmonary artery anastomosis and is preferred to the Potts procedure, which is an aorta–pulmonary artery anastomosis, because it can be undone at the time of the definitive open-heart surgery. Both procedures are palliative and are done

to increase blood flow to the lungs. At a future time when the palliative measure is no longer effective, open-heart surgery is done to repair the VSD and resect the pulmonary stenosis.

Tricuspid Atresia

Atresia of the tricuspid valve is a congenital defect in which there is a complete closure of this valve, an interatrial septal defect, a hypoplastic right ventricle, and a normal mitral valve and left ventricle (Fig. 34-14). Blood flows to the lungs from either the left ventricle through a VSD to the pulmonary artery or through a patent ductus arteriosus. All the blood from the systemic circulation is shunted from the right atrium through an interatrial communication (usually a patent foramen ovale) to the left atrium and eventually into the left ventricle, which functions as a single, common ventricle.

The prognosis for children with this defect is very poor. Many die in the neonatal period, and 80 percent of those who do not have surgery die before the age of 3 years.

These infants are cyanotic at birth with dyspnea, polycythemia, clubbing, and hypoxia occurring early. The physical examination may reveal no murmur, and the second sound is pure. The characteristic cyanosis is severe unless the pulmonary artery arises from the left ventricle. Cyanosis may then be mild or absent because of the increased pulmonary flow. However as the pulmonary resistance increases, the cyanosis increases progressively. Congestive heart failure may occur.

An ECG tracing reveals left ventricular hypertrophy, and chest x-rays show that the pulmonary vascular markings are diminished. A cardiac catheterization is done to obtain base-line data. If the ASD is not adequate, the defect may be enlarged by the Rashkind procedure.

Palliative surgery may be performed to increase pulmonary blood flow if hypoxic episodes occur. In infants under 6 weeks of age, a side-to-side anastomosis between the ascending aorta and right pulmonary artery is done. In older infants and children the Glenn procedure, a side-to-end anastomosis of the superior vena cava to the right pulmonary artery is performed. A complete surgical correction is not possible at this time; the palliative efforts are made to sustain life.

Ebstein's Malformation

In Ebstein's malformation there is an obstruction to the filling of the right ventricle because malformed cusps of the tricuspid valve adhere to the ventricular septum, causing tricuspid regurgitation (insufficiency). With the blood flow obstructed, there is a large right-to-left shunt through the patent foramen ovale or a small ASD with resultant cyanosis. The right atrial mean pressure may be normal or elevated, while the right ventricle and pulmonary artery pressures are normal. The symptoms presented vary, but the neonate or infant is usually mildly cyanotic and dyspneic and in congestive heart failure.

The ECG is characterized by tall, wide, bizarre P waves, and the x-rays reveal an enlarged heart. Fluoroscopy studies and angiocardiography are included in the diagnostic work-up.

Prognosis   While the prognosis depends on the degree of obstruction to blood flow, it is poor in the presence of other lesions, marked cyanosis, and extreme cardiomegaly. Death is usually due to arrhythmia, emboli, or congestive heart failure.

When the tricuspid regurgitation is mild, palliation is excellent. Medical management encompasses the problems of right-sided failure, arrhythmias, and complications of associated right-to-left shunting, especially brain abscesses. The development of bacterial endocarditis is also a dreaded complication.

Several methods of surgical correction have been attempted, including a bypass of the right side of the heart, reconstruction of the tricuspid valve, and prosthetic replacement. The latter has been the most successful. However, at the present time there is no one best corrective procedure available.

ACQUIRED CARDIAC CONDITIONS IN CHILDREN
Acute Rheumatic Fever

Rheumatic fever, a collagen disease, is an important cause of heart disease in children. It is difficult to determine its incidence accurately since the diagnostic criteria vary and the disease is not a reportable one in the United States. Even with the increased treatment available for infection, rheumatic fever still occurs and affects approximately 0.5 percent of school-age children.

Acute rheumatic fever is a systemic inflammatory disease that usually develops 10 or 14 days to 6 weeks (if reinfection occurs) following a group A, β-hemolytic streptococcus infection, and it is found most often in children between the ages of 7 and 14 years. The diagnosis is based on the application of the modified Jones criteria for acute rheumatic fever. The presence of two major criteria or one major and two minor criteria strongly suggests that the child

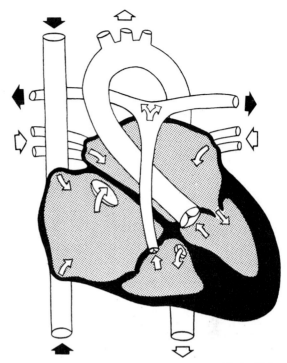

Figure 34-14   Tricuspid atresia. *(From Ross Clinical Education Aid #7, Ross Laboratories, Columbus, Ohio.)*

has acute rheumatic fever. Major criteria include migratory polyarthritis, carditis, chorea, erythema marginatum, or subcutaneous nodules. The minor criteria consist of a fever, a previous streptococcal infection, arthritis, leukocytosis, an elevated erythrocyte sedimentation rate, a positive C-reactive protein, a prolonged P-R interval, prior history of rheumatic fever, and the presence of inactive heart disease.

There appears to be an inherited tendency or familial predisposition to rheumatic fever since children of rheumatic parents contract acute rheumatic fever more readily than do children of nonrheumatic parents. It also seems to occur more frequently in the lower socioeconomic groups where overcrowding, poor nutrition, and poor hygienic conditions contribute to a higher incidence of this acquired disease. There is a seasonal variation; rheumatic fever is more common in the spring on the East coast and in the winter on the West coast of the United States. Recurrences of rheumatic fever are frequent after reinfection with streptococci.

Since rheumatic fever occurs in school-age children, this disease is often diagnosed during a routine school physical examination. Early diagnosis is difficult because major signs and symptoms are absent and complaints may be vague. General symptoms such as malaise, pallor, loss of weight, and loss of appetite are frequently associated with rheumatic fever; however, the course of illness varies and may not include all the symptoms mentioned. The most typical lesions of rheumatic fever occur in the connective tissue of the arteries, subcutaneous tissue, and the heart.

While inflammation of the pericardium, myocardium, and valves occur, the mitral and aortic valves are the most susceptible to damage. The carditis, evident within 2 weeks, is manifested by tachycardia, cardiac enlargement, cardiac murmurs, and a change in the sound of prior murmurs. Occasionally, increased venous pressure, edema, and dyspnea occur as compensatory symptoms. Also, a friction murmur is audible at times.

The myocardial lesion primarily involved in rheumatic fever is the formation of *Aschoff's bodies*. With the inflammation present, there is a cellular response to the altered collagen common to the perivascular connective tissue, and the result is the formation of nodules known as Aschoff's bodies. With aging this lesion becomes more fibrous.

For obvious reasons, rheumatic changes in the heart are of great concern. The endocardial changes consist principally of vegetation (blood, platelets, and fibrin) that develops on the valves of the heart. These seem to localize on the atrial surface of the mitral valve and the ventricular surface of the aortic valve. The valves are swollen, edematous, and distorted. The myocardium is the site of Aschoff's bodies, especially in the left atrium and the ventricles. The pericardium, if involved in the process, characteristically manifests serofibrinous pericarditis, varying from the mild to the predominantly exudative form. This may cause cardiac tamponade.

The clinical picture for children with rheumatic fever is variable. The onset may be acute, but a multitude of other factors are involved. In about 50 percent of the children with rheumatic fever the parents describe a cold or sore throat 10 days to 6 weeks before the onset of illness. This illness may have been treated with an antimicrobial agent either transiently or in an inadequate dosage. The severity of the respiratory infection may have been average and its duration usually no more than 2 to 4 days. Other children may experience a low-grade fever, complain of abdominal pain, or have spontaneous nosebleeds or dyspnea on exertion for a period of time.

The acute attack of rheumatic fever may follow the infection and consist of (1) a fever of 38 to 39°C (100.4 to 102.2°F), (2) leukocytosis, (3) elevation of the erythrocyte sedimentation rate, (4) mild or occasionally severe anemia, and (5) lassitude, irritability, and moderate weight loss. After the acute phase, the child may then experience some of the specific manifestations of rheumatic fever—arthritis, carditis, or chorea. Other symptoms may include epistaxis, abdominal pain, and skin manifestations.

Arthritis, the most common complaint of children with rheumatic fever, involves several joints simultaneously or in succession. The involved joints are tender, swollen, and painful to move and remain in this condition as the disease runs its course in 3 weeks or less.[27] Usually the large joints such as the knees, ankles, wrists, and elbows are involved. The older child has more severe joint involvement than the younger child, and the pain is so intense that the weight of a blanket may be unbearable. Sometimes the arthritis of rheumatic fever is confused with "growing pains," which are worse at night and relieved by massage. The child with rheumatic fever cannot bear to have his joints manipulated because of the intense pain.

Cardiac involvement is usually accompanied by a change in the quality of the pulse. Definite evidence of carditis almost necessitates the diagnosis of rheumatic fever in children. Although statistics do not exist, carditis is probably seen in about 50 percent of the cases, and it is found in nearly all fatal cases.

Rheumatic fever is responsible for the majority of organic mitral valve lesions and eventually causes mitral stenosis in most cases. For the evaluation of carditis, a knowledge of the condition of the child's heart before the onset of the present illness is of great importance. If a new murmur is identified, the likelihood of carditis is strong. Apical systolic murmurs can be considered significant only if they last through at least half of systole. Apical diastolic murmurs, always significant, are commonly found in acute carditis at a time when no organic mitral stenosis is present.[28] The origin of the murmur is not clear, but it is thought to be due to relative mitral stenosis caused by dilatation of the left ventricle.

Pericarditis may occur and can be detected by a friction rub. The heart sounds in acute carditis often lose their luster and become distant, dull, and muffled with the development of a large effusion. Poor cardiac pulsations as well as the feeble heart sounds may be evident and should be noted by the nurse. A ventricular diastolic gallop is commonly present in acute rheumatic carditis.

Carditis usually causes permanent changes and can be fatal. Congestive heart failure is a common manifestation, and distended neck veins, hepato-megaly, pulmonary rales, low urinary output, and even pitting edema are seen. An astute nurse may identify the ventricular diastolic murmur before the appearance of these frank symptoms of congestive heart failure. Almost axiomatically, any child with rheumatic heart disease who is in failure has active carditis. This phenomenon is in contrast to adults in whom congestive heart failure may be an outcome of mechanical stress placed on the heart as a conse-quence of valvular lesions caused by childhood rheu-matic heart disease.

Electrocardiographic tracings may be of help in evaluating the degree of cardiac involvement in this disease. The changes, however, may be transient. Prolongation of the P-R interval (first degree block) and the presence of the Wenckebach phenomenon (second degree block) are the most frequently de-scribed abnormalities. However, the presence of these abnormalities alone does not necessarily mean active carditis.

Chorea, or St. Vitus dance, involves the nervous system and is manifested by muscular twitchings, weakness, and purposeless movements. These signs may be insidious. At first the child may show evi-dence of not concentrating in school, exhibiting mood swings, being hyperirritable, and demonstrat-ing other signs of inappropriate behavior. Jerky, in-voluntary movements become evident. This involve-ment may begin 2 to 6 months after the initial infec-tion, and it affects girls much more frequently than boys. The muscular weakness can be so extreme that the child cannot sit up or even talk. The symptoms gradually subside after a period of time.

The skin manifestations of rheumatic fever are erythematous areas with irregular borders, sharply demarcated and often of a transient nature. Ery-thema marginatum is often seen with carditis.

Rheumatic nodules are a major and specific manifestation of rheumatic fever. These subcuta-neous nodules attached to tendon sheaths have a symmetrical distribution over the scapula, elbows, edge of the patella, the vertebrae, and the occiput. They are painless and freely movable under the skin. Although they may be found in other conditions, they occur in severe or chronic forms of rheumatic activ-ity. They may last a few days or a few weeks.

Severe nosebleeds also occur in about 10 per-cent of the patients with acute rheumatic fever. These nosebleeds are not associated with trauma. Queries related to nose-picking should be made when taking the history because it is the common-est cause of epistaxis in childhood.

Abdominal pain is seen in a small number of children with acute rheumatic fever. If accompanied by general signs of inflammation, acute appendicitis may be suspected. Acute appendicitis may be the initial admitting diagnosis of children with acute rheumatic fever.

The major aim of therapy is to prevent perma-nent cardiac damage, the only long-term serious complication of acute rheumatic fever. Bed rest dur-ing the acute febrile part of the illness is standard, especially in the presence of carditis. A gradual in-crease in activity is begun once the sedimentation rate has returned to normal and the signs of inflam-mation have subsided. This period may extend to 6 to 12 weeks. Careful observation for recurrence of signs and symptoms, especially those of a cardiac nature, is of utmost importance for the nurse. Man-agement, if successful, can prevent valvular damage or minimize progression of existing valvular damage. Improvement of cardiac function and general symp-tomatic relief during the acute phase is an important goal.

Some patients in the acute phase do not feel acutely ill and, therefore, are a problem to maintain on bed rest. Other children withdraw while they are sick. Still others become belligerent and may re-quire great patience on the part of the family or nurse caring for the child. Since the child can exhibit all types of behavior (rebellion, withdrawal, etc.) during the acute phase of rheumatic fever, it is very impor-tant for the nurse to understand and anticipate the needs of these children, particularly during the bed rest phase. This child needs distractions to keep him from becoming restless and bored. Some physicians believe that rather than insisting the child remain on complete bed rest that he be allowed limited activity. If this child is being cared for at home, he should be located close to the bathroom and telephone and have passive types of games available until there are no specific limitations placed on his activity.

The first priority in chemotherapeutic treatment is eradication of the streptococcal infection, fol-lowed by long-term chemoprophylaxis. Penicillin is the drug of choice except for those children sensi-tive to the drug. In such cases, erythromycin is selected. It is given in an oral form unless the child has had previous episodes of carditis or rheumatic fever; then parenteral antibiotics are given. The length of therapy varies, but those patients with severe valvular involvement are usually maintained on life-long prophylaxis.

Since there does not appear to be any evidence that carditis can be prevented by the utilization of corticosteroids, these medications are generally used when patients present symptoms of congestive heart failure. Short-term studies seem to indicate that corticosteroids do not reduce the incidence of murmurs;[29] however, additional research is needed. If they are used, cushingoid symptoms can be expected. The combination of steroid therapy and stress may lead to the development of gastric ulcers.

While aspirin does not appear to alter the duration of the rheumatic attack, it does contribute to the child's comfort, especially when he is febrile or joint pain is present. The massive doses of salicylates formerly given to patients are no longer being used. The signs of aspirin toxicity and the effects of salicylates on the clotting time are important concerns. Since aspirin reduces a patient's fever, relieves his joint pain, and lowers his sedimentation rate, a nurse must carefully evaluate and record the child's response to this therapy. The medications selected, their dosages, and the duration of use vary. They are highly individualized to meet the needs of patients who present with a wide variety of symptoms.

Since the patient may have a fever, fluid intake should be carefully recorded. The child should not be allowed to become dehydrated; at the same time, excessive fluids which would augment the congestive heart failure and fluid retention should be avoided. Skin turgor should be observed to evaluate hydration.

If chorea develops, the patient must be protected from injury since the possibility of convulsions exists. Side rails should be padded, the nails should be trimmed, and an assessment of the need for restraints should be made. The patient must be continuously observed. Any increase in choreic movements should be noted. The child's temperature needs to be taken rectally. Sedation may be necessary.

These children experience extreme frustration because of mood swings or lack of control over their movements. Most children do not understand their outbursts of anger or mood changes and therefore may need assistance. Such frustration may lead to anxiety or additional emotional stress, which increases choreiform movements and causes exhaustion.

The possibility of recurrence is real. Therefore the nurse should play a vital role in follow-up care. Teaching the child and his family why the medications should be continued, the clinic visits kept, and the affected child protected from family members with respiratory infections or sore throats are points which should be emphasized. The American Heart Association recommends that all patients who currently have or have had acute rheumatic fever should be placed indefinitely on a program of prophylaxis.

Such a recommendation markedly reduces the frequency of recurrences of acute rheumatic fever.

This long-term treatment and hospitalization is an emotional and financial burden on the child and his family. Health team members must be cognizant of family needs, including those which can best be met by the public health nurse, social worker, or nutritionist. The local branch of the American Heart Association should be a primary community resource.

Prognosis The prognosis in rheumatic fever varies. Carditis is the most severe and possible fatal complication; therefore, the nurse's main role is to maintain a balance between the body's needs and the supply of blood the weakened heart is able to deliver. This involves decreasing the child's activity, being cognizant of symptoms of heart failure, and, in general, creating a restful situation for the heart. When treatment is instituted promptly and there is a good response, the prognosis is favorable. Usually there is a better prognosis if the first attack occurs in an older child.

Atherosclerosis*

Although *atherosclerosis*, a condition characterized by fatty deposits on the walls of arteries, has been associated with middle-aged and older adults, the atherosclerotic process is beginning to receive attention from those concerned with the prevention of cardiovascular conditions in children. In the near future, the nurse can expect to have an active role in the nursing management and health maintenance of children who are at risk of developing this disorder.

Fatty streaks can be seen as early as 6 months of age in the endothelium of the aorta. The need for the continued investigation of hypercholesterolemia and its identification in children is important because it is known to be a hereditary metabolic disease. Its incidence exceeds phenylketonuria and galactosemia, two conditions for which newborns are routinely screened.

Primary familial hypercholesterolemia is considered the most significant of the hyperlipoproteinemias with regard to the later development of premature cardiovascular diseases. The condition is known to be inherited as an autosomal dominant trait, or it

* The writers wish to acknowledge the assistance of Major Peter Freis, M.D., U.S. Army Medical Corps, Walter Reed Army Medical Center, Washington, D.C., for his assistance in the preparation of this section. The information presented here is adapted from a paper he delivered at the 10th Annual Uniformed Services Pediatrics Seminar in Biloxi, Mississippi, March 25–29, 1974.

may result from a combination of genes which carry the trait. Incidence is estimated to be as high as one in every 400 persons in the United States.

Laboratory tests usually show an increase in low density lipoprotein (LPL) on lipoprotein electrophoresis, which may or may not be accompanied by a cholesterol elevation. Screening for cholesterol and triglyceride determinations on children at the age of 5 years who have a family history of premature cardiovascular disease (a myocardial infarction before age 50) was recommended by the American Academy of Pediatrics in 1971. All siblings of hyperlipoproteinemic patients should also be tested, regardless of their age. A fasting serum cholesterol above 240 mg/100 ml is considered abnormal in a screening test. Early assessment and periodic reevaluation appear to be the most important measures in the identification and management of atherosclerotic processes in children.

Bacterial Endocarditis

Bacterial endocarditis is a febrile illness which is frequently difficult to diagnose. It may occur without preexisting heart disease, but it usually occurs as a complication of congenital or rheumatic heart disease or following a systemic infection. Bacterial endocarditis has been classified as acute or subacute; however, the former is seldom seen in pediatrics. When it occurs, the acute form is usually fatal; therefore, the subacute type of endocarditis will be discussed.

Subacute bacterial endocarditis (SBE) is an infectious disease caused by *Streptococcus viridans* in a majority of cases, with other types of streptococci, staphylococci, or gram-negative organisms implicated in the remainder. The infection involves abnormal heart tissue, especially rheumatic lesions or congenital heart defects. It may develop (1) in the presence of an atrioventricular communication such as a patent ductus arteriosus, (2) as a complication of coarctation of the aorta, or (3) in cyanotic patients, especially those with a previous pulmonary anastomosis when the infection is on the anastomosis.

The greatest incidence occurs in conjunction with dental problems, genitourinary procedures, localized foci of infection, general surgery, criminal abortion, or following cardiac surgery.

The lesions in this disease consist of so-called vegetation, composed of fibrin, leukocytes, and bacteria, which adheres to the valvular or endocardial surface. As a result of the turbulent blood flow, portions of these vegetations may dislodge and embolize either to the lungs or the systemic circulation. Emboli formation, therefore, is the most characteristic manifestation of this disease.

Signs of subacute bacterial endocarditis are subtle and may be overlooked. There is usually an insidious onset with a fever, lethargy, general malaise, and anorexia. Splenomegaly and retinal hemorrhages may be present. *Splinter hemorrhages* (longitudinal black, splinter-shaped hemorrhagic areas involving the distal third of the nail) and *Osler's nodes* (reddish-purple, raised nodules with white centers found in the distal pads of fingers or toes) are evidence of embolic phenomenon.

An ECG reveals a prolonged P-R interval and changes in the T wave. Cardiomegaly is evident on x-ray. Laboratory studies indicate an elevated erythrocyte sedimentation rate, leukocytosis, anemia, albuminuria, and sometimes a microscopic hematuria. A murmur is often present and changeable in character, and the heart action is forceful and rapid with an occasional gallop rhythm.

It is essential to identify the causative organism; therefore, multiple blood cultures are obtained routinely. While the treatment depends on the organism cultured out, it generally involves the administration of large doses of antibiotics for a prolonged period of time. For example, if *S. viridans* is the culprit, penicillin may be given intravenously for up to 6 weeks. Combinations of drugs, such as streptomycin and penicillin, may be used. The causative agent determines the selection, and an individualized treatment schedule is devised for each patient.

Long-term follow-up care is imperative, and blood cultures are a part of each subsequent examination. If a repairable cardiovascular anomaly is present, corrective surgery is considered. In those children with a congenital heart defect or prior rheumatic infections, antibiotics should be administered routinely when a dental procedure or surgery is performed or when an acute respiratory infection is present.

Prognosis Chemotherapeutic advances have improved the prognosis of subacute bacterial endocarditis. It continues to be a very serious inflammatory process, the outcome of which depends on the length of time the infection is present before the diagnosis is made.

Pericarditis

Pericarditis is an inflammation of the pericardium which may be caused by rheumatic fever, collagen diseases, pyogenic microorganisms, trauma, or certain severe hereditary anemias. The cause may also remain unknown. The involvement of the pericardium may be of the dry and fibrinous type or one in which an effusion develops. The latter may be serous, exudative, hemorrhagic, or purulent in nature. Should the infection be acute, the exudative effusion may initiate the development of fibrosis and chronic constrictive pericarditis, which compresses the heart and restricts returning blood flow and cardiac contractibility.

In pericarditis without effusion there is an acute sharp pain which is relieved by sitting up, turning to the side, or leaning forward. It is made more intense by moving, coughing, or laughing. Pain is identified in the infant by his persistent crying and restlessness. Older children may complain of referred pain to the tip of the shoulder, the neck, or the left arm. A friction rub is heard at any point over the precordium and it varies in intensity according to changes in position.

With pericardial effusion there is pain, a cough, and possibly dyspnea. X-rays reveal cardiac enlargement. While a friction rub is present, the heart sounds are also usually muffled. On x-ray the lung fields may be congested if the patient is in heart failure. A complication of pericarditis with effusion, in addition to chronic constrictive pericarditis, is *cardiac tamponade.*

Cardiac tamponade occurs because there is compression of the heart by fluid within the pericardium which hinders venous return, restricts the heart's ability to fill properly, and produces increased systemic and pulmonary venous pressure and decreased cardiac output. These comments pertain only to tamponade associated with rapid onset. When fluid accumulates slowly, a compensatory measure allows the walls to stretch gradually and avoids cardiac tamponade.

A nurse who observes a patient with a rapid accumulation of pericardial fluid observes an acutely ill child who appears to be very anxious and who has cold and clammy extremities indicative of shock. There is peripheral edema, the neck veins are probably distended, and the pulse is rapid and difficult to palpate. *Pulsus paradoxus,* a fall in the systolic blood pressure during inspiration greater than the normal 5 to 10 mmHg, is an invaluable indication of tamponade.

In confirming the diagnosis, cardiologists use a variety of diagnostic aids including the intravenous injection of carbon dioxide, echocardiography, radioactive scanning, or angiocardiography. Time and the available equipment influence their decision making, for this situation is one in which treatment is an urgent life-saving measure.

Should this complication develop, the pericardial fluid must be removed by paracentesis. It is a nursing responsibility to gather all the resuscitation equipment, including the defibrillator, for utilization should the need arise. The patient is monitored continually during the procedure and for a period of time after the aspiration. As the fluid is removed, the patient's status improves dramatically; however, diligent surveillance is imperative as the condition may recur. These patients are frequently placed in intensive care units where careful observation and monitoring of vital signs, especially blood pressure and venous pressure, can be done easily. The fluid which is removed is studied to determine the cause of its accumulation and prevent its recurrence. The chemotherapy which may be instituted is determined by the causative organism or precipitating factor.

Primary Myocardial Disease

There are several common forms of myocardial disease which are inflammatory in nature, or result from diseases of connective tissue or systemic infection. Rheumatic fever is the most frequent cause, but other problems caused by the presence of bacteria, viral agents, rickettsia, collagen disorders, or some infiltrative process may precipitate myocardial involvement. Specific causative diseases include glycogen storage disease, progressive muscular dystrophy, Coxsackie virus, and Friedreich's ataxia. Severe anemic, metabolic, or endocrine imbalance may also result in a secondary myocarditis.

Generally, the onset is sudden with a temperature increase, rapid pulse, and dyspnea. Cardiomegaly is seen on x-ray, and signs of heart failure may be present. The heart sounds are of poor quality —dull, muffled, or indistinct.

Treatment is symptomatic and aimed at controlling the underlying cause. Should heart failure be present, a cardiotonic regimen is started.

Prognosis The prognosis is usually good but depends on the extent of involvement. The development of residual myocardial fibrosis may account for the myocardial insufficiency seen later in life.[30]

NURSING MANAGEMENT OF THE CHILD UNDERGOING HEART SURGERY
Preoperative Period

To prepare children and parents adequately for cardiac surgery, children are usually admitted to the hospital approximately 3 to 5 days prior to the surgical procedure. The presurgical evaluation includes a history, physical examination, and diagnostic tests. The diagnostic procedures completed before surgery include an electrocardiogram, phonocardiogram, chest x-rays, cardiac catheterization, angiocardiography, and pulmonary function tests. (See the section on diagnostic procedures in this chapter.)

Results of blood tests are used for preoperative assessment and as a basis for comparison in nursing and medical management postoperatively. Essential tests are complete blood count, hemoglobin, hematocrit, bleeding and clotting studies, prothrombin time, blood urea nitrogen, serum electrolytes, and blood typing and cross-match. Several units of blood will be reserved for use in the operative and postoperative periods. The white blood cell count is checked to determine the absence of infection. The preoperative urinalysis, and the pH and specific gravity in particular, provide important reference criteria for comparison in the assessment of kidney function postoperatively.

Preoperative Nursing Assessment This assessment begins with the admission procedures and is an essential component of the total preoperative evaluation. Measurements of height, weight, and vital signs are made upon admission. Thereafter, the temperature, pulse, respirations and blood pressure are measured and recorded three or four times a day. The child's preoperative range of vital signs will be used as a standard of reference in evaluation of the child's physiologic status during and after surgery. Since the child must be free from fever and infection before surgery, any elevation in temperature or other symptoms of infection should be reported to the surgeon promptly.

The nurse should make sure the child is weighed daily, on the *same scale,* and at the same time each day. The early morning is the preferred time for recording daily weight. The height and weight measurements will be used to calculate the child's body surface area in determining dosage of medications and anesthesia and to identify the child's fluid, blood, and nutritional requirements during and after surgery.

Because any existing fluid and electrolyte imbalance must be corrected to the greatest extent possible before surgery, the preoperative record of intake and output is an essential assessment tool which must be complete and accurate.

The nursing history, obtained through interview of the child and parents upon admission, provides information necessary to plan individualized pre- and postoperative care. Pertinent factors such as the child's level of understanding, usual routines, his preferences, and any special needs should be discussed during this interview. The initial interview and history also allow the nurse to assess the child's and the parents' behavior and the patterns of parent-child interaction. These nursing observations often provide an indication of the degree of the child's and parents' anxiety concerning the anticipated surgery.

Preparation of the Child and Parents This preparation for the preoperative, operative, and postoperative periods is a mandatory nursing responsibility. The teaching, counseling, and emotional support of the child and parents initiated by the nurse during the first contact with the family is essential throughout the child's hospitalization.

Preparing the parents The nurse should provide opportunities for the parents to discuss their child with the nurse at a time when the child is not present to help establish a rapport with the parents. The nurse can use this time to assess the *parents'* needs in relation to their child's hospitalization and surgery.

The nurse should recognize that anticipation of their child's surgery, with its benefits and risks, is likely to be very stressful for the parents and that they may need the nurse's assistance in order to verbalize their questions and feelings. Despite overwhelming concern, many parents are reluctant to ask the nurse for time to answer their questions. Rather than assume that parents do not need to confer with the nurse because they seem informed, the nurse should initiate conferences with them as often as necessary. Expression of the parents' concerns about their child and the forthcoming surgery can be facilitated if the nurse provides ample time, privacy, and a relaxed atmosphere for the discussions. The parents should be encouraged to ask questions, and the questions should be answered succinctly, accurately, and in sufficient depth.

In preparing the parents for the child's surgery, the nurse should ask them what they already know and what they have already told their child about the hospital and the operation. The nurse can then elaborate on what the parents already know, and correct misinformation or misunderstanding they might express. Visual aids should be used whenever possible because quite frequently the parents' anxiety interferes with their accurate perception of the nurse's teaching.

When the nurse feels that the parents are ready,

details of all pre- and postoperative procedures their child will experience can be explained. If the nurse and parents plan and carry out the child's care together, the benefit to the child is likely to be greater than if the parents and nurse support the child independently of each other. The nurse should encourage the parents to participate in their child's preparation for surgery as much as possible if they feel comfortable taking part.

It is important to assure the parents that a nurse will always be with their child in the operating room and following his operation. In many hospitals, the nurse who cares for the child before surgery accompanies him to the operating room and remains with the child until he is under anesthesia. This practice is considered to be effective in reducing the parents' and the child's apprehension. It is also beneficial for the family to meet the operating room, recovery room, and special care unit nurses before the day of surgery. The preparation of children and parents may include a visit to these special areas.

The nurse must thoroughly explain all postoperative treatments and procedures the child is likely to receive as well as the complex machines, tubes, drainage apparatus, and infusion bottles that will surround their child after the operation. The parents should be given as much detail as they are ready to accept. Photographs and diagrams should be used when the parents cannot see the actual equipment. If the nurse does not prepare the parents with a realistic version of their child's postoperative appearance, they may be stunned or unduly frightened when they first see the child. The nurse should also tell the parents that although their child may appear very ill when surrounded by all the equipment, he will be having frequent postoperative treatments and exercises which are essential to his recovery.

The nurse should explain to the parents that thorough preparation for surgery that is geared to their child's level of understanding and paced according to his readiness to learn is important for the child's physical and emotional well-being before the operation and his successful recovery after surgery.

Preparing the child   The child's preparation for cardiac surgery begins a few days before the operation. Initiating preparation early tends to promote the child's cooperation during the actual procedures because the child has had a chance to "practice" what he will do, and the routines and equipment will be somewhat familiar to him.

All preoperative instruction must be individualized according to the child's informational and emo-

tional needs. His age, previous knowledge of his condition, and his previous experiences with hospitalization and surgery must be considered by the nurse in planning a teaching approach. Principles which should govern teaching-learning activities for the child include (1) building on the child's previous information; (2) proceeding from the simple to the complex; (3) presenting nonthreatening activities before those which might be threatening for the child; (4) utilizing short teaching and practice sessions; (5) pacing the introduction of new information according to the child's readiness; (6) giving reasons for treatments and activities in simple, but truthful, terms; and (7) using miniature models, dolls, diagrams, photographs, and actual equipment, when appropriate, as much as possible. A discussion of techniques which will help the nurse plan appropriate preparation for the child is presented in Part 3.

Turning, coughing, and deep breathing   The nurse should explain that after the child wakes up, a nurse will help him turn from his back to his side, and he will be asked to take deep breaths and cough deeply. The nurse can demonstrate each exercise for the child and then ask the child to imitate them. The child will probably need to repeat the postoperative exercises several times during the first session, and he should "practice" them every day with the nurse or his parents. Blowing bubbles and blowing up balloons can make deep breathing fun for the child.

The nurse may need to spend considerable time teaching the child to cough *deeply,* not just in his throat. If the child coughs only in his throat, he will not be able to raise the mucus which accumulates in the bronchi and trachea after anesthesia. In order to teach him to cough properly, the nurse can tell the child to take a deep breath and to make the cough come from "down deep inside" while he lets the air out. During the practice sessions, the child should sit upright and lean forward slightly (the position which will be assumed for coughing postoperatively), and the nurse should place both hands on the child's chest as if "splinting" the chest. If the child is coughing properly, the nurse should feel the chest expansion during inspiration and the thoracic wall vibrations during the cough. The child should be told that it will be harder to cough deeply after the operation because his chest will hurt, but the nurses will help him by holding their hands or a pillow against his chest.

Chest physical therapy   Chest physical therapy and postural drainage are often used to promote adequate respiratory function postoperatively. The treatments are frequently initiated 2 or 3 days preoperatively in order to improve respiratory function before surgery and to familiarize the child (and parents) with the procedure. If chest physiotherapy is planned for the child after the operation but not initiated prior to surgery, the nurse or a physiotherapist should demonstrate the techniques at least once during the preoperative period. The reader is referred to the section on chest physiotherapy in Chapter 33.

Inhalation therapy   The child is likely to receive humidified oxygen via tent, croupette, or, if the child is older, by mask. Intermittent positive pressure breathing treatments may also be prescribed. The child should see and handle the equipment. The machines should be turned on for a short time so the child can become accustomed to the sound and the feeling of the oxygen flow and the positive pressure gusts. If the child will be placed in a mist tent, the fog in the tent will diminish his ability to see out. This can be extremely frightening for the child upon awakening, and it might also cause the child to become disoriented or restless. It is advisable to set up a tent with mist and encourage the child to explore sight and sound from the inside of the tent during the day or evening before surgery.

Water-seal chest drainage   The child should be informed that when he awakens there will be a large bandage on his chest and one or two tubes which will come through the bandage from his chest. The child should be told that the tubes should never be pulled. The nurse should explain that the tubes will be attached to special bottles that collect air and blood but that the tubes will be long enough for him to sit up and turn in his bed. It should be emphasized that the chest tubes are temporary and will be removed by the doctor a few days after the operation. The nurse can also give the child a simple explanation of the removal of the tubes if he asks how the tubes will come out.

Infusions and angiocatheters   In explaining the cutdown or angiocatheters that will be used for infusions and to measure arterial and central venous pressures, the nurse can tell the child that he will have small tubes in his arms and legs when he wakes up and that the doctors and nurses will give him sugar water and medicines through the tubes until he is allowed to eat again. The nurse should tell him that the tubes will not hurt and that they will be removed when he starts to get better.

Cardioscope   The electrocardiogram leads will often be familiar to most children because of repeated tests, but the child should be informed that he will awaken with lead wires on his arms and legs. The nurse should show the child a model or photograph of the monitor that will be used. Because the cardioscope-pacemaker-defibrillator monitor is much larger than the usual electrocardiogram machine, its size may be threatening for the child.

Immediate Preoperative Preparation   In most hospitals, routine preoperative preparation is not extensive and is best done on the day or evening before surgery. Explanation of the skin prep, if the surgeon prescribes one, and the enema can be done a short time before the nurse does the treatment.

The child should be told that he will not be able to eat anything after a specified time during the night. The nurse should explain to the child that he will receive injections before he goes to the operating room that will make him feel sleepy. The means of transport to the operating room, i.e., stretcher or the child's own bed, and who will accompany him should be discussed. The child should also be told if he must wear a hospital gown instead of his own pajamas. If at all possible, the parents should be encouraged to come to see the child on the morning of surgery. If they plan to be present, the child should be told that he can see them in the morning.

The nurse should tell the child that he will probably feel sore when he wakes up and that he should tell the nurse when he feels sore so the nurse can give him medicine to take some of the "hurt" away.

The *skin preparation* of children who will have cardiac surgery varies with institutions and surgeons. In some hospitals, skin preparation is limited to a scrub with an antibacterial skin cleanser which is done in the operating room. Some surgeons prefer to begin skin preparation on the evening before surgery or a few days before surgery. The nurse is responsible for insuring that the proper number of scrubs, baths, or showers, usually with an antibacterial agent, have been carried out as specified by the surgeon.

The older child is usually given an *enema* on the evening before surgery in order to prevent postoperative abdominal distention which would cause him discomfort and possibly interfere with reexpansion of the lung. Solid food and most liquids are usually withheld for 12 hours prior to the induction of anesthesia, but the child should be permitted to have water up to 6 or 8 hours before induction in order to maintain adequate hydration. Because the ratio of water to total body size is very high in the young infant, neonates and infants up to 6 months of age should be given feedings of clear glucose water until 4 hours before induction.[31]

The nurse caring for the child undergoing cardiac surgery will be responsible for administration of certain *medications.* Children are usually placed on a series of prophylactic doses of antibiotics in order to prevent postoperative infection, especially endocarditis, which is a serious and potentially catastrophic complication. In order to achieve a satisfactory blood level of the antibiotic, the first dose of a broad spectrum antibiotic or two antibiotics, one for gram-positive and one for gram-negative organisms, is usually administered intramuscularly on the evening before surgery. Therapy is continued for 4 or 5 days.

Sometimes children who will be placed on cardiopulmonary by-pass (heart-lung machine) during surgery will receive *heparin* preoperatively to prevent the formation of intravascular thrombi. Heparin is an extremely potent anticoagulant, and the nurse must use the utmost care in preparing the correct dosage of this drug. Therapy with heparin is directed toward achieving a coagulation time which is two to three times the normal Lee-White coagulation time of 9 to 12 minutes.

Digitalis, a drug commonly used to treat infants and children in congestive heart failure, is known to adversely affect cardiac rhythms during surgery.[32] The usual dose of digitalis is withheld on the day of surgery. If necessary, therapy may be resumed postoperatively.

Infants and children usually receive minimal or no *preanesthetic medication* prior to cardiac surgery to avoid inducing the side effect of cardiorespiratory depression. Infants may receive a small intramuscular dose of *atropine sulfate* which helps to minimize production of secretions and prevents bradycardia, which could occur as an adverse effect of endotracheal intubation. In addition to atropine sulfate or *scopolamine,* older children may be given a small dose of a mild barbiturate which is sufficient to make them quiet and relaxed when arriving in the operating room. It is very important that the nurse administer these preoperative medications at the time designated. The anesthesiologist usually times the administration of the preanesthetic medications so that anesthetic induction can be performed when the action of the medications is at its peak.

Intraoperative Period

It is estimated that 60 percent of infants with congenital heart defects who are not treated surgically die within 1 year, and one-half of these infants do not survive for 1 month.[33] Therefore, cardiovascular surgery may be cited as a significant means of reducing infant mortality due to congenital heart defects. Although surgical treatment of congenital heart defects may be performed on persons of all ages, the majority of operative procedures are performed on infants and young children.

Cardiovascular surgery in children may be either *corrective* or *palliative.* Corrective surgery is attempted if the mortality rate for the procedure is acceptable in relation to the severity of the child's condition. The objective of surgery for coarctation of the aorta, patent ductus arteriosus, and vascular ring is correction of the defect. Palliative surgery, which largely consists of closed-heart procedures, is most often performed on high-risk newborns because they do not tolerate the cardiopulmonary by-pass required for open procedures well. The objective of palliative surgery is to improve the existing hemodynamics sufficiently to allow the child's survival until the corrective surgery can be performed. Examples of palliative cardiac surgery are (1) creation of a shunt to the pulmonary artery from the aorta for tetralogy of Fallot; (2) atrial septectomy (Blalock-Hanlon operation) for transposition of the great vessels; and (3) pulmonary artery banding for ventricular septal defects. Although palliative, the Blalock-Hanlon operation is currently the only surgical treatment for tricuspid atresia.[34] Children who had palliative surgery as infants are usually scheduled for corrective surgery when they reach 4 or 5 years of age.

The anesthesiologist determines the *anesthetic agents* that will be used during surgery. This decision is based on preoperative evaluation of the child's general condition, the heart defect, other physiologic alterations which exist, and drugs which the child has received. No particular agent is considered superior to others, but anesthesiologists seem to prefer inducing amnesia with a small dose of a rapid-acting barbiturate hypnotic, followed by a muscle relaxant and inhalation anesthesia which is administered via endotracheal tube. Infants under 1 year of age do not usually receive the hypnotic agent. Regardless of the agents used, the anesthesiologist will be concerned with delivery of a light, smooth level of anesthesia. Deep anesthesia is definitely contraindicated.

As with cardiac catheterization, maintenance of adequate *body temperature* of the child, especially the small infant, is of critical importance during cardiovascular surgery. Before surgery on premature infants and neonates, the circulating nurse in the operating room should see that the infant's extremities are wrapped in absorbent cotton and that there is a stockinette cap on the child's head. These should be applied *before* the child is removed from the incubator. A radiant shield should be used to warm the child during cutdowns and other preliminary procedures. The infant should be placed on an Underwriters' Laboratory–approved warming pad that is electrically grounded. The circulating nurse should raise the thermostat of the operating room to 78 or 80°F (25.6 or 26.7°C) for all procedures done on neonates and small infants. The body temperature of children of all ages will be monitored via electronic rectal probe during surgery. Some institutions use plastic drapes which adhere to the child's skin as an aid in conserving body heat. The nurse is also responsible for seeing that *all* intravenous fluids, blood transfusions, and irrigating solutions are warmed before use. Thermic blankets may be used if necessary. Young children who are having open-heart surgery will receive the additional benefit of thermoregulation of heat exchange during cardiopulmonary by-pass. In some children it may be desirable to induce *hypothermia* during by-pass in order to reduce the child's oxygen needs during surgery.

During the surgical procedure, several indicators of physiologic status are observed carefully. *Heart rhythms* are monitored on a cardioscope. The *heart sounds* are auscultated by an esophageal stethoscope. An indwelling angiocatheter and auscultation are used to monitor *arterial blood pressure*. A catheter inserted into the inferior or superior vena cava measures *central venous pressure*. Samples for *blood gas* determinations are taken at frequent intervals. If the child is having surgery which requires cardiopulmonary by-pass, electroencephalogram leads are applied in order to identify the development of cerebral anoxia during the surgery.

Use of a Foley catheter in infants and small children may be waived during surgery; the incidence of kidney failure related to cardiac surgery in children is low, and the insertion of a catheter may unnecessarily subject the child to risk of infection. A pediatric urine collection device with attached drainage tubing and a urimeter is usually sufficient to monitor kidney function during the operative procedure.

Extracorporeal circulation, also called cardiopulmonary by-pass, is a system used in open-heart surgery whereby a heart-lung machine oxygenates venous blood which has been removed from the body and returns the freshly oxygenated blood to the arterial circulation. The use of extracorporeal circulation diverts blood from its usual route through the heart and lungs to permit the surgeon a relatively dry field. Extracorporeal circulation is established by inserting a cannula in the inferior and superior vena cavae through a small incision in the right atrium; the cannula diverts venous blood to the machine. Oxygenated blood from the machine is released into circulation by an arterial cannula.

Before instituting by-pass, the extracorporeal circuit is usually primed with heparinized blood for surgery on infants. A 5 percent dextrose and water solution, which may also be heparinized, is used to prime the machine prior to surgery on children. The rate of blood flow during by-pass is calculated on the basis of the child's total body surface area. The bloodless heart will continue to beat during the surgery unless the surgeon needs to stop the heart contraction by inducing temporary ventricular fibrillation. Although machines used for extracorporeal circulation differ mechanically in the method of oxygenation employed, the underlying principle and technique of arterial and venous cannulation are the same with different models.

Maintenance of *blood volume* of the infant or child is a critical factor during cardiac surgery. *All* blood lost or removed for blood tests is replaced, volume for volume.

The hours during which their child is in the operating room are emotionally tense and upsetting ones for parents. It is perhaps the ominous unknown which creates much of the parents' burden as they await the completion of their child's operation. This time of uncertainty for them may be viewed as a crisis because there is likely to be a striking imbalance between the emotional magnitude of the situation and the parents' limited immediate coping resources.[35]

Since the nurse is virtually the only contact between the parents and their child at this time, the nurse should place a high priority on supporting the parents. In a crisis, it is the quality and timing of the intervention, not the quantity, that is important. Therefore, even if the nurse can spend only short intervals of time with the parents, this will be valuable in helping them sustain the stress of the waiting period. The nurse's verbal intervention need not be extensive in order to be therapeutic for the parents. Brief progress reports about the child, even if only to assure them that he is doing as expected, are most effective in helping the parents move toward healthy resolution of this brief crisis.

Postoperative Period

After the incision is closed and the wound is dressed, a portable chest x-ray is taken before the child leaves the operating room. He is also weighed immediately after the procedure. This measurement will serve as a guide for blood and fluid replacement postoperatively. Some children may be extubated in the operating room if their general condition is good. If respiratory function is weak, the endotracheal tube will not be removed until later.

In hospitals where there is a special care nursery, the neonate will usually go directly to that unit following surgery. Before transfer to a special care or intensive care unit, infants and older children may go to the recovery room.

Nursing Management Continuous, astute observation and meticulous attention to supportive care measures characterize the postoperative nursing management of children who have had cardiovascular surgery.

The *vital signs* should be checked every 15 minutes for the first 24 hours. The nurse must be alert to even subtle alterations because serious impending complications are often first manifested by changes in the child's vital signs. The cardioscope is used to monitor the *heart rate* and *rhythm.* In addition to measurement of *arterial blood pressure* by auscultation, the child will usually have a catheter inserted through the femoral or brachial artery which is used for the measurement of *systemic intra-arterial blood pressure* and is monitored on an oscilloscope. The intra-arterial blood pressure should closely correspond to the arterial blood pressure that is heard on auscultation. A sharp difference between these pressures might indicate an alteration in peripheral vascular resistance. In addition to the arterial catheter, the child may also have a catheter leading to the left atrium if surgery was performed to correct an atrial defect or if the child had an open-heart procedure.

The *central venous pressure* is a recording of the amount of pressure in the right atrium. It assesses the balance between blood being pumped into systemic circulation and the venous return to the heart. The central venous pressure catheter is usually inserted through the right cephalic or basilic vein. The normal right atrial pressure is approximately 0 mmHg.

The intra-arterial and central venous pressures should be evaluated in relation to each other. If the contraction of the left ventricle becomes weak or the patient goes into shock, the central venous pressure is likely to rise while the intra-arterial pressure will drop. However, if the patient is hypovolemic in the presence of shock, the central venous pressure may not rise and may even decrease. An *increase* in the central venous pressure and a decrease in the intra-arterial pressure is also characteristic of cardiac tamponade.

An increase in the central venous pressure without a drop in the intra-arterial blood pressure could indicate an increasing blood volume. The nurse should remember that after surgery to correct tetralogy of Fallot it is common for the central venous pressure to rise temporarily. This rise seems to be a physiologic response related to a need for increased pressure in order to fill the right ventricle after the recent surgery.[36] The cardiovascular pressure readings should be observed frequently during the first hours after surgery. These measurements provide valuable information about the adequacy of cardiac output when they are correlated with blood gases, pH, and the urinary output.

The nurse must ensure that the child has a *patent airway* at all times. Suctioning of respiratory secretions may be necessary during the early postoperative period. Many children respond to cardiac surgery so well that they do not require respiratory assistance or even an oropharyngeal airway in the early postoperative period. Most children, however, will usually receive humidified oxygen by tent, hood, or mask. When blood gases show that the child can maintain adequate oxygen tension on room air, the oxygen may be discontinued. A heated nebulizer should be used after the oxygen is discontinued in order to humidify the inhaled air and to reduce viscosity of the pulmonary secretions.

Children who have poor respiratory ventilation will be placed on a respirator until they can establish effective ventilation unassisted. The endotracheal tube is usually left in place for 1 or 2 days if the child is on a respirator. A temporary tracheostomy is performed if the child needs respiratory assistance for a longer period. In order to prevent the child from fighting the respirator, small doses of morphine sulfate may be given at intervals. Despite its effect on the respiratory center of the brain, morphine sulfate is considered a safe drug for administration to infants and young children on respirators.[37]

Measures which are employed to promote adequate respiratory function include intermittent positive pressure breathing treatments, chest physiotherapy, postural drainage, and frequent coughing, turning, and deep breathing exercises. The nurse should institute and maintain an hourly schedule for the turning, coughing, and deep breathing. These exercises will be quite painful for the child, and he will need much encouragement from the nurse, no matter how well he "practiced" before surgery. Administration of the prescribed analgesic and splinting the child's chest with the nurse's hands or a pillow will make these treatments easier for the child to endure. Blood gas determinations are frequently made as a means of assessing the quality of ventilation.

One or two tubes are placed in the pleural cavity before the incision is closed. The purpose of these tubes, often called thoracotomy tubes, is to reestablish negative intrapleural pressure that is necessary for lung reexpansion. Negative pressure is created by submerging the tube a few centimeters below water in a sterile glass bottle. Both air and fluid, including blood, can be expected to drain through the tubes. When there are two chest tubes, the uppermost tube is likely to drain air while the lower tube usually drains fluid.

Water-seal chest drainage may be instituted with either a one, two, or three-bottle system. Three variations of water-sealed systems are shown in Fig. 34-16. Some hospitals may use a commercially manufactured system made of plastic which is compact and portable.

Certain measures and precautions are essential to the successful nursing management of the child who has thoracotomy tubes and water-seal drainage. It is most important to check the entire system frequently to *make sure there are no leaks*. If the water seal becomes disrupted, the lungs will collapse. The nurse should begin with inspection of the site of the tubes and *check every inch of tubing* between the patient and the bottles.

All rubber stoppers should be secured by adhesive tape. The glass tubes should be inspected for cracks or breakage, and the nurse should verify that the correct tube is submerged in the water. In order to prevent accidental breakage of the bottles and loss of the water seal, the bottles should be placed in a protective basket or they should be taped to the floor. Each bottle should bear the following warning: *do not empty*.

Two rubber-shod clamps for each chest tube must be secured to the bed linen and within the nurse's reach at all times. In the event that the nurse discovers a leak in the system or a break of the water seal, *both* clamps should be applied to the tubes immediately, as close as possible to the child's chest wall. There should be no tension on the tubes; sufficient tubing is provided to allow for the child's movement.

Each tube should have a thick piece of gauze coated with a liberal amount of petrolatum jelly placed with the petrolatum side *up* on the adhesive side of a wide piece of tape. This emergency "dressing" is kept at the bedside and within the nurse's reach at all times. In the event that a chest tube becomes dislodged accidentally, the nurse must cover the site with the gauze immediately and notify the surgeon.

There should be a *fluctuating column of water* in the submerged tube. Fluctuation is expected during inspiration, expiration, and coughing. The fluctuation indicates that the tubes are patent and that the system is working properly. If the nurse notes an absence of the fluctuation, the entire system should be checked to make sure the tubes are not kinked or compressed. At times, a blood clot may obstruct the tube, and the nurse may use a "milking" or stripping action in order to dislodge the clot. This procedure must be done with extreme care in order to prevent dislodging the tube by accident. One hand should be used to hold the tube securely while the other hand strips the tube with short, smooth strokes. The nurse should begin milking the tube at the child's chest and proceed toward the bottle. If milking is unsuccessful, the surgeon should be notified. He may elect to irrigate the tube with sterile saline. If the tubes have been in place a few days, absence of fluctuation may be an indication that the lungs have expanded.

At no time should the bottles be as high as or higher than the level of the child's chest. During transportation, the tubes should be clamped with the two rubber-shod clamps and the bottles should be carried *below* the level of the child's chest. The tubing should not be allowed to loop down below the top of the bottles. After allowing sufficient tubing to permit the child's turning in bed, the nurse should coil the excess tubing smoothly and wrap the coils with a piece of adhesive tape. A tab of adhesive tape should then be pinned to the bed linen. In order to prevent fluid which has already drained from the pleural cavity from flowing back into the cavity, the child should only be turned from his back to the side with the chest tubes until the surgeon removes the tubes.

The nurse must observe and record the *character* and *amount* of all thoracotomy tube drainage. Although the total volume of the drainage from the pleural cavity in children is not expected to be very large, the nurse should expect the largest amount of drainage during the first 12 hours after surgery. Drainage following cardiovascular surgery is expected to be bloody, but the nurse must be attentive to the character of the drainage to discriminate between expected drainage and the copious, fresh red blood of a hemorrhage. The nurse needs to remember that children who have had repair of tetralogy of Fallot or repair of transposition of the great vessels will usually have more bloody drainage than children who have had other procedures. At the same time, however, the nurse should also remember that hemorrhage from the thoracotomy tubes is the most common postoperative complication after these two procedures.[38]

An increase in the rate of bright red drainage and restlessness and alterations in the child's vital signs suggest the possibility of hemorrhage. The surgeon can determine the severity of hemorrhage from the thoracotomy tubes by comparison of the total blood drained, the hourly rate of bleeding, the rate of blood transfusion, and the presence of blood in the pleural cavity that is detected by chest x-ray. If it is determined that the child is hemorrhaging, he will be returned to the operating room immediately.

The amount of drainage from thoracotomy tubes should be recorded at hourly intervals or more frequently if the rate of drainage is rapid. The nurse can ascertain the rate and amount of drainage by placing a dated piece of adhesive tape in a vertical position on the bottle which will collect drainage from the pleural cavity. If the bottle is already calibrated to indicate volume, the tape should be placed next to the calibrations for greatest accuracy, as shown in Fig. 34-15A. If the bottle is not precalibrated, the volume must be determined, and a vertical tape with volume calibrations must be applied to the bottle, as shown in Fig. 34-15B. If the thoracotomy tube is submerged in water, the nurse must remember to indicate the initial water level as soon as the patient is received from the operating room (Figs. 34-15A and B).

Daily portable chest x-rays are taken to determine the amount of lung reexpansion. The chest x-ray will also identify hemorrhage into the pleural cavity which may elude drainage through the thoracotomy tube. The lungs usually reexpand in 2 or 3 days after surgery. When the surgeon determines that the lungs have reexpanded, the thoracotomy tubes are removed and an airtight petrolatum jelly gauze dressing and bandage are applied.

The child's body *temperature* is either monitored electrically during the early postoperative period or measured by the rectal or axillary method every 4 hours. Some elevation in temperature is expected postoperatively; but if the child's temperature exceeds 102°F (38.8°C) external hypothermia may be used to reduce the fever. Persistent elevation of temperature suggests infection; blood cultures are done to identify the bacterial agent so treatment can be instituted promptly.

Fluid and electrolyte balance is carefully regulated by use of intravenous infusions, strict intake and output, measurement of weight daily, and frequent blood tests. The administration rate of all fluid infusions and transfusions must be carefully monitored by the nurse. The surgeon will usually specify a fluid administration rate which is adequate to maintain circulating blood volume but which is not rapid enough to produce fluid overload and heart failure. Pediatric infusion sets equipped with a burette that holds no more than 100 ml of fluid should be used. The site of all infusions should be checked frequently and the surrounding skin examined for evidence of phlebitis.

The nurse must keep a scrupulous fluid *intake and output* record. In addition to recording urinary output, it is important to include drainage from all tubes, especially the thoracotomy tubes. The nurse must not forget to include the amount of blood drawn for laboratory studies on the output record. The child should be *weighed daily* on a bed scale.

The output *rate, specific gravity,* and *pH* of the child's urine are important physiologic indices after cardiac surgery. The child should excrete at least 30 ml of urine per hour. A decrease in the urinary output may indicate kidney failure, and it usually accompanies shock due to hypovolemia or inadequate cardiac output. Hourly urine samples are measured and tested for specific gravity and pH. A specific gravity of below 1.010 should be reported to the surgeon; this is a sign that the kidneys have diminished ability to concentrate urine. A high specific gravity (above 1.025) may be found when the urinary output is low. Normally, the urinary pH should be slightly acidic. In metabolic acidosis, the urinary pH is usually low; it may rise in the presence of alkalosis.

In addition to their use as indicators of the adequacy of ventilation, *blood gas* measurements, such as P_{O_2}, P_{CO_2}, and pH, are used to identify alterations in the child's metabolic acid-base balance. It is not uncommon for metabolic acidosis, as identified by pH of the blood, to result from inadequate peripheral oxygen perfusion in the postoperative period. When present, metabolic acidosis is usually treated with sodium bicarbonate. Postoperative respiratory acidosis, if mild, is usually not treated. Of the *serum electrolytes,* potassium and sodium are watched most closely. Rapid shifts in the extracellular fluid, with resultant loss of potassium from the intracellular fluid, are a common cause of cardiac arrhythmias postoperatively. *Hyponatremia,* a deficiency of sodium, is sometimes encountered after extracorporeal circulation when dextrose and water were used to prime the machine. Treatment consists of limiting water intake and administering diuretics.

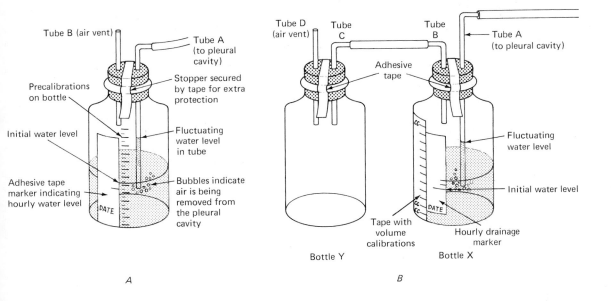

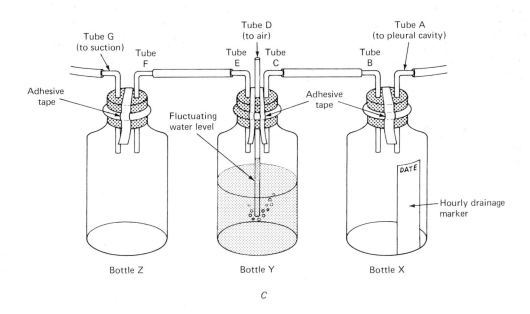

Figure 34-15 Water-seal drainage systems. *(A)* The one-bottle gravity system is the most basic water-sealed system. Note that tube A, from the patient's pleural cavity, is submerged in water. This type of system is used when the pleural cavity is expected to drain air and only a small amount of fluid. (Some surgeons may elect to attach tube B to suction apparatus.) *(B)* The two-bottle gravity system operates on the same principle as the one-bottle system. This system is used when a large amount of fluid is expected to drain from the pleural cavity. If bottle X becomes full, the excess fluid will transfer to bottle Y via tubes B and C. This will prevent fluid from reentering the pleural cavity. Bottle Y is called the "trap" bottle. (Some surgeons may elect to attach tube D to suction apparatus.) *(C)* In the three-bottle suction system, bottle X is *empty.* This permits accuracy in noting the amount and type of fluid drainage from the pleural cavity. The amount of negative pressure transferred to the patient is determined by the distance to which tube D is submerged in the water. In some instances, tube A would also be submerged in water. This provides an additional safeguard to the patient in the event that bottle Y becomes damaged.

The general physiologic status of the child can be evaluated by certain other blood studies following surgery. These most often include hemoglobin, hematocrit, prothrombin time, partial thromboplastin time, platelet count, bleeding and clotting time, serum bilirubin, and blood urea nitrogen.

The child may be *positioned* on his back until the endotracheal tube or airway are removed. The semi-Fowler's position is usually preferred after the child awakens because it facilitates drainage from the chest tubes and may make breathing easier for the child. During the early postoperative period, passive range of motion exercises should be performed by the nurse four times a day. As the child regains strength, he should be encouraged to do the exercises himself until he becomes fully ambulatory.

Angiocatheters, altered coagulation patterns, and blood transfusions predispose the child to the development of postoperative phlebitis and thrombi. Therefore the nurse must frequently assess the color, temperature, and pulses of the child's extremities.

Children who have had cardiovascular surgery are given a minimum of medications. During the first postoperative days, the child may be given small doses of an analgesic. Prophylactic antibiotic therapy which was instituted before surgery is continued. Children who had cardiac failure prior to surgery or those who develop symptoms of failure after surgery are treated with digitalis and diuretics.

Today, many surgeons feel that children who are having cardiovascular surgery do not require a nasogastric tube for gastric decompression unless severe nausea and vomiting or abdominal distention occur. After the bowel sounds return, the child is started on ice chips and then placed on a diet which gradually progresses from clear liquids to solids as his condition permits. Carbonated beverages should be avoided.

Complications of Cardiac Surgery The most common and serious complications to which the nurse should be alert involve the cardiovascular system and the respiratory system and are likely to occur during the first few postoperative days. Vigilant observation by the nurse is essential for early detection and treatment of postoperative complications.

Shock may be a manifestation of underlying hypovolemia, hemorrhage, or cardiac tamponade. In addition to treatment of the precipitating cause, the child should be treated with sodium bicarbonate and given blood and respiratory assistance if necessary.

Hemorrhage can occur after any procedure but is seen more frequently in children who have had long procedures during which the extracorporeal circulation was primed with a heparinized fluid. Protamine sulfate is administered to counteract the effects of the heparin. Hemorrhage may also be a complication after repair of cyanotic congenital heart defects because these patients have been observed to demonstrate prolonged bleeding times.[39]

Cardiac tamponade may occur as a result of the pressure effects of clotted and unclotted blood which is confined in the mediastinal space.[40] It usually occurs after several hours of undetected bleeding. Cardiac tamponade should be considered if the nurse notes malfunction of the thoracotomy tubes. It may be accompanied by a decrease in the blood pressure and a narrowing pulse pressure. If the patient is not hypovolemic, the central venous pressure will be elevated. Signs suggestive of cardiac failure may also be evident. The nurse who observes signs which might indicate cardiac tamponade should notify the surgeon immediately.

Heart failure and *low cardiac output* are different manifestations of the same problem. The first time it develops in a child after surgery, failure may be due to overload of the ventricles as a result of the new hemodynamic pattern. Heart failure may extend into the postoperative period in children who had failure before surgery.

The trauma of surgery increases the possibility of *cardiac arrhythmias*. Children who have had long surgery under cardiopulmonary by-pass, a ventriculotomy and/or atriotomy, digitalis therapy, or potassium imbalance seem most susceptible. Temporary venous pacing may be instituted for these transient disorders.

Heart block is the most common complication after repair of an ostium primum atrial septal defect. It is thought that it results from injury to the conduction system during suturing of the defect.[41] It is usually transient, but permanent heart block can occur. A permanent pacemaker is inserted for permanent heart block.

Hemolytic anemia is common in almost all patients who have had open-heart procedures. It is believed to be related to damage of red blood cells during cardiopulmonary by-pass.[42] If the hematocrit is low, the child is given a transfusion of whole blood or packed cells.

Inadequate ventilation, tenacious secretions, pulmonary edema, or hemorrhage can result in *atelectasis.* Removal or treatment of the cause and administration of intermittent positive pressure breathing and bronchodilators may be used to alleviate this complication.

Pneumothorax, the collection of air in the pleural cavity, may occur postoperatively after the lung has reexpanded. Pneumothorax may occur as a result of a leak in the water-seal drainage system, or it may develop spontaneously. In small neonates and premature infants, pneumothorax tends to recur after correction of a patent ductus arteriosus.[43] Pneumothorax may result in the shift of the heart and the other lung toward the empty space in the mediastinum called *mediastinal shift.* There may be a sharp pain when the pneumothorax occurs, which causes the child to cry out suddenly. He may then become dyspneic and restless. Treatment consists of reinsertion of thoracotomy tubes and reinstitution of water-seal drainage.

Pulmonary edema may be associated with left-sided heart failure after surgery. It is the most common complication of repair of total anomalous venous drainage and the Mustard operation.[44] Treatment is directed toward modifying the effects of the postoperative hemodynamics.

There are two conditions which are characteristic complications of cardiac surgery: *postcardiotomy syndrome* and *postperfusion syndrome.* The *postcardiotomy syndrome* may occur as early as the end of the first postoperative week and as late as several months after surgery. It is characterized by a sudden fever, carditis, and pleurisy that may or may not be accompanied by effusion. It usually subsides after rest and treatment with saliclylates, but it can recur.[45, 46] The onset of the *postperfusion syndrome* usually occurs somewhere between the third and twelfth week after surgery. There is fever, malaise, and splenomegaly. The white blood cell count can range between 3,000 and 15,000 per milliliter. Most of these cells are atypical lymphocytes. Postperfusion syndrome, too, is treated with salicylates and rest.[47, 48] Without alarming the parents, the nurse should outline the symptoms of these conditions and instruct them to notify the physician if the child should develop them after he goes home.

The Convalescent Period

After the early postoperative period, the nursing management is largely focused on helping the child gain strength and in preparing the entire family for his discharge from the hospital. If the child has an uneventful postoperative course, he may be discharged about 7 to 10 days after surgery and allowed to resume full activity in 1 or 2 months.

Planned activity and rest periods and visits from siblings as well as parents are important for the convalescent child. It is also advisable to allow older children to have occasional short visits from schoolmates and peers. These activities are helpful in easing the child's transition to home and community after a long hospitalization.

The convalescent period should also be one during which the child starts to move from the dependent role he necessarily assumed during hospitalization, and possibly before, to one of more independence. Many of the child's former limitations are removed by the surgery, and most activity limitations will eventually be lifted. The child and parents will need the nurse's assistance in becoming comfortable in dealing with the child's newly acquired capacities. They will need to learn how to help the child pace his activities in order to prevent fatigue. The child who formerly had many restrictions will need much encouragement and support of the nurse and parents as he attempts new activities.

The nurse should confer with the parents concerning their plans for the child after discharge. They are likely to need some assistance in comfortably allowing their child to engage in new activities and to exercise the amount of independence appropriate for his age. The hospital nurse can also facilitate the child's transfer to home and to the community by initiating a referral to the community health nurse and by providing the school nurse with a summary of the child's hospitalization and present condition. The nurse might also suggest that the parents investigate the informal parents' discussion groups which are sponsored by the American Heart Association in some communities as a helpful resource for them after the child goes home.

REFERENCES

1 American Academy of Pediatrics, Committee on Hospital Care, *Care of Children in Hospitals,* 2d ed., Evanston, Ill., 1971, p. 91.
2 Richard D. Rowe and Ali Mehrizi, *The Neonate with Congenital Heart Disease,* W. B. Saunders Company, Philadelphia, 1968, pp. 4 and 30.
3 Ibid., p. 30.
4 Charles S. Ho, L. Jerome Krovetz, and Richard D. Rowe, "Major Complications of Cardiac Catheterization and Angiocardiography in Infants and Children," *Johns Hopkins Medical Journal,* 131(3):247–258, September 1972.
5 Eugene Braunwald and John Ross, Jr., "Methods of Study" in Robert E. Cooke (ed.), *The Biologic Basis of Pediatric Practice,* McGraw-Hill Book Company, New York, 1968, p. 329.
6 John D. Keith, Richard D. Rowe, and Peter Vlad, *Heart Disease in Infancy and Childhood,* 2d ed., The Macmillan Company, New York, 1967, p. 76.
7 Gerard Van Leeuwen, *A Manual of Newborn Medicine,* Yearbook Medical Publishers, Inc., Chicago, 1973, p. 201.
8 Rowe and Mehrizi, op. cit., p. 30.
9 S. Gorham Babson, and Ralph C. Benson, *Management*

of High Risk Pregnancy and Intensive Care of the Neonate, The C. V. Mosby Company, St. Louis, 1971, p. 248.

10 Rowe and Mehrizi, op. cit., p. 30.

11 Ho, Krovetz, and Rowe, op. cit., p. 249.

12 Van Leeuwen, op. cit., p. 200.

13 Eugene Braunwald and Richard Gorlin, "Total Population Studied, Procedures Employed and Incidence of Complications," in Eugene Braunwald and Harold J. Swan (eds.), Cooperative Study on Cardiac Catheterization, The American Heart Association, New York, 1968, p. 17.

14 Abraham M. Rudolph, "Complications Occurring in Infants and Children," in Eugene Braunwald and Harold J. Swan (eds.), Cooperative Study on Cardiac Catheterization, The American Heart Association, New York, 1968, p. 61.

15 Ibid., pp. 64–65.

16 Sheldon B. Korones, High-Risk Newborn Infants: The Basis for Intensive Nursing Care, The C. V. Mosby Company, St. Louis, 1972, p. 167.

17 Waldo Nelson, Victor C. Vaughn, and R. James McKay, Textbook of Pediatrics, 9th ed., W. B. Saunders Company, Philadelphia, 1969, p. 1066.

18 H. Ekert and M. Sheers, "Preoperative and Postoperative Platelet Function in Cyanotic Congenital Heart Disease," Journal of Thoracic and Cardiovascular Surgery, 67(2):184–190, February 1974.

19 Nelson, Vaughn, and McKay, op. cit., p. 316.

20 Harold Abramson, Resuscitation of the Newborn Infant, The C. V. Mosby Company, St. Louis, 1973, p. 153.

21 Nelson, Vaughn, and McKay, op. cit., p. 316.

22 Ibid.

23 Eugenie F. Doyle, "Congestive Heart Failure in Infancy and Childhood," in Henry L. Barnett (ed.), Pediatrics, 15th ed., Appleton-Century-Crofts, New York, 1972, p. 1422.

24 Keith, Rowe, and Vlad, op. cit., p. 213.

25 W. Rashkind and W. W. Miller, "Creation of an Atrial Septal Defect without Thoracotomy," Journal of the American Medical Association, 196:991, 1966.

26 E. Ching, J. W. DuShane, D. C. McGoon, and G. R. Danielson, "Total Correction of Cardiac Anomalies in Infancy Using Extracorporeal Circulation," Journal of Thoracic and Cardiovascular Surgery, 62:117, 1971.

27 J. Willis Hurst, R. Bruce Logue, Robert C. Schlant, and Nanette Kass Wenger, The Heart, 3d ed., McGraw-Hill Book Company, New York, 1974, p. 828.

28 E. R. Bland, P. D. White, and T. D. Jones, "Development

of Mitral Stenosis in Young People with Discussion of Frequent Misinterpretation of Middiastolic Murmur at Cardiac Apex," American Heart Journal, 10:995, 1935.

29 Hurst, Logue, Schlant, and Wenger, op. cit., p. 837.

30 Sidney Blumenthal, "Infections of the Heart," in Henry L. Barnett (ed.), Pediatrics, Appleton-Century-Crofts, New York, 1972, p. 1428.

31 Nelson, Vaughn, and McKay, op. cit., p. 313.

32 Janet B. Wonderlich, Anesthetic Management, in Donal M. Billig and Marshall B. Kriedberg (eds.), The Management of Neonates and Infants with Congenital Heart Disease, Grune & Stratton, New York, 1973, pp. 29–30.

33 Denton A. Cooley and Grady L. Hallman, Cardiovascular Surgery during the First Year of Life, in Richard H. Egdahl and John A. Mannick (eds.), Modern Surgery, Grune & Stratton, New York, 1970, p. 326.

34 Grady L. Hallman, The Heart, in Paul F. Nora (ed.), Operative Surgery: Principles and Techniques, Lea & Febiger, Philadelphia, 1972, p. 324.

35 Gerald Caplan, Principles of Preventive Psychiatry, Basic Books, Inc., Publishers, New York, 1964, p. 39.

36 Nelson, Vaughn, and McKay, op. cit., p. 1015.

37 Robert N. Reynolds, Postoperative Respiratory Care, in Donal M. Billig and Marshall B. Kriedberg (eds.), The Management of Neonates and Infants with Congenital Heart Disease, Grune & Stratton, New York, 1973, p. 41.

38 Hallman, op. cit., pp. 330 and 334.

39 Ekert and Sheers, op. cit.

40 W. Gerald Austen, Cardiac Surgery, in Committee on Pre- and Postoperative Care, American College of Surgeons, A Manual of Preoperative and Postoperative Care, 2d ed., W. B. Saunders Company, Philadelphia, 1971, p. 319.

41 Hallman, op. cit., p. 326.

42 Austen, op. cit., p. 332.

43 D. Alton Murphy, Eugene Outerbridge, Les Stern, Gordon M. Karn, Wanda Jeiger, and Jose Rosales, "Management of Premature Infants with Patent Ductus Arteriosus," Journal of Thoracic and Cardiovascular Surgery, 67:221–228, 1974.

44 Eoin Aberdeen, "Pulmonary Artery Constriction," in W. P. Clelland (ed.), Operative Surgery 2: Thorax, J. B. Lippincott Company, Philadelphia, 1968, pp. 209 and 218.

45 Nelson, Vaughn, and McKay, op. cit., p. 1015.

46 Austen, op. cit., p. 330.

47 Ibid., pp. 330–331.

48 Nelson, Vaughn, and McKay, op. cit., p. 1015.

35

THE HEMOPOIETIC SYSTEM

PATRICIA ELLIS GREENE and
LAURA MARIA BLOOMQUIST COOPER*

EMBRYOLOGY AND FUNCTION OF BLOOD COMPONENTS

The circulating blood consists of two portions: the liquid plasma and the formed elements. The formed elements are the *erythrocytes*, or red blood cells, the *leukocytes*, or white blood cells, and the *thrombocytes*, or platelets. These elements perform most of the functional activities of the blood. The erythrocytes function primarily in the transport of oxygen and carbon dioxide between the tissues of the body and the lungs. The leukocytes form the most significant part of the body's defense against infections, while the thrombocytes, along with portions of the plasma, provide a mechanism for the coagulation of blood.

Hemopoiesis

The production of the formed elements of the blood, hemopoiesis, is one of the earliest functions of the human embryo. Several theories have been put forth to explain the origin of the formed elements. One theory is that a single primitive cell, the hemocytoblast, has the potential to give rise to the other formed elements. A precursor of the primitive cells, the angioblast, can be found in the embryo as early as the blastocyst stage of development. A contrasting theory is that each of the formed elements has a separate precursor or primitive cell distinct from all other cells. According to this theory, the erythroblast would be the precursor of the erythrocyte. This pattern would be similar for the other formed elements.

Hemopoietic activity occurs in successive locations beginning by the second week of embryonic life. The blood islands, which give rise to the primitive blood cells, can be found in two locations. The blood islands first appear in the wall of the yolk sac. By the fourth week, they also appear in the mesenchyme tissue spread throughout the embryo. In both areas, the blood islands differentiate in a similar manner. The peripheries of the blood islands form primitive channels of the vessels of the circulatory system. The centers of the blood islands form primitive blood cells, the precursors of the erythrocytes, megakaryocytes, and granulocytes. The primitive cell is a particular derivative of the mesenchyme of the embryo. By the sixth to the eighth weeks, hemopoietic activity reaches a peak in the mesenchyme and begins to specialize in certain areas. The hemo-

* The authors gratefully acknowledge the assistance of Gerald E. Bloom, M.D., in the preparation of this chapter.

poietic activity of the yolk sac has diminished by the eighth week, although the yolk sac continues to function in other ways until later in fetal life.

From the second month until midfetal life, the liver is the most active of all the structures involved in hemopoiesis. Clusters of erythrocytes, megakaryocytes, and granulocytes form in the mesenchyme between the liver cells. These cells are much smaller than the large, nucleated cells preceding them. The liver is the principal source of erythropoiesis in the fetus until the bone marrow takes over this function. Shortly after the liver becomes active, the spleen becomes another site for erythropoiesis and leukopoiesis. These functions reach a peak and diminish as lymphopoiesis becomes the major function of the spleen around the fifth month of fetal life.

The bone marrow becomes active around the fourth month, beginning with leukopoiesis and gradually assuming the erythropoietic activity which was previously a function of the liver and spleen. Bone marrow appears as early as the sixth week of development, but it does not become active until after the peak of activity in the liver and spleen. Two to three weeks after birth, the bone marrow becomes the main site of hemopoietic activity. In the early period of hemopoiesis, there is considerable overlap of functions among the sites of activity. Each site reaches its peak and diminishes as another site assumes the function of blood production. During early childhood, all the bones are filled with red marrow. Gradually, hemopoiesis becomes limited to

the marrow of the ribs, the sternum, and the bodies of the vertebrae, which remain the major centers for erythropoietic and granulopoietic activity through out the lifetime. (See Fig. 35-1.) Although no longer active in hemopoiesis, the mesenchyme of the liver and spleen retain the potential for the formation of blood. In periods of stress, they may become active to compensate for a loss of blood formation elsewhere in the body.

Erythrocytes

The erythrocytes are the blood's circulating red cells or corpuscles (Fig. 35-2). The early red cell, the erythroblast, is a large, nucleated cell which undergoes a series of changes bringing it to the functioning, nonnucleated, biconcave disk form of the mature erythrocyte. The red cells are produced in successive sites in the fetus until erythropoiesis is carried out exclusively by the red bone marrow. The erythroblast, formed in the bone marrow, is the precursor of the normoblast, which then gives rise to the reticulocyte and the erythrocyte. The reticulocyte is nearly as mature as the erythrocyte and is normally present in the circulation in small numbers. Erythropoiesis is very active in the fetus; thus an increased number of immature erythrocytes are released into the circulation of the fetus.

Blood samples drawn from the 3-month-old fetus contain about 90 percent reticulocytes. The percentage decreases to 15 to 30 percent at 6 months and 4 to 6 percent at birth. The adult level

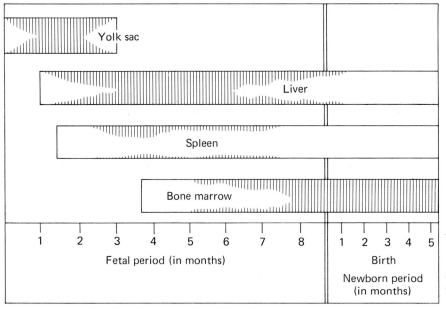

Figure 35-1 Developmental changes in hemopoietic sites. The shaded areas indicate periods of hemopoietic activity in various sites. *(Adapted from Kleihauer, Archiv fur Kinderheilkunde, Supplement 53, 1966a, Stuttgart.)*

reached by the first week of extrauterine life, ranges from 0.5 to 1.6 percent. An elevation of the number of circulating reticulocytes is an indication that an accelerated red cell production is occurring in an attempt to meet an increased need for red cells, such as to replace those destroyed by hemolysis. *Hemolysis* is the destruction of red cells liberating *hemoglobin* (discussed below) from the cell into the plasma of the blood. A depression of the number of circulating red cells, concurrent with a decreased hemoglobin, is known as *anemia*. The normal red cell count of the full-term newborn ranges between 5 and 6 million cells/cu mm of blood. By the end of the first year of life the average has decreased to 4.6 million/cu mm. The average red cell count in the teenager is 5.4 million cells/cu mm for males and 4.8 million cells for females. Table 35-1 gives the average normal blood values at different ages.

The main function of the erythrocytes is the transport of oxygen from the lungs to the tissues and the transport of carbon dioxide from the tissues to the lungs. This activity is contingent upon the most important component of the erythrocyte, the hemoglobin. The outer membrane of the red cell functions to maintain the homeostasis of the cell by the transport of water and electrolytes.

Hemoglobin A unique substance, hemoglobin is composed of a simple protein, *globin*, attached to an iron-containing pigment, *heme*. The heme is the substance which gives the red coloration to the oxygenated erythrocytes. Furthermore, heme gives hemoglobin the ability to bind with oxygen and car-

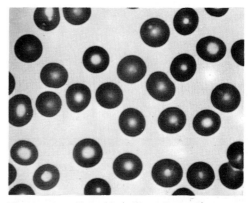

Figure 35-2 Normal erythrocytes as they appear under magnification. The hemoglobin is evenly centered in the biconcave disk of the cell. *(From A. M. Mauer, Pediatric Hematology, McGraw-Hill Book Company, New York, 1969, p. 25.)*

bon dioxide for transport. Three types of hemoglobin develop sequentially in the fetus. The predominating type present in the earliest part of embryonic development (until the second month) is a very primitive substance called *embryonic hemoglobin*. This form completely disappears by the third month of gestation as the fetal hemoglobin becomes more dominant. Fetal hemoglobin reaches a peak of about 90 percent of the hemoglobin produced and then begins to decrease after the sixth month of fetal life. At birth, 45 to 90 percent of the newborn's hemoglobin is of the fetal type. Adult hemoglobin is present in increasing amounts, replacing the fetal type by the first year of life. (See Fig. 35-3.) Some fetal hemo-

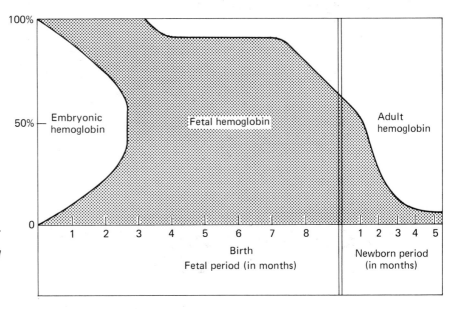

Figure 35-3 Types of hemoglobin produced during fetal and neonatal development. *(Adapted from Kleihauer, Archiv fur Kinderheilkunde, Supplement 53, 1966a, Stuttgart.)*

Table 35-1 THE AVERAGE RANGE OF NORMAL BLOOD VALUES MEASURED AT DIFFERENT AGES

Component	Premature	Full-term	2 days	7 days	14 days	2 mo
Hemoglobin, Gm/100 ml	13–18	13.7–20	18–21.2	196	13–20	13.3
RBC/cu mm, in millions	5–6	5–6	5.3–5.6	5.3	5–5.1	4.5
Nucleated RBC, %	5–15	1–5	1–2	0*		
Hematocrit, Gm/100 ml	45–55	43–65	56.1	52.7	30–66	38.9
WBC/cu mm, in thousands	15	9–38	21–22	5–21	5–21	5–21
Neutrophils, %	40–80	40–80	55	40	36–40	36–40
Eosinophils, %	2–3	2–3	5	5	2–3†	
Lymphocytes, %	30–31	30–31	20	20	48–53	48–53
Monocytes	6–12	6–12	15	15	8–9	8–9
Immature WBC, %	Over 10	3–10	5	0*		
Platelets/cu mm, in thousands	50–300	100–350	400	400	300–400	300–400
Reticulocytes, %	Up to 10	4–6	3	3	0.5–1.6†	

* Not normally found in the circulating blood after this age.
† Remains approximately the same for succeeding age levels.

globin may be present through the entire lifetime of the person.

Hemoglobin is synthesized by the cytoplasm of the erythropoietic cells. These cells have the potential to produce both kinds of hemoglobin; however, fetal hemoglobin is favored before birth, and the adult type is favored after birth. Fetal hemoglobin is easily distinguished from adult hemoglobin by its greater resistance to alkali denaturation as well as a greater solubility, particularly in phosphate buffers. This distinction becomes a valuable determinant for the diagnosis of problems of feto-maternal transfusion occurring during the progress of a pregnancy and labor. A fundamental feature of the fetal hemoglobin-containing erythrocyte is its greater tendency to take up oxygen at lower oxygen tensions, such as that in the fetal circulation, and its greater discharge of carbon dioxide. This feature of fetal hemoglobin is valuable to the erythrocyte during intrauterine life because of the dependency on the maternal circulation for oxygen–carbon dioxide transport.

Hemoglobin in the cord blood of the newborn has a concentration of 16.6 to 17.1 Gm/100 ml of blood. By the second year of life, the hemoglobin concentration has dropped from its initial high concentration to 11 Gm/100 ml. The hemoglobin concentration averages between 11 to 13 Gm/100 ml until puberty, when the concentration rises to an average of 14 Gm/100 ml for females and 16 Gm/100 ml of blood for males.

The red blood cell has a life-span of approximately 120 days. After this period of circulation, it becomes fragmented and is destroyed by the process of *phagocytosis* (a function of certain leukocytes) in the spleen, liver, and red bone marrow. During this process, iron is salvaged from the hemoglobin and returned to the bone marrow for storage and for production of new hemoglobin. The remainder of the hemoglobin, the globin and the iron-free particles, is excreted into the reticuloendothelial system, spleen, lymph nodes, bone marrow, liver, and connective tissues; where separation into the globin protein and the degradation to bilirubin occurs.

Bilirubin This substance is a pigment, specifically a waste product formed from the hemoglobin. The two types of bilirubin are the direct type, or conjugated bilirubin, which becomes elevated in the blood following intra- or extrahepatic obstruction of the bile ducts, and the indirect type, which rises as a result of degradation of the erythrocytes and excessive destruction of hemoglobin such as occurs in the hemolytic anemias. When the bilirubin level in the blood becomes elevated, a condition known as *hyperbilirubinemia*, the pigment stains the body tis-

3 mo	6 mo	1 yr	2 yr	4 yr	8–12 yr	Adult	
						Male	Female
9.5–14	10.5–14	11–12.2	11.6–13	12.6–13	11–19	14–18	12–16
4.3–4.5	4.6	4.6–4.7	4.7–4.8	4.7–4.8	4.8–5.1	5.4	4.8
28–41	33–42	32–40	34–40	36–44	39–47	42–52	37–47
6–18	1–15	4.5–13.5	9–12	8–10	8	5–10	5–10
30–35	30–45	40–50	40–50	50–55	55–60	35–70	35–70
						2–3	2–3
55–63	48–60	48–53	48–50	40–48	30–38	30–35	30–35
7	5	5	5–8	5–8	5–8	5–8	5–8
360	250–350†					250–350	250–350
						0.5–1.6	0.5–1.6

sues, skin, and sclera, producing a tinge of color referred to as *jaundice*. A normal amount of circulating bilirubin is 0.2 to 1.4 mg/100 ml of blood. Hyperbilirubinemia occurs when the amount of circulating bilirubin reaches 15 to 20 mg/100 ml of blood.

Leukocytes

Classification   The leukocytes, or white blood cells, are nucleated cells, larger in size than the erythrocytes. There are five kinds of white cells, each serving distinct functions for the body and each identifiable by distinct characteristics. The leukocytes are classified into granular and agranular types by the presence or absence of granular substances in the cytoplasm. Granulocytes are of three types: neutrophils, eosinophils, and basophils. Nongranular leukocytes are of two types: monocytes and lymphocytes. As was the case with red blood cells, immature precursors of white cells are found in the circulating blood in certain disease states and have diagnostic significance. The precursor of the granulocytes is the myeloblast, which forms the myelocyte and finally the mature granulocyte. The precursor of the monocyte is the monoblast. The lymphocytes and the granulocytes form in the lymphatic tissue of the lymph nodes and spleen, tonsils, thymus, bone marrow, and Peyer's patches of the gastrointestinal tract and liver. Monocytes originate and develop in the myeloid tissue of the red bone marrow, in the lymph nodes, and in the spleen.

At birth the number of circulating white blood cells is high with a range of 9,000 to 38,000 cells per cu mm of blood. By the end of the first year of life, the range begins to decrease to 8,000 to 10,000 per cu mm of blood. Severe depression of the white cells, leukopenia, is seen in certain infections. Leukocytosis, an increase in the number of white cells, frequently accompanies such disorders as leukemia. The life-span of the leukocytes is generally unknown. Some granulocytes live for 24 hours, others as long as 30 days. It is known that leukocytes survive both in the intravascular area of the circulating blood and in the extravascular tissues. The pulmonary circulation also serves as a reservoir for the leukocytes. Leukocytes that have reached the end of their life-span are removed by the lungs, liver, spleen, kidneys, gastrointestinal tract, and striated muscle fibers.

Phagocytosis   The most important function of the leukocytes is the protection of the body against infection. Phagocytosis is the process by which the leukocytes ingest and consequently destroy foreign particles and bacteria which invade the body, as well as fragmented cells in the bloodstream. Phagocytosis is the function of the neutrophils, concentrating on the bacteria. The neutrophils are known as *microphagocytes* in contrast to the macrophagocytes, the monocytes, which concentrate on the ingestion of the larger foreign particles and fragmented cells. The eosinophils become active in phagocytosis with the invasion of animal parasites like the trichinae. The eosinophils are also active in allergic states such as asthma. When the basophils undergo degranulation during an anaphylactic reaction, heparin and histamine, contained in the cytoplasm of the cells, are released. The lymphocytes are active in the formation of antibodies, an element of the immunologic system of the body. The lymphocytes are closely associated with *gamma globulin*, one of the proteins of the blood plasma. Gamma globulin, a substance formed in the lymphatic tissue and in the liver, is released during inflammatory reactions by the degradation of the lymphocytes. See Table 35-2 for a delineation of the leukocytes and their individual functions.

Thrombocytes

The thrombocytes, or blood platelets, are the smallest of the blood's formed elements. These non-nucleated, granular bodies are fragments of the megakaryocytes, the precursor of the thrombocytes evident in the second month of embryonic life. The platelets function in homeostasis and in storage of certain metabolic substances; in addition, they have some role in the process of phagocytosis and an integral role in the *coagulation* process. When the integrity of the vessel wall is destroyed, the platelets adhere to the inner surface, forming a plug which slows and stops the flow of blood, thereby minimizing blood loss. In addition, degradation of the platelets causes the release of a platelet factor which interacts with other substances in the blood plasma to form a fibrous clot at the site of the injury (see Fig.

35-4). The platelets simultaneously release serotonin, a vasoconstrictor, which further contributes to the slowing of the blood flow from the injured site. The normal quantity of platelets in the newborn ranges from 100,000 to 350,000 cells/cu mm. A level of platelets below 100,000 cells/cu mm is a characteristic of the disorder known as *thrombocytopenia*.

Plasma

The liquid portion of the blood, plasma, is the medium by which the formed elements are transported in the blood vessels. The constituents of plasma function in the maintenance of homeostasis by the transport and distribution of nutrients, hormones, certain chemicals, and waste materials. About 90 percent of the plasma is composed of water. When needed, the plasma can draw from the body tissues storing excess water. Approximately six to eight percent of the plasma is the protein substances albumin, gamma globulin, fibrinogen, and prothrombin. Albumin serves an osmotic function in the regulation of the volume of plasma in the blood vessels. Gamma globulin's intimate role with the lymphocytes was discussed earlier in the chapter. Fibrinogen and prothrombin are essential to the coagulation process. The remaining 1 to 2 percent of the constituents are glucose, amino acids, inorganic salts, gases, waste materials, and hormones.

Blood Volume

The volumes of plasma and of formed elements determine blood volume. A premature newborn has a blood volume of about 108 ml/kg of body weight or, for example, approximately 540 ml in the case of the 5-lb (2.27 kg) premature. A newborn at term has a volume of 85 ml/kg, or approximately 640 ml for the average 7½-lb (3.4-kg) newborn. The difference in the blood volumes is due to the increased amount of

Figure 35-4   Coagulation process.

Platelet factor
 +
Antihemophilic factors ——————$with\ Ca^{++}$—————→ release of plasma
 +   prothromboplastin
Other blood coagulation factors

Prothrombin
 + ——————$with\ Ca^{++}$—————→ thrombin
Plasma thromboplastin

Fibrinogen
 + —————→ fibrin —————————→ clot formation
Thrombin

Table 35-2 IDENTIFICATION, CHARACTERIZATION, AND FUNCTION OF LEUKOCYTES

Type of leukocyte	Identification		Percent in the blood	Major function of the cell	Disorders causing alteration from normal
	Nuclei	Cytoplasm			
Granulocytes Neutrophils	Nonsegmented or segmented with 2–5 lobes	Granules stain pink or violet with neutral dye	4–5 (nonsegmented) 60–65 (segmented)	Microphagocytosis: phagocytosis of bacteria	Splenectomy
Eosinophils	2 oval-shaped lobes	Granules stain reddish orange or deep red with acid dye or eosin	1–4	Phagocytosis of animal parasites (trichinae)	Splenectomy, eosinophilic leukemia or leukemoid reaction, Hodgkin's disease, acute infectious lymphocytosis (recovery phase)
Basophils	Round or kidney-shaped	Granules stain bluish black with basic dye	0–0.5	Release of heparin and histamine	Splenectomy, Hodgkin's disease, chronic myeloid leukemia, polycythemia vera, chronic hemolytic anemia
Nongranular leukocytes Lymphocytes	Large, round, or oval	Thin layers of cytoplasm with no granules	20–35	Antibody formation and release of gamma globulin	Infectious mononucleosis
Monocytes	Large, oval, or kidney-shaped	Abundant cytoplasm with no granules	5–10	Macrophagocytosis: phagocytosis of foreign particles and fragmented cells	Infectious mononucleosis, Hodgkin's disease, acute infection, or bacterial invasion (recovery phase)

plasma in the premature. By the third month of life, the blood volume of the neonate decreases to 75 to 80 ml/kg, remaining relatively consistent during the life-span.

Lymph

A fluid, lymph is closely interrelated with the circulation of the blood and the lymphocytes. It is derived from the blood plasma; thus it has a similar content of water and solutes. Lymph plays an integral role in the body's defense against infections as the concentration of leukocytes may be as high as 40,000 cells/cu mm. These cells are mostly lymphocytes formed in the lymphoid tissue. An increased production of lymphocytes, as in the leukemia disorders, produces an enlargement of some lymph nodes where the lymphocytes are formed. The lymphatic system is anatomically interrelated with the cardiovascular system.

Blood Groups and the Rh Factor

The erythrocyte is singularly important in the blood groups and the Rh factor. A substance on the surface of the red cell is responsible for *agglutination*, or clumping, of the red cells in the presence of an *antibody*, or an *agglutinin*. This substance is known by its characteristics as an *agglutinogen*, or an *antigen*, which makes possible the agglutination of red cells. Karl Landsteiner was the Nobel Prize winner whose work led to the formation of the international ABO system of classifying blood groups, basing the classification on compatibility. The ABO system was first noted in 1900 when anti-A and anti-B serums were used to identify the A and B antigens.

The ABO System   In this system there are four blood groups: A, B, AB, and O. The blood group is determined genetically by the pairing of parental genes. There are six possible genotypes: AA, AO, BB, BO, AB, and OO. It is impossible to distinguish between the AA and AO and BB and BO genotypes of the A and B groups, respectively. The blood groups develop in the embryo along with the early red cells. By the second or third month of fetal development, it is possible to detect the A and B isoagglutinogens, an antibody factor transferred from the maternal circulation.

Blood from two persons is considered compatible when agglutination does not occur in the presence of the antibody. The antibody in the plasma makes it possible for the plasma to agglutinate or cause clumping of the red cells. The A blood group has the A antigen and the anti-B antibody, while the opposite B antigen and anti-A antibody are present in the B blood group. The AB blood group has both the A and B antigens and neither antibody; thus it is compatible with any other blood group when it is the recipient. The O blood group contains both the anti-A and anti-B antibody but neither antigen. The O blood group is considered a universal donor as it is compatible when given to any other blood group (refer to Table 35-3).

The Rh Factor   Landsteiner and Weiner in 1940 discovered the Rh factor from their experiments with rhesus monkeys, from which the name Rh is derived. The blood of the rhesus monkey, when injected into a rabbit, caused agglutination of the rabbit's red blood cells. This phenomenon was also demonstrated in human blood. The Rh factor was identified as an important cause of certain hemolytic reactions occurring during blood transfusions. Levine and others in 1941 related the Rh factor to the erythroblastosis fetalis phenomenon (to be discussed later in this chapter).

The *Rh factor* is an antigen contained in the outer membrane of the erythrocyte. Its function and nature are generally unknown. There are several antigens in the Rh system, the most important of these being the D antigen. The presence or absence of this antigen gives rise to the Rh-positive or Rh-negative identification. The incidence of D antigen

Table 35-3 ABO SYSTEM OF ANTIGENS AND ANTIBODIES FOR DETERMINING BLOOD COMPATIBILITY

Blood group	Antigen	Antibody	Compatibility	
			Can be donor to type	Can receive from type
A	A	Anti-B	A or AB	A or O
B	B	Anti-A	B or AB	B or O
AB	A and B	No antibodies	AB	A, B, AB, or O
O	No antigen	Anti-A and Anti-B	A, B, AB, or O	O

or Rh-positive blood among Caucasians is 85 percent. Rh-negative blood is generally less common in persons from other racial groups. Several other antigens have been identified; however, they are only rarely involved in hemolytic disorders. These antigens are the Kell, Sutter, Duffy, Lewis, Lutheran, and Kidd groups, whose factors have occasionally been demonstrated in erythroblastosis fetalis.

HEMATOLOGIC DEVIATIONS AND DISEASES IN THE PREMATURE AND NEWBORN

In the assessment of the premature and newborn suspected of hematologic deviations, the nurse needs to be cognizant of the events surrounding the maternal-fetal interaction. Infections, ingestion of drugs, dissimilar parental blood groups (particularly the Rh factor), a prolonged labor with a rupture of membranes early in the course of labor, and unusual vaginal bleeding may be forewarners of several different hematologic problems. Anticipation of jaundice, anemia, or acute blood loss producing shock is possible by the thorough understanding of the history of the newborn.

The nurse is the interpreter for the newborn, who can communicate in so many diverse ways the message that something is not quite right in its body. The nurse should determine significant findings from a knowledge of the normal pattern of behavior and should note where the premature or full-term newborn's behavior falls on the continuum progressing from a normal to a severe deviation. He should become familiar with the uniqueness of each newborn so as to adequately and accurately interpret the meaning of the deviant behavior, which he is often the first person to detect. Observation is the primary mode of assessing the status of the newborn, particularly regarding the deviations resulting from a hematologic disorder.

Deviations Related to the Maternal-Fetal Interaction

The hemopoietic system, the cells produced by this system, and the functions which they serve are subject to interferences and pathologic deviations affecting the fetus in utero and the premature and full-term newborn. Most often these deviations are related to the interaction of the mother and fetus during the pregnancy. An intimate and active communication is made possible by means of the placenta and the blood circulating through it. All the elements essential for fetal growth and development are supplied by the mother through her blood. The iron store necessary for hemoglobin production is drawn from the mother's supply. The nutrients needed for cell growth and maturation are provided by the maternal circulation. Gaseous exchange occurs as a result of the communication between the fetal and maternal circulations.

Isoimmunization The fetus, considered as an accepted transplant during the pregnancy, can be at risk of being rejected at any time. The immunologic system is one manner by which the body rejects the transplant. This rejection occurs when the body develops antibodies against the blood or cells of the transplant. *Isoimmunization*, the formation of antibodies against the blood cells of the fetus, should be differentiated from *autoimmunization*, formation by the body of antibodies against a disease and leading to immunity. Isoimmunization is the major cause of hemolytic anemia in the premature and the newborn. It occurs when an antigenic substance on the surface of the fetal red cells is transferred to the maternal circulation, where antibodies are produced, creating a reaction known as *sensitization*. Later, these antibodies cross the placental barrier and attach themselves to the fetal red cells, where agglutination occurs. Agglutination elicits hemolysis, which removes the erythrocytes from the fetal circulation, producing an anemic state.

Erythroblastosis Fetalis One form of hemolytic anemia is known as *erythroblastosis fetalis*, deriving its name from the frequent manifestation of the nucleated erythroblast cells in the blood released from the liver, spleen, and bone marrow to compensate for the massive hemolysis occurring during the disease process. The most common form of erythroblastosis is an incompatibility of the ABO blood groups, occurring in about two-thirds of the erythroblastotic newborns. The Rh factor (D antigen) incompatibility, producing a more severe and sometimes fatal reaction, causes less than a third of the cases.

Pathogenesis The Rh factor incompatibility results when a woman who is Rh-negative carries an Rh-positive fetus. The fetal Rh antigens leak into the maternal circulation in minute amounts, where antibodies are formed against the Rh-positive antigen. The first baby will rarely be affected by this sensitization, but subsequent babies probably will have a reaction because of the presence of the anti-D antibodies. ABO incompatibility is not as active an antibody formation process as the Rh antibody formation. The mother has blood group O; the fetus, blood group A or B. Blood leakage allows antibody formation against the A or B antigens of the fetus. The first baby, as well as the other babies, may be affected by this sensitization.

Prevention of Rh incompatibility As methods of prevention make its occurrence less frequent Rh incompatibility has become almost an historic disease. RhoGAM, an Rh(D) gamma globulin, administered within 72 hours after the termination of the pregnancy in which the Rh-negative mother carried or delivered an Rh-positive baby, can prevent the development of antibodies that would cause complications in the next pregnancy. RhoGAM is administered only if the mother with the Rh-negative blood also has a negative Coombs' test. (See Fig. 35-5.)

Clinical manifestations Hydrops fetalis, the most severe form of erythroblastosis fetalis, begins in the fetal stage of development. It is characterized by severe anemia and generalized edema, or *anasarca*, due to cardiac failure, as well as hepatosplenomegaly. There is no jaundice, as the bile pigments are still being excreted through the placenta into the maternal circulation. Premature births are common; however, most of the hydropic newborns are stillborn. Those who do survive rarely live for more than a few hours. The most common form of erythroblastosis fetalis is *icterus neonatorum*, a severe jaundice occurring early in the newborn period. Icterus neonatorum is characterized by jaundice evident a few hours after birth and within the first 24 hours. Anemia, petechiae, and hepatosplenomegaly are also prevalent. Hyperbilirubinemia, an increase in the bilirubin level, is expected with this disease, because of a rising rate of destruction of erythrocytes and a concurrent low capacity of the hepatic system to conjugate and excrete the bilirubin. A milder form of erythroblastosis presents only with jaundice and anemia.

Kernicterus This condition is a complication of hyperbilirubinemia in which unconjugated bilirubin enters the brain tissues, staining the basal ganglions, as well as other areas, and destroying the brain cells. Early signs of this disease include either depression or excitation. Excitation is manifested by the appearance of twitching, high-pitched crying, opisthotonos, hypertonia, and generalized seizure activity. Depression is characterized by poor feeding habits 36 hours after birth, lack of sucking and rooting reflexes, hypotonia, lethargy, an absent Moro reflex, and eventual coma. Death is common as a result of either severe depression or excitation. Serious impairment of mental and motor functions is apparent in the growth and development of those infants who survive the disease.

Diagnosis In the premature and full-term newborn, laboratory tests are performed to determine the status of the blood and disease process. The direct *Coombs' test*, a test of the antiglobins or antibodies on the red blood cells of the newborn, is done on the blood taken from the cord at birth. The Coombs' test will be positive only if the mother is Rh-negative and the newborn is Rh-positive. The direct Coombs' test, when ABO incompatibility is suspected, is usually negative if the mother has type A, B, or O blood. A positive Coombs' test is generally indicative of erythroblastosis. Testing of the blood also shows a reduced hematocrit with an increased number of normoblasts or nucleated, immature red blood cells. A characteristic of ABO incompatibility, but not of Rh incompatibility, is the appearance of spherocytes in the blood, as well as the presence of the normoblasts. *Spherocytes* are sphere-shaped erythrocytes which are smaller and thicker than normal erythrocytes and demonstrate an increased osmotic fragility. They are mature in contrast to the reticulocytes. The reticulocyte count is usually above the normal range, sometimes reaching 40 to 50 percent in a severe manifestation of the disease.

Treatment The objectives of the treatment for the premature and newborn affected by erythroblastosis are to control or prevent the development of cardiac failure and related edema, to control or prevent hyperbilirubinemia and the subsequent danger of the development of kernicterus, and to control anemia. The development of cardiac failure is associated with the severe anemia caused by the hemolysis of the erythrocytes.

Exchange transfusion Treatment is accomplished by the use of an exchange transfusion and phototherapy. The *exchange transfusion* removes the red cells that are normal and not sensitized. It also removes some of the bilirubin causing the jaundice. Generally, the exchange transfusion is indicated when the rising bilirubin levels in the blood reach 15 mg/100 ml of blood in the premature and 20 mg/100 ml of blood in the term newborn. An exchange transfusion may be necessary because of other manifestations, such as severe anemia, edema, hepatosplenomegaly at birth, and petechiae, as well as indications from previous pregnancies, such as an infant born with severe erythroblastosis fetalis or a stillborn, hydropic fetus. The newborn's activity level and his feeding habits are important considerations in the decision to do an exchange transfusion, as early

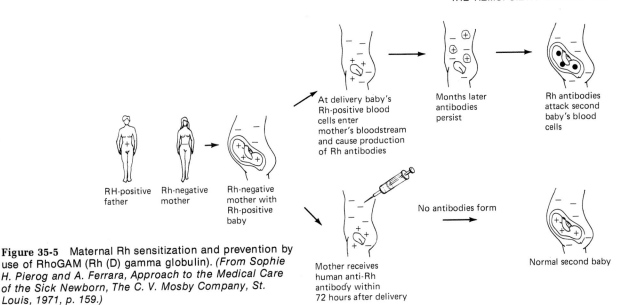

Figure 35-5 Maternal Rh sensitization and prevention by use of RhoGAM (Rh (D) gamma globulin). *(From Sophie H. Pierog and A. Ferrara, Approach to the Medical Care of the Sick Newborn, The C. V. Mosby Company, St. Louis, 1971, p. 159.)*

signs of kernicterus alter the activity and feeding habits.

In Rh incompatibility, fresh whole Rh-negative blood is used for the transfusion. The blood is matched with either the infant's own type or type O blood. The donor blood for ABO incompatibility needs to be type O and should not be the infant's type. A cross match to the mother's serum further reduces the risks of the transfusion in both types of incompatibility.

The procedure is performed through a cannula placed in the umbilical vein of the newborn still accessible for several hours after birth. The amount of donor blood used is approximately 500 ml to twice the amount of the newborn's blood volume. The transfusion is often referred to as a *double-volume exchange*, as twice the newborn's blood volume is exchanged. The exchange transfusion will replace and clear about 85 percent of the newborn's blood. Depending on the weight of the newborn and his subsequent blood volume, 5 to 20 ml of the newborn's blood is alternately removed and replaced with fresh whole blood.

The nurse has a great responsibility during the procedure, as there are many dangers inherent in the exchange transfusion which can be prevented or checked before serious difficulties arise. Since it takes at least an hour to complete, the newborn must be kept warm and have his temperature monitored. *Acidosis*, an abnormal decrease in blood pH, can result from the stress of being too cold. The vital signs and heart and respiratory rates must be moni-

tored throughout the procedure, in order to detect any deviation from the normal. The monitoring is frequently accomplished with the use of a cardiac or vital signs monitor attached to the newborn. A careful record of the amount of blood exchanged must be kept. This record helps prevent system overload from the excessive infusion of donor blood or shock from too-rapid removal of the newborn's blood. System overload can put the newborn into cardiac failure or result in cardiac arrest. The use of old blood (more than 48 hours old) can result in cardiac arrest from the elevated potassium level in the donor blood, as well as produce acidosis, as the donor blood pH is often less than 6.8. The normal pH of blood in the newborn ranges from 7.35 to 7.44. A range of 6.8 to 7.8 is still compatible with life. Hypocalcemia, which contributes to an irregular cardiac rhythm, is prevented by the infusion of 1 ml of 10 percent calcium gluconate after each 100 ml of blood exchanged. The lines or tubing of the transfusion set must be kept tightly closed during the exchange to prevent the admission of air. An air embolus can result in death or serious impairment of the brain cells.

A transfusion can also be performed in utero to provide support for the fetus in risk of hydrops after the twenty-eighth but before the thirty-fourth week. The main attempt is to correct the anemia produced by the hemolysis of the red cells. The transfusion is performed by inserting a needle into the mother's abdomen and into the amniotic sac, where adult red cells are injected into the peritoneal cavity of the fetus. The red cells will be absorbed by the circulation of the fetus. When the diagnosis of fetal hydrops is established, a transfusion is unable to correct the effects of the disease process.

Phototherapy A second method of treatment is *phototherapy*, the use of an artificial blue light which lowers the bilirubin levels in the skin and blood serum. (See Fig. 35-6.) Phototherapy operates on the principle of photooxidation of the bilirubin to other products which are then excretable. The newborn is placed under the light with the entire skin area exposed for 24 to 48 hours. The temperature must be monitored to ensure that the newborn is maintaining a normal temperature and is not suffering cold stress from the exposure. The newborn may develop loose stools during the therapy. It is essential that the newborn's eyes be protected from the light, as purulent conjunctivitis may result from prolonged exposure. The protection is provided through a blindfold made from a cloth or sterile cotton eye pads secured over the eyes; it should be checked and replaced at regular intervals. Some newborns with Rh incompatibility do not respond as well to phototherapy as to other methods of treatment such as an exchange transfusion. The success of phototherapy is generally measured by the decrease of the bilirubin level in the blood.

Jaundice The presenting clinical manifestation of the hemolytic anemias in the premature and newborn, jaundice, is caused by an elevation of the bilirubin level in the blood. There are numerous related disorders presenting with jaundice as shown in the outline below (adapted from Korones[1]):

1 Jaundice due to hemolysis of the intravascular system
  a Erythroblastosis fetalis related to Rh or ABO incompatibility
  b Polycythemia
  c Abnormalities of the erythrocytes
    (1) Hereditary spherocytosis
    (2) Hereditary elliptocytosis
    (3) Pyknocytosis
    (4) Hereditary nonspherocytosis hemolytic disease
    (5) Pathology of the hemoglobin
  d Chemically induced abnormalities
    (1) Enzyme deficiencies (glucose 6-phosphate dehydrogenase)
    (2) Vitamin K deficiency
    (3) Maternal ingestion of drugs (e.g., naphthalene)
2 Jaundice due to hemorrhage into enclosed places
  a Hematomas
  b Hemorrhage into body organs (e.g., liver or spleen)
  c Intraventricular hemorrhage and other hemorrhages into the scalp and cranium
3 Jaundice due to infectious causes
  a Bacterial
    (1) Pyelonephritis and urinary tract infections
    (2) Congenital syphilis
    (3) Septicemia
  b Nonbacterial
    (1) Toxoplasmosis
    (2) Cytomegalovirus
    (3) Rubella
    (4) Herpes simplex
    (5) Coxsackie virus
    (6) Neonatal hepatitis
4 Jaundice related to other causes
  a Physiologic jaundice of the newborn
  b Heinz body anemia of the premature
  c Hypoxia of diabetic mother
  d Respiratory distress syndrome
  e Prematurity
  f Breast milk ingestion syndrome
  g Transient familial tendency for hyperbilirubinemia
  h Biliary atresia
  i Hypothyroidism

The most important consideration in differentiating the disorder of which jaundice is a symptom is the time when it begins. During the first 24 to 48 hours, the development of jaundice is most indicative of the hemolytic disease process of the Rh or ABO or other blood group incompatibilities. After that period, the jaundice may be simple physiologic jaundice, a normal occurrence in neonatal life that does not require intensive therapy. Physiologic jaundice, between the second and fifth day of life, is related to a delay in the enzyme system of the liver, particularly in premature newborns. The enzyme system converts indirect to direct bilirubin, which is then excreted by the liver. Physiologic jaundice is also related to the increased destruction of red blood cells, common immediately after birth.

In order to recognize jaundice early, it is imperative that the newborn be observed frequently during the first 24 to 48 hours to assess his color and appearance. Adequate light is essential for the examination. Sunlight or ordinary daylight is best, for it eliminates many of the distortions of artificial lighting. The color of the lights and clothing or blankets surrounding the infant may influence the appearance of the skin. Yellow makes it difficult to compare the jaundiced skin to normal coloration. Pink colors often cause a yellowish tint. Blue light or colors make jaundice appear black. In the premature and newborn with darker skins, examination and detection of color differences is even more difficult, requiring an acutely trained eye and critical evaluation and comparisons. During examination of an infant, a simple *blanching* of the skin of the forehead or cheeks or other areas can reveal a jaundiced color. Blanching is done by pressing the skin for a second with the forefinger and then releasing the pressure to observe the blood return and color of the area. In jaundice due to the hemolytic anemias the skin has a

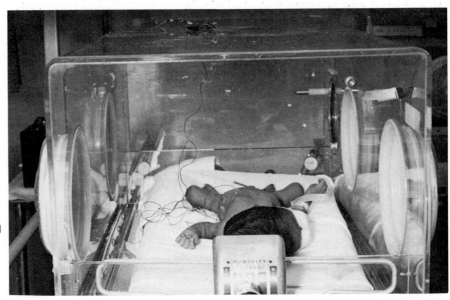

Figure 35-6 The jaundiced newborn undergoing phototherapy for hyperbilirubinemia. The newborn's eyes are covered to prevent the development of acute conjunctivitis. The newborn's entire skin area is exposed to provide maximum therapy from the light.

yellowish color because of the presence of unconjugated, indirect bilirubin. In contrast, in liver disorders and septicemia the conjugated bilirubin produces a greenish skin tint.

Nursing management The nursing assessment of the premature or full-term newborn in whom erythroblastosis fetalis is suspected is based upon factors ascertained from the maternal-fetal history, specifically the presence of dissimilar blood groups, a maternal negative Rh, or evidence of previous sensitization, in addition to factors observed in the newborn's color, activity level, vital signs, and blood chemistries. The nurse should observe the newborn to detect the early development of jaundice, pigmentation of the urine, pallor of anemia, edema, cyanosis, and the signs of central nervous system involvement, i.e., depression, excitation, or convulsions associated with kernicterus. Interpretation of the observations made leads to a nursing diagnosis of the manifestations characteristic of erythroblastosis fetalis. Prompt reporting to the physician of these manifestations and deviations in vital signs is crucial to nursing intervention. Prevention of upper respiratory infections, a frequent complication associated with a severe manifestation of the disease, is a responsibility to be met by means of constant attention given to the newborn's position, change of position, aeration of the lungs, and feeding habits which avoid aspiration into the lungs. In addition, the nurse must maintain the newborn's hydration, nutrition, and body warmth, even during such a procedure as an exchange transfusion or phototherapy.

Immune Thrombocytopenia

Pathogenesis An immune reaction similar to that which is responsible for the development of erythroblastosis fetalis can also cause thrombocytopenia. This immune reaction is a rare occurrence. The fetal platelets crossing the placental barrier interact with the maternal platelets to form antibodies against the fetal platelets. The antibodies enter the fetal circulation and destroy the fetal platelets.

Clinical manifestations In this disorder the clinical manifestations are similar to those of thrombocytopenia from other causes (to be discussed later). The only exception is that intracranial hemorrhage may occur more frequently in the immune reaction.

Diagnosis A diagnosis is made by laboratory tests including a platelet count. The platelet count will be below 100,000 cells/cu mm. The presence of platelet antibodies also is indicative of an immune reaction.

Treatment The usual method of treatment for an immune reaction is an exchange transfusion, like that done for Rh and ABO incompatibilities. The exchange transfusion will remove defective platelets and clear the blood of platelet antibodies. Corticosteroids are also used.

Immune Leukopenia Immune leukopenia is an uncommon occurrence in the newborn period. However, it is also analogous to the isoimmunization causing erythroblastosis. Antibody formation in the maternal circulation increases the rate of leukocyte removal from the fetal circulation and gradually produces a gross reduction of the marrow reserve of the leukocytes. The usual method of treatment for immune leukopenia is an exchange transfusion.

Hemolytic Anemia

Heinz Body Anemia in the Premature

Pathogenesis   One form of hemolytic anemia in the premature newborn is known as *Heinz body anemia*. The Heinz body is an abnormality of the erythrocyte in which there are particular intracellular inclusions in the membrane of the cell indicating a hemolytic process.

Clinical manifestations   Heinz body anemia is characterized by jaundice appearing between the first to fifth day. Anemia develops by the second to third week when the jaundice is less evident.

Diagnosis   A diagnosis is made by an examination of the blood smear. Prior to the development of anemia, the blood smear shows an increasing number of Heinz bodies. The unusual appearance of the Heinz bodies revealed by a staining process is shown in Fig. 35-7. Differential diagnosis is more difficult when anemia increases.

Treatment   As in other anemias, Heinz body anemia is often treated by simple transfusion of whole blood or *packed cells* which are secured from whole blood by removing most of the plasma. A rising level of bilirubin, with the appearance of jaundice, may necessitate the use of phototherapy or an exchange transfusion.

Nursing management   In assessing the premature newborn who is jaundiced, the nurse needs to recognize that this newborn is more likely to be jaundiced because of a greater immaturity of the hepatic system than the full-term newborn. Consequently, prompt reporting of jaundice and a concurrent rising level of serum bilirubin will lead to early differential medical diagnosis and treatment before anemia can develop. Frequent observation of the premature newborn's color, vital signs, and blood chemistries must be made.

Hemolytic Anemia as a Result of Infection

Pathogenesis   Hemolytic anemia in the premature and newborn can occur as a result of viral or bacterial infections transmitted to the fetus from the mother. The viruses, which are the cause of blood cell de-struction, anemia, and jaundice, are rubella, cytomegalic inclusion disease, Coxsackie virus, and herpesvirus. Sepsis, toxoplasmosis, and congenital syphilis also cause hemolysis. These infections are most often transmitted across the placenta at any time during the pregnancy. Another route of contracting bacterial infections is by way of the vaginal canal and cervix. A prolonged period of labor, with premature rupture of the membranes, for more than 24 hours before delivery can also contribute to the development of perinatal infections.

Clinical manifestations   The development of *chorioamnionitis*, an acute inflammation of the fetal side of the placenta and amniotic sac, accompanies perinatal infections. Anemia begins to develop in the fetus from the hemolysis instigated by the infections. Jaundice is not apparent until several hours after birth.

Diagnosis   The maternal history is important in the anticipation and detection of infection, as well as in the diagnostic procedure. Examination of the blood of the newborn will show the decreased level of red cells and the increased bilirubin level. Cultures of the blood, eyes, cord, skin, and other sites can indicate bacterial growth or viral invasion.

Treatment   The therapy for anemia resulting from infections is best directed toward the specific bacteria or virus causing the infection and resultant anemia. This therapy is the utilization of antibiotics specific to the infectious agent. The anemia, if particularly severe, can be treated with a simple transfusion of packed cells to increase the number of red cells. The development of hyperbilirubinemia may require an exchange transfusion.

Nursing management   A primary nursing responsibility is the prevention of infection during both the perinatal and newborn periods. A clean environment helps prevent the infectious process. Since bacterial infections can be acquired during the labor period after the rupture of membranes, it is essential that the equipment used and the persons coming in contact with the mother be free from infection. This precaution needs to be carried over to the newborn period. A clean environment in the nursery can prevent contamination from equipment, persons providing care, and other newborns who may have infections.

Observation of the newborn's color and activity level, particularly as related to the hemoglobin and hematocrit at birth, and a history of perinatal infection are essential to the nursing assessment. Deviations in the vital signs and the development of edema, jaundice, or extreme pallor are important factors to be considered in planning nursing intervention.

Hemolytic Anemia as an Inherited Disorder

Pathogenesis Hemolytic anemia may be caused by disorders that are inherited. These disorders, which accelerate the destruction of erythrocytes, become evident during the newborn or neonatal period and may persist into infancy. Among these disorders are congenital spherocytosis, elliptocytosis, nonspherocytosis or other disorders of the erythrocytes, and enzyme deficiencies such as glucose 6-phosphate dehydrogenase (G-6-PD) and pyruvate-kinase deficiency.

Clinical manifestations Jaundice associated with hyperbilirubinemia is one of the presenting symptoms during the first few hours to the first week of life. Pallor and anemia will also be evident.

Diagnosis A laboratory analysis of the blood reveals an unusual shape to the erythrocytes, such as an elliptic shape in the disorder elliptocytosis. Spherocytes may also be present. If the disorder is due to an enzymatic deficiency of the erythrocytes, this will be detected by laboratory tests. A diagnosis is also made by considering the family history, which may or may not reveal a prior occurrence of the disease.

Treatment Severe anemia is treated with a transfusion to provide functional red cells. An exchange transfusion may be indicated with the development of hyperbilirubinemia. Phototherapy is also indicated as an alternative or additional treatment for hyperbilirubinemia.

Anemia from Blood Loss

The premature and newborn can suffer from acute and chronic blood loss producing anemia. (See Table 35-4.) The chronic blood loss can occur slowly during fetal life as a result of *feto-maternal* or *feto-fetal* transfusion or as a result of hemorrhage into an enclosed place in the body. The acute blood loss producing shock can also occur from the transfusion or hemorrhage, as well as from traumatic ruptures or tears of the cord or placenta.

Acute Blood Loss

Clinical manifestations The premature or newborn in shock from acute blood loss appears at birth to be extremely pale and cyanotic with gasping respira-

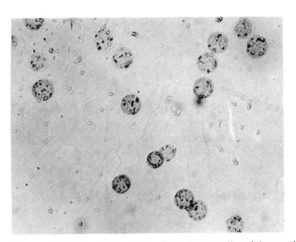

Figure 35-7 The Heinz body. The abnormality of the erythrocyte produces anemia, most commonly in the premature newborn. (*From A. M. Mauer, Pediatric Hematology, McGraw-Hill Book Company, New York, 1969, p. 74.*)

tions and retractions. He is not active and has a very weak cry. He is also tachypneic or breathing rapidly and may have tachycardia or an accelerated heart rate. (In the full-term newborn, the range of the apical pulse is 110 to 150 beats taken for a full minute. The premature newborn tends to have a slightly higher pulse. Respirations range from 30 to 40

Table 35-4 COMMON CAUSES OF FETAL AND NEONATAL BLOOD LOSS

1 Obstetric accidents causing acute blood loss
  a Cord
    (1) Traumatic rupture of the normal cord
    (2) Rupture of a vessel aneurysm or varix
    (3) Traumatic tearing of the vessels with the insertion of instruments during delivery
  b Placenta
    (1) Placenta previa
    (2) Abruptio placenta
    (3) Accidental incision into the fetal side of the placenta during a cesarean section
    (4) Rupture of a multilobular placenta
2 Transfusions causing acute or chronic blood loss
  a Feto-maternal transfusion
  b Feto-fetal transfusion in identical twins
3 Hemorrhage into enclosed places causing acute or chronic blood loss
  a Intracranial
  b Cephalohematoma
  c Bleeding into scalp
  d Pulmonary
  e Rupture of the liver or spleen
  f Retroperitoneal
  g Gastrointestinal

Source: Adapted from S. B. Korones, *High-Risk Newborn Infants*, The C. V. Mosby Company, St. Louis, 1972, pp. 162–163.

breaths and must be counted for a full minute as the respirations tend to be irregular, particularly in the premature.) This classic picture of shock may have manifestations similar to those of asphyxiation; therefore, it is essential to distinguish between the symptoms of shock and those of acute respiratory distress or asphyxiation. Indicators helpful in this differentiation are described in Table 35-5. The newborn who is asphyxiated has a low heart rate from oxygen hunger, has slow, labored, or absent respirations, and is cyanotic. He responds readily to oxygen therapy. In contrast, the newborn in shock has an accelerated heart rate unless he is suffering from oxygen hunger, in which case his heart rate decreases. He has accelerated respirations. He is also cyanotic; however, he does not respond to oxygen therapy as the asphyxiated newborn does.

Diagnosis The blood values in the newborn who is anemic from acute blood loss remain within normal limits for a period of hours after birth and are not valid determinants in making a diagnosis. Edema, hepatosplenomegaly, increased reticulocytes, decreased hemoglobin, decreased erythrocyte count, and jaundice, the classic indicators of anemia, are not present unless the blood loss has occurred over a longer period of time or is related to hemolytic anemia. The determination of the cause of the blood loss and the identification of the symptoms as those of shock are most important in diagnosing acute blood loss.

Treatment For acute blood loss, treatment consists first of reacting to the state of shock by raising the blood volume. Whole blood is used to transfuse the newborn as this raises the blood volume while replacing the loss of erythrocytes. Plasma may be given prior to the transfusion with whole blood when the loss of blood has been particularly severe. If the newborn is hypoxic, clearing the airway and administering oxygen are essential. Assisting the respirations may also be necessary.

Chronic Blood Loss Chronic blood loss occurs over a longer period of time than does acute blood loss. It results from a transfusion of fetal blood into the maternal circulation or into the circulation of the twin in monochorionic pregnancies.

Clinical manifestations The newborn can present the picture of shock at birth if the blood loss has been particularly severe. More commonly, signs of iron deficiency anemia are present at birth: the newborn has a critical hemoglobin (lower than 7 to 8 Gm/100 ml) and pallor of the skin and mucous membranes.

In the phenomenon of twin-to-twin or feto-fetal transfusion, an abnormal communication of the usually separate circulations of the two fetuses results in a shunting of blood from one twin to the other. (See Fig. 35-8*A* and *B*.) One twin will be anemic, the other *plethoric*, that is, with a larger than normal blood volume. The anemic twin is small in size, has a pale appearance, and exhibits signs of hypotension. There is a decreased amount of amniotic fluid. The plethoric twin is reddish in color, prone to hemorrhage, hypertensive, and has signs of an enlarged heart and hepatosplenomegaly. There is an increased volume of amniotic fluid in the plethoric twin's amniotic sac. Heart failure, pulmonary congestion, and hyperbilirubinemia are common in the plethoric twin. The intensity of the appearance of each twin is dependent on the amount of shunting and the length of time over which it has occurred.

Diagnosis There are two indications of feto-maternal transfusion. First, fetal hemoglobin and fetal red cells will be found in the maternal circulation. The presence of fetal hemoglobin can easily be demonstrated by the resistance of fetal hemoglobin

Table 35-5 DIFFERENTIATION OF SHOCK FROM BLOOD LOSS AND ASPHYXIATION IN THE PREMATURE AND FULL-TERM NEWBORN

Determinants	Shock from blood loss	Asphyxiation
Cardiac rate	Tachycardia (over 160 beats per min) unless severely hypoxic	Bradycardia (under 80 beats per min) from hypoxia
Respiratory rate	Tachypnea (over 50–60 breaths per min)	Apnea or extremely slow and labored respirations
Color	Cyanotic	Cyanotic
Response to oxygen therapy	No response	Rapid response

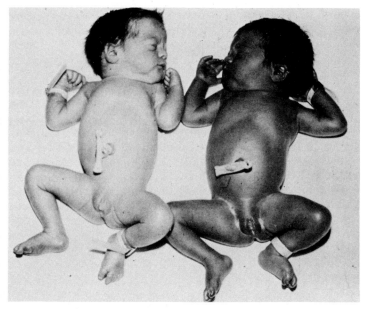

A

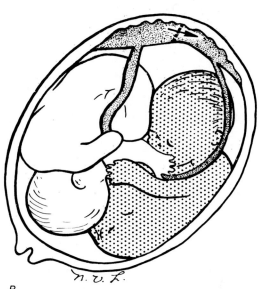

B

Figure 35-8 The feto-fetal transfusion syndrome in identical twins. *(A)* Identical twins as they appear 6 hours after birth. The plethoric twin is the darker, larger twin on the right. The hematocrit is 87 percent in the plethoric twin, in contrast with 32 percent in the anemic, smaller twin. *(B)* Drawing of a monochorionic placenta of twins with transfusion syndrome. The anemic twin's (right) thin umbilical cord is attached to the pale half of the placenta. The plethoric twin's thick, engorged umbilical cord is attached to the thick, congested portion of the placenta. The single placenta contains an unbalanced arteriovenous shunt at the vascular equator (broken line). *(From C. Pochedly and S. Musiker, "Twin-to-Twin Transfusion Syndrome," Postgraduate Medicine, 47(3):173–174, March 1970.)*

to alkali denaturation. Second, if the fetus and mother are not of the same blood group, fetal erythrocytes indicative of another group will be present.

A difference in the hemoglobin levels of the twins greater than 5 Gm/100 ml of blood is indicative of feto-fetal shunting process. The amount of amniotic fluid in each amniotic sac is also important in determining that the shunting has occurred.

Treatment   The treatment is based on the degree of the anemia. A transfusion of packed cells may be given immediately after birth or later, depending on the level of the hemoglobin and the presence of other signs, such as an extreme pallor. The hemoglobin should be brought at least to the level of 12 Gm/100 ml of blood. Supplemental iron given with the diet is also helpful in restoring the hemoglobin level. It is used when the hemoglobin level drops following aggressive therapy, such as transfusion. An exchange transfusion can be done in which the volume removed is replaced with a volume of packed red cells. This method keeps the blood volume constant while rapidly raising the hemoglobin and hema-

tocrit. The plethoric twin is treated with an exchange transfusion in which the volume removed is greater than that replaced with a volume of packed red cells. This method lowers the blood volume while maintaining the hemoglobin at a high level. When the hemolysis of red cells produces hyperbilirubinemia, an exchange transfusion or phototherapy is used.

Nursing Management   The nursing assessment of the anemic newborn suffering from blood loss is based upon the determinants that are used to distinguish shock from asphyxiation. These are the respiratory rate, the heart rate, the color, and the response to oxygen. Since the blood values change more slowly, they are not adequate determinants to be used in the assessment. Blood loss producing shock requires accurate observation to ascertain the acuteness of the situation. The premature suffers more from blood loss than does the full-term newborn; therefore, blood loss and the resultant shock should be considered as a greater emergency in the premature. Once the nursing diagnosis has been documented by the determinants, intervention is planned involving immediate steps to notify the physician and begin treatment to correct shock. Nursing intervention includes providing warmth, placing the newborn in shock position with his head lower than his extremities, and monitoring the vital signs and color at frequent intervals to evaluate response to treatment.

The nursing assessment of twins from a monochorionic pregnancy in the presence of any evidence of a shunting process (feto-fetal transfusion) is a comparative assessment of the twins. Observation is made of the differences in color, size, vital signs, and hemoglobin values. The anemic twin must be observed for the possibility of impending shock. The plethoric twin is observed for signs of the development of cardiac failure precipitated by systemic overload. Nursing intervention is planned to provide warmth, constant surveillance of the vital signs, evaluation of quality as well as the rate of respiration and pulse, and observation of the color and activity of the newborn. It is necessary to protect the plethoric twin from any danger of trauma which could produce abnormal bleeding.

Polycythemia

Pathogenesis An increase in blood volume and red cell concentration, or *polycythemia*, can result from an abnormal transfer of maternal blood into the fetal circulation during the pregnancy, a prolonged emptying of the placenta into the newborn immediately after delivery, or an increased production and circulation of red cells to provide adequate oxygen for the body tissues. Many cases are idiopathic, having no demonstrable cause. If the hematocrit is significantly high, there is a danger of thrombosis and infarction in vital areas such as the brain or heart.

Clinical Manifestations The newborn with polycythemia appears much like the plethoric newborn as described above. Respiratory distress is a common consequence of the increased blood volume. Convulsions and cardiac failure may also result from systemic overload.

Diagnosis The diagnosis is made by the laboratory analysis of the blood to determine the hematocrit and hemoglobin levels, both of which will be elevated. A hematocrit of over 70 percent and a hemoglobin of greater than 23 Gm/100 ml mean that difficulties are more likely to occur.

Treatment The treatment, as in the treatment for the plethoric twin, is concerned with decreasing the blood volume to lessen the risks from systemic overload. Heparin or other anticoagulants are used to decrease the danger of coagulation within the blood circulation and the risk of thrombosis.

Nursing Management The nursing assessment of the polycythemic newborn is similar to that utilized with the plethoric twin. When anticoagulants are used, nursing intervention must include the prevention of injury and the observation of any sites from which blood samples are taken. Hematomas can easily develop at these sites when proper care is not given. Direct pressure to stop the flow of blood must be maintained for a longer period of time than necessary with normal blood. The development of respiratory distress is prevented by frequently changing the newborn's position. Aspiration during feedings must also be prevented.

Hemorrhagic Disease of the Newborn

Pathogenesis *Hemorrhagic disease of the newborn* is related to deviations in the coagulation mechanism of the blood plasma. It is limited to the first few days of the newborn period. Hemorrhagic disease is caused by a deficiency of vitamin K upon which the prothrombin and other coagulation factors of the blood plasma are dependent for their production in the liver.

Clinical Manifestations Hemorrhaging in the form of oozing from the cord, hematuria, and gastrointestinal bleeding are common, appearing between the second and fifth days. Petechiae and ecchymoses appear on the body and extremities of the newborn. Anemia can result from continuous and prolonged oozing of blood. The stools may be tar-colored, or the newborn may have a bright red emesis when the gastrointestinal bleeding is extensive.

Diagnosis A prolonged prothrombin time and partial thromboplastin time are the most significant of the laboratory values. The clotting time is found to be normal. The platelet count and the red cell counts continue to be normal.

Treatment Vitamin K, administered prophylactically after birth, is effective in the prevention of the deficiency at most health agencies. Vitamin K is also the choice method of treatment. One milligram vitamin K administered intravenously begins to take effect in about 4 to 6 hours, controlling the hemorrhagic problem.

Nursing Management The nursing assessment of the newborn suspected of hemorrhagic disease is based upon observations for any evidence of unusual bleeding. The sclera, skin, cord, urine, and stools are observed for blood or oozing. Nursing intervention is planned to avoid the danger of trauma and its consequent bleeding. As with the polycythemic newborn being treated with anticoagulants, there is a risk in taking blood samples. The nurse should try to prevent the development of hematomas as well as excessive loss of blood.

Thrombocytopenia Purpura

Pathogenesis Thrombocytopenia purpura is a deficiency of platelets caused by infections acquired during fetal life or during the newborn period. It may be associated with disseminated intravascular coagulation (DIC). Giant congenital hemangiomas can also cause this disorder.

The infections causing thrombocytopenia purpura are congenital syphilis, cytomegalovirus, toxoplasmosis, herpes virus, septicemia, and rubella. These infections are acquired in a similar manner to infections causing hemolytic anemia, which may be a concurrent problem in the thrombocytopenic newborn. Thrombocytopenia may be induced by the maternal ingestion of drugs during the pregnancy. The drugs, which destroy the platelets in both the mother and fetus or cause antibody formation against the fetal platelets, are the thiazides, sulfonamides, and quinine. An immune reaction is also possible, as discussed earlier, although this form rarely occurs. The giant hemangioma is a tumor that traps and destroys the platelets.

Clinical Manifestations The hemorrhagic condition of thrombocytopenia produces extravasated blood which, when broken down, elevates the bilirubin in the blood, producing jaundice. Ecchymoses and petechial lesions are characteristic of the disorder.

Diagnosis A diagnosis is made by screening the newborn's history, that is, the maternal-fetal interaction, for the ingestion of certain drugs, for infections, and for disorders occurring concurrently with the pregnancy, such as systemic lupus erythematosus. Laboratory tests will reveal a platelet count below 100,000 cells/cu mm. A bone marrow examination may also be done to detect the presence of megakaryocytes associated with an immune reaction or the lack of these cells indicative of the onset of aplastic anemia (discussed later) which can follow thrombocytopenia. DIC is characterized by the depletion or consumption of the platelets, fibrinogen, and clotting factors of the plasma, so that a group of distorted, fragmented platelet cells appears in the blood smear.

Treatment The administration of fresh whole blood is the main therapy for severe anemia caused by the hemorrhages. Platelets, in the whole blood, replace the depleted supply in the newborn's blood. Anticoagulants, specifically heparin, are administered when thrombocytopenia is associated with DIC. Heparin works to stop the defibrination process and allows the coagulation mechanism to be restored to its normal functioning. Irradiation or surgical removal are the alternatives available in the treatment of the hemangioma. Irradiation reduces and eliminates the tumor.

Nursing Management The nursing assessment of the newborn with a reduction in platelets is based upon observations of the color and vital signs to detect the development of jaundice, ecchymoses, and petechial lesions. The nurse needs to be cognizant of factors in the maternal-fetal interaction which would indicate a tendency for the development of thrombocytopenia. It is important for the nurse to protect the hemangioma from trauma and provide for cleanliness and good skin care in the area being irradiated to prevent excessive skin breakdown. It is also important to provide warmth and adequate hydration and nutrition.

HEMOPOIETIC DEVIATIONS AND DISEASES IN THE INFANT
Anemia

Anemia, the most common hemopoietic disorder of childhood, results from a reduction in the number of red blood cells, a lowered concentration of available hemoglobin, or both. The anemias may be divided into two categories: those resulting from impairment in production of red blood cells and those resulting from increased destruction or loss of red blood cells.

Clinical Manifestations The clinical features of anemia are related to the decrease in the oxygen-carrying capacity of the blood. Signs and symptoms may be nonspecific—irritability, weakness, anorexia, decreased exercise tolerance, and lack of interest in surroundings. When the hemoglobin level falls below 7 to 8 Gm/100 ml, cardiac compensatory adjustments occur, and pallor of the skin and mucosa may develop. When anemia is severe, the skin may assume a waxy, sallow appearance. Cardiac decompensation occurs, and congestive heart failure may develop with symptoms of tachycardia, tachypnea, shortness of breath, dyspnea, edema, and hepatomegaly. A peculiarity of infants is their ability to adjust to the stress of anemia unusually well. It is not uncommon for an infant to maintain a hemoglobin as low as 4 or 5 Gm/100 ml and manifest no signs or symptoms. Older children also demonstrate an ability to tolerate low hemoglobin levels, particularly if their anemia develops gradually.

Diagnosis and Treatment The diagnosis and treatment of anemia vary with the etiology of the disorder. Specific therapy will be discussed later in the chapter when specific disorders are described. Transfusion of packed cells may be used with several types of anemia. When cardiac compensatory adjustments occur, the blood volume is increased to enhance profusion of tissues. The volume of whole blood required to supply the necessary quantity of red blood cells may overload the child's circulatory system. When packed cell transfusions are prepared, the erythrocytes are spun down and the bulk of fluid and other formed elements are left behind. This type of transfusion enables the child to receive a high concentration of erythrocytes in a small quantity of fluid.

Nursing Management The nursing assessment should include determination of the child's current functional level. An estimation of his exercise tolerance and level of frustration should be made. Factors which may contribute to the disease process should be investigated. A thorough dietary history (to be discussed in more detail with iron deficiency) should be taken. Possible toxic agents in the environment, such as chemicals and drugs, should be identified. A close observation of the interaction of family members may reveal what influence they have on the child's adjustment to the limitations of his disease. Do they automatically assist him when he needs assistance, or must he ask for help? Is he allowed to participate in activities when he is able, or is he restricted?

The nurse who is attuned to early signs of irritability, fatigue, and frustration in the child should be prepared to make necessary adjustments in the environment. The irritable infant must have his needs met promptly. Crying may cause further fatigue. Disruptive treatments and procedures should be scheduled together to allow for uninterrupted periods of rest. When caring for an older child, careful selection of activities in which he can engage without frustration is essential. When he begins to show signs of fatigue, sedentary activities such as handcrafts and coloring should be presented. When possible, he should be given several alternatives and allowed to choose. A short attention span should be anticipated.

Fear of hospitalization can be exaggerated by fear of separation from mother. Allowing the mother to participate actively in the child's care may reduce this fear. Explanation of procedures and exploration through play may reduce anxiety and fear in the older child. When intrusive procedures are necessary, allowing him to participate in the preparation for the procedure by wiping the area with alcohol and applying the adhesive cover may help him maintain some control of the situation.

Anemic children are often anorectic. Infants should be fed slowly and offered frequent small feedings if necessary. The child should be rewarded for positive attempts to eat. The older child may wish to participate in the selection and preparation of the food. Simple tasks, such as helping the younger children prepare their meal trays, may stimulate his eating. Tiring activities and unpleasant procedures and treatments should not be scheduled at mealtime.

The nursing responsibilities to a child receiving a transfusion are great. The child should be monitored closely for signs and symptoms of a transfusion reaction. A change in the child's vital signs may be the first indication of incompatibility. Other signs and symptoms for which the nurse should observe are pain, tightness in the chest, chilling, an urticarial rash, and a decrease in urinary output. When a transfusion reaction is suspected, the transfusion should be stopped at once and the physician should be notified. It is advisable to administer transfusions with a double setup in which both blood and an intravenous solution are connected by a stopcock. With this arrangement fluid is available to maintain the patency of the intravenous line in the event that the transfusion must be stopped. The untransfused blood should be saved and returned to the blood bank.

If possible, a child's parent should remain with the child during the procedure. The nurse should explain the procedure to the parent and elicit his or her assistance during the preparation, if it is appropriate to do so. The infusion site should be securely immobilized in a position that is comfortable for the child. He should be provided with familiar comforting objects and diversionary activity during the procedure.

Infusion of the blood may be difficult and tedious, but transfusions should be administered slowly to prevent volume overload and to protect the child's small, fragile veins. The cells may clog the tubing, and it may be necessary to intermittently flush the tubing with an intravenous solution.

Anemias Resulting from Impairment in Production of Red Blood Cells

Iron Deficiency Anemia

Pathogenesis Iron deficiency anemia is the most common type of anemia in childhood. It occurs most commonly between the ages of 6 and 24 months. Prior to this time the child's iron requirements are usually met by the reserves acquired during fetal life. A positive iron balance in childhood is dependent on several factors. Possible causes of iron deficiency include

1 Insufficient supply: dietary deficiency, inadequate stores at birth
2 Impaired absorption: diarrhea, malabsorption syndrome
3 Excessive demands: growth requirements, chronic illness
4 Blood loss: hemorrhage, parasitic infection

Clinical manifestations The clinical features of iron deficiency are similar to those mentioned in the general discussion of anemia. When children with iron deficiency acquire infections, their condition is aggravated by a decreased absorption of iron. It has been suggested that *pica*, a hunger for and ingestion of unsuitable substances, such as clay or starch, may result from and contribute to iron deficiency.

Diagnosis The clinical findings of pallor combined with the history of an iron-deficient diet are suggestive of iron deficiency anemia. The characteristic appearance of the stained blood smear is that of many small red cells or *microcytes* that are pale or *hypochromic*. This central pallor of the cells indicates the marked deficiency of hemoglobin.

Treatment Iron salt preparations are administered orally in most cases. Ferrous sulfate is most often used because it is both inexpensive and effective. A rapid response in the hemoglobin is expected when therapy is begun, but the child is continued on oral iron for 4 to 6 weeks after normal blood values are established to replenish body stores. If insufficient dietary supply is the cause of the deficiency, a change in dietary habits is essential. Milk is a relatively poor source of iron. Many infants and children who drink large quantities of milk do so to the exclusion of other foods which contain more iron. When this is the case, milk intake should be limited to 1 quart per day. Foods high in iron, such as meat, fortified cereal, vegetables, and fruit, should be introduced to the diet.

Nursing management The nursing assessment should focus on the child's dietary habits. Information should be obtained regarding the type and quantity of food eaten, the methods of feeding used, and the child's reaction to eating. The nurse should assess the parents' understanding of dietary requirement and nutritional value of foods.

Diet teaching can be a delicate matter. The nurse must be aware that dietary habits are influenced by cultural and socioeconomic factors. In some cultures a fat, chubby baby is considered a reflection of good mothering. Babies who are fed nothing but milk and carbohydrates for the first year of life may be fat and appear healthy to the mother. It is difficult for her to appreciate the need for a change in dietary habits. Mothers may resist including iron-containing foods in their babies' diet because they are more expensive or unfamiliar.

It is important to explain the reasons for diet change to the parents in language they can understand. Visual aids and pictures may be helpful. Explanations and suggestions may need to be repeated several times. The nurse may investigate with the parents sources of inexpensive iron-containing foods which are available in their community. A plan should be implemented to introduce new foods to the baby's diet. The baby may better tolerate frequent small feedings. The environment should be free of stress at feeding time, and he should be fed in the presence of other children or family members if possible. It is important that the nurse be accepting of the family's cultural habits and patterns but stress the rationale for the change in a nonjudgmental way.

The infant may resist transferring from an exclusive milk diet to one that includes new, unfamiliar foods. When this is the case, it is important to consistently limit the amount of milk offered, and to continue gently offering foods even if the infant rejects them. He will eventually turn to the new foods to satisfy his hunger.

When oral iron therapy is used, the parent should be warned that the stools will be darker. If liquid preparations are used, they should be administered carefully, because if the iron touches the child's teeth, they may become stained. The nurse should stress to the parent the importance of continuing the iron therapy according to the physician's plans. Many parents are tempted to discontinue the therapy when a good response is obtained.

Hypoplastic Anemia or Blackfan-Diamond

Pathogenesis Hypoplastic anemia, also called congenital pure red cell anemia, is characterized by a failure of erythropoiesis without a depression of leukocytes or platelets. Though the etiology of the disease is unknown, several theories including a genetic basis have been proposed.

Clinical manifestations The disease presents insidiously with symptoms of anemia usually present before the child is 1 year of age. The course of the disease may be one of persistent, progressive anemia requiring frequent transfusions. Spontaneous, permanent remissions occur in approximately one-fourth to one-third of the patients between 1 and 13 years of age.

Diagnosis The red blood cells are normochromic and normocytic, but there is a virtual lack of erythropoietic activity in the blood and bone marrow. Red blood cell precursors are reduced in the marrow, and reticulocytes are markedly diminished.

Treatment Supportive measures include long-term administration of transfusions of packed cells to patients who fail to respond to therapy. Corticosteroids are used, and approximately 50 percent of the patients will respond to therapy and will show signs of spontaneous erythropoiesis. The corticosteroids are usually administered on a staggered schedule instead of daily to minimize the drug's effect on growth. Patients who fail to respond to therapy may die of the complications of chronic anemia and repeated transfusions.

Nursing management The approaches included in the discussion of anemia should be employed with the child with hypoplastic anemia. In addition, the nurse should prepare the parents for the side effects of corticosteroid therapy including appetite and behavior changes, weight gain, predisposition to infections, and possible hypertension.

Anemias Resulting from an Increased Destruction or Loss of Red Blood Cells

Hereditary Spherocytosis

Pathogenesis Hereditary spherocytosis is a congenital hemolytic anemia. Occasionally cases present with no evidence of a familial pattern. The cases are presumed to be new mutations. The basic physiologic defects are a spherocytic shape of the erythrocyte and an increased osmotic fragility. The spleen represents an unfavorable environment for these abnormal cells. Circulation through the spleen results in sequestration and destruction of the erythrocytes.

Clinical manifestations The manifestations of the disease can be extremely variable among patients and in individual patients at different times. The signs and symptoms of anemia and hemolysis may be noticed early in infancy. The most serious complication of the disease is the occurrence of aplastic crises which are associated with a transient cessation of hemopoiesis. The crises are rare and usually self-limiting. The episodes may last a week and are accompanied by increasing pallor, fever, shortness of breath, and weakness.

Diagnosis Finding the characteristic morphologic abnormality of the red cell confirms the diagnosis. Examination of the stained smear will reveal a varying number of the characteristic spherocytic erythrocytes. The osmotic fragility of the cells can be established by placing them in hypotonic saline solution; water will enter the spherocytic cells, and they will rupture.

Treatment The major form of therapy, splenectomy, results in a clinical cure—although the morphology of the erythrocyte remains unchanged, the sequestration and destruction of the cells terminate. The splenectomy is not usually done before the child is 4 to 5 years of age, because of the potential risk of overwhelming bacterial infections encountered in younger splenectomized children. Most children are able to maintain a hemoglobin of 7 to 8 Gm/100 ml until the splenectomy can be performed.

Nursing management The nursing intervention appropriate for an anemic child is discussed above and for a child undergoing surgery is discussed in various chapters in Part 3.

Sickle-Cell Hemoglobinopathies

Pathogenesis The sickle-cell hemoglobinopathies are hereditary disorders characterized by the presence of an abnormal type of hemoglobin in the red blood cell. The basic defect is a substitution of valine for glutamic acid in the sixth position of the beta polypeptide chain of the hemoglobin molecule. This structural change facilitates the sickling phenomenon. In the presence of deoxygenation a stacking of sickle hemoglobin molecules occurs, and the cell assumes an irregular shape. The abnormally shaped cells increase blood viscosity, and viscosity results in stasis and sludging of the cells and further deoxygenation. Deoxygenation leads to further sickling, eventual occlusion of small vessels, and tissue ischemia, with infarction and necrosis occurring.

The sickling phenomenon takes place when the oxygen tension in the blood is lowered. Decreased oxygen tension may be triggered by infection, dehydration, exposure to cold, or physical or emotional stress. (See Fig. 35-9.)

Sickle trait is a heterozygous occurrence of the sickle gene resulting in a combination of normal adult hemoglobin and sickle hemoglobin in the red blood cell. *Sickle-cell anemia* is a homozygous occurrence of the sickle gene resulting in a severe hemolytic anemia. (See Fig. 35-10.)

Clinical manifestations　Clinical manifestations of sickle trait are rare. Discovery of the trait is often incidental or a result of a screening effort for purposes of genetic counseling or military induction. Occasionally severe hypoxia resulting from shock, exposure to low oxygen content, or surgery may result in discovery of sickling. Clinical manifestations of sickle-cell anemia occurring in infancy include frequent infections, failure to thrive, irritability, pallor, hepatosplenomegaly, jaundice, and growth retardation. Periods of well-being may be interrupted by periods of sickling crisis. Manifestations rarely occur before 6 months of age and may not occur until the child is 2 to 3 years of age. Older children may complain of joint, back, and abdominal pain, headache, nausea and vomiting, and frequent infections, particularly of the respiratory tract.

The possible complications of sickle-cell anemia include aplastic, hyperhemolytic, and sequestration crises. The vascular occlusion or thrombotic crises, the most common complications of the disease, are responsible for a majority of the multitude of defects acquired by the child with sickle-cell disease. The thrombotic crises may involve any area of the body: Soft-tissue swelling and pain result from vascular occlusion in the area of a large joint. The "hand-foot" syndrome (Fig. 35-11) is a complication seen in children under 2 years of age. Characteristically this syndrome is accompanied by pain, fever, swelling of soft tissue of the hands and feet, and infarction of the underlying bones. The complication is self-limiting, and complete healing can be expected. Vital organs such as the lungs, kidneys, liver, brain, and eye may be involved, and serious complications can result.

Diagnosis　Several methods of detecting and diagnosing the presence of the sickle hemoglobin in the red blood cell are available. Examination of a stained

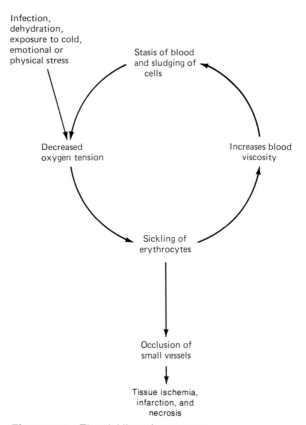

Figure 35-9　The sickling phenomenon.

blood smear may reveal a few sickled cells. These cells are, however, found only in the blood of persons with sickle-cell anemia. The sickle-turbidity tube test is available for use in screening situations. A drop of blood obtained from a finger stick is placed in a tube containing a measured amount of test reagent. The solution is mixed and allowed to stand for 5 minutes. The appearance of the solution determines the results of the test. Some commercial preparations used in this test allow a distinction between sickle trait and sickle-cell anemia, and others do not. This distinction can be made with a hemoglobin electrophoresis. This method separates the various types of hemoglobin, making it possible to identify the type and amount of hemoglobin present.

Treatment　Administration of oral and intravenous fluids is essential. Dehydration causes decreased blood volume, sludging, increased blood viscosity, and further sickling. Fever, which may accelerate dehydration, can be controlled with antipyretics. Crises are usually accompanied by severe pain

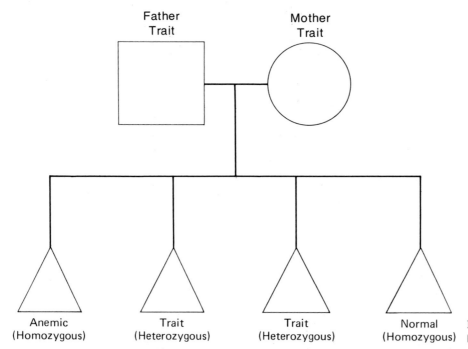

Father
Trait

Mother
Trait

Anemic
(Homozygous)

Trait
(Heterozygous)

Trait
(Heterozygous)

Normal
(Homozygous)

Figure 35-10 The inheritance pattern of sickle-cell disease.

which persists for several days. Analgesics should be used appropriately to control the pain.

Hypertransfusion of packed cells may be used during thrombotic crises when involvement of vital organs may be life-threatening. Raising the hemoglobin to high levels diminishes bone marrow production of additional sickle cells and dilutes the existing sickle cells with normal transfused erythrocytes. This decreases the viscosity of the blood, but the complications of long-term hypertransfusion contraindicate using this approach routinely.

Some recent studies have covered the development of more effective therapy and evaluation of the use of urea and cyanate solutions. These agents are highly experimental at the present time, and few data are available to document their usefulness. Further evaluation is necessary before this type of therapy can be considered for use except in an experimental environment.

Incidence and prognosis Sickle-cell disease is found primarily in blacks. Its incidence in Caucasians is extremely low. These occasional cases are thought to be the result of distant intermarriages or new genetic mutations. The incidence of sickle trait and sickle-cell disease in the black population is 1:10 and 1:400, respectively.

The prognosis for patients with sickle-cell anemia is generally grave. Death usually occurs in childhood or early adult life. Occasionally patients with sickle-cell anemia experience only few and minor complications. Patients with sickle trait can expect to live a normal life-span uncomplicated by the defect.

Nursing management The nursing assessment should determine the source of pain, if possible, and measures which may comfort an irritable infant or child. Measures to be considered include holding or rocking the infant, singing to him, or reading stories. Providing familiar objects and persons may be helpful. Bathing the child in warm water or applying local heat or massage may reduce the pain.

In many situations, measures which may comfort the patient must be selected by trial and error. When effective measures are identified, they should be recorded and shared with the entire nursing staff.

It is important to assess the environment to identify factors which may aggravate the sickling process and to provide optimal surroundings for the patient. He should be warm, well hydrated, free from stress, and protected from infection.

An evaluation of the parents' understanding of the disease and the genetic implication is essential. The goal of genetic counseling is to inform the child's parents of the genetic implications of the disease. If they request information about birth control measures, it should be made available to them.

Thalassemia (Cooley's Anemia or Mediterranean Anemia)

Pathogenesis Thalassemia is a hereditary disorder in which there is an impaired ability to form adult hemoglobin. Red cell production is less affected, and consequently the individual red cells contain markedly diminished amounts of hemoglobin. The erythrocytes produced are fragile, abnormally shaped, and easily destroyed. The erythropoietic system attempts to compensate for the defect by producing abnormally high amounts of fetal hemoglobin. This disorder is found primarily in persons of Mediterranean descent, but cases occur in most racial groups. The heterozygous state, thalassemia minor, is associated with mild anemia. Children carrying this trait are usually asymptomatic.

Clinical manifestations Thalassemia major or Cooley's anemia, the homozygous form of the disease, results in a severe progressive hemolytic anemia which presents in the second 6 months of life. The signs and symptoms of severe anemia discussed earlier accompany this disease. Marked splenomegaly causes a protrusion of the child's abdomen. In an attempt to compensate for the hematopoietic defect, the marrow becomes hyperplastic, the marrow space enlarges, and skeletal changes result. The most prominent example of this process is the characteristic "mongoloid" or "rodent-like" appearance of the child's facies. (See Fig. 35-12.) Growth retardation resulting from chronic anemia becomes apparent in later childhood.

A combination of the cardiac decompensation associated with anemia and the myocardial fibrosis caused by *hemosiderosis* produces cardiac failure in the older child. Hemosiderosis is an accumulation of the iron-containing substance *hemosiderin* which results from the phagocytic digestion of erythrocytes. This deposit of iron is an inevitable complication of frequent transfusions. The characteristic muddy yellow complexion seen in these children results from a combination of jaundice, hemosiderosis, and pallor.

Diagnosis The diagnosis of thalassemia major is usually suspected in a severely anemic child of Mediterranean extraction when the characteristic clinical finding and blood picture are considered. The characteristic blood picture is one of hypochromic, microcytic erythrocytes, which are distorted in shape, and numerous target cells and nucleated red blood cells. The diagnosis is confirmed by the child's electrophoretic pattern which reveals predominance

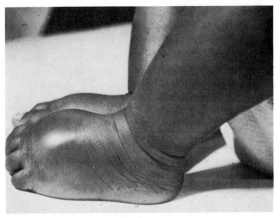

Figure 35-11 The appearance of the feet in the "hand-foot" syndrome in infants with sickle-cell disease. *(From A. M. Mauer, Pediatric Hematology, McGraw-Hill Book Company, New York, 1969, p. 94.)*

of fetal hemoglobin and small varying amounts of normal adult hemoglobin.

Treatment and prognosis There is no specific treatment for thalassemia. Frequent transfusions are required to maintain a functional hemoglobin level. If the child's spleen begins to sequester red cells abnormally and the demands for transfusion are increased, a splenectomy may be indicated. The

Figure 35-12 The characteristic facies of a child with thalassemia major. *(From A. M. Mauer, Pediatric Hematology, McGraw-Hill Book Company, New York, 1969, p. 137.)*

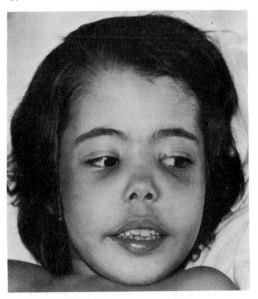

incidence of postsplenectomy infections is high in these patients, and prophylactic antibiotic therapy is often used.

The child's prognosis depends on the severity of the disease. Some patients do relatively well with few transfusions. Others require transfusions with increasing frequency. If the child lives to adolescence, his disease may become less severe. Most children succumb to complications of anemia, infection, or frequent transfusion before adolescence.

HEMATOLOGIC DEVIATIONS AND DISEASES IN THE TODDLER
Hemophilia

Pathogenesis Hemophilia is an inherited coagulation disorder. The most common forms of the disease, classic hemophilia (hemophilia A, or factor VIII deficiency) and Christmas disease (hemophilia B, or factor IX deficiency), account for 95 percent of the hemophilias, with classic hemophilia accounting for 84 percent of the total.

Classic hemophilia and Christmas disease are transmitted in a sex-linked recessive manner, generally from an asymptomatic carrier mother to an affected son. Affected children are unable to produce sufficient amounts of the coagulation factor involved. Children with less than 1 percent of the plasma factor are considered severe hemophiliacs. Children with 1 to 5 percent or more of the factor may have a mild to moderate form of hemophilia. These children may be free of spontaneous bleeding and require replacement therapy only with surgery or trauma. Figure 35-4 depicts the role of antihemophilic factors in blood coagulation.

Clinical Manifestations The disease is characterized by recurrent episodes of hemorrhage. The bleeding may be spontaneous or caused by slight injury. The specific manifestations depend on the area involved. Certain types of bleeding are characteristic of particular age groups. In infancy, prolonged hemorrhage may occur following circumcision or immunization. As the child progresses to the toddler state and experiences frequent falls, bleeding into soft tissues and from mucous membranes becomes more common. Injuries of the nose and mouth cause most of these bleeding episodes.

The school-age child with severe hemophilia must cope with the most debilitating complication of the disease, *hemarthrosis*, or bleeding into a joint. The child may first notice pain, tenderness, and limitation of motion. As bleeding progresses, the joint may become swollen and warm. Muscle spasms and

changes in soft tissue structure occur, resulting in the formation of flexion contractures. Recurrence of bleeding causes further degenerative changes which may lead to permanent fixation of the joint.

Hematuria and gastrointestinal bleeding are more common in the adolescent. School-age children and adolescents may experience frequent episodes of epistaxis. Fortunately, bleeding within the central nervous system is a rare complication.

Diagnosis A history of congenital bleeding disorder in a male child which appears in other maternal male relatives will lead the physician to a diagnosis of a coagulation disorder. A number of coagulation studies including screening tests and specific factor assays can be done to determine which clotting factor is deficient. An essential part of the diagnosis is the establishment of the severity of the disorder, which is related to the level of the affected factor.

Treatment Protection from injury is an important aspect of treatment. With infants, the crib and playpen may be padded. When the child begins to walk, his environment should be as free of hazards as possible. Removal of large, hard toys and sharp pieces of furniture such as end tables provides a much safer area for him to explore.

When bleeding episodes occur, local and systemic measures are employed to arrest the process. Local measures may include application of ice bags and pressure to the affected area. When the site of bleeding is accessible, the area may be packed with hemostatic agents. The child should be at complete rest with the affected part immobilized. Joints should be elevated and supported in a slightly flexed position.

Plasma replacement therapy should be started immediately. Infusion of fresh plasma or concentrates of the deficient factor will raise the plasma factor level sufficiently to allow hemostasis. Use of cryoprecipitate is often the treatment of choice. It is a relatively inexpensive concentrate, and it is easily prepared from fresh plasma. Hemarthroses may require continuation of replacement therapy for 3 to 4 days.

When bleeding into a joint has been controlled, active range of motion to the level of pain should be instituted. Motion of the joint facilitates absorption of the blood and may prevent contracture of the tissues. Cautious ambulation may begin in 48 hours. Surgical management of the affected joint may be necessary. Aspiration of residual blood under sterile conditions and application of traction with splints and casts are two of the orthopedic approaches used.

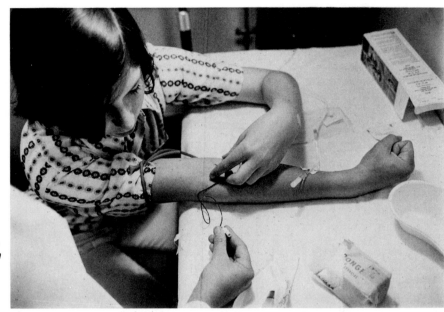

Figure 35-13   A child administering his cryoprecipitate. *(From Elaine Sergis and Margaret W. Hilgartner, "Hemophilia," American Journal of Nursing, 72(11):2020, 1972.)*

The cost and inconvenience of frequent infusions have promoted the development of home management programs. In these programs, patients and their families are taught to administer their own infusions. The goals of the program are prompt effective control of bleeding episodes and greater independence of the patient from the hospital and the health care team.

Patients soon learn to recognize the earliest symptoms of bleeding. Home care programs allow them to institute therapy minutes after they are aware of bleeding. Early institution of therapy permits earlier control of bleeding, fewer complications, and less interruption of normal activity. In some cases where the disease is severe and frequent transfusions are required to control bleeding, the patients are placed on prophylactic infusion programs. They are instructed to administer therapy routinely two to three times a week. The goal of this approach is maintenance of adequate levels of the clotting factor and prevention of bleeding. The prophylactic approach may be used to eliminate the risk of bleeding when the patient is participating in aggressive rehabilitative physical therapy programs and must be able to engage in active exercise. Some institutions report that children as young as 5 and 6 years of age are administering their own cryoprecipitate. (See Fig. 35-13.)

The team approach to treatment of hemophilia is essential. Ideally the team should consist of the child and his family, a pediatrician, a hematologist, an orthopedist, a dentist, a physical therapist, a psychologist, a social worker, and a nurse. Coordination of the efforts of all members of the team should provide smooth, comprehensive management of this complex disease and afford the patient the opportunity to function as a healthy, independent individual.

Nursing Management   The child's functional ability may vary considerably from time to time. During bleeding episodes he may be in extreme pain, and any movement may cause more pain and possibly more bleeding. When the bleeding has been controlled, his range of motion can be established by trial and error. Anemia caused by blood loss may decrease his activity tolerance. The nursing assessment should define the amount and kind of activity and exercise the child can tolerate and what assistance those caring for him should supply.

An assessment of the child's environment should be made to identify hazardous objects. Removing toys from the path of an unsteady toddler may prevent unnecessary falls.

Success in a home transfusion program is dependent upon the family's attitude. The nurse is often in the best position to assess the family's readiness to approach this endeavor. By allowing the parent to assume increasing amounts of responsibility in caring for the hospitalized child and observing his reaction to this responsibility, the nurse can evaluate the parent-child interaction and adjustment to the situation. If the child is an out-patient, the nurse may delegate to the parent some of the preliminary procedures of the transfusion, such as preparing the area with alcohol and applying the tourniquet.

As the family becomes more involved in the home transfusion program, more instruction and support will be needed. The nurse should anticipate repeating instructions several times and should convey acceptance of the parents' fears and hesitancies. The family must be alerted to notify some member of the medical team if any questions or unexpected complications arise. It is advisable to provide the family with a pamphlet explaining in detail the transfusion procedure, the indications for transfusion, and the complications.

The young child who may not be familiar with the hospital may be frightened by the strange new environment. He may be in pain or frightened by a bleeding episode. His parents' fear and anxiety are easily communicated to him. Supporting the child's parents and making it possible for them to remain with the child is an essential nursing function at this time. The first objective may be to prepare for and administer the infusion as soon as possible, but the nurse should never be too rushed to explain what he and the other members of the team are doing to the child. If restraints are necessary, they should be explained, and the child should be made as comfortable as possible.

Optimal positioning is essential. During a bleeding episode, the child should be at rest and comfortable with the site of bleeding immobilized. The child can tell the nurse how he will be most comfortable and direct those moving him accordingly. When bleeding is controlled and mobilization has begun, the child may need considerable encouragement and positive reinforcement for his efforts. He may hesitate to move for fear of increasing his pain. The nurse should *never* forcefully move a joint.

The process of accepting hemophilia as a chronic illness is a complex one for the child and his family. The genetic aspects of the disease have obvious implications. Many mothers experience feelings of guilt and resentment. Fathers and siblings resent the child's limitations. The constant threat of hemorrhage interferes with many family activities and stands between the child and his peers who are able to lead active lives. Sergis suggests that maternal overprotection may be a component in the development of two-behavior patterns commonly seen in hemophiliac children: passive-dependence and risk-taking.[2] A fine balance between meeting the child's needs for protection from injury and allowing inde-

pendence must be established. Many families who have worked together in home infusion programs have profited from discussing these problems among themselves. Fortunately, these programs have afforded the hemophiliac and his family a degree of independence from the hospital that was never possible before.

HEMOPOIETIC DEVIATIONS AND DISEASES IN THE PRESCHOOLER
Leukemia

Pathogenesis Leukemia is a malignancy of unknown etiology affecting the blood-forming organs. The disease is characterized by a replacement of the normal marrow elements with abnormal accumulations of leukocytes and their precursors. The classification of the disease refers to the type of white blood cell which is predominant in the bone marrow and peripheral blood. Approximately 90 percent of the cases of childhood leukemia are classified as acute lymphocytic or lymphoblastic leukemia (ALL). The majority of the remaining cases are acute myelocytic or myeloblastic leukemia (AML). Myeloblastic leukemia is less responsive to therapy, and the patients suffering from it have a graver prognosis than do those with ALL. When the cell type found is very immature and cannot be differentiated into the lymphocytic or myelocytic series, the term *stem cell leukemia* may be used.

Clinical Manifestations The most common signs and symptoms of leukemia include fever, abdominal and bone pain, anorexia, lethargy, pallor, hepatosplenomegaly, lymphadenopathy, malaise, petechiae, and ecchymoses. These findings may be present at the time of diagnosis and may recur periodically as the disease progresses.

The clinical features may be related to the disease process itself or to the therapy used. Those related to the disease fall into four main categories. *Anemia* results from erythropoietic failure and from blood loss. The complications of anemia experienced by the child with leukemia are similar to those discussed in the infancy section earlier in this chapter.

The leukemic patient's white blood cells are generally immature or abnormal and provide inadequate resistance to *infection*. Localized infections such as oral and rectal ulcers are often the cause of pain and loss of function. The threat of developing an overwhelming viral, fungal, or bacterial infection is always present. These systemic infections are the cause of death in 60 to 80 percent of the children with leukemia.

Hemorrhage is usually the result of an insufficient number of platelets. There appears to be a synergistic relation between thrombocytopenia and infection. Occasionally a child with a low platelet count may not manifest signs of bleeding until he develops an infection. In most cases thrombocytopenia alone may account for the bleeding.

Leukemic invasion of any organ system in the body can result in alteration or failure of that organ system. The central nervous system is a common site of leukemic infiltration. Symptoms associated with this complication include headache, vomiting, visual changes, and convulsions. When meningeal infiltration occurs, the child may experience pain with flexion of the neck. Infiltration of the lungs, kidneys, and bones may also occur.

The clinical features related to the therapy are as significant as those related to the disease itself. The problem of infection is accentuated by (1) myelosuppression, a suppression of the cellular elements of the marrow, (2) depressed immunologic function caused by chemotherapy, and (3) superinfection caused by antibiotic therapy. Antibiotic therapy destroys normal flora as well as pathogenic organisms. When this occurs, other pathogenic organisms which were previously controlled by the normal flora are able to grow, and superinfection develops. When therapy is instituted and large numbers of cells are rapidly destroyed, *hyperuricemia* may result. If there is crystallization of the uric acid and obstruction of the renal tubules, renal function may be impaired. Hyperuricemia can be effectively controlled with increased fluid intake and administration of allopurinol.

Clinical Course   The untreated disease progresses rapidly, with death occurring within weeks to months after diagnosis. However, the introduction of chemotherapy in 1947 has drastically changed this prognosis for most leukemic patients. Utilization of chemotherapeutic agents enables greater than 90 percent of children with newly diagnosed cases of ALL to achieve an initial *remission*. When the disease is diagnosed, chemotherapy removes the abnormal cells, allowing the normal marrow elements to return. The appearance of less than 5 percent abnormal cells in the peripheral blood and bone marrow is considered a remission. Increasing numbers of children are being maintained in their initial remission states in excess of 5 years. These children have received chemotherapy for 2 to 3 years, then treatment was discontinued with no recurrence of disease.

If the child's leukemic cells become resistant to the drugs being used, the abnormal cells return and a *bone marrow relapse* occurs. Appearance of abnormal cells in the spinal fluid, an indication of central nervous system invasion, is termed a *central nervous system relapse*. CNS relapses are frequently followed by bone marrow relapses. The duration of remissions is variable. There is a tendency for successive remissions to become increasingly shorter. A child may experience several remissions and recurrent relapses before he succumbs to complications of the disease.

Diagnosis   The diagnosis of leukemia is established by a stained smear of peripheral blood and bone marrow aspirate which reveals the typical picture of replacement of normal marrow elements with abnormal cells. The child's course is followed closely with frequent (usually weekly) evaluations of his peripheral blood. The policy for reexamining the child's bone marrow at specific time intervals varies from one institution to another. The aspirate is most often taken from the posterior iliac crest or the lower thoracic or lumbar vertebral spinous processes. Tibial aspirations are performed on children under 2 years of age. Sterile surgical technique is used. The skin is washed well with an iodine solution and alcohol, and the area is draped with sterile towels. Local anesthesia may be used. The aspiration can be done rapidly if the child is immobile. He will experience pain when the periosteum is penetrated and when the marrow is aspirated. The nurse has an important role in assisting the patient during a marrow aspiration. He must prepare the patient by explaining the procedure to him. Children are often most concerned with the position they will have to assume and the number of injections that will be necessary. They often tolerate the procedure with greater ease when they are permitted to remain in a sitting position. They must understand that it is essential for them to be still and that someone will help them remain still by holding them in the correct position. The nurse must convey to the child acceptance of his expression of fear and anger. Providing a means of talking about the experience through play, storytelling, or role playing may be helpful (see Fig. 35-14).

Treatment   The goal of therapy is eradication of leukemia cells and restoration of normal marrow function. The drugs included in Table 35-6 can be used in a variety of combinations to induce and maintain a remission. Side effects of chemotherapy are experienced by all children, but the severity of these side effects varies from one child to another.

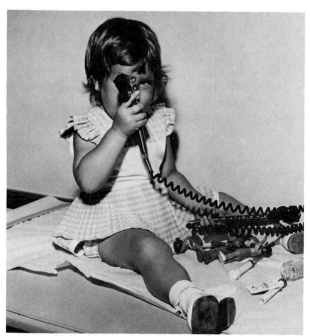

Figure 35-14 A child using play as a means of exploring traumatic hospital procedures.

Those most often encountered include appetite fluctuations, alopecia, development of cushingoid features, nausea, vomiting, myelosuppression, infection, and mucous membrane ulceration.

Supportive therapy is essential during periods of bone marrow inbalance. Early recognition of infection and prompt institution of appropriate measures can be life-saving. Antibiotics are used aggressively to combat the infectious process. Transfusion is used to counteract the complications of anemia and thrombocytopenia. Packed red blood cells are generally transfused in place of whole blood to avoid volume overload. The use of platelet concentrations is a relatively new procedure which has helped to control the hemorrhagic manifestations of thrombocytopenia. The nursing responsibilities related to transfusion are discussed in the infancy section of this chapter. Other measures used to combat complications of leukopenia include protective isolation, placement in a germ-free laminar air-flow unit,[3] and administration of white blood cell transfusions. Treatment of central nervous system leukemia includes irradiation of the cranium and possibly the spinal axis and intrathecal administration of chemotherapy. The high incidence of CNS involvement and the resulting bone marrow relapses have prompted physicians in many centers to incorporate a prophylactic course of therapy into their treatment protocols. Children receive CNS treatment soon after their first remission is established. Inclusion of this course of prophylactic therapy has resulted in a significant lengthening of remissions. Side effects of the CNS therapy include alopecia and possible marked anorexia, nausea and vomiting, headache, and hyperpigmentation of the skin in the radiation port.

Nursing Management A child with leukemia can experience extreme changes in his state of wellbeing within a short period of time. At the time of diagnosis he may be asymptomatic or have a few minor complaints, or he may be critically ill. When therapy is begun, the disease process may be reversed with surprising rapidity. As the disease progresses, the child may or may not experience severe toxicity to the drugs used. The potential for leukemic infiltration of any organ system in the body is always present. The nursing assessment must be extensive to determine the effects these factors have on the child's functional level. Frequent reassessments are necessary to detect changes in the patient's needs.

The nurse should examine the patient several times each day for early signs and symptoms of infection. He should inspect the child's mouth and skin for signs of infection such as redness, swelling, drainage, and tissue warmth. Any evidence of infection should be reported to the physician at once.

Certain problems are common in childhood leukemia and should be considered when planning for nursing care. All families are faced with the task of understanding and adjusting to a chronic, fatal illness. The nursing implications of this aspect of the disease are discussed in Chapter 29.

Normal eating patterns are often interrupted by fluctuations of appetite and mechanical difficulties with chewing and swallowing. One of the side effects of steroids is a marked increase in appetite. The child and his family generally welcome this change from his previous anorectic state. When the steroids are discontinued, his appetite tapers off rapidly before it returns to pre-illness levels. Some children maintain a poor appetite throughout their illness owing to the disease and/or side effects of medications.

When the child is experiencing a loss of appetite, a behavior modification approach may be helpful. All too often the child's hesitation to eat becomes a focus of the entire family's attention. If attention is paid to the child's attempts to eat and he is ignored when he refuses to eat, he may respond to the positive reinforcement and make a greater effort to eat. High-caloric preparations which are available commercially provide an excellent means of supplying daily requirements. Some preparations are available in pleasant fruit flavors and supply as much as 295 calories per 4 fl oz.

A pleasant environment can encourage the anorectic child to eat. Eating in a group, either with the family at home or with other children in the hospital, may be desirable. Preparing the child and his family for changes in appetite may reduce their anxiety about this phenomenon. Oral intake of food has long been associated with well-being and survival. Family members who have not adjusted to the implications of the illness feel helpless and frustrated. The child's refusal to eat accentuates these feelings of helplessness, particularly for the mother who may identify providing nourishment as an essential part of her role.

Painful mouth ulcers or infections of the oral cavity may prevent the child from chewing or swallowing. Ulcers may be caused by medications. Children taking methotrexate frequently develop lesions of the oral and gastrointestinal mucosa. Infection of these lesions with enteric gram-negative organisms is not uncommon. The lesions may become necrotic, and large portions of tissue may be sloughed. Other common lesions are oral candidiasis and gingivitis. When thrombocytopenia and hemorrhage develop, there may be oozing from the gums. The child is discouraged from eating by the pain and unpleasant taste in his mouth (see Fig. 35-15). When oral lesions are present, soft foods and cold foods may be tolerated better.

The nurse must accurately assess the patient's oral hygiene and make an appropriate plan for mouth care. Several approaches are possible. A soft-bristled toothbrush should be used. If lesions are neither extensive nor painful, the child can continue to use a toothbrush but should avoid brushing the lesion. When brushing is contraindicated, rinsing the mouth with a mouthwash/water solution may be substituted. This solution should be applied to the teeth with a cotton-tipped applicator and the debris rinsed with water if possible. If the mouth is severely affected and the mouthwash will not be tolerated, rinsing with water will be of some help. The child may specify the water temperature he desires. A dilute solution of hydrogen peroxide and water may be swabbed on the teeth with a cotton-tipped applicator occasionally, but it should not be used frequently. The use of regular rinsing is much more desirable to prevent the crusting and caking of debris. When oral lesions are present, the use of

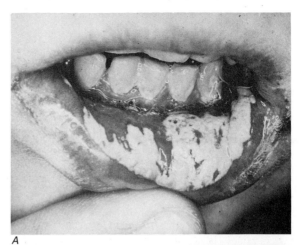

A

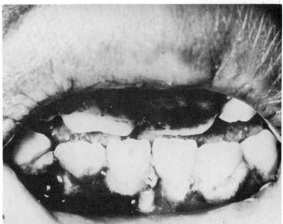

B

Figure 35-15 Oral lesions seen in children with leukemia. (A) Oral candidiasis or thrush. (From W. T. Hughes and S. Feldman, "Infections in Children with Leukemia," Hospital Medicine, 8(12):68–69, 1972.) (B) Bleeding of the gums.

straws and other sharp eating utensils should be avoided.

When possible, the anorectic child should be allowed to participate in the selection of his diet. He will, of course, need supervision, but allowing him some form of control may stimulate his interest in eating.

Many children develop constipation while taking vincristine. If the child is very ill, the measures which facilitate normal bowel function such as exercise and intake of foods high in bulk may not be realistic. It is important that the child maintain an adequate fluid intake. Laxatives are generally administered routinely if constipation develops. The doctor should be notified if there is any indication that a child taking vincristine is becoming constipated, as this is

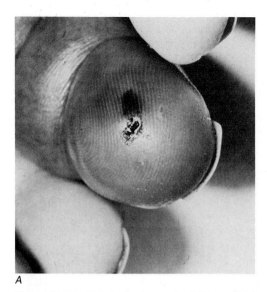
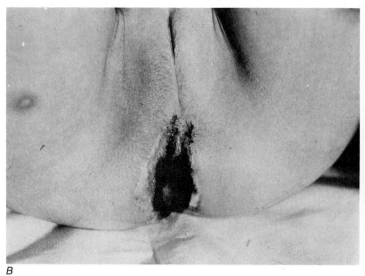

A   *B*

Figure 35-16   Skin lesions seen in children with leukemia. *(A)* Cellulitis resulting from a finger puncture. *(From W. T. Hughes and S. Feldman, "Infections in Children with Leukemia," Hospital Medicine, 8(12):68–69, 1972.) (B)* A perianal lesion in a child with pseudomonas sepsis.

often the first sign of neurotoxicity to the drug. An alteration of the dosage of the drug may be necessary.

The development of rectal ulcers is not uncommon. They may result from mucosal damage by chemotherapy or infection, particularly with pseudomonas organisms. The ulcers may begin as small tender erythematous areas and progress to large necrotic lesions (see Fig. 35-16*A* and *B*). It is important to examine the neutropenic child's perirectal area routinely for any early signs of these lesions. If antibiotic therapy is started immediately, the infectious process may be controlled. The policy at many institutions is to avoid taking rectal temperatures on leukemic patients to prevent possible trauma to the gastrointestinal mucosa. The perianal area should be washed well with pHisoHex and water to remove any feces or urine. It is not advisable to apply ointments to the area if skin breakdown has occurred, as these agents tend to trap bacterial organisms. Positioning the child so that there is no pressure on the lesion and applying a heat lamp four times a day may promote healing.

Thrombocytopenic bleeding is a frequently encountered complication. The child may have numerous ecchymoses and petechiae which can appear in any area of the body. Bleeding into soft tissue provides an excellent medium for infection. Efforts must be made to prevent bleeding, so protecting the child from injuries is essential. Intramuscular injections are avoided during this period of time.

Physical changes in appearance are inevitable for the child with leukemia. Some changes are related to the side effects of medications; others are caused by the weight loss and wasting of chronic illness. It is important for the nurse to prepare the child and his family for these changes and assist them in coping with their feelings as they arise. Young children may cope with their feelings through play and story-telling. The nurse should facilitate play activities for the child and take advantage of opportunities to communicate with him through play. Older children, who are concerned about hair loss, may be interested in selecting and wearing a wig or cap. Many mothers of young children are more concerned about these changes than the child himself. They may be embarrassed by comments made by friends and strangers and feel guilty about their reactions. Reassuring the family that these feelings are shared by other parents and that the nurse understands and accepts their feelings is most helpful.

During periods of exacerbation of the disease the child is often irritable and in pain. Those caring for him should be sure to move him gently. Bone and soft tissue involvement may make any sudden movement painful. Careful positioning can relieve tension on these areas. Providing a quiet, pleasant environment may promote comfort and rest. The nurse should support the family members and enable them to remain with the child as much as possible. Fear of separation from parents is of major concern to the pre-school-age child.

If the child is able to participate in diversional activities, he may enjoy selecting the activities in which he is most interested. The nurse should take advantage of every opportunity to allow the child to control his environment. It is important to avoid exposing him to activities he will be unable to accomplish.

When the disease is controlled, the child may return to normal activities. His family should be encouraged to treat him as a normal child when possible. It is difficult for parents to discipline and make demands of a child who has a potentially terminal illness, but the child will feel most secure in an atmosphere that approaches the one with which he was familiar before he became ill. The nurse may be in contact with persons in the community who will be involved with the child as he returns to normal activities. Teachers and ministers are frequently in close contact with the child. They often have fears and misconceptions about the illness which the nurse can dispel.

Implementation of an appropriate nursing care plan should be a joint effort of the child, his family, and the nurse. The family should be allowed to participate in the care and to assume as much responsibility as they are comfortable with. Suggesting specific tasks that the mother can do may reduce her feelings of helplessness and anxiety.

The nursing plan should include provisions for meeting the nurse's needs. There should be adequate opportunity for the nurse to explore his feelings about death with members of the staff who are able to offer support. Nurses' feelings of helplessness may be reduced by the development of a structured nursing care plan which specifies concrete solutions to nursing problems.

The availability of effective chemotherapy and supportive therapy has made the return to normal activity a reality for the child with leukemia. Deviations from normal are always a threat to the child. In many situations, such as drug toxicity, the cause of the deviation can be eliminated. The nurse's role in the management of the illness is to detect these deviations and initiate appropriate measures aimed at eliminating the cause.

HEMOPOIETIC DEVIATIONS AND DISEASES IN THE SCHOOL-AGE CHILD
Aplastic Anemia

Pathogenesis Aplastic anemia is a disease of the bone marrow characterized by a profound depression of the production of the formed elements of the blood—red blood cells, white blood cells, and platelets. This disease may be congenital or acquired. Fanconi's anemia is the eponym given to the congenital form of the disease. Abnormalities of the skeletal and renal structures, the central nervous system, and skin pigmentation are associated with the syndrome.

Approximately half the cases of acquired aplastic anemia are related to drug, radiation, or chemical exposure. Chloramphenicol, sulfonamides, phenylbutazone, DDT, benzene, radiation, and chemotherapeutic drugs are considered to be possible etiologic agents. The remaining cases of acquired aplastic anemia are of idiopathic origin.

Clinical Manifestations The clinical features of the disease are related to the marrow depression. They closely resemble the complications of myelosuppression seen in the leukemic patient. Hemorrhagic manifestations of thrombocytopenia are often the first signs of the disease. Severe anemia and bacterial infections subsequently develop. If acute episodes of infection and bleeding can be controlled, approximately one-half of the children will respond to therapy. Most of the children who fail to respond die of these complications within 6 to 15 months of diagnosis. When a patient responds to therapy, the progressive course of improvement may take from several months to several years. The first sign of improvement is an increase in the production of red cells. Next, the white count increases and returns to normal. Platelets are the last cells to respond, and thrombocytopenia may persist for several months.

Treatment A first step in controlling the disease is recognition and removal of any toxic agent with which the child is in contact. Essential supportive measures include transfusion of packed cells and platelet-rich concentrations and administration of appropriate antibiotics.

The drug therapy used is a combination of corticosteroids, usually prednisone, and androgens—hormones which stimulate the development of male secondary sex characteristics. This drug combination is continued for a prolonged period of time. Response to therapy may not be evident for 2 to 4 months.

Bone marrow transplantation has been tried as a therapeutic measure. At the present time unrelated donor transplants are not successful because of complications of graft rejection. When transplantation is done, multiple marrow aspirations are taken from the donor under general anesthesia. The patient receives the marrow by intravenous infusion.

Nursing Management Many of the complications of anemia, infection, and bleeding seen in the child with leukemia are also seen in the child with aplastic anemia. He is irritable, weak, listless, and anorectic. His normal patterns of eating and elimination may be interrupted by painful oral and rectal lesions. Hemorrhagic and infectious lesions may appear on any part of his body. Many of the skin care, mouth care, and comfort measures described above for the care of the child with leukemia can be used. The school-age child may wish to assume more responsibility for making decisions about and carrying out his own care than the younger child. The nurse should assess the child's ability and desire to participate in his own care and offer assistance when it is appropriate to do so.

The task of adjusting to aplastic anemia is complicated by the uncertainty of the prognosis. During the first few months of the illness it cannot be determined if the child will respond to therapy or fail to respond and die of complications. The child and his family anxiously await the results of each blood test. This uncertainty reinforces the feelings of denial experienced by many family members who are accepting a chronic fatal illness. It is important to avoid unrealistically encouraging the family. The greatest harm in denying the possibility of eventual death is that the child and his family may not feel free to discuss their feelings of fear and anger in an atmosphere of unquestionable hope.

When bone marrow transfusions are to be part of the therapy, parent or sibling donors are preferred. All potential donors are typed for compatibility. This event can create a number of stressful situations. Incompatible family members as well as compatible donors may blame themselves for treatment failure. Parents are faced with another difficult decision. Many express hesitation to subject a well sibling to the trauma of marrow extraction in the face of possible treatment failure.

In addition to the side effects of corticosteroid therapy discussed in the leukemia section of this chapter, the child must cope with masculinizing effects of androgen therapy. This task is particularly difficult for girls. Physical changes most frequently encountered include increased growth of facial and body hair, deepening of the voice, flushing of the skin, and development of acne. The school-age child is often self-conscious about these changes. It is essential that he be warned that they will develop and reassured that they will disappear when the medication is discontinued. When the child returns to school and association with peers, he must cope with their curiosity. It may be helpful for the nurse to contact the child's teacher. Explaining the physical changes and complications of the disease and therapy may allay the teacher's fears and correct misconceptions.

The Purpuras

The group of disorders known as the purpuras is characterized by bleeding into the skin. Bleeding from mucous membranes and other organs and tissues may also occur. Purpuras can be classified as nonthrombocytopenic (normal platelet count) or thrombocytopenic (a reduced number of platelets). Nonthrombocytopenic bleeding is related to a defect of small vessel or platelet function. Anaphylactoid purpura, or Henoch-Schönlein syndrome, is the most common nonthrombocytopenic purpura. The syndrome is an acute allergic response of unknown cause characterized by a confluent purpuric rash involving the lower extremities and the buttocks, pain and swelling of the joints, abdominal pain, and renal involvement.

Idiopathic thrombocytopenic purpura is the most common of the thrombocytopenic purpuras of childhood. The disease is characterized by a reduction in the number of platelets, usually to less than 40,000/cu mm, with resultant bleeding into the skin, mucous membranes, and subcutaneous tissues.

Idiopathic Thrombocytopenic Purpura

Clinical manifestations A majority of the cases are acute and self-limiting. The onset of the disease is sudden and often follows a viral infection. With these cases, a spontaneous remission will occur. The length of time from diagnosis to remission varies from a few weeks to 1 year. Most children recover within the first 6 weeks. Approximately 10 percent of the children develop a chronic form of the disease, but most of these eventually recover.

The most common hemorrhagic manifestations are petechial and ecchymotic lesions of the skin and bleeding from the nose, oral mucosa, gastrointestinal tract, kidneys, and vagina. Rarely, intracranial hemorrhage may occur.

Treatment Transfusions of fresh blood and platelet concentrates may be administered to replace and control blood loss. Corticosteroid therapy is often employed to reduce the severity of the hemorrhagic manifestations and hasten the remission of the disease. If thrombocytopenia persists beyond 6 months, a splenectomy may be performed. Approximately 85 percent of children with chronic cases of the disease will recover after splenectomy.

Nursing management During periods of active bleeding the child should be observed closely for signs and symptoms of shock and intracranial hemorrhage. Bleeding is frightening for the child and his family. The nurse should reassure them that the blood loss can be controlled with transfusions. It may be helpful to remind them that the large, numerous bruises on the child's body are not painful. Epistaxis may be persistent and troublesome. When routine compression and packing measures are not successful at controlling the bleeding, the nose may be packed with a hemostatic substance or a small wedge of salt pork.

Protection from injury is important during periods of thrombocytopenia. Slight falls may precipitate hemorrhage into internal organs. The child may return to school, but he should avoid body contact sports. It is generally advisable that he not participate in physical education.

Spleen Trauma and Splenectomy

Pathogenesis Traumatic laceration to the spleen, causing intraperitoneal hemorrhage, is the most common reason for splenectomy in childhood. Occurrence increases with age, as the child's involvement in sports and more adventuresome play increases. A blunt blow to the abdomen can occur in auto accidents, fights, falls from trees or playground equipment, contact sports, and sledding accidents. The blow may produce symptoms and perhaps other injuries, such as bruises and bone fractures. Often, though, the injury is mild, with no external signs, and almost overlooked until symptoms develop.

Clinical Manifestations Abdominal pain and tenderness in the upper left quadrant is accompanied by nausea and vomiting. Pain in the left shoulder may occur. Additional symptoms are those of blood loss: increased pulse, perspiration, pallor, falling blood pressure. A slowly falling hemoglobin may be indicative if splenic trauma is not readily diagnosed. The spleen may be enlarged and palpable as a mass in the left upper quadrant.

A peritoneal tap will produce blood, but a negative tap does not mean laceration is not present. Abdominal and chest x-rays will assist in differential diagnosis. A serum amylase test will be high in pancreatitis (which produces similar symptoms) but normal in lacerated spleen.

Nursing Management Preoperative preparation for splenectomy depends largely on the illness of the child and on the urgency of the situation. The most important measure is evaluation of the child's condition, to which perceptive nursing observations may contribute greatly. Blood transfusions may be necessary to stabilize the condition of the child with splenic laceration. The child may have other injuries which must be considered in preparation for surgery. Platelets and fresh whole blood can be used during surgery performed for idiopathic thrombocytopenic purpura to maximize hemostasis. Gastric compression is the other measure required preoperatively.

Regardless of the reason for the surgery, it is usually simple and without complications. The postoperative course follows closely that of uncomplicated appendectomy.

Although not confirmed by immunologic studies, many clinical studies show a high incidence of serious, overwhelming infection in the 2 years after splenectomy. Infants, in particular, are susceptible to septicemia, meningitis, and meningococcemia, but children are also most predisposed to infection. When infections do occur, the mortality rate is higher than might be expected.

HEMATOLOGIC DEVIATIONS AND DISORDERS IN THE ADOLESCENT
Hodgkin's Disease

Pathogenesis Hodgkin's disease is a malignancy of the lymphoid system characterized by the occurrence of solid tumors in the lymph nodes; they may appear in many nodes in distant areas of the body. A variety of histologic patterns of malignant cells can be identified, but the occurrence of a unique type of cell, termed a *Reed-Sternberg* cell, is considered by most pathologists to be essential for the diagnosis of Hodgkin's disease.

Though the disease is uncommon in childhood, it may occur in children between the ages of 4 and 12 years. There is a significant increase in the number of cases in children 11 years of age, with the peak incidence occurring between 15 and 29 years of age.

Clinical Manifestations The manifestations of the disease are generally related to lymph node enlargement. The nodes are characteristically painless, firm, and movable in the surrounding tissue. The most serious complication of node enlargement is tracheobronchial compression and subsequent airway obstruction when the mediastinum is involved. Compression of the esophagus may inhibit swallowing.

Infiltration of nonlymphoid organs is rare, but when it occurs, specific complications related to the organ system result. Systemic reactions including fever, pruritis, rash, night sweats, anorexia, lethargy, weakness, and general malaise are common.

Anergy, a diminished sensitivity to specified antigens, accompanies the disease, particularly in the later stages. Infection is a major complication of this phenomenon. Viral, bacterial, and fungal infections may be widely disseminated and overwhelming.

Diagnosis and Treatment Accurate treatment is dependent upon an accurate diagnostic evaluation of the disease. A surgical biopsy of an affected node is done to determine the type of cell which is involved. A lymphangiogram may be done to detect metastatic nodal involvement. Using local anesthesia, a radiopaque contrast material is injected into a lymphatic vessel on the dorsum of the foot. Nodal enlargement and architecture can be visualized on x-ray. If abdominal involvement is suspected, an exploratory laparotomy and splenectomy may be done. Multiple biopsies are done at the time of surgery. A staging system is used to classify the extent of the disease. The following criteria are commonly used for staging Hodgkin's disease.[4]

Stage I	Disease limited to a single lymph node group with the exclusion of the mediastinum and abdomen.
Stage II	Disease in one or more lymph node groups, contiguous or noncontiguous but limited by the diaphragm to either the upper or lower half of the body.
Stage III	Disease above and below the diaphragm with involvement limited to lymph nodes, the spleen, or Waldeyer's Ring.
Stage IV	Systemic involvement of organs other than those listed above (bone marrow, lungs, kidneys, liver, gastrointestinal tract, and central nervous system).

A classification of *A* (no symptoms) or *B* (symptomatic) refers to the absence or presence of systemic symptoms described above.

Generally, patients with more advanced stages of the disease receive more aggressive therapy and have a graver prognosis. Standard therapy programs include radiation and chemotherapy. Prednisone, vincristine, cyclophosphamide, procarbazine, and nitrogen mustard are chemotherapeutic agents commonly used. This therapy regime can cause the side effects discussed earlier, such as appetite fluctuations, peripheral neuropathy, constipation, alopecia, cystitis, nausea and vomiting, and bone marrow suppression (see Table 35-6.)

The mean survival time after diagnosis is between 2 and 3 years. Children with stage I disease at the time of diagnosis have a significant chance of living more than 5 years.

Nursing management Caring for an adolescent with a chronic and potentially fatal illness is a difficult task for many nurses. The adolescent is used to assuming the responsibility of planning his activities and caring for himself. With Hodgkin's disease he must cope with the limitations of the disease itself as well as the toxicities of the therapy. Many of his previous activities are too strenuous. The side effects of therapy impose embarrassing changes of appearance on his already rapidly changing body. A major developmental task of adolescence is establishment of emotional and physical independence. The limitations of the disease force the adolescent to rely on family members and medical and nursing personnel for assistance with basic activities of daily living. The task of facing this change of life style and possible death force him to turn to others for emotional support as well. The nurse is frequently uncomfortable in this situation. The patient's hesitancy to ask for help is often met with the nurse's hesitancy to offer help.

It is more difficult to talk about illness and death with the adolescent. Though he may have a realistic understanding of death, his family may feel the need to protect him from the truth to prevent him from worrying.

It is usually most helpful if the nurse conveys to the adolescent a willingness to talk about his illness if he wishes to do so. He will feel more secure if his questions are answered honestly and directly.

When possible, the adolescent can plan activities around his therapy schedule. Many patients receiving therapy in the morning can expect a few hours of nausea and vomiting immediately following the treatment but will recover by afternoon. If chemotherapy is given on the same day each week, he can leave that day free in his schedule in anticipation of side effects.

At the time of diagnosis the adolescent should be approached in a direct, open manner. The diagnostic procedures such as the biopsy, lymphangiogram, and exploratory laparotomy may be much less stressful if he knows what to expect.

It is wise to encourage the adolescent to take part in his care as much as possible. If he is experiencing night sweats, it may be advisable to supply him with a change of bed clothes at night so that if he awakens with moist clothing, he can solve the problem himself and not have to call the nurse for assistance.

Table 35-6 DRUGS USED IN THE TREATMENT OF ACUTE LEUKEMIA

Drugs/category	Method of administration	Mechanism of action	Side effects/toxicity
Prednisone: adrenocorticosteroid	Oral	Influences transcription of messenger RNA to protein synthesis	Increased appetite, weight gain, fluid retention, striation, immunosuppression, growth arrest, psychosis, hypertension
	I.V.; infiltration causes necrosis of tissue; verify patency of vein *before* infusion	Mitotic arrest	Nausea, alopecia, constipation, adynamic ileus, neurotoxicity, myelosuppression
6-Mercaptopurine (Purinethol): antimetabolite, purine antagonist	Oral	Blocks purine synthesis	Nausea, vomiting, myelosuppression, mucous membrane ulceration
Methotrexate: antimetabolite, folic acid antagonist	Oral or I.V.; infiltration causes blistering and tissue necrosis; verify patency of vein *before* infusion	Blocks purine and pyrimidine synthesis	Nausea, vomiting, myelosuppression, mucous membrane ulceration, hepatotoxicity
Cytosine arabinoside (Cytosar): antimetabolite, pyrimidine antagonist	I.V.; anticipate severe nausea and vomiting during or soon after infusion	Inhibits DNA synthesis	Severe nausea and vomiting, myelosuppression, mucous membrane ulceration, alopecia
Cyclophosphamide (Cytoxan): alkylating agent	Oral or I.V.; patient should be well hydrated at time of administration and for 48 hr to decrease side effects of cystitis	Reacts with essential intracellular functional groups	Alopecia, nausea, vomiting, dizziness, myelosuppression, cystitis
Daunomycin: antibiotic	I.V.	Blocks RNA production	Myelosuppression, cardiotoxicity
L-Asparaginase: enzyme	I.V.; observe closely for signs of hypersensitivity; emergency equipment should always be available	Destroys the supply of asparagine available to neoplastic cells	Nausea, vomiting, lethargy, somnolence, fever, hypersensitivity, hepatotoxicity, hypoalbuminemia, coagulopathy
Allopurinol: xanthine-oxidase inhibitor	Oral	Blocks formation of uric acid, an end product of oncolysis	Inhibits the degradation and inactivation of 6-mercaptopurine

Source: Adapted from Kjell Koch et al., "Chemotherapy in Childhood Malignancies," *Journal of the Florida Medical Association*, 58(11):25, 1971.

Infectious Mononucleosis

Pathogenesis Infectious mononucleosis is an acute infectious disease now thought to be caused by a member of the herpesvirus group called *EB virus*. Epidemiologic observations suggest that the organism is transmitted with oral contact and exchange of saliva rather than casual exposure. The incubation period is between 4 and 14 days. Though the disease may occur in children of any age, it is rarely seen in infants. The age of peak incidence is between 17 and 25 years.

Diagnosis and Clinical Manifestations Examination of the peripheral blood reveals an increase in the number of lymphocytes and the appearance of an atypical form of lymphocyte. Clinical symptoms, which may develop insidiously, include fever, sore throat, malaise, headache, fatigue, and lethargy. Lymph node enlargement and splenomegaly are common. Symptoms may last for 2 weeks.

Complications are uncommon, but those reported include hepatitis, rupture of the spleen, secondary infection, and involvement of other organs.

Treatment The disease is self-limiting, and no specific therapy has been shown to be effective in controlling the uncomplicated disease process. Symptomatic relief of pain with analgesics and fever with antipyretics is indicated. Bed rest during the acute febrile stage of the disease is advised. The patient's activity should be governed by his fatigability. He should be observed closely for evidence of superinfection, so that appropriate antibiotics may be administered.

Nursing Management An important goal of nursing care is to make the patient as comfortable as possible. Coordination of feedings and administration of analgesics may make it easier for the patient with a sore throat to swallow and help him rest more comfortably after eating. Maintenance of an adequate fluid intake is often difficult. The patient is uncomfortable, irritable, and not eager to swallow. Cool, bland fluids which are often best tolerated may not be available to the college-age patient recovering in a dormitory room. If student volunteers are available, it is advisable to have someone visit the patient as often as possible to replenish his supply of liquids.

The adolescent is often involved in numerous school and extracurricular activities. The nurse may help him rest more comfortably by assisting him in making necessary arrangements to continue his activities in bed or to return to them when he recovers.

REFERENCES

1 S. B. Korones, *High-Risk Newborn Infants*, The C. V. Mosby Company, St. Louis, 1972, pp. 171–172; G. B. Odell, "Postnatal Care," in R. E. Cooke (ed.), *The Biologic Basis of Pediatric Practice*, McGraw-Hill Book Company, New York, 1968, p. 1502.
2 Elaine Sergis and Margaret W. Hilgartner, "Hemophilia," *American Journal of Nursing*, 72(11):2013, 1972.
3 Charlotte Isler, "The Cancer Nurses: How the Specialists Are Doing It," *RN*, 35(2):28–37, 1972.
4 C. B. Pratt, "Management of Malignant Solid Tumors in Children," *Pediatric Clinics of North America*, 19(4): 1141–1155, 1972.

BIBLIOGRAPHY

Babson, G. S.: *Management of the High-Risk Pregnancy and Intensive Care of the Neonate*, The C. V. Mosby Company, St. Louis, 1971.
Barnes, A. C.: *Intra-uterine Development*, Lea & Febiger, Philadelphia, 1968.
Crosby, Marion H.: "Control Systems and Children with Lymphoblastic Leukemia," *Nursing Clinics of North America*, 6(3):407–413, 1971.
Feldman, Doneta B., Sell, Elsa J., Gray, J. K., and Lazzara, A.: *Manual of Newborn Care of Grady Memorial Hospital*, Emory University, Atlanta, 1972 (unpublished).
Foster, Sue: "Sickle Cell Anemia: Closing the Gap between Theory and Therapy," *American Journal of Nursing*, 71(10):1952–1956, 1971.
Harper, P. A.: *Preventive Pediatrics*, Appleton-Century-Crofts, Inc., New York, 1962.
Herrmann, Judith, and Light, I. J.: "Infection Control in the Newborn Nursery," *Nursing Clinics of North America*, 6(1):55–65, 1971.
Hughes, W. T., and Feldman, S.: "Infections in Children with Leukemia," *Hospital Medicine*, 8(12):67–75, 1972.
Isler, Charlotte: "Care of the Pediatric Patient with Leukemia," *RN*, 35(4):30–35, 1972.
Koch, Kjell, Bloom, G. E., and Wolfson, S. L.: "Chemotherapy in Childhood Malignancies," *Journal of the Florida Medical Association*, 58(11):24–35, 1971.
Lazerson, J.: "The Prophylactic Approach to Hemophilia A," *Hospital Practice*, 6:99–109, 1971.
Leifer, Gloria: *Principles and Techniques in Pediatric Nursing*, 2d ed., W. B. Saunders Company, Philadelphia, 1972.
Lucey, J. F.: "Neonatal Jaundice and Phototherapy," *Pediatric Clinics of North America*, 19(4):827–839, 1972.
Marlow, Dorothy R.: *Textbook of Pediatric Nursing*, W. B. Saunders Company, Philadelphia, 1969.
Mauer, A. M.: *Pediatric Hematology*, McGraw-Hill Book Company, New York, 1969.
Mengel, C. E., Frei III, E., and Machman, R.: *Hematology: Principles and Practice*, Year Book Medical Publishers, Inc., Chicago, 1972.
Nelson, W. E., Vaughn III, V. C., and McKay, R. J.: *Textbook of Pediatrics*, 9th ed., W. B. Saunders Company, Philadelphia, 1969.

Pierog, Sophie H., and Ferrara, A.: *Approach to Medical Care of the Sick Newborn*, The C. V. Mosby Company, St. Louis, 1971.

Pochedly, C.: "Sickle Cell Anemia: Recognition and Management," *American Journal of Nursing*, 71(10):1948–1951, 1971.

Reed, Barbara, Sutarius, Janet, and Coen, R.: "Management of the Infant during Labor, Delivery and the Immediate Neonatal Period," *Nursing Clinics of North America*, 6(1):3–14, 1971.

Roach, Lora B.: "Assessment: Color Changes in Dark Skin," *Nursing '72*, 2(11):19–22, 1972.

Segal, S.: "Oxygen: Too Much, Too Little," *Nursing Clinics of North America*, 6(1):39–53, 1971.

Smith, C. H.: *Blood Diseases of Infancy and Childhood*, 3d ed., The C. V. Mosby Company, St. Louis, 1972.

Van Eys, Jan: "Home Management of Hemophilia A," *Journal of the Tennessee Medical Association*, 64(5): 407–410, 1971.

Whipple, Dorothy V.: *Dynamics of Development: Euthenic Pediatrics*, McGraw-Hill Book Company, New York, 1966.

White, Dorothy Wats: "Living with Hemophilia," *Nursing Outlook*, 12:36–39, 1964.

THE GASTRO-INTESTINAL SYSTEM

ROSE MARY SHANNON

The gastrointestinal system (the digestive tract or the alimentary canal) has the major function of moving food through the body. The process features *digestion* (the chemical and physical breakdown of foods into simpler molecular units), *absorption* (the passage of digested foods into the circulatory system), and *elimination* (the passage out of the body of undigested and undigestable material). The liver, spleen, and pancreas serve more varied functions.

EMBRYOLOGY OF THE GASTROINTESTINAL SYSTEM

During the third week of gestation, the cephalic, caudal, and lateral folds incorporate the dorsal part of the yolk sac into the embryo, forming the primitive gut. This gut is divided into three parts: the foregut, the midgut, and the hindgut. Blood is supplied by three branches of the dorsal aorta: the celiac, the superior mesenteric, and the inferior mesenteric arteries.

Foregut

The derivatives of the foregut include (1) the pharynx and its structures, (2) the lower respiratory tract, (3) the esophagus, (4) the stomach, (5) the duodenum as far as the point of entrance of the common bile duct, (6) the liver and the pancreas, and (7) the biliary apparatus.

The *esophagus* and the trachea become separate partitions of the embryonic tracheoesophageal septum very early. The very short esophagus elongates rapidly, reaching its final length by 7 weeks. Its endoderm proliferates almost to the point of obliterating the lumen. Recanalization then occurs. Striated muscle of the esophagus is innervated by the vagus nerves, while its smooth muscle is supplied by a visceral plexus.

The *stomach* initially appears as a fusiform dilatation of the caudal part of the foregut which soon enlarges and broadens ventrodorsally. Since the dorsal border grows faster than the ventral section, it produces the greater curvature. As the stomach acquires its adult shape, it rotates 90° in a clockwise direction around its longitudinal axis, acquiring its adult position, with the lesser curvature on the right, the greater curvature on the left. The rotation results in a blood supply from the left vagus nerve to the anterior stomach wall and from the right vagus nerve to the posterior wall. It is suspended from the dorsal wall of the abdominal cavity by the dorsal mesentery or dorsal mesogastrium. As the embryo lengthens, the caudal part of the septum transversum thins and becomes the ventral mesentery or ventral mesogastrium, attaching the stomach and duodenum to the ventral wall of the abdominal cavity.

Isolated clefts develop between the cells of the dorsal mesogastrium and coalesce to form a single cavity, the *lesser peritoneal sac.* It lies dorsal to the stomach and to the right of the esophagus. As growth continues, the cranial end is cut off by the diaphragm. Then, the lesser sac communicates with the main peritoneal cavity (or greater peritoneal sac) through a small opening, the *epiploic foramen* or the *foramen of Winslow.*

The caudal part of the foregut and the most cephalic part of the midgut grow rapidly and form a C-shaped loop that projects ventrally, the *duodenum.* The junction of the two is at the apex of the duodenal loop. Since it is derived from both the foregut and the midgut, the duodenum is supplied by branches of the celiac and superior mesenteric arteries. The lumen of the duodenum is obliterated by epithelial growth but is recanalized in the second month.

The *liver* and *biliary apparatus* arise as a bud from the most caudal part of the foregut. The largest cranial part becomes the liver, a small caudal portion expands to form the *gallbladder.* Proliferating endodermal cells give rise to interfacing cords of liver cells and to the epithelial lining of the intrahepatic portion of the biliary apparatus. As the liver cords penetrate the septum transversum, they break up the umbilical and vitelline veins, forming the hepatic sinusoids. The fibrous and hemopoietic tissue and Kupffer cells of the liver are derived from the splanchnic mesenchyme. The right and left lobes begin equal in size, but the right lobe becomes much larger. During the sixth week, hemopoiesis begins, giving the liver a bright red appearance and causing the large size of the fetal liver.

The *extrahepatic biliary apparatus* is first occluded and then recanalized as it grows. The stalk of the gallbladder becomes the *cystic duct,* while the stalk connecting the hepatic and cystic ducts to the duodenum becomes the *common bile duct.* Initial attachment is ventral until the duodenum rotates so that the entrance of the common bile duct is on the dorsal wall of the duodenum. Bile pigment begins to form during the thirteenth to sixteenth weeks and enters the duodenum, giving its contents (meconium) a dark green color.

The ventral mesentery, a thin membrane, gives rise to (1) the *lesser omentum,* passing from the lower to the ventral border of the stomach (gastrohepatic ligament) and from the liver to the duodenum (duodenohepatic ligament), (2) the *falciform ligament* extending from the liver to the anterior abdominal wall, through which the umbilical vein passes, and (3) the *visceral peritoneum* of the liver, which covers the liver except for the crown-shaped area in direct contact with the diaphragm.

The *pancreas* develops from dorsal and ventral pancreatic buds in the most caudal part of the foregut. The dorsal bud is larger, appears first, and grows into the dorsal mesentery, forming the main bulk of the pancreas. The ventral bud begins near the duodenum and is carried dorsally to fuse with the dorsal bud when the duodenum rotates, forming the inferior head of the pancreas. The main pancreatic duct develops from an anastomosis of the ducts of both buds. The endoderm forms a network of tubules; acini develop at the ends of these tubules. Islets of Langerhans develop from groups of cells which separate from the tubules and begin to secrete insulin at about 20 weeks.

The *spleen* develops its characteristic shape early from a mass of mesenchymal cells between layers of dorsal mesogastrium. As the stomach rotates, the left surface of the mesogastrium fuses with the peritoneum over the left kidney. The mesenchymal cells differentiate, forming the capsule, connective tissue framework, and the parenchyme of the spleen. It is a hemopoietic organ in fetal life and continues lymphocyte and monocyte production through life.

Midgut

The derivatives are (1) the small intestines except the duodenum to the point of the common bile duct entrance, (2) the cecum and appendix, (3) the ascending colon, and (4) the proximal part of the transverse colon. The blood supply is from the superior mesenteric artery.

Herniation, rotation, return, further rotation, and fixation of the midgut occur during its development. As the midgut elongates, it forms a ventral V-shaped intestinal loop which "herniates" into the umbilical cord as a result of a shortage of space in the abdomen due to the large fetal liver and kidneys. Within the umbilical cord, the midgut loop rotates 90° counterclockwise around the axis of the superior mesenteric artery. During the tenth week, the intestines return rapidly to the abdomen, undergoing a *further* 180°-counterclockwise rotation, for a total of 270°, placing the bowel in its permanent position.

The midgut loop has two limbs, a *proximal*

limb, which forms intestine, and a *distal limb,* which undergoes little change except for the development of the cecal diverticulum. Lengthening of the proximal part of the colon gives rise to the *hepatic flexure* and *ascending colon.* As the intestines assume final position, the mesentery of the ascending colon fuses with the parietal peritoneum and disappears, making it retroperitoneal. The other intestinal divisions retain their mesenteries attached from the duodenojejunal junction downward to the ileocecal junction. The duodenum and the head of the pancreas also become retroperitoneal.

The cecal diverticulum, a conical pouch on the distal limb, appears in the fifth week. The distal end of this blind sac forms the *appendix.* As the colon elongates, the cecum and the appendix descend and become fixed in position, with variation in the position of the appendix.

Hindgut

The derivatives of this area are (1) the distal part of the transverse colon, (2) the descending colon, (3) the sigmoid colon, (4) the rectum, (5) the upper portion of the anal canal, and (6) part of the urogenital system. The hindgut is supplied by the inferior mesenteric artery. The change in blood supply from the superior (supplying the midgut) to the inferior indicates the junction between the segment of the transverse colon derived from the midgut and the segment derived from the hindgut. The descending colon becomes retroperitoneal when its mesentery fuses with the peritoneum of the left dorsal abdominal wall and disappears. The hindgut extends from the midgut to the cloacal membrane, which is composed of endoderm of the cloaca and ectoderm of the anal pit (or proctoderm).

The urorectal septum across the cloaca develops caudal extensions as it grows, which produce folds in the lateral walls of the cloaca. These folds fuse, dividing the cloaca into (1) the *rectum* and *upper anal canal* dorsally and (2) the urogenital sinus ventrally. Fusion of the urorectal septum and the cloacal membrane forms the anal membrane. Changes in the ectoderm around this membrane form a shallow pit, *the anal pit.* The anal membrane, at the bottom of the pit, ruptures at the seventh week, opening the anal canal and establishing communication between the gastrointestinal tract and the amniotic sac. The anal canal is derived from the hindgut (upper two-thirds) and the anal pit (lower one-third). Arterial blood supply, lymphatic and venous drainage, and the nerve supply differ for the two parts, delineated at the pectinate line (the site of the fetal anal membrane).

PHYSIOLOGY OF THE GASTROINTESTINAL SYSTEM

The *esophagus* lies posterior to the trachea and heart and extends from the pharynx to the stomach, piercing the diaphragm in its descent from the thoracic to the abdominal cavities. It is a collapsible tube whose only function is to allow passage of food and fluids from the oropharynx to the stomach.

The *stomach* lies in the upper left quadrant of the abdomen. The cardiac sphincter muscle functions at the entrance to the stomach, and the pyloric sphincter muscle controls the opening into the duodenum. Its mucous lining is arranged in temporary longitudinal folds called *rugae,* which allow for distention. Numerous microscopic tubular glands are embedded in the gastric mucosa. Those glands that line the body and fundus secrete most of the gastric juice, which is composed of mucus, enzymes, and hydrochloric acid. The surface epithelial cells secrete mucus, while parietal cells secrete hydrochloric acid, and chief cells secrete the enzymes.

The stomach (1) serves as a reservoir for food until it can be partially digested and moved on, (2) secretes gastric juice, (3) secretes an unknown "intrinsic factor," necessary for the absorption of vitamin B_{12}, (4) by contractions of its muscular coat, churns food into small particles and moves it into the duodenum, and (5) carries on a limited amount of absorption of some water, alcohol, and some drugs.

The inner mucosa of the *small intestine* lies in permanent circular folds, (valvulae conniventes) from which extend inward, microscopic fingerlike projections (villi). These villi greatly increase the surface available for digestion and absorption. Beneath the surface lie microscopic glands of Lieberkühn, which secrete digestive enzymes, and, in the duodenum, Brunner's glands, which secrete mucus. The intestines also contain clusters of lymph nodes (Peyer's patches) and numerous single lymph nodes (known as *solitary nodes*), where the absorbed nutients enter the lymphatic circulation.

The three main functions of the small intestine are (1) completion of the digestion of foods, (2) absorption of the end products of digestion into the blood and lymph, and (3) secretion of hormones which help to control the secretion of pancreatic juice, bile, and intestinal juice.

Glands and solitary nodes are located in the submucosal layers of the *large intestine.* Small sacs (haustra) give the mucosal wall a puckered appearance. The main functions are absorption of water, an undetermined part in absorption of fats, and elimination of wastes.

The *liver* is a vital organ and the largest gland in the body. Its functions include secreting bile (a pint a day), which facilitates digestion and absorption of fat and removal of some waste products, and metabolizing all three food types. In carbohydrate metabolism the liver carries on the processes of glycogenesis, glycogenolysis, and gluconeogenesis, all essential in the homeostasis of blood sugar. Liver cells also carry out fat catabolism. Liver cells perform an essential function in protein anabolism by synthesizing blood proteins—prothrombin, fibrinogen, albumins, and many globulins—which are important in blood clotting, water balance, and maintenance of normal blood pressure and circulation.

The *gallbladder* stores and concentrates bile which enters the hepatic and cystic ducts. During digestion, the gallbladder contracts, ejecting the concentrated bile into the duodenum.

The *pancreas* (1) secretes the digestive enzymes found in pancreatic juice, (2) from beta cells secretes insulin, the hormone with major control over carbohydrate metabolism, and (3) from alpha cells secretes glucagon which is important in carbohydrate metabolism.

Two kinds of digestive changes, *mechanical* and *chemical,* are necessary for absorption to occur. Mechanical digestive changes are those that change the physical state of foods to minutely dissolved particles, propel them forward in the digestive tract, and facilitate absorption. *Mastication,* which occurs in the mouth, breaks up food and mixes it with saliva. The movement of food out of the mouth into the pharynx, esophagus, and stomach is termed *deglutition* or swallowing. Deglutition occurs in three stages. Firstly, a ground, rolled bolus of food soaked with saliva is directed to the back of the mouth by the tongue and forced into the pharynx. Secondly, the bolus is directed by reflex control into the esophagus. The tongue prevents it from reentering the mouth. Automatic raising of the soft palate bars it from the nasal passages. The muscles of the pharyngotympanic tubes prevent entrance to the middle ear and pharynx. Elevation of the larynx and movements of the arytenoid cartilages protect the trachea. Thirdly, stimulation of the esophageal mucosa by the food bolus initiates the reflex of esophageal peristalsis, which moves the food into the stomach.

Emptying of the stomach requires between 1 and 4 hours for the average meal. As small amounts of gastric contents become liquefied, very small amounts are ejected about every 20 seconds into the duodenum until a certain amount accumulates. Emptying of the stomach is controlled by an enterogastric reflex. Fats and sugars in the intestine stimulate the mucosa to release enterogastrone into the blood which inhibits gastric peristalsis. Proteins and acids initiate reflex emptying of the stomach, stimulating vagal nerve receptors in the intestinal mucosa.

Churning occurs in the stomach, the small intestine, and the haustra of the large intestine. This process mixes food and digestive juices thoroughly, bringing all food in contact with the mucosa. Peristalsis in the stomach and the entire length of the intestine propels the contents along.

Mass peristalsis begins in the descending colon, moving the remaining intestinal contents into the sigmoid colon and rectum. Emptying of the rectum, *defecation,* is a reflex action brought about by stimulation of receptors in the rectal mucosa by distention, along with the complex interaction of colonic peristalsis, action of the anal sphincters, and voluntary straining.

Changes in the *chemical composition* of food result from hydrolysis. Enzymes present in the digestive juices catalyze the hydrolysis.

Carbohydrate digestion varies according to the complexity of the compound, since carbohydrates are saccharides. Polysaccharides, starches, contain many saccharide groups and must be hydrolyzed to disaccharides by enzymes known as *amylases,* found in saliva (ptyalin) and pancreatic juice (amylopsin). Disaccharides are hydrolyzed to monosaccharides by sucrase, lactase, and maltase, found in intestinal juice (succus entericus). Monosaccharides (glucose, fructose, and galactose) are absorbed directly.

Protein digestion is facilitated by enzymes called *proteases* which catalyze the hydrolysis of the large protein molecule into intermediate compounds (proteoses and peptides) and then into amino acids. The main proteases are pepsin in gastric juice, trypsin in pancreatic juice, peptidases in intestinal juice.

Fat digestion must be facilitated by *emulsification* of the fats since they are insoluble in water. Bile emulsifies fats in the small intestine. The main fat-digesting enzyme is pancreatic lipase.

Vitamins, minerals, and water are absorbed in their original form. Residues of digestion (cellulose, undigested fats, and undigested connective tissue and toxins from meat proteins) resist digestion and are eliminated from the body.

Complicated reflex and chemical (hormonal)

mechanisms control the *flow of digestive juices* so that they are secreted when they are needed and in the needed amounts. Chemical, mechanical, olfactory, and visual stimuli initiate reflex secretion of saliva. Gastric secretion is initiated partly by the same reflex mechanism. The hormone gastrin, released by gastric mucosa in the presence of partially digested proteins, controls the gastric secretion, while enterogastrone mentioned before inhibits the secretion. Pancreatic secretion is controlled chemically by the hormones secretin and pancreozymin and by some reflex action. Secretin is released when hydrochloric acid, protein, and fat digestion products act on the duodenal mucosa and stimulate the pancreas. Pancreozymin stimulates enzyme production by the pancreas.

Secretin also stimulates the liver to secrete bile. The ejection of bile from the gallbladder is controlled by a hormone cholecystokinin, which is formed by the intestinal mucosa when fats are present in the duodenum.

Regulation of the secretion of intestinal juice is not fully understood. It is thought that hydrochloric acid and food products stimulate the intestinal mucosa to release a hormone enterocrinin into the blood, which stimulates intestinal secretion. Neural and reflex mechanisms also may play a part.

Absorption is a process which takes place by a passive component (of diffusion, filtration, and osmosis) and by an active transport mechanism not clearly understood. Carbohydrates (as monosaccharides) and proteins (as amino acids) are absorbed into the intestinal capillaries and enter the portal vein circulation. Fats, as glycerol and as fatty acids, and bile salts together in a water-soluble substance enter the lymphatic circulation.

PROCEDURES USED AS ADJUNCTS TO PRIMARY TREATMENT
Biopsies

Biopsies of the *mouth, esophagus,* and *stomach* are rarely necessary in children; however, they are obtained when degeneration of the area exists or when a neoplasm is suspected.

Liver biopsy is performed frequently in children when deterioration of liver tissue is suspected, as in biliary atresia, portal hypertension, and neoplasms of the liver. The child does not receive food or fluids immediately before the procedure, and he is usually given a sedative or analgesic. Immobilization is imperative for a safe, successful procedure, but it may be difficult to achieve in the young child. Older children usually co-

operate if the procedure is explained fully. The child may be asked especially to hold his breath at the time the needle is inserted. Manual immobilization of the abdomen must usually be done with infants or very small children. If all the equipment is prepared in advance, the nurse can concentrate on supporting or positioning the child.

In this procedure a subcostal or intracostal incision is made and a Silverman needle, a Roth-Turkel needle (sometimes with syringe suction), or a Menghini needle is inserted. A small tissue sample is then obtained for microscopic study. Hemorrhage, a most frequent and dangerous complication, can be avoided if the patient is properly restrained and if moderate pressure is applied for 5 to 10 minutes after the procedure has been completed.

Biopsy of the *small intestine* is seldom necessary unless it is done as part of an operative procedure to identify obscure enteropathies. A modified Crosby capsule, adapted for pediatric use, is best with children. The tube may be weighted with a mercury bag to facilitate insertion. A cooperative infant often initiates sucking when the tip of the tube is touched to his mouth and will swallow quickly. The child between 2 and 5 years, or an irritable, uncooperative infant, will need sedation before the capsule is passed. Children over 5 years can be given Nupercaine lozenges. The tube is advanced 5 to 10 cm beyond the stomach mark once the tube is in the stomach. After the child is placed on his right side, it may take 30 to 40 minutes for the tube to advance into the duodenum by peristalsis. It must be taped to the cheek securely when it is in place.

A Birmingham capsule or a multiple biopsy tube may be used instead. Most children are unable to swallow for a few hours afterward, necessitating positioning on the abdomen or side, possible nasopharyngeal suctioning, and close observation.

A *large intestine* biopsy is important in diagnosis and differentiation of ulcerative colitis, Crohn's disease, tumors, or Hirschsprung's disease. Except when performed during abdominal surgery, a lower intestinal biopsy is done through a sigmoidoscope. It can be done as a suction biopsy using the Crosby modified capsule or, most commonly, by (nonsuction) rectal biopsy (pinch) forceps. Occasionally, in diagnosis of Hirschsprung's disease, an open rectal examination, with biopsy, is performed under anesthesia. There may be some rectal bleeding following this procedure. Hemorrhage and perforation are rare. Nothing, including

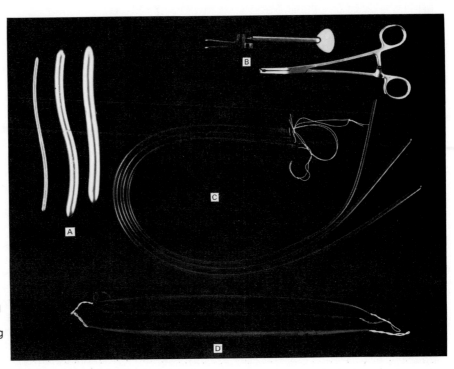

Figure 36-1 Instruments used in the treatment of esophageal and anal disease. (*A*) Hager dilator. (*B*) Gross spur-crushing clamp. (*C*) Mercury dilator. (*D*) Tucker dilator.

a thermometer, is inserted into the rectum for approximately three to five days.

A *rectal biopsy* is done with the child frequently under anesthesia and in lithotomy position. The mucosa is everted and mobilized, and a section of both layers of muscle is taken, using biopsy forceps. A closure with catgut sutures is made.

Dilations

The purpose of dilating either the *esophagus* or the *anus* is to prevent scar tissue contractions which form strictures or to stretch already contracted tissue. The esophagus may contain scar tissue at the anastomotic lines of a tracheoesophageal fistula repair and colon interposition. Scarring may be an aftermath of lye ingestion. The anus may require dilation because of stenotic or membranous imperforate anus or as a postsurgical procedure following a pull-through operation for an imperforate anus or Hirschsprung's disease.

Esophageal dilation is accomplished by using Tucker or mercury dilators. *Tucker dilators* (Fig. 36-1*D*), hard rubber tubes tapered at both ends, have nylon cord loops (about 20 in. long) attached to each tapered end. A gastrostomy must be present since a thin nylon cord is threaded through the nostril, toward the stomach, and the end leaves the stomach through the gastrostomy. The gastrostomy end of the nylon cord is knotted to the end entering the nostril, making a complete circle. During dilation, the knot is untied and the string at the nostril is tied to the well-lubricated dilator while a new length of string is tied to the other end. When the dilator is pulled down through the esophagus emerging through the gastrostomy, the new string remains in place. The ends are knotted as before, and the string is used for the next dilation. These dilations are done on a regular basis (every few days) for minor strictures until a large-sized dilator passes easily. The average size of the Tucker dilators used in pediatrics ranges from 8 to 36.

Mercury dilators (Fig. 36-1*C*) are long, nontapered rubber tubes weighted with mercury on the insertion end. They are used for dilation when no gastrostomy is present. In many cases, anesthesia is necessary to perform the procedure because of fear, uncooperativeness, discomfort, gagging, and coughing by the child. However, when support and assistance are given during these procedures, the patient may learn to swallow the tube with a minimum of fear and discomfort. The dilator is threaded down slowly and withdrawn immediately. This type of dilation may need to be carried out for long periods of time, especially after severe lye burns of the esophagus. The child is able to eat soon after these procedures.

Hager dilators (Fig. 36-1A), used for anal dilation, are smooth, conical metal instruments, varying from size 2 to 32. The ends are rounded, with each end a different size so that the dilator increases in diameter as it is inserted. Efforts should be made during the procedure to prevent tension and subsequent tightening of the anus by the child. The dilator is warmed and lubricated. When in position, it is held in place for a few minutes or longer. The next largest size is used when no resistance is encountered. This procedure may be necessary on a daily basis for up to 2 weeks postoperatively. It may be continued at home by finger dilation or with a wax candle of appropriate diameter. An alternative is to have the child return to the doctor for weekly or periodic dilations. Anal stenosis following pull-through surgery may reoccur, in complicated cases, 1 to 2 years after surgery, requiring short courses of dilator or manual dilation.

Endoscopy

Esophagoscopy is a diagnostic aid and a treatment tool. Esophagoscopy is necessary diagnostically to determine the extent of esophageal varices and in treatment to sclerose the varices. The procedure is used to determine the extent of scarring after surgery or lye ingestion and the presence of stenosis or esophagitis. Dilation with mercury dilators for scarring and stricture can be done through an esophagoscope. Since the procedure is done under general anesthesia, preoperatively the child is given nothing by mouth for 6 to 8 hours and medicated accordingly. Usually a normal diet is resumed after the child has recovered from anesthesia.

Proctoscopy and *sigmoidoscopy* are used as diagnostic aids in some diseases of the bowel such as Hirschsprung's disease or rectal polyps. Repeated examinations may be necessary in evaluating treatment, as with patients with ulcerative colitis.

The instruments used are rigid hollow tubes with illumination within the unit. Adult sizes are used with larger children, while the size used for infants is only 14 cm in length. A flexible sigmoidoscope is used for viewing beyond the rectum. Biopsy and excision of rectal polyps can be done with this instrument. The knee-chest position is desired, although the infant may be placed on his back with his thighs abducted to his flanks. The

nurse holding him should stand at his head. Efforts are directed at relaxing the child to make the procedure less painful and visualization successful. An older child needs a complete explanation of what is to be done. Most children do not need analgesics. Bowel preparation is avoided because it may cause mucosal changes, negating the diagnostic value of the examination. The discomfort disappears as soon as the procedure is over, and the child returns to his previous activity and diet.

Gastric Intubation

A nasogastric tube may be necessary in order to instill medication or feedings; remove gastric contents; obtain gastric secretions for diagnostic tests; remove amniotic fluid in the neonate; and for preoperative and postoperative decompression.

A polyetheylene French catheter of the smallest diameter which will function for the purpose is preferred; however, a straight rubber French catheter may be used. A double-lumen tube has proved to be the least irritating to mucosa. Measurement for insertion orally or nasally is the same: the length from the tip of the child's nose to the earlobe and down to the xiphoid process. This length can be marked on the tube by tape or indelible marking pen. The tip is lubricated with lubricating jelly before insertion. Oily substances should not be used because of the danger of oil aspiration. Inserting the tube is smoother if the tube is rolled into a tight circle, which allows the plastic material to follow the natural contour of the oro- or nasopharynx into the stomach. As the tube is gently but steadily threaded, there should be no resistance; however, the child will experience gagging. Swallowing water may help the older child pass the tube more easily. Difficult passage, resistance, choking, coughing, or color change are indications for withdrawing the tube for reinsertion.

Escape of air via the tube as it reaches the stomach is not heard with the small-lumen tubes used for infants. The placement of the tube can be tested by aspirating stomach contents (which are replaced) or by instilling 1 to 3 cc (ml) of air with a syringe into the tube as the nurse listens with a stethoscope for the air rushing into the stomach. Parents may be taught to put the open end of the tube under water, which will produce constant air bubbles when the tube is misplaced in the respiratory tract.

If the tube is to remain in place, it should be taped *flat* as it leaves the naris. Under *no* circumstances should the tube be pulled up and against the tip of the naris or against nasal mucosa where it will cause irritation and tissue breakdown. Narrow adhesive tape fits around the tube and across the cheeks in one strip, thereby preventing the tube from slipping out of place. It should be changed frequently, every 2 to 5 days.

Gavage feeding is an important procedure in supplying adequate nutrition to infants too small and to any child too ill to tolerate oral feedings. Infants with respiratory distress, cardiac anomalies, or nasopharyngeal anomalies may need tube feedings. On occasion, the fluid given for nutrition is objectionable in taste to a child (such as an elemental diet fluid) or must be given in a constant flow via drip or a feeding pump (as for severe malnutrition or burns). Oral insertion of the tube for feeding causes less irritation, less chance of aspiration, and less adverse gag reflex. Preparation should always include a recheck of tube position, aspiration of stomach contents and replacement, and aspiration of air from tubing. Often, for premature babies, the amount of aspirate retained in the stomach from the previous feeding is subtracted from the amount to be given, avoiding distention of the stomach. The feeding should be given slowly. It is ideal to hold the baby and allow him to suck on a pacifier, thereby simulating a normal feeding so that he does not lose the satisfaction of bottle feedings. If he cannot be held, he should be positioned on his side or abdomen with his head slightly elevated. He will need to be burped during and after the feeding.

Flushing the tube with sterile water after a feeding makes it cleaner, patent, and a poorer medium for bacterial growth. Oral and nasal hygiene are necessary preventatives against upper respiratory and ear infections.

When *gastric lavage* is utilized to remove undesirable materials from the stomach, the child is positioned on his side with his head low in anticipation of vomiting. Insertion of a *nasogastric tube before surgery* prevents vomiting and decompresses the intestine, making it easier to handle during surgery. Immediately following surgery, there is no peristalsis, and bowel function is static. Therefore *postoperative decompression* is necessary to prevent abdominal distention caused by swallowed air and gastric and intestinal secretions. Abdominal distention elevates the diaphragm, placing tension on abdominal and intestinal wounds and creating unnecessary complications. If the tube is blocked, the child may vomit and aspirate. Maintaining tube patency is a nursing responsibility; it is irrigated with a specified amount of saline solution every 2 hours. The nurse must check for position, flow, and contents returned and note unusual fluctuation in the amounts for each measured period of time (for example, between irrigations).

Drainage may be accomplished by attaching the tube to intermittent machine suction, gravity drainage, or in-the-bed level drainage. Continual suction will damage stomach mucosa, and it is never used. The tube should not be clamped unless ordered by the doctor for specific periods to test the child's tolerance. These nasogastric tubes are removed when bowel function returns. Some indicators are passage of stool, flatus, and diminished amounts of fluid drained.

Gastrointestinal Fluid Replacement

Diarrhea and vomiting, primary clinical manifestations of gastrointestinal disease, lead directly and commonly to states of dehydration and electrolyte imbalance. Intraabdominal surgery complicates these problems. In addition to a malfunction caused by an abnormality within the gastrointestinal tract itself, increased loss of water and electrolytes may occur following anorexia, starvation, poor or improper feeding practices, malabsorption due to a systemic disease, or the administration of chemicals or medications for other reasons. Vomiting and diarrhea are common to conditions such as infectious diarrhea, diabetic ketosis, adrenal crisis, infections, and disturbances of the mucosa of the intestine.

Since gastrointestinal intake and output of water account for a large exchange of water, its loss and the subsequent dehydration is rapid. When oral intake is inadequate to balance the loss, further dehydration results. Body water loss in an infant is more rapid than in an older child. In the presence of diarrhea, fluid requirement may be as much as three times the normal daily requirement. Symptoms occur when there is acute loss of 5 percent of the body weight as water. It is considered severe at 10 percent, with peripheral vascular collapse occurring at 15 percent. A fatal level is 20 percent. It may take 36 to 48 hours to reverse dehydration, and the volume administered is the sum of daily maintenance requirement plus dehydration factor.

The degree of imbalance is dependent upon the composition of the gastrointestinal fluids being lost. Gastric fluid loss occurs through vomiting, gastric suction, or a fistula. Intestinal fluid loss happens in the presence of intestinal suction, fistula, ostomies, and diarrhea. The most common modes of loss must be accurately and adequately measured for purposes of monitoring and replacement. However, loss from fistulas is not measurable, and accurate estimation of severe vomiting is a difficult measurement. Fluid loss is replaced volume for volume.

All gastrointestinal losses, particularly those from diarrhea, contain moderate to large amounts of sodium. The large intestine reabsorbs water as well as salt as sodium and chloride and exchanges potassium and bicarbonate. The small intestine fluid (containing digestive secretions) is high in bicarbonate and sodium and relatively lower in chloride and potassium. Sodium loss is high in the presence of vomiting because gastric mucus contains high concentrations of sodium, and production of the mucus is stimulated by vomiting, adding to sodium loss.

Sodium replacement in parenteral fluid therapy is dependent upon the degree of sodium loss in comparison with water loss and the size of the patient, which will determine the speed with which the loss is replaced. Therapy aimed at correcting dehydration is planned on average deficits for water, sodium, and chloride. The degree of sodium loss in proportion to water loss can be determined by serum sodium, and will indicate the type of dehydration under treatment (isonatremic, hyponatremic, or hypernatremic). Water and electrolyte deficit are estimated as mild, moderate, or severe and are combined with maintenance therapy when given.

Potassium deficiency, as with sodium, may result from a greatly reduced intake as in fasting, due to the body's subsequent breakdown of body fat and protein. Diarrhea, particularly when prolonged, produces high potassium loss. Hypocalemia (decreased potassium) may cause, as well as be the result of, vomiting, creating a vicious circle. The administration of potassium after 24 hours of parenteral fluid therapy is a usual practice. Initially, during therapy for diarrhea and/or vomiting, it is not administered for the first 12 to 24 hours until urine excretion is established as normal.

Diarrhea is the foremost cause of water and electrolyte loss in pediatrics. There are three main physiologic disturbances in diarrhea: dehydration, imbalance in acid-base status with acidosis, and shock, which occurs when dehydration is severe enough to produce circulatory disturbances. The two important variables to be considered when initiating therapy are the volume of body fluids and their osmolality. Since the composition of intes-

tinal fluids resembles the composition of extracellular fluid, diarrheal dehydration is a loss of extracellular water and electrolytes, which gives rise to clinical signs of thirst, cold extremities, poor skin turgor, and loss of body weight. The latter is useful in assessing water loss and replacement for short periods of time. In addition, fluid replacement must include estimates of normal body needs and ongoing losses (such as continued diarrhea). Because the sodium content of the body and its accompanying chloride determines the distribution of body water, an increase or decrease in sodium in the plasma or serum reflects changes in the extracellular fluid. These proportions (or osmolarity of body fluids solute concentration) are important in determining the extent of dehydration and shock. In about two-thirds of diarrheal dehydration, loss of salt is in proportion to loss of water. When water loss is higher than sodium loss, *hypernatremic* dehydration results. This condition may be seen when any factor increases water loss (such as fever, hyperventilation, or dry hot environment). Very small and very young infants are especially likely to develop hypernatremic dehydration. In situations where water intake has been stopped suddenly while loss continues, this form of dehydration may develop.

A small number of patients may develop hyponatremic dehydration in diarrheal disease when the child is given sugar water, weak tea, or other fluid which contains no appreciable amounts of salt (electrolytes).

Potassium losses in diarrheal stool are great, and when diarrhea has been present over 24 hours they can be significant. Replacement is usually made on the basis of an average because deficits are hard to measure, even with a serum potassium blood level. Lowered calcium levels may occur in the presence of potassium loss.

The first phase of diarrheal therapy restores circulation by use of albumin, plasma, or blood, if shock is clinically evident. The second phase restores body fluids to an acceptable volume. The solution given always contains sodium and chloride. Additions of bicarbonate or other solutions, such as lactate solutions, depend on the complexity of the child's condition. This takes about 24 hours in isotonic dehydration, but it should be done over 48 hours in hypernatremic dehydration. Most often, in isotonic dehydration, the deficit may be restored in the first 6 to 8 hours. During the third phase, early recovery, parenteral fluid may be continued while oral electrolyte or a glucose solution with electrolytes is begun. Milk feedings, which increase stool frequency and volume, should not be given until the fourth phase, late recovery. Reintroduction of milk should be done slowly, in small amounts, and adjusted according to the presence of diarrhea.

Abnormal postoperative fluid losses usually occur through the gastrointestinal tract in the form of diarrhea or vomiting. Routines should include measurement of volume, electrolyte content studies, and simple tests using Labstix guaiac tablets and Clinitest tablets, when such losses are expected or are present, in order to plan for minimizing the effects of the losses.

Pediatric abdominal surgery includes complex conditions which interfere with or prevent postoperative oral alimentation or cause unpredictable gastrointestinal loss. Extensive resection of the gastrointestinal tract results in partial or complete failure of carbohydrate, fat, amino acid, water, electrolyte, vitamin, and mineral absorption, in varying degrees. Immediate postoperative attempts toward normal gastrointestinal function may be unsuccessful or fluctuate radically. Cautious introduction of formula, fluids, and foods and careful notation of any changes in bowel signs are essential nursing activities.

Disaccharidase deficiencies are common in infants and toddlers, necessitating a completely milk-free diet. Banana powder, soy products, or carbohydrate-free formulas are used. Fat intolerance is more of a problem in older age groups, and fat-controlled diets are indicated. In some cases, oral elemental liquid diets serve as a temporary bridge between hyperalimentation and a more normal oral diet. Nursing observations and assessments during this time are valuable in reestablishing a normal feeding pattern. The parents, especially the mother, must learn the diet peculiarities of the infant or child, normal daily food requirements which fit into the child's diet framework, signs of diet intolerance, and ways to control it. These children are subject to frequent, unexplained bouts of diarrhea and are supersensitive to common childhood gastrointestinal illnesses. Very recent studies have indicated that the effects of deficiencies resulting from the loss of portions of the gastrointestinal tract may be significant and may not be apparent until years later.

Multiple surgical procedures, such as are required in correction of extensive congenital anomalies of the gastrointestinal tract, put off resumption of normal function. Recovery after each operation is incomplete, resulting in an infant or a child who is unable to ingest or absorb sufficient nutrition. Intravenous therapy or hyperalimentation for a longer period than usual may be a necessary part of the postoperative management.

Peritonitis causes additional fluid and electrolyte loss (internal or "third-space" loss) which is particularly difficult to manage. An abnormal leak of plasma proteins into the abdominal cavity occurs because of the large inflamed peritoneal surface. Water and extracellular electrolytes are lost secondarily to this leak. Most patients show a mild to moderate respiratory alkalosis; thus sodium chloride rather than sodium bicarbonate should be used in replacement. If losses are severe, overt circulatory collapse may occur. Replacement is based on the amount of clinical dehydration, calculation of loss in relation to body weight, and careful monitoring of the circulatory status.

The most common cause of metabolic alkalosis in pediatrics is *protracted vomiting* of gastric juices, predominantly hydrochloric acid, as in pyloric stenosis. In addition to the hydrochloric acid there are small amounts of sodium and potassium in gastric juice, both as chloride salts. Loss of gastric juice causes a large loss of hydrogen and chloride and small losses of sodium and potassium, resulting in metabolic alkalosis and hypochloremia. However, infants who vomit from causes other than pyloric stenosis may have a blood pH which is alkaline, normal, or acid. When a child vomits with an open pylorus, the vomitus will be a mixture of gastric acid and alkaline small-intestinal fluids (pancreatic juice, succus entericus, and bile). It is possible that the concomitant loss of these two fluids will balance each other. When metabolic alkalosis does occur, further potassium and sodium losses result as the kidney responds in attempts to restore balance. These losses come from body stores, since, because of the vomiting, there is no replenishment from the diet. Changes in body composition occur which reflect the metabolic alkalosis, potassium depletion, and variable degrees of dehydration.

Body compensation to metabolic alkalosis is respiratory, but it is often unpredictable, irregular, or not present. It is important to rehydrate the infant, repair potassium depletion, and correct the alkalosis. Withholding oral feedings and eliminating vomiting will control the primary cause of alkalosis. Intravenous fluid therapy must include maintenance requirements and restoration of any fluid losses, chloride (to expand the fluid lost extracellularly), and potassium. It may take several days to prepare an infant with pyloric stenosis and resultant metabolic imbalance for surgery.

Hyperalimentation[1]

Central venous hyperalimentation provides protein and calorie intake sufficient to sustain life and to promote growth in the absence of adequate gastrointestinal tract function. In particular, it is used for children with congenital bowel anomalies, extensive burns, and intractable diarrhea. To be effective, the fluid must contain protein (amino acids in the form of protein hydrolysate), calories (generally as hypertonic dextrose solution), water to maintain hydration, vitamins, minerals, and electrolytes.

High concentration makes it extremely irritating to blood vessel walls. The silastic catheter through which the fluid is given must be placed into a vein large enough that sclerosis and thrombosis do not occur and blood flow is rapid, so that the solution is diluted before it enters peripheral circulation. The catheter is inserted through the jugular vein and threaded down to the superior vena cava at the level of the right atrium, in a surgical procedure. Occasionally, the brachial artery may be used. The catheter is secured subcutaneously by sutures at the insertion site, which may be on the chest, the neck, or immediately posterior to the ear.

An intravenous pump must be used at all times since the fluid will not drip by gravity through the filter at the slow rate required for small children and the possibility of blood backup and clotting in the silastic catheter is great. If necessary, it is possible to run the fluid without a pump in large, older children. The pump must be one which provides a continuously closed system. A micropore filter specific for this use must be placed between the end of the silastic line and the intravenous tubing, to filter out bacteria and harmful materials. Medications given through the filter tend to block it so that a T connector may be used between the filter and the silastic line to facilitate administration and to prevent any interruption of the line.

The child usually is begun on a 10 percent dextrose concentration of hyperalimentation fluid, given in a volume equal to the child's basic fluid requirement. Increases to a 15 percent solution and, finally, to 20 percent are made as the child indicates tolerance for each progressive concentration. If the child remains on hyperalimentation, he receives a 20 percent concentration, but the amount

of fluid given is increased according to the child's weight gain. Under normal circumstances, discontinuation of hyperalimentation is done gradually, in reverse of the process just described, as the child is able to tolerate and thrive on normal gastrointestinal alimentation. Oral alimentation is begun and progresses simultaneously as hyperalimentation is decreased.

Hyperalimentation solution is ordered at the rate of 135 to 150 ml/kg/day (approximately 104 to 115 kcal/kg/day). Given at a constant ordered rate, the solution allows the metabolic system to function at full capacity at all times. The child is receiving as much fluid and glucose as he can tolerate. Because of the high osmolality of the concentrated dextrose, a sudden increase in the infusion rate will cause hyperglycemia and osmotic diuresis which may result in dehydration, seizures, and coma. Variations in flow should not exceed 10 percent of the ordered rate per hour; higher rates should be reported immediately to the physician. The nurse cannot compensate by a rate change for any fluid lost or gained in previous hours.

Hyperalimentation fluid must be mixed by specially trained personnel under optimum sterile conditions. The fluid can be refrigerated after mixing and should be discarded after a maximum of 5 days, a date which should be indicated on the fluid label.

Since hyperalimentation fluid is rich in life-supporting nutrients, it is also an excellent culture medium for yeast and bacteria. The chance of sepsis is greatly increased when a child is receiving hyperalimentation fluid through an indwelling catheter, but in most cases it is preventable. Strict attention must be paid to routines for proper care and use of the line and fluid.

Adherence to daily nursing routines which monitor patient response and maintain a high level of sterility and cleanliness are vital for the use of hyperalimentation. Dextrostix, urine and stool Labstix, Clinitest on stool, exact intake and output, and daily weights are the common and routinely used daily monitoring tools. Frequency of Dextrostix testing varies from every 4 hours to daily, according to doctor's orders. Findings below 45mg/100 ml or above 175 mg/100 ml are generally considered abnormal, and further action should be taken. All aspects of hyperalimentation should be checked for explanation. Hypoglycemia may be caused by a leak in the tubing or a sudden decrease in infusion rate, while hyperglycemia can be precipitated by a sudden increase in infusion rate, or it may be the first symptom of sepsis. A nursing plan for rotation of sites for blood samples should be formulated and kept at the bedside. Nursing measures should be taken to prevent extra tissue trauma to these sites and to promote healing.

Findings for urine Labstix should be negative, although traces of protein and pH of 5 to 6 may occur. Positive glucose may indicate intolerance of fluid or an osmotic diuresis due to fluid overload. Stool testing is especially important in diarrhea when a pH of 8 or higher represents loss of electrolytes and possible acidosis. After the child has begun feedings, stool testing with Clinitest tablets may indicate poor absorption of dextrose. All these findings are recorded on special charts so that fluctuations or deviations in the pattern can be seen readily.

Monitoring by means of regularly scheduled blood tests is routine. Complete blood count and differential, urea, nitrogen, electrolytes, calcium, phosphorus, and total protein are done biweekly or triweekly as long as hyperalimentation continues. To enhance the fluid contents and provide complete nutrition, iron and vitamin K supplements are given intramuscularly. Head and chest circumferences, done weekly on the same day, are recorded and compared with weight changes to determine the child's development rate.

Although all procedures and care of the child should be carried out to minimize chance of infection, the daily changes both of the dressing over the line site and of the entire intravenous apparatus, including the fluid, are important means of preventing infection. The nurse performs the dressing changes using complete sterile technique. Solutions and antibiotic ointments used vary from hospital to hospital, but iodine preparations have been found to be very effective. The site is exposed first, carefully, without tension on the line, and examined. Loose sutures, redness, edema, or sediment must be reported to the doctor. Sediment, in particular, usually indicates infection. The nurse also checks the line for kinking, undue tension, or small leaks before applying antibiotic ointment and the sterile dressings. Reapplication of the dressing includes small, nonbulky gauze and arrangement of the line so it is looped several times, but not kinked, and in optimum position for taping of the filter. The dressing is always taped occlusively and reinforced when necessary.

Change of fluid and tubing is best done in coordination with dressing change, once a day, or anytime new fluid is being given. The entire setup is connected and primed with fluid before connection to the child's line. A hemostat with padded prongs (kept at the bedside) is used to occlude the line during the change so that no air is drawn into it. Thus, the change must be quick. Used filters are cultured on designated days of the week as another precaution against infection.

The silastic line should be used only for infusion of hyperalimentation or specifically ordered fluids, all of which must have the same percentage of dextrose as the patient requires. Infusion of blood or blood products or withdrawal of blood specimens cannot be done without harm. On rare occasions, a blood culture may be withdrawn by the doctor if line infection is suspected. Due to the location of the line in the vena cava, clot formation, blood loss, air embolism, and perforations in the silastic tubing are life-threatening to the child. Aspiration and irrigation of the line when clots are present is done only by a doctor. Any break in the line, which may result in blood loss or air intake during the inspiratory phase of respiration, must be occluded immediately with the padded hemostat mentioned above. Further steps to reestablish a closed line must include cleaning of the open ends, gentle withdrawal of air from the line (if present), and repair of any breaks in the line. The line must be cut sterilely below the break and a sterile medicut reinserted. Further monitoring for any complications of blood loss or air embolism must also be instituted.

Infants and young children must be restrained adequately at all times to avoid the possibility of contamination, damage, or withdrawal of the silastic catheter. Restraint should be secure to the bed and allow the child as much arm movement as possible but not enough to reach the tubing from any angle. For older children, line taping and positioning must be done so that their mobility does not endanger it.

Since the children usually are not receiving oral feedings and are restrained to some degree, they are subject to more delays in normal development than the average child hospitalized in early life. Besides maternal separation, they are deprived of oral satisfaction and learning experienced during feedings, and, equally important, the attention, stimulation, and body contact shared between mother and child, especially the infant. Loss of sucking reflex and withdrawal are not uncommon when a baby is sustained on hyperalimentation for a prolonged period of time. Hand-mouth-eye contact develops simultaneously in the infant and can be delayed or abnormal. Mobility deprivation in the older child has a great adverse effect.

For these reasons, a comprehensive nursing

care plan should be instituted for each of these patients and changed to reflect the child's needs. Parents should be impressed with the importance of their visits, and encouraged to hold and cuddle younger children. Age-appropriate substitutes for oral satisfaction, such as pacifiers, whistles, and "blowing" activities, should be part of the plan. If possible, one or two persons should be chosen to care for the child. Infants should be up in an infant seat, playpen, or swing when they are awake. Sensory stimulation should be moderate but varied.

Peripheral hyperalimentation is used when the child needs to be maintained on intravenous fluids for a short time or when normal alimentation needs to be supplemented. Because superficial veins are especially fragile, a 10 to 15 percent solution is the highest concentration which can be used. Therefore, the child cannot gain weight as he can on central hyperalimentation. In general the same procedures and precautions are followed. Since any dextrose solution is dangerously irritating to human tissue, the nurse must frequently evaluate the condition of the skin around the needle to detect infiltration. Severe infiltrations cause tissue sloughing and frequently require skin grafts.

Surgical Openings ("Ostomies")

Cervical esophagostomy is a procedure done for types of esophageal atresia in which there is a proximal blind esophageal pouch. The end of the pouch is exteriorized at the base of the neck so that naso- and oropharyngeal secretions drain to the outside. The preferred location is on the left side, because of the approach used for the subsequent anastomosis of the colon. Repositioning, in a separate surgical procedure, must be done if the esophagostomy is placed on the right. The procedure enables definitive surgery to be postponed until a better time.

Initially, a plastic catheter may be placed into the stoma to facilitate drainage for the first few days or longer. After removal, a soft piece of toweling or absorbent material is placed over the opening to collect the secretions. Saliva is not irritating to the skin, and excoriation does not occur if the area is cleaned regularly and the toweling changed. A thin coating of petroleum jelly may be used on the skin around the stoma.

An accompanying gastrostomy is necessary for feeding the child. At any age the child should be introduced to oral foods and fluids (formula, if an infant) which will drain from the esophagostomy after they are chewed and swallowed. Some doctors may prefer to give only sugar water. These oral "feedings" are given at the same time as the gastrostomy feedings, so that the child may relate satiation of hunger and fullness in his stomach to the sensations of chewing and swallowing. Oral feedings have been found to relax the pyloric sphincter, promoting digestion. If this is not done, the child will need to relearn the eating process, which often he resists. Description of the technique which may be used to resume oral feedings when the child resists is given in discussion of esophageal atresia below.

Gastrostomy is a common component of operative management of gastrointestinal diseases. It provides the means for earlier postoperative nutrition and for decompression of the stomach. A gastrostomy makes it possible to avoid the potential hazards of prolonged nasogastric intubation and to prevent esophageal reflux. It acts as a safety and outlet valve when vomiting occurs. Reflux of air and gastric contents into the tube when the baby strains or cries prevents additional pressure in the stomach.

The tube is placed halfway down the greater curvature of the stomach and is secured by a purse-string suture, after which the stomach itself is sutured to the anterior peritoneum, creating the Stamm gastrostomy. A mushroom catheter, size 16 to 18, with the tip cut off, is preferred over a Foley catheter since the balloon of the Foley is large, crowding the stomachs of small children and possibly being caught and pushed into the duodenum by the strong peristaltic waves, creating an obstruction. The tube must be fixed firmly to the skin by means of tape or by use of a cut nipple and silk suture. Should the mushroom catheter pull out, it is replaced with a short Foley catheter. Infection may occur postoperatively at any time, particularly if skin excoriation is extensive. Steps to prevent skin breakdown vary, but they are based on keeping the area clean and dry. No dressings are used, and petrolatum, ointments, karaya gum powder, or lamp treatments daily may help. Continuous firm fixation of the catheter and prevention of pull on it aid in minimizing widening of the skin opening and subsequent leakage which occurs in a long-term gastrostomy. Once this situation has occurred, nutrition, skin, and general maintenance problems of the gastrostomy are magnified and may require surgical revision, closure, or another means of feeding.

Immediately after the surgical procedure the gastrostomy is placed on gravity drainage for about 24 hours, with the child in a 45° semiupright position. The tube may be irrigated with saline solution, or air may be instilled to prevent gastric distention depending on the doctor. The fluid drained is collected into a tube and floor bottle, a bag, or a test tube, depending on the amount and the gravity pull desired. Machine suction may pull the opposite stomach wall, therefore it is not a desirable method.

Feedings begin after the tube has been attached to a syringe and elevated to the top of the incubator or a short distance above the child in a bed. Progression takes place from, at first, lowering the gastrostomy to straight drainage between feedings; next, to continuously elevating the tube; and eventually, to clamping the tube between feedings. Glucose water is the first fluid given, followed by dilute formula. A slow, regular rate of instillation of the feeding is achieved by varying the height of the tube. When elevated, the height of the fluid column is the maximum pressure that can be exerted upon the stomach. Mechanical or manual force should never be used. A Y tube is used by some for simultaneous decompression during feeding. For optimum feeding, the child, if an infant, should be held and given a pacifier. In many cases, when oral feedings are begun, they are given concurrently with the gastrostomy feedings, which are gradually decreased as oral feedings are increased in amount.

For a time after feeding becomes totally oral, the gastrostomy may be maintained in the event it is needed again. Within 7 to 10 days after the tube is removed, the opening will close by contracture. In a few cases, surgical closure is necessary.

Colostomy and *ileostomy* are stages in treatment of specific pediatric intestinal diseases. They are most often temporary, enabling definitive treatment to be delayed until the child grows and more complex procedures may be done, as with imperforate anus and Hirschsprung's disease. Extensive ulcerative colitis may require a permanent ileostomy, while temporary ileostomy is done for meconium ileus. As with adults, either may be necessary when widespread malignant tumors or irreparable intraabdominal trauma is present.

Sigmoid colostomy with a single stoma is the most common procedure. A colostomy for Hirschsprung's disease is placed in the transverse colon when the diseased portion is large. Divided or loop colostomy is done when the distal bowel segment must be available for preparation for definitive surgery or when an outlet for drainage is needed, as in Hirschsprung's disease.

Since most colostomies are done on smaller children, irrigation is not a factor in management, but prevention and treatment of skin excoriation around the stoma is a problem. A collection bag is not desirable for infants and very young children since the bag does not adhere well. It slides over the stoma repeatedly and contributes to the development of stoma stenosis or retraction. Small squares of tissue, cut with an opening to fit over the stoma, prevent stool from touching the skin and aid in easy removal of stool. A cloth diaper, folded lengthwise, holds this in place, and it is not bulky under clothing. Older children wear a type of disposable bag, the type with a karaya seal ring being most desirable.

A collection bag must be used as soon as an ileostomy begins to function to prevent the skin breakdown which appears quickly as a result of the high amount of digestive enzymes in the liquid stool. The bag must be one which fits snugly around the stoma and allows no stool to contact the skin.

A variety of products or combinations of products are used to prevent as well as heal skin excoriation. The most frequently used are a form of karaya (powder, gum paste), Silicote ointment, a form of zinc oxide, and a product provided by the company that supplies the bag. Although exposure to air and a treatment light is successful treatment for colostomy-induced breakdown, it will only produce further excoriation with ileostomies. Changes of either bag or dressing must take place more frequently with infants for several reasons: skin breakdown is more frequent; the bag or dressing does not stay in place as well; and infant elimination is more frequent than with older children.

Problems with specific foods, clothing, leakage, and odor occur with children as with adults and must be met as they occur. Dehydration from diarrhea occurs quickly with either colostomy or ileostomy but is especially dangerous with the latter. A child should be involved in caring for his ostomy and in handling problems it causes, at his own age level. For example, a 10-year-old may be capable of complete care and awareness of his diet; a 3-year-old may help with the cleaning and dressing change. This approach will ensure a healthier child who cooperates in maintaining optimum functioning of his ostomy.

GASTROINTESTINAL DISEASES IN THE INFANT
Newborn Surgical Emergencies

Congenital Diaphragmatic Hernia This disease represents one of the most acute emergencies in the newborn period. A mortality of 25 to 40 percent is influenced by prompt diagnosis and treatment based on complete recognition of the presenting problems. There is no predilection of either sex or race. Mortality rises rapidly in treatment of the youngest and smallest infants and is highest in the first 24 hours after birth. In a majority of cases, the herniation is into the left side of the chest, resulting in a hypoplastic left lung.

The infant has a large (barrel) chest in comparison with its small (scaphoid) abdomen, due to the location of the abdominal viscera in the chest. Breath sounds are absent, particularly on the left, heart sounds are displaced to the right, and the chest is dull to percussion. Tachypnea, nasal flaring, and chest retraction, usually present, become more pronounced with crying. The most definitive sign in diagnosis is dextrocardia in a child who has spasmodic attacks of cyanosis and difficulty in feeding due to dypsnea. Classic signs of intestinal obstruction may also be present. Generally, death is attributable to severe oxygen deprivation (see Fig. 36-2).

Diagnosis is confirmed by x-rays and provides the basis for distinguishing this disease from lung cysts, lung hamartoma, paralysis of the diaphragm secondary to phrenic nerve involvement, and *eventration* of the diaphragm (a weakness but not an opening in the diaphragmatic wall which results in an elevation of that section so that it protrudes into the chest). Gas-filled bowel and stomach can be seen in the thorax, with collapse of the lung and displacement of the mediastinum.

Surgical and nursing management Immediate relief of respiratory distress is attained by administration of oxygen in high concentrations and by gastric decompression. Positive pressure ventilation by mask adds to the distress by adding to the air and pressure in the stomach and bowel already present. Tracheal intubation is necessary if positive pressure ventilation is indicated. The nurse elevates the baby's head in semi-Fowler's position and places him on the affected side so that the unaffected lung may expand.

Surgery is performed immediately. A transabdominal approach is used when intestinal obstruc-

tion is present or even suspected. Otherwise a transthoracic approach is used. Water-seal chest suction for 2 to 3 days relieves the pneumothorax resulting from the operation. Since spontaneous pneumothorax or pneumothorax of the unaffected lung also may occur, positive pressure ventilation is often used routinely for several days following surgery. Chest physiotherapy is begun and continued through the acute postoperative period. Since a nasogastric tube with constant suction is maintained till peristalsis occurs, intravenous therapy must be used.

Nursing focus at this time must be on the respiratory effort of the baby. The nurse is alert to signs of respiratory complications and to the possibility of hemorrhage. In addition to maintenance of the treatments given above, the nurse makes frequent changes in the position of the baby and carries out nasopharyngeal suction at necessary intervals to assist him in reestablishing normal respiration.

In the convalescent period, focus of nursing care shifts to the problems of feeding. These babies are often lethargic, not interested in feeding, and, if coaxed, gag easily and vomit. A schedule which allows flexibility to take advantage of his readiness to eat and his appetite at each feeding (with a ceiling limit on the amount he may take) is best. The nurse uses feeding techniques which eliminate swallowing of air and compression of the baby's stomach by poor positioning in the arms. Frequent burping is essential. Development of a hiatal hernia is a common occurrence in the convalescent period.

The baby's parents can be overwhelmed, particularly by the speed with which surgery must be done, the severity of the symptoms, the high mortality rate of the disease, and the mass of mechanical aids, including respirator, which they see around their tiny baby. The infant's mother must participate in his care, especially feedings, so that she may learn the best technique of feeding the infant, achieving success before his discharge.

Esophageal Atresia with Tracheoesophageal Fistula Rapid diagnosis is extremely vital to the child with one of the six types of esophageal atresia. Estimates vary that from 85 to 95 percent of cases have both esophageal atresia and tracheoesophageal fistula, variations of types II, III, and IV. The remainder have one or the other defect present, as in types I, V, and VI. Complications occur frequently, and prognosis depends directly on the speed of treatment, which often has a prolonged and tortuous course.

Types and clinical manifestations The classic picture of an infant with this anomaly is one who has excessive amounts of mucus, sometimes bubbling from his nostrils, and is choking, sneezing, and coughing. Cyanosis occurs particularly at feeding time (of diagnostic importance). The feeding is often expelled through the nostrils immediately. Respiratory difficulty and cyanosis are relieved temporarily but noticeably by suctioning of the nasopharynx. Progressive recurrent abdominal distention, because air travels in and out of the stomach through the fistula, may be present.

Types of esophageal atresia which occur, with particular characteristics of each, are shown in Fig. 36-3. Types I, IV, and V are rare. With type II, the infants often die before diagnosis and treatment occur. Type III occurs most frequently, and type VI is next in incidence.

Type III, atresia of the esophagus with a fistula from the lower pouch and a blind upper pouch, occurs in an estimated 85 percent of cases. This type is described as a "classic picture" of the disease. Aspiration takes place through overflow of the upper pouch (as in type I) but also results from reflux of gastric secretions through the fistula into the bronchi, which can be more serious. The reflux results when intrathoracic pressure is increased (from crying, for example), causing air to rush into the lower esophagus via the fistula and into the stomach, which becomes distended and produces vomiting.

Gastrostomy and constant drainage of the upper pouch may be used to postpone more definitive surgery for up to 2 weeks if the child is too ill for complex surgery. Ligation of the fistula is done then, and the completion of correction varies.

Type VI, stenosis of the esophagus without fistula or atresia, is more common than other types except type III. The narrowing, which generally oc-

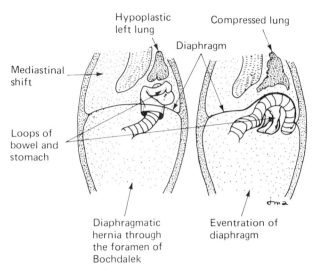

Figure 36-2 Comparison of pathologic anatomies of diaphragmatic malformations.

curs two-thirds of the way down the esophagus, may cause complete obstruction with symptoms similar to those of atresia or may be mild, causing obstruction to solid food only. As the baby begins chopped food, he becomes a fussy eater and may vomit undigested food. Aspiration may take place if vomiting is frequent.

Symptoms are often diagnostic along with an inability to pass a nasogastric catheter and to obtain stomach contents. When the catheter coils in the mucus-filled pouch, the fluid obtained must be recognized as saliva and not gastric secretions.

Confirmed diagnosis of the presence of esophageal atresia and differentiation of types depends on x-ray when a radiopaque catheter is inserted into the blind pouch which shows on film. Radiopaque contrast material is not used unless abso-

Figure 36-3 Types of esophageal atresia. Type I, esophageal atresia with no fistula; blind pouches. Type II, lower esophageal atresia, fistula from upper pouch. Type III, esophageal atresia, blind upper pouch, fistula from lower pouch. Type IV, esophageal atresia with fistulas from both pouches. Type V, no esophageal atresia; connecting fistula. Type VI, esophageal stenosis.

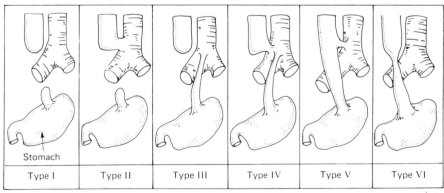

lutely necessary because of aspiration dangers, but upper gastrointestinal barium swallows are needed to confirm diagnosis of types V and VI. Fistulas are not constantly patent, making diagnosis of their presence more difficult.

The wide variation and combinations of approaches in treatment reflect the differences in the six types and also the accepted philosophy of treatment of this defect, known as *staging* (repeated operations separated by periods of time, waiting for growth). In particular, staging is the approach for premature babies, critically ill babies, ones who have major associated anomalies, and those in which a wide disparity between the blind ends of the esophagus in size or in distance exists. The degree of aspiration pneumonia will also be a determinant. Ligation of the fistula must always take place immediately except in type III. If possible, primary end-to-end anastomosis of the esophagus is performed at the same time. Some surgeons also do a gastrostomy as a supportive measure, while others do not.

If the surgery is deferred, there are three existing methods to prevent the oral secretions from accumulating in the blind pouch. Most common is the use of a double-lumen nasogastric tube which ends in the blind pouch and is attached to constant suction. The tube is changed daily to ensure patency. A lesser known method is the use of an *esophageal frame,* a metal frame similar to a Bradford frame but small enough for an incubator, used with a canvas cover which contains an opening for the baby's face, shoulder rests, and canvas restraint straps. The baby is placed face downward in Trendelenburg's position so that mucus drains out of the mouth and nose by gravity. Gastrostomy feedings are used in both methods. The time interval allows for growth of the esophageal blind segments so that primary anastomosis may be possible, although esophageal reconstruction may still be the final outcome. When the patient's condition is stable, a surgeon may attempt elongation of the proximal pouch by *bougie* treatment, using mercury-weighted dilators or firm catheters inserted briefly each day to stretch the esophagus.

The third method in use is cervical esophagostomy, done when the child's respiratory problems are too severe, when the need for esophageal reconstruction is unavoidable, or when the first two methods of management prove unsuccessful in controlling secretions. Tracheostomy may be an additional supportive operation the child must endure if respiratory complications are too severe.

Reconstruction of the esophagus (esophageal replacement, colon transposition, or colon transplant) is performed when there is too wide a gap between the proximal and distal pouches of the esophagus in esophageal atresia without fistula and when a leak occurs in the primary anastomosis. Until the child is as old as 6 months or more to about 2 years of age, he must be maintained by cervical esophagostomy to handle saliva and by gastrostomy feedings, with small oral feedings if at all possible. Clear liquid diet and succinylsulfathiazole are used to clean the colon, but enemas or laxatives are avoided because of possible adverse effects.

The procedure involves, in this order, left thoracotomy to prepare esophageal pouches and to measure the length of the colon needed; laparotomy in which the segment of colon needed is divided at its proximal and distal ends and then anastomosed to form continuous colon once more; the colon to be transplanted is brought, complete with blood supply, through a surgical hole in the diaphragm near the hiatus and joined to the esophageal pouches. Water-seal chest drainage is continued for 7 to 10 days, the most common time for anastomatic leaks to occur.

Postoperatively, the nasogastric catheter decompresses the stomach by water-seal suction for 2 to 3 days to prevent strain on the suture line. The gastrostomy tube is open and elevated even after the catheter is removed, and oral fluids are begun immediately in gradually increasing amounts and strengths. Ischemia, which causes total breakdown of the transplant, is the most common complication.

The colon has a propulsive action but adapts soon to functioning in unison with the esophagus, which has peristaltic action, thereby accounting for the large amounts of burping the baby does in the first few weeks and the uncomfortable sensations he seems to feel which cause him to be fussy without obvious reason. His breath often has a strong stool odor in the first postoperative month.

Nursing management   Immediately upon diagnosis, constant suction through a double-lumen catheter ending in the blind pouch should begin. Close observation of respiratory behavior will demonstrate any need for additional suctioning of the nasopharynx. The nurse should be especially alert for indications of respiratory effort: retraction, circumoral cyanosis, "fussing," open mouth, and nasal flaring. Oxygen, humidity, and warmth via incubator are important preoperatively and for several weeks postoperatively. Intravenous fluids are begun before surgery and are often changed to hyperalimentation.

The best position for the baby varies, but it is important. When gastric reflux is present (types III to VI), elevation to 20 or 30° is best. The doctor may determine the position to be used when a fistula opens from the upper pouch. The baby also may be placed flat or very slightly prone in Trendelenburg's position. He should be kept *flat* after anastomosis but *elevated* if catheter drainage of the pouch is being done (to promote pooling of secretions at the catheter tip) or after cervical esophagostomy. Hyperextension of the neck should be avoided since it places tension on any existing suture line.

For nasopharyngeal suctioning postoperatively, the nurse must use a catheter marked so that it will not be inserted too near the anastomosis. Suctioning as frequent as every 5 to 10 minutes may be necessary the first day. Nursing judgment must be acute in determining the need since suctioning may increase the edema already present from the surgery. Regular oral hygiene prevents bacterial growth in the abundant secretions.

In catheter drainage of the pouch, the nurse must observe its patency and maintain suction at a low, intermittent level. Depending on the procedures of the hospital, the nurse may be responsible for changing the tube. When the esophageal frame is used, the face needs to be wiped and cleaned frequently.

Nursing planning must take into consideration the physical restrictions placed on the baby with this defect as well as the social and emotional opportunities he lacks. The treatment for esophageal atresia extends over the entire first year, a crucial time in development.

Following anastomosis, gastrostomy feedings are instituted after determining the volume of gastric contents by aspiration with syringe. Feedings should be given slowly or dripped in every 2 to 3 hours. Oral feedings are begun after about two weeks if a gastrostomy is present or after about a week if the surgeon does not perform a gastrostomy. They should be given slowly so that the baby expends as little effort as possible, and may be completed by gastrostomy should the baby tire. The nurse should use techniques which prevent any possibility of coughing, choking from too much milk, or regurgitating from too much air. Some infants may be slow, lethargic eaters, although others are vigorous. A slightly elevated position is usually best for feeding. Developing complications may become evident during feedings.

Initial oral feedings are difficult, for the baby has never experienced eating. The process may take 2 to 4 or 5 weeks for older children to establish. Emphasis must be on patient, gentle, frequent, and pleasant feedings rather than on a rigid schedule of certain amounts. The most effective nursing action is to develop and follow a written care plan built around the child's reactions to and behavior during attempts at oral feeding. The baby then has a chance to use his energy on adapting to the disturbing experience rather than on a "hodgepodge" of various approaches. His mother can be especially effective if she is encouraged and helped to feel at ease in feeding.

Complications are common and often severe enough to require extended treatment. Most frequent in occurrence is *stricture* at the sites of anastomosis, in the months following primary esophageal anastomosis or esophageal reconstruction. One or two dilations under anesthesia may be sufficient to eliminate it; regularly scheduled dilation with Tucker dilators will be necessary if the stricture is persistent. Signs of stricture (refusal of feedings, pronounced coughing, and dysphagia) should be reviewed with the parents prior to discharge after anastomotic surgery.

Prognosis for eventual complete recovery or even recovery at all depends on innumerable factors. Infants may have a frequent "brassy" cough and a lowered resistance to respiratory infections in the first 6 months to 2 years of life.

Imperforate Anus   Prompt surgical management is essential for an infant with imperforate anus. The anomaly occurs equally in both sexes and is seen infrequently in nonwhites. Other major anomalies occur in 40 to 50 percent of cases, while an equal percentage have associated genitourinary tract anomalies. Cloacal deformities have a high incidence. Esophageal atresia with tracheoesophageal fistula is associated more frequently with imperforate anus than with other gastrointestinal tract anomalies.

Anatomic types, clinical manifestations, and diagnosis   There are four types of imperforate anus: type I, stenosis (in about 5 percent of cases); type II, membraneous (10 to 15 percent); type III, agenesis, high and low (75 to 80 percent); and type IV, atretic (less than 5 percent). (See Fig. 36-4.)

Agenesis, with wide variations, consists of normal outward anal appearances, abnormal anal mus-

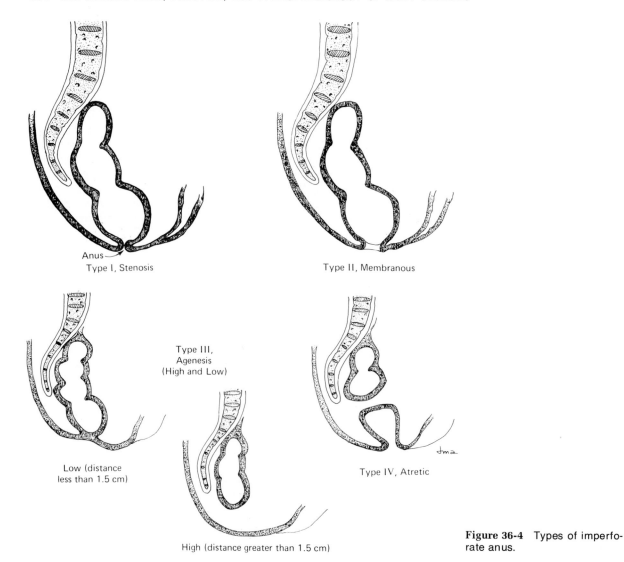

Anus
Type I, Stenosis

Type II, Membranous

Type III,
Agenesis
(High and Low)

Low (distance
less than 1.5 cm)

Type IV, Atretic

High (distance greater than 1.5 cm)

Figure 36-4 Types of imperforate anus.

culature, inadequate innervation of the area, and associated fistulas of the agenetic type because development of the rectum is minimal or nil. In low agenesis, there are 1.5 cm or less between the blind end of the colon and the anal dimple; in high agenesis, there are more than 1.5 cm, an important distinction. A dimple exists at the site where the anus should be, and there may be puckering of the surrounding skin, an indication of the presence of sphincter muscles. However, there may be neither puckering nor dimple; the anal area may be rather flat between the buttocks. In severe cases, the buttocks, also, may be completely flat, usually a good indication of poor levator ani development.[2] There is a high incidence of fistular development between the rectum and genitourinary tract.

Diagnosis is often made on newborn examination or by an observant nurse. At 2 to 3 days of age, symptoms related to low-bowel obstruction develop: abdominal distention and vomiting. Respiratory difficulty, dehydration, *tympanites,* and *borborygmus* occur as the disease remains untreated.

Definitive diagnosis is made by x-ray using the Wangensteen-Rice method. The infant is held down while the abdomen is filmed. Gas in the colon rises to reveal an outline of the rectal pouch, giving an indication of its position with relation to the anal membrane.

In surgical and nursing management of low agenetic types, corrective surgery is an anoplasty, either a perineal "cutback" anoplasty or a Y-V–plasty, done under general anesthesia. A Hager dilation regimen is instituted as soon as initial healing takes place. Nursing objectives focus on prevention of suture line infection and promotion of healing. Generally, the diaper is left off and the suture line cleaned, using cotton-tipped applicators and hydrogen peroxide, or the solution named by the doctor, after each stool. Nothing is inserted into the rectum. The baby's position is alternated, side to side, to decrease tension on the suture line. Feedings are begun in 1 to 2 days.

In surgical and nursing management of high agenetic and atretic types, a *transverse,* divided colostomy is done immediately. Later, at age 6 to 12 months, the infant has a sacroabdominoperineal pull-through operation, the primary procedure. The location of the blind pouch of the rectum in relation to the pubococcygeal line, seen on roentenogram, is important in determining the surgical approach.

The surgeon must evaluate and consider many factors: innervation of the external and internal sphincters, neuromuscular deficits if present, fistulas, size of the external opening to be created, and the levator muscle sling (the main mechanism for rectal continence in imperforate anus) in order to correct the defect optimally. Even if the anatomic deficiencies prevent successful surgery, bowel control can be managed via the "perineal colostomy" created and bowel habit training.

Nursing care postoperatively is the same for both the colostomy and pull-through. Intravenous fluids and nasogastric suction are necessary until feedings are begun. The infant rarely needs oxygen and nasopharyngeal suctioning longer than 1 or 2 days postoperatively. After a colostomy, the baby is fed when stooling has started. Oral feedings following a pull-through are not begun until peristalsis resumes, stooling occurs, and initial healing has taken place. The baby usually eats eagerly, and vomiting is unusual. Parents need to learn both colostomy care and rectal dilation procedures they will use after the pull-through. Their anxiety, which may increase because of expectation of a wait of months or years for final assurance that normal bowel function has been achieved, demands understanding from the nurse.

Factors which determine prognosis Normal bowel control is achieved after treatment in stenotic, membraneous, and low agenetic types. Mortality is

low and normal functioning is possible in the majority of cases. Success in closing fistulas of all types is high. The success of the abdominoperineal pull-through operation depends on accurate placement of the rectum within the puborectalis sling without tearing or overstretching of the sphincter mechanism. Assessment of the surgery is done between the ages 4 to 6 years. If bowel control is not optimum, the child may be treated by release or transplant of the anal muscles, electrical stimulation of muscles, or reexploration with replacement of the rectum in the puborectalis sling.

Even though assured of complete bowel control, the parents approach toilet training with trepidation. If the child has less than optimum control, toilet training may be unsuccessful or very stressful for both parents and child. The family then faces uncertainty of when and whether the child will achieve control. Cleanliness, odor, and perineal breakdown are continuing problems. Inability to control his bowel movements is a serious handicap to the child in socialization and school attendance.

Intestinal Atresias Atresia along the intestinal tract is the most common cause of intestinal obstruction in the newborn. Incidence of *duodenal* and *ileal* atresias is highest, but the *jejunum* is affected frequently, the *colon* least frequently. Atresia of the bowel is an interruption in continuity which may take the form of a septum in the lumen of the bowel, stenosis, complete atresia of varying lengths, separated blind ends of bowel, or multiple atresias.

Often, there are associated congenital anomalies. Specifically, a large number of infants with duodenal atresia have Down's syndrome, and many with those two anomalies have congenital heart defects.

Occurrence is not genetically linked but arises from maldevelopment of the bowel in the second to third months of fetal life. Generally the cause of duodenal atresia is thought to differ from that of other intestinal atresias. The duodenal lumen is first obliterated and then reestablished as fetal bowel development occurs. The atresia results when the lumen of the duodenum is not reestablished. Atresias of jejunum, ileum, and colon are caused by interruptions to the vascular supply of the embryonic bowel.

Classic symptoms of newborn intestinal obstruction are vomiting of green bile (because the obstruction is below the *ampulla of Vater*), abdominal distention, and absence of stooling in the first 24 hours. Polyhydramnios is usually present at delivery of the infant with intestinal obstruction. The higher the obstruction, the earlier the symptoms appear. The intestine may rupture before birth and seal over, creating a sterile peritonitis with small calcified deposits scattered throughout the abdomen.

Characteristics peculiar to duodenal atresia Abdominal distention will be less than with other atresias or nonexistent, but reflux of duodenal secretions may cause obvious distention in the epigastric area and more vomiting than with other types. Infants with duodenal atresia often pass normal stool. A huge, distended stomach and a "double bubble" of distended duodenum appear on x-ray.

Characteristics peculiar to jejunal and ileal atresia The presentation of atresia of the jejunum (Fig. 36-5) proximal to the duodenum is identical to that of duodenal atresia. An infant with jejunal atresia of any segment may have stools; with ileal atresia he will not. Plain, erect x-ray shows dilated loops of proximal bowel and small unused distal bowel. Barium enema may show a microcolon.

In a rare instance, atresia of a huge segment of bowel, including jejunum and ileum, may occur. Although extensive resection is done, survival is extremely uncertain because it is not known exactly how much bowel must be present for adequate function to take place. At least 10 to 12 cm is the minimum length for survival beyond the immediate postoperative period.

Treatment of duodenal atresia Two different procedures for anastomosis can be used after dissection of the affected portion is done. Duodenoduodenostomy, joining the proximal and distal portions of the duodenum, is the procedure chosen when possible. A side-to-side anastomosis between the dilated duodenum and the first loop of jejunum (duodenojejunostomy) may be done instead. In most cases, a gastrostomy is created during surgery, and the *Waterson method* for postoperative feeding (jejunostomy feedings) is initiated. A small feeding tube, which emerges from the gastrostomy opening, extends through the stomach and across the anastomosis, ending at least 10 cm beyond the anastomosis. Feedings may begin earlier in the postoperative period via this tube while use of the new anastomosis is avoided until it heals. Postoperatively, gastric decompression is continued for about ten days because of prolonged free reflux of duodenal contents into the stomach.

Treatment of jejunal and ileal atresia The first step in surgical correction is excision of the atretic segment and of the distended segment of bowel proximal to the atresia, necessary because it lacks adequate peristalsis. Direct anastomosis of proximal and distal segments (jejunojejunostomy, jejunoileostomy, or ileoileostomy) can be done. In each, leakage or obstruction from filling of the blind pouches adjacent to the anastomosis is the most likely complication. A gastrostomy is almost always created.

Nursing management Vomiting and *aspiration of vomitus* are the greatest dangers in both the preoperative and postoperative periods and require alertness by the nurse. He must take preventive measures such as positioning, maintaining patency of nasogastric or gastrostomy tubes, nasopharyngeal suctioning, and observation for aspiration. Intravenous fluids are begun prior to surgery and continued afterward. For many infants, especially premature ones, those in critical condition, or those requiring extensive resection, hyperalimentation is used. Oxygen with humidity may be required after surgery.

Gastric decompression is done by nasogastric catheter before surgery and, in most cases, by gastrostomy after surgery. The gastrostomy tube is clamped and removed later, often after discharge. Resumption of feedings is gradual. Feeding problems of vomiting, low intake, lack of interest in feeding, abdominal distention after feedings, and sometimes diarrhea may occur. The infant may need special formulas which are predigested or nonallergic in content. Banana powder formula, in particular, is often used if feeding problems continue.

If a Waterson feeding tube is present in the infant, the nurse must use careful handling and slow feeding to prevent slipping of the tube in the intestine or pulling the tube out of place completely. During and after the feeding, he watches for signs which indicate that the tube is out of position, such as vomiting, unusual distention, milk seepage, or milk in the gastrostomy tube.

Episodes of diarrhea occur intermittently and may be severe enough to necessitate intravenous therapy for a few days. The nurse must observe stool size, frequency, and consistency, particularly in relation to increases in feedings. Stool monitoring for protein content and sugar absorption is done also by use of Labstix and Clinitest tablets. Guaiac testing determines presence of bleeding. Powdered charcoal, fed to the baby and timed for appearance in the stool, aids in determining the speed of peristalsis in the bowel.

Meconium Ileus The infant with meconium ileus is critically ill at birth or within a few hours after birth. It is the most severe form of cystic fibrosis, affecting about five to ten percent of those children. A deficiency or absence of enzymes normally released into the intestine by the pancreas and abnormalities of mucus-secreting glands cause meconium to be viscous, tarry, and impacted, obstructing the terminal ileum. If the obstruction is severe, the baby may be born with perforated intestine, gangrene, and meconium peritonitis.

These infants are pale and lethargic, vomit, have abdominal distention, and may exhibit signs of shock. They pass no meconium. Doughy loops of the intestine may be palpated, and a small, tight, funnel-shaped rectum is present. On x-ray examination, granular patterns—a "ground-glass" appearance (Neuhauser's sign)—caused by air bubbles trapped in the meconium are seen.

Diagnosis may be difficult because the symptoms and radiologic findings are similar to those for other intestinal obstructions. A family history of cystic fibrosis completes a positive diagnosis. The blood electrolytes and blood gas levels may be abnormal and depend on the severity of the infant's condition. A sweat test is not reliable in a newborn, but it is done after 1 month as an additional method of confirming the diagnosis.

A laparotomy is always necessary. Preoperatively, decompression of the stomach and speed in preparing the baby for surgery are important. The baby may have respiratory distress because of abdominal distention and peritonitis. He is positioned so that the abdomen is not compressed and the chest is slightly hyperextended. Oxygen is administered, and nasopharyageal suction may be necessary. Intravenous fluids or hyperalimentation are employed.

In the mildest cases, the surgeon performs manual extraction of the meconium followed by irrigation of the intestine through an *enterotomy,* then closes the abdominal incision. In the majority, a *Roux-Y anastomosis* with a temporary ileostomy is done. The ileostomy is created at the point in the intestine where sticky meconium begins. The proximal loop of the intestine (the nonaffected part) is sutured below the ileostomy to form a continuous intestine below the surface, facilitating irrigation of the intestine postoperatively. The ileostomy will shrink to close without surgery later. Occasionally, a double-loop ileostomy is done which must be

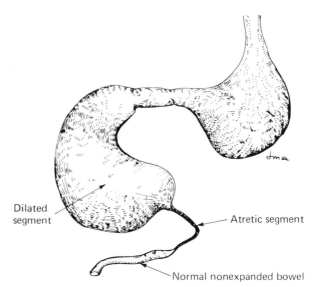

Dilated segment

Atretic segment

Normal nonexpanded bowel

Figure 36-5 Jejunal atresia.

closed later. Often, the intestine is resected before these procedures if perforation, gangrene, or extreme cyanosis and distention of the intestine are present. Another form of surgery is the *Mikulicz enterotomy,* a resection of the intestine with an ileocolostomy which must be closed later.

Postoperatively, the nurse focuses on minimizing or preventing pulmonary complications, performing the ileostomy irrigations, reestablishing normal feedings and elimination, and educating the parents. The baby receives oxygen, humidity, chest physiotherapy, and nasopharyngeal suctioning. The humidity and chest physiotherapy are continued at home; parents need to learn these techniques. A nurse should change the infant's position frequently and observe his responses to handling and care.

Irrigations of the ileostomy are started within a few days after surgery and done once or twice a day initially. They are continued until normal gastrointestinal function is established. Hydrogen peroxide, pancreatic enzyme solution, or acetylcysteine (a surface-tension reducer) is utilized. Pancreatic enzyme may produce a chemical colitis and all may be irritating to the intestine or the skin and may cause electrolyte imbalance. The nurse performing the irrigations must be alert to the possibilities of leakage around the anastomosis or ileostomy. Abdominal and perineal skin should be protected and the area cleaned thoroughly after each irrigation.

Feedings are started later, and pancreatic enzymes must be included in the formula. The infants sometimes have difficulty in starting feedings, with vomiting, small intake, diarrhea, and irritability. However, with nursing patience and persistence in a normal feeding schedule, the baby becomes a good eater.

Necrotizing Enterocolitis This is a highly lethal syndrome of newborn infants, primarily premature infants. The incidence of perinatal complications, especially hypoxia at birth and the presence of ruptured membranes at 24 hours or earlier, is significantly high in newborns who develop this disease. Necrotic lesions may be present in any part of the intestine below the duodenum, but are most common in the lower ileum, the ascending and transverse colon, or both.[3] Their presence is characterized by frequent mucosal ulcerations, pseudomembrane formation and inflammation, *pneumatosis intestinalis* (extraluminal or intramural air bubbles and strips), and perforation.

The onset, which occurs in the first 2 to 3 weeks of life, is characterized by jaundice and apnea, followed by delayed gastric emptying, vomiting, abdominal distention, and gastrointestinal bleeding, sometimes with bloody diarrhea. As the disease fulminates, symptoms of intestinal perforation or overwhelming septicemia develop prior to death.

The cause is unknown; however, the clinical manifestations and surgical findings indicate that a diminished blood flow to the intestines has occurred.[4] Sex and race have not been proved significant.

Treatment has remained nonspecific and symptomatic. Constant gastric decompression by nasogastric tube is important. Antibiotic therapy is instituted, although choice of antibiotics varies and there is some speculation that it is ineffective or hastens progression of the disease. Intravenous therapy, especially hyperalimentation, is used to maintain fluid and nutritional needs during the course of the illness. Anastomosis is done for intestinal perforation and removal of affected bowel.

Nursing management Acute, continuous nursing observation is essential, and it is accompanied by immediate report of even minute changes in the infant's appearance, behavior, or specific disease symptoms. It is essential that the nurse prevent additional stress by maintaining an environment in which temperature, oxygen, humidity, intravenous fluid flow, and gastric decompression are constant and stable. Minimal handling enhances the nonstressful environment. The degree and frequency of

apnea require blood gas and blood pressure monitoring and at times mechanical respirator assistance. Parents can be given little positive reassurance, for therapy consists of careful monitoring and waiting. Since very few infants have survived, little is known about later complications and the future health of the child.

Omphalocele and Gastroschisis Both omphalocele and gastroschisis are defects immediately apparent at birth in which abdominal viscera protrude through an abdominal wall defect and are lying out on the abdomen (Fig. 36-6). In differentiation of diagnosis, gastroschisis is located below and separate from the umbilicus and has no sac or covering, while the omphalocele is centrally located, includes the umbilicus, and is covered originally by a sac, although the sac may disintegrate in utero.[5] It is a rare defect, and other abnormalies may be present. The risk of infection supersedes all other problems.

Omphalocele results from failure of fusion of the abdominal lateral folds by the tenth week of fetal life. *Gastroschisis* is due to the failure of embryologic tissue to mature in the abdominal layers, leaving a defect. The majority of both defects involve primarily intestine. An underdeveloped abdominal cavity is a codefect. The sac of omphalocele (a transplant avascular membrane) is easily ruptured, either in utero or during birth, causing an immediate emergency and high mortality. If rupture occurs, the intestines become thickened, matted, and edematous, a primary cause of other complications. There may be respiratory difficulty, pneumonia, signs of sepsis, or peritonitis.

Infection control is instituted immediately after birth by covering the sac or exposed abdominal organs with sterile towels or sponges saturated with normal saline. These coverings are kept wet, covered with dry sterile towels to maintain sterility of the inner dressings, and changed when loosened for examination. Sterile gloves are always used. Antibiotic therapy is begun before surgery and continued until the danger of infection has subsided.

Another primary consideration is to prevent tension on the area. Positioning, turning, and restricting behavior (arm restraints) must be done cautiously. Since it may be necessary to do treatments and take x-rays in the incubator, handling may be awkward, and two people may be necessary. Supportive therapy, such as gastric decompression, is usually begun immediately.

When a very small defect occurs, the surgi-

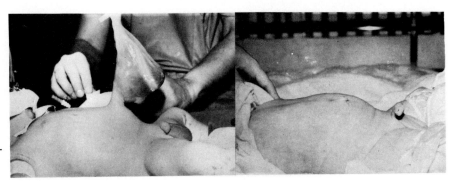

Figure 36-6 Baby with ompha-locele. (*Left*) Before surgery. (*Right*) After surgical repair.

cal treatment can be complete closure of the muscle wall, with return of the bowel, to the abdominal cavity. In most cases, the defect is too large and requires several stages of treatment. In all the basic approaches to closure, a gastrostomy often is done.

For moderate-size omphaloceles, skin flaps from both sides of the defect are joined over the omphalocele until the abdominal cavity has enlarged. Later, between about 10 months to 2 years, a ventral umbilical herniorrhaphy is done as the final stage. In addition to the basic focus of nursing care emphasized above, supportive measures such as intravenous fluids, nasopharyngeal suctioning, the use of an incubator, humidity, and, in some cases, oxygen are crucial. Hyperalimentation has been increasingly valuable in maintaining nutrition optimal for rapid healing and resistance to infection. Postoperatively, gastric decompression takes place via gastrostomy, and gradually feedings via the gastrostomy begin. Oral feedings, which begin when healing is well established, may be marred only by occasional vomiting.

In the presence of larger defects, the most conservative method is painting the omphalocele sac with an aqueous solution of Mercurochrome or another antiseptic and albumin-coagulating solution, such as silver nitrate. These measures are employed when the omphalocele is unruptured, intraabdominal pressure is low, and peritonitis is not present. They are continued until granulation and skin growth occur and the sac has contracted sufficiently to perform a skin flap closure. The eschar formed is hard and inflexible around the edges, and, until union with the skin edges is completed, small amounts of abdominal fluid may leak. This therapy is continued while observation is constant; however, increased leakage or the appear-

ance of a gap may necessitate treatment of a more drastic nature. An ever-present danger during this treatment is mercury poisoning, evidenced by edema, bright red spots of skin on body surface other than that being painted, and central nervous system signs such as lethargy and seizures. The presence of mercury in the urine may exist before clinical signs appear, so urinalysis monitoring is essential. The nurse must apply the solution by swab, usually daily, thoroughly but sparingly to avoid painting surfaces which do not need painting. Feedings are not given until after the eschar is completed. The infant lies on sterile towels, and sterile gloves and materials are used in handling the omphalocele.

Creating an artificial celom (sac) is recent and proving successful for ruptured omphaloceles. The sac, Dacron sheeting coated with silastic and, sometimes, with knitted Telfa, is sutured to the skin or the full thickness of the abdominal wall which surrounds the omphalocele. It is suspended to the top of the incubator by a rubber band (to allow flexibility) fastened to a tongue blade placed over the opening in the incubator top. The bag is shortened every 1 to 3 days, as the abdominal viscera reenter the cavity, thereby permitting a skin-flap closure in 7 to 10 days. Antibiotic solution and, sometimes, silver nitrate are dripped continually onto the prosthesis to combat infection. Sterile handling and basic supportive care are required. Feedings via gastrostomy may be started before the skin-flap procedure if the child's condition is stable.

During the convalescent period, intermittent bouts of gastroenteritis, vomiting, or low intake may occur. Feeding techniques required for intestinal atresia are frequently needed.

Mortality is highest in the first few days. While

complications are more frequent than for many other diseases, if closure of skin is achieved, the child usually does well.

Diseases of Higher Incidence in the Infant

Cleft Lip and Cleft Palate Occurring together or separately, with many variations, cleft lip and cleft palate require a long-term interdisciplinary approach for optimum treatment. The defects create problems with feeding, upper respiratory and ear infections, speech, dental formation, and self-image.

The defects are generally considered hereditary, although no exact pathogenesis has been found, and the defect may appear without a familial history. However, the occurrence of the defect in the family makes possible a prediction, by percentage, of the likelihood of future occurrence (Table 36-1). The two anomalies are not always present together. Cleft lip has a higher incidence in males, while cleft palate is more common in females.

In the fifth to the eighth weeks of fetal life, the maxillary and premaxillary processes which form the upper lip fail to fuse, creating a cleft lip. The defect usually occurs with a cleft palate, which results when the palatal processes do not fuse, 1 month later. The cleft lip can be *unilateral* or *bilateral*. A *midline* cleft is extremely rare. The extent of the defect varies from a slight indentation to a widely opened cleft. An *incomplete* cleft may be only notching of the vermillion border or may extend to the nostril.

The *complete* cleft involves the alveolus to some degree, and the nostril is distorted to one side. The floor of the nose and upper gum may also be deformed. Any combination of these malformations may occur.

The defects of a cleft palate are usually diverse. The cleft may involve the *soft palate* with the

tissues of the uvula, or it may include the *hard palate* and, sometimes, the nose. The cleft occurs in the midline of the soft palate, but it may exist on one or both sides of the hard palate. It always extends front to back. The cleft palate forms a passageway between the nasopharynx and the nose, causing feeding and respiratory difficulties and susceptibility to infection. It is more difficult to repair than the lip. A palatal defect may occur without an accompanying lip anomaly.

Surgery to close the lip is done as early as possible. Many surgeons follow a "rule of 10"; that is, the baby should weigh 10 lb, be 10 weeks of age, and have 10 Gm of hemoglobin preoperatively. Palate surgery is postponed until about 12 to 18 months. Too early a repair may harm tooth buds; with a late repair, undesirable speech patterns may be established and the palatal structure may be too rigid. Surgery for revisions of repair, correction of nose deformities, and reconstruction of the nasopharynx for speech improvement (a *velopharyngeal flap operation*) are frequently necessary.

Problems in the period from birth to lip closure Feeding is the most immediate and most apparent problem. The infant cannot maintain closed suction around the nipple in his mouth nor use mouth movement adequately to pull on the nipple because of the open palate. However, he has a strong desire to suck, and the sucking motions are present, thereby providing success in nipple feeding before lip closure. A soft but regular *crosscut* nipple is best, although a premature-type nipple may be needed for very small babies. The nipple is placed in the usual position in the mouth, *not in the cleft*, so that he can use his sucking muscles as strongly as possible. The bottle should be disposable or have a soft base so that the individual feeding the infant can maintain gentle, steady pressure on the base of the bottle. Because sucking and swallowing are an integrated process in a baby's feeding, this method prevents choking, coughing, and other difficulties in feeding. Since the baby swallows more air than normal, burping must be frequent. Being fed in a sitting or semisitting position adds to the baby's success in swallowing and prevents choking. Caution must be taken to refrain from constantly removing the nipple from his mouth because of the noises he makes or the fear of choking, for the baby becomes more upset and crying adds to the problem. He will take longer to feed than most babies. A small amount of water should be given after a feeding to rinse the mouth. Once the nurse has in-

Table 36-1 PERCENTAGE RISKS IN INCIDENCE OF CLEFT LIP AND CLEFT PALATE

Affected	Risks for offspring, %
1 child	4–7
1 parent	2
1 child and 1 parent	11
1 child and 1 sibling	10

Source: Audiovisual aid to teaching used by the University of Pittsburgh School of Nursing, Pediatric Nursing Department.

stituted a successful feeding pattern, the process should be taught to the baby's mother.

Precautions against infections are necessary, since ear and upper respiratory infections are frequent. Not feeding the infant lying down and not confining him to lying on his back for long periods decrease ear infections, since the pharyngeal opening of the eustachian tube is often in an abnormal position. The baby breathes through his mouth, and mouth care is necessary to prevent dry, cracked lips. There is no need for restraining the arms before surgery.

The presence of an unsightly defect causes guilt, fear, misunderstanding, and, at times, revulsion on the part of parents. The hereditary factor may lead the parents to feel that they caused the defect. They need accurate, emphatic reassurance that the defect causes no malfunctioning of the remaining gastrointestinal tract or accompanying brain damage. They will need nursing assistance in becoming confident in feeding their infant.

Surgical and nursing management of cleft lip After surgery the baby may be restless, irritable, and fussy, wanting to be held much of the time in the first few days. He has a difficult time adapting to the small airway and to the excess mucus which may be a temporary result of the surgery. The latter is especially true during feedings. The nurse must evaluate the respiratory distress and observe for swelling of the tongue, mouth, and nostrils. Crying adds to his distress and puts a strain on the suture line. Often, a mist tent is used postoperatively to minimize respiratory distress and hemorrhage, which constitute the two greatest complications after cleft-lip closure.

A second area of nursing concern involves the positioning and restraining required after surgery. The suture line must be protected from blows, rubbing, pressure, and sucking. A curved metal Logan bow, taped down on either side of the suture line and over the lip, is put in place after surgery. The baby must wear elbow restraints at all times to prevent him from putting hands or objects into his mouth. A chain of safety pins from the wrist of the restraint to the diaper pin on each side will keep him from rubbing the lip with his arms. These restraints should be removed every 4 hours. Since the baby can lie only on his back, it is best to seat him in a plastic infant seat as much as possible for variety, comfort, and entertainment. He also may have difficulty sleeping if he is accustomed to sleeping on his abdomen. If he is able to roll over, he will need to be restrained by a wide

cloth pinned across his body when lying on his back. Measures such as placing him out where there is activity, holding him when he is fussy, or hanging toys within his sight and within reach of his restrained arms will help to alleviate the effects of all these restrictions.

Feedings must be given by a rubber-tipped medicine dropper which is always placed to the side of the mouth and away from the suture line. The baby is prevented from sucking on the dropper. This method of feeding is continued for about three weeks until the lip is completely healed and breast or bottle feedings are resumed. Dropper feeding is often a frustrating, tiring effort for the baby, especially at first. He cannot suck, he cannot get the formula as fast as he would like, and he swallows more air. Small, frequent feedings may help. Clear liquids are given on the first postoperative day, then milk feedings are resumed. Strained foods can be added to the milk and dropper feedings, if allowed by the surgeon. The baby will be more content if his hunger is satisfied. The nurse should place the formula within easy reach and feed the baby at a regular, fairly fast pace, the pace at which the baby would suck, adding to his contentment at feeding time and preventing suture line stress. After a feeding, sterile water should be utilized to rinse out the mouth.

Immediately after feedings, the suture line is cleaned with cotton-tipped applicators and one-half strength hydrogen peroxide. Prevention of crusts (with prevention of strain on the suture line) is a major nursing focus. They can cause uneven healing and scarring of the suture line. A collection of exudate and milk on the suture line may also lead to infection and separation of the line, marring the lip repair. The Logan bow serves to hold a narrow strip of fine mesh gauze over the suture line. This material is constantly moistened with normal saline, until all sutures are removed, thereby preventing crust formation. The gauze is removed before feeding and a new strip is applied after feeding so that it does not lie on the suture line saturated with milk. The tapes which hold the Logan bow must be kept clean and dry. Appropriate care should be taught to parents.

Surgical and nursing management of cleft palate Closure of the palate is done before speech begins, if possible, because if it is not, the gutteral tone due to the open palate may remain even after repair, when normal speech is possible. The palate may require one repair, as in the case of a soft-palate defect, or a two-stage repair, requiring two operations when a severe defect is present. Preoperatively, in addition to basic preparation, bleeding and clotting times are determined because hemorrhage or excess bleeding is a frequent postoperative complication.

Postoperatively, since the child is older than one who has had surgery for cleft lip, he is more active and more aware of his pain and restraint. These children are placed on their abdomens to facilitate drainage of mucus and blood. Mist tents moisten the mucous membranes of the oropharynx, which become dry because of mouth breathing.

After the first day, the child may be up with elbow restraints in place. Techniques which make feeding more enjoyable are utilized. Paper cups are used. Straws, plastic cups or glasses, and eating utensils are never used because they may harm or even perforate the suture line. Sterile water rinses are done after feedings. The patient resumes a full diet in 3 to 4 weeks.

Closure of the palate is more difficult and subject to more strain and infection than is closure of cleft lip. Sucking, blowing, talking, laughing, or putting objects in the mouth may cause strain on the repair.

Even after these repairs have been completed, long-term care for dental correction and establishment of proper speech is necessary. Revisions of lip repair, nostril correction, or the velopharyngeal flap may need to be done as late as 8 or 9 years of age.

Diarrhea and Gastroenteritis Diarrhea is one of the symptoms most frequently seen in pediatrics. It is a disturbance in intestinal motility and absorption, interfering with water and electrolyte absorption and accelerating the excretion of intestinal contents. The most important criteria for identification are an increase in frequency of stooling, a change in consistency (watery), and the appearance of green-colored stools. Diarrhea may be a primary disease entity or an associated symptom of another disease. (See Table 36-2.) The majority of diarrhea conditions are classified as infectious. Viral gastroenteritis is the most widespread and self-limited. Adenoviruses and enteroviruses, including Echo and Coxsackie viruses, have been isolated as causative agents in viral diarrhea affecting all age groups. Shigellae and salmonellae, bacterial pathogens, are also responsible for diarrhea at any age. Children under 2 years of age may frequently be infected by pathogenic *Escherichia coli*. The incidence of all infectious diarrheas is affected by health, nutrition, hygiene, climate, and seasonal variation.

Acute nonspecific gastroenteritis (viral) Usually identified by seasonal occurrences, viral gastroenteritis is highly contagious and may be widespread. Often, since the disease is brief, self-limiting, and mild, the causative agent is presumed to be viral and the virus is not actually identified by laboratory methods. Onset is sudden, usually beginning with vomiting for 6 to 24 hours, accompanied by fever. Diarrhea, which follows, lasts 3 to 10 days, often producing a distended abdomen, crampy severe abdominal pain, and increased bowel sounds. Since the child is not in a toxic condition, symptomatic treatment is usually all that is necessary.

Gastroenteritis due to pathogenic Escherichia coli When diarrhea occurs in infants, the gram-negative bacteria *E. coli* is suspected immediately as the causative agent. It is sporadic and is often identified with frequent, rapid-spread outbreaks of diarrhea in newborn nurseries and in infant areas of institutions.

The organism grows in the entire intestinal tract, producing congestion and petechiae of the mucosa and intestinal dilation. Diagnosis is made by stool culture. The onset may be gradual or sudden—the latter is usually more severe. Children with mild disease may have green, liquid diarrhea, with fever and irritability for only a few days. In the majority of cases, projectile vomiting and explosive, green, liquid diarrhea are the presenting symptoms. Abdominal distention is marked. Because of the rapid loss of fluid into the gastrointestinal tract, the child may be very ill, displaying the following signs of dehydration and acid-base imbalance: high fever, rapid, shallow breathing, hollow eyes, and a depressed fontanel. Length of the illness depends on the promptness of treatment, but it may linger for weeks.

The disease is carrier-passed, and prevention is extremely important. In newborn nurseries or pediatric infant areas control measures should be implemented immediately and should include: (1) isolation of an infant with diarrhea or a history of diarrhea followed by stool culture, (2) observation of other children as symptoms occur, and (3) strict handwashing techniques and special handling of diapers, stool, food, and formulas. Such procedures should be maintained until stool cultures are negative.

Salmonellosis and shigellosis Bacterial gastroenteritis caused by *Salmonella* or *Shigella* organisms occurs sporadically or in epidemics. It is a mild, self-limiting disease affecting children under 5 years of

Table 36-2 CAUSES OF DIARRHEA IN CHILDREN

Acute diarrhea	Chronic diarrhea

Otherwise well child
  Antibiotics
  Contaminated foodstuffs
  Dietary indiscretions
  Parasites
  Poisons
 	
Sick child
  Enteral
    Appendicitis
    Bacterial gastroenteritis
    Carbohydrate intolerance
    Hirschsprung's disease
    Inflammatory bowel disease
    Milk protein allergy
    Necrotizing enterocolitis
    Nonspecific gastroenteritis (viral)
    Pseudomembranous enterocolitis
 	
  Parenteral
    Upper respiratory tract infection (otitis media)
    Urinary tract infection
	Otherwise well child
	  Carbohydrate intolerance
	  Dietary indiscretions
	  Irritable colon syndrome
	  Milk protein allergy
	  Parasites
	  Polyposis
	
	Sick child (not thriving)
	  Abetalipoproteinemia
	  Acrodermatitis enteropathica
	  Carbohydrate intolerance
	  Carcinoid tumors
	  Celiac disease
	  Chronic pancreatitis
	  Cystic fibrosis
	  Enterokinase deficiency
	  Exocrine pancreatic hypoplasia
	  Familial chloride diarrhea
	  Ganglioneuroma
	  Hyperthyroidism
	  Immune deficiencies
	  Inflammatory bowel disease
	  Lymphangiectasis
	  Maternal deprivation
	  Polyposis
	  Protein calories malnutrition
	  Short-bowel syndrome
	  Stagnant loop syndrome
	  Whipple's disease
	  Zollinger-Ellison syndrome

age. The most common mode of transmission is food, especially eggs, meat, shellfish, and milk. During food preparation, one contaminated food may infect another. The food itself may be contaminated, initially by the handler in a meat-packing plant, canning factory, poultry plant, restaurant, home, or institution kitchen. Direct transmission can occur from household pets such as dogs, cats, turtles, and parakeets. *Salmonella* organisms have been found in water traps, air, and dust.

The mucosa of the stomach and small intestine is inflamed and edematous. *Peyer's patches* show edema and superficial ulceration. The gastroenteritis begins with vomiting, fever, and diarrhea, the latter being watery, with large amounts of pus and mucus. There may be nausea with severe abdominal pain. Symptoms are gone in several days.

Salmonellosis and shigellosis are diseases reportable to the health department. Household contacts must be investigated. The presence of carriers or other members of the family with symptoms is high. Younger children are especially vulnerable. A carrier, one who has either been asymptomatic or recovered from the disease, still excretes microorganisms for 3 to 4 weeks or as long as 2 months. Teaching the family about stool handling, food handling, and common modes of transmission must be thorough and immediate. Stool cultures and medical examinations should be conscientiously done at intervals.

The four major groups of the *Shigella* bacterium are responsible for shigellosis or bacillary dysentery. The clinical picture for transmission, manifestations, incidence, and control are identical to that of salmonellosis except for the colon, which is affected in shigellosis. Shigellae can be transmitted by carrier flies as well as modes already mentioned. The incidence is higher in warm months and in warm climates. When sigmoidoscopy is done, petechiae, swelling, acute inflammatory exudates, shallow irregular ulcerations, and sloughing of gray membranous material can be seen. One strain of *Shigella* is neurotoxic, and others produce endotoxins which have neurotoxic activity. Therefore, a child with even milder disease may have convulsions, and meningismus may be present. Convalescence is longer than that for salmonellosis. A picture of low fever, intermittent diarrhea, and failure to thrive may last for weeks.

Nursing management Since the child's status deteriorates rapidly, the most immediate need is the replacement of fluid and electrolyte losses. The patient is not given anything to eat in order to rest the bowel. Readiness for oral fluids is determined by a decrease in number of stools or progress toward firmer consistency. The baby is initially given small amounts of clear fluids. Prepared electrolyte solutions may be used to replace loss and to maintain electrolyte balance even if diarrhea has not subsided. With improvement, the child may be advanced to milk feedings, or full fluids for the older child. In a baby a temporary decrease in dissacharide tolerance may be evident, and a lactose-free formula may be ordered. Older children return to a full diet within a few days after cessation of symptoms. Medications are not usually prescribed, for they may mask symptoms.

Parenteral fluids are required in the majority of hospitalized patients. Due to a reduction in plasma volume secondary to water and electrolyte loss, the child may exhibit signs of shock. Normal saline or a balanced lactate solution is given to correct volume. The rate and composition are changed so as to maintain normal hydration and correct the electrolyte deficit (based on an estimate of weight loss). If the child is in severe acidosis, sodium bicarbonate is given initially.

Nursing observations must be accurate when monitoring fluid and electrolyte loss. The baby should be weighed daily or twice daily in severe cases. Additional fluid loss is determined by weighing the infant's vomitus and used diapers. Labstix, guaiac test, and Clinitest tablets on stools provide further data on the status of the patient.

Isolation should be instituted for all cases of bacterially caused diarrhea. The family needs to be taught the necessary hospital measures for isolation, especially of the stool.

Recovery, even in a severely ill baby, is rapid and evident in his behavior. The baby or child becomes active, alert, and playful, and his appetite returns.

Intractable diarrhea A puzzling, irreversible, self-perpetuating diarrhea develops in some infants beginning soon after birth. Onset may be gradual or rapid. The mortality rate is high, and often the child deteriorates despite hospital treatment. Repeated negative stool cultures and diarrhea of more than 2 weeks duration point to the diagnosis.

The pathology is that of widespread inflammation and necrosis of intestinal mucosa the entire length of the bowel, with thinning (rather than the more common inflammatory reaction of thickening) of the bowel wall. The problem may appear secondary to any one of the causes of diarrhea noted in Table 36-2. A battery of screening studies includes abdominal x-rays, barium enema x-ray, blood, urine, and stool cultures, stool test for ova and parasites, a sweat test, blood smear, stool fat absorption, serum electrophoresis, and blood acid-base tests, elimination of cow's milk from the diet, repeated testing of the stool for pH and reducing substance (to rule out disaccharide intolerance), and repeated guaiac tests for blood.

The child may have other gastrointestinal signs, such as vomiting and abdominal distention. A continuous untreated condition results in shock and death. The child has malnutrition with continued weight loss. Treatment consists of a long period of resting the bowel until normal functioning resumes, with accompanying supportive measures. Restoration of fluid and electrolyte loss and acid-base balance must be immediate by intravenous fluids and drugs. The child is given nothing by mouth and receives parenteral hyperalimentation, usually for 4 weeks or longer. Albumin, plasma, and whole blood may be given intermittently. Antibiotics are not given routinely. When oral feedings are resumed, milk proteins and lactose are eliminated, and a monosaccharide- or carbohydrate-free formula is given. *Lactobacillus* cultures in granular form are given to aid in resumption of normal bowel activity.

A major area of nursing focus is monitoring of the baby's condition by use of the stool tests mentioned above and careful output measurement in addition to routine nursing procedures and astute observation. The nurse can prevent later complications in the feeding and developmental areas by providing the stimulation and human contact essential to the baby's well-being. Otherwise the infant becomes inactive and withdrawn, loses the ability to make eye contact, and stops cooing or smiling. Without nursing intervention, the child spends much of the time "curled in a ball," sucking voraciously on his fingers to the point of extreme excoriation. When oral feeding is resumed, it is extremely difficult to entice him to suck on a nipple because he prefers the fingers.

There are several other causes of diarrhea of which a nurse should be cognizant. Staphyloccal food poisoning causes symptoms similar to infectious diarrhea; however, it is self-limiting. Diarrhea may also occur as a response to several antibiotics. Malnutrition may lead to altered mucosa, abnormal motility, changed bacterial flora, defective disaccharidose activity, and ultimately diarrhea. Dietary diarrhea may occur from overfeeding, a change in the composition of a baby's formula, transition from breast to bottle feeding, the introduction of new foods, and, in older children, the ingestion of spices or irritating foods. In allergic diarrhea, the incitant may be milk protein or lactose.

Hiatus Hernia In children hiatus hernia, a protrusion of the stomach through the esophageal hiatus, is considered a congenitally caused defect because the hiatus is *abnormally wide.* The majority of hernias are the *sliding* type which has no accompanying peritoneal sac, as the *rolling* type does. Most hiatus hernias are small.

It is more frequent and more severe in males. There is often a history of vomiting in the family, although no established familial pattern has been found. Associated abnormalities such as pyloric stenosis, abnormalities of the glottis and trachea, mental retardation, and Down's syndrome have been found.[6]

Forceful vomiting begins between 1 week and 1 month of age. The baby has no dysphagia, and there is no change in elimination patterns. As vomiting continues, the vomitus may contain old blood. The vomiting causes anemia, weight loss, dehydration, and malnutrition if unchecked. Vomiting stops first during the day, and by 9 months to 1 year of age, it no longer occurs.

If the condition is complicated by the development of esophagitis or esophageal stricture, dysphagia is present, and vomiting is more severe and occurs for longer episodes. Aspiration pneumonia is a frequent complication.

Diagnosis is based on barium x-ray of the upper gastrointestinal tract which shows the distended stomach above the diaphragm and the reflux occurring. When surgery is contemplated, an esophagoscopy is done.

Medical management of the defect is preferred and relatively simple. The child is fed in an upright position, and the formula or milk is thickened with dry instant baby cereal or baby food. After the feeding, the baby is kept upright for about ½ hour. Seating the baby in a plastic padded infant seat may be useful until the baby is about one year old or until he no longer vomits.

Surgery is necessary if symptoms continue unabated, especially if weight loss occurs and if severe esophagitis or ulceration in the esophagus develops. The simplest procedure is *gastropexy,* performed via a laparotomy. After the hiatus hernia is reduced, the esophagus is brought down to a correct length below the diaphragm and the stomach is "tacked" in place so that tension prevents any "sliding" upward. For some children, specifically for those under age 2 years, the repair of the hernia is preceded by *retrograde dilation* of an esophageal stricture. Hager dilators are passed upward through a small incision in the stomach wall. After closure of the incision, a gastropexy is done. *Fundus plication,* which is used less frequently, can be done by a thoracic or abdominal approach. After the hernia is repaired, the fundus of the stomach is folded around the lower esophagus and sutured in place. If esophagitis, ulceration, and subsequent complications continue despite less radical treatment, *colon replacement* of the esophagus will need to be undertaken.

The postoperative course follows closely that of simple thoracotomy or laparotomy.

The child will have underwater chest drainage and basic respiratory therapy for a few days. Gastric decompression by nasogastric tube and intravenous fluids will be used until feedings are begun. Complications do not usually occur.

Feedings remain the major focus in nursing planning. Depending on the surgeon, feedings are resumed within a few days after surgery. The child will need small, frequent feedings and much patience. He is slow, inconsistent, tires easily, and, at times, refuses to eat. The most effective approach to feeding the baby with hiatus hernia following surgery is a written care plan, followed by all, which focuses on his behavior in various positions "in arms," with different nipples, or at different times of the day. He often needs a very soft "premie" nipple. The plan also should consider finger foods for the older child. The mother should be included in feeding attempts, and information should be shared with her. It is especially discouraging for her to find any difficulty with feeding after surgery which she had hoped would eliminate the problem.

Recurrence of the hernia is common, but the symptoms are usually milder than before. Later, after the symptoms disappear, signs of esophageal stricture may develop.

Hirschsprung's Disease Also termed *megacolon* or *aganglionosis* of the large intestine, Hirschsprung's disease is identified and treated in infancy. It appears almost totally in Caucasian males but may occur in blacks and is familial, with two or three children sometimes affected in one family. The diseased bowel is most frequently located in the rectosigmoid area.

The specific cause of Hirschsprung's disease is a congenital absence of the *parasympathetic* nerve ganglion cells in the mesenteric *plexus* of the distal bowel. Affected bowel is unable to transmit coordinated peristaltic waves and to pass fecal material along its length. The *normal* portion of intestine proximal to it becomes hypertrophied and greatly dilated from the effect of peristalsis and the fecal mass which accumulates. The fecal mass impedes reabsorption of water and essential minerals through the colonic mucosa.

The usual presence of a transition area containing normally and abnormally innervated areas between the dilated bowel and the unused, narrow bowel creates a *conical* or funnel-shaped appearance, a diagnostic sign of the disease (Fig. 36-7). The transitional segment is often narrow, uneven, or "patchy," skipping areas of bowel. Defecation is controlled by the parasympathetic nervous system to which the internal and external sphincters, the anus, and the lower colon respond in a coordinated manner.

In the neonate, delay in the passage of meconium or the signs of intestinal obstruction are primary clinical manifestations. In older infants, who constitute a great majority of cases, the initial symptom is *obstinate constipation.* Intermittent, progressively increasing abdominal distention is present, and large fecal masses may be palpated. In later stages, if undiagnosed, the child looks chronically ill and has malnutrition, nausea, lethargy, anemia, and respiratory embarrassment on effort. The foul odor of breath and stool is striking. The presence of diarrhea may indicate enterocolitis and a rapidly worsening condition, accompanied by dehydration and electrolyte imbalance.

Barium enemas and abdominal x-rays should be done before treatment is begun. Attempts to clean, alter, or deflate the distended bowel may delay diagnosis. While a history and radiologic findings are conclusive, with less obvious clinical manifestations a full-thickness rectal biopsy is essential for diagnosis.

Since medical management of the disease is ineffective, creation of a transverse or sigmoid colostomy is the initial procedure done for most children. It serves to deflate and clean the bowel prior to further surgery, to enable the child's nutritional and general body condition to improve, and to postpone definitive surgery until more optimal age for a very small infant. Frozen-section biopsy at the colostomy site and in individually selected areas of the colon is done to gain more accurate knowledge about the extent of the problem. Prior to the colostomy procedure, the child receives stool softeners, liquid diet, and neomycin by mouth and instillation rectally. Removal of stool is done manually and by colonic irrigations.

Basically, each of the three major definitive operations consists of dissection of the dilated (not functional) bowel and the segment of aganglionic bowel and then anastomosis. They may be understood best by briefly describing the main steps of each which differ.

Swenson's pull-through After resection of the distended segment, the aganglionic portion and the rectum are everted through the anus. Then the normal bowel is brought down and sutured (a) as the aganglionic segment is excised and, finally, the normal bowel is sutured (b) to the anus and trimmed. The anastomosis *features two layers* (muscle and mucosa) and *pelvic dissection.*

Duhamel pull-through Following resection of the distended segment, a space is made retrorectally. The end of normal bowel is pulled into this space and through an incision made in the posterior rectal wall, then sutured side by side to the rectum. Two Kocher clamps or a Gross spur-crushing clamp, placed on the common wall, are left for 5 to 8 days until the wall sloughs. This anastomosis is done *intraabdominally,* avoiding the dangers of pelvic dissection, and retains an *intact external sphincter.*

Soave procedure This approach utilizes an *anorectal mucosa-exising* technique and *self-anastomosis* by the *bowel.* Intraabdominally, the seromuscular layer of the entire length of affected bowel is separated from the (inner) mucosal layer beginning at the proximal normal bowel downward while the same is done from the anus upward till the entire outer layer forms a "tube" detached from the inner bowel. The "tube" is brought out through a previously excised "circle" of anal tissue (internal and external sphincters) to the point of normal bowel but *not sutured.* The protruding bowel consists of aganglionic bowel and the distal distended portion. A rectal tube is inserted and left for 15 to 20 days till auto-anastomosis takes place. Protruding bowel is cauterized, under anesthesia. To avoid abdominal infection, no intraabdominal excision is used. The colostomy may be closed at the same time in any of the three, but complications may be avoided in some cases by waiting about two months and closing it separately. Long-range prognosis depends on the child's ability to return to normal diet, to thrive without more than usual susceptibility to gastrointestinal infection, and to achieve anal continence.

Nursing management To assist in rapid *diagnosis,* the nurse should make objective detailed written and verbal reports of the child's behavior, using knowledge of symptoms of the disease, in particular, observations of gastrointestinal tract manifestations (such as stooling, vomiting, abdominal distention), and indications of abdominal pain. Conversation with the parents, especially the mother, may elicit information about the disease which did not emerge in the doctor's history, especially since any child's behavior in feeding and stooling varies a great deal and the mother may attach no significance to these variations.

Rehydration and improvement of *nutrition,* although based on doctor's orders, are largely functions of nursing persistence preoperatively and postoperatively. After diagnosis of Hirschsprung's disease, intravenous fluids may be administered. These fluids are continued postoperatively until the operative area and/or bowel are ready for feedings, a few days after colostomy and 10 days or more after pull-through. Gastric decompression by nasogastric tube is carried out. The replacement of electrolytes in the fluid is always necessary because of the loss due to intestinal dysfunction and vomiting.

Some children will be allowed to take clear fluids or may be on a low-residue diet preoperatively. A variety of small, frequent feedings are offered. Normal diet can be resumed gradually postoperatively. These children are frequently "picky" feeders and have trouble establishing good eating habits. They have poor appetites, eat slowly, or become uncomfortable with abdominal distention after eating. The nurse must use judgment and initiate changes in the feeding technique. He should be aware that certain foods, given to a child, will mimic gastrointestinal symptoms (such as red jello, which will color the stool blood-red, and large amounts of some fruits, which may cause slight diarrhea).

A primary area of concern in gastrointestinal disease is *reestablishment* of *normal elimination.* Generally, elimination after surgery, including colostomy, will be diarrheic and flatulent. Observations of the infant (evidence of pain on elimination, abdominal distention, behavior during feeding) and accurate descriptions of early stools or alterations in the stool are especially important in determining whether the child is having normal progression toward formed stools. Diarrhea stools are measured by liquid container or by weighed diapers and are replaced in equal amounts in intravenous or oral fluids to prevent dehydration. Stool testing methods such as Labstix, guaiac, or Clinitest tablets should also be

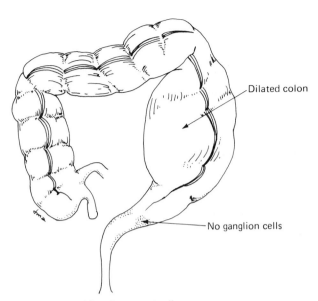

Figure 36-7 Hirschsprung's disease.

done till stools are considered normal. These data determine presence of sugar and blood which indicate abnormal intestinal function.

Perineal and anal excoriation always accompanies pull-through operations and diarrhea. Careful cleaning, frequent changing, and the use of ointments are usually adequate to minimize the occurrence and to heal the diaper area.

Hirschsprung's disease and many gastrointestinal diseases have an *emotional impact* due to peculiarities in their manifestations and treatment as well as to the effects any illness causes. Postoperatively the baby may be irritable, crying for long periods, not comforted easily, and pale and sick looking. The numerous "attachments" (nasogastric tube, rectal tube in Soave pull-through) mean less handling, less activity, and immobilization in bed. Therefore the effects of this immobility must be recognized.

Feeding fulfills emotional needs as well as physical needs. The need to suck is often overwhelming to a baby. Deprivation for long periods can cause him to be unhappy and fussy or withdrawn. A pacifier may be used, or the infant may be held as if he were being fed. The satisfactions which an older child gets from feedings must be remembered, and substitutions given to him.

The nurse must give the parents practical help and steps for colostomy care, perhaps for gastrostomy care, and for dilations of the anus if they are to be done at home.

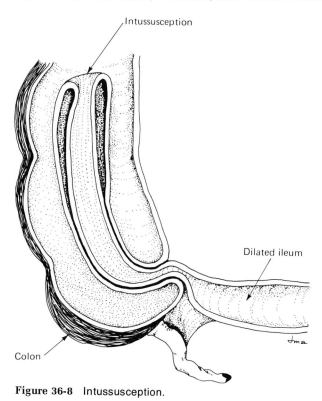

Figure 36-8 Intussusception.

Intussusception   Intussusception is the invagination or telescoping of a portion of the small intestine or colon into a more distal segment of the intestine (Fig. 36-8). It is rare in infants under 6 months of age and occurs equally in infants between 6 to 12 months and children between 1 and 2 years of age. It affects Caucasian males most frequently.

The cause is unknown, but it may be related to disturbances in intestinal motility (such as cystic fibrosis, infection, or recent abdominal surgery or injury). Generally, acute enteritis, Meckel's diverticulum, polyps, cysts, and malrotation are cited as predisposing factors in occurrence of the illness.

The onset is sudden in an otherwise healthy child. Symptoms are vomiting, paroxysmal colicky abdominal pain, and stools which resemble "current jelly" (brown, bloody, mucoid material). The baby responds to the pain by loud, shrill crying, paleness, and pulling his legs up sharply. A sausage-shaped mass along the course of the ascending or transverse colon can be palpated, and an x-ray of the abdomen demonstrates a "staircase pattern" of air in the bowel, confirming the diagnosis.

Nursing management   During the first 24 to 48 hours, barium enema is used to reduce the telescoped bowel by hydrostatic pressure. Symptoms abate immediately, normal feedings are resumed within 24 hours, and the baby is discharged. If symptoms continue, surgery is indicated. During surgery, manual reduction is usually successful. Intestinal resection may be necessary if the lesion is irreducible or the intestine has been irreparably damaged. Preoperatively and postoperatively, the nurse must manage intravenous fluids and nasogastric decompression, position the infant, and care for the suture line to prevent infection and reduce the stress factor.

Malrotation and Volvulus   Within the intimate and interdependent development of the abdomen, a high small-bowel obstruction may develop from three separate but related abnormalities. Malrotation of the colon, volvulus of the midgut, and adhesive bands which constrict the duodenum are most commonly found together (Fig. 36-9). This combination affects mainly newborns, then infants under 6 months of age, and last, children older than 6 months.

During the tenth week of fetal life, the cecum normally rotates into the lower right quadrant while the mesentery of the ascending colon fixes to the posterior abdominal wall. If the cecum remains in the upper right quadrant, it has malrotated, pulling the duodenum out of position and causing partial obstruction. Duodenal bands fix the cecum to the abnormal site. Since the mesentery remains unattached or not firmly attached, the small intestine twists (volvulus) around the base of the mesentery, causing a strangulation of the bowel, occluding the superior mesenteric blood vessels. Symptoms are due to the occlusion as well as the bowel obstruction.

Bile-stained vomitus, pain, and diminished or absent stools are the primary symptoms. Mucus and blood may seep from the rectum because of strangulated bowel. The infant exhibits signs of shock or infection. A high obstruction causes greater loss of pancreatic and gastric secretions and bile so that the baby is more likely to have rapid electrolyte imbalance, determined by blood gas levels and blood electrolyte levels. The volvulus may be palpable. Upper gastrointestinal films and barium enema aid in differentiating this illness from duodenal obstruction or high intestinal atresia.

Surgical and nursing management   The Ladd procedure, a definitive operation for this condition, consists of reducing the volvulus, dividing the bands compressing the duodenum, and mobilizing the cecum. Resection is necessary if ischemia or necrosis is present in the bowel.

Management includes intravenous fluids and gastric decompression, until peristalsis and normal stooling take place. Feedings are begun then and increased gradually. The nurse must observe for complications of abdominal surgery.

Pyloric Stenosis This condition occurs predominantly in male infants, and frequently in first-born children. Heredity or familial predisposing factors have not been proved to be significant, but the incidence in offspring of mothers who had the disease as infants is high. Vomiting begins soon after birth or in the following 4 to 6 weeks. It may be gradual and intermittent or sudden and severe. In a small number of infants, the onset of vomiting begins as late as 2 to 3 months of age. Peristaltic waves passing left to right are visible during or immediately after a feeding. In the majority of cases, the hypertrophied pylorus, about the size of an olive, can be palpated in the upper right quadrant. If the vomiting continues untreated, dehydration, malnutrition with weight loss, and alkalosis result. A conclusive diagnosis is made by x-ray which demonstrates gastric retention with an elongated and narrow antrum of the pylorus.

Initially, spasm of the circular muscle around the pylorus occurs followed by a progressive hypertrophy which develops in a day or two. Various studies attribute cause of the spasm to degeneration of the nerves of the stomach and pylorus; failure of development of either the nerves or the muscle itself; tonic contraction of the muscle. The definitive treatment for pyloric stenosis is the Fredet-Ramstedt procedure. The hypertrophied muscles are split down to, but not through, the submucosa and parallel to the pyloric lumen. The procedure is done immediately if the infant is well hydrated and in electrolyte balance. Intravenous fluids and often gastric decompression are begun prior to surgery and continued for 1 or 2 days postoperatively. In moderate to severe cases, preoperative treatment also includes monitoring blood gas and blood electrolyte levels at 4- to 8-hour intervals until the infant's condition is stable enough for surgery. Within 2 days after surgery, oral feedings are introduced beginning with 5 percent glucose and water. After progression to full-strength formula, amounts are increased every few feedings up to a normal amount for age. Some vomiting may occur postoperatively.

Some physicians treat the disease medically by

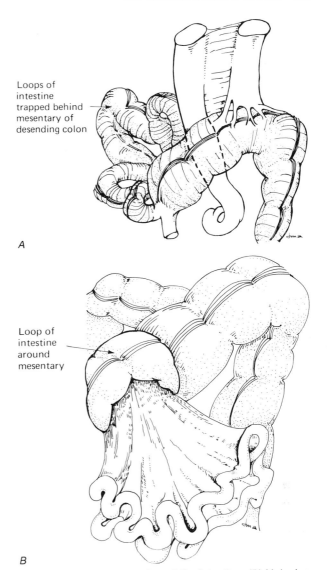

Loops of intestine trapped behind mesentary of desending colon

A

Loop of intestine around mesentary

B

Figure 36-9 (*A*) Malrotation of the intestine. (*B*) Volvulus.

antispasmodic drugs; changes in amount, frequency, and thickness of feedings; and changes in position of the infant after feeding. If there is no improvement, surgery is performed.

Nursing management Preoperative and postoperative nursing emphasis should be on careful control of intravenous fluids, gastric decompression, and observations of the baby's response to treatment. However, a major nursing responsibility involves reinstitution of oral feedings. A nurse's observations will help the physician determine the baby's readiness for increases in amount and strength of feedings. The nurse should burp the baby when necessary, and the nipple selected for use should not allow the flow of milk to be too fast. Positioning after feeding is not a major factor in retention of the formula.

Since the mother has become negatively conditioned to the baby's constant vomiting, she is hesitant and nervous about feeding him, which may contribute to a higher postoperative incidence of vomiting. It is important that she participate in hospital feeding.

Diseases of Lower Incidence in the Infant

Chalasia of the Esophagus Infrequently, between about the third to tenth days of a baby's life, the cardiac sphincter muscle fails to function, causing it to be relaxed and patent constantly and beginning a period of prolonged, repeated nonprojectile vomiting. The vomiting is more pronounced when the baby is lying down. Often, he is hungry afterward. Pressure on the baby's abdomen produces reflux into the esophagus. Aspiration of vomitus may complicate the problem. Constant irritation by gastric contents erodes the esophagus to the extent that peptic esophagitis may develop.

Treatment consists of offering thickened feedings and placing the baby in an erect position for ½ hour after each feeding, usually in an adjustable plastic seat. After 6 weeks to 2 months, treatment may be discontinued with no recurrence.

Annular Pancreas In rare instances, fusion of anterior and posterior pancreatic tissue during fetal development forms a ring of pancreatic tissue around the duodenum. It is frequently associated with duodenal atresia or stenosis in the newborn or may constrict the duodenum causing obstruction. The common bile duct may also be blocked by the ring. Clinical manifestations are those of high intestinal obstruction with jaundice if the bile ducts are affected. Associated abnormalities may be present.

Surgical division of the ring has been unsuccessful, and a high number of cases develop pancreatic fistulas. A bypass operation (duodenojejunum) relieves the obstruction but does not interfere with gastric functions. This operation is also used to correct any existing duodenal stenosis or atresia.

Nursing management of both preoperative and postoperative care is the same as that of babies with intestinal atresia. Recovery is complete in most cases with no further problems.

Biliary Atresia Congenital atresia of the bile ducts results from one of several anatomic fetal malformations such as complete failure of the bile ducts to develop, bile ducts which are ribbonlike and unopened, or the development of bile ducts which end in a blind pouch. Bile builds up in the liver because it lacks passage to the intestine.

Persistent jaundice in a newborn is the primary symptom. An elevated *direct bilirubin* test distinguishes liver disease from blood incompatibilities. The infant has clay-colored stools and darkly pigmented urine, both more striking in biliary atresia. A rose bengal test is always positive with biliary atresia. If diagnosis and treatment of biliary atresia are delayed longer than 2 months, the liver may be permanently damaged.

The diagnostic test must be exploratory laparotomy with liver biopsy and x-rays of the bile ducts during surgery. If the bile duct ends in a blind pouch, the surgeon is able to suture the end to the intestine, which will relieve the jaundice, but it is not definitive surgery. Liver transplantation is still unproved but may be an answer for treatment in the future.

Nursing management Nursing observation can help greatly in diagnosis. The nurse observes and records color and consistency of stools, tests them for bile, and may need to save them for examination by the doctor or the laboratory. The nurse must bear in mind that the urine's dark pigment may discolor the stool. He may need to take steps to separate the two by urine collection. Preoperatively, the baby is fed orally and maintained on intravenous fluids. Injections of vitamin K are given to prevent excess bleeding.

Postoperatively, nasogastric decompression and intravenous fluids are continued for only a few days till feedings can be resumed. The risk of pulmonary infections is higher with biliary atresia, and so the nurse must reposition the baby frequently and do nasopharyngeal suctioning when needed. Itching of the skin is extreme, but it may be soothed by lotions. The nurse may need to cover the baby's hands with mittens and keep his fingernails trimmed to prevent him from excoriating his skin with scratching. These babies are very irritable and uncomfortable. They require extra comfort, holding, and gentleness from the nurse.

Although these children may live for several years, there is no treatment to prolong life. They may return to the hospital frequently for relief of ascites, infections, or gastrointestinal bleeding due to esophageal varices.

Curd Obstruction Lower intestinal obstruction which appears in normal newborns 5 to 14 days after normal feeding and stooling have been established is a recent finding. The obstruction is caused by an extremely sticky milk curd in the lower ileum (a lacto-bezoar). It is postulated that modern newborns are breast fed less and are given early feedings high in fat, protein, and calories. The infants have a slight, transient absorption deficit which produces symptoms if they are given highly concentrated feedings.

In a few cases, repeated enemas are effective. In most cases, a laparotomy with wash-out of affected intestine is necessary. The nursing approach to care of the babies preoperatively and postoperatively is the same as with other intestinal obstructions. The infants recover completely and are not affected in later life.

Pierre Robin Syndrome The occurrence of Pierre Robin syndrome is higher in families with a history of cleft palate but the chance of a familial pattern is small compared with that of cleft lip or cleft palate. The syndrome has three features: cleft palate, a tongue which falls back on the pharynx (*glossoptosis*), and an underdeveloped mandible. Diagnosis can be made on the basis of physical appearance along with the symptoms of obstruction during respirations. Obstruction occurs especially during inspiration, since the tongue lies against the posterior pharyngeal wall and the epiglottis and is pulled back and down during inspiration. Choking, cyanosis, struggling, and severe retraction in intercostal spaces and substernal and suprasternal areas result. The respiratory problem is more acute when the infant is quiet because of the flaccidity of the tongue.

Nursing management The anatomic features account for the two most immediate objectives in care, establishment of feeding and adequate respiration. Generally, these problems involve nursing management.

The baby is placed in a prone position in the bed so that the tongue and jaw fall forward. The nurse must position the baby's neck at varying degrees of hyperextension and elevate his upper trunk slightly to achieve better positioning of his head. Subtle differences in positioning for each baby give him maximum aid in respiration for the first 5 to 7 days of life. He may require nasopharyngeal suction whenever large amounts of thick mucus are present.

In a minority of cases, traction to hold the tongue forward may be required for the first week of life. It is accomplished by silk suture through the tip of the tongue pulling the tongue forward by means of weights on the end of the suture or by securing the end of the suture string on the baby's chest or chin. It is important to observe for hermorrhage, slipping, or cutting of the tongue by the suture and for infection.

The nurse uses a feeding technique which considers the cleft palate, the glossoptosis, and the respiratory effort. The baby is able to take oral feedings from a bottle. He is fed in a vertical position, often very slightly forward, so that he must push his jaw forward to suck (*orthostatic feeding* position). As his head rests in the nurse's hand, he can use gentle finger pressure at the attachment of the mandible on one or both sides to aid in bringing the jaw forward. The baby eats slowly, tires easily, and must be allowed to suck at his own pace. Since a cleft palate is present, this infant's feeding technique should be similar to babies with that defect. The nurse plays an important role in helping parents realize that the baby's respiratory difficulties can be minimized or eliminated through the use of techniques and precautions described.

Within 3 or 4 months, the mandible grows to accommodate the tongue, and by 1 year of age its appearance is normal, except in very severe cases. Weight gain is often slow and ear infections may occur frequently because of the cleft palate. Speech and dental correction may also be needed in the early years of the child's life because of the cleft palate.

Omphalitis The umbilical cord may become contaminated owing to prematurely ruptured maternal membranes during the birth process or severance of the cord, resulting in infection of the cord and umbilical area in the newborn. A local swelling with redness, tenderness, and, often, seropurulent discharge develops. Similar symptoms on other areas of the trunk indicate spread of the infection.

If the infection travels through the patent lumen of the obliterated umbilical arteries, lower abdominal wall infection, peritonitis, and septicemia result. Infiltration of the portal vein and inferior vena cava may cause umbilical vein thrombosis and extrahepatic portal obstruction. Lymphatic vessels carry the infection to the lower or upper abdominal wall and lower thoracic area, resulting in extensive cellulitis.

For these reasons, treatment must be vigorous and thorough to cure the infection. Mild cases may be treated effectively with silver nitrate applicators two or three times and regular cleansing. For moderate to severe infection, hospitalization is necessary to administer intravenous antibiotics which are continued until the symptoms have subsided. Warm saline compresses may be used. Drainage of abscesses and excision of necrosis may be necessary. The nurse must review with the parents the regular cleansing which will be required after discharge while helping to alleviate any feeling of the mother that the infection "is all her fault."

Rumination In this illness there is no pathologic condition in the gastrointestinal tract, but vomiting is the presenting symptom. It has a psychologic cause and is the result of a disturbed mother-infant relationship. Vomiting takes place in numerous very small amounts of clear watery fluid over several hours after feedings or during the entire time between feedings. It is accompanied by finger sucking, pacifier sucking, or active movements of the mouth (such as churning tongue). Often the older baby appears to be gagging himself, and he may stop when vocal disapproval is shown by the adult. A frequent report from the mother is that the child "reswallows" his vomitus. Subsequently, there may be chronic malnutrition with "starvation stools" and weight loss. Constant irritation of the nasopharyngeal area and the presence of the vomitus in the nasopharynx give rise to the symptoms of chronic upper respiratory problems. In older babies, if the condition continues unabated, esophagitis and a patent cardiac sphincter, which allows a reflux of stomach contents, develop, presenting further problems (see Fig. 36-10).

The disease may be recognized by a combination of negative test results for other causes of vomiting plus improvement under therapy for rumination. A dual approach of working with the child and with the mother is instituted. Therapy for the child is aimed at providing those elements missing to make eating a satisfying experience and at substituting acceptable hand and mouth pleasures (cooing, smiling, sucking, tactile experience) for the unacceptable hand-mouth activity of rumination. Intensive therapy will produce changes including cessation of vomiting in 7 to 10 days.

GASTROINTESTINAL DISEASES IN THE TODDLER AND PRESCHOOLER
Diseases of Higher Incidence

Foreign Bodies in the Gastrointestinal Tract During the inquisitive years of toddlerhood, children frequently ingest objects which cannot be digested. Pins, parts of toys, and buttons are the items most commonly swallowed. Most objects pass spontaneously from the gastrointestinal tract, but objects which are long or sharp may present serious difficulty. The child should be hospitalized for ingestion of any sharp object. *Bezoars,* thickly matted masses of materials whose structure makes digestion impossible, are more troublesome foreign bodies.

After ingestion, the child does not necessarily experience dysphagia, although the object remains in the esophagus. The most common areas in the gastrointestinal tract where objects lodge are the esophagus at the cricopharyngeal level, the aortic level, and the upper diaphragmatic area. These objects can be removed easily by esophagoscopy under general anesthesia after being visualized on chest roentgenogram. After 24 hours observation, the child is usually discharged.

If the object lodges in the stomach, the child can be observed for passage. It should pass through the pylorus in 5 days or less. Surgical intervention may be necessary if x-rays reveal retention within any area of the gastrointestinal tract. Bobby pins and long objects have particular difficulty passing through the duodenum because of its U shape. Coins and other large objects may remain at the pylorus or the ileocecal valve. The appendix and the rectum are two other common areas of difficult passage. Objects in the rectum are accessible to proctoscopy. The child's stool should be checked carefully during this time. Repeat roentgenograms monitor the passage.

There are three types of bezoars which develop in the stomach or, less frequently, the small bowel. *Phytobezoars* consist of vegetable matter. *Trichobezoars,* the most common, are balls of hair, occur in girls more than boys, and are the result of *pica.* This type frequently is seen in children who are emotionally disturbed or severely retarded. In both types, the child complains of vague abdominal pain, vomits, and develops anorexia which leads to weight loss. A laparotomy for removal is necessary. If pica is the primary problem, investigation and treatment directed toward its elimination should be undertaken in otherwise normal children. The third type, *lactobezoars,* has been described under "Curd Obstruction" above.

Nursing management Many times, especially since the predominant age group is under 5 years, the hospitalization and procedures are more upsetting than the object itself, a fact that should guide the nurse in caring for the child. Preparation before surgery and care afterward are largely according to the

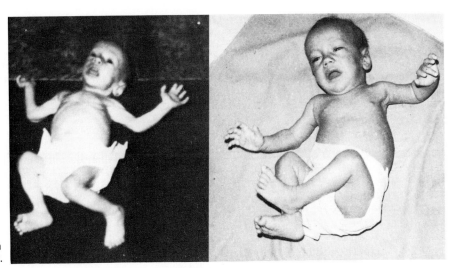

Figure 36-10 Rumination. (*Left*) Baby 1 week before admission. (*Right*) Same baby on day of discharge 3 weeks later.

operative procedure, and observation for complications plays an important role. Humidity by croup tent or mask may be needed if esophagoscopy is done. After abdominal surgery, intravenous fluids and nasogastric tube for gastric decompression are used for 1 to 3 days, generally before oral fluids may be started. Resumption of normal activity is fairly rapid. The child's parents often feel guilty, and they need to know that medical personnel do not consider it their fault. Since the child is well to begin with, recovery is fast and complete.

Intestinal Parasites[7]   The intestinal parasites found commonly in North America are classified under two types: Protozoa and helminths, the latter including roundworms and tapeworms.[8] Southern areas have the highest incidence. Preschoolers seem most susceptible to all types, with the exception of pinworms. Fecal contamination of food, soil, water, and hands begins each infestation, although cycles differ with different types. Hospitalization occurs infrequently.

Protozoa   *Amebiasis* occurs only in subtropical areas and, particularly, in areas of poor sanitation. After ingestion of contaminated material, the organisms remain in the large intestine, causing diarrhea and blood-streaked stools. A stool smear can verify its presence. Treatment by the drug metronidazole is effective.

Nematodes (roundworms)   In general, roundworms cause symptoms of gastroenteritis. *Ascariasis* occurs mainly in Southern areas. Infection with *Ascaris* starts with the eggs, which are present in topsoil

contaminated with feces. After the eggs are ingested, they hatch in the duodenum. The larvae pass through the intestinal wall into the bloodstream, are carried via the portal system to the liver, are carried to the lungs, and migrate up to the epiglottis. After they are swallowed, they remain and develop into adults in the small intestine, causing colicky pain. The child may eliminate a worm, pencil size, in vomitus or stool. Complications are rare but may develop because of the bulk of the roundworm (intestinal obstruction, acute appendicitis, intussusception, or intestinal perforation) or to unusual extraintestinal migration of larvae (pneumonia, jaundice, or hepatomegaly). Treatment with piperazine citrate once and again 2 days later eliminates the parasite.

Oxyuriasis, or pinworm infection, is found most commonly in schoolchildren. After initial infestation, the 2- to 12-mm worm attaches itself to the mucosa of the cecum and appendix. Females migrate at night down the intestine, crawl outside, and deposit their eggs on the perianal area and perineum. Since the most common and persistent symptom is anal pruritis, the eggs are carried back to the mouth, are ingested, hatch in the duodenum, and pass to the cecum. Local perianal infection, vaginitis, and salpingitis may develop from scratching of the anus. Diagnosis is confirmed by collection of pinworms with the clear cellulose tape method (placing the tape on the perianal area less than a minute, preferably at night or early morning), then examination on a slide covered with toluene under a microscope. The entire family must be treated and observe thorough personal hygiene. The mother may help the child refrain from scratching by frequent washing of the anal area and using a spray especially to prevent itching. If drug treatment is necessary, pyrvinium pamoate is used in one dose and another dose 2 weeks later or piperazine citrate daily for 7 days.

Whipworm (*Trichuris trichiuria*), a roundworm, is very small, transparent, and lives only in human beings. After ingestion, eggs hatch in the duodenum, migrate to the cecum, and attach themselves to the wall causing an inflammatory reaction at the point of each attachment. It occurs more frequently in ages 1 to 4 years and in malnourished children. Mild cases may remain asymptomatic and need no treatment. More severe cases have gastrointestinal symptoms, diarrhea in particular which may become chronic. The worms will appear on stool smear and may be visually apparent on proctoscopic examination. The drug thiabendazole, given two times a day for 2 days, is used for moderate to severe cases. A 0.1 percent solution of hexylresorcinol may be given as an enema, the amount depending on the child's size.

Cestodes (tapeworms) When human beings ingest meat infected with encysted larvae of the beef tapeworm (*Taenia saginata*) or the pork tapeworm (*T. solium*), they develop *taeniasis*. The ingested larvae hatch in the small intestine where they attach themselves to the wall. Clinical manifestations are diarrhea, "hunger pain," increased appetite, loss of weight, and eosinophilia. The tapeworms are very long and may cause obstruction if they mass in the intestinal lumen. Segments may break off and obstruct the appendix. The pork tapeworm may cause more serious complications when the larva migrate extraintestinally and form cysts in other tissues, especially eye, brain, and muscle causing permanent damage (cysticercosis).

The drug of choice is quinacrine orally or by duodenal tube which gives a greater concentration of the drug in the intestine. Four doses, 10 minutes apart, are administered. Saline in large amounts to flush the gastrointestinal tract is given about 2 hours later. Another drug, niclosamide, in a single dose may be used for treatment of beef tapeworm but not pork, since the drug renders the tapeworm digestible and digestion of the pork tapeworms may release eggs whose larval stage will cause cysticercosis. Prevention relies on thorough cooking of meat and adequate sanitation.

The fish tapeworm, *Diphyllobothrium latum,* is even longer than the beef and pork tapeworms and infests man through ingestion of raw fish. Eggs incubate in contaminated water and are eaten by water fleas which transmit the larvae to fish. Macrocytic anemia is a common finding in the infected per-son. Other symptoms and treatment are the same as those given above.

The nurse's role, especially that of the office nurse, public health nurse, and school nurse, is one of teaching good personal and environmental hygiene, emphasizing the reasons for its importance.

Lye Ingestion, Corrosive Esophagitis, and Gastritis
The ingestion of any strong chemical or highly acidic or alkaloid material will cause immediate inflammatory reaction or damage (burns, ulcerations) to the mucosal lining of the upper gastrointestinal tract. Probably the most common material ingested is lye, although, in the last few years, awareness of the problem has influenced a change in content of alkaloid products, and the most dangerous ones with high lye content are no longer made. Cleaning products, liquid or powder, for any purpose, should be placed out of reach of children, preferably in a locked cupboard because they are the products which most commonly cause corrosive esophagitis. Recent studies support the theory that ingestions of obviously nonedible chemicals are accidents with a psychologic base.

As the child swallows, after ingestion, he experiences immediate burning pain in his mouth and throat, and chest if contact takes place further into the esophagus as it does with liquid. He is usually unable to swallow afterward. If the material is powdered, damage may be limited to the oropharyngeal area only. Crystal forms dissolve in the mouth, combining with saliva and causing burns for the few minutes after ingestion. If the child is given water after crystal ingestion, it may add to the problem.

Treatment Immediate action is to neutralize the action of the chemical. Admission to the hospital is necessary to determine the extent of the burns. The child is given pain medication and placed in a humidity tent. Fluids and foods are withheld until an esophagoscopy can be done. If burns are not extensive, antacids are given frequently and regularly. Steroids are used to decrease inflammation and scarring. The length of steroid treatment varies with the severity of the burns. If the child can eat, he is allowed only fluids, clear or full liquid, until inflammation is under control. Then he is advanced to soft, nonabrasive foods or to a normal diet. Bed rest is not necessary. If the child is unable to swallow, he must be positioned so that saliva runs out, and he may need careful suctioning. Soothing ointments and creams may be used on the external burns of the mouth.

Mercury dilation is instituted to prevent esophageal stricture as soon as inflammation has subsided. In severe burns, regular dilation may continue for months or years to combat unpreventable stricture. A gastrostomy may be necessary in severe cases. Colon interposition, as used for esophageal atresia, is done when other treatment proves unsuccessful.

In most children, the burns are not extensive and treatment is limited to the immediate treatment with, perhaps, a short course of dilation. Even in mild cases, the child is frightened, the parents guilt-ridden and shocked, and both need understanding.

Corrosive gastritis Only a small number of children who swallow chemicals develop gastritis. Large amounts of ferrous sulfate and calcium chloride, especially, cause severe reactions. As the chemical enters the stomach, it causes immediate pyloro-spasm followed by edema and superficial ulcers. The child's vomitus is often blood streaked, and he has abdominal pain. The treatment is the same as that for peptic ulcer and may include intravenous fluids and antibiotics. In severe cases, obstruction of the intestine or perforation of the stomach and peritonitis may occur (see Chap. 16).

Meckel's Diverticulum As a result of incomplete obliteration of the yolk stalk which feeds the embryo in early weeks of fetal life, portions of the stalk remain and create several abnormalities in the gastrointestinal tract. Meckel's diverticulum, an outpouching on the terminal ileum, is the most common (Fig. 36-11). Adhesive bands (Meckel's bands) also may join the diverticulum to the umbilicus. Occasionally, a fistula follows the same path to the umbilicus as the bands.

The abnormality often remains asymptomatic and is discovered incidental to treatment for other illness. Painless rectal bleeding is the major symptom, often massive. If bleeding progresses, the child may bleed into shock. Meckel's diverticulum may cause intestinal obstruction, perforation, and peritonitis. Decision to operate is based on the extent of bleeding evidenced. Generally, excision by wedge resection of the intestine at the location of the diverticulum and anastomosis is the procedure of choice. In instances of massive bleeding, blood transfusions are necessary.

Nursing management The principle nursing concern is observation to prevent hemorrhage and

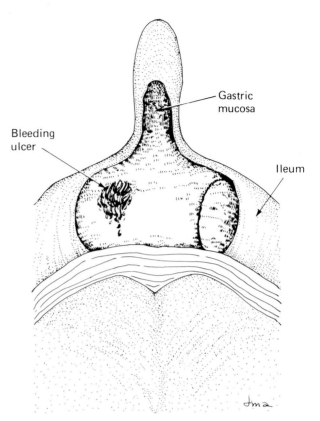

Figure 36-11 Meckel's diverticulum.

shock. Vital signs, blood pressure, skin color, and volume of blood in the stool are important gauges of the child's condition. Labstix and guaiac tests performed by the nurse on each stool can determine the amount of blood present. In the immediate postoperative period, the child will need gastric decompression by nasogastric catheter and intravenous fluids until eating is resumed. Other precautions, observations, nursing techniques, and reassurance to the parents are those of any intestinal operation. Recovery is usually complete with no further problem and no recurrence.

Polyps of the Intestine Generally, polyps in a child are not premalignant and occur most commonly in the colon, although they can occur in other sections of the intestines. Symptoms are extremely rare in infancy and most common in preschool and school-age children. Bright red rectal bleeding, either frank or as spots on the stool, with no pain in an apparently healthy child is a diagnostic manifestation. Intermittent diarrhea and mucus from the rectum also may occur. The cause is idiopathic.

Diagnosis is made by proctoscopy, although barium enema is used if polyps are obscure and hard to see. Simple excision is accomplished through a sigmoidoscope under anesthesia. Some doctors feel that the presence of polyps in scattered positions suggest a developing polyposis and the child should be observed for a few years. All polyps should be removed before the age of 15 since adult polyps are often precancerous. Polyps high in the intestine may require laparotomy for excision.

Physical care of the child is minimal since hospitalization is usually no longer than 2 days. If the hospital has a short-term (less than a day) surgical unit, the child will be admitted there. The child will be allowed up and have a normal diet by the end of the day and usually has no pain. On admission, he and his family may be exceptionally apprehensive because of the rectal bleeding which they see. They need to know what will be done and, especially, that bleeding will not appear after surgery.

Focus on nursing treatment will vary depending on the surgery done, whether simple excision, colectomy, or more extensive surgery. Hemorrhage after excision is the most frequent, as well as the better known, complication of any laparotomy or resection. The nurse's assistance in helping the child and his family learn to adjust his roughage-controlled diet, to care for an ileostomy, if present, and to allow the child to live as normally as possible is most valuable to them.

Portal Hypertension with Esophageal Varices[9] The first sign of portal hypertension, the result of blockage in the portal venous system, most often appears in early childhood. Since venous blood from the digestive system empties first into the portal system which then carries it to the inferior vena cava, any blockage in this system will impede this flow of blood. The veins that normally empty into the portal system become engorged, dilated, and tortuous as the blood they carry backs up and attempts to find *collateral* pathways to the vena cava. The veins in the esophagus develop esophageal varices which may bleed massively and suddenly or may ooze small amounts over a period of time.

The site of the obstruction and the extent of liver damage are factors which influence the prognosis and management. The most common cause of portal hypertension in children is *extrahepatic* obstruction caused by congenital stenosis of venous channels, adhesions constricting the vessels, or thrombosis of splenic or portal veins. The principle *intrahepatic* cause is cirrhosis of the liver. Death in children with this disease is most often due to hepatic coma.

Esophagoscopy and barium swallow roentenogram will confirm the diagnosis and aid in determining the extent of the esophageal varices. A splenoportogram, done under anesthesia, identifies the obstruction site and aids in planning further management of the disease. Tissue obtained by needle biopsy of the liver is normal in extrahepatic and abnormal in intrahepatic obstructions. A battery of liver function tests further determines the extent of liver damage.

About 75 percent of children with portal hypertension and esophageal varices have their first bleeding episode before 7 years of age.[10] Children who have extrahepatic obstruction experience earlier and more frequent bleeding. Large, tarry stools may be the first indication that bleeding has begun, followed by hematemesis. The clinical manifestation most associated with esophageal varices is massive vomiting of bright red blood. The causes may be (1) gastric acid eroding the varices in the lower esophagus, (2) irritation of the varices by bulky or rough-textured food, (3) an increase in pressure in the area of the varices, perhaps from coughing, or (4) ingestion of aspirin.

Any bleeding must be treated immediately. The stomach should be irrigated with large amounts of iced normal saline via a nasogastric tube and bulb syringe. A decrease in or cessation of bleeding should be apparent during or soon after the irrigation. This treatment may be repeated, but, if bleeding continues, the *Sengstaken-Blakemore tube* is necessary (Fig. 36-12).

Since the tube has inflatable balloons, it must be tested for function before it is inserted through the nares. Once in place, the tube remains for 24 to 48 hours before there is danger of ulceration. The tube must be tightly taped so that it does not slip up (airway obstruction or esophageal rupture) or slip down (eliminating pressure on the cardiac sphincter and lower esophagus). A form of traction may be used to maintain the position. If the tube is to be left in place for a longer period of time, it must be deflated every 6 to 8 hours for about 10 minutes, and deflated for several hours before removal.

The procedure is frightening to the smaller child and very uncomfortable even for the older child. Thorough explanation and much reassurance must be given to the patient. No sedatives are given in the presence of bleeding, and so the nursing approach is doubly important. With the tube in place, the child cannot swallow his saliva, and therefore it is expectorated or suctioned out. Positioning him on his side is important. Elevating the head of the bed relieves the discomfort of the tube. Restraint may be

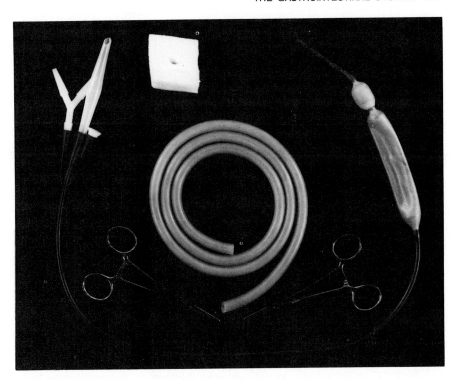

Figure 36-12 Sengstaken-Blakemore tube used to treat esophageal varices.

necessary. Antibiotics are administered prophylactically. Sometimes the posterior pituitary hormone, *Pitressin,* is administered intravenously to produce vasoconstriction.

Conservative treatment and nursing management Since symptoms occur early and operative procedures for shunting are more successful in the older child, management is aimed at medical maintenance, for as long as possible, particularly in children under 6 years of age. Admission to the hospital is usually due to bleeding, and is supported by administration of blood, intramuscular vitamin K, and iron preparations. If the blood ammonia level is very high, a *low-protein,* low-fat, high-carbohydrate diet is given. The amount of diet protein is increased as the child's condition stabilizes and bleeding is controlled. Some doctors prefer bland, soft foods, in an attempt to prevent bleeding. The child in hepatic coma will need hyperalimentation and other intravenous fluids, central venous pressure lines, regular monitoring of vital signs, liver function tests, and determination of blood gases and electrolytes. Nursing observation should include describing a child's orientation to his surroundings and behavior as well as his level of consciousness.

As the child convalesces, activity, fluids, salt, and diet will all be restricted, according to his condi-

tion. To protect the child from upper respiratory tract infection, the physician may limit activities including where and when he can go outside his home. With such restrictions, the child may become uncooperative, negative, demanding, or withdrawn. The nurse can help by talking to him on his own level about his illness and the reasons for the restrictions, and helping him to voice his anger about them. Recovery to the point of adequate health is possible but depends on the age at which symptoms develop, the severity of the secondary manifestations (liver damage and esophageal varices), and the success of the surgical procedure when it is done. Injection of the varices with a sclerosing solution under esophagoscopy may temporarily control bleeding, but future attempts to establish shunting will be difficult because of obliterated blood vessels. A transthoracic ligation of the esophageal varices is temporarily effective for controlling the bleeding in a child who is too young, too ill, or unsuitable for a shunt procedure.

Surgical intervention The *portocaval anastomosis* is the most successful shunting procedure in children over 5 years and the procedure of choice for intrahepatic obstruction. The portal vein is anastomosed side to side or end to side of the inferior vena cava, so that blood bypasses the liver. Indications for performing the surgery are hemorrhage from varices, large esophageal varices (even though not bleeding), and increasing ascites.

The most successful intervention for extrahepatic obstruction is the *splenorenal anastomosis* when the proximal end of the divided splenic vein is anastomosed to the side of the left renal vein. In children under 10 years of age, the splenic veins are too small and will thrombose, and so the operation is done only for older children. Indications for surgery are repeated hemorrhage, esophageal varices, splenomegaly, and hypersplenism. When shunts are not possible, colon replacement with esophagogastrectomy (resection of the esophageal varices) is a last resort.

Diseases of Lower Incidence

Acute Hydrops of the Gallbladder   Still unusual but increasing in incidence, acute dilation of the gallbladder without gallstones or an obvious inflammatory disease occurs, generally, in the late preschool-age period but can occur in infancy and the school-age period. The symptoms are the same as those of many acute obstructive gastrointestinal conditions, and diagnosis is often made at the time of surgery. A mass in the upper right quadrant is present in more than half the cases.

The cause is unknown. The gallbladder is large, distended, and edematous, and various degrees of inflammation are present. The bile is sterile. Anatomic abnormality of the cystic duct has been suggested as a cause. Other findings point to an infectious process which causes decreased drainage of the gallbladder or actual kinking of the cystic duct. Enlargement of adjacent lymph nodes often accompanies the condition.

Various types of treatment have been used. Simple aspiration, cholecystotomy drainage of the gallbladder (the preferred treatment), and cholecystectomy have all proved successful. The postoperative course is usually uncomplicated, and, following drainage procedures, gallbladder function returns to normal.

Nursing management   Preoperative preparation and postoperative care are the same as for any acute abdominal surgery. Feedings and activity can be gradually resumed within a few days. Cholecystotomy drainage may present a challenge to the nurse because the patient is often too young to understand or too frightened to leave the tubing undisturbed unless the nurse takes time and effort to help

him. Since children are inclined to be active even in bed, the nurse must take special precautions to maintain a sterile and intact dressing and to prevent the tube from being pulled out. Very active hand play and as much body mobility, including walking, as can be arranged are much more effective than constant restraints. The concerns of the child's parents will be alleviated by the knowledge that, once the acute convalescence is over, he will have no further problem.

Celiac Disease[11]   Gluten enteropathy, commonly called *celiac disease* or *sprue,* is a symptom complex resulting from generalized malabsorption. It is most common in children between 18 months and 2 years of age. The inability to absorb rye or wheat gluten might be hereditary, or it may result from a constitutional tendency, may be environmentally caused, or both. Theories of the cause range from an enzyme deficiency in the child's body to an immunologic response to the alcohol fraction of gluten or the inability to absorb the water-insoluble protein fraction of wheat.[12]

The two most common and most prominent symptoms are diarrhea between the ages of 6 to 12 months and failure to thrive. The stools, which are definitive for the disease, are huge, pale, bulky, foul-smelling, and greasy. They often *float* in water, whereas normal stools sink. The combination of calorie loss from diarrhea and anorexia, a result of the decreased absorption in the bowel, produces a rapid deceleration in increase in height and in weight. The child has a grossly distended abdomen and muscle wasting of the limbs and buttocks, in contrast to a rounded face. Abdominal pain and vomiting are part of the complex in some children. The chronic illness produces an irritable, difficult-to-handle child. The child may have peripheral edema and finger clubbing due to anemia and hypoproteinemia. Vitamin and mineral deficiencies may cause osteomalacia, rickets, and tetany in a small number of children.

A battery of tests may be necessary to establish the diagnosis. Barium x-ray of the small intestine shows changes in the intestine and mucosa and will eliminate other abdominal pathology as the cause. Bone age is retarded on x-ray or may show deficiency changes.

Stool examination for volume, consistency odor, and density is a most important test. Stool cultures, stool smears, and chymotrypsin test on stool are all normal. A 3-day fecal-fat collection shows a high degree of fat malabsorption, 20 to 35 percent of intake remaining in the stool as opposed to 10 percent as the upper limit for normal stool.[13] Liver function tests and sweat test (for cystic fibrosis) are normal. Glucose tolerance and D-xylose tolerance tests show poor absorption because of the overall malabsorptive ability of the bowel. Blood test results include low serum protein, low hemoglobin and serum iron, and slightly decreased serum immunoglobins.

Nursing management   At first, treatment must be aimed at symptoms as well as basic pathology. A gluten-free diet is prescribed, and lactose is omitted until repair of the intestinal mucosa takes place. Since the child is severely malnourished and anorexic, small frequent meals are most successful. The changes in the mucosal lining are reversible, and most children outgrow the intolerance to gluten. Symptomatic treatment may include vitamin injections, iron preparations, and magnesium and calcium gluconate for tetany. Electrolyte imbalances are corrected. In severe disease, corticosteroids are used to hasten mucosal repair.

The chronic illness, irritability, and anorexia present problems for nursing focus. The nurse must use time, patience, and ingenuity to provide increased calories and protein and to help the child in gaining the development achievements he may lack. In teaching parents, emphasis on the cause of the problem and the need for maintaining the specific diet are imperative issues for successful management.

GASTROINTESTINAL DISEASES IN THE SCHOOL-AGE CHILD AND ADOLESCENT
Diseases of Higher Incidence

Appendicitis Inflammation with infection of the vermiform appendix is one of the most common conditions requiring surgery in children from age 2 years and older. It is rare in infants and very common in school-agers and adolescents. Males are affected in higher numbers than females. The incidence rises in the spring, perhaps because of the greater incidence of gastroenteritis at that time of the year.

The appendix is a vestigial remnant located on the cecum just beyond the ileocecal valve and has no recognizable function. The lumen becomes blocked, causing inflammation of the walls of the appendix and stasis of fecal material within, and infection develops. The obstruction is common, usually caused by a fecalith. As the infection progresses, pressure within the appendix may cause perfora-

tion. Interference with the blood supply increases the possibility of gangrene. When the appendix ruptures, generalized peritonitis occurs in younger children, and a more localized or walled-off abscess in older children (because of a longer omentum which aids in preventing spread).

Early recognition of appendicitis prevents rupture and its complications. Pain is *always* present so that any child with abdominal pain is immediately suspected of having appendicitis. The disease may begin with the child's complaint of a "stomach ache." The pain is persistent and progressive and quickly localizes in the right lower quadrant, midway between the umbilicus and the ileac crest (McBurney's point). The pain and an elevated white blood cell count are conclusive for diagnosis of appendicitis. After the onset of pain, nausea and vomiting are accompanying signs. Fever is not necessarily present.

Appendectomy is the definitive procedure. Preoperatively, the child is allowed nothing to eat or drink. Vomiting may be controlled by a nasogastric tube attached to suction. Lavage of the stomach will be necessary if the child has eaten recently. Narcotics are given for pain, or the preoperative medication for surgery will be pain-relieving if surgery is imminent. The haste of hospitalization and surgery combined with the pain is frightening. Short, simple information about what is being done with opportunity for questions is most reassuring, along with the knowledge that the pain will be eliminated. The parents are often very apprehensive, sometimes out of proportion to the "simple" surgery being done, because they have had no opportunity to prepare themselves and because they often fear there is something more seriously wrong.

Postoperative recovery is rapid and usually trouble-free. Intravenous fluids, gastric decompression, and nothing by mouth are continued until peristalsis is established, in 1 to 2 days. The child is usually allowed out of bed and to sit about 12 hours after surgery or the next day. Diet and activity rapidly return to normal. After discharge, the child may return to school in 1 to 2 weeks. Sports and strenuous activity such as bicycle riding are restricted for several more weeks. Antibiotics are given routinely. Besides general assistance and encouragement in his progression to recovery, nursing observations for the development of abscess or peritonitis are most important. The signs may be vague and variable, such as irritability, reluctance to move, prolonged complaints of postoperative pain, and poor appetite rather than definite pain, fever, and more apparent illness, which develop later in abscess formation.

Therefore, this behavior should be recorded and reported as it is noticed.

Ruptured Appendix and Peritonitis If the appendix has ruptured, the child will be sicker and the course of recovery longer. Penrose drains are placed in the incision at the time of surgery in an attempt to drain the exudate and prevent abscess formation or to drain the abscess if one is present. The child should lie in semi-Fowler's position so that the exudate will collect in the lower abdomen. Frequent positioning of the child on his right side will facilitate drainage through the drains. If drainage is successful, the drains will be "advanced" regularly till they can be removed, often in 1 to 2 weeks. It is the nurse's responsibility to maintain sterile, dry dressings to prevent further complications and to minimize discomfort and odor.

If an abscess develops, an incision and drainage by laparotomy must be done after it localizes. The Penrose drain procedure must be utilized again, and the doctor may order irrigations of the incision, using antibiotic or germicidal solutions if the infection is persistent. In very severe cases, an abscess develops more than once and requires repetition of the entire course of treatment. During this time, antibiotic therapy by intravenous fluid drip is maintained. The nurse should be aware of the many reasons for the depression and irritability which the child displays. He begins to feel he will never get better; this psychologic effect alone requires much patience and support from the nurse.

Chronic Inflammatory Bowel Disease[14] *Ulcerative colitis* generally occurs between the ages of 10 and 19 years. The incidence is highest in whites, Jews, and persons in upper socioeconomic groups. Genetic and environmental factors seem to contribute to its development. Frequently other family members have a history of bowel disease, as well as rhinitis, asthma, eczema, and other allergies.

Emotional disturbance is known to exacerbate ulcerative colitis in many cases. Affected children tend to be dependent and emotionally fragile and to have personality disturbances. Their mothers are often overprotective, dominating, and self-centered.

Suspicion that an inflammatory bowel disease is present is verified by upper gastrointestinal barium x-ray study and barium enema x-ray. A rectosigmoidoscopy is a necessary part of a diagnostic work-up, with either a mucosal section or full-thickness biopsy. Anemia due to blood loss is present. Decreased serum albumin reflects the presence of chronic inflammation and protein-losing enteropathy. Colon malabsorption in ulcerative colitis causes an abnormal fecal-fat test and sometimes lowered D-xylose tolerance.

Ulcerative colitis may take one of two courses. A *remitting* course is most frequent, in which severe and frequent exacerbations are seen early in the disease and complete remission may occur after a few years. The other course is that of a *chronic, continuous* disease. Intestinal symptoms are mild, but chronic malnutrition and anemia are constant. Neither complete remission nor severe exacerbations occur. The severity of the attacks and the scarcity of early symptoms are not helpful in predicting the future course of the disease.

Findings on x-ray early in the disease may be nonspecific with superficial ulcerations and thickening of the bowel wall. The colon is affected in all cases and, generally, the rectum. Chronic disease is noted by a complete disappearance of haustral markings, shortening of the colon, and thickening of the bowel wall to a degree that a diagnostic feature of the disease is "lead-pipe" colon.

The risk of carcinoma is significantly high in children who have ulcerative colitis before 20 years of age and in patients who have had the disease 10 years or more. The highest risk occurs in those in whom the total colon is involved, and susceptibility increases with the length of the disease.[15] A biopsy indicates epithelial changes (*metaplasia*), pointing to those patients at risk. Since these carcinomas are poorly differentiated and metastasize early, the child should receive frequent x-ray and endoscopic examinations.

Nursing management Hospitalization during acute exacerbations is necessary if the attack is severe or dehydration and signs of complications occur. Hospitalization often is helpful in providing better observation of the child during the attack and a closer view of interrelationships between the adolescent and his family. Time during hospitalizations can be utilized by a nurse in helping them adjust to and understand the illness. Communication between doctor and nurse must be constant to provide consistent information and approach and, thus, decrease the stress involved.

A high-protein, high-carbohydrate, normal-fat, high-vitamin diet is preferred. If malabsorption is a problem, a lactose-free diet may be used in addition. During acute attacks, the child may need fluid or blood volume replacement. The child is given nothing by mouth if he is vomiting. Hyperalimentation, especially in the long convalescence after surgery, improves the child's nutritional condition and rests the bowel. Small frequent meals, flexibility in times of meals, allowing the child to choose his own foods, and use of appropriate snack or "fun" foods are successful nursing interventions in combating anorexia.

Bed rest is required in acute attacks, although activity is allowed, according to the child's ability. Children with ulcerative colitis may engage in normal play and school during remissions. Since these children are dependent and passive, they may need encouragement in self-help and in participation in play. The nurse must be alert to opportunities for small acceptable amounts of activity and provide a variety of these opportunities. Progress in increasing activity, interest, and participation is never sudden and full but slow and fluctuating.

A number of drugs may be used with many variations in combinations. Antidiarrheal agents, opiates (used sparingly in acute attacks), anticholinergic drugs to reduce rectal spasm, and aspirin for discomfort are supportive drugs. Salicylazosulfapyridine helps to relieve symptoms in acute attacks and is a deterrent to further exacerbations but produces many gastrointestinal side effects, and dosage must be adjusted. Adrenocorticotropic hormone (ACTH) and parenteral corticosteroids are given to reduce the inflammatory reaction and may be given by enema in acute rectal involvement. They are discontinued when clinical improvement occurs. Immunosuppressive drugs may be used. Broad-spectrum antibiotics are used after surgery.

Psychotherapy in conjunction with medical and surgical treatment has influenced the success of treatment. Its value is becoming recognized increasingly. When medical management is not enough to control ulcerative colitis, when the bowel has carcinomatous degeneration, or when there is total colonic involvement, a total colectomy may be necessary. The ileostomy created may add further complications. Since resection of the bowel for regional enteritis is much less successful because of recurrence in formerly normal bowel, it is reserved for severe cases. Often, the disease reappears first at the site of the anastomosis. Colectomy when the disease affects only the colon is successful because disease of the small intestine may expand to the colon but disease of the colon does not expand to include the small intestine.

Table 36-3 A COMPARISON OF CLINICAL MANIFESTATIONS OF ULCERATIVE COLITIS AND REGIONAL ENTERITIS

Manifestations	Ulcerative colitis	Regional enteritis
Initial symptoms	Good health till onset Painless passage of bloody stools, often in early morning Change in bowel habits with constipation	Growth retardation often before gastrointestinal signs Resembles gastroenteritis or acute appendicitis Early systemic signs: arthritis, uveitis, stomatitis, erythema nodosum Fever, often of unknown origin
Most frequent symptoms	Severe diarrhea Abdominal pain: less severe crampy, sensation to defecate induced by eating, relieved by defecation Anorexia in acute stage Dehydration Malnutrition, retarded maturation, includes secondary sex characteristics Mucocutaneous lesions of skin, eyes, joints Signs of inflammation (chills, low evening fever, leukocytosis)	Abdominal pain, crampy, severe, induced by eating, relieved by defecation if colon involved; periumbilical, often in right lower quadrant Anorexia: may be severe Diarrhea: not always present, acute, severe; mucopurulent indicates severe rectosigmoid disease; bleeding is rare; early morning or nocturnal urge to defecate Chronically ill, muscle wasting Peripheral edema, early, if present
Symptoms indicative of severe disease	Nausea and vomiting Nocturnal urge to defecate Abdominal distention (toxic megacolon or impending perforation) Anal fissure Chronic hepatitis Fatty infiltration of liver due to chronic malnutrition	Nausea and vomiting Clubbing of fingers Perirectal disease: abscess, fistula

The complexity of medical and surgical treatment establishes close continuous observation, monitoring, and reporting as a major nursing emphasis. The response of the child to treatment and drugs as the disease progresses, development of complications, and his emotional response to his environment are all interrelated factors requiring astute judgment by the nurse. The personality of the child may tempt the nurse to encourage too much dependency or may be offensive to a nurse who feels that the child should be more independent and active than he is. These latter feelings may be combined, particularly, with strong negative ideas that the child's dependency is fostered too much by his mother and family, in general. Although the nurse can find small ways acceptable to the child and his mother, if he requires too much alteration in their relationship during hospitalization, the resultant stress may affect the disease adversely. The mother must be allowed to participate in the child's care even beyond the extent that the nurse prefers.

About one-half of children with ulcerative colitis may lead relatively normal lives with mild or infrequent exacerbations. A severe, initial attack or total colon involvement may produce a guarded prognosis. Extension of the disease to nonaffected colon occurs very early in the development of the disease if it occurs at all. The most difficult to manage is the chronic continuous type, since carcinomatous changes are frequent and medical management is not successful. The patient with ulcerative colitis may die from fulminating disease, hemorrhage, intestinal complications, sepsis, or cirrhosis.

Neoplasms of the Gastrointestinal Tract Considered as a group, neoplasms (cysts, hyperplasia, and tumors) are not common in children. However, with the exception of appendicitis and trauma, neoplasms account for many *newly developed* surgical problems in the older child. The most frequent symptom common to all abdominal tumors is abdominal discomfort or pain and a palpable abdominal mass. Generalized gastrointestinal related manifestations usually follow, especially anorexia, nausea and vomiting, weight loss, fatigue, pallor, and a change in bowel habits, particularly diarrhea. Rectal bleeding is present in a few instances. Nonmalignant tumors may present symptoms only by mechanical interference (due to their growth) with other abdominal structures, tumors such as liver hamartoma, liver cyst, and pancreatic cysts. When a tumor is suspected, surgical exploration is a necessity. Before the operative procedure, diagnostic measures to ascertain location, involvement with surrounding structures, and size are done. In spite of these measures, findings at surgery are frequently unexpected.

Nursing management Since the clinical manifestations of abdominal tumors mimic many frequent childhood illnesses, vague complaints delay diagnosis and complicate the course of the disease. Most benign tumors and less extensive malignant tumors for which an intestinal resection is done require the care given for abdominal laparotomy. If an extensive resection is done, the care includes close observation for infection, hemorrhage, fistulas from the operative site into the peritoneum or to the surface, or malfunctioning of the bowel due to surgery (as evidenced by diarrhea, cramping, and other intestinal signs). Hyperalimentation may be used, and gastric decompression by nasogastric tube may be required for a longer period. The nurse can expect these children to be sicker, to require more supportive measures, and to be quiet, withdrawn, and inactive. Such behavior requires the nurse to find opportunities for the child to participate in any play for which he has the strength, thus encouraging him to be more active.

Should a malignancy be present, a course of radiation treatment usually follows surgery. In rare cases, when the tumor has involved many structures, radiation therapy may be done before surgery as well as afterward. These treatments may begin when the child is still in the hospital and continue after discharge. Side effects include lethargy, anorexia, vomiting, and weakness; however, these problems disappear when radiation is completed. Efforts to minimize these secondary effects are part of the nursing emphasis. Frequent small meals and a flexible schedule that allows the child to eat when and what he wants often assists the child in improving his nutritional state. Radiation destroys white blood cells temporarily, so that the child should be protected against infection and may need reverse isolation. Nursing management should include keeping him from close contact with children with infection, thorough handwashing, and close attention to sterile and clean techniques in his treatments.

Since these children are generally older and understand much of what is happening, even if they are not told of the malignancy, it is difficult to know how much of the child's reactions after surgery (lethargy, weakness, inactivity) are due to response of his body to the tumor and treatment and how much is caused by emotional reaction. The parents become anxious to the point where their behavior with the child may change, producing fear and anxiety in him. They may overreact to procedures or care given, which may be misinterpreted by the nursing or medical staff. Opportunities for questions should be made available to parents, for the diagnosis is devastating. Even the knowledge that a benign tumor has been found causes them anxiety because tumor is often equated with "cancer."

There is much controversy about how much and what the child should be told. Close communication and exchange of observations of the child's behavior and conversation between the doctors, the nurses, and the parents are necessary to provide a consistent, reassuring approach to the child. Evasiveness tends only to increase the child's anxiety. Teen-age and pre-teen children, especially, may develop hostility, apathy, acting-out behavior, or other extremes due to the stress of "fearing but not knowing."

Diseases of Lower Incidence

Cholecystitis and Cholelithiasis Cholecystitis, acute and chronic, either with or without stones, and cholelithiasis, alone, are unusual illnesses in childhood. Most frequently, the clinical picture is one of chronic cholecystitis with cholelithiasis. Other aspects of the clinical picture are a familial incidence of gallbladder disease, occurrence in a large majority of females, an average age of 8 to 10 years, and a high incidence of overweight. It is extremely rare in infants. At times, symptoms arise first in the pregnant adolescent. Abdominal pain, in the upper right quadrant or midepigastrium when localized, accompanied by nausea and vomiting, is the primary symptom. Periumbilical pain in the disease is peculiar to children and is confusing in diagnosis. Tenderness of the abdomen is not present. Intolerance to fatty foods is less than in adults, while jaundice is more common. Perforation of the gallbladder due to cholelithiasis occurs but with less acute symptoms of shock than in the adult, a fact important for the nurse to remember for observation.

Although no cause has been established, there seem to be some basic abnormalities of the biliary system which predispose to disease and an infection which leads to the acute phase. Associated systemic illness is not uncommon. If surgery is not indicated, precise diagnosis may not be made for some time. Cholecystography assists in diagnosis once the illness is suspected.

Definitive surgery is a cholecystectomy, which is usually uncomplicated and has a safe postoperative course. No specific postoperative practices or limited diet are usually needed, and the general principles of care in a laparotomy are followed.

Peptic and Duodenal Ulcers Ulcers in children, which are increasing in incidence, occur at all ages and in both sexes, but there is a significant rise in numbers and in proportion of males affected in the adolescent population. It is thought that the hormones produced in puberty or the environmental factors which contribute to stress in males account for this rise. Especially in older children and adolescents, emotional factors play an important role in development and can frequently be identified in the child's history. However, a definite causative factor is not found. In younger children, stress ulcers generally develop secondary to primary disease or trauma. The most frequent are meningitis, sepsis, shock, central nervous system disease, burns, surgical treatment for congenital gastrointestinal malformations, cystic fibrosis, and gastroenteritis. Children receiving corticosteroids are especially vulnerable to stress ulcers and there is usually a family history of ulcers.

Neonatal ulcers, which have a high mortality, are rare, almost always severe, and need emergency treatment. The ulcers are generally gastric. Massive hemorrhage, perforation, or both are the presenting symptoms, which may be sudden. Frequent causative factors include hypoxia at birth and difficult labor and delivery. Medical treatment is preferred, but, because of perforation, surgery is done often, ranging from simple closure to partial gastrectomy.

Ulcers in *infants* are also unusual but occur following gastroenteritis or meningitis as the most common causative factors. The clinical picture is that of a poor eater, with vomiting, crying spells, abdominal distention, and, sometimes, failure to thrive or hematemesis. Incidence of perforation and hemorrhage is also higher than in older children. Medical treatment is less successful because of the incidence of complications. Diagnosis is very difficult in this age group.

In children of age 1 to 7 years, vague abdominal pain or "hunger pains" is a common symptom. The relationship of pain to meals is more frequent but not always similar to the adult pattern. The child may be anorexic or have peculiar eating habits.

The manifestations of *children over 7 years,* and especially in *preadolescence* and *adolescence,* are those typical of the adult pattern. Exacerbations are more common and develop more often than in younger age groups.

The diagnosis of ulcers in children must be differentiated from other abdominal illness, and a gastric analysis is not usually helpful. The ulcers frequently do not show on x-ray, but duodenal scarring or irritability will be apparent. If an ulcer is suspected and treatment is begun, in the absence of evidence of any other illness, the good response to treatment may be the only basis for diagnosis.

Conservative treatment is the administration of antacids, sometimes every 1 to 2 hours in severe or acute cases. Antispasmodics and antisecretory drugs may be used also. In the presence of large amounts of bleeding, the approach may follow that for bleeding esophageal varices. The child will not be fed until acute bleeding subsides. A bland soft diet, progressing from liquids to semisolids, follows and is used also in less acute cases. The ulcers generally heal spontaneously on this regimen, and bed rest is not usually needed. After healing, the child's diet will include many additional foods, those specifically causing pain being excluded. Coffee, tea, beef bouillon, spices, and carbonated beverages should be omitted. Nutrition, the content and pattern of daily eating, represents a major nursing focus. Teaching for both the child and his parents will be more effective if the nurse plans quiet periods of discussion rather than just telling them the diet.

In many older children, psychotherapy or a form of psychiatric help in adjusting to their environment is required or is of value in preventing recurrences, because of the causative presence of stress.[16] Recognition of this aspect by the nurse and support of the coping methods of the child and parents, without prejudgment, during hospitalization is an important contribution to healing. Acute ulcers generally heal rapidly. In a high number of children who have chronic ulcers, the problem continues into adulthood or recurs then.

REFERENCES

1 Most of this section was prepared by Donna Jones, R.N., Assistant Head Nurse, Infants' Unit, Children's Hospital of Pittsburgh.
2 K. Sukarochana and W. B. Kieswatter, "Imperforate Anus," *General Practitioner,* vol. XXXVIII, October 1968, pp. 91–92.
3 R. J. Touloukian, W. E. Berdon, R. A. Amoury, and T. V. Santulli, "Surgical Experience with Necrotizing Enterocolitis in the Infant," *Journal of Pediatric Surgery*, 2(15): 390, October 1967.
4 Ibid., p. 398.
5 J. A. Haller, Jr., and J. L. Talbert, "Skin Defects," *Surgical Emergencies in the Newborn,* Lea & Febiger, Philadelphia, 1972, p. 121.
6 W. T. Mustard et al., "The Esophagus," *Pediatric Surgery,* Year Book Medical Publishers, Inc., Chicago, 1969, p. 394.
7 This section includes material from A. Silverman, C. C. Roy, and F. J. Cozzeto, "Intestinal Parasites," Chap. 16, *Pediatric Clinical Gastroenterology,* The C. V. Mosby Company, St. Louis, 1971.
8 Ibid., p. 242.
9 The pattern of organization of this section was adapted from Anne Altshuler, "Esophageal Varices in Children," *American Journal of Nursing,* vol. 72, no. 4, April 1972.
10 Ibid., p. 690.
11 Laboratory test information is adapted from Silverman et al., op. cit., pp. 158–163.
12 Ibid., p. 157.
13 Ibid., p. 160.
14 The general overview of pathology and clinical manifestations in this section is from Silverman et al., ibid.
15 Ibid., p. 207.
16 M. Baida, J. A. McIntyre, and M. Deitel, "Peptic Ulcer in Children and Adolescents," *Archives of Surgery,* vol. XC, July 1969, p. 18.

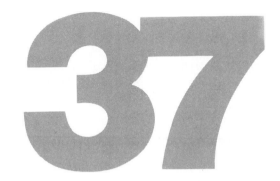

THE REPRODUCTIVE SYSTEM

JANE COOPER EVANS
and CHRISTINA M. GRAF

The primary organs of the reproductive system are the *gonads*—the *ovaries* in the female and the *testes* in the male. The gonads with their internal and external accessory structures make reproduction possible. The main function of the ovaries and testes is the production of *gametes*, or sex cells: *spermatogenesis*, the production of sperm by the testes, and *oogenesis*, the production of ova by the ovaries.

The secondary function of the gonads is the production of gonadal hormones, which affect the reproductive structures and other body structures, as well. The reproductive system is closely involved with and affected by other body systems, both in development and in functioning.

EMBRYOLOGY

Sex determination, the tendency of the organism to develop as either male or female, occurs at the time of fertilization and is dependent on the specific chromosomal constitution of the fertilizing spermatozoon. *Sex differentiation*, the development of organs and structures specific to either the male or the female sex, occurs during the early embryonic period. The differentiation of the gonads is based on the genetic complement of the embryo. Presence of the Y chromosome causes differentiation of the gonads as testes. Absence of the Y chromosome, with either an XX or XO chromosomal pattern, causes differentiation of the gonads as ovaries. However, differentiation of the accessory structures of the reproductive tract and of the external genitalia depends on the presence or absence of the testes. Therefore, a genetically male embryo will, with gonadal agenesis, develop female characteristics.

Undifferentiated Stage

In the earliest, undifferentiated stage of development, the organism is *bipotential*; that is, the embryo has neither male nor female characteristics and may develop either.

The gonads arise on the urogenital ridge as a proliferation of the coelomic epithelium. The early, indifferent gonad is composed of a *cortex* and a *medulla*; although the gonad is bipotential, the components are unipotential, that is, the cortex can develop only as an ovary and the medulla as a testis. The primordial sex cells originate in the yolk sac near the allantois and migrate to the developing gonad.

The internal accessory structures develop from

the mesonephric (Wolffian) ducts in the male and the paramesonephric (Müllerian) ducts in the female. The mesonephric ducts are the common outlets of the mesonephric tubules in the early stages of renal system development. The paramesonephric ducts develop along the posterior abdominal wall of the embryo. Both sets of ducts are present in the embryo in the undifferentiated stage. However, as differentiation progresses, the paramesonephric ducts in the male and the mesonephric ducts in the female degenerate and remain as vestigial structures.

The external genitalia begin to develop in the sixth week, with the genital tubercle arising as a swelling between the umbilical cord and the cloacal membrane. The genital tubercle elongates to form the phallus, with a glans at its end. Urethral folds develop posteriorly to the phallus, surrounding the urethral groove which is the opening of the urogenital sinus. Finally, genital swellings appear around the urethral folds.

Differentiated Stage

Sex differentiation in the male begins at about the seventh week, as the testes develop from the medullary portion of the gonad, and the gonadal cortex correspondingly regresses. The sex cords, which have surrounded the sex cells, become separated from the coelomic epithelium and develop into U-shaped *seminiferous tubules.* The free ends of these tubules form the *straight tubules*, and the primordial sex cells within the seminiferous tubules form the *spermatogonia.*

The mesenchyme forms a dense, fibrous layer, the *tunica albuginea,* the covering of the testes. The mesenchyme also produces the *interstitial (Leydig) cells*, which reach a peak at about seventeen weeks, then regress almost totally until, at puberty, they once more proliferate. The proliferation of the interstitial cells during the fetal period coincides with the development of the accessory structures. These structures, the duct of epididymis, the vas deferens, the seminal vesicles, and the ejaculatory duct, form from the mesonephric ducts as they develop caudally to the prostatic urethra.

The phallus in the male continues to elongate and, as it does, pulls the urethral folds together to cover the urethral groove and form the penile urethra which eventually opens onto the tip of the glans penis. The prepuce grows from the base of the glans penis to its tip. The genital swellings fuse to form the scrotum.

The testes originally lie in the posterior abdomen. By the third month, because of the development of the trunk and the abdominal structures, their position is close to the inguinal ring. The inguinal canal develops from a peritoneal sac, the processus vaginalis, which passes through the abdominal wall to the genital swellings. Usually during the eighth month the testes migrate through the inguinal canal to the scrotum.

The development of the ovaries occurs later than that of the testes, with predominance of the gonadal cortex and regression of the medulla. The sex cells with surrounding sex cords appear as disorganized clumps, then develop as oocytes and, with the cords, form primordial *graafian follicles* at about eighteen weeks. The oocytes proliferate, reaching a peak of perhaps 7 million at about seven months. The mesenchyme of the ovary forms the *ovarian stroma*, the connective tissue which supports the ovary.

The paramesonephric ducts grow caudally, joining at the midline in the pelvic cavity to form a single strand. The lumens of the ducts are divided by a septum which subsequently disappears, forming the cavity of the uterus and the cervix. The upper juncture of the ducts forms the fundus of the uterus. The portion of the ducts above the juncture forms the fallopian tubes, with fimbriae lying close to the ovaries.

As the caudal end of the fused paramesonephric ducts reaches the urogenital sinus, cellular proliferation forms the vaginal plate which develops a lumen and enlarges to form the vagina. The hymen appears as a membrane at the junction of the vaginal plate and the urogenital sinus.

The phallus in the female bends toward the anus and forms the clitoris. The genital folds and the genital swellings develop as the labia minora and the labia majora, surrounding the vestibule, which is the lower portion of the urogenital sinus.

Differentiation is generally complete by the twelfth week, with the external genitalia of the fetus recognizably male or female.

PHYSIOLOGY
Hormonal Functions of the Male Reproductive System

Hormonal control of the reproductive system, in both the male and the female, is centered in the hypothalamus (see Fig. 37-1). The hypothalamus is influenced by a number of elements such as heredity, environment, circulating reproductive hormones, and neural humors to increase or decrease its secretion of *gonadotropic hormone releasing factors.*

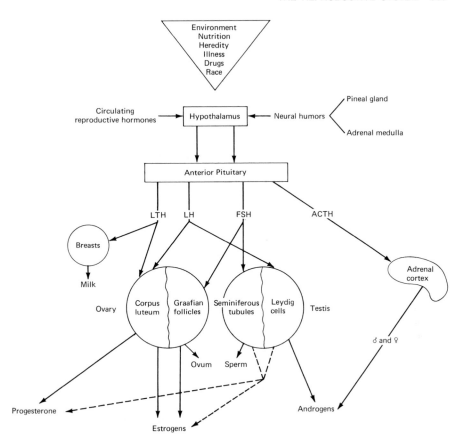

Figure 37-1 Hormonal factors affecting the reproductive system.

These factors are the follicle-stimulating hormone releasing factor (FSHRF) and the luteinizing hormone releasing factor (LHRF), and their action stimulates the anterior pituitary or adenohypophysis to release follicle-stimulating hormone (FSH) and luteinizing hormone (LH), respectively. The chemistry of these releasing factors is unknown at this time; however, their existence is evident.

FSH in the male is responsible for the growth and development of the seminiferous tubules of the testes and for spermatogenesis. LH, sometimes referred to as *interstitial-cell stimulating hormone* (ICSH) in the male, is responsible for the development of the Leydig cells and the subsequent production of androgens and estrogens. LH is also required for the development of the seminal vesicles and the prostate, and for their subsequent contribution to semen production and ejaculation.

Male sex hormones are called *androgens*, whether they are produced by the testes or the adrenal cortex. *Testosterone*, however, is considered to be the prime androgen because it is secreted in a much greater quantity than any others that have

been identified. Androgens are responsible for the growth and development of the male sex organs, the penis, scrotum, and testes, and for the development of the secondary sex characteristics including pubic, axillary, and facial hair; deepening of the voice; increase in length and density of bones; muscular growth; seborrhea and development of the sweat glands; increase in the thickness of the skin; increase in the texture (ruggedness) of the subcutaneous tissue; darkening of the skin from melatonin deposits; increase in basal metabolic rate up to 15 percent; and increase in the amount of circulating hemoglobin and red blood cells (see Table 37-1).

The anterior pituitary produces a third gonadotropic hormone, luteotropic hormone (LTH), but at this time its function in the male reproductive system is unknown.

Spermatogenesis Spermatogonia (germ cells) are present at birth, but are inactive. *Spermatogenesis*, or the production of spermatozoa from spermatogonia, actually begins at puberty. After puberty, under the influence of FSH, the germ cells, through rapid mitotic division, continue to proliferate through old age with little reduction in activity.

Spermatogenesis may be divided into three stages: mitosis and meiosis of the spermatocytes; maturation and storage of the spermatozoa; and emission, ejaculation, or degeneration of spermatozoa.

Mitosis and meiosis   Spermatogonia increase in size to become *primary spermatocytes*, which reproduce their 46 chromosomes autocatalytically to 92 chromosomes; then, stimulated by FSH, they undergo mitotic division into *secondary spermatocytes* containing 46 chromosomes each (see Fig. 37-2). The secondary spermatocytes divide through meiosis into *spermatids* containing 23 chromosomes each. In this fashion, each spermatogonium generates four spermatids. This germ cell division in the male differs from that of the female in that both mitosis and meiosis take place within a few hours to a few weeks. In the female, however, mitosis is completed prior to birth, and meiosis in a given cell takes place just prior to its release from the graafian follicle. Another difference between the male and the female is that each primary spermatocyte can develop into four mature spermatozoa, but each primary oocyte will develop only one mature ovum. (The other three polar bodies which develop from the oocyte have minimal cytoplasm and degenerate as a result.)[1]

Maturation and storage   After the meiotic phase, each new spermatid still has a simple epithelioid cell structure which matures into a highly differentiated spermatozoon by attaching to the *Sertoli cells* (sustentacular cells of the germinal epithelium). From the Sertoli cells, the new spermatids derive the hormones or enzymes and nutrient material necessary to develop the head, neck, body, and tail of mature spermatozoa.

Once the spermatozoa develop from the spermatids in the seminiferous tubules, they pass into the epididymis. At this point they are nonmotile and incapable of fertilization; yet, within 18 hours, they become mobile and capable of penetrating the ovum. Some small number of spermatozoa are thought to remain in the epididymis, but most spermatozoa are stored in the vas deferens and its ampulla. They can be stored and retain their fertility for as long as 42 days, though with average sexual activity, storage is not longer than a few days and sometimes a few hours.

Emission, ejaculation, or degeneration   Especially during puberty, and for some time thereafter, young males are prone to nocturnal emissions. These emissions are thought to be the result of a buildup in the secretion of spermatozoa, seminal secretions, and prostate secretions which are released during sleep, possibly in connection with the normal erotic dreams of the adolescent male. In some normal adolescent males, masturbation is frequent enough to eliminate the need for nocturnal emissions.

Ejaculation is a complex process which results from reflex mechanisms integrated in the sacral and lumbar regions of the spinal cord and is initiated by either psychic or actual sexual stimulation. The first stage is erection, effected by parasympathetic impulses which dilate the arteries of the penis and constrict the veins. Arterial blood then enters the sinusoids of the erectile tissue under high pressure, causing the penis to become rigid and elongated. Penetration into the female vagina is then possible. Intense stimulation of the glans penis along with psychic stimuli causes the release of sympathetic impulses from the spinal cord at the level of the 1st or 2d lumbar vertebra through the hypogastric plexus to the genitals. Peristaltic contractions are initiated in the testes, the epididymis, and the vas deferens, causing the ejaculation of spermatozoa into the internal urethra. Rhythmic contractions of the prostate and seminal vesicles discharge fluid which, when mixed with spermatozoa, becomes semen. The process of ejaculation as described thus far is properly called *emission*. The pudendal nerve impulses sent from the cord to the skeletal nerves at the base of the penis cause rhythmic pressure increases and the eventual expulsion of the semen out the urethra. This latter process is more appropriately termed *ejaculation*.

Once spermatozoa have been ejaculated into the female vagina, their life-span is 24 to 72 hours. With the assistance of myometrial contractions, they must ascend the uterus and enter the fallopian tubes in order to penetrate the ovum which has traveled to the outer ampulla of the tube. Although over 100 million spermatozoa are deposited in the vagina, approximately one million manage to enter the cervix, and, of these, only a few thousand are able to navigate the uterotubal junction, so that 100 or fewer spermatozoa actually reach the tubal ampulla and the ovum. Only one spermatozoon is required to fertilize the ovum.

It has been speculated that spermatozoa and fluid degenerate and are reabsorbed in the absence

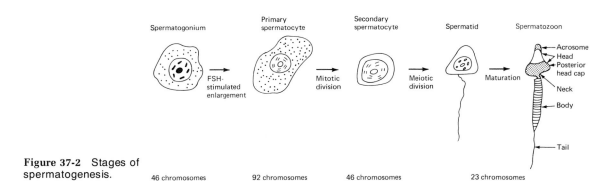

Figure 37-2 Stages of spermatogenesis.

Spermatogonium — 46 chromosomes
Primary spermatocyte — 92 chromosomes
Secondary spermatocyte — 46 chromosomes
Spermatid — 23 chromosomes
Spermatozoon — Acrosome, Head, Posterior head cap, Neck, Body, Tail

FSH-stimulated enlargement → Mitotic division → Meiotic division → Maturation

of emission or ejaculation. The aspiration of degenerating spermatozoa seems to support this theory. It has also been suggested that spermatozoa are discarded through emission into the urine at the end of their life cycle. Spermatozoa have been found in male urine on occasion. The life cycle of spermatozoa from the first mitotic division of the primary spermatocyte is estimated to be between 64 and 74 days.

Spermatogenesis can be affected by a number of physical factors. It has been established that spermatogenesis will not take place in the absence of FSH. Orchitis secondary to mumps or gonorrhea may cause scarring of the seminiferous tubules and subsequent sterility if the infections are severe. Another factor which affects spermatogenesis is temperature. The optimum temperature for production and storage of spermatozoa is lower than the normal temperature of the abdominal cavity. Scrotal temperature averages 2.2°C lower than the abdominal cavity temperature, but may range from 1.5 to 2.5°C lower. Temperatures substantially higher than this will retard spermatogenesis temporarily and sometimes permanently. The body attempts to compensate for changes in temperature by relaxation and dangling of the scrotum away from the body in hot weather and retraction of the scrotum and testes against the body in cold weather.

Table 37-1   ACTION OF THE GONADAL HORMONES

Hormone	Source	Action in the male	Action in the female
Androgens*	Leydig cells, adrenal cortex	Development of testes, scrotum, penis; voice change; pubic and axillary hair; seborrhea; skeletal and muscular growth; thickening of skin; deposits of melatonin in skin; increase in hemoglobin and RBC; increase in basal metabolic rate	Development of clitoris and labia majora; pubic and axillary hair; seborrhea; skeletal and muscular growth
Estrogens†	Graafian follicles, corpus luteum, seminiferous tubules, Leydig cells	Osteogenesis	Development of uterus, tubes, cervix, vagina, external genitalia; breast development (stromal tissue, fat deposits, ducts); distribution of body fat; osteogenesis
Progesterone†	Corpus luteum, seminiferous tubules, Leydig cells	Acne	Endometrial secretions; breast development (lobules, alveoli); voice changes; increased body temperature; acne

* Action in female not clearly understood.
† Source and action in male not clearly understood.

Hormonal Functions of the Female Reproduction System

The development and functioning of the female reproductive system, as of the male reproductive system, is controlled by a complex, interacting system of hormones derived mainly from the hypothalamus, the anterior pituitary, and the gonads (see Fig. 37-1). The same hypothalamic hormones in the female stimulate the anterior pituitary to produce three gonadotropic hormones: follicle-stimulating hormone (FSH), luteinizing hormone (LH), and luteotropic hormone (LTH). FSH stimulates the growth of the ovary itself and, more specifically, the growth of the primordial follicle. LH acts synergistically with FSH to cause rapid growth of the follicle with ovulation. LTH affects the development of the corpus luteum after ovulation. LTH also has a second effect, that of stimulating the breasts to produce milk, and is often called *lactogen* or *lactogenic hormone.*

Stimulated by the gonadotropic hormones, the ovary produces two types of hormones: *estrogen* and *progesterone* (see Table 37-1). Estrogen is responsible for the proliferation of cells of the reproductive organs and related structures. Thus the changes at puberty in the uterus, fallopian tubes, and vagina, the growth of the labia minora and majora, and the development of secondary sex characteristics are a result of circulating estrogens. These hormones also exert an effect on the skeletal system, causing a growth spurt at the time of puberty and an earlier closure of the epiphyses than occurs in males. During the normal menstrual cycle, estrogen acts on the uterine endometrium to cause cell proliferation.

Progesterone is secreted by the corpus luteum during the latter half of the menstrual cycle. Progesterone acts synergistically with estrogen and produces secretory changes in the endometrium, preparing it for the implantation of a fertilized ovum. This hormone also causes secretory changes in the breast, affecting the lobules and alveoli to make them capable of secreting milk. (Note that progesterone does not cause lactation, which is a function of LTH, but only develops the capacity for lactation.)

The interaction of the pituitary hormones and the ovarian hormones is affected by a feedback mechanism. Increasing levels of FSH stimulate the ovary to produce estrogen and the primordial follicles to develop into mature graafian follicles. LH enhances this development and promotes ovulation. Following ovulation, the corpus luteum secretes large amounts of estrogen and progesterone. These circulating hormones exert a negative feedback effect on the anterior pituitary, causing a decrease in FSH and LH production. As the corpus luteum degenerates, decreasing levels of estrogen and progesterone are accompanied by increased secretion of FSH and LH. The third gonadotropic hormone, LTH, is not affected in this manner, but acts in a reciprocal manner with FSH and LH: when the anterior pituitary secretes increased amounts of FSH and LH, secretion of LTH is decreased and vice versa (see Fig. 37-3).

The Menstrual Cycle In the maturing female, a rhythmic cycle develops which results in the maturation and release of a single ovum from the ovary, and in the preparation of the endometrial lining for the implantation of a fertilized ovum. The cycle repeats itself on an average of every 28 days (except during pregnancy), although it may vary from 20 to 45 days as a normal cycle.

Ovarian cycle The primordial follicle, composed of germ cell and surrounding granulosa cells, begins to grow slowly under the stimulation of FSH. Initially, this growth involves the ovum itself, then causes the growth of theca cells around the granulosa cells. The additional secretion of LH causes a more rapid growth of the follicle with a corresponding increase in the production of estrogen.

With each cycle, as many as 20 primordial follicles may begin to mature; generally, one follicle supersedes the others and ovulates, while the others degenerate. In this mature graafian follicle, the ovum with surrounding cells has moved to one pole of the follicle and, on about the fourteenth day of the cycle, is expelled by the follicle, to be drawn in by the fimbriated ends of the fallopian tube.

In the next few hours, the cells of the follicle enlarge and acquire a distinctly yellow color, the whole becoming a corpus luteum. The corpus luteum is sustained by increased production of LTH from the anterior pituitary, and produces large amounts of estrogen and progesterone. About the eighth day following ovulation, the corpus luteum begins to involute and by about the twelfth day following ovulation has ceased functioning. This process of involution is associated with decreasing levels of LTH and decreasing production of estrogen and progesterone. With the decrease in the production of gonadal hormones comes an increase in the secretion of FSH to stimulate the primordial follicles and repeat the cycle.

Endometrial cycle At the beginning of the cycle, the uterine endometrium desquamates and is, as a result, very thin. The estrogens produced by the developing follicle stimulate the endometrium to increase in number of cells. This *proliferative phase* continues until ovulation and the development of the corpus luteum. The endometrium enters the *secretory phase* and is affected by both estrogens and progesterone. The estrogens continue to affect cell proliferation. Under the influence of progesterone, the epithelial glandular cells develop and secrete small amounts of epithelial fluid.

With the involution of the corpus luteum and the rapid decrease of estrogens and progesterone, the epithelium again desquamates and menstruation occurs.

Fertilization If the ovum released from the follicle is fertilized, the pattern of the cycle is interrupted. The early fertilized ovum develops trophoblastic cells which produce a hormone, chorionic gonadotropin. This hormone prevents the involution of the corpus luteum, which then continues to produce estrogens and progesterone. The gonadal hormones sustain the development of the endometrium, which is necessary for the development of the placenta and other fetal tissues, and neither menstruation nor follicular activity occurs.

NURSING APPROACHES IN THE CARE OF THE NEWBORN AND INFANT

Examination of the external genitalia of the newborn includes observations of size, configuration, color, and symmetry. At birth, the penis of the male is approximately 3 to 4 cm (1.2 to 1.6 in.) in length. The prepuce (foreskin) is adherent and not retractable. During the first months after birth, the prepuce becomes less adherent and can be manually retracted. Beyond about four months of age, an adherent prepuce is considered pathologic, and the adhesion must be surgically corrected.

The urinary meatus of the newborn is generally not discernible at the tip of the glans. Therefore, the infant's voiding should be observed to ascertain the position of the meatus and to determine possible occlusion of the meatus by the prepuce. The scrotum of the newborn is symmetric, and the skin thickened, wrinkled, and pigmented. The testes can usually be palpated in the scrotum, and their size and consistency determined.

The clitoris in the normal female infant is only a few millimeters long. The labia minora are usually

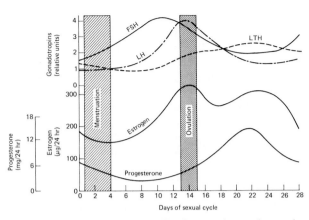

Figure 37-3 Approximate cyclic changes in ovarian and pituitary secretion of the different hormones involved in the female sexual cycle. *(Reprinted from A. C. Guyton, Textbook of Medical Physiology, 4th ed., W. B. Saunders Company, Philadelphia, 1971, p. 965.)*

more prominent than the labia majora, but will become smaller in the first few weeks after birth. The labia are symmetric and can be completely separated. The urinary meatus is usually not visible, but the vaginal orifice is easily seen and normally appears reddened.

The reproductive system is inactive in the newborn. The testes contain primary spermatogonia, but spermatogenesis will not begin until puberty. Unlike the testes, the ovary produces no additional oocytes after about the seventh month of fetal life. The ovary of the newborn contains perhaps as many as 1 to 3 million oocytes; by 7 years of age, this number will be reduced to approximately 300,000.

In the examination of the newborn infant during the immediate postnatal period, a number of minor deviations may be noted which are transient, require no treatment, and are not properly regarded as abnormalities.

Pseudomenstruation is a vaginal discharge of small amounts of bloody material, resulting from placental transfer of maternal hormones which affect the endometrium of the infant's uterus. The same transfer of hormones may affect the breast tissue of either the male or the female infant, causing *breast engorgement* with or without drainage of small amounts of milk-like fluid. Examination of the genitalia may demonstrate *edema of the vulva or scrotum* as a result of placental transfer of hormones. Edema is also seen in infants of a breech delivery and is caused by the trauma of delivery.

Undescended testes are not an uncommon finding on physical examination of the newborn.

Although the testes generally migrate to the scrotum during the eighth month of fetal life, descent may not occur until 1 to 2 months after birth. If the testes are not present in the scrotum, they may descend when warm, moist compresses are applied to the infant's scrotum or lower abdomen, or when he is put, sitting, in a basin of warm water. If the testes do not descend with warming, gentle pressure exerted on the lower abdomen may push them into the scrotum.

These conditions are not indications of abnormality and require no treatment. It is important that the nurse discuss the condition and its cause with the parents to allay any undue concern on their part. The parents should, however, be aware that any discharge, engorgement, or edema which occurs beyond the immediate neonatal period is abnormal and requires prompt medical attention.

In the normal newborn, the primary focus of nursing care in relation to the reproductive system is in maintaining the cleanliness and integrity of the genitalia. The parents are taught adequate hygienic measures for the infant, including thorough washing of the area after each voiding or stool and separation of the labia, or gentle retraction of the prepuce, for adequate cleansing.

Conditions Requiring Immediate Diagnosis and Treatment

Hermaphroditism Sex determination and differentiation have been previously discussed, and to these a third element of sexual maturation may be added: sex assignment. *Sex assignment* is the combination of physical and psychologic factors which determines a person's subjective sex, the gender role which he assumes. The physical determinants—gonadal functioning, external genitalia, and secondary sex characteristics—have already been discussed. Just as important, however, are the psychologic determinants.

Often the first question asked after the birth of a baby is, "What is it, boy or girl?" Once that question is answered, the infant receives innumerable stimuli which reinforce the male or female designation. Names, clothes, colors, toys are all geared to distinguish sex. Parental and societal expectations, even during the newborn period, differ for boys and girls. As the child develops and grows, he becomes aware of the differences, internalizes this awareness, and conducts himself accordingly. His own expectations and behavior thus become relatively consonant with the gender role defined at birth.

Because of the overwhelming social and psy-chologic implications, reassignment of sex role after the initial designation will be difficult and embarrassing both for parents and child, and may have serious psychologic consequences for the child. Therefore, it is essential that sex designation be accurate. Detailed and precise evaluation of the infant's genitalia is most important. An abnormally small penis, hypospadias, and undescended testes may raise a question about the sex of an apparent male. If only one of these three signs is present, the true sex will almost invariably be male. If more than one is present, further investigation is indicated. An enlarged clitoris, partially or completely fused labia, or labia which are pigmented and thickened may raise the question of true sex in an apparent female.

Ambiguous genitalia and development associated with chromosomal abnormalities are discussed in Chapter 39. Some specific conditions, however, deserve discussion here.

A *male pseudohermaphrodite* is a person who has testes but whose external genitalia are female or ambiguous. This condition occurs with rare forms of congenital adrenal hyperplasia, Reifenstein's syndrome (a hereditary condition marked by hypospadias, hypogonadism, and gynecomastia), or, less rarely, testicular feminization syndrome (discussed later in this chapter in the section on adolescence). Infants with incomplete virilization of the external genitalia (e.g., hypospadias with otherwise normal male genitalia) are *not* considered to be pseudohermaphrodites.

In the *female pseudohermaphrodite,* ovaries are present, but external genitalia are male or ambiguous. The most common cause of this is congenital adrenal hyperplasia (see Chap. 39). Masculinization of the external female genitalia may also be caused by placental transfer of androgenic hormone from a mother who has a virilizing ovarian tumor or who has been treated with testosterone. It has also been noted that administration of synthetic progesterone (chemically similar to testosterone) to a mother with threatened abortion may cause masculinization of her female infant's external genitalia. If ambiguous genitalia are caused by maternal transmission of androgenic substances, little treatment is needed except for surgical repair of fused labia and of the vaginal outlet.

True pseudohermaphroditism is a rare condition in which the gonads consist of both ovarian and testicular tissue, and the external genitalia exhibit varying degrees of ambiguity. The cause is as yet unknown, and the chromosomal patterns vary.

Several diagnostic tools are available for determining the true sex of the infant with ambiguous external genitalia: buccal smear to determine presence of chromatin; urethroscopy and x-ray visualization to detect vaginal or cervical structures and presence of the urogenital sinus; 17-ketosteroid excretion in the urine which may indicate adrenal cortical hyperplasia; chromosomal studies to determine genetic sex; and laparotomy to visualize the gonads and internal structures.[2] The sex designation is generally that to which the external genitalia most closely correspond, rather than that indicated by the gonads. Subsequent surgical reconstruction is done as indicated to reinforce this designation.

As has been stated, it is important that an early diagnosis and designation of sex be made. The infant himself is psychosexually undifferentiated, and, until about two years of age, sex reassignment can be effected with little psychologic damage. However, the parents of the infant with ambiguous genitalia are frequently confused and distraught, especially if the designation of the infant's sex must be delayed or changed. Explanation of the embryologic origin of the genitalia may help them to understand the ambiguous development. Once sex designation is made, the parents' approach to the infant may be affected by their seeing the child as a "boy-girl" rather than boy or girl. They need an opportunity to discuss their feelings and concerns and must be encouraged and assisted to consider the infant totally as boy or girl. They will have questions about the child's future ability to develop normally, to have adequate sexual relations, and to reproduce. The physician can be expected to discuss these questions with the parents and review any corrective surgery to be performed. The nurse can give the parents continued support and reiterate the physician's explanations.

Sarcoma Botryoides   Malignant tumors or masses of the reproductive tract generally occur less frequently in children than in adults. Sarcoma botryoides, although it is rare, is seen more frequently in infants and young children than in older children or adults. This sarcoma arises generally from the vagina and appears as a polypoid, grapelike mass, brownish pink in color. Because of the necrosing tendency of the tumor and its extreme friability, early symptoms are vaginal bleeding and a malodorous discharge and may include expulsion of a piece of the tissue mass. The tumor grows rapidly, and protrusion of the grapelike mass from the vagina may be the initial symptom observed. The tumor is highly malignant, and rapid dissemination may involve other organs of the pelvic cavity.

Treatment of sarcoma botryoides is an aggressive surgical attack which includes radical hysterectomy and vaginectomy. Pelvic exenteration may be necessary, depending on the extent of the metastasis. Radiation therapy alone is not effective, but has been used in conjunction with surgical treatment. However, prognosis for the child with sarcoma botryoides is poor.

Nursing care of the patient with sarcoma botryoides begins with early recognition of symptoms. The nurse and the parents must be alert to any signs of vaginal bleeding or discharge on the infant. Support for the parents following diagnosis of the condition is important. The extent of the surgery, the adjustment in the care of their infant following surgery, and the poor prognosis of the disease can so overwhelm the parents that they may be unable to function effectively until they have an opportunity to examine their feelings and reactions. The nursing care of the infant prior to and following surgery will be dictated by the extent of the surgery; specific measures have been discussed in Chapter 24. Particularly if any form of pelvic exenteration is performed, the parents will need help in learning how to care for their child following discharge. Referral to a community health nurse is also important, both to provide for the care of the infant at home and to enable the parents to receive continuing support.

Conditions Requiring Subsequent Diagnosis and/or Treatment

Inguinal Hernia   An *inguinal hernia* is a protrusion of the hernial sac through the wall of the abdomen, the inguinal opening, or into the scrotum (sometimes referred to as a *scrotal hernia*). Inguinal hernias may be present at birth, or they may appear at a later age. They are more common in males than in females and are discovered more often on the right than on the left, although they may be bilateral.

Normally, the processus vaginalis precedes the testis in its retroperitoneal descent from the genital ridge into the scrotum during the eighth fetal month. The upper section atrophies, and the lower section forms the tunica vaginalis around the testis. When the upper section fails to atrophy, an inguinal hernia frequently results.

The hernial sac may extend all the way into the scrotum or may stop at the inguinal ring. It usually remains empty for awhile, but may fill with peritoneal fluid, a gonad, or intestine at any time. As a rule, the child is 2 to 4 months old before enough abdominal pressure develops to force an entry into the hernial sac. When the infant cries or strains, or when the older child coughs, stands, or strains, a mass will appear in the groin. This hernial mass can usually be reduced back into the abdominal cavity by gentle manipulation. Many times, by rubbing together the sides of the empty hernial sac, the nurse can elicit the "silk-glove" sensation, which is diagnostic of hernia.

In addition to these symptoms, if intestine is herniating into the sac, the child will be fretful and anorexic and will exhibit other symptoms of partial intestinal obstruction such as pain, difficulty in defecating, and perhaps local pressure. If the intestine becomes trapped in the sac, complete obstruction occurs with strangulation of the bowel, gangrene, bowel rupture, and perhaps death, unless there is surgical intervention. The child vomits, may have abdominal distention, local tenderness, fever, and cessation of bowel movements.

Sometimes an ovary in female infants prolapses into the hernial sac. Whether this ovarian herniation is transient or becomes incarcerated, immediate surgical correction is indicated to prevent damage to the ovary. If strangulation has already occurred, the ovary is permanently damaged, but immediate surgery is still indicated to prevent gangrene.

Surgical repair as soon as possible is the treatment of choice for inguinal hernias. Sometimes a bilateral repair will be performed on a child with a unilateral hernia because of the high frequency of subsequent hernia on the unaffected side. However, surgeons differ on their preference regarding this approach.The surgical repair involves extracting the herniated tissue and transfixing the neck of the processus vaginalis at the internal ring. This surgery is relatively simple and is well tolerated by children and small infants.

Preoperative nursing care of the child with an inguinal hernia is directed toward keeping the infant from straining, as he does when he cries or attempts to pass a constipated or an irritatingly loose stool. Straining may aggravate or induce strangulation; therefore, diet should be geared to regulating stools, and the child should be kept as happy and as quiet as possible. Playing strenuously or crying because he cannot have anything to eat before surgery may precipitate dehydration in the child. As a general rule, an infant can be allowed clear fluids until approximately 2 hours prior to surgery. It is therefore important for the nurse to ensure that the infant receives some fluid 2 hours prior to surgery to prevent dehydration, provided that fluids are not otherwise contraindicated.

Preoperative teaching is directed toward the parents to relieve their anxiety. They should understand that the surgery is far less complicated in the infant than in the adult, and that the infant will be awake and playing a few hours after surgery. Postoperatively, the child may have his diet as tolerated and be as active as he desires. Use of a pediatric urine collector will help to keep the wound dry and free of contamination.

Umbilical Hernia   An *umbilical hernia* is a protrusion of omentum or small intestine through a congenital weakness or opening of the umbilical ring. It is a soft swelling of tissue covered by skin and may look like a finger protruding from the umbilical area when the child cries, coughs, or strains. It may occur in any race, but is more common in the Negro race. It usually appears before the age of 6 months, and, unless it is unusually large, it will generally vanish spontaneously by the age of 1 year. It is normally easily reduced by manipulation but may strangulate on rare occasions. No treatment is recommended unless it does strangulate or unless it becomes progressively larger after the age of 2 years. Then a surgical repair of the umbilical ring is indicated. If the surgery is performed, a pressure dressing is applied to the umbilical area after surgery, and this dressing must be kept in place as well as dry and clean. Nursing care is otherwise essentially the same as that for inguinal hernia.

Phimosis   A tightening of the prepuce over the penis so that the foreskin cannot be retracted is termed *phimosis*.This is the normal condition of the prepuce in the newborn and, unless the urinary meatus is occluded, requires no treatment. The foreskin will not be retractable for several weeks after birth. If the meatus is occluded, or if phimosis occurs later in life, *circumcision*, surgical removal of the prepuce, is indicated. In the Jewish faith, ritual circumcision is performed on all male infants on the eighth day of life.

The routine circumcision of all newborn male infants is a much-debated procedure. Proponents feel that it is beneficial in providing for greater cleanliness and as prevention against future development of phimosis. They also note the decreased incidence of cervical carcinoma among women whose husbands have been circumcised. Opponents feel that the penis after circumcision is more prone to ulceration, which may lead to meatal stenosis. They also question the validity of the statistical evidence related to cervical carcinoma.

Since circumcision is a surgical procedure, it requires the consent of the parents. They should be given sufficient information to make an informed decision. If circumcision is performed, the infant is closely observed following the procedure for signs of excessive bleeding. Petrolatum gauze may be applied to the penis for several days to promote healing. The infant should also be closely observed for adequacy of voiding, for quality of the urinary stream, and for presence of blood in the urine. The mother is taught to maintain cleanliness of the area, to apply the gauze, and to observe for signs of infection or excessive bleeding.

If the infant is not circumcised, the mother is instructed in cleanliness of the area. The prepuce must not be forcibly retracted. However, when it becomes less adherent, it can be gently and briefly retracted in order to clean the area. Prolonged retraction of the prepuce can cause interruption of the blood supply to the glans.

NURSING APPROACHES IN THE CARE OF THE TODDLER AND PRESCHOOLER

Assessment of the reproductive system in the toddler or preschooler is the same as that for the infant, except that careful explanations to the child, as well as to his parents, are required for each step in the examination. When attempting to palpate the child's abdomen, it is helpful for the examiner to enlist his aid by cupping the child's hand in his own. This reduces the child's anxiety, makes him feel that he is helping, and does not interfere with the examiner's fingers. The child is more likely to relax his abdomen. When the nurse examines the young girl's vagina, he may also enlist her help to hold the labia apart. The nurse may use distraction in dealing with the toddler's anxieties.

To examine a young boy for descent of the testes, it is helpful to have him climb onto the examining table with as little help as possible and to assume a cross-legged "tailor" sitting position. Climbing causes abdominal pressure which forces normally retracted testes into the scrotum, and the "tailor" sitting position traps them by flattening the inguinal canal. Descent of the testes may also be achieved by having the child take a warm bath, or cough and strain, and then assume the "tailor" sitting position. The *cremasteric reflex* (retraction of the testes into the abdomen) is not present at birth, but the nurse or physician may prevent this response when examining the older child by placing his fingers across the upper portion of the inguinal canal, thereby obstructing the ascent of the testes when the scrotum is examined.

In the male at this age, the stretched penis should measure between 4 and 7 cm (1.6 and 2.8 in.). In the female, the labia minora are very small and flat, and the labia majora are puffy but proportionate to the perineum. As part of the examination, the labia should be palpated for lumps. The unestrogenized vaginal opening is somewhat more red than the rest of the genitalia.

The child should also be examined for precocious breast development, abdominal masses, unusual or disproportionate enlargement of the genitalia, and discoloration of the genitalia.

Separation from his parents is interpreted by the child under 4 years of age as desertion or punishment, and results in fears of attack and feelings of helplessness. However, the psychologic meaning of illnesses and treatments seems to have greater potential effects on the 4- to 8-year-old than separation from the parents. Anxiety, regression, and depression may result from fears of body mutilation (castration) and misinterpretation of painful treatments or surgery as punishment for real or imaginary transgressions. Nursing care must include reassuring the child that he is not being punished, explaining everything at his level of understanding, and, if possible, arranging for the parents to stay with him in the hospital.

Play may be useful therapy in preparing the child for surgery and in helping him work through his feelings about what is done to him. Preoperative teaching of the parents is more effective if all parents whose children are having surgery get together and learn as a group what to expect before and after surgery. It has been found that parents taught in groups ask more questions, have better rapport with the nurses, are more supportive of each other while the children are in surgery, are less anxious, and are more helpful in keeping the child on his postoperative regimen.

Diseases or Deviations

Hydrocele   A *hydrocele* is a fluctuant mass of fluid within the processus vaginalis and is often associated with inguinal hernia. It may be communicating or noncommunicating, and is sometimes difficult to differentiate from a hernia. It is a flexible, but tense, translucent mass below the spermatic cord.

A *noncommunicating hydrocele* occurs when peritoneal fluid is trapped in the testicular tunica vaginalis during the closure of the processus vaginalis. No treatment is necessary because the fluid is usually reabsorbed slowly during the child's first year of life. A *communicating hydrocele* occurs when the processus vaginalis remains open, allowing peritoneal fluid into the spermatic cord or into the canal of Nuck in females. It may enlarge as the day progresses and the activity of the child forces peritoneal fluid into the cord or canal. Supine relaxation at night allows the fluid to flow back into the peritoneal cavity, making the hydrocele smaller in the morning. The hydrocele may be present at birth or may appear sometime later. Since it is evidence of a patent processus vaginalis and an invitation for an inguinal hernia, surgery is the treatment of choice. The procedure involves opening the inguinal canal and removing the hernial sac.

The nursing care for a hydrocele and its repair is the same as for an inguinal hernia.

Cryptorchidism   Failure of one testis or both testes to descend into the scrotum is termed *cryptorchidism.* It occurs unilaterally four times as often as it does bilaterally. The testis may be *internal,* i.e., within the inguinal tract or the abdomen, or *ectopic*, i.e., located superficially in the inguinal pouch, in the femoral area, or in the perineum at the base of the penis.

Undescended testes are present in 3 percent of the term male newborn population and in 20 percent of the premature male population. By the age of 1 month, 50 percent of these have descended spontaneously, and, by 1 year, 80 percent descend into the scrotum. Some of the testes that fail to descend in early childhood will do so spontaneously during puberty.[3]

The cause of cryptorchidism is poorly understood. It is known that both the testes and the ovaries develop from the same point on the genital ridge; that the stimulus which causes the testes to move from the abdomen into the scrotum is the testosterone secreted by the male fetus; and that descent into the scrotum usually begins during the eighth fetal month. The known causes of nondescent are (1) mechanical interference with the passage of the testes into the scrotum; (2) a deficiency of gonadotropin; and (3) defective testes. The mechanical interference may be associated with undeveloped genital ducts or internal duct anomalies such as vaginal pouch remnants, fibrous bands, adhesions, or a short spermatic cord. When gonadotropins are deficient, there is not enough production of testosterone to stimulate or complete the descent.

The treatment of simple cryptorchidism is controversial and ranges from surgical intervention prior to the age of 6 years to no treatment at all. Conservative treatment is usually preferred to surgery, since the majority of testes will descend spon-

taneously by puberty. The frequently recommended treatment is a short course of chorionic gonadotropin given intramuscularly. When the testes have not descended by the age of 8 and sometimes 10 years, chorionic gonadotropin is given for 6 to 8 weeks. The dose varies from 500 units intramuscularly three times a week for 6 to 8 weeks to 1,000 to 5,000 units three times a week for 3 weeks. If signs of testicular descent appear during the initial course, a repeat course may be given after 10 weeks. If there is no indication of improvement during the initial course of treatment, surgery is indicated.

Orchiopexy is the surgical procedure to correct cryptorchidism and consists of dissecting the testis and spermatic cord from the surrounding tissue and transplanting the testis through the inguinal canal. The testis is then secured in place with a suture to a rubber band attached to the thigh with adhesive tape. The rubber band serves to maintain the position of the testis in the scrotum, but is not meant to apply pressure. There is as much risk of injury to the testes from surgical intervention as there is from no treatment whatsover,[4] but some physicians feel that surgery should be performed before the age of 6 years because that is the age at which the testicular tubules begin to develop. Many physicians, however, feel that the damage to the tubules from the body temperature to which they are exposed is slight before the age of 8 or 10 years and prefer postponing surgery until then.

Abdominal testes are often defective and are associated with other genital abnormalities such as inguinal hernia or hypogonadism. Malignancy is common in testes that remain in the abdomen after puberty. Therefore, surgical removal of abdominal testes is indicated when biopsy reveals defective testes. Sterility always exists when the testes remain in the abdomen, whether because of the associated abnormalities or because of the exposure of the testes to normal body temperature (2.2°C higher than the normal scrotal temperature) for an extended period of time. Higher temperatures retard spermatogenesis and may damage the tubules to the extent that sterility is permanent.

Case-finding occurs with the older child during an examination or when anxious parents (or the child himself) approach the nurse. It is wise to reassure the child and his parents that testes present in the scrotum at birth, or testes that descended at some point thereafter, often ascend and may even reside out of the scrotum at intervals during childhood. A warm bath followed by coughing or straining will frequently achieve descent in the older child. Referral to a physician is in order if warming, coughing, and straining do not achieve descent. In addition to the referral, the nurse must deal with the parents' anxieties, usually centering on concerns about sterility, homosexuality, or cancer. The parents may not feel comfortable in verbalizing their concerns; they may even feel that the child is defective and inadequate, and may not tell the child about his condition and pending treatment. In most cases, contrary to his parents' belief that he is ignorant of the problem, the child is aware that his scrotum is not normal, but has a feeling that the problem should not be discussed. Sometimes he will deny the existence of a problem.

As soon as a child is admitted for orchiopexy, the nurse should assess what he knows about his condition and pending treatment and what his anxieties are. The attention that has been focused on his scrotum will heighten his concerns about genital mutilation. He should be reassured that his penis will not be involved in the surgery, that it will be only his scrotum. (The nurse should be sure that the child understands this terminology or should use the terminology with which he is familiar.) He should be told to expect the rubber bands, and that they will be removed within 5 to 7 days. He should be told to expect some swelling of his scrotum after surgery and perhaps ice packs around the scrotum for several hours after surgery. His activity should be normal after anesthesia, and he should not have much pain. His fluid preferences should be ascertained so that his favorite fluids can be offered after surgery to restore his fluid balance. If the child is of school age, plans should be made that will allow him an opportunity to see or converse by phone with his friends, as separation anxiety may be more closely related with peers at this age.

Postoperatively, particular attention should be given to prevention of infection by keeping the suture line clean and free of fecal material. The child should be taught to wipe posteriorly after bowel movements, and care should be taken not to place too much pressure on the rubber band securing the testis in the scrotum. Antibiotics are sometimes administered to prevent infection.

Torsion of the Testis   This condition is an idiopathic twisting of the vascular pedicle of the appendix testis or the spermatic cord, which interferes with the normally rich blood supply to the testis. There may be no symptoms during the neonatal period, or there may be enlargement and tenseness of the testis with a unilateral red or bluish discoloration and swelling of the scrotum. The older child may com-

plain of discomfort with the swollen testis. Later, there may be severe pain, exquisite tenderness, lower abdominal pain, fever, nausea, and vomiting. These are signs of infarction and necrosis of the testis.

Surgical correction is the treatment for torsion of the testis. Unless it is necrotic, the testis is not removed but is attached to the scrotal tissue. If the testis is removed, a prosthesis may replace it for psychologic reasons and for cosmetic effect.

Nursing care is centered around relieving pain and distracting the child from his pain and discomfort both preoperatively and postoperatively. The mother's help is invaluable here, especially in relieving the excessive separation anxiety of the toddler. The nursing history should reflect the child's favorite pastimes and also indicate his terminology for his penis and scrotum.

Preoperative teaching should be geared to the child's level of understanding. Support for the scrotum may be helpful in relieving the pain, but may also be intolerable because of the tenderness.

Postoperative nursing care is again directed toward relieving the discomfort now aggravated by surgery. Ice bags may be applied to the scrotum immediately after surgery to reduce swelling, but may not be tolerable. Care should be taken to prevent wound contamination, but the child may be as active as he desires.

NURSING APPROACHES IN THE CARE OF THE SCHOOL-AGE CHILD

There is a great deal of asynchrony or asymmetry in the physical development of the school-age child which may make nursing assessment difficult. This asymmetry may be of more concern to the parents, but can also be a concern of the child. One breast normally develops more rapidly than the other, and one side of the scrotum is usually larger than the other. The rapid weight gain and fat accumulation in the male which precedes the growth spurt of puberty may be a source of anxiety to the boy and to his parents because the penis appears to be disproportionate in size. If the stretched penis is between 5 and 11 cm (2.0 and 4.3 in.), it is normal. Careful, factual explanation is required to reassure the parents and the child.

Separation anxiety related to parents may not be a problem for the child in this age group, but some anxiety in relation to separation from peers is engendered when the child is hospitalized. Oedipal anxieties are usually dormant, and genital surgery is not usually so traumatic for him as it is for the preschooler or for the adolescent. Castration fears are likely to be present, however, and careful explanation and repeated reassurances are important, even for the child who does not ask for them.

Postoperatively, the school-age child is not usually so active as the preschooler, nor so accepting of necessary procedures. He may react more aggressively and needs as much independence as possible.

The school-age child is concerned about his body image. He fears genital inadequacy, loss of body control or mastery, and muscular weakness. Verbal reassurance is beneficial, but play which allows him to release pent-up energy and anxiety is more effective. It is important to the hospitalized child to be assigned to a room with others of the same age and sex.

Diseases or Deviations

Precocious Puberty   There is considerable variation in the ages at which puberty occurs. Generally, however, it is accepted that 8 years in females and 10 years in males is the earliest age at which sexual maturation normally begins. Maturation prior to that time is termed *precocious puberty.*

True precocious puberty involves the early activation of the hypothalamic-pituitary-gonadal axis. Sexual development includes the growth and functioning of the gonads as well as the appearance of secondary sex characteristics. This may be caused by a central nervous system lesion, or it may be idiopathic. The most frequently occurring type is idiopathic precocious puberty, and diagnosis is made after eliminating organic problems as the cause.

In *pseudoprecocious puberty,* the initial release of gonadotropins does not occur. Although secondary sex characteristics appear, the gonads do not develop, and ovulation or spermatogenesis does not take place. Pseudoprecocious puberty may be caused by gonadal or adrenal tumors, or by the administration or accidental ingestion of gonadal hormones.

Precocious puberty can develop at any time during infancy, early childhood, or the early school-age period, and is seen more frequently in females than in males. Sexual maturation generally follows the normal sequence, although it may be greatly disorganized. Menarche in females has been observed as early as 1 year, and pregnancy recorded as early as 5½ years. In males, spermatogenesis has occurred at 5 to 6 years.

In both sexes, and with either pseudoprecocious puberty or true precocious puberty, growth spurt and bone development evolve as a result of the increase in gonadal hormone levels. This increase also causes early closure of the epiphyses. Therefore, the child with precocious puberty will be taller than average during childhood, but in adulthood will be shorter than average. In all children, intellectual and psychosexual development parallel chronologic age rather than sexual development.

The child with precocious puberty is evaluated carefully to determine cause. Brain scan, skull x-rays, and electroencephalogram may be done to discover the presence or absence of central nervous system lesions. Ovarian tumors are usually easily noted on abdominal or bimanual palpation. Testicular tumors are also easily discovered by palpation. Discussion of adrenal tumors may be found in Chapter 39. Accurate history with attention to the opportunity for ingestion of hormones is also important. When the cause is known, treatment is directed toward the primary disturbance.

If no organic disturbance is noted, precocious puberty is then diagnosed as idiopathic. Progesterone has been used in treating idiopathic precocious puberty, but, although menstruation ceases and breast development is retarded, no effect has been noted on bone growth and development.

With no treatment, these children will develop normally, except for their accelerated sexual development, and will have no residual effects other than short stature. However, it is important that a child with diagnosed idiopathic precocious puberty be reevaluated for central nervous system lesion or, more rarely, gonadal tumors which were not demonstrated on initial examination.

Both the child and the parents may be concerned and embarrassed about the child's early maturation. Since the parents will be of greatest help to the child, it is important that the nurse assist them to understand their own and their child's reactions. Medical explanations may have to be reiterated and clarified for the parents.

The child will need some explanation, in terms he can understand, about what is happening to his body. These should be given calmly and factually, with no overtones of disapproval or reproof. Sometimes the child with precocious puberty will develop feelings of inferiority because he is different from other children. His shyness and tendency to withdraw may be intensified by the teasing of other children who have not yet developed sexually. If the child understands that he is not really different but only growing more rapidly, and that the other children will develop as he is, he may be more comfortable with his precocity. Some of the physical changes which make the child appear different can be minimized by clothing styles which make these changes appear less obvious. The child will need to learn the hygiene measures associated with pubertal development.

Finally, the parents of the child with precocious sexual development must understand clearly that his intellectual, emotional, and social development does not parallel his physical development. Therefore, it is important that the child be protected from situations in which older children or adults might take advantage of his sexual precocity.

Premature Thelarche and Adrenarche *Premature thelarche* is the development of breast tissue, either bilaterally or unilaterally, in the young child prior to the onset of puberty, but unaccompanied by the development of other signs of precocious puberty. Since the breasts begin normal development at about 8 years of age, premature thelarche must, by definition, appear before this and may occur in a child as young as 1 to 2 years of age.

Premature thelarche generally appears as disks of breast tissue around the nipple area, which may be associated with tenderness. The breasts may grow for a time, then arrest in development or even regress somewhat. There is, however, no development of the nipple and pigmentation of the areola.

Premature adrenarche (pubarche) is the development of pubic hair prior to the onset of puberty, unaccompanied by the development of other signs of precocious puberty. Occasionally, the development of axillary hair is associated with pubarche.

These conditions, when they occur in the absence of other signs of precocious puberty or organic disease, are benign and require no treatment. The nurse should assist the parents to understand this, and to treat their appearance calmly to avoid arousing undue concern in the child.

Vulvovaginitis This is an inflammatory condition of the vulva and the vagina, common to both young girls and to adolescents. The combined terminology is used because vulvitis rarely occurs without subsequent inflammation of the vagina, and vice versa. It is prevalent in young children because the unestrogenized vaginal mucosa has a neutral pH, is thin and taut, lacks glycogen and lactobacilli, and is therefore highly susceptible to infection.

The most common cause of vulvovaginitis is a bacterial infection which may result from poor local hygiene with contamination by feces, urine, or unclean fingers; insertion into the vagina of such foreign bodies as hairpins, stones, nuts, pennies, and wads of toilet paper; and gonorrhea acquired from inadvertent indirect contact with discharge from an infected adult, attempted intercourse, or sexual abuse. Vulvovaginitis sometimes occurs when organisms associated with respiratory disease are transferred to the genital area by fingers contaminated by nose-picking or finger-sucking.

The vulvovaginitis resulting from poor local hygiene is usually of nonspecific or mixed bacterial origin, but it may be caused by a virus, a fungus, or pinworms. Since it is difficult to isolate a single causative organism, the treatment of choice is good local hygiene. If necessary, local application of estrogen creams is instituted to reduce the susceptibility of the vaginal mucosa. A broad-spectrum antibiotic may be administered intramuscularly if the infection is severe or if it is associated with a respiratory infection.

When the condition continues, a foreign body in the vagina should be suspected. Once the foreign body is removed and the vagina irrigated, no further treatment is necessary. The acute inflammation should subside within 3 days, and the infection should be gone within 1 to 3 weeks. The treatment for gonorrheal vulvovaginitis includes determination and elimination of the source of infection and administration of aqueous procaine penicillin G intramuscularly. Nursing care is primarily directed toward case-finding, environmental and patient cleanliness, and support and teaching of both the patient and her family.

The nurse must be familiar with the symptoms of vulvovaginitis (see Table 37-2), being frequently the first health professional to discover it. The mother may approach the nurse because she has noticed a vaginal discharge, red, swollen vulva, and excessive crying and irritability, with one or more of the other signs and symptoms. If the child is old enough, she may complain of pain with walking, sitting, voiding, or defecating, and a sensation of itching or burning. In the hospital, the nurse should be alert for vulvovaginitis in any child admitted with an infection, especially respiratory. Children contaminate their fingers with exudate and transfer the infection to the highly susceptible vulvovaginal area. Gonorrheal vulvovaginitis also spreads easily in institutions and is often not immediately diagnosed. Therefore, any child with vulvovaginitis should have her own thermometer and bedpan, and the personnel should be instructed to exercise extra care in handwashing.

Good local hygiene is the primary nursing goal. This involves gentle but thorough cleansing of the area after each bowel movement and at least twice

Table 37-2 VULVOVAGINITIS IN CHILDREN

Cause	Most common signs and symptoms	Treatment
Nonspecific bacteria	Erythema; edema; excoriation; maceration; poor local hygiene; scratches; scant vaginal discharge	Good local hygiene, followed by local application of estrogen cream; if no response, broad-spectrum antibiotic intramuscularly
Foreign object	Erythema; edema; excoriation; profuse, bloody, foul, purulent vaginal discharge	Removal of foreign object; vaginal irrigation; good local hygiene
Gonorrhea	Erythema; edema; excoriation; maceration; profuse, purulent, yellow, creamy vaginal discharge	Elimination of source; aqueous procaine penicillin G intramuscularly

daily with a castile soap. However, if the inflammation is severe, vegetable oil is preferable to soap as a cleansing agent. Since the mother is the best person to bathe the child who cannot bathe herself, the mother should be taught to cleanse the area thoroughly from front to back, rinse well, and blot, rather than rub, dry. The area should be left open to the air to complete drying, and cornstarch may be applied to reduce friction. Panties should be made of loose-fitting white cotton to avoid irritation from dye or constriction. As soon as she is old enough, the child should be taught to wipe herself from front to back after voiding and defecating and during bathing.

A poor state of health may contribute to the child's susceptibility to vaginitis, and the nurse may have to work with both the child and her parents to improve nutrition and overall health status. It may be necessary to involve the dietitian to help the family with meal planning and the purchase of food.

Finally, depending on age, both the child and her mother are usually concerned about the presence of a vaginal discharge. This requires support, explanation, reassurance, and teaching by the nurse. The parents may need to know that their child is not a "bad girl" because she placed a foreign object in her vagina. She was simply indulging in ordinary childhood exploration and manipulation similar to placing objects in the ear or nose. However, if there is a recurrence, further investigation may be needed to rule out emotional disorders.

Acute Testicular Injury Injury of the scrotum and testes are common in young males over the age of 2 years. Falls on playground equipment and bicycle bars are the most frequent cause. There is exquisite pain at the time of the injury. Later there is usually pain and red or bluish discoloration of the scrotum where the injury occurred, sometimes accompanied by swelling. Pain and a history of injury are the essentials of diagnosis. Contusion is the usual result

of such an injury, and no treatment is required. Support to the scrotum may be helpful, and ice may be applied immediately after the injury to decrease the contusion.

If the contusion is severe, necrosis may result. The symptoms then resemble those of necrosis caused by torsion of the testis, and surgical removal of the affected testis is necessary.

Support of the scrotum is helpful, and warm baths may be soothing and increase the rate of absorption of the contusion after bleeding has stopped. Prolonged hot baths are contraindicated in a child who has reached puberty, since this prolonged exposure to high temperatures may cause sterility. Parents are usually concerned that the child will become sterile as a result of the testicular injury, so nursing care is designed to relieve this anxiety. In rare instances where surgery is required, the nursing care is the same as that for torsion of the testis.

Malignant Conditions of the Reproductive Tract Prior to adulthood, malignant conditions of the reproductive tract occur rarely. *Teratomas* are tumors containing several types of tissue and may be either malignant or benign. Testicular teratomas may be asymptomatic, with unilateral scrotal enlargement that may be mistaken for hydrocele. Ovarian teratoma may be palpated as an asymptomatic mass, or may be diagnosed following episodes of abdominal pain, nausea, and vomiting. These episodes are caused by torsion of the ovarian pedicle. If the teratoma is benign, removal of the affected gonad is sufficient. Malignant teratomas require more extensive and agressive treatment.

Carcinoma of the cervix is infrequently seen and is generally an adenocarcinoma. Symptoms may include vaginal discharge or abnormal vaginal bleeding. Surgical treatment will vary from local excision to extended hysterectomy, depending on the extent of the involvement. Recently, *adenocarcinoma of the vagina* and sometimes of the cervix has been observed in girls whose mothers received stilbestrol during their pregnancies.[5] These patients may have vaginal bleeding or discharge, or may be asymptomatic. Diagnosis is made on vaginal examination, since vaginal cytology may be negative. Surgical treatment generally involves removal of the vagina, cervix, and uterus.

Although these tumors are seen relatively infrequently, success of treatment depends on early diagnosis and prompt intervention. The presenting symptoms may not excite particular concern: for example, irregular vaginal bleeding which can be a symptom of vaginal adenocarcinoma may be erroneously diagnosed as the irregular cyclic functioning common to many adolescents after menarche. Therefore, it is important that the nurse encourage the parents to seek medical evaluation for their child whenever abnormal bleeding, vaginal discharge, enlarged scrotum, or other symptoms are noted.

Considerable anxiety will be aroused in the parent and in the child (depending on his age) when the diagnosis is established and surgery discussed. The nurse can assist the parents and the child by providing an opportunity for them to discuss their concerns and by reiterating and reinforcing the physician's explanations. They will have questions about the effect of the surgery on the child's future sexual activity and reproductive functions. Unilateral gonadectomy will have no effect on reproductive functions, since the other reproductive organs, including one gonad, remain intact. More extensive surgery will have an effect, however, and this should be explained clearly.

Nursing care of the child prior to and following surgery is according to the principles of gynecologic or urologic nursing care, adapted, of course, to the age of the child. Following hospitalization, referral to the community health nurse can provide the child and the family with continued care and support. Care of the terminally ill child and his family is discussed in Chapter 29.

NURSING APPROACHES IN THE CARE OF THE ADOLESCENT

At any stage along the way, the nurse may be called upon to give the adolescent the ego support he so desperately needs. The nurse can reassure the teenager that his development and its attendant anxieties are normal, and can sometimes prepare him for the next stages of his development.

The adolescent needs accurate, honest information about his developing body. The nurse should not assume on the basis of his approach that he understands. Frequently the adolescent has received little basic sex education, but has exchanged erroneous information and misconceptions with his peers. However, he may be unwilling to admit ignorance, feeling that this reflects negatively on himself. Therefore, the nurse must determine the extent of his knowledge and build on that, reassuring him by his approach that his curiosity is normal and his interest in learning laudable. Sex education should not be limited to anatomy and physiology or what might be termed basic mechanics of the reproductive system. The adolescent also should understand his own behavior and the behavior of others, and should learn to communicate and establish effective relationships with others. The nurse then becomes one of many—including parents, teachers, social workers, and doctors—who can assist the adolescent to understand the foundations upon which he will base his future behavior and relationships.

Illness or surgery which involves the reproductive system can cause particular anxiety in the adolescent. He is very much aware of his developing sexuality, and anything which seems to impinge upon this can be threatening to his self-image. It is important for the nurse to respect the characteristic shyness and need for privacy of this age group. Every procedure performed should be explained in detail to the patient, drapes should be used during examinations, and the nurse should remain in the room when the doctor performs a physical examination on an adolescent female. Findings should also be discussed, as the adolescent is prone to wild imaginings. Again, the nurse should not assume that the adolescent understands because he asks no questions.

The pelvic examination can be frightening for the adolescent girl, particularly if her mother or an older sister conveys anxiety about this procedure. The nurse who will be present during the examination can, by a calm and reassuring manner and continued explanations, help to allay the girl's fears. Usually the adolescent will be more comfortable if her mother is not present during the examination.

Diseases or Deviations

Imperforate Hymen The hymen is a membrane of epithelial tissue which develops at the juncture of the urogenital sinus and the vaginal plate. If the lumen fails to appear, the hymen is *imperforate*.

The imperforate hymen is usually detected prior to puberty, and will generally cause no difficulty during early childhood. With menarche, however, the cyclical uterine discharge will cause an accumulation of blood in the vagina (hematocolpos), in the uterus (hematometra), and eventually in the tubes (hematosalpinx). Initially, this may not cause noticeable discomfort, but may present as a pelvic mass or, more rarely, with the initial complaint of flank pain due to urinary retention. However, the increase of accumulated blood may be accompanied by a gradual increase in pelvic discomfort.

Diagnosis is made on noting the bulging, intact hymen in a patient who has supposedly not reached menarche. Treatment consists of surgical incision of the hymen or, preferably, excision of a portion of the hymen, with release of the accumulated blood. There is generally no damage to the reproductive tract as a result of the accumulation.

The adolescent girl is very conscious of her developing body and may be particularly concerned about surgical procedures involving the genital area. She should have a clear understanding of what is to be done and of the indications for the surgery. She should understand that, following surgery, she will menstruate in a relatively normal cycle, and that this condition will not interfere with her ability to have satisfactory sexual experiences or to conceive and bear children. Following surgery, mild analgesics or warm sitz baths may relieve any transient discomfort.

Amenorrhea   The absence of menses is termed *amenorrhea*; it may be either primary or secondary. In *primary amenorrhea,* menarche does not occur; in *secondary amenorrhea,* menses cease at some time after menarche. Secondary amenorrhea is a normal condition during pregnancy and lactation and after menopause; primary amenorrhea prior to the age of puberty is also normal. Excepting these, amenorrhea is a symptom of some underlying disorder which must itself be discovered and treated.

Since menstruation is related to delicate hormonal balance as well as to the integrity of the reproductive organs themselves, disorders which interfere with the functioning of the hypothalamus, the pituitary, the ovaries, or the uterus and vagina may produce amenorrhea. If primary amenorrhea is associated with the development of secondary sex characteristics, the absence of menarche suggests a defect in the anatomic structure of the uterus and/or vagina, or imperforate hymen. Primary amenorrhea associated with little or no development of secondary sex characteristics suggests disturbances in the hormonal interaction resulting from genetic defects such as adrenogenital syndrome, testicular femini-

zation, or gonadal dysgenesis. Intracranial lesions and pituitary failure may also cause primary amenorrhea.

Secondary amenorrhea likewise can be related to a variety of causative factors. Again, organic brain disease may be a cause, as may ovarian neoplasm or polycystic ovary. Nutritional and psychologic disturbances apparently affect hypothalamic functioning, although the exact mechanism is unknown. Sudden weight gain or "crash" dieting, emotional disturbances, and psychiatric illness may be associated with secondary amenorrhea. Recently, it has been found that discontinuance of oral contraceptives, if they have been taken over a long period of time, may produce amenorrhea.

The adolescent with amenorrhea may be considerably concerned and anxious about her continued failure to menstruate. Since amenorrhea is frequently a symptom of a physical disturbance, the nurse must encourage the girl to obtain medical evaluation. The nurse will be able to support the adolescent through the physical examination and necessary diagnostic tests. Subsequent nursing care will depend on the specific diagnosis.

Dysfunctional Uterine Bleeding   A universally accepted definition of the term *dysfunctional uterine bleeding* has not yet been developed. For the purposes of this text, dysfunctional uterine bleeding in the adolescent is considered to be irregular, prolonged, or excessive bleeding not associated with disorders of the reproductive system, systemic disease, or pregnancy or its complications.

In the adolescent, dysfunctional uterine bleeding is generally a result of idiopathic anovulation. Because ovulation fails to occur, there is no formation of a corpus luteum or production of progesterone. Consistent, elevated levels of estrogen maintain the proliferative phase of the endometrium until the endometrium can no longer support this and breakthrough bleeding occurs. The bleeding episodes may be irregular in occurrence, in duration, and in amount, and are generally not accompanied by pelvic pain.

Diagnosis of dysfunctional uterine bleeding is generally made on the basis of history, physical examination, and diagnostic testing to rule out organic cause. When the diagnosis has been established, treatment for the majority of adolescents may be primarily directed toward maintaining good health both physically and psychologically until the cycle readjusts itself. Anovulation is frequently associated with inadequate nutrition and psychologic stress.

Therefore, a well-balanced diet, rest, and relaxation are essential. Supplemental iron may also be given for associated borderline anemia.

Health teaching is an important element in the nursing care of the adolescent with dysfunctional uterine bleeding. She must understand the normal menstrual cycle and the factors which may affect it. She must realize that adequate activity and exercise, as well as adequate rest, are important in maintaining a normal cycle. The adolescent can also be helped to understand what constitutes good nutrition, and to adjust her eating habits accordingly. She should be encouraged to keep an accurate record of her menstrual cycle and assisted in distinguishing between normal and abnormal menstrual bleeding.

If the bleeding is particularly heavy, hormonal therapy may be introduced. Large doses of progesterone, often combined with small doses of estrogens, will stop the bleeding. When the bleeding ceases, the dosage of progesterone is decreased for several weeks, then discontinued. It is then necessary to cycle the girl on oral progesterone for 3 to 4 months, or dysfunctional bleeding will recur. After this, the hormones are discontinued and the patient closely observed in the expectation that the system will have regulated itself. The girl should understand the purpose of the hormonal therapy and should be encouraged to report any unusual side effects which she may experience.

When dysfunctional bleeding fails to respond to more conservative management, dilatation and curettage may be necessary to control hemorrhage. Following surgery, the patient should be closely checked for excessive vaginal bleeding. If vaginal packing has been inserted following surgery, this may cause discomfort and difficulty in voiding. The discomfort is usually relieved with mild analgesics; more severe or persistent pain may indicate uterine perforation and should be reported immediately. The difficulty in voiding is usually overcome when the patient is able to get out of bed to the bathroom. The vaginal packing is generally removed within 24 hours following surgery, and the girl is again closely observed for excessive bleeding.

Dysmenorrhea Painful menstruation, or dysmenorrhea, may be either primary or secondary. *Secondary dysmenorrhea* is a symptom associated with a specific organic cause, such as pelvic inflammatory disease or endometriosis, and the treatment is directed toward the primary disease entity.

Primary dysmenorrhea is seen more frequently in adolescent girls than secondary dysmenorrhea, and is painful menstruation in the absence of obvious organic disturbance. It is associated with ovulatory cycles, as contrasted with the usually painless bleeding of anovulatory cycles in dysfunctional uterine bleeding. The specific cause of primary dysmenorrhea is not clear, but theories have been advanced relating it to hormone imbalance, cervical obstruction, uterine hyperplasia, poor posture, and neurogenic and psychogenic disturbances.[6]

The symptoms of dysmenorrhea occur at the time of the onset of menses, or just prior to or following the onset. The quality of pain may be sharp or dull, cyclic and cramplike, or steady and less intense. There may be associated anxiety symptoms (headache, fatigue, irritability) or gastrointestinal symptoms (nausea, vomiting).

In the absence of a specific cause, treatment of primary dysmenorrhea is largely empiric. Mild analgesics (aspirin, Darvon, Empirin), amphetamines (Edrisal), and simple exercises may be prescribed in conjunction with general means used to allay concerns and anxieties associated with this period of development. Diuretics may be prescribed if accompanying signs of premenstrual tension and fluid retention are present. Recently, the use of synthetic hormones—the oral contraceptives—has been successful in treating primary dysmenorrhea. With the use of estrogen alone or of estrogen and progesterone in combination, an anovulatory cycle can be produced. Less frequently, surgical intervention in the form of uterine sounding or presacral neurectomy has been used with varying degrees of success.

Simple means which may relieve dysmenorrhea include short periods of rest, nonstrenuous activities to occupy time and attention, and warm baths. Attention at all times to good posture and general exercise to improve muscle tone will help decrease discomfort during menstruation. The nurse should caution the girl to take medications only as prescribed.

Delayed Puberty When there is no evidence of sexual development in a female by the age of 15, or in a male by the age of 17, delayed puberty is said to exist. Based on the average age of puberty and the mean standard deviation of 2.5, delayed puberty exists in a 12.5-year-old female when there are no breast buds or strands of pubic hair, and in a 14.5-year-old male when there is no increase in the size of the external genitalia or strands of pubic hair.

Delayed puberty is caused by gonadal deficits (hypogonadism), gonadotropin deficits, or simple idiopathic delayed sexual maturation. It is more common in males than in females, and causes more psychologic problems in males than in females.

A number of factors influence the onset of puberty. Research indicates that puberty can occur later in children who have had little opportunity to mix and socialize with the opposite sex.[7] It is postulated that social cues, expectations, and pressures hasten the onset of puberty. Children rise to meet expectations, and there is a great deal of pressure from parents and peers to take an interest in the opposite sex. Children are bombarded with sex-oriented advertising designed to affect the conscious as well as the subconscious mind. All these factors may influence higher central nervous system centers to initiate the onset of puberty.

Poor nutrition retards the onset of puberty, as do drugs such as reserpine, and illnesses such as debilitating infections, regional ileitis, lesions or neoplasms of the hypothalamus, pituitary, or gonads, and undetected hypothyroidism.

All the above factors, along with unknown neural humors (unidentified cerebral chemical substances) and unknown higher central nervous system centers, affect the hypothalamus and the anterior pituitary to initiate or retard the release of gonadotropins and thereby initiate the onset of puberty.

Gonadal deficits include gonadal dysgenesis, anorchia congenita, rudimentary ovaries or testes, chromosomal disorders such as Klinefelter's and Turner's syndromes, and endocrine disorders such as adrenal hyperplasia and testicular feminization. Gonadotropin deficits include Kallman's and Laurence-Moon-Biedl syndromes, isolated gonadotropin deficiency, and more commonly panhypopituitarism. Other factors which may affect the functioning of the hypothalamic-pituitary-gonadal axis and cause delayed puberty are nutritional deficiencies and chronic systemic disease such as cardiac disease, diabetes mellitus, anemias, respiratory disease, malabsorption syndrome, severe renal disease, and collagen disease. A diagnosis of simple idiopathic delayed puberty can be made only when endocrine and cytogenetic diagnostic studies have been performed and both gonadal and gonadotropin deficits are ruled out.

There is a direct correlation between the adolescent growth spurt and sex changes, so that pathologic delayed puberty is often ruled out if there has been no spurt in physical growth. (See Chap. 39.) It is true that pathology is more likely in cases where there is a growth spurt but no secondary sex changes; however, the psychologic effects of severely retarded puberty warrant treatment whether

or not a growth spurt has occurred. If the bone age is in line with height and there is a family history of late sexual maturation, reassurance of the adolescent and his family based on normal laboratory reports may be all the treatment necessary. However, in any case of simple delayed puberty, the patient, his family, and the health professionals should collaborate to determine whether gonadal hormonal therapy (estrogen and progesterone or testosterone) should be given. This treatment results in satisfactory development of secondary sex characteristics and will frequently initiate true puberty. For this reason, hormonal therapy is usually given for 1 year and then interrupted for a year to allow puberty to develop. Therapy is especially indicated in an adolescent who is withdrawn, acting out, or failing in school, or who shows evidence of developing severe psychologic problems.

The psychologic problems of the late maturer claim the major portion of the nurse's attention. Frequently the nurse is the first person approached by the anxious adolescent or his parents. Although the nurse may obtain a history of familial retarded sexual maturation and find evidence of a growth spurt and pubic hair, he should still refer the patient to a physician for diagnostic evaluation. Reassurance that maturation is taking place, although slowly, should include sharing the facts with the adolescent and his family. The nurse can emphasize the positive signs—the appearance of pubic hair or breast buds, enlargement of the genitalia, or the growth spurt. Factual evidence is more convincing and reassuring than unsupported statements that "everything will be all right; development will start soon."

Other nursing care includes (1) demonstrating an active interest by listening to the adolescent; (2) discussing and emphasizing his assets; (3) encouraging and supporting his participation in school and peer activities (physically nonthreatening activities such as team manager, coach's assistant, editor of the paper, or fashion consultant to increase the adolescent's stature with his peers); and (4) allaying the anxiety of his parents as much as possible.

Testicular Feminization This condition is a form of male pseudohermaphroditism in which the external genitalia are completely feminized. Internal structures are absent except for the testes, which may be located in the labia, the inguinal canal, or the abdomen. The cause is unknown, but it has been suggested that an inborn enzymatic error reduces endorgan response to androgens.

Occasionally, the testes are palpated on routine

examination of the girl or discovered during abdominal surgery. Usually, however, diagnosis is not made until puberty, when the adolescent presents with primary amenorrhea. Feminine secondary sex characteristics develop, but because of lack of end-organ response to androgens, pubic and axillary hair is scanty or absent. Pelvic examination reveals the vagina to be shortened, ending in a blind pouch. The testes may be palpated as an abdominal, inguinal, or labial mass. Buccal smear is chromatin-negative, and chromosomal pattern is male.

Any attempt at reassignment of sex can precipitate severe psychologic problems in the adolescent, since gender role has been well established. Therefore, all therapeutic measures are directed toward reinforcing the feminine identity. The testes exert a feminizing effect and are left in place through puberty. Once secondary sex characteristics have developed, the testes are removed because of the high incidence of neoplasm of the gonads in testicular feminization. Following surgery, the patient is maintained on estrogen therapy.

Usually these girls can have normal intercourse, but will not menstruate and cannot bear children. This knowledge can create feelings of inadequacy in the girl, and the nurse can assist her to explore these feelings and to assess them realistically.

Venereal Disease   This is a communicable disease which is contacted through direct sexual activity. Several types of venereal disease have been identified, but the most prevalent are gonorrhea and syphilis. Both are caused by anaerobic organisms which cannot survive outside a warm, enclosed environment such as the human body provides. Gonorrhea occurs considerably more frequently than syphilis, but the effects of untreated syphilis are far more serious. Syphilis and gonorrhea are similar in their mode of transmission, but they are totally different diseases which can be present or contracted simultaneously. Treatment of one will not necessarily cure the other.

Venereal disease is a major health problem among adolescents and young adults. In one state alone, 70 percent of the new cases reported in 1972 occurred in the 15- to 25-year age group. Reported cases almost doubled in the 5-year period from 1965 to 1970, and have been increasing by 10 to 15 percent each year since then.[8]

There is evidence to link the increase in venereal disease with increases in sexual promiscuity. Sweden, with its permissive attitude toward sexual promiscuity, has the highest venereal disease rate in the world. China, under the influence of Mao Tse-tung's puritanical thoughts on promiscuity and prostitution, has virtually no venereal disease.

However, another factor probably more closely related to the increased incidence of venereal disease is the change in common methods of contraception. The use of a condom during intercourse protects the penis from direct contact with infecting organisms in the female genital tract, and protects the vagina from similar direct contact with infecting organisms in the male genital tract. The use of foams and other local agents prior to intercourse lowers the pH of the vagina and decreases (but does not eliminate) the risk of infection. However, oral contraceptives and intrauterine devices, more frequently in use now, provide no such protection. In fact, oral contraceptives raise the pH of the vagina, increasing its susceptibility to infection by removing the protection of the normally acid pH. A woman taking oral contraceptives has a 100 percent chance of infection from a single exposure to an infected partner, whereas a woman not taking oral contraceptives has only a 40 percent chance of infection.

Also involved in the increased incidence of venereal disease is the attitude of both health professionals and lay people. Since the diagnosis and treatment of venereal disease is almost totally effective, this problem is not so aggressively attacked as are other diseases. The attitudes among the health professionals that "It's someone else's problem," or "It's curable, so it isn't really a problem," have been conveyed to the public. In addition, because venereal disease frequently raises questions of morality, people may be reluctant to talk about or to hear about the problem. Therefore, although more consideration is being given to venereal disease in professional and lay literature, there is still widespread apathy about it. Effective venereal disease education must take into account the facts that penicillin-resistant strains of *Neisseria gonorrhoeae* are developing all over the United States, that debilitating complications can result from these diseases, and that realistic preventive measures do exist.

Many people are reluctant to seek treatment for venereal disease, and this may be particularly true for the adolescent. In some states, an adolescent cannot be treated without the consent of his parents. If the adolescent anticipates negative or punitive parental response, he may prefer to forego treatment. Venereal disease is a reportable communicable disease, and health departments use follow-up and testing of the patient's sexual contacts as a method of case-finding. Because the person may be concerned about protection of confidentiality, either he may decide not to seek treatment or the physician may decide not to make the report.

Venereal disease has reached epidemic proportions. The means are available to control this problem, but until ignorance and apathy are overcome, it will persist.

Gonorrhea (GC, clap, gleet, strain, morning dose) is a submucous infection caused by *N. gonorrhoeae.* The incubation period is usually 2 to 8 days. The initial manifestations in the male are a thick, purulent discharge from the penis (the discharge later becomes thin and watery), and a burning sensation with urination. The bladder, prostate, and other genitourinary organs may then become involved. The penis is red, swollen, and sore when the tissue around the urethra is infected. Increased burning, urgency, and urinary frequency are signs of bladder infection. Urethral scarring, stenosis, or occlusion may occur if the inflammation is severe. An inflamed scrotum is hard, swollen, painful, and heavy, and permanent sterility may result from scarring of the tubules and/or the epididymides on both sides.

Females rarely exhibit any definitive symptoms of gonorrhea in the early stages of the disease. If symptoms are present, they may include a vague feeling of fullness, a light, purulent, yellow vaginal discharge, and discomfort or ache in the abdomen, all of which are easily misinterpreted. Later, the Bartholin glands may become swollen and inflamed, making sitting or walking painful. The discharge may spread the infection to the urethra and the bladder, causing burning, urgency, and urinary frequency, or it may spread to the anal area, causing itching and a slight discharge. More frequently, however, anal gonorrhea in males or females causes no symptoms whatsoever. (This asymptomatology, along with increased mobility and promiscuity, may account for the high incidence of gonorrhea in male homosexuals.) Symptoms of pelvic inflammatory disease may be the first noticeable symptoms of gonorrhea in the female. Severe abdominal pain, high fever, and vomiting are indications that the fallopian tubes are infected. If this infection becomes chronic, there may be dyspareunia, low back pain, anemia, abnormal menstruation, and eventually scarring of the tubes with permanent sterility.

Untreated gonorrhea in either the male or the female may eventually result in arthritis, heart disease, and death through gonococcal invasion of the bloodstream.

Fluorescent-tagged antibody methods are the most accurate means of diagnosing gonorrhea in either the male or the female. A Gram-stained smear of penile discharge is useful in diagnosing the male patient, but a similar smear of vaginal discharge is not valid in the female patient.

Aqueous procaine penicillin G, 2.4 million units given in one or more doses, is the treatment of choice. Oral tetracycline or other broad-spectrum antibiotic is given for penicillin-resistant strains of gonococci or to allergic patients. A new cell-fractionalization technique has been developed in the Midwest to aid in isolating *N. gonorrhoeae* antigens. Once the antigens have been isolated, a vaccine against gonorrhea can be developed.[9] This is of particular importance in view of the rapidly developing antibiotic-resistant strains of gonococci.

Syphilis (syph, lues) is caused by *Treponema pallidum,* a spirochete which enters the body during coitus or through cuts and other breaks in the skin or mucous membranes. The incubation period is usually 21 days but can be anywhere from 10 to 90 days.

The first external sign of syphilis is a chancre which appears at the site of the infection (genital, anal, or oral). It may resemble a pimple or papule initially, then ulcerate, and later indurate. It lasts about six weeks, then disappears with or without treatment. The chancre represents the primary stage of syphilis. During this time, serologic tests will be negative, since the body has not developed sufficient reagin. However, the organism is present in the fluid of the lesion and can be visualized microscopically.

The secondary stage of syphilis begins 6 weeks to 6 months after the infection and lasts up to 2 years. During this stage, the untreated person develops skin rashes, mucous membrane patches, alopecia, general malaise with headaches, low-grade fever, chronic sore throat, and swollen lymph glands. The symptoms may appear intermittently during this period. Serologic testing is positive.

Without treatment, the latent stage of syphilis develops about 2 years after infection and may last for several years or several decades. There are no symptoms during this stage, although serologic testing will be positive. The disease is still contagious during the first 2 years of this stage; later, it is generally noncommunicable.

The late stage of syphilis occurs between 4 and 20 years after the initial infection, and in some infected persons it may not occur at all. It does, however, present the most serious symptoms. There is destruction of bone tissue, degenerative skin lesions called *gummas,* paresis, blindness, heart disease, and severe crippling or paralysis.

Serologic testing, particularly the VDRL slide

test, is most frequently used to diagnose syphilis. Virus infection or recent vaccinations may produce a false-positive result, and the use of the FTA-ABS (fluorescent treponemal antibody absorption) test will differentiate between false- and true-positive results. *Treponema pallidum* can also be visualized microscopically, and this is the only accurate method of diagnosing primary-stage syphilis.

The most effective treatment for syphilis continues to be penicillin given in total dosage of 2.4 to 4.8 million units. Penicillin-resistant strains of *T. pallidum* have not been identified; however, patients who are allergic to penicillin have been successfully treated with 30 to 40 Gm total dosage of either tetracycline or erythromycin. Research is also in progress to develop a vaccine against syphilis, but this is not yet completed.[10]

In any setting, the nurse is in an important position to educate the public about venereal disease and its prevention, thereby helping to curb the epidemic. Community and school health nurses can be particularly involved in case-finding, referral, and preventive education. Many adolescents who suspect they have venereal disease will go to a nurse rather than to their parents. This is particularly true in those large cities where free clinics, staffed by nurses and other health professionals donating their time and skills, have been set up.

It is extremely important that the nurse help the adolescent feel at ease. He should be assured that the information he gives will be kept confidential, although an epidemiologic investigation must be done. The nurse should determine why the adolescent thinks he has venereal disease and what he knows about the disease. Misinformation should be corrected and knowledge gaps filled in. He should be referred for treatment and epidemiologic follow-up.

Emotional problems are an important aspect of the nursing care of the adolescent with venereal disease and are the most frequently neglected aspects of his care. Any basic emotional problem the adolescent may have is amplified when it becomes known that he has contracted venereal disease. There may be problems in relations with parents, difficulty in communicating with parents and peers, an exaggerated need for affection, and anxiety over sexual impulses and sexual identification. The nurse should try to understand the adolescent's problems from his point of view and, within the realities of the situation, help him to find appropriate solutions. He can support the adolescent, pointing out his assets, and encouraging him in overcoming his problems. It is of utmost importance that the nurse be open, honest,

able to listen, and, particularly, nonjudgmental and accepting in his approach to the adolescent with venereal disease. Too often, an attitude of moral righteousness and condemnation on the part of health professionals makes it impossible for the adolescent to seek or accept help.

Ideally, all young people should be required to take courses in family life and sex education that include factual, nonmoralistic presentations on venereal disease. The nurse will find it helpful to accumulate reading material, pamphlets, and visual aids which are useful either to the adolescent or to an anxious parent. Further information should be available for the adolescent who contracts venereal disease, not only to inform him about the disease, but also to assist the nurse in teaching him to care for himself without infecting those with whom he comes in contact.

Bathing the genitals with soap and water, urinating before and after intercourse, wearing condoms during intercourse, and using vaginal spermatocides prior to intercourse are all means of reducing the chances of contracting venereal disease in the future. It should be pointed out, however, that douching may force disease organisms into the vagina rather than have any beneficial antiseptic effect on invading organisms.

Finally, the adolescent must understand that treatment for venereal disease does not protect him against reinfection. Symptoms which develop after treatment require medical attention just as did those symptoms which originally brought him to seek help.

Rape Illicit carnal knowledge of a woman by force and without her consent constitutes rape. Three elements are necessary in a legal sense: penetration by the male organ at least to the labia or vulva; force, which may be physical or through threats or intimidation; and lack of consent of the woman. In some situations—where the woman is younger than the age of consent or is mentally retarded, for example—lawful consent cannot be given, and intercourse is then termed *statutory rape.*

The incidence of rape is rising, and is probably higher than statistics would indicate because fear and shame may prevent the woman's reporting the attack. Although rape is reported in all age groups, it occurs more frequently with the adolescent.

Because the sequelae of rape can include numerous difficulties for the girl—pregnancy, venereal disease, emotional trauma, legal action—the evaluation of a girl who has been raped includes a detailed history both of the specific incident and of her previous medical history and sexual activity. Careful examination is performed, which includes general observation and examination for bruises, abrasions, and other evidence of injury. Vaginal examination is performed to determine the extent of injury to the genital organs and to obtain specimens for laboratory examination for spermatozoa. It is important also to include evaluation of the girl's emotional state, which may range from extreme agitation and hysteria to total lack of affect.

Treatment is initially directed toward obvious injuries requiring immediate attention. After thorough evaluation, less urgent treatment of injuries, such as suturing of minor lacerations, is done. Evaluation and treatment must also take into consideration the possibility of pregnancy or disease. A pregnancy test is done immediately to determine whether the girl was pregnant prior to the rape. This will then be repeated should she not menstruate according to her normal cycle. A regimen for postcoital contraception may also be prescribed. Antibiotic therapy for syphilis and gonorrhea is instituted.

The psychologic reactions to rape may be particularly severe. Initially, the girl may be very disturbed and overwrought. She may then enter a period of apparent adjustment, during which she does not discuss the incident and, in fact, uses denial as a means of coping with her feelings. After several weeks or perhaps months, this may give way to a period of depression and engender the need to verbalize her feelings and concerns before the emotional problems can be resolved.

The girl who is brought to the emergency room or doctor's office because she has been raped may be very agitated, frightened, and ashamed. The nurse's attitude must be supportive and nonjudgmental if he is to be of help to the patient. The nurse will be present during the examination and treatment, and his observations of the patient's physical and emotional status should be accurately and completely recorded.

Primarily, however, the nurse will direct his efforts toward supporting the patient during this time. Procedures and treatments should be explained in detail, in terminology appropriate to the girl's level of understanding. The patient's description of the incident and the events surrounding it may be confused and disorganized. Using appropriate interviewing techniques, the nurse may assist the patient to bring order to her recollections. The nurse can also give the patient an opportunity to express her feelings and concerns. In some hospitals, the chaplain's service has instituted a program to work with rape victims and can be extremely helpful to the girl in working through her feelings.

The girl's subsequent adjustment to the emotional trauma of rape, as well as the effectiveness of any treatment, may be affected by the attitude of her parents. If they exhibit little or no concern about the incident, they will be unable to understand or to assist the girl in coping with her feelings and problems. Punitive parents may simply enhance the fear and guilt which she experiences and make a healthy adjustment impossible. Revengeful parents may be so filled with their own rage at the person responsible that they may be unable to consider the girl's feelings. Overprotective parents may delay any healthy readjustment by reinforcing the girl's own denial or by limiting normal social activity.

It is important, then, that the nurse observe and evaluate the parent-child relations and discuss with the parents their own feelings and reactions. The parents as well as the patient should have a clear understanding of the treatments and procedures necessary.

Ideally, the girl and her family should be followed by the nurse in the community after initial treatment. It is necessary that the nurse receive adequate information from the referring agency in order to provide continuity of care.

Patients and family will be most receptive to nursing contact during the first few days after the attack,[11] as they are most in need of emotional support at this time. The nurse will have the opportunity to assess the family's strengths and weaknesses, and assist them to cope with their feelings. In his discussions, he may be able to add to the history already obtained, particularly in reference to previous emotional disturbance.

Concerns at this time will center around the possibility of pregnancy and venereal disease. The nurse should emphasize the need for continuing prescribed treatment and should assist the girl in obtaining necessary medical follow-up, including further testing for pregnancy and disease. The girl may be emotionally upset at this time and need to reiterate and elaborate on the events which have taken place. Patients with more severe or prolonged disturbance, especially those with a history of previous disturbance, must be referred for more intensive counseling and therapy. The incident itself and the fact of its being reported to the police may arouse feelings of guilt in both the parents (What should I have done to prevent this?) and the child (What did I do to provoke this?). These have to be discussed and considered in order to be resolved.

After the initial crisis period, the girl may be less receptive to the nurse as she enters the period of denial. However, it is important that the nurse continue to follow the patient and to make himself available when the patient feels the need to talk about her experience and work through her feelings.

Should court proceedings be instituted, the trial can be an additional source of trauma for the girl. The necessity to review the events among strangers and the attempts of a defense attorney to imply complicity on the girl's part may arouse further guilt feelings in the girl. This may precipitate a period of depression, and the nurse can assist the girl to verbalize her feelings and to deal with them realistically. Unless the girl is able to resolve the emotional problems associated with rape, this experience may interfere with future heterosexual relationships.

Incestuous rape is often not reported. Usually this involves the girl's father, sometimes an older brother or uncle. The girl may fear reprisals from the relative, or may feel guilty because she enjoys some aspect of the relations, and therefore may not seek help. However, when incestual rape is discovered, every effort must be made to protect the girl. This may include removing her from the home situation. Repeated incestual experiences will seriously impair the girl's ability to establish future heterosexual relations, and she may need intensive psychotherapy. Ideally, therapy should also include the family.

Pregnancy Adolescence is usually a crisis state to which a person brings certain strengths and abilities enabling him to cope with the demands of the crisis. Pregnancy, also a normal crisis state, when superimposed on adolescence, requires of the person skills and strengths not yet developed and, at the same time, deprives the individual of some which have been available to him. This is true for both the adolescent girl and the adolescent boy, whether they are married or unmarried.

The adolescent, in his development toward a mature, healthy, well-integrated adult, must relinquish his dependence on his family, establish satisfactory relations with the opposite sex, and decide what he wants to do with his life. His involvement with his peer group helps him to cope with the conflict between independence and dependence, giving him an opportunity to be simultaneously different and the same. Schooling is important not only because of its contribution to future plans but also for its social value in establishing heterosexual relationships. At the same time, rapid physical changes make him particularly conscious of his developing body.

Adolescents differ somewhat in their response to their developing sexuality. Adolescent girls see intercourse as a means to obtain affection, accept-

ance, and identity. Their sexual experiences tend to be an outgrowth of romantic love and the ideals which they attach to it. For the adolescent boy, intercourse with orgasm is an end in itself. He has fewer notions of romantic love, and affection for him is a means to an end. However, both adolescent girls and adolescent boys are alike in that they have not yet developed a capacity for intimacy and mature love. They are still working toward developing their own identity and independence and determining the direction of their lives.

Under these circumstances, then, the teen-age marriage is likely to be relatively unstable. The participants have assumed a responsibility for which they may be ill-prepared. Pregnancy in such a situation can be an additional responsibility with which they are unable to cope.

The adult pregnant woman who is married and desires her pregnancy generally has numerous strengths in the acceptance of pregnancy, in the degree of maturity she has attained, and in the stability of her environment with a husband, a home, and a reasonable degree of financial security. These assets enable her to cope with some of the demands of pregnancy: physical changes, increased dependency needs, and role change.

The pregnant adolescent girl has few of these strengths. She may deny the fact of her pregnancy, and this denial may be facilitated if she has a frequently irregular menstrual cycle. She is still struggling for the maturity which the older woman has attained. If she is unmarried, her main source of support is the family from whom she is trying to break away. If she is wed, as has been noted, her marriage is likely to be unstable and financial security doubtful.[12] Her pregnancy compounds the problems of adolescence, too. If social sanctions do not isolate her from her peer group, school regulations may. As her pregnancy progresses, physical changes enhance her concerns about her body image.

Medically, the pregnant adolescent is considered to be at higher risk than her older counterpart. She is more prone to complications, particularly prematurity and possibly toxemia, and, in the younger (under 15 years) adolescent, contracted pelvis. The complications are not solely a function of her age, however, for environment, nutrition, drugs, and the extent of prenatal care can also play a part. Nutrition among teen-agers is generally less than ideal: fad diets and erratic eating habits are common. The "drug scene" has become a part of the teen-ager's life; although the extent of the effects of these drugs is not fully known, many drugs are known to have a detrimental effect on the infant. Finally, the pregnant teen-ager is more likely to delay seeking prenatal care because of her wish to deny the pregnancy, fear of the reactions of family or friends, ignorance of available facilities, or a host of other reasons. It is ironic that these girls, who are most in need of adequate care and assistance, are frequently the least likely to receive it.

The pregnant adolescent, with limited resources upon which to draw, is subjected to such stresses that it is not surprising that her instinct is to deny the situation. When the pregnancy is confirmed, her first decision may be whether to continue with the pregnancy. Whether or not the girl elects to terminate the pregnancy, she faces a number of stresses and will require the cooperative efforts of various professional disciplines to receive optimal care. The nurse as a member of this team can assist the teen-ager to identify her needs and find realistic solutions to her problems.

As the adolescent progresses through her pregnancy, she will experience all the physical and emotional changes that the adult pregnant woman experiences, but may have less information and understanding regarding them. However, she will be as concerned about her welfare and her baby's welfare, and about those things which will affect them. She should be encouraged and assisted to obtain medical evaluation, with an understanding of what is done and why it is necessary. Nutrition is also important, although the pregnant teen-ager may not know what constitutes an adequate diet and may need information about it. Similarly, if the girl understands the potential harmful effects of drugs on her unborn infant, she is more likely to be cautious in using them.

Many teen-agers have little knowledge of reproduction and have learned what little they know from equally ill-informed friends. The nurse should first determine the extent and accuracy of the girl's knowledge and build from there. Fear of labor and delivery is common to all pregnant women, and may be intensified in the uninformed adolescent. The nurse will need to explore this topic repeatedly.

If the adolescent is wed, or if she is unwed and decides to keep her baby, she will need further help in planning for the care of the infant. Films, books, and discussions centered around the various aspects of child care as well as around normal growth and development will be helpful to her.

Another area of need centers around the developmental characteristics of adolescence. The normal concerns of adolescence, discussed in Chapters 14 and 28, are made more difficult to resolve by the impact of pregnancy at this time. Since many states and communities refuse to permit a pregnant girl—married or unmarried—to remain in school, she is effectively deprived of one of her primary sources of support, her peer group. Recently, an increasing number of programs have been developed which enable pregnant girls to continue their schooling either on an individual basis or, more frequently, in groups. The group setting, although it separates the girl from her nonpregnant peers, has many advantages. In particular, it creates the opportunity for the girls to learn and draw support from others with similar problems and concerns and from the professionals who work with them.

For the adolescent who is attempting to resolve a conflict between independence and dependence, the increased dependency needs of pregnancy may be particularly difficult to handle. She can be helped to understand the dependence that is a function of pregnancy, and, at the same time, to progress toward independence. This is done by aiding her to make intelligent decisions based on accurate information, as well as through continued education and training for the future.

Body image is a particular concern during adolescence, and, again, the physical changes occurring during pregnancy can have an added impact on the girl. Her fears may be colored by the tales she has heard, and she may have repeated questions about breast changes, stretch marks, and regaining her figure. It cannot be stressed too often that the availability of accurate, honest information and the opportunity to discuss her fears and concerns are of primary importance to the pregnant adolescent in coping with her crisis.

The adolescent expectant father is also without strengths which he will need to cope with the pregnancy. Within marriage, his financial resources may be severely limited by the lack of extensive training or education needed to ensure an adequate income. Like the adolescent girl, his knowledge of conception, pregnancy, and childbirth may be meager. The emotional changes and increased dependency needs of a pregnant woman may be totally baffling to him, making it difficult for him to provide the support and help which his wife may need. The adolescent expectant father, therefore, needs assistance in increasing his knowledge and understanding of pregnancy, and in planning for his expanded family.

The adolescent unwed mother Some problems are encountered in the unwed adolescent that are not seen in the married pregnant adolescent. The social stigma attached to unwed pregnancy is still very obvious and contributes to the girl's difficulty in accepting the pregnancy and seeking prenatal care. School regulations, as noted previously, reinforce this. Attitudes of friends or family may range from studied indifference to overt hostility. All these, in addition to her own feelings about unwed pregnancy in general, may contribute to an extreme sense of guilt. She needs the opportunity to express and explore these feelings in order to maintain or regain feelings of self-esteem.

She may face the decision of whether to marry, and this decision may be influenced more by family and social concerns than by an objective evaluation of the alternatives. She must be helped to understand the alternatives available to her and to consider the possible consequences of each course of action.

One particularly difficult decision which the adolescent unwed mother faces is whether to keep the infant or to place it for adoption. This should be her own decision, but, in order to make it, she must be helped to understand all ramifications of each alternative. If she keeps the infant, how will she care for it? What financial resources does she have? Will she live alone or at home, and is this desirable or feasible? What will be the effect on the child of growing up without a father? How can these various problems be realistically solved? If she places the infant for adoption, what will be the effect of this on the baby, on herself, and on her family? There is no universally correct answer to this dilemma. However, with thorough consideration of all aspects of this problem, the girl is more able to choose the better solution for herself and for her infant. (One possible consequence of the group setting for pregnant teenagers should be mentioned in connection with this question. An important factor in a girl's decision whether to keep her baby or place it for adoption may be peer pressure. If most of the girls in a particular group are keeping their babies, it may be very difficult for one girl in the group to decide to place her baby for adoption. The opinion of her peers may seem to be more important than the other factors she considers. If she does make a different decision, she and the group may need help in understanding their reactions.)

If the girl decides to place her infant for adoption, she faces additional problems after delivery. Whether or not she sees the baby in the hospital —and again there is no single right answer to this question—the separation will engender grief at the loss of the infant. It is important that the nurse understand this and help the mother through the grieving process. Indeed, the adolescent may need to review all the steps which led her to make the decision,

a decision difficult to make before the baby is born but often more difficult to carry out after birth.

It is important that the pregnant adolescent have access to adequate information regarding contraception to prevent future unwanted pregnancies. Once a girl has become sexually active, she is likely to continue to be so. The younger she becomes pregnant, the more likely she is to have repeated pregnancies in a shorter period of time. The choice of contraceptive method must be made on an individual basis. In general, intrauterine devices which are small enough to be tolerated without pain by the younger patient may be less effective in controlling conception. Oral contraceptives may cause further disruption of the menstrual cycle in a girl with a history of irregular or infrequent menstruation. These and other factors must be considered before one method can be chosen for a particular girl.

Discussion of contraception may give rise to a variety of feelings among pregnant adolescents. Some girls may feel that the use of contraceptives makes sexual activity seem preplanned and thus less meaningful. Some may resist the implication that they will continue to be sexually active. Some may see the use of contraceptives as an indication that they cannot be "good" because "good girls don't do that" and therefore would not need contraceptives. Discussion should focus not merely on which method does what. It is more important that the girl understand what influences her behavior and what means she has of controlling it.

In relation to this, it is important to try to determine why the pregnancy occurred. It is rare that a girl becomes pregnant because she does not understand even the most rudimentary aspects of intercourse and conception. The pregnancy may occur as a result of a relation which was meaningful to her. The adolescent unwed mother frequently comes from a disordered family background, and she may have become pregnant in an attempt to receive affection, emotional support, or security. While the original situation exists which impelled the girl to seek pregnancy as a solution, the availability of contraceptives will not necessarily prevent subsequent pregnancies. However, with a greater self-insight, the girl can make an intelligent decision regarding her behavior which may or may not involve the use of contraceptives.

The adolescent unwed father In any discussion of pregnancy or the care of the pregnant woman, the expectant father is often included as an afterthought. The adolescent unwed father is rarely even an afterthought: he is almost totally forgotten unless he is sought for marriage to the unwed mother or for financial support for the child. He is believed, often erroneously, to have no feeling for the child and mother, no interest in their future, and no rights as far as the child is concerned. He is assumed to wish to escape any responsibility for the pregnancy, although the responses he may receive from adults (anger on the part of the girl's parents and disapproval or disappointment on the part of his parents) rather than his own feelings may engender this reaction.

Little has been done to improve our understanding of the adolescent unwed father. He may, like the unwed mother, be seeking affection and security. However, Pannor,[13] in reporting research in California, provides some additional insight. The unwed father is usually not irresponsible and uncaring: unwed pregnancy frequently arises from a situation that was meaningful to both the boy and the girl. Initially, the unwed father may have difficulty in accepting the fact of his fatherhood. Once this is accepted, however, he generally demonstrates concern for the child and wants to act responsibly if given opportunity and assistance.

The unwed father can be encouraged to give emotional support to the girl, which is beneficial to both. He may also become involved in decisions regarding the possibility of marriage or the future of the child. Like the unwed mother, he may have limited knowledge about reproduction and contraception. He should also be made aware of his legal rights and responsibilities, which vary according to state law. It is more important, however, that assumptions about the adolescent unwed father be discarded, that he be approached as an individual with needs and concerns in the situation, and that he, like the unwed mother, be given an opportunity to use the crisis as a means of personal growth.

The family of the adolescent unwed mother   During and following pregnancy the adolescent unwed mother needs support. Frequently, however, family relationships are already disordered, and her pregnancy merely compounds an already troubled situation. The girl may anticipate angered and hostile reactions to her pregnancy, and may in fact receive them. Assistance may be limited to attempts to persuade the girl to terminate the pregnancy, to marry the father of the child, or to hide the pregnancy and place the infant for adoption.

Smith,[14] in working with the mothers of pregnant teen-agers, has outlined a sequence in the transition to the role of grandmother. Consideration of these steps may give some insight into the impact of adolescent pregnancy on the family.

The initial process by which the mother learns of her daughter's pregnancy may seem accidental. Like her daughter, the mother tends to overlook obvious signs and symptoms in an attempt to deny the pregnancy. Once the fact of the pregnancy is established, her reaction may indeed be one of anger, but may also be coupled with feelings of guilt (What did I do wrong?) and sadness (She'll miss the fun of growing up). Attempts may be made to force the girl into termination of pregnancy or marriage.

As the pregnancy progresses, some degree of equilibrium is established, and the fact of the pregnancy becomes at least tolerable. The girl's mother may enter into plans for the care of the infant, if it is not placed for adoption. Apparently during the third trimester, however, the reality of her situation becomes more apparent to the expectant grandmother. The pronounced physical changes in her daughter and the obvious activity of the infant contribute to her changed feelings. During this period, the girl and her mother may become closer, sharing the experiences of their separate pregnancies.

The birth of the baby does not necessarily complete the transition. Particularly if the infant is in the home with the mother and the grandmother, it may be difficult for the adolescent's mother to relinquish her role and to assist her daughter in developing in a mothering role.

The responses and modes of adjustment of the father and siblings of the adolescent unwed mother have received little attention, and similar research on their concerns is needed. With an understanding of the anticipated reactions of the family of the unwed mother, the nurse is better able to plan his care of the family and to assist them in coping with the crisis. Although the nurse is able to use such information as a basis for planning care, he must adapt the plan of care to the individual family situation. In an already disordered family, strengths may be so limited that the pregnant teen-ager finds little or no support. It is important, therefore, to evaluate the family relations and build on their strengths in order to help the girl and her family to cope with the problems of pregnancy. The parents as well as the girl need an opportunity to express their concern and explore their feelings. They, too, need adequate and accurate information in order to make their own decisions and to assist their daughter in making hers.

REFERENCES

1 T. W. Glenister, F. E. Hytton, and M. G. Kerr, "Human Reproduction," in R. Passmore and J. S. Robeson (eds.), *A Companion to Medical Studies,* vol. I, 2d ed.,

Blackwell Scientific Publications, Ltd., Oxford, 1969, pp. 37.10–37.11.
2 A. J. Schaffer and Mary Ellen Avery, *Diseases of the Newborn*, 3d ed., W. B. Saunders Company, Philadelphia, 1971, pp. 459–460.
3 H. K. Silver, R. W. Gotlin, and D. O'Brien, "Endocrine Disorders," in C. H. Kempe et al. (eds.), *Current Pediatric Diagnosis and Treatment*, Lange Medical Publications, Los Altos, Calif., 1970, p. 517.
4 Mohsen Ziai, *Pediatrics*, Little, Brown and Company, Boston, 1969, p. 119.
5 A. L. Herbst and R. E. Scully, "Vaginal Cancer in Young Females," *Audio Digest Foundation Obstetrics and Gynecology*, 20(2), 1973.
6 D. Sloan, "Pelvic Pain and Dysmenorrhea," *Pediatric Clinics of North America*, 19(3):675–676, 1972.
7 D. Hubble (ed.), *Pediatric Endocrinology*, F. A. Davis Company, Philadelphia, 1969, p. 168.
8 Texas State Health Department, Venereal Disease Morbidity Statistics, 1972.
9 Sharon Golub, "V.D., The Unconquered Menace," *RN*, 33(3):39, 1972.
10 Ibid., p. 39.
11 C. R. Hayman and Charlene Lanza, "Sexual Assault on Women and Girls," *American Journal of Obstetrics and Gynecology*, 109(3):483, 1971.
12 Marion Howard, "Comprehensive Community Programs for the Pregnant Teenager," *Clinics of Obstetrics and Gynecology*, 14(2):473–474, 1971.
13 R. Pannor, "Teen-age Unwed Father," *Clinical Obstetrics and Gynecology*, 14(2):466–472, 1971.
14 Eleanor Smith, "Transition to the Role of Grandmother as Studied with Mothers of Pregnant Adolescents," *ANA Clinical Sessions*, Appleton-Century-Crofts, Inc., New York, 1970, pp. 140–148.

BIBLIOGRAPHY

Adams, Paul L.: "Delayed Sexual Maturation in Boys," *Medical Aspects of Human Sexuality*, 6(4):34 pp. ff., 1972.
Ahern, Cheryl: "I Think I Have VD," *Nursing Clinics of North America*, 8(1):77–90, 1973.
Altchek, A. (ed.): "Symposium on Pediatric and Adolescent Gynecology," *Pediatric Clinics of North America*, 19(3):507–819, 1972.
Baker, G. E.: "Delayed and Precocious Puberty," *Audio Digest Foundation Pediatrics*, 19(8), 1972.
Bender, S. J.: *Venereal Disease*, Wm. C. Brown Company Publishers, Dubuque, Iowa, 1971.
Blake, Florence E., Howell, F. W. and Waechter, E. H.,: *Nursing Care of Children*, J. B. Lippincott Company, Philadelphia, 1970.
Brown, R. C.: "Ovarian Tumors in Childhood and Adolescence," *Postgraduate Medicine*, 50(6):230–235, 1971.
Caldwell, J. G., "Congenital Syphilis: A Non-Venereal Disease" *American Journal of Nursing*, 71(9):1768–1772, 1971.
Charles, D. (ed.): "Menstrual Disorders," *Clinical Obstetrics and Gynecology*, 12(3):691–827, 1969.
Cooke, R. E. (ed.): *The Biological Basis of Pediatric Practice*, McGraw-Hill Book Company, New York, 1965.
Cornell, Elizabeth B., and Jacobson, Linbania: "Pregnancy, the Teenager and Sex Education," *American Journal of Public Health*, 61(9):1840–1845, 1971.

Coulter, M. D., and Hayles, A. B.: "Precocious Puberty," *Advances in Pediatrics*, 17:125–138, 1970.
Danies, W. A., Jr.: *The Adolescent Patient*, The C. V. Mosby Company, St. Louis, 1970.
Davis, Lucille, and Grace, Helen: "Anticipatory Counselling of Unwed Mothers," *Nursing Clinics of North America*, 6(4):581–590, 1971.
Evard, J. R.: "Rape: The Medical, Social and Legal Implications," *American Journal of Obstetrics and Gynecology*, 111(2):197–199, 1971.
Federman, D. D.: "The Assessment of Organ Function—The Testis," *New England Journal of Medicine*, 285(3):901–903, 1971.
Fitzpatrick, Genevieve M.: *Gynecologic Nursing*, The Macmillan Company, New York, 1968.
Fluker, J. L.: "Syphilis," *Practitioner*, 209(11):605–613, 1972.
Freedman, A. M., and Kaplan, H. I.: *The Child: His Psychological and Cultural Development*, vol. I, Atheneum Publishers, New York, 1972.
Gellis, S.: "Undescended Testicles," *Pediatric Conferences with Sydney Gellis*, W. B. Saunders Company, Philadelphia, 1971.
Grant, J. A., and Heald, F. P.: "Complications of Adolescent Pregnancy," *Clinical Pediatrics*, 11(10):167–169, 1972.
Guyton, A. C.: *Textbook of Medical Physiology*, 4th ed., W. B. Saunders Company, Philadelphia, 1971.
Hammar, S. L., and Eddy, Jo Ann: *Nursing Care of the Adolescent*, Springer Publishing Co., Inc., New York, 1966.
Hayman, C. R., Lewis, Frances R., Stewart, Wm. F., and Grant, M.: "A Public Health Program for Sexually Assaulted Women," *Obstetrical and Gynecological Survey*, 23(2):204–206, 1968.
Howells, J. G. (ed.): *Modern Perspectives in Adolescent Psychology*, Brunner Mazel, Inc., New York, 1971.
Huffman, J. W. (ed.): "Gynecology of Adolescence," *Clinical Obstetrics and Gynecology*, 14(4):961–1108, 1971.
Jones, H. P., and Heller, R. H.: *Pediatric and Adolescent Gynecology*, The Williams & Wilkins Company, Baltimore, 1968.
Marlow, Dorothy R.: *Textbook of Pediatric Nursing*, 4th ed., W. B. Saunders Company, Philadelphia, 1973.
Massay, J. B., Garcia, Celso-Ramon, and Emich Jr., J. P.: "Management of Sexually Assaulted Women," *Obstetrical and Gynecological Survey*, 27(3):190–192, 1972.
Nelson, R. M.: "Abnormal Adolescent Menstruation," *Audio Digest Foundation Pediatrics*, 18(17), 1972.
Nelson, W. E. (ed.): *Textbook of Pediatrics*, 9th ed., W. B. Saunders Company, Philadelphia, 1969.
Shaw, Bernice L.: "When the Problem Is Rape," *RN*, 35(4):25–28, 1972.
Snell, R. S.: *Clinical Embryology for Medical Students*, Little, Brown and Company, Boston, 1972.
Summitt, R. L.: "Differential Diagnosis of Genital Ambiguity in the Newborn," *Clinical Obstetrics and Gynecology*, 15(1):112–140, 1972.
Taylor, E. S.: *Essentials of Gynecology*, 4th ed., Lea & Febiger, Philadelphia, 1969.
Wallace, Helen M. (ed.): "Human Reproductive Problems of the Adolescent," *Clinical Obstetrics and Gynecology*, 13(2):325–488, 1971.
Wallach, E. E. (ed.): "Dysfunctional Uterine Bleeding," *Clinical Obstetrics and Gynecology*, 13(2):363–488, 1970.
Williams, R. H.: *Textbook of Endocrinology*, 4th ed., W. B. Saunders Company, Philadelphia, 1968.

THE URINARY SYSTEM

DEBORAH B. DEAN and PATRICIA J. PHILLIPS

EMBRYOLOGY OF THE URINARY SYSTEM

Embryologic development of the urinary system begins within the first weeks after conception and progresses through three stages (Fig. 38-1). Embryologically the tubules of each stage of development arise from the intermediate mesoderm which later becomes the nephrogenic cord. The pronephros represents the earliest and most rudimentary stage. This structure makes its appearance at about the third week of gestation and degenerates in several weeks without ever functioning.

The second stage of development begins the fourth week of gestation. The ureter of the pronephros forms the mesonephric duct which stimulates the formation of the mesonephros. This kidney gradually forms about 40 pairs of tubules and glomeruli. The mesonephros is functional in the elimination of nitrogenous waste products until the end of the fourth month. As the metanephric kidney begins to function, the mesonephric duct system degenerates except for portions in the male which develop into the vas deferens, ejaculatory duct, and ducts of the epididymis and the ureteral buds, which in both sexes develop into the metanephros, the final kidney. Incomplete or faulty development of the ureteral buds accounts for many anomalies found in the ureters, renal pelvis, and collecting tubules.

Each ureteral bud forms a primitive renal pelvis which branches to form the major and minor calyces, ducts of Bellini, and collecting ducts in the renal pyramids. As the ureteral buds grow, S-shaped clefts develop in the surrounding mesoderm. One end of the cleft lies adjacent to a branch of the ureteral bud. This end eventually becomes continuous with the ureteral bud and forms the collecting ducts. The other end, a primitive nephron, forms a capillary network which develops into the glomerulus. As the cleft grows, the proximal and distal tubules and Henle's loop are formed. This union forms a continuous channel from Bowman's capsule to the bladder. If union develops inadequately, obstruction to urinary flow results.

After the thirty-fifth week of gestation no new nephrons are formed; therefore, the number present at birth remains the same throughout life unless the child is born prematurely. In this case he may still be actively producing nephrons. Otherwise, the postnatal growth of the kidney occurs from cell hypertrophy, lengthening of the tubular system, and increases in vascular and connective tissues.

Circulation is supplied to the developing kidney by multiple branches from the aorta. During the process, some of these branches degenerate and others merge so that at term a single renal artery and single renal vein supply each kidney.

Between the sixth and seventh weeks of gestation, the formation of the lower urinary tract begins. The urorectal septum divides the cloaca into the anterior and dorsal segments. The anterior segment, the urogenital sinus, represents the primordium of the bladder, female urethra, and lower part of the vagina. As the bladder enlarges, the ureters become incorporated in the bladder wall.

The male urethra is formed by a process of fusion of lateral folds over the urethral groove. If the fusion of the groove is incomplete, hypospadius results.

About the third month of gestation the fetal kidney begins to secrete urine. The amount of urine excreted increases as gestation progresses and represents an increasing proportion of the amniotic fluid volume. If there is an absence or scanty amount of amniotic fluid, the kidneys have either failed to develop or are nonfunctional.

At birth the tubules are short and narrow, and the epithelium of the glomeruli and tubules is thick. These structural and functional immaturities prolong glomerular filtration and tubule absorption. By 5 months of age the glomeruli and tubules are structurally mature, and between the ages of 12 and 18 months the epithelium of the glomeruli and tubules becomes as thin as in the adult.

RENAL PHYSIOLOGY

The urinary system consists of the kidneys, ureters, bladder, and urethra. The kidney removes wastes from the body, maintains body fluid homeostasis, excretes hormones, and plays a role in metabolism. The kidneys of the healthy newborn are qualitatively able to perform these functions despite renal immaturity. However, when illness of the newborn or prematurity intervenes, special considerations must be made for the functional limitations of the kidney, particularly in the areas of drug therapy, types of formula prescribed, and administration of parenteral fluid.

Urine Production and Maintenance of Fluid and Electrolyte Balance

Glomerular Filtration   Glomerular hydrostatic pressure, colloid osmotic pressure of the blood, and the hydrostatic pressure of the fluid in the capsule result in glomerular filtration. The anatomic structure of the afferent and efferent arterioles which supply blood to the glomerular capillaries creates glomeru-

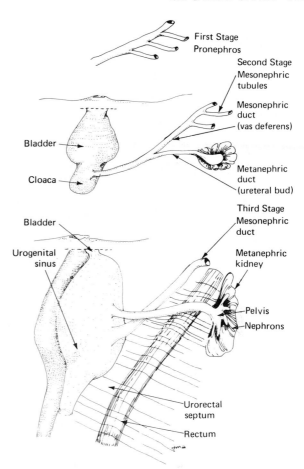

Figure 38-1   Schematic representation of the three embryonic kidneys in the human fetus and the embryonic development of the collecting system.

lar hydrostatic pressure (Fig. 38-2). This pressure forces water and solutes in the blood to be filtered into Bowman's capsule (see Fig. 38-3). The capillary pressure in the glomeruli is greater than anywhere else in the body because the afferent arterioles are wider than the efferent arterioles. This difference in size produces resistance and consequently pressure. The glomerular hydrostatic pressure is the major force that drives fluid out while the hydrostatic osmotic pressure of the capsule and the colloid osmotic pressure exert an opposing force.

Tubular Reabsorption and Secretion   The amount o glomerular filtrate is reduced by about 98 percent as the fluid and solutes are reabsorbed by the cells in the tubules, particularly the proximal tubules. Reabsorption occurs by osmosis, diffusion, and active transport. In active transport substances such as

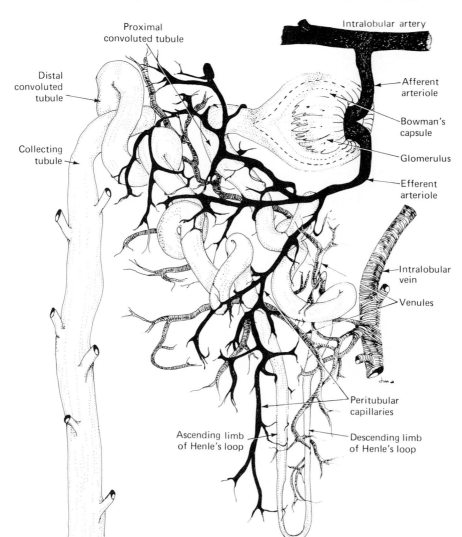

Proximal
convoluted tubule

Distal
convoluted
tubule

Collecting
tubule

Intralobular artery

Afferent
arteriole

Bowman's
capsule

Glomerulus

Efferent
arteriole

Intralobular
vein

Venules

Peritubular
capillaries

Ascending limb
of Henle's loop

Descending limb
of Henle's loop

Figure 38-2 Blood supply to
the nephron unit. Note that the
blood flows through the intralobular artery, afferent arteriole,
glomerulus, efferent arteriole,
peritubular capillaries, venules,
and intralobular vein.

glucose and electrolytes are moved by energy
against a concentration or pressure gradient. Reabsorption is also selective since substances necessary to the body are recaptured and waste products
are eliminated. (See Fig. 38-3.)

The active transport of sodium ions in the
proximal tubules influences the movement of chloride ions and water. As the sodium ions are reabsorbed, chloride ions follow by diffusion. The resultant momentary hypertonicity of the blood
initiates the movement of water by osmosis from the
tubules. The reabsorption of the water is referred to
as *obligatory water reabsorption.* This process
satisfies the body's needs to maintain homeostasis.

Antidiuretic hormone (ADH) controls the amount
of water that is returned to the blood. ADH acts on

the cells of the distal tubules producing facultative
reabsorption. The amount of ADH secreted by the
posterior pituitary is influenced primarily by an increase in plasma osmotic pressure and a decrease
in extracellular volume. ADH production is also
stimulated by exercise, emotional stress, pain, and
drugs (see Fig. 38-4).

Water reabsorption is also influenced by *aldosterone,* a hormone secreted by the adrenal cortex.
It causes sodium to be reabsorbed in the distal
tubules. As stated earlier, the movement of sodium
obligates a certain quantity of water to be reabsorbed.

Tubular secretion occurs in the distal and collecting tubules. In this process potassium and hydrogen ions are secreted by active transport into the

tubular filtrate from the blood. The amount of potassium secreted depends on the amount of total body potassium, aldosterone activity, acid-base balance, and composition of the urine. Ammonia through diffusion is also added to the filtrate in the tubules (see Fig. 38-3).

Production of Hormones

The kidney produces erythropoietin, a hormone that stimulates the production of red blood cells when hypoxia is present. In chronic renal failure, anemia results because of reduced production of erythropoietin. The kidney also releases renin, which controls the secretion of aldosterone.

Metabolic Role of Kidney

Recent research demonstrates that metabolic conversions occurring in the kidney may affect the entire body. Normal calcium absorption is dependent on a metabolite of vitamin D. This metabolite is produced exclusively in the kidney. Recently it has also been shown that the kidney participates in gluconeogenesis during periods of prolonged fasting.[1]

DIAGNOSTIC PROCEDURES

The nurse should be well versed in the diagnostic procedures that are included in a genitourinary work-up. While his assistance will be needed in the performance of some procedures, the nurse's role in preparing the child and explaining the tests to him is of primary importance. Similarly, parents may be confused and anxious over the barrage of procedures scheduled for their child. Although the physician may initially explain each diagnostic test and its purpose, the nurse is in an excellent position to reiterate and expand those explanations and to include details regarding the child's anticipated feelings and familiar people who will be nearby.

Urinalysis

The nurse must be familiar with the components of the routine urinalysis. A freshly voided specimen collected in the early morning is ideal for urinalysis since the formed elements are preserved best when the urine is concentrated and acidic. The practice of plying young children with drinks of water to obtain a specimen as quickly as possible is rightly condemned. Very dilute urines are unsuitable for examination because red cells quickly undergo lysis in dilute urine, and the dilution itself may obscure significant abnormalities. For example, a 2+ reaction

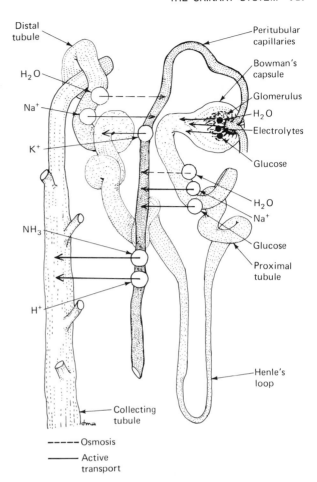

Figure 38-3 Diagram of glomerular filtration, tubular reabsorption, and tubular secretion.

for protein in a concentrated urine may appear as only a trace reaction if the urine is dilute.

Urinalysis routinely includes determination of pH and specific gravity, tests for the presence of protein and reducing substances such as blood, glucose, and ketones, and microscopic examination for cells, casts, bacteria, and crystals.

pH Nitrazine indicator paper changes through a range of colors from yellow to dark blue over the normal urine pH range of 4.0 to 8.2. The pH is usually acid, 5.0 to 6.0, in the fasting state. Elevation of pH beyond 8.0 or 8.2 suggests that either the patient has a urinary infection because of a urea-splitting organism such as *Proteus* or the specimen has been allowed to stand at room temperature for several hours, permitting a luxuriant growth of contaminating bacteria within the container. Control of urine pH is an important factor in obtaining the maximum

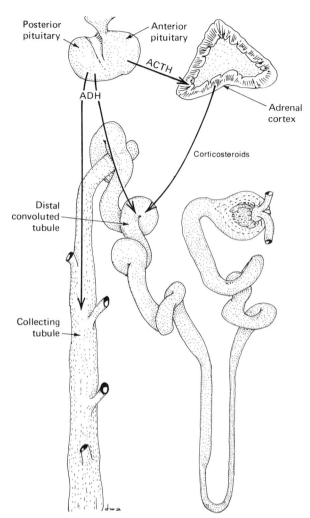

Figure 38-4 Hormonal influence on tubular reabsorption. Adrenocorticotropic hormone (ACTH) stimulates the adrenal cortex to secrete glucocorticoids, which then stimulate the distal tubules to reabsorb sodium and excrete potassium.

therapeutic value from certain antibiotics and urinary disinfectants. Kanamycin and streptomycin, for example, are most effective if urine pH is kept in the alkaline range.

Specific Gravity The specific gravity (sp. g.) of an early morning concentrated specimen is normally 1.024 to 1.030 and is measured roughly by a hydrometer or more accurately by a total solids meter that utilizes a single drop of urine. During diuresis, specific gravity may fall to 1.000 or 1.001. This test provides an estimate of the kidneys' ability to concentrate and dilute urine, *a function that is lost early in renal disease.*

Protein, Blood, Glucose, and Ketones The dipstick test for these substances (using reagent papers) is very convenient for the screening of large numbers of specimens, for testing at home, and for testing when the available urine volume is small. Positive findings of these substances are termed proteinuria (1 +), hematuria, glucosuria, and ketonuria.

Microscopic Examination With practice and supervision, the nurse can learn to examine centrifuged sediment or uncentrifuged concentrated urine for red blood cells, white blood cells, casts, bacteria, and crystals.

12- or 24-Hour Urine Collections A diagnostic urine collection of 12 or 24 hours may be ordered. The nurse should explain collection techniques to the child, parents, and nursing staff and should supervise the collection carefully. These 12- or 24-hour collections are often required to determine (1) quantitative protein excretion (any amount in excess of 200 mg/24 hours is considered abnormal); (2) the rate of excretion of red cells, white cells, and casts in the urine—an Addis count (normal values are 600,000/12 hours for red blood cells, 1 million/12 hours for white blood cells, and 10,000/12 hours for casts); and (3) *rarely,* urine electrolyte concentrations (specifically, sodium and potassium).[2] The nurse should know the procedure for collection, such as whether the specimen should be kept on ice or whether buffered Formalin should be added to the container as a preservative, and should anticipate situations normally encountered with children. For example, a child who needs to have a bowel movement during the collection period should be asked to urinate first so that the specimen is not contaminated or discarded with the stool.

The collection period is begun just after the child has voided (this specimen being discarded) and is completed with the collection of the specimen voided 12 or 24 hours later. *Timed collections always begin and end with the bladder empty.* Infants and young children rarely void "by the clock," so the nurse should know that a 13-hour or 22-hour specimen *is* satisfactory, provided that the dates and exact times of starting and ending the collection period are recorded on the collection bottle and accompanying identification cards.

Collection of complete 12- or 24-hour specimens from active infants of either sex is far from easy but can be accomplished if the nurse is given a few guidelines. When not being held by an attendant or parent, the infant may need to be mildly restrained in the supine position using soft cotton bandages around wrists and ankles; restraints are secured to the crib frame beneath the mattress, *not* to the side rails. After the skin around the meatus and perineum has been cleansed of powder and/or ointment and thoroughly dried, an adhesive plastic collecting bag (disposable colostomy pouch) is prepared for use. A small circular opening in the adhesive plate should be made for boys; an oval opening should be cut for girls. The bag is then fitted into place. Special care is needed to ensure that the adhesive surface is pressed firmly onto the skin posteriorly to avoid leakage and fecal contamination, especially in female infants.

In order to remove individual specimens collected in the bag during the 12- or 24-hour period without removing the bag each time or undoing the closure at the bottom of the pouch (which often loosens the adhesive seal on the child's perineum), a small piece of polyethylene tubing is inserted into the bag through a small hole in one of the upper corners. Individual voidings are aspirated with a regular syringe (minus the needle). The collection device should be checked repeatedly, every 30 minutes, throughout the collection period. Informed parents are often invaluable in the proper execution of these procedures.

Renal Function Tests[*][3]

Serum BUN and Creatinine Urea and creatinine are nitrogenous wastes that are normally removed by the kidney. Their concentration in the blood increases as kidney function becomes impaired, and they are used as yardsticks of improvement or deterioration of the patient's condition. Creatinine is derived from muscle creatine. The plasma concentration, which is normally less than 1 mg/100 ml in children, is unaffected by changes in the diet or in the daily fluid intake. The blood urea nitrogen (BUN), which is normally less than 20 mg/100 ml, varies according to the protein and fluid intake and is therefore a less specific index of change in renal function than is the plasma creatinine. Nevertheless, the BUN is widely used in pediatrics because of its ease of determination and the additional reflection it provides of the child's state of hydration. Plasma creatinine determination is routinely done on patients with known renal disease or in those cases where the significance of an elevated BUN is uncertain. The BUN and creatinine concentrations do not become consis-

tently elevated above normal until the kidneys' filtration rate is reduced by about 60 percent. Hence, they provide only a crude index of renal function. Clearance measurements must be used to determine lesser degrees of renal impairment.

Urea and creatinine clearance tests "Clearance" refers to the volume of plasma that is completely "cleared" of some particular substance in 1 minute. One must assume that the substance, a certain plasma constituent, is freely filtered at the glomerulus so that its concentration in the filtrate is not so different from that in the plasma; further, one must assume that the tubules neither reabsorb the substance nor add to it by active secretion. Thus, clearance is a means of expressing the rate of urinary excretion of a given substance in terms of a certain volume of plasma—the volume of plasma that contains the same total amount of the substance as appears in the urine in 1 minute.

In clinical testing with children, one determines the clearance of urea and/or creatinine, substances normally present at a relatively stable concentration in the plasma which can be measured in timed urine specimens by simple chemical methods. Urea clearance may vary due to the following two factors: rate of urine flow (more urea diffuses back out of the tubule when urine flow is sluggish) and plasma BUN variability as a function of diet and fluid intake. The clearance of endogenous creatinine is unaffected by diet, fluid intake, and rate of urine flow. However, both determinations may result in wide errors if the nurse is not careful to ensure complete emptying of the bladder with each voiding, especially if collection periods are short. Credé techniques (using the hand to apply external pressure on the bladder to express urine) and temporary catheterization may be indicated in children with neurogenic bladders or ileal conduits.

Given an initial good flow of urine in the child, two 2-hour collection periods can provide accurate clearance information; one 2-hour period serves as a "check" on the other (both in urine flow and plasma value concentrations of urea and creatinine). Moreover, if both urea and creatinine clearances are determined simultaneously, values for the two substances, expressed as "percents of normal" (normal creatinine clearance = 110 ml/min/1.73 sq m; normal urea clearance = 70 ml/min/1.73 sq m) can be compared as a further "check" on accuracy.

Urine concentration test The maximum specific gravity (or osmolality—another way of expressing concentration) that the child can achieve after a

---

[*] The following discussion is taken almost exclusively from James's *Renal Disease in Childhood* and from the clinical work of Dr. George A. Richard, J. H. Miller Health Center, Gainesville, Fla.

period of fluid deprivation is a simple and reliable test of kidney function. The specific gravity of the urine in a normal child after 12 hours of fluid deprivation will usually exceed 1.024. As renal function deteriorates, the tendency is for normal concentrating and diluting ability to be lost, so that urine from a patient with severe renal deficiency has a relatively fixed specific gravity (around 1.010). A concentration test is conveniently run overnight, although fluid restriction for infants is generally less than 12 hours. For the older child, no fluids are given after supper; the child voids, discards this urine, and notes the time. Twelve or more hours later, or whenever the child awakes for the day, the first specimen obtained would be suitable for concentration determination. Ideally, the second specimen of the morning prior to any fluid intake would be even more accurate in such determination since that urine is most certainly not residual.

Clean-Voided Specimen

The method of collecting clean-voided specimens from infants and children is discussed under urinary tract infections later in this chapter. For children with neurogenic bladders, the same basic techniques are applied, but the nurse or parent may have to use Credé techniques. The nurse can anticipate a poor stream and should not collect any urine that has "dribbled" over the skin. In some of these same instances, the physician will prefer to use a suprapubic bladder tap (Fig. 38-5) or to introduce a temporary catheter into the bladder. Likewise, for children with ileal conduits (see the section on surgical treatment later in this chapter) the nurse will clean and dry the child's stoma as she would the external genitalia, having first manually expressed as much "trapped" urine from immediately within the conduit as possible. A sterile catheter is introduced into the stoma, and the draining urine is collected in a sterile basin.

The nurse may be responsible for "planting" clean-voided urine on Testuria, a handy screening media. A commercial adaptation of the filter paper dipstick is used to inoculate a small agar plate, which is then incubated at 37°C (98.6°F) overnight. Although actual identification of bacterial type is not possible, Testuria does provide a screening test for bacterial presence and for colony count. A range of 0 to 2 colonies is considered negative, or minimal contaminant. A range of 3 to 25 colonies is suspicious, corresponding to the 10,000 to 100,000 bacteria/ml range, and the culture should be repeated. A finding of more than 25 colonies is considered positive, equal to or greater than 100,000 or 10^5 bacteria/ml of urine. All positive Testurias are then forwarded to the main clinical laboratory for identification and various antibiotic sensitivity tests.

Common X-Ray Procedures

In general, x-ray studies are used to determine the size, shape, and position of the kidneys and details of their blood supply. In addition, kidney function can be roughly determined according to how well each kidney concentrates and excretes radiopaque contrast media.

Intravenous Pyelogram (IVP)   The intravenous pyelogram is a widely used study of the upper urinary tract; it is especially valuable in the diagnosis of suspected structural anomalies in the collecting systems and in assessing the extent of pyelonephritis. The IVP can also provide information concerning the separate function of each kidney. Severe impairment of the kidneys' filtration rate (BUN > 40 mg/100 ml), however, prevents good visualization, as does water or solute diuresis.

While exact procedures for preparation vary with location, some period of prior fluid restriction is generally indicated in children. Usually an antecubital vein is the site of injection of diluted contrast material, although intramuscular injection in small infants may be an alternative. (The concentration of contrast material by the kidney is generally less when using this method, but may be sufficient to provide critical information.) The total number of films taken, the interval between films, and the positioning of the patient are determined by the pediatrician and radiologist, depending on the needs of the individual situation. Generally the young child reacts most to the "shot" and to being required to lie still for some minutes.

The only absolute contraindication to an IVP is a previous severe sensitivity reaction to the contrast material, and such reactions are rare. Generally, a preliminary test dose of 1 ml of contrast media is injected intravenously, and the child is observed closely for 30 to 60 seconds. If there are no adverse signs, the full dose is injected. While allergic reactions are very uncommon in infants and small children, the incidence of sensitivity reaction, such as urticarial hives and wheezing, increases in school-age children and adolescents, especially if the child has a history of asthma. Such sensitivity reactions can be well controlled by an intravenous dose of diphenhydramine (Benadryl), and the drug should always be readily available.

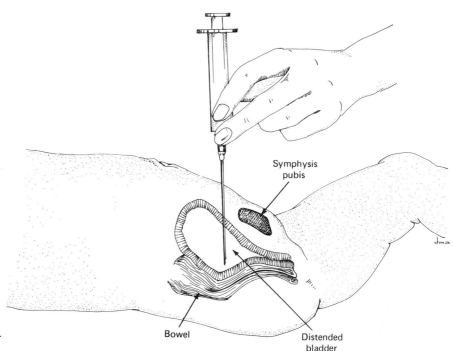

Figure 38-5 Suprapubic aspiration.

Labels in figure: Symphysis pubis — Bowel — Distended bladder

Cystogram or Cystourethrogram The voiding cystourethrogram (VCUG) is used to study the bladder and the contour of the urethra during voiding and to demonstrate the presence of vesicoureteral reflux. The patient is catheterized and the bladder is slowly filled with contrast material so that its size and outline can be determined. The capacity of the bladder ranges from 75 ml in newborns to 300 ml in older children. In older children, the catheter is removed and the patient is encouraged to void. (Actual moving pictures or a cine technique may be used to provide a dynamic record of the act of urination.) Small infants will start to urinate spontaneously whenever bladder filling reaches the point of discomfort. X-ray films are taken at close intervals to outline the urethra for evidence of any obstruction and to demonstrate vesicoureteral reflux, evident either when the bladder is filling or only during urination. A final film is taken to demonstrate whether the bladder has emptied completely and whether there is evidence of refluxed contrast media in the renal pelvis.

Because a VCUG involves catheterization (the part of the procedure which children find most objectionable), it is not used indiscriminately. Indeed, it is contraindicated in the presence of acute urinary tract infection because of the risk of spreading infection to the kidney by reflux or of initiating bacteremia. The astute nurse should know the patient's status regarding active infection, right down to the most recent Testuria and/or microscopic examination of clean-voided urine prior to the procedure. In the presence of active infection or the suspicion of it, the risks of this procedure do outweigh the benefits.

The nurse can help the child relieve postcatheterization discomfort by forcing fluids and applying cold compresses to the urinary meatus as necessary. The nurse may also suggest to the parent that the child be placed in a tub of warm water and be allowed to void for the first time in the tub.

Cystoscopy A urologic procedure done under general anesthesia, cystoscopy remains the most direct means of studying the anatomy of the lower urinary tract and a prerequisite to retrograde pyelography. Cystoscopic findings are related to factors such as ureteral-orifice size, shape (normal, cone, stadium, horseshoe, golfhole), and location (lateral or proximal in trigone of bladder) and to abnormalities of function such as reflux.

Some major indications for cystoscopy and possible retrograde pyelography include:

(1) situations where there is absent or imperfect visualization of one or both collecting systems by intravenous pyelography; (2) unexplained hema-

turia where the source of bleeding and its cause must be determined, for example, cystitis, stone, or tumor; (3) suspected ectopic opening of the ureter, persistent reflux, or suspected ureterocele; (4) unexplained anuria where bilateral ureteral obstruction is suspected; (5) cases of suspected unilateral renal or renal vascular disease where the urine from each kidney must be examined separately; and (6) cases of recurrent urinary tract infection with a normal or doubtfully abnormal intravenous pyelogram and cystogram.[4]

Because this procedure involves general anesthesia, the nurse should preoperatively prepare the patient in deep breathing and coughing techniques; colorful balloons at the bedside are excellent reminders. Early ambulation is an added plus. The physician will order frequent checking of vital signs throughout and forced fluids upon full recovery from the anesthesia; similar comfort measures as for postcatheterization (as discussed in the section on cystograms above) may be employed with the physician's support.

Renal Biopsy

Percutaneous needle biopsy of the kidney often provides critical information on which the physician can base a diagnosis or prognosis in children with clinically established renal disease. Serial biopsies, along with clearance tests of renal function, are helpful in assessing the progress of children with persistent nephritic processes and may help in determining the choice of therapy and its value. Diagnostic renal biopsy is generally recommended in the following situations:

1 Unexplained hematuria or proteinuria
2 Nephrotic syndrome that is unresponsive to steroid therapy
3 Systemic lupus erythematosus
4 Persistent glomerulonephritis
5 Acute renal failure of unexplained cause
6 Unexplained hypertension

The biopsy procedure itself may be explained to parents and children as a diagnostic study involving the removal of a small piece of kidney tissue (about the size of a pencil lead) for examination under the microscope and for special staining. These techniques are helpful in determining the type and severity of disease within the kidney and may be helpful in guiding appropriate treatment. The nurse should stress that although the child remains awake, lying on his stomach during the procedure, his back is "put to sleep" so that only distinct deep *pressure* will be felt at the moment of securing the tissue itself. For young, highly anxious children, however, the physician may request that supplemental anesthesia be available.

Prerequisites to biopsy are signed parental consent, x-ray evidence that two kidneys are indeed present, and laboratory studies indicating that red blood count and blood-clotting mechanisms are normal.

The child is premedicated usually with meperidine (Demerol), 1 mg/kg body weight, and pentobarbital (Nembutal), 2 mg/kg body weight. After careful cleansing of the skin, a solution of 1 percent xylocaine is used intradermally and deeply to numb the biopsy site. Fluoroscopy is an extremely useful adjunct in guiding placement of the biopsy needle after initial localization of kidney cortex. Although a sterile pressure bandage may be applied afterward, the incision through which the biopsy needle passes is just a nick—less than 2 cm.

After the biopsy, strict bed rest with no exceptions is maintained for at least 12 hours; the child may lie on his back or abdomen. The nurse will check regularly and frequently for bleeding from the bandage site and will monitor pulse and blood pressure as ordered (every 15 minutes times 8; every half-hour times 4; every hour times 4; then every 3 hours). The child and parents are requested to force fluids to a specified amount, depending on body weight; they are also requested to save all voided urine at the bedside so that it can be checked visually and with reagent dipsticks for bleeding. Some flank tenderness and guarding is common for 24 to 48 hours after the biopsy and may reflect a small amount of perirenal bleeding.

Absolute contraindications to biopsy are the presence of a solitary kidney or a hemorrhagic tendency. Relative contraindications include very small kidneys, advanced renal failure, and severe hypertension. It appears that the hazard of bleeding increases under these circumstances, and the small fibrotic kidney is difficult to localize and take a biopsy from. The major reported complication from the biopsy procedure is bleeding, which may occur externally in the urine or may be concealed internally as a perirenal hematoma. The published series of biopsies in children suggest that the incidence of serious complications in the child is lower than that seen in the adult patient.[5]

URINARY PROBLEMS IN THE NEWBORN AND INFANT

Knowledge of embryologic development provides the nurse with a better understanding of how congenital or structural anomalies occur. According to several authorities 5 to 10 percent of all infants are born with a malformation of the urinary tract. In comparison, 1 percent of all infants are born with congenital malformations of the heart.[6] Fortunately, many of the urinary tract deformities are clinically unimportant, and many others are surgically correctable.

The majority of urinary tract anomalies are asymptomatic; however, some of these may be detected because of the significant correlation between anomalies of the urinary tract and other congenital anomalies. The following are some of the anomalies commonly associated with urinary tract malformations:

1 Low-set malformed ears
2 Chromosomal disorders, especially D and E trisomy
3 Absent abdominal muscles
4 Anomalies of the spinal cord and lower extremities
5 Imperforate anus or genital deviation
6 Wilms' tumor
7 Congenital ascites
8 Cystic disease of liver
9 Positive family history of renal disease (hereditary nephritis, cystic disease)[7]

The anomalies which are symptomatic present a challenge to the nurse since early diagnosis is needed to prevent renal damage. Some of the symptoms to observe in the infant are:

1 Abdominal mass in neonatal period
2 Unexplained dehydration, acidosis, or anemia[8]

Infantile Polycystic Disease

This disease, an autosomal recessive trait, presents in infancy or early childhood. The child has enlarged kidneys filled with cysts at birth and often has floppy, low-set ears, prominent epicanthal folds, beaklike nose, and a small chin. This appearance is commonly referred to as Potter facies. An intravenous pyelogram is peculiar to this disease in that the contrast media is retained by the kidneys for a day or more.

If the infant survives, the treatment program centers around progressive renal failure, with dialysis and transplantation as possibilities. Since the disease is hereditary, the parents need to be counseled concerning the risk of future offspring.

Wilms' Tumor

One of the most common malignant tumors in children, Wilms' tumor is classified as an embryoma. In two-thirds of the cases the parents note an abdominal mass. An intravenous pyelogram demonstrates how the mass distorts rather than displaces the collecting system.

The tumor is treated with a combination of surgery, radiation therapy, and chemotherapy. Preoperatively radiation therapy may be used to reduce the size of the tumor, and a chemotherapeutic agent administered. The nurse is responsible for posting a sign on the patient's crib warning against abdominal manipulation which increases the danger of metastasis. Postoperatively, radiation therapy and chemotherapy are used to prevent or treat pulmonary metastasis. The highest survival rates are obtained in infants under 1 year of age.

Obstruction of the Collecting System

A partial or complete obstruction of the ureters or urethra results in destruction of the nephrons. James reports that experiments have shown 50 percent permanent decrease in filtration rate in total obstruction of 1 week.[9] Chronic obstructive disease not only causes a decrease in filtration rate but also hydronephrosis, an increase in length and width of the ureters, and hypertrophy of the bladder.

Early treatment in obstructive disease is imperative to prevent irreversible destruction of the nephrons. However, the success of surgical intervention in the treatment of obstructive disease is questionable.

Obstruction of Ureteropelvic Junction

Obstruction at the ureteropelvic junction, the most common obstructive deformity, results from pressure by a blood vessel on the ureter, narrowing of the ureter, or abnormal insertion of the ureter into the renal pelvis. The child may be asymptomatic, or he may present with abdominal pain, nausea, vomiting, elevated blood pressure, or recurrent urinary tract infections. An intravenous pyelogram demonstrates the narrow ureteropelvic junction and hydronephrosis.

If the obstruction is complete, the treatment is surgical. However, if there is partial obstruction with nonprogressive hydronephrosis, the conservative approach is the treatment of choice, since there is little evidence that surgery is successful. If the kidney is severely damaged, a nephrectomy may be done.

Duplication of Ureters and Pelvis

Duplication of a ureter results when the ureteral bud (see Fig. 38-1) branches prematurely. The deformity is more prevalent in girls and may be unilateral or bilateral. The treatment is conservative if there is no reflux and both ureters are normal. If reflux exists, surgical intervention is necessary.

Ureterocele

Frequently associated with duplication, ureterocele is an enlargement of the lower end of the ureter. Because the ureteral opening is usually stenotic, hydronephrosis and hydroureter are present. The treatment of this condition is surgical.

Exstrophy of the Bladder

Exstrophy results from failure of the anterior portion of the cloacal membrane to develop (see Fig. 38-1). It is characterized by varying degrees of exstroversion of the bladder and frequently is accompanied by other anomalies such as epispadias, inguinal hernias, and undescended testes.

Treatment is aimed at preserving renal function, preventing complications of incontinence, constructing a penis in the male, and improving the appearance of the child. Since bladder reconstruction has had limited success, urinary diversional surgery appears to be the treatment of choice.

Because of the bladder eversion there is continuous bathing of the mucosa and surrounding abdominal skin with urine. This condition requires immediate and meticulous nursing intervention to prevent skin breakdown and ulceration of the bladder mucosa. Fine-mesh gauze impregnated with petrolatum can be applied to prevent irritation and promote comfort to the sensitive bladder mucosa, and various barrier creams can be applied to the surrounding skin for protection. Frequent diaper changes and meticulous skin care, particularly after each stool, also aids in preventing skin breakdown and infection. These neonates have typical newborn needs; however, they have a tendency to be irritable and fussy. The causes of their fussiness should be identified since this behavior aggravates their hernias and predisposes them to rectal prolapse.

Until surgery is performed, the parents assume responsibility for their baby's care. Seeing the defect, cleaning the affected area, and feeding the baby are difficult procedures for them to do. They need encouragement, support, and time in which to assimilate and demonstrate the teaching that is done.

Epispadias

Epispadias, a congenital anomaly in which the urethral meatus is located on the dorsal surface of the penis, rarely occurs as an isolated condition, but is more commonly seen as a component of exstrophy of the bladder. The defect occurs five times more frequently in males. The mild cases of epispadias in females require no surgical intervention; however, the condition in males should be repaired between 2 and 3 years of age for functional and cosmetic reasons.

Epispadias is classified according to the position of the urethral meatus. In the least severe form the meatus is located in the dorsum of the glans. When the meatus is located along the dorsum of the penis, the epispadias is considered to be more severe (see Fig. 38-6). In this type the penis is curved dorsally, is flattened, and is smaller than usual. In the most severe type the penis is short and blunt, and the urethral meatus is present at the penopubic junction. Generally, incontinence accompanies this degree of epispadias, the prepuce hangs from the ventral surface, and the symphysis pubis is widened.

The kind and amount of surgical intervention depend upon the severity of the deformity. If chordee is present, it is released to correct the abnormal dorsal curvature. The urethral meatus is relocated in the glans, and the prepuce is transferred from the ventral surface to the dorsal.

Hypospadias

Hypospadias is an anomaly whereby the urethral meatus is located on the ventral surface of the penis (see Fig. 38-7). The meatus most frequently ends in the shaft of the penis or near the glans. Less common cases in which the meatus is found in the scrotum or in the perineum are more severe. Chordee accompanies most cases of hypospadias. This condition results from normal tissue being replaced by a tough band of fibrous tissue which bends the penis ventrally.

Hypospadias is treated surgically by a multistage or a one-stage procedure. In the one-step procedure an extension of the urethra is formed from a skin graft, and the chordee is released. When the multistage approach is used, the chordee is released initially, and urethroplasty is done in one or more future operations. For a detailed discussion on the surgical procedures used to correct hypospadias and epispadias, a urology textbook would be helpful.

Initially, it is important for the nurse to observe the newborn's voiding pattern. A meatotomy may be required if there is an abnormal voiding pattern. At the time of repair a perineal urethrotomy, a suprapubic tube, or a Foley catheter is utilized to divert urine from the operative site. Keeping the incision dry and free from trauma are extremely important factors in the success of the repair.

RENAL PROBLEMS IN THE TODDLER
Childhood Nephrosis

The nephrotic syndrome is a clinical entity with multiple causes resulting from a variety of disease states and nephrotoxic agents. Nephrosis may be found in patients of all ages but is most common in its "pure" form in toddlers and preschoolers.

The clinical terms *nephrosis, childhood nephrosis,* or *idiopathic nephrotic syndrome* can be used interchangeably to describe that disease which develops in the absence of any obvious precipitating cause or underlying disease. Older names for this disorder are *pure nephrosis* or *lipoid nephrosis.*[10]

The nurse recognizes the nephrotic child by his generalized edema (if untreated) or by his mild to pronounced cushingoid features (if undergoing steroid therapy). The nephrotic child is usually accompanied by anxious parents for whom the nurse must care as well. Parents' questions, at the outset, generally deal with "the cause of this" and "the difference between nephritis and nephrosis."

Childhood nephrosis is less common than acute glomerulonephritis. The prevalence of nephrosis is approximately 7 cases per 100,000 children below the age of 5 years.[11] There is a preponderance of affected boys over girls. The disease is seen worldwide, with no racial or geographic determinant.

The most common age of onset for nephrosis is between 1½ and 2½ years, while acute nephritis is most common between 4 and 7 years of age and is uncommon in children under 2 years of age. The peak period of onset is during late infancy, but idiopathic nephrotic syndrome may be seen in older children, adolescents, and adults.

Most parents are distressed to hear that the exact cause of childhood nephrosis is yet unknown. However, the chief pathogenetic feature common to all varieties of nephrotic syndrome *is* known: increased glomerular membrane permeability to large molecules so that considerable quantities of plasma proteins escape into the urine. Albumin is lost in greatest quantity because of its high plasma concentration and relatively low molecular weight. "The nature of the 'leak' in the filter is not understood. No distinct breaks or discontinuities in the basement membrane of the glomerular capillaries can be seen,

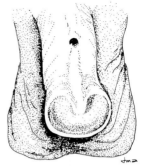

Figure 38-6   Penile epispadias with dorsal chordee.

even with the electron microscope, and it seems likely, therefore, that the leakage of proteins results from some molecular change in the filtering membrane itself."[12]

James proposes a schema for the pathogenesis of the nephrotic syndrome which is sequential, though unproved experimentally (Fig. 38-8). From this schema, one can identify the specific criteria suggested for defining the nephrotic syndrome.[13] Values in parentheses are arbitrary.

1   Proteinuria: Protein in the urine (3.5 Gm/24 hours or more) or proteinuria in excess of 0.1 Gm/kg body weight per day, which is prerequisite to the development of the other manifestations of the syndrome. This finding alone serves to establish the diagnosis of the syndrome for clinical purposes.[14]
2   Hypoalbuminemia: Low blood levels of albumin. The plasma albumin concentration falls as albumin is lost in the urine and is not balanced by the synthesis rate in the liver (3 Gm/100 ml or less in serum).
3   Hyperlipidemia: High blood levels of lipids (300 mg cholesterol/100 ml or more in serum).
4   Edema.

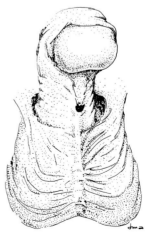

Figure 38-7   Midpenile hypospadias and chordee.

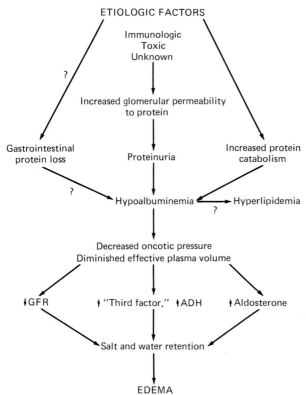

Figure 38-8 Schema for pathogenesis of the nephrotic syndrome. *(From J. A. James, Renal Disease in Childhood, 2d ed., The C. V. Mosby Company, St. Louis, 1972, p. 197.)*

Examining the phenomenon of edema in nephrosis more closely, James poses an interesting explanation. He suggests that edema

> represents a *compensatory* phenomenon, the purpose of which is to maintain the plasma volume at a safe level despite a great reduction in the plasma osmotic pressure. *If edema formation did not occur, the nephrotic child would be in serious difficulties from circulatory insufficiency.*[15] [italics added]

Indeed, the nephrotic child is usually brought to the pediatrician because of "swelling." Parents may first notice periorbital edema in the child which does not subside; they may say that the child's shoes or trousers have been difficult to fasten or the child has shown a sudden weight gain. Physiologically, extracellular fluid collection *does* occur in the child's peritoneal cavity, legs, and external genitalia (labia or scrotum). The skin over his abdomen may become stretched and shiny, with veins prominent; the devitalized skin in this region and previously mentioned

edematous areas has a characteristic waxy pallor and frequently breaks down because of increased interstitial fluid pressure and poor tissue tone. The child may have rectal prolapse, herniation, and/or hydrocele for similar reasons.

Progressive wasting of the skeletal muscles may take place because of the continuous, voluminous drain of plasma protein nitrogen into the urine which is not adequately replaced by dietary nitrogen. Like the child who is suffering exclusively from protein malnutrition, the chronic nephrotic patient's wasted, sticklike extremities and prominent rib cage are in sharp contrast to his distended abdomen (Figs. 38-9 and 38-10).

The parent also notices a decreased frequency of the child's urination and "foamy" or "frothy" looking urine. Despite his appearance, the child with nephrosis appears to feel relatively well, although he tires easily and his appetite is poor. His blood pressure is normal or slightly lower than average. He may, however, be anxious and embarrassed by his edematous, unattractive appearance; nurses, doctors, and other health care workers would do well to avoid thoughtless remarks for this child's sake.

Having received the diagnosis, parents next question the natural course of nephrosis: "How long will it last? Will my child remain this severely affected?" Parents need to know that childhood nephrosis is a chronic disease; they should think of the condition in terms of months or years rather than days or weeks and that, however successful the initial treatment may be, medical supervision will have to be continued for at least 2 to 3 years because of the risk of exacerbation.

The duration and severity of any child's clinical course is variable. At one extreme is the child who undergoes spontaneous or steroid-induced diuresis after one edematous episode and experiences no relapse; at the other extreme is the child who remains persistently swollen, fails to respond to steroids and other drugs, and dies of progressive renal disease in 2 to 3 years. The majority of cases of nephrotic children lie in between, experiencing any number of remissions and exacerbations over a period of 1 to 10 years (Fig. 38-11). These children generally recover but may have compromised renal function for life.

It may be helpful and hopeful to point out to parents that the response to therapy in adults and children is considerably different. Estimates are that 54 percent of all children, as opposed to 21 percent of adults, have complete remission either on steroids or without treatment.[16] In addition, it is well recognized that most children with nephrotic syndrome have minimal or *no* pathologic changes in renal biopsy specimens.[17] The occurrence of hypertension and hematuria in children is infrequent but denotes a poorer prognosis.

Active nephrosis can have its complications. The child with generalized edema is unusually susceptible to intercurrent infections; this susceptibility is not solely attributable to reduced serum gamma globulin. Prophylactic treatment with extraneous gamma globulin does not seem to reduce the frequency of infection significantly. Indeed, edema fluid in living tissue is an excellent culture medium which offers little resistance to the spread of infection.

Prior to the introduction of effective antibiotics, peritonitis (pneumococcal) was the principal cause of death in nephrotic children. Other fatal infections were cellulitis, septicemia, and pneumonia. Deaths from bacterial infection in nephrotic patients are now rare, thanks to intensive, appropriate antibiotic treatment when necessary. Furthermore, children can be maintained edema-free with steroid therapy. However, the nephrotic child *is* as susceptible as any child to the common viral respiratory infections, and these intermittent infections frequently appear to precipitate exacerbations of edema.

Complications related to edema buildup may include ascites and respiratory distress. Diuretic therapy is usually effective in relieving this massive edema, and paracentesis is rarely needed. A common problem among nephrotic children may be loose bowel movements, probably resulting from intestinal malabsorption secondary to edema of the bowel wall. Nursing management includes (1) reassuring the child that the frequent bowel movements are "not his fault" and will probably subside as his edema decreases and (2) maintaining immaculate skin care to prevent excoriated buttocks and perineum.

Medical and Nursing Management

Activity The nephrotic child, considering his age and developmental level, will generally pace his own activity and set his own limits satisfactorily. Ambulation to prevent osteoporosis and participation in school or play activities are desirable for the child's sense of well-being. The aim is the prevention of excessive fatigue. However, bed rest is indicated and generally not resisted by the child during (a) acute infections and (b) when the child is undergoing a rapid diuresis. Once edema has been lost, nephrotic children may resume the full activity of their normal companions with mild caution against "overdoing it."

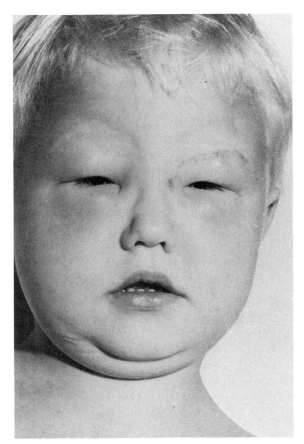

Figure 38-9 Child with active nephrosis. Note the severe periorbital and facial edema. *(Courtesy of S. Hellerstein, M.D., Children's Mercy Hospital, Kansas City, Mo.)*

Diet Children with active nephrosis are renowned for their poor appetites. Thus, physicians, dietitians, nurses, and parents must pool their knowledge of the child to formulate a diet that is both nutritionally adequate and well tolerated. (Nutritional information gathered from the parents and child by the nurse in an initial nursing history or nursing interview may prove vital in this respect if the parents are not always available.) Most physicians will agree that there is obviously no benefit in a diet the child consistently refuses, no matter how desirable it may be in theory.

"Salt restriction is necessary because the edematous nephrotic child retains almost all of the salt given to him as edema fluid. Salt retention and the accumulation of edema fluid represent a necessary homeostatic adjustment to hypoproteinemia in nephrosis so that it is undesirable to eliminate salt from the diet completely."[18] On practical grounds, few children will tolerate the general tastelessness of an extremely low-sodium diet, and it is impossible to

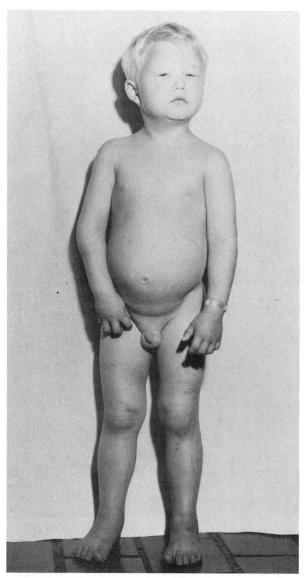

Figure 38-10   Full-length view of the child in Fig. 38-9. Note edema of the abdomen, scrotum, arms, legs, and feet. *(Courtesy of S. Hellerstein, M.D., Children's Mercy Hospital, Kansas City, Mo.)*

severe and incapacitating edema, in whom any further increase in fluid accumulation might precipitate respiratory embarrassment.[19] Once diuresis has occurred, the previous moderate restriction on sodium is advocated, but parents may allow the child bacon, crackers, and other salty treats occasionally.

A high-protein diet (much milk, meat, and eggs) would be desirable in nephrotic children to offset their persistent negative nitrogen balance and tissue wasting due to heavy proteinuria, but toleration for such a diet is again a problem. A compromise diet containing 2 to 3 Gm protein/kg. body weight per day is satisfactory.[20]

While edematous nephrotic children retain sodium, they excrete potassium and ammonia as the principal urinary cations. Their diet should therefore include extra potassium in the form of juices, fruits (oranges, bananas, grapes), and milk. Concomitantly, fluid restriction is imposed only in extreme edematous phases; restriction is based on the child's previous day's urine output plus estimated insensible losses by way of the skin and lungs. When careful monitoring of fluid intake and urine output is desired, the nurse can often enlist the aid of the young patient by means of a simple bedside picture chart; the child feels he is actively participating in his care and exercising some control over his own restrictions in this manner.

Skin care   The potential skin care problems of edematous nephrotic children have been mentioned. Ulceration occurs most readily over the scrotum, perineum, and buttocks where deterioration is aided by pressure, immobility, and exposure to urine and the proteolytic action of loose stools. *Prevention* of breakdown of the skin is the key word for the nurse, in planning a meticulous program of skin care which includes frequent diaper changes, careful washing and drying of the exposed skin and skin folds with mild soap and water, and the liberal use of nonallergenic powder or cornstarch. Improvisation of a nonconstricting scrotal or labial support from soft cotton batting may be needed. If, despite precautions, the skin breaks down, powder and ointment should be discontinued; careful washing should continue, and the skin should be exposed to freely circulating air. Heat lamps should be used with utmost care to avoid burns. Some physicians favor the use of zinc oxide paste on resistant denuded areas to protect the skin against further irritation by urine and stool. Until the precipitating state of edema is relieved through diuresis, healing of severely ulcerated areas will usually not occur.

Femoral venipunctures[21]   and   intramuscular

prevent *completely* the accumulation of edema by dietary salt restriction. Hence, sodium intake is generally only moderately restricted to 1 to 2 Gm daily. Excessively salty foods are prohibited and extra added salt in cooking or at the table is deleted; however, regular foods (bread, butter, milk) rather than the salt-free varieties are allowed. The use of very low sodium diets (300 mg salt daily) is reserved for the short-term treatment of patients who present with injections in the buttocks should be avoided.[22] In addition to the risk of infection, clinical evidence suggests that a hypercoagulable state exists in the nephrotic syndrome and that fibrinolysis is impaired. Hypovolemia, stasis, and infection, in addition to direct injury to the vessel wall by such procedures as femoral venipuncture, may favor thromboembolism.

Infection   Prevention of infection has much in common with psychologic support and education of parents and their affected and nonaffected children. Until recent years, virtual isolation of the nephrotic child, whether edematous or not, was the rule, due to hazards of intercurrent infection. With the advent of better drugs and cognizance of the emotional deprivation and parental anxiety fostered by these restrictions, medical teams realized that the advantages of "normalcy" often outweigh the hazards. General recommendations now are that the young nephrotic child be kept away only from large gatherings (parties, Sunday school classes), especially during periods of increased respiratory infections. For the older nephrotic child, the benefit of attending regular school classes generally outweighs the risk of increased exposure to infection, but this decision must be made on an individual basis by the physician. Prior to the child's discharge from the hospital, nurse and parents should begin to plan for his being tutored at home if he is unable to resume regular schooling.

Routine antibiotic prophylaxis is not generally used with nephrotic children because of risks of superimposed infections of *Candida, Pseudomonas,* and other resistant organisms. (An exception might be oral penicillin G in nephrotic children who come from families with other young children and a high risk of cross infection.)

Support for parents and patients   Confronted with explanations of their child's disease and the many details of his daily management whether in the hospital or at home, parents may understandably appear bewildered and overwhelmed, requiring continuing psychologic support and education from the nurse, physician, and other team members. Parental behavior and verbal expressions denoting excessive feelings of guilt, denial, overindulgence, and other potentially harmful attitudes should be recognized, respected, and approached honestly by the nurse and physician. Empathy, respect, and a willingness to become involved to assist parents in working through their own solutions to problems are prerequisite skills for any nurse working with parents of children with chronic disease. It is often helpful, at

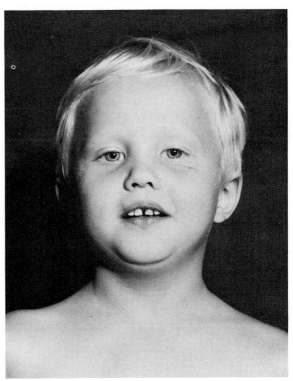

Figure 38-11   The same child shown in Figs. 38-9 and 38-10 after 1 month of corticosteroid therapy. *(Courtesy of S. Hellerstein, M.D., Children's Mercy Hospital, Kansas City, Mo.)*

the outset, to ask both child and parents, individually or together, what their understanding of the condition is. The nurse's response to their answers should promote understanding and optimal attitudes about the disease. To the common question, "What is the difference between nephritis and nephrosis?" one can respond that the diseases are not the same but are closely related in affecting the kidney and that both are considered forms of an old term, Bright's disease. Since Bright's disease is often believed to be universally fatal, one should add that nephrosis is a chronic form of Bright's disease occurring in children. The outlook for recovery is reasonably good. Again, chronicity refers to medical care and supervision for months, perhaps years—a fact which should be repeated.

Psychologic support for the child will actively involve parents and the nurse on a daily basis. Behavioral or verbal expressions of anxiety over hospitalization and separation, depression, change in body image, and fear of a permanent disease state and death are likely in various forms from all nephrotic children. To pretend these factors do not directly influence the child's progress is to deny the child that progress. The nurse must practice listening and observational skills, respect the child's right to his feelings, and allot sufficient time and energy to demonstrate caring daily. The child often suggests ways to solve his own problems and to facilitate independence and participation in his own care.

Corticosteroid treatment Corticosteroids have become the mainstay of a nephrotic child's medical management, offering a brighter prognosis for the child and cooperative responsibilities for nurse and parents.

> The goals of corticosteroid therapy are, first, to relieve edema and other manifestations of the nephrotic state, and, second, to keep the child in a state of clinical and chemical normality for as long as possible or until spontaneous healing of the underlying disease takes place (maintenance treatment). Successful treatment with corticosteroids results in the disappearance of all the clinical, biochemical, and morphologic abnormalities of the nephrotic syndrome and therefore represents a much more effective therapeutic approach than the use of albumin infusions or diuretics, which merely control the amount of edema without affecting the basic disease process.[23]

The exact mode of action of corticosteroids in nephrosis is unknown. Though all corticosteroid preparations (cortisone, hydrocortisone, prednisone, prednisolone, triamcinolone, dexamethasone, and others) are equally effective in inducing remissions when given in equivalent dosage, prednisone is generally the drug of choice because it has less tendency to induce salt retention and potassium loss.

The initial course of steroid treatment to induce remission (relieve edema) involves a dosage of prednisone of 60 mg/sq m body surface area per day in four divided doses for 4 weeks, followed by prednisone 60 mg/sq m in a single dose every other day for 4 weeks. Treatment is then stopped abruptly without tapering.[24] Potassium supplementation is not needed providing the child is drinking milk and fruit juices and providing that a potassium-losing diuretic is not being used.[25] While the child is under the close supervision of the physician, the nurse should advise the parents of symptoms to report: additional weight gain, headaches, nausea, fever, or evidence of infection. The nurse should carefully monitor the child's weight and blood pressure (using the appropriate size cuff and noting the child's posture, that is, standing or recumbent) during hospitalization or frequent office/clinic visits. The nurse, in conjunction with the physician, will also monitor serum sodium, potassium, bicarbonate, and blood urea nitrogen (BUN) at the beginning of therapy and at regular intervals thereafter, noting major changes. If the child develops evidence of infection, hypertension (140/100 mm Hg), or electrolyte imbalance, he will no doubt be admitted to the hospital without delay; advance preparation for these eventualities is often helpful to parents.

Diuresis usually begins between the eighth and fourteenth day of treatment, and is designated by a decrease in proteinuria, a shift of urine pH from acid to alkaline, and a gradual increase in urinary output with corresponding loss of weight.[26] To the child's joy, he may lose up to 8 pounds of edema fluid in a single day! During this phase, he should be on bed rest except for elimination. The child's activity and appetite generally improve markedly with the onset of diuresis. Steroid treatment continues daily for 10 to 14 days after diuresis occurs, at which time proteinuria will be absent or greatly reduced and serum albumin concentration will be nearing normal.

At this time the regimen of maintenance steroid therapy (60 mg/sq m body surface in a single dose every other day for 4 weeks) is begun. It is designed to suppress exacerbations until spontaneous recovery occurs. The rationale for alternating therapy hinges on reducing the undesirable side effects of the steroids and in possibly not suppressing the child's own adrenal production *in toto.*[27]

Parents, with assistance and support from the nurse, will test the child's first morning urine specimen for protein with a reagent strip (Albustix) and record the results daily or twice weekly. Specifications for resuming daily steroid treatment and/or increased dosage with evidence of increasing proteinuria (more than "trace" or 1+ protein) will again vary with physicians, but the nurse should know and explain the physician's orders on an individual basis. Usually the appearance of consecutive 2+ reactions in a child who is otherwise well and whose urine previously showed no proteinuria is considered evidence of a relapse.

> Relapses are treated with a two-week course of steroids given daily, followed by a two-week course of steroids given every other day in the previously mentioned dosage. Two relapses, that is, three episodes of the nephrotic syndrome within a single year, are considered to qualify the case as a frequent-relapse or steroid-dependent case, and cyclophosphamide treatment is initiated.[28]

Clinical features correlating with a poor therapeutic response to steroids include: early infancy or near adult age group, duration of nephrotic syndrome for more than 6 months, hypertension, azotemia, significant hematuria, relatively low serum cholesterol, and "unselective" proteinuria.[29]

Previously recommended treatment plans emphasized the importance of long-term maintenance therapy in preventing relapses after the initial treatment had relieved edema. Wider recognition of the steroid-dependent group of children, increasing concern about the side effects of long-term steroid therapy, and the advent of cytotoxic drug therapy have combined to swing the pendulum back toward shorter courses of steroid therapy.[30]

Steroid therapy has its common, bothersome, but not serious side effects; it also has some severe but rare complications. (See Table 38-1.) The nurse should remember to reassure patients and parents that nearly all persons treated with steroids develop Cushing's syndrome (clinical manifestations of hyperadrenocorticism) to some degree. Children may be alarmed by the flushing and rounding of the face (moon facies), appearance of a pad of fatty tissue over the base of the neck (buffalo hump), abdominal distention, striae, liver enlargement, greatly increased appetite with accompanying weight gain, and increased body hair (hirsutism). Acne may be aggravated in adolescents. Though cushingoid features cause distress and embarrassment, they tend to become less prominent when intermittent maintenance therapy is begun and will disappear entirely within 2 to 3 months after the steroid treatment is stopped.

Serious side effects and uncommon complications of steroid therapy include the "masking" of infections (chickenpox could prove fatal), peptic ulceration, growth suppression, cataracts, precipitation of diabetes mellitus, thromboembolism, intracranial hypertension, and adrenal suppression and insufficiency. The latter factor is most worrisome because the frequency of permanent adrenal suppression in children who have received long-term steroid therapy for nephrosis is unknown. Parents should thus be alerted to this "stress factor" and should never discontinue the child's steroid therapy without the physician's knowledge and consent. Sudden fatal adrenal insufficiency could develop without warning if the child is exposed to stressful situations such as infection, anesthesia and surgery, or

Table 38-1 SIDE EFFECTS OF CORTICOSTEROIDS IN PHARMACOLOGIC DOSES

Body system	Common	Uncommon
Cardiovascular	Plethora	Thromboembolism
Hematologic	Leukocytosis	Hypertension*
Gastrointestinal	Hepatomegaly	Peptic ulceration
	Abdominal distention	Pancreatitis
Endocrine	Adrenal suppression, sometimes persistent	Diabetes mellitus (reversible or irreversible)
Eye		Cataracts
Skin	Poor healing, striae	Panniculitis
	Moniliasis	
	Hirsutism	
Central nervous system		Pseudotumor
		Seizures
Psychiatric	Depression	Psychosis
	Hyperactivity	
Bone	Osteoporosis	Compression fractures
	Delayed growth	Avascular necrosis
Immunologic	Decreased resistance to infection	Exacerbation of tuberculosis
	Decreased febrile response to infection	Fatal chickenpox
General	Obesity	Edema*
	Increased appetite	Hypokalemia and alkalosis*
	Azotemia if renal function impaired	

* Commonest with ACTH, cortisone, and hydrocortisone.
Source: From J. A. James, *Renal Disease in Childhood*, 2d ed., The C. V. Mosby Company, St. Louis, 1972.

injury. Reportedly, however, adrenal suppression of measurable degree does not occur with every-other-day therapy.

Unresponsiveness to steroids Unfortunately steroids cannot be hailed as the "miracle drugs" of nephrosis since not all children respond favorably to steroid therapy. On the basis of therapeutic response, patients with the nephrotic syndrome may be classified into three groups:

1 Steroid-sensitive: Children *may* respond to a single short course of steroids without evidence of relapse after cessation of therapy. Less than 10 percent of children with idiopathic nephrotic syndrome fail to undergo a remission during the initial course of steroid therapy,[31] and up to 40 percent of such children may be in this group.[32]
2 Steroid-dependent: Some children respond incompletely; i.e., proteinuria is decreased but not absent, edema subsides somewhat. These children tend to relapse on lowered dosages of steroids and require further supportive treatment (i.e., diuretics, diet). They tend to have frequent relapses over many years and therefore receive large amounts of steroids, resulting in cushingoid features and growth retardation.
3 Steroid-resistant: Approximately 10 to 25 percent of children and a much higher percentage (70 to 80 percent) of adults become resistant to steroid treatment or cannot be maintained in remission without developing serious side effects from steroid therapy.

For the latter group, recognition of long-term toxic effects of corticoids, as well as the therapeutic failures, have prompted a revival of interest in immunosuppressive drugs [i.e., azathioprine (Imuran), cyclophosphamide (Cytoxan), methotrexate]. Cyclophosphamide in conjunction with prednisone and then by itself has proved promising in providing longer remissions.[33] The nurse should be aware of toxic reactions to cyclophosphamide: suppression of bone marrow (white blood cell count below 3,000 cells/cu mm), intercurrent fulminating bacterial or viral infections (measles and chickenpox), ulceration of gastric mucosa, alopecia, hemorrhagic cystitis, and others.

Attempts to predict any particular child's clinical course and final outcome regarding childhood nephrosis is difficult. The overall statistics show that roughly 70 percent of the patients recover completely, 5 percent die from infections and other intercurrent diseases, and 25 percent become unresponsive to steroid therapy and continue to show proteinuria and a variable amount of edema.[34-36]

The natural history of lipoid nephrosis, as modified by steroid therapy, was studied in 61 children who were between 1 and 6 years of age at onset. The average period of follow-up observation was 13.7 years. A relapsing course was evident early; complete resolution was likely in the absence of relapse during the first 2 to 3 years after onset. "These data indicate that the nephrotic syndrome in preschool-age children is not a benign disease despite the high responsiveness to treatment. . . . Recurrences will be experienced by the majority of patients for many years. However, the incidence of progression to renal failure remains low and in most children there is a marked reduction in activity by adolescence."[37] Late relapses are usually brought under control quickly with a short course of steroid therapy, and it is justifiable to be moderately optimistic about the future if the child remains free of all signs of the disease for longer than a year.[38] In any event, the nurse should expect to share with the child and his family the ups and downs of a chronic condition that will, it is hoped, eventually resolve.

Urinary Tract Infections

The seriousness of urinary tract infections in children is best appreciated when long-term effects are considered (Fig. 38-12). For over 25 years, medical investigators have emphasized the recurrent nature of urinary tract infections and their tendency toward chronicity, with distortion of anatomy and function of the kidney and potential progression to renal failure. Moreover, in the past decade, concepts of cause, natural course, and treatment of these common infections have been in a state of constant flux.

The nurse in a pediatrician's office or in pediatric outpatient clinic cannot fail to be impressed by the sheer number of children diagnosed as having a "UTI." The staff nurse or clinical specialist cannot fail to be impressed by the tenacity of infection in children with chronic, recurrent pyelonephritis and the crippling sequelae. Traditionally, the responsibility for the care of children with urinary tract infections has been shared by the general practitioner, pediatrician, and the urologist. Today the nurse is assuming an expanded role in the care of these patients by carefully collecting specimens, planting "screening" cultures, interpreting growth results, and helping supervise home-medication regimens. Furthermore, the radiologist provides important additional information in determining whether the kidneys are functioning normally and whether there is unobstructed flow of urine throughout the urinary tract. Thus, nurse, pediatrician, urologist, radiologist, and parent must communicate continually and consistently against a background of change and conflicting recommendations to ensure optimum care for the affected child.

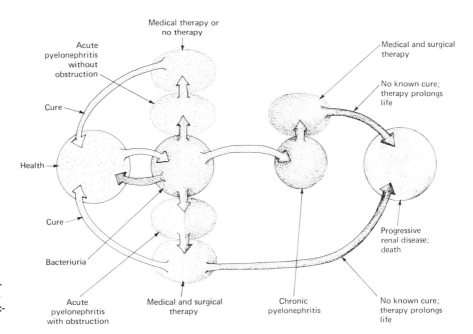

Medical therapy or no therapy

Acute pyelonephritis without obstruction

Medical and surgical therapy

No known cure; therapy prolongs life

Cure

Health

Cure

Bacteriuria

Acute pyelonephritis with obstruction

Medical and surgical therapy

Chronic pyelonephritis

No known cure; therapy prolongs life

Progressive renal disease; death

Figure 38-12   Schematic diagram demonstrating the seriousness of urinary tract infections in children.

In order to understand urinary tract infections, one must become familiar with current terminology. *Bacteriuria* means simply growth of bacteria in the urine. Since bladder urine is normally sterile, a positive urine culture implies either (1) there is active bacterial growth in the urinary tract, or (2) contamination has occurred from passage through the urethra or from the outside surroundings.

The term *significant bacteriuria* is used when the urine is shown by culture to contain more than 100,000 (10^5) bacteria per milliliter. Significant bacteriuria in a specimen collected under proper aseptic precautions is highly suggestive of infection within the urinary tract, although significant bacteriuria may be found in individuals who have no clinical symptoms or signs of urinary tract infection. This is known as *asymptomatic bacteriuria*. It reflects an abnormal state of affairs within the urinary tract, somewhat comparable to a latent infection or carrier state.[39]

Clinically, the nurse may see patients whose diagnoses utilize traditional terminology, which attempts to localize symptoms. The patient having bacteriuria with urgency, frequency, and dysuria has symptoms suggesting infection in the *lower* urinary tract, i.e., cystitis. Those patients with bacteriuria and back pain, chills, fever, and vomiting have symptoms suggesting infection of the *upper* urinary tract, i.e., acute pyelonephritis. Chronic pyelonephritis re-

fers to actual renal disease *believed* to be caused by bacterial infection in the kidney, either past or present.[40] Because of the difficulties in localizing the site of infection from clinical findings alone and because infection spreads easily within the tract, many authorities prefer to use the general term *urinary tract infection* (UTI) without further qualification.

Urinary tract infection in children is often closely associated with *vesicoureteral reflux;* this term refers to the retrograde flow of bladder urine up into the ureters, a phenomenon which can be demonstrated radiologically. The demonstration of reflux implies that the valve mechanism normally guarding the vesicoureteral (bladder-ureteral) junction is incompetent, possibly owing to the edema and inflammation caused by infection (Fig. 38-13). When reflux occurs, urine goes up the ureters during voiding and returns to the bladder when voiding has stopped. Therefore, residual urine results, and a pool for further infection exists. Reflux may be slight or gross, transient or persistent, unilateral or bilateral—depending on clinical evidence of infection and/or radiologic evidence of obstructive uropathy.

Landmark studies have been performed by Kunin,[41] who initially surveyed a large population (approximately 4,000) of apparently healthy schoolchildren between the ages of 6 and 18 years and determined the incidence of significantly positive urine cultures in specimens obtained by the clean-catch technique. Significant bacteriuria (i.e., count of 100,000 bacteria/ml of urine) was found in 1.2 percent of the girls and 0.03 percent of the boys, a preponderance in the girls of over 30:1. The prevalence of bacteriuria varied with age and race, being significantly commoner in Caucasian girls before puberty and in Negro girls after puberty. None of the girls with bacteriuria was troubled with enough symptoms that she sought medical advice, and the majority were asymptomatic. Further results suggest that girls with bacteriuria are very likely to experience recurrences of bacteriuria after a course of treatment with an appropriate antibacterial drug (75 percent relapse within 2 years).[42]

Certain anatomic and physiologic factors have been identified relating to susceptibility and/or resistance to urinary tract infection and are described below.

Protective Factors

Periodic removal of bacteria by urination   Although urine at body temperature is a good culture medium, under normal circumstances the bladder urine is repeatedly flushed away in the act of micturition. However, a film of urine always remains behind, and ample time may exist for rapid multiplication before the next voiding. While some investigators state that the beneficial effects of a high fluid intake in patients with UTI are attributable to more frequent flushing of the urinary tract, others maintain that voiding is not a very efficient mechanism for ridding the bladder of bacteria. Even in the absence of reflux, the physical characteristics of flow within the urinary tract are such that it is possible for organisms lying close to the wall of the ureter to move in a retrograde manner against the descending stream of urine.[43] Other protective factors must be highly interrelated.

Urinary acidity   Urine is normally slightly acid (pH 6), and most urinary pathogens multiply less rapidly in an acidic growth medium. (Drugs and diet may also enhance acidity.)

Mucosal defense mechanism   "It has been shown experimentally that bacteria placed in direct contact with exposed, intact bladder mucosa are lysed within a few minutes. Close contact is essential, and lysis will not take place if there is much residual urine present. The nature of the lytic substance is not known. It is nonspecific, and it is not an antibody."[44]

Circulating antibodies   Specific antibodies against infecting organisms appear in the serum of patients with pyelonephritis and in the serum of animals with experimentally induced pyelonephritis.[45]

Susceptibility Factors

Catheterization and instrumentation   Bacteria in the lower urethra are inevitably introduced into the bladder whenever an instrument or catheter is passed (risk of iatrogenic bacteriuria). "The incidence of bacteriuria approaches 100 percent if a catheter is left in place for 3 or 4 days unless special precautions are taken"[46] (i.e., strict asepsis in catheterization and maintenance of a closed drainage system).

Obstruction   Obstruction to the flow of urine at *any* level within the urinary tract (intrarenal, ureteral-pelvic junction, ureteral, vesicoureteral junction, vesicular, urethral) is the commonest factor predisposing to infection. Often such obstructive lesions can be corrected surgically. Obstruction prevents complete emptying; similarly, a pattern of incomplete emptying leading to infection results from neurologic lesions that disturb the normal pattern of bladder contraction and relaxation constituting the voiding mechanism (i.e., the "neurogenic bladder").

Short female urethra   Considerable clinical evidence suggests that the ascent of bacteria within the urethra represents the most common pathway of infection of the urinary tract. In the male, the length of the urethra and the antibacterial properties of prostatic secretion at puberty are effective barriers to invasion by this path. In female children, however, the urethra is less than 2 cm long and opens directly into a contaminated area. Tight clothing, poor hygiene, and local inflammation caused by pinworm infection, for instance, may increase the chances of ascending infection.

Collection of Clean-voided Urine Specimens   One of the nurse's most important functions in working with children suspected of having a UTI, then, is his participation, whether supervisory or directly, in the screening process, i.e., the aseptic collection of a clean-voided urine specimen. Culture of a properly collected urine specimen using quantitative colony count technique is the definitive diagnostic test for urinary tract infection. The collection of clean-catch specimens is described below.

Girls   Explain to the child that, with her help, you wish to collect some urine (using, from the nursing history data, the child's name for urine such as "peepee"). Ask the parent to accompany you to the bathroom if the child wishes. Have the child assume her normal sitting posture on the toilet (likewise on a bedpan if necessary, ensuring privacy), then ask her to spread her legs widely. Spreading the child's labia with a gloved hand, the nurse or parent then cleanses the vulva and meatus using generous amounts of benzalkonium chloride 1:750 solution on sterile cotton or gauze using single strokes from front to back. The cleansed area is then dried carefully with sterile gauze or cotton. Careful drying is important, as infecting bacteria may not grow if the urine specimen is contaminated with an antiseptic. Keeping the labia spread, the nurse or parent should encourage the child to begin to void. Only *after* the stream has started should one attempt to catch the midportion of urine in a sterile widemouthed container so that it does not touch the child's skin or clothing at all. Upon collection of the specimen, thank the child for her help and cooperation.

Boys Using similar preliminaries and normal voiding posture, the nurse or parent should cleanse the glans penis and meatus in the same fashion as described above. In uncircumcised male children the foreskin must be retracted with gloved hand and the glans gently cleansed. It may be impossible to retract the foreskin in newborn infants or in boys with phimosis, and force should not be used; the doctor should be notified. With foreskin remaining retracted, the boy should be requested to void, and the urine specimen is obtained. The child should receive praise for his cooperation. Adolescent boys should collect their own midstream specimen adequately, given a sufficient explanation.

Infants Commercially available sterile collection bags are used to collect specimens from infants of both sexes. After the preliminary cleansing and drying, the bag is applied (spreading labia in girls), and the baby is comforted and given clear fluids by bottle.

These measures often stimulate urination, and in any case, the bag is less likely to become dislodged if the baby is content and not kicking and screaming. Restraints on the legs are necessary only if the baby has to be left alone with the bag in place, for example, in a hospital room. A firmly pinned diaper helps to keep the bag in place. The baby must be watched carefully and the collection bag removed as soon as the baby voids; if no specimen has appeared after 45 minutes, the cleansing procedure must be repeated and a new bag applied.[47]

Properly collected bag specimens often yield negative culture results. However, in uncircumcised male infants, and other unusual cases of bag urine, growth in culture is often significant and of mixed

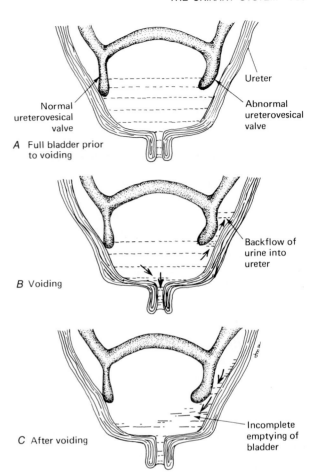

Figure 38-13 Vesicoureteral reflux. (*A*) Note the incompetent valve on the right and competent valve on the left. (*B*) During voiding, urine is refluxed into the right ureter. (*C*) After voiding, the urine returns from the right ureter to the bladder.

flora; hence, evidence of infection is *not* clear-cut and therapy open to question. In such cases where contamination is questionable, the physician or nurse clinician may prefer to do a suprapubic (percutaneous) bladder tap. (See Fig. 38-5.) A sterile needle is introduced directly into the bladder, and urine is aspirated for culture. The procedure is safe and is painless when properly done,[48] although the nurse should alert parents to the procedure and respect their decision to stay with or leave the child momentarily.

In all the above cases, specimens for culture must either be plated out within 30 minutes or they must be refrigerated, because bacterial multiplication in the urine proceeds rapidly at room temperature; the number of organisms doubles every 15 or

20 minutes. Specimens may be stored for as long as 48 hours at refrigerator temperature (8°C, 46.4°F) without significant change in the bacterial count.[49]

The bacteria commonly responsible for infection in the urinary system are *Escherichia coli,* one or more species of *Klebsiella, Enterobacter, Proteus,* and *Pseudomonas,* and various enterococci, all normal constituents of the fecal flora. These organisms are not equally significant as causes of UTI. *E. coli* is the causative organism in about 85 percent of acute infections of the bladder and kidneys in patients in whom no obstruction exists and neither antimicrobial agents nor instruments have been used. In contrast, patients who have been treated with antimicrobial drugs or who have been subjected to urologic procedures are more likely to have *Proteus, Pseudomonas,* or enterococci as the offending organisms. The percent of all UTI caused by *Staphylococcus aureus* is small.[50]

Medical and Nursing Management The clinical manifestations of urinary tract infections have already been discussed in part and vary greatly depending on the age of the child, site of infection, and severity of infection. In the newborn, symptoms of acute pyelonephritis are nonspecific and may easily be mistaken for gastroenteritis or bacterial sepsis.

Acute pyelonephritis in toddlers and older children characteristically has an acute onset with high fever, costovertebral angle (CVA) tenderness unilaterally or bilaterally, vomiting, and dysuria. Febrile convulsions are not unknown. Vomiting, anorexia, and loose stools may lead the physician to diagnose gastroenteritis. The mother, if prompted, may recall helpful observations that the child urinates excessively (polyuria), screams when he urinates (dysuria), or passes foul-smelling urine. In cases of unexplained illness of a young child, a urinalysis with microscopic examination should be routine.

In older children with recurrent UTI, symptoms generally include pallor, listlessness, and anorexia over a period of time. Exacerbations of infection may cause the child to pass cloudy, odorous urine; to complain of burning and discomfort during urination; and to relapse to nocturia or enuresis when he previously remained dry. It is important to check the blood pressure since hypertension may develop early in children with infected, dysplastic kidneys.

The child with cystitis more often will complain of severe lower abdominal pain, burning on urination, and urgency or enuresis but will lack signs of systemic disturbance such as fever and vomiting. Frank hematuria may occur.

The medical aims of treatment of children with UTI are to clear up the primary infection, to correct surgically any congenital or acquired obstruction in the urinary tract, and to reduce by long-term follow-up the number of clinical or bacteriologic exacerbations. Nursing care encompasses and furthers these goals as well as provides supportive, symptomatic care for the child and parents.

Since antibacterial drug therapy is the mainstay of treatment, the nurse should become familiar with those bactericidal or bacteriostatic agents most used, the dosages, their common side effects and adverse reactions. Among the more frequently used drugs are sulfisoxazole (Gantrisin), nitrofurantoin (Furadantin), streptomycin, kanamycin, and colistin. (J. A. James' *Renal Disease in Childhood* has in Table 6-2 a good summary of antibacterial drugs used in urinary tract infections.) Antibiotic treatment should be guided by the results of urine cultures and sensitivities whenever possible, as well as by the clinical response to treatment. The nurse will assist in obtaining initial and follow-up urine specimens for culture and will relay pertinent information as to the child's response to the drug therapy. Initial symptoms will generally disappear within 48 to 72 hours of the start of antibacterial treatment. A repeat urine culture will be negative at this time if an effective antibacterial agent has been selected.

The hospitalized child may require intravenous fluid therapy until the infection and fever are brought under control. If "forcing fluids" is prescribed, not only to prevent dehydration but also to ensure frequent flushing of the bladder, an oral fluid plan specified in cubic centimeters per 8-hour period may be worked out with the child's cooperation and posted at the bedside. Allotments for waking hours take precedence, and equivalent measures for the child should be shown (for example, 1 large drinking glass = 240 cc).

Once a child's symptoms and bacteriuria are controlled, decisions must be made concerning the duration of treatment, which varies from 2 to 6 weeks or more, the duration of follow-up cultures, and the desirability of further diagnostic studies.

The nurse involved with a pediatric renal service is in an excellent position to do valuable nursing research in areas not yet explored, perhaps by devising an "epidemiologic" approach to data gathering by means of a clinic worksheet (Fig. 38-14). This author, with the encouragement of Dr. George Richard at the J. H. Miller Health Center, Gainesville, Fla., undertook a pilot study to investigate the effect, if any, of tub bathing versus shower or sponge bathing on the subsequent appearance of bacteriuria in female volunteer subjects. While the unpublished results are available, the small sample size ($N = 25$) prohibits any conclusions. If urinary tract infections and their sequelae constitute a large and perplexing problem in preventive medicine, then it seems that the nurse involved in renal pediatrics should have a fertile field for investigation in the hope of adding new nursing knowledge in this area.

RENAL PROBLEMS IN THE PRESCHOOL AND SCHOOL-AGE CHILD
Glomerulonephritis

Acute glomerulonephritis or poststreptococcal glomerulonephritis is predominantly a disease of childhood and is the most common form of glomerulone-

Figure 38-14 NURSING WORKSHEET USED TO COLLECT PATIENT DATA IN A PEDIATRIC RENAL/GU CLINIC*

Date: _____ Return app't.: _____

Nursing interview #: _____ Age: _____

My child's diagnosis is: _____

To me, this means: _____

In my understanding, the purpose for the present clinic visit is: _____

My child is also having a problem in addition to or as a result of the above medical problem, in the area of (check one or more of the following if applicable):

1 Eating
  a eats too little _____
  b eats too much _____
  c nausea, vomiting _____
  d salt restricted _____
  e hard to swallow or chew _____
  f change in eating habits _____
2 Fluid intake
  a drinks too much _____
  b drinks too little _____
3 Sleeping
  a trouble falling asleep _____
  b waking up at night _____
  c dreams, nightmares _____
  d needs extra naps _____
4 Toileting
  a urinating
    (1) wets bed at night _____
    (2) no bladder control _____
    (3) burning _____
    (4) urinates very often _____
    (5) urinates only in "dribbles," small amount _____
    (6) blood in urine _____
    (7) protein in urine _____
  b bowel movement
    (1) constipation _____
    (2) diarrhea _____
    (3) no bowel control _____
    (4) pain _____
5 Medications
  a steroid (i.e., prednisone) _____
  b antibiotic _____
  c blood pressure medicine _____
  d acid-base solution _____
  e other _____
6 Breathing
  a gets short of breath _____
  b sore throats _____

7 Skin
  a sores on arms or legs _____
  b swelling around eyes or of fingers, ankles _____
  c color _____
8 Senses
  a seeing _____
  b hearing _____
  c speaking _____
  d headaches _____
9 Motor activity
  a problem with crawling or walking _____
  b restricted at home _____
  c restricted from physical education at school _____
10 School
  a having learning problems _____
  b staying out of school _____
11 Home
  a gets special attention _____
  b problem getting along with brothers/sisters _____
  c problem getting along with playmates _____
  d overdependent, clings to parents _____
  e problem adjusting to new situations _____
12 Self
  a too small for age _____
  b too large for age _____
  c disturbed about appearance (overweight, "puffy" cheeks, etc.) _____
  d disturbed about way he/she urinates—"Not like other kids" _____
  e disturbed about odor, leaking, or dribbling urine _____
13 Other (parents)
  financial _____
  insurance _____

If any of above areas is checked, please describe the problem(s) more fully here:

Nursing approach:

Other questions I would like to discuss with the doctors:

* Scoring guide:
+1: Seen only as a slight problem which minimally interferes with child's activities of daily living and the total family pattern.
+2: Problem definitely exists: some disruption of child's activities of daily living and total family pattern.
+3: Severe problem hindering child and rest of family.
+4: Urgent problem for which professional help is actively being sought.
Source: From Deborah Dean, Vanderbilt University, Nashville, Tenn.

phritis in children. Almost all cases of acute glomerulonephritis are related to a previous infection with "nephritogenic strains" of group A beta-hemolytic streptococci. Following the initial streptococcal infection, there is a latent period of 7 to 14 days before the appearance of symptoms. During this period the child feels well, and the urine is normal. It is generally believed that the renal injury results from an antigen-antibody reaction which is stimulated by the initial streptococcal infection.

Acute glomerulonephritis occurs most frequently in children from 2 to 6 years of age, with the peak age being 5 years. Boys are affected more often than girls in a ratio of 3:2. The risk of developing nephritis after a streptococcal infection is probably 1:100. The risk also varies with the prevalence of nephritogenic strains of streptococci within any community and the likelihood of cross infection. Therefore, the disease is more frequently seen in children from low-income families where housing and nutrition are substandard. The initial streptococcal infection most commonly associated with acute glomerulonephritis in the northern part of the United States is the sore throat which is more prevalent during the winter and spring. In the Southern states impetigo and infected insect bites are a leading cause.[51]

Community, clinic, and school nurses are in an excellent position to detect possible carriers of beta-hemolytic streptococci. In suspected cases, throat and suspicious skin lesions should be cultured, and carriers of beta-hemolytic streptococci should be referred to a physician for treatment with penicillin.

Acute Phase During the acute phase of glomerulonephritis, the kidneys are moderately enlarged, the glomerular tufts fill Bowman's space, and the capillary loops are obliterated by edema and proliferation of the lining endothelial cells. This cellular swelling and proliferation obstructs the glomerular capillaries, reducing the glomerular filtrate and the amount of sodium and water that is passed to the tubules for reabsorption. As a result, the cardinal clinical features of acute glomerulonephritis are edema, hypertension, and circulatory congestion.

The presenting symptoms during the acute or edematous phase are usually periorbital edema (Fig. 38-15) in the morning and a decreased amount of cloudy, brown urine. The brown color indicates that blood is mixing with urine in the bladder. The edema usually spreads to the feet but rarely progresses beyond a moderate degree. The child appears lethargic and pale and has a poor appetite. The pulse rate is decreased, and the blood pressure is increased, the range being 120 to 180/80 to 120.[52]

Microscopic examination of the urine reveals numerous red blood cells, leukocytes, epithelial cells, and casts. The urine gives a positive chemical reaction for free blood pigments. In 50 percent of the children with acute glomerulonephritis, there is a moderate elevation in BUN and creatinine levels. The BUN elevation rarely exceeds 100 mg/100 ml. Urine protein usually shows a 3+ to 4+ reaction, but rarely is more than 3 Gm excreted daily.[53]

During the acute phase the child may have a reduction in hemoglobin and hematocrit. Such a change is classified as *transient anemia* and requires no treatment. The chest x-ray during the edematous phase is characteristic and may furnish a diagnosis. The film reveals cardiac enlargement and pulmonary vascular congestion. The acute phase of glomerulonephritis usually lasts 7 days but may persist for 3 weeks. Increased urinary output and a subtle decrease in body weight alert the nurse to the first signs of improvement. Within several days urine volume increases greatly and may be as much as 3 liters/24 hours. As diuresis progresses, the blood pressure begins to drop, and the child's appetite and sense of well-being return to normal (Fig. 38-16). However, proteinuria of 1+ to 2+ may persist for a few weeks, and microscopic hematuria for as long as a year.[54]

During the acute phase of glomerulonephritis the major complications are hypertensive encephalopathy, cardiac failure, and, very rarely, acute renal failure. Even though these complications infrequently occur, the nurse needs to be alert to their presenting signs and symptoms.

Medical and Nursing Management The treatment for acute glomerulonephritis is nonspecific; unless the patient has severe edema, hypertension, or oliguria (less than 400 ml/24 hours), he can be treated at home.[55] Recovery is spontaneous in almost all cases, if in the acute phase there is intelligent use of dietary and fluid restrictions and drug therapy.

The amount of activity allowed is directly proportional to the severity of clinical manifestations. If the patient is not hypertensive, he may have bathroom privileges and be up for meals. However, the patient with hypertension and circulatory congestion needs strict bed rest to decrease the risk of cardiac failure. Bed rest also increases glomerular filtration and prevents great fluctuations in blood pressure. Most children with acute glomerulonephritis limit their own activity and seldom rebel against the period of confinement.

Circulatory congestion, hypertension, and edema result from the salt and water retention; therefore, the patient's salt and fluid intake need to be closely monitored by the nurse and dietician so that they remain within the functional capacity of the diseased kidneys.

During the edematous phase *all* patients with acute glomerulonephritis should be weighed daily. Weight change is the best index of overall fluid balance. A meticulous record of amount of urinary output and description of color should be kept by the nurse as a means of monitoring the degree of oliguria and hematuria. A 24-hour intake and output sheet at the patient's bedside will ensure the most accurate charting.

Dietary restrictions also depend upon the severity of the presenting clinical manifestations. In all patients with hypertension or edema the intake of sodium is restricted (300 mg), and for those with mild hypertension a diet of no added salt is allowed. When a sodium-restricted diet is necessary, the nurse can make the diet more palatable and successful by obtaining a diet history from the patient and/or family. Until the patient is voiding at least 200 ml of urine/24 hours, he should be on a limited potassium intake. If the BUN is elevated above 100 mg/100 ml, a low-protein diet is advisable.[56] All dietary restrictions can be lifted once diuresis has occurred.

Medical treatment of patients with acute glomerulonephritis will usually include an adequate course of penicillin unless the patient has already been treated prior to admission. During the convalescent period, penicillin therapy is usually not recommended. However, if a child is returning to an environment where there is a high risk of cross infection, he may be placed on prophylactic penicillin for a month or two.

Treatment of Complications   If there are no signs of encephalopathy, antihypertensive therapy is withheld. If the diastolic blood pressure rises above 100 mm Hg or if symptoms of encephalopathy appear, antihypertensive treatment should be instituted. The form of therapy most generally used is a combination of parenteral reserpine and intramuscular hydralazine. The effect of the treatment occurs within an hour and is effective for 6 to 8 hours. Anticonvulsant and antihypertensive therapy are given if the patient convulses. If signs of cardiac failure occur, the child is usually digitalized (see Chap. 34) and placed on a no-salt diet; antihypertensive therapy is initiated. Acute renal failure occurs rarely, but if the daily output of urine remains below 200 ml, the child is placed on a treatment regimen for severe oliguria.[57]

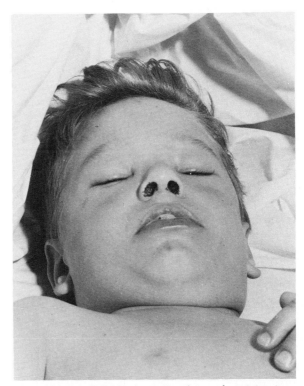

Figure 38-15   Child in the acute phase of poststreptococcal glomerulonephritis. Note the periorbital edema. *(Courtesy of S. Hellerstein, M.D., Children's Mercy Hospital, Kansas City, Mo.)*

Convalescent Period   The convalescent period begins at the completion of diuresis and the resolution of hypertension. During this phase the child feels well and wants to be active. It is practically impossible to enforce bed rest and medically unnecessary. Three or four days before discharge the child should be observed closely for gross hematuria and weight gain. The child will be dismissed on indoor activities and will be able to return to school in 2 weeks if there is no recurrence of hematuria or hypertension. Since microscopic hematuria may persist for a year or more, it is generally recommended that the child refrain from competitive sports and strenuous activities until the urine is completely free of red blood cells.

Prognosis   Poststreptococcal acute glomerulonephritis in young children is generally a benign disease, and the prognosis is usually considered to be good. Death during the acute phase is very uncommon, and some authorities have reported 100 percent recovery from the disease. However, the older age groups do not share this excellent prognosis as

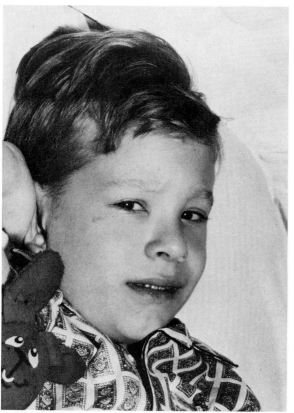

Figure 38-16 The same child shown in Fig. 38-15 after several days of diuresis. Note the decrease in periorbital edema. *(Courtesy of S. Hellerstein, M.D., Children's Mercy Hospital, Kansas City, Mo.)*

a significant percentage develop chronic renal disease.

RENAL PROBLEMS IN THE ADOLESCENT
Chronic Glomerulonephritis

Chronic glomerulonephritis, used here exclusively in its clinical rather than its histologic context, describes any idiopathic, progressive form of renal disease whose clinical picture of proteinuria, hematuria, and hypertension indicates major involvement of the glomeruli. Excluded from the chronic nephritis group are patients with clinically identical renal disease caused by familial glomerulonephritis, lupus erythematosus, Henock-Schönlein purpura, and focal glomerulonephritis. Each of these diseases has specific clinical, laboratory, or histologic findings that define it as a separate disease entity.

While controversy and research continue con-

cerning the pathogenesis of chronic nephritis, two hypotheses are prevalent: (1) It always represents a complication of previous acute nephritis, and (2) it is a separate disease, unrelated to acute nephritis.

Adolescents presenting with chronic nephritis show varied symptoms. On the one hand, the child may feel entirely well, and proteinuria is discovered on a routine physical; on the other hand, a child may first manifest unexplained gross hematuria, with hypertension and edema, or with unexplained renal failure. The natural progression of the disease is also highly individual, varying from latent to subacute to rapidly progressive or malignant processes.

No laboratory findings are specifically diagnostic of chronic nephritis. Serologically, the ASO titer is generally low or normal; in addition, cultures of the throat do not show any beta-hemolytic streptococci. Urinalysis usually reveals moderate to heavy proteinuria (2+ to 3+), intermittent gross hematuria, abnormal sediment (red cells, white cells, and cellular casts), and, as the disease progresses, a fixed specific gravity (sp. g.) of only 1.010 to 1.014. The normal kidney will concentrate to 1.024 sp. g. or higher after a period of fluid deprivation. Abnormalities in blood chemistry will be reflected in BUN, serum creatinine, and electrolyte imbalances, if at all.

Although clinical diagnosis of chronic glomerulonephritis is made from the history, physical examination, and laboratory findings, a renal biopsy is essential in order to determine the histologic type of the disease and its possible termination by drug treatment. Diagnostic biopsy would be considered in all children with nephritis that begins acutely and persists for 2 to 3 weeks without improvement, despite therapy; likewise, biopsy is indicated before any patient diagnosed as having chronic nephritis is started on treatment with cytotoxic drugs.

Of all renal pediatric patients, adolescents seem to benefit most from a factual discussion of what a biopsy entails (often with visual aids such as slides and diagrams); they gain support and control from the nurse who attempts to make the "unknown known." Of course, the amount and detail of explanation varies with the child's expressed needs.

In addition to assisting with the diagnostic aspects such as specimen collections, the nurse plans the care of a patient with chronic glomerulonephritis to revolve around his daily activities and needs. Normal activity and school attendance is advocated versus bed rest, except during flare-ups with edema and hypertension. The clinic nurse may need to help the adolescent boy or girl find viable substitutes for strenuous competitive and/or contact sports (such as managing a team or playing in a band).

The need for hospital admission in chronic glomerulonephritis is similar to that of acute glomerulonephritis and nephrotic syndrome, i.e., when the patient has severe edema, acute or uncontrolled hypertension, oliguria, severe electrolyte imbalance, and severe intercurrent infection. Usually no dietary restrictions are imposed unless the patient is edematous, hypertensive, or azotemic. For edema and hypertension, a no-added-salt diet (1 to 2 Gm of sodium/day) is prescribed; if the BUN exceeds 50 to 60 mg/100 ml (normal 8 to 15 mg/100 ml), a protein-restricted diet similar to that used for chronic renal failure (0.5 Gm protein/kg body weight with protein-containing essential amino acids) may be indicated. Supplemental vitamins and minerals may be ordered.

Intercurrent infection often causes exacerbations of edema, hematuria, and electrolyte imbalance in adolescents with chronic nephritis. Vigorous antibiotic therapy may be instituted. The nurse will want to reassure the adolescent that the transient edema altering his or her appearance is often a function of intercurrent infection and/or hypertension and may subside with appropriate drug treatment. Thiazide diuretics along with reserpine and hydralazine are generally the drugs of choice.

Despite disappointing clinical results, corticosteroids in combination with cytotoxic drugs are used in the medical treatment of chronic nephritis. The value of steroids is not known clearly, but they may reduce the incidence of bone marrow depression and produce undesirable side effects. Use of immunosuppressive therapy in chronic renal disease has been a direct outgrowth of work in renal homotransplantation. The previously prevailing rationale was that if rejection of homografts could be delayed or prevented by these drugs, perhaps the precipitous downhill course of certain kinds of chronic nephritis could be altered. However, actual clinical trials show that the failure of immunosuppressive therapy to alter the course of a supposedly immunologically determined disease is in contrast to its success in suppressing transplant rejection and frequent relapses in the minimal change disease type of the nephrotic syndrome. The implications are either that the immune reaction in glomerulonephritis is of a type that cannot readily be suppressed or, more probably, that nonimmunologic factors are responsible for the progression of the disease, if not its cause.[58] The principal drugs in use are 6-mercaptopurine, azathioprine, and cyclophosphamide; the latter two can be given by mouth. While the mode of action of these drugs is unknown, they exert antiproliferative and anti-inflammatory effects and effect immunosuppression.

If immunosuppressive drug therapy is initiated, preliminary bone marrow examination and weekly or biweekly complete blood counts should be obtained and noted by the nurse as well as by the physician; for example, a neutrophil count of 1,000 cells/cu mm would be an indication for stopping treatment temporarily. The nurse should alert both adolescent and parents to the potential threat of a mild infection which could fulminate under the umbrella of depressed immune defenses. Ulceration of oral mucosa, alopecia, and hemorrhagic cystitis are specific complications of cyclophosphamide treatment. The alopecia may become total and terribly embarrassing to the adolescent; the nurse may suggest the interim use of wigs or turbans, while reaffirming that the hair grows in again when the drug is stopped. Serious side effects of these drugs are largely dose related.

The psychologic aspects of management in such a chronic disease with an uncertain prognosis are extremely important. Any existing weaknesses or strains in the parent-child relation will no doubt surface. While parents may exhibit guilt, denial, and overindulgence, the adolescent may react with aggression and/or withdrawal. Depression over the illness and the possibility of death may be dealt with overtly or covertly by the adolescent and his parents; confrontation with these issues may be wished for and feared at the same time. Perhaps by merely giving verbal recognition to the existing state of tense ambivalence, the nurse can initiate open communication between parents and child and between medical personnel and child—thereby enabling all concerned to cope more effectively with the energy and resources available.

Although the prognosis for children with chronic nephritis is serious, progression of the disease is extremely variable. Some children remain clinically well for years, with minimal signs of deterioration in kidney function. Moreover, advances in hemodialysis and transplantation make it possible to manage much more effectively the patient whose disease has progressed to the point of chronic renal insufficiency. Newer drug therapy may also serve to curb the downhill course in its early stages. Hope grows with each year's research and progress in the field of chronic renal disease.

Other Forms of Renal Disease in Adolescence

Alport's Syndrome The renal manifestations of *familial glomerulonephritis* are identical to those of idiopathic chronic glomerulonephritis, but the disease follows a *familial pattern,* and progressive *nerve deafness* is a frequently associated finding. Both sexes can be affected, but the severity of renal involvement and deafness is much greater in males. The progression of familial nephritis is not altered by corticosteroid or cytotoxic drug therapy. Hence, symptomatic and supportive treatment for chronic nephritis is all that can be offered at this time. The adolescent's normal patterns and activities should be as unrestricted as possible; hearing assessments and appropriate management for hearing loss should be included in the care plan. Family members should be counseled by a geneticist, if possible, concerning the genetic implications of the disease, since the pattern of inheritance is not always predictable.

Medullary Cystic Disease   *Juvenile nephronophthisis* is another progressive familial disease of the kidneys that causes death in late childhood or adolescence. Outstanding features of the disease are (1) familial incidence (two or more siblings may be affected); (2) insidious onset of chronic renal insufficiency; (3) polyuria with low, fixed specific gravity; (4) absence of proteinuria and hypertension until the late stages of the disease; azotemia before development of proteinuria, a most unusual sequence; and (5) anemia and, in some cases, persistent hypokalemia.[59] While the cause of juvenile nephronophthisis is unknown, the pattern of inheritance is consistent with an autosomal-recessive trait. No specific treatment is known that will alter the natural course of the disease, and so management is the same as that for chronic nephritis and renal insufficiency. Hypokalemia may be corrected by supplemental potassium salts, 3 to 4 mEq/kg body weight per day.

Systemic Lupus Erythematosus   One other condition, not familial, which has renal complications in adolescence as part of the overall systemic disease process is *lupus erythematosus*. Of unknown etiology, systemic lupus erythematosus (SLE) is characterized by the development of numerous autoantibodies directed toward components of the patient's tissues, and reactions involving these antibodies are responsible for most of the clinical and laboratory findings.

> The manifestations of lupus in children cover an extremely wide range of organ systems. The commoner symptoms and signs include skin rashes (particularly a malar rash of the classic "butterfly" type), joint pains and arthritis, fever, hepatosplenomegaly and generalized adenopathy, inflammation of the serous membranes with effusions, anemia and thrombocytopenia, hyperglobulinemia, and signs of renal involvement. The disease is very much commoner in girls than in boys, and it is rarely seen in children under the age of 6 or 7 years. At least 75 percent of children with lupus erythematosus have some degree of renal involvement.[60]

Upon biopsy, foci of necrosis and hypercellularity are found within the glomeruli. The systemic symptoms of lupus (skin rash, joint pains, and fever) can be greatly suppressed by high dose corticosteroid therapy, but the effectiveness of steroids in controlling the progression of the renal lesions is less pronounced. Currently, azathioprine is the alternate drug of choice, often in conjunction with prolonged low-dose steroids. Diuretics and antihypertensives may be added to the regimen in light of edema and high blood pressure. Because patients with lupus appear to be unusually susceptible to infections, prolonged treatment with steroids and azathioprine which suppress the body's resistance to systemic infection, is not without hazard. Lupus erythematosus in the child carries a more serious prognosis than in the adult, largely because of the elements of renal failure and infection. Each child's progression is variable, and experience with cytotoxic drugs in lupus is still too limited to allow assessment of prolonging survival time.

MEDICAL TREATMENT

While the child with progressive, chronic renal failure, whatever the cause, has more in his favor today than at any time in history, he still may reach a point in the course of his disease when conservative management fails and more aggressive treatment is indicated. Such treatment may be medical or surgical.

Peritoneal Dialysis

Dialysis can be an effective procedure for correcting body fluid homeostasis and preserving life in the child whose renal function is so severely limited that he would otherwise die. For the child in acute renal failure due to sudden illness or trauma, poisoning, drug intoxication, or other cause, dialysis may be the supportive, interim treatment of choice, used to tide him over the period of oliguria; for the uremic child in chronic renal failure, however, dialysis may represent a more permanent commitment to the full gamut of treatment available—long-term hemodialysis and preparation for homotransplantation.

Long-term dialysis is recommended (1) when glomerular filtration is less than 1 or 2 ml per minute and the patient cannot survive on an 18-20 Gm protein diet without [uremic] symptoms; (2) when there are persistent symptoms from uremia; a BUN exceeding 150 mg per 100 ml, creatinine over 15 mg per 100 ml, potassium above 6 mEq per liter, and plasma bicarbonate less than 16 mEq per liter, despite good dietary control; in the presence of persistent edema, hyponatremia, hypertension, and congestive cardiac failure; and when there is peripheral neuropathy or multiple and frequent complications.[61]

Of the two types of dialysis, peritoneal dialysis has become a relatively safe and readily available procedure—often done repeatedly to keep the child either (1) comfortable for as long as possible or (2) in a holding pattern, prior to acceptance in a long-term hemodialysis and homotransplantation program. While the financial, moral, logistic, and technical problems of the latter will be discussed more fully in following sections, the technique of peritoneal dialysis, generally the method of choice in children at present, is presented here.

Dialysis is based on the physical principle that small molecules (crystalloids) in a volume of fluid will diffuse through a semipermeable membrane from an area of greater concentration to an area of lesser concentration of that solute. Undesirable solutes, such as urea and potassium, are removed through this process.

When the flow of dialyzing fluid is increased from 1 to 3.5 liters/hour, urea clearance increases from 12 to 30 ml/minute. Further increments in clearance may be obtained with higher flow rates, but such rates are uncomfortable to the pediatric patient and hard to achieve clinically. Heating dialysis fluid from 20° to 37°C (from 68° to 98.6°F) causes dilatation of peritoneal vessels and increases urea clearance by 35 percent. It also prevents body chilling and additional discomfort in the patient. Hypertonic solutions (4.5 or 7 percent glucose) increase urea transport and may be used to remove fluid in overhydrated or edematous patients. The standard dialysis solution, however, contains 1.5 Gm glucose/100 ml and has osmotic concentration only somewhat significantly higher than the plasma (370 mOsm/kg versus 290 mOsm/kg)—a differential which prevents absorption of unduly large amounts of fluid from the peritoneal cavity. When the preceding *hypertonic* solutions are used, a careful record must be kept of the patient's weight and of the amount of fluid ex-

changed to prevent hypovolemia; the volume of fluid returned at the end of each exchange will exceed the volume infused by 100 to 200 ml. Permeability of the peritoneum is increased by heat, hypertonic solutions, infection, and experimental surface-active agents.

Dialysis Procedure Adolescents often benefit from talking directly or by telephone with peers who have undergone peritoneal dialysis; they seem to rely heavily on having a radio and magazines at the bedside to get them through the procedure. Younger children often cling to favorite stuffed toys or a blanket and depend on parents' presence at the bedside.

Premedication [chlorpromazine (Thorazine) or meperidine (Demerol)] may be ordered at the discretion of the physician, depending on the age and status of the child. The nurse should encourage the child to void or assist in catheterization of the urinary bladder under aseptic conditions if the child cannot void spontaneously. (The latter is a precaution to avoid accidental bladder perforation.) The anterior abdomen is then scrubbed a few centimeters below the umbilicus in the midline and prepared as for a surgical procedure. Strict asepsis *must* be maintained, since peritonitis is the most serious and most common complication. The mother may want to hold both the child's hands during the initial steps of the procedure. The first bottle of warmed dialysis fluid with administration set attached is hung at the bedside, ready for use.

Unless the child presents with ascites, the peritoneal cavity is routinely filled with dialysis fluid before an attempt is made to insert the peritoneal catheter. The risk of perforating the bowel or deeper structures is reduced, and the return of free fluid when the catheter is inserted attests to its proper placement in the peritoneal cavity. This preliminary filling is accomplished through an 18-gauge needle inserted near the midline at the site chosen for subsequent insertion of the catheter. (The site will have been injected with Novocain by this time.) Generally, about two-thirds of the estimated exchange volume, about 600 cc, will be allowed to run in through the needle, leaving the remainder to run in through the catheter after its insertion.

Commercially available stylet-catheters are gauged for appropriate size, hence making a smaller hole in the peritoneum and resulting in less fluid leakage. Under strict asepsis, the stylet-catheter is pushed by the physician through a small (1 cm) horizontal skin incision into the peritoneal cavity, using firm but controlled pressure until there is a distinct feeling of "give," when the peritoneum is entered. The stylet is then removed, and fluid will escape from the end of the catheter. The total perforated length of the catheter must lie in the peritoneal cavity. The infusion set is then connected to the catheter, and the remaining fluid allowed to run into the peritoneal cavity. Sometimes a skin suture wrapped tightly around the catheter is needed to prevent its slipping. Antibiotic ointment and small dressings are placed over the wound, and the whole is firmly taped in place.

From this point, the nurse's chief responsibility lies in monitoring infusions and exchanges, charting accurately, and assessing the child's comfort. While the volume of fluid infused during each exchange should distend the abdominal cavity, it should not cause pain. (The average volume tolerated is about 60 to 80 ml/kg body weight.)[62] The dialysate is run in over a 15-minute period, allowed to equilibrate for 45 to 60 minutes, and then drained in 10 to 15 minutes. Based on falling levels of urea and creatinine and restoration of normal serum concentrations of sodium, potassium, chloride, and bicarbonate, dialysis will continue from 24 to 72 hours.

Technically, the nurse is responsible for several aspects of the ongoing dialysis procedure. Figure 38-17 shows a typical peritoneal dialysis flowsheet, which should be examined during the following discussion.

The standard dialysis solution has an electrolyte composition similar to extracellular fluid but contains no potassium or urea. The child should be weighed carefully before, during, and after dialysis at specified intervals, using the same bedside scale and same conditions (amount of clothing, blankets, independent weight of catheter estimated, etc.). Body weight acts as a check on the record of volume infused, volume recovered, and cumulative fluid balance kept at the bedside.

Vital signs noted frequently (every 1 to 4 hours) correlate with the state of circulation and fluid depletion or overload, electrolyte imbalance, etc. Example: Tachycardia and hypotension might indicate acute volume depletion. Bleeding would also have to be ruled out, should those symptoms develop. A rise in body temperature may herald the onset of peritonitis. As a precaution, the nurse may be ordered to change the fluid administration set for a new one after each four to six exchanges, since the inside of the tubing may become contaminated during the bottle changes and other manipulations. More adequate filter systems to remove bacteria are being devised, however.

Routinely, 1,000 units of heparin are added to each of the first three bottles of dialysate. The amount of anticoagulant is not sufficient to interfere with systemic blood clotting but does help to prevent small clots from plugging the drainage holes in the tip of the catheter. The overall infusion procedure is

Figure 38-17 TYPICAL PERITONEAL DIALYSIS FLOWSHEET

PERITONEAL DIALYSIS FLOWSHEET

Patient:
Hospital #:

Age:
Beginning weight: 12.5 kg
Height:

Date:

Surface area: sq m

Time	Bottle	Volume, ml In	Volume, ml Out	Cumulative fluid balance*	Medications added	Vital signs, weight, remarks
11:00 A.M.	1	1,000			1,000 U heparin	P: 120; BP: 140/100 Blood-tinged fluid returned
12:15 P.M.	1		900	−100		
12:30 P.M.	2	1,000			1,000 U heparin	
1:40 P.M.	2		950	−50		P: 140; BP: 134/88 Weight: 12.6 kg
2:00 P.M.	3	1,000			1,000 U heparin	
3:20 P.M.	3		1,100	+100		P: 160; BP: 150/100 Dr. King notified

* Minus sign (−) means more fluid in than out (patient retaining excess).
 Plus sign (+) means more fluid out than in (patient losing fluid).
Source: From Deborah Dean, Vanderbilt University, Nashville, Tenn.

less uncomfortable to the patient and more efficient if the fluid is brought to body temperature in a basin of warm water.

Initially, the dialysis fluid may contain no potassium, especially if the patient's serum potassium is over 7 mEq/liter. "Since the correction of acidosis by dialysis promotes the net movement of extracellular potassium ions into the cells, the serum potassium concentration may fall rapidly during the dialysis procedure. If it falls below 3.5 mEq/liter, 4 mEq of potassium chloride solution should be added to each liter of fluid infused, or the modified dialysis solution containing 4 mEq/liter of potassium should be substituted."[63] The nurse should be alert to complaints of muscular weakness, cramping, and dizziness in the patient.

Because of the possibility of nausea and vomiting, it is wise to limit oral intake to ice chips and a very little fluid during the first 24 hours of dialysis. Later, sour ball candy may help satiate the child. Mouth care and lemon swabs to keep lips moist will make the child feel better.

Complications of peritoneal dialysis include bleeding and leakage, inadequate fluid return, puncture of the bowel or bladder, and infection (peritonitis.)

Hemodialysis (Extracorporeal)

The technique of peritoneal dialysis, which is well established as the dialytic method of choice in children at present, has been discussed in great detail. However, much of the technical information currently published regarding artificial-kidney dialysis (extracorporeal hemodialysis) will no doubt be outdated a year from now. Thus, a more basic discussion of principles and problems involved in chronic dialysis seems in order. (Because long-term hemodialysis and homotransplantation in children must be considered in a complementary rather than competitive relation, see the section on surgical treatment below for a more thorough discussion of the implications of both.)

In extracorporeal hemodialysis, the dialysis procedure is conducted outside the patient's body by means of an artificial kidney (Fig. 38-18). The patient's arterial blood is pumped through a dialysis apparatus at the bedside, and exchange of solutes between the plasma and the bath fluid takes place across a dialyzing membrane according to the same principles previously described. The "cleansed" venous blood is then returned to the patient. Artificial-kidney dialysis has been shown to be about four times as efficient as peritoneal dialysis in remov-

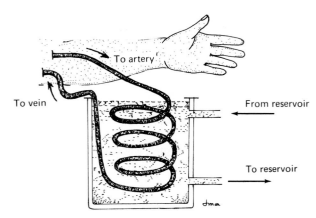

Figure 38-18   Artificial-kidney dialysis. The child's blood is circulated through a cellophane coil suspended in a bath of appropriate composition. *(From J. A. James, Renal Disease in Childhood, 2d ed., The C. V. Mosby Company, St. Louis, 1972, p. 333.)*

ing dialyzable poisons and drugs from the body fluids; that is, 6 hours of artificial kidney dialysis is equivalent to 24 hours of peritoneal dialysis. However, prerequisites of a relatively large volume of blood and arterial size large enough to provide the rate of flow necessary for efficient dialysis are limiting factors in the small child. Smaller, more efficient dialyzers having less internal resistance and requiring less blood for priming are being developed, but they are still limited in application.

The important technical advance that has made chronic dialysis possible for both adults and children is the Scribner shunt, "an external loop made of Silastic, connecting cannulae placed in a major artery and vein in the forearm or leg. This creates a permanent arteriovenous shunt, and once established, it is a relatively simple matter to disconnect the loop and attach the cannulae to the arterial and venous sides of an artificial kidney as often as needed."[64] Also, a subcutaneous arteriovenous shunt can be created surgically. At a minimum, twice-weekly dialysis periods of 6 to 8 hours are required.

The problems of maintaining functioning shunts are much greater in children. In a study of 22 children maintained on chronic dialysis, the most common severe complication was infection and clotting of the arteriovenous shunt. Femoral shunts were placed in 10 of the children, and one resulted in ischemic damage to the leg with partial loss of motor function.[65] Hypertension, anemia, convulsions, rickets and osteitis fibrosa (effecting growth failure), and delayed or absent sexual maturation were other clinical findings seen recurrently.

Serious questions center around the problems of case selection, expense, and resources in chronic dialysis programs even for adults; for children, the questions of benefit versus detriment are paramount.

SURGICAL TREATMENT

Surgical interventions in children are necessary to (1) relieve cases of severe obstructive or nonobstructive uropathy so that ensuing renal damage from reflux, inadequate urinary drainage, and infection may be prevented; (2) bypass nonfunctional areas in the urinary tract (i.e., diversion of urinary stream into a loop of ileum necessitated by neurogenic bladder); (3) remove diseased or totally nonfunctioning kidneys (unilateral or bilateral nephrectomy); and (4) transplant functional kidneys from donor to recipient.

Ureteral Reimplantation

An example of the first type of surgical intervention is reimplantation of the ureters. Normally the ureters pass obliquely through the muscle of the bladder wall so that a flap valve is formed to prevent any backflow of urine into the ureters when the bladder contracts and empties. Reflux of urine into the ureters and renal pelvis on one or both sides during voiding indicates that the ureterovesical valve mechanism is incompetent. Armed with such diagnostic findings from cystogram and cystoscopy, the pediatric urologist may intervene surgically to reimplant the ureter(s) more obliquely into the bladder and to lengthen the submucosal tunnel so as to enhance the anatomic arrangement of distal ureteral and trigonal smooth muscle fibers.[66] The urologist would, of course, defer surgery until the urinary tract has been adequately drained by means of indwelling catheter, suprapubic cystotomy, or nephrostomy tubes, and cleared of infection; if possible, by the use of appropriate antibiotics, and until kidney function has improved to the extent possible.

The child who has had a ureteral reimplantation should be treated pre- and postoperatively as any child who undergoes a major surgical procedure. Of special import after the operation are the bilateral ureteral splints (small polyethylene tubes) from each ureter and the suprapubic tube from the bladder. Each tube is attached to a separate closed drainage system which must be kept sterile and free of obstruction, kinks, or compression; the purpose of these tubes is to facilitate drainage and promote healing by support and decompression. The nurse will want to note the character (bloody, clear) and amount or absence of urine from the separate ureteral and bladder tubes every 1 to 2 hours, depending on the policy of the hospital. Ambulation is a challenge for both nurse and child, but can and should be accomplished with proper care and assistance. Unfortunately, not all problems of infection and inadequate drainage can be completely solved by ureteral reimplantation, since normal drainage depends upon the normal peristaltic activity of the ureter and pelvis. This drainage is usually impaired to some degree by previous infection, tortuosity, and scar tissue.

Ileal Conduit Surgery

A second type of surgical intervention, ileal conduit surgery, makes it possible to drain urine from the kidneys by entirely bypassing the bladder. While children treated by means of such surgery have a long history of kidney or bladder difficulties, not all have this procedure for the same reason. The operation, in some cases a lifesaving one, is recommended when there are serious difficulties with the muscles or nerves controlling the bladder, congenital malformations of the urinary tract, obstructions, chronic infections, scarring, or other associated findings. Whatever the problem, all children who need ileal conduit surgery share a serious impairment of their urinary tract function; they and their parents also share a great need for explanation and preparation for surgery as the operation is a major and generally irreversible one, causing change in the child's appearance and body function.

In the operation, a small segment of the ileum, only a few inches long, is resected. The remaining ends of small intestine are rejoined, and the child is left with a normal digestive tract. The separated section of intestine is made to function in a new way: one end of the section is sutured closed. A small opening is made in the child's abdominal wall, usually laterally and a little below the waistline. The open end of the segment is brought through this opening, folded back, and attached to the outside of the abdominal wall to form a stoma. (See Fig. 38-19.)

To conclude the operation, the ureters are severed near the bladder and attached to the segment of the ileum that has been surgically separated. Thus, urine then drains into the ileal conduit.

From the ileal segment, urine continually drains into a rubber or plastic collecting pouch which must be worn over the stoma. (See Fig. 38-20.) While the pouch is worn at all times, it must be emptied at intervals and periodically cleaned and replaced. A

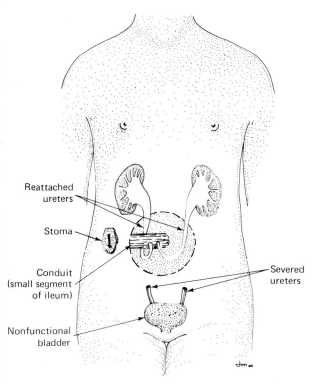

Reattached
ureters

Stoma

Conduit
(small segment
of ileum)

Nonfunctional
bladder

Severed
ureters

Figure 38-19   Anatomic drawing of an ileal conduit. *(From Joanne Bluestone, Your Child and Ileal Conduit Surgery, Charles C Thomas, Publisher, Springfield, Ill., 1970.)*

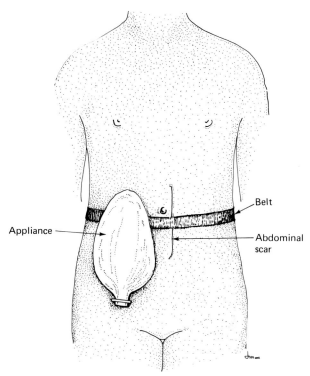

Appliance

Belt

Abdominal
scar

Figure 38-20   Position of the permanent appliance after an ileal conduit procedure. *(From Joanne Bluestone, Your Child and Ileal Conduit Surgery, Charles C Thomas, Publisher, Springfield, Ill., 1970.)*

small valve on the bag enables a child to control going to the bathroom as readily as his or her friends.

"All told, the ileal conduit surgery, together with the appliance that must always be worn, imposes few limitations on the child's activities. In fact, the operation greatly increases the possibility of an active life for the child who has previously been seriously ill."[67]

In retrospect, most parents and children agree with the preceding statement. However, when facing the procedure preoperatively, they also express reluctance, if not hostility, to such a change of body image. Grief, guilt, and despair are normal emotions on the part of child and parent, expressed openly or in indirect ways. Early fear and depression are part of the emotional storm which may have more long-term implications: Will ileal surgery impair the boy's masculinity or athletic ability? Will it affect his future sexual capacity? Will a daughter remain attractive? Can she marry and have children? The nurse may anticipate such feelings and questions and encourage appropriate discussion. Ileal conduit surgery itself has no effect on the sexual organs or childbearing, although other factors of the child's condi-

tion may. The nurse may help initiate discussion of such questions for the parents with the child's physicians. The child's reaction to surgery and his acceptance of his bodily changes will be affected greatly by the manner in which his mother and father handle their own feelings. Awkwardness, shame, and secretiveness are "contagious." Hence, parents do well to (1) learn as much as they can about the surgery, (2) talk about their worries, and (3) get all the help they can.

The nurse is in an excellent position to assist parents and children throughout the hospitalization period if he himself is well-versed in the preparation and procedures involved with ileal conduits. Certainly it is the nurse's responsibility to assist parents and children with learning the techniques of appliance application and removal and hygiene measures *during* the hospitalization. The references at the end of the chapter delineate these measures clearly and give suggestions for adapting to an active life (the child at school, traveling, etc.). The nurse may also initiate contact among able families who have undergone the procedure to assist "new" children and parents, either personally or by correspondence, in an each-one-teach-one fashion. Truly, the nurse has great potential as a member of the health team for helping shape a family's adjustment to ileal conduit surgery.[68]

Kidney Transplantation

Finally, when extended hemodialysis and homotransplantation are offered to pediatric patients, surgical intervention is ultimately part of the picture. In the actual surgery, the donor kidney is removed and perfused with cold saline to clear it of blood and to reduce the temperature of the graft to 4° to 10°C (39.2° to 50°F). It is then implanted without delay into the iliac fossa of the recipient; the main renal artery and vein are connected to the iliac vessels, and the ureter is implanted into the bladder of the recipient. Bilateral nephrectomy is carried out on the recipient before or during the transplantation procedure when there is severe hypertension or when the underlying disease is polycystic disease or chronic pyelonephritis. The recipient must, of course, be maintained on dialysis until urine formation in the transplant begins—which may be hours or weeks.

Immediately after surgery the child is started on immunosuppressive drug therapy, usually a combination of prednisone and azathioprine, to counteract the major threat of rejection phenomena in the graft. Signs of rejection may occur immediately or be delayed for some months; such signs are falling urine output, fever, rising BUN and creatinine, and, on biopsy, infiltration of the kidney with lymphocytes.

Concomitantly, the child receiving large doses of steroids and immunosuppressives is a prime candidate for generalized infection, especially of fungal and viral origin. (More transplant patients succumb to infection than rejection processes.) Other clinical complications may include (1) recurrence of glomerulonephritis in the transplanted kidney in patients whose original disease was chronic glomerulonephritis and (2) transplant lung, which results from cross reactivity between antikidney antibodies and antigens in the lung.

The most successful transplants are those between identical twins, since the problem of rejection does not arise. The next most successful are those in which kidneys are transplanted between related individuals. In general, it appears that siblings are most likely to be the best match, parents are somewhat less compatible, and more removed relatives even less. Transplants from unrelated donors and from donor cadavers, performed immediately after death of the donor, are even less likely to be successful. Only one of many moral or ethical issues, therefore, is the alternative to a child whose parent or mature sibling, both in age (21 years or older) and outlook, is *not* a suitable donor either medically or by his or her choice.

In light of such "iceberg" dilemmas, the findings of Korsch, Fine, Grushkin, and Negrete are of great importance.[69] In their study, 40 children, 2 to 18 years of age, had received 45 renal grafts from 13 live, related donors and 32 cadaver donors. At the time of reporting, 32 children were alive 1 to 42 months after transplantation with functioning grafts. Two children were returned to hemodialysis, and six children had died. In the immediate posttransplant period, three children developed psychiatric problems, and five children actually stopped taking their immunosuppressant drugs. Figures 38-21 to 38-24 illustrate the emotional and social adjustment of child and family as they encounter the various landmarks in the course of end-stage kidney disease, hemodialysis, and homotransplantation.

Figure 38-21 represents the downhill course as kidney function deteriorates to the point of renal failure. At this stage depression and withdrawal are characteristic responses of child and family. Furthermore, if the presence of renal disease is an unexpected shock, acceptance of the hopeless condition of the kidney and the need for dramatic, swift treatment may be blocked by extreme denial. Parents especially may be required to cooperate with a program of peritoneal dialysis or hemodialysis and sometimes nephrectomy before they are really ready even to accept the diagnosis of kidney disease as such, and most certainly before they are psychologically ready to accept the fact that the child's kidneys are indeed so bad that bilateral nephrectomy is necessary.

For the child himself, the need for peritoneal dialysis for symptom relief is often seen as a desperate measure. Finding the procedure uncomfortable and even painful, some adolescent patients claim it is so humiliating and intolerable that they would rather die than undergo it repeatedly.

Figure 38-22 represents the time of insertion of the Scribner shunt. Although some complications and setbacks are apt to occur in the course of hemodialysis, in general this period is one of renewed hope and rehabilitation for child and family. Just as drastic changes in parental attitudes and behavior have been observed as the possibility of hemodialysis and extended life for the child is introduced, so are dramatic personality changes frequently seen in the child himself. He may literally blossom, once his

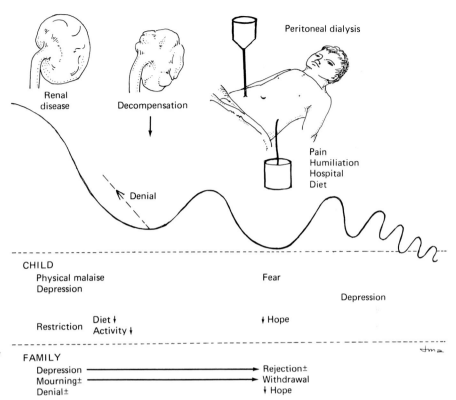

Figure 38-21 *(Adapted from Barbara Korsch et al., "Experiences with Children and Their Families during Extended Hemodialysis and Kidney Transplantation," Pediatric Clinics of North America, 18(2):630, May 1971, W. B. Saunders Company, Philadelphia.)*

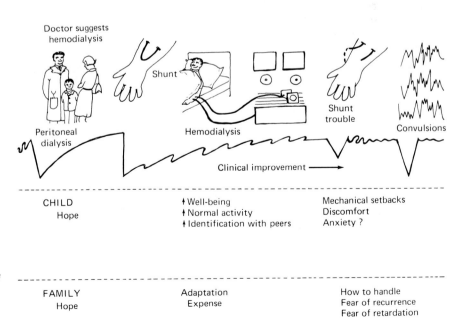

Figure 38-22 *(Adapted from Barbara Korsch et al., "Experiences with Children and Their Families during Extended Hemodialysis and Kidney Transplantation," Pediatric Clinics of North America, 18(2):630, May 1971, W. B. Saunders Company, Philadelphia.)*

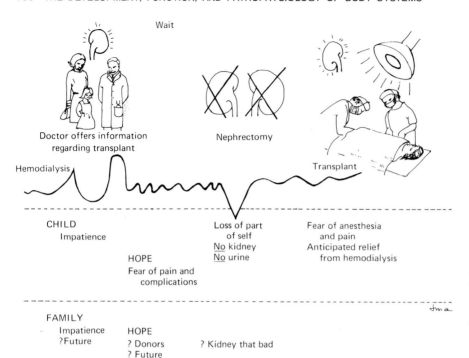

Figure 38-23 *(Adapted from Barbara Korsch et al., "Experiences with Children and Their Families during Extended Hemodialysis and Kidney Transplantation," Pediatric Clinics of North America, 18(2):630, May 1971, W. B. Saunders Company, Philadelphia.)*

physical sense of well-being is restored and he is less frightened.

Figure 38-23 shows the physiologic and psychologic preparation for homotransplantation. The anticipation of the transplant is at first invested only with hope and magic; then other concerns intervene to present a more realistic picture. Removal of the child's own kidneys in preparation for the transplant, though logical from the medical view, is almost always hard to take for the child and family. The step implies such a final, negative verdict concerning the state of the child's own kidneys that there are usually some questions in the parents' minds as to whether the physician was absolutely justified in the need for removal. The child no doubt mourns the loss of part of himself; he is troubled by his subsequent complete inability to urinate on his own and with the incumbent, even more complete, dependence on "the machine." The transplant itself is a time for mixed feelings for all concerned. Parents and staff may have gnawing doubts beneath their superficial enthusiasm and optimism. The child is usually preoccupied with immediate anxieties and physical discomforts.

Figure 38-24 represents features of the experience with dialysis and transplantation that are anticipated least clearly. Parents and professionals may look to the moment of transplantation as the moment when the miracle will be achieved and when a well-functioning kidney will cause the child to return to good health and complete rehabilitation. Instead, Korsch et al. have learned that some of the more severe trials for patient, family, and staff occur in the posttransplant period: surgical complications, rejection crises, intercurrent infections, delay or interruption in the course of spontaneous urine production, even fears arising from news items concerning the failing of a heart transplant in far-off Africa. Continued vigilance for serious complications must be tempered with efforts at reassurance and promotion of normal life patterns for child and family—an almost impossible combination.

Steriod medication is a double-edged sword for all patients. The interference with growth, combined with a tendency to cause excess appetite, weight gain, and cushingoid appearance, become psychologic problems; however, temporary refusal to continue medication seriously endangers the functioning of the transplanted kidney.

Parents tend to overprotect their children following kidney transplantation even if the kidney is functioning extremely well. There is fear of injury and trauma to the transplanted kidney. One pathetic feature of the posttransplantation experience is that many children feel that if they try hard enough and are "good" enough, the functioning and longevity of

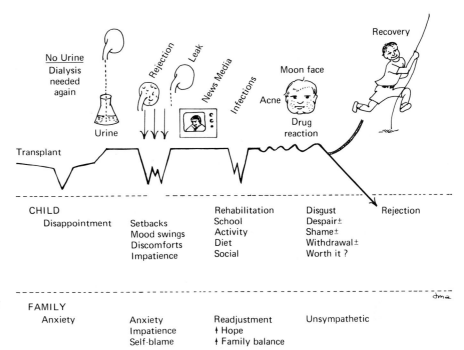

Recovery

No Urine
Dialysis
needed
again

Rejection

Leak

News Media

Infections

Acne

Moon face

Drug
reaction

Urine

Transplant

CHILD
Disappointment

Setbacks
Mood swings
Discomforts
Impatience

Rehabilitation
School
Activity
Diet
Social

Disgust
Despair±
Shame±
Withdrawal±
Worth it ?

Rejection

Figure 38-24 *(Adapted from Barbara Korsch et al., "Experiences with Children and Their Families during Extended Hemodialysis and Kidney Transplantation," Pediatric Clinics of North America, 18(2):630, May 1971, W. B. Saunders Company, Philadelphia.)*

FAMILY
Anxiety

Anxiety
Impatience
Self-blame

Readjustment
↑ Hope
↑ Family balance

Unsympathetic

the transplanted kidney will be enhanced. The reverse, of course, is that if rejection or complications occur, the children feel in large measure responsible because of some misbehavior or noncompliance with medical advice on their part.

In those instances in which the transplanted kidney had to be removed because of rejection, the children have been returned to hemodialysis and have had to repeat the whole series of experiences diagrammed in the four figures (Figs. 38-21 to 38-24). Obviously, the second time around, a very different psychologic situation is presented. The authors feel it is too early to formulate impressions, except perhaps to state that the clinical course for those few children prepared successfully for the second transplant has not been as arduous as had been anticipated by the staff. Perhaps the exaggerated fears in the professional mind had their roots in an awareness of having failed the child in previous attempts.

Korsch et al. do contend that an extremely important lesson has been that the timetables, priorities, and value systems of the professional team members are often greatly at variance with those of the patients involved in the program. The fact that nephrectomy is seen as a step forward by team members, whereas to child and family it is perceived primarily as a loss and as a setback, is but one example of the many occasions when the professional team

has learned to explore first how a particular experience or treatment is perceived by the parents before assuming that they will accept it on the terms in which it has been offered to them.

CONCLUSION

As increasingly dramatic methods for prolonging life and interfering drastically with the natural history of renal disease in children are developed, one hopes that all members of the medical profession are taking a critical look at what is gained for children and their families. It is of paramount importance that while knowledge increases in technical, scientific, and physiologic areas, simultaneous attention is paid to the emotional and social implications of kidney diseases and the new treatment programs for sick children and their families. Nurses are in a pivotal position for collecting information and for accomplishing such advancements in the health care team.

REFERENCES

1 J. A. James, *Renal Disease in Childhood,* 2d ed., The C. V. Mosby Company, St. Louis, 1972, p. 27.
2 James, op. cit., 1968, pp. 51 and 59.
3 James, op. cit., 1972, pp. 13–15 and 62–65.
4 James, op. cit., 1968, p. 69.
5 Ibid., p. 72.

6 James, op. cit., 1972, p. 78.
7 Ibid., p. 84.
8 Ibid.
9 Ibid., p. 97.
10 James, op. cit., 1968, p. 196.
11 M. B. Rothenberg and W. Heymann, "The Incidence of the Nephrotic Syndrome in Children," *Pediatrics,* 19:446, 1957.
12 James, op. cit., 1968, p. 197.
13 F. Smith et al., "The Nephrotic Syndrome: Current Concepts," *Annals of Internal Medicine,* 76:463, March 1972.
14 James, op. cit., 1972, p. 196.
15 James, op. cit., 1968, p. 198.
16 Smith et al., op. cit., pp. 463–477.
17 J. Churg, R. Habib, and R. H. White, "Pathology of the Nephrotic Syndrome in Children," *Lancet,* 1:1299–1302, 1970.
18 James, op. cit., 1968, p. 212.
19 Ibid.
20 Ibid., p. 213.
21 R. B. Goldbloom, D. A. Hillman, and T. V. Santulli, "Arterial Thrombosis Following Femoral Venipuncture in Edematous Nephrotic Children," *Pediatrics,* 40:450, 1967.
22 James, op. cit., 1972, p. 209.
23 James, op. cit., 1968, p. 215.
24 James, op. cit., 1972, p. 213.
25 Ibid., p. 214.
26 Ibid., p. 216.
27 L. Soyaka and K. Saxena, "Alternate Day Steroid Therapy for Nephrotic Children," *Journal of the American Medical Association,* 192:225, 1965.
28 James, op. cit., 1972, p. 213.
29 Smith et al., op. cit., p. 464.
30 James, op. cit., 1972, p. 213.
31 James, op. cit., 1968, p. 221.
32 Smith et al., op. cit., p. 472.
33 Ibid., p. 473.
34 D. Cornfield and M. W. Schwartz, "Nephrosis, A Long-Term Study of Children Treated with Corticosteroids," *Pediatrics,* 68:507, 1966.
35 G. C. Arneil, "164 Children with Nephrosis," *Lancet,* 2:1103, 1961.
36 James, op. cit., 1968, p. 223.
37 N. J. Siegel et al., "Long-Term Follow-up of Children with Steroid-Responsive Nephrotic Syndrome," *Journal of Pediatrics,* 81:251, 257, August 1972.
38 James, op. cit., 1968, p. 224.
39 Ibid., p. 129.
40 M. Kory and S. O. Waife (eds.), *Kidney and Urinary Tract Infections,* Lilly Research Laboratories, Indianapolis, 1972, p. 13.
41 C. Kunin, I. Southall, and A. Paguin, "Epidemiology of Urinary Tract Infections," *New England Journal of Medicine,* 263:817–823, Oct. 27, 1960.
42 C. Kunin, R. Deutscher, and A. Paguin, "Urinary Tract Infection in School Children; an Epidemiologic, Clinical, and Laboratory Study," *Medicine* (Baltimore), 43:91, 1964.
43 James, op. cit., p. 136.
44 James, op. cit., 1972, p. 133.
45 James, op. cit., 1968, p. 131.
46 James, op. cit., p. 135.
47 James, op. cit., 1972, p. 130.
48 L. Saccharow and C. Pryles, "Further Experience with the Use of Percutaneous Suprapubic Aspiration of the Urinary Bladder: Bacteriologic Studies in 654 Infants and Children," *Pediatrics,* 43:1018, 1969.
49 James, op. cit., p. 130.
50 Kory and Waife, op. cit., pp. 15–16.
51 James, op. cit., 1972, pp. 177–178.
52 Ibid., p. 180.
53 Ibid., p. 181.
54 Ibid., p. 188.
55 Ibid., p. 189.
56 Ibid., p. 190.
57 Ibid., p. 192.
58 Ibid., p. 239.
59 James, op. cit., 1968, p. 273.
60 James, op. cit., 1972, p. 295.
61 F. Wang, "Conservative Management of Chronic Renal Failure," *Medical Clinics of North America,* 55:151, January 1971.
62 James, op. cit., 1972, p. 337.
63 Ibid., p. 339.
64 James, op. cit., 1968, p. 345.
65 M. Holliday, D. Potter, and R. Dobrin, "Treatment of Renal Failure in Children," *Pediatric Clinics of North America,* 18(2):620, May 1971.
66 R. L. Dale et al., "Ureteral Reimplantation; a Study of the Simple Pull-Through Technique in Normal and Dilated Ureters," *Journal of Urology,* 106:198–203, August 1971.
67 Health Education Department, The Children's Hospital Medical Center, Boston, *Your Child and Ileal Conduit Surgery,* Charles C Thomas, Publisher, Springfield, Ill., 1970, p. IX.
68 Ibid.
69 B. Korsch, R. Fine, C. Gruskin, and V. Negrete, "Experiences with Children and Their Families during Extended Hemodialysis and Kidney Transplantation," *Pediatric Clinics of North America,* 18(2):625–637, May 1971.

BIBLIOGRAPHY

Anthony, Catherine P., and Kolthoff, Norma J.: *Textbook of Anatomy and Physiology,* 8th ed., The C. V. Mosby Company, St. Louis, 1971.

Cobbs, C., and Kaye, D.: "Antibacterial Mechanisms in the Bladder," *Yale Journal of Biology and Medicine,* 40:93, 1967.

Cooke, R. E. (ed.): *The Biologic Basis of Pediatric Practice,* McGraw-Hill Book Company, New York, 1968.

Cox, C. E., and Heinman, F.: "Experiments with Induced Bacteria Vesical Emptying and Bacterial Growth on the Mechanism of Bladder Defense to Infection," *Journal of Urology,* 86:739, 1961.

Dunea, G.: "Peritoneal Dialysis and Hemodialysis," *Medical Clinics of North America,* 55:155–175, January 1971.

Edelmann, C. M. (ed): *Pediatric Clinics of North America,* 18(2), May 1971, W. B. Saunders Company, Philadelphia.

Greisheimer, Esther M., and Wiedeman, Mary P.: *Physiology and Anatomy,* 9th ed., J. B. Lippincott Company, Philadelphia, 1972.

Horton, C. E., and Devine, C. J.: *Clinical Symposia, Hypospadias and Epispadias,* Ciba Publications Section, Summit, N.J., 24(3), 1972.

Jeter, Katherine: *Management of the Urinary Stoma,* Department of Urology, College of Physicians and Surgeons of Columbia University Squier Urological Clinic, Columbia-Presbyterian Medical Center, New York, 1970.

——— and Bloom, S.: "Management of Stomal Complications Following Ileal or Colonic Conduit Operations in Children," *Ostomy Quarterly,* 10(2), 1973.

Lenneberg, Edith S., and Werner, Miriam: *The Ostomy Handbook,* United Ostomy Association, Inc., Los Angeles, Calif., 1973.

Nelson, W. E.: *Textbook of Pediatrics,* 8th ed., W. B. Saunders Company, Philadelphia, 1964.

Norden, C., Greene, G., and Kass, E.: "Antibacterial Mechanisms of the Urinary Bladder," *Journal of Clinical Investigations*, 47:2689, 1968.

Patten, B. M.: *Human Embryology,* 3d, ed., McGraw-Hill Book Company, New York, 1968.

Whipple, Dorothy V.: *Dynamics of Development: Euthenic Pediatrics,* McGraw-Hill Book Company, New York, 1966.

Suggested References for Parents and Patients

Bluestone, Joanne: *Your Child and Ileal Conduit Surgery,* Charles C Thomas, Publisher, Springfield, Ill., 1970.

Jeter, Katherine: *Count Your Blessings*, Department of Urology, College of Physicians and Surgeons of Columbia University Squier Urological Clinic, Columbia-Presbyterian Medical Center, New York, 1970.

Norris, Carol: *All about Jimmy,* United Ostomy Association, Inc., Los Angeles, Calif., 1973 (coloring book to explain a child's ostomy to him).

THE ENDOCRINE SYSTEM

MILDRED FENSKE

EMBRYOLOGY OF THE ENDOCRINE SYSTEM
Pituitary Gland

The *pituitary gland* or *hypophysis* arises from ecto-dermal tissue. The primordia of the anterior and posterior portions of the pituitary are easily seen by the fourth week of embryonic life. The anterior portion, which is derived from the lining of a primordium known as *Rathke's pocket,* undergoes more striking and extensive changes than the posterior portion, which arises from the infundibular process or the embryonic head. The infundibular process eventually evolves into the *pars neuralis.*

Originally, Rathke's pocket is superficially located as an extension of the stomodeum situated on the ventral surface of the head. As Rathke's pocket elongates, its closed end is affixed to the infundibular process. Eventually, the stock from which this primordium arises narrows (at about 6½ weeks) and finally disconnects from the stomodeum. The stomodeal portion of the hypophysis forms a double-layered cup around the pars neuralis. The rostral part of its outer layer thickens rapidly and assumes a glandular appearance. This structure is destined to be the *pars distalis* or anterior lobe. The inner layer fuses with the pars neuralis and is known as the *pars intermedia.* A pair of lateral buds arises on either side of the infundibular stalk and forms a collarlike structure about its neck, destined to become the *pars tuberalis.* This stage is reached about eleven weeks after conception. It is not known when endocrine production begins in fetal life.

Thyroid Gland

About the end of the fourth week, the primordium of the *thyroid gland* arises between the first and second pharyngeal pouches and very soon is bilobular. Once it disconnects from the pharyngeal floor, it moves downward. During its migration, diverticulae which have broken loose from the fourth pharyngeal pouches merge with the lateral lobes of the median thyroid precursor. During the seventh week, the structure has reached the level of the laryngeal primordium. The thyroid precursor expands in size, and, in the third month, vascular connective tissue forms. During the fourth month, thyroid follicles are formed from colloid. The surrounding connective tissue gradually differentiates into the fibroelastic tissue of the stroma. This connective tissue is highly vascular and thus facilitates the passage of hormones into the bloodstream.

Parathyroid Glands

The *parathyroid glands* arise in two pairs: one pair from the third pharyngeal pouches (parathyroids III) and the other from the fourth pharyngeal pouches (parathyroids IV). Parathyroids III are closely associated with the thymic primordium. Each breaks away from the third pharyngeal pouches during the seventh week and begins a downward migration. By the eighth week each structure is distinct, but parathyroids III remain attached to the thymic primordium until they eventually lie caudal to parathyroids IV, having been embedded in either connective tissue next to the thyroid or the tip of the thymus. Parathroids IV develop in close association with the diverticulae which are incorporated with the lateral lobes of the median thyroid precursor. They either adhere to the thyroid capsule or become embedded in thyroid tissue. Eventually, parathyroids IV assume a position caudal to parathyroids III on the underside of the thyroid. Parathyroid hormone activity is thought to be present by the thirteenth week of gestation.

Thymus Gland

Thymic primordia do not appear until the latter part of the sixth week. Initially they have small cleftlike lumens which greatly enlongate by the seventh week and are soon lost. The primordia then rapidly increase in bulk. Each distal tip moves toward the other and makes contact by the middle of the eighth week, as they migrate downward in the neck and under the sternum into the mediastinum. Fusion remains superficial. During the third month, they begin to lose their likeness to other young glands as they develop *thymic (Hassall's) corpuscles* from epithelial cords. Epithelial remnants are separated through an ingrowth of mesenchyme which, late in the third month, begins to evolve into reticular connective tissue and the precursors of lymphocytes. The gland now rapidly becomes a lymphoid organ. It eventually is lobulated as the fetus is approaching term. The cortex of each lobule contains lymphoid tissue, and the medulla is populated with lymphocytes. It increases in weight from 12 to 15 Gm at birth to 30 to 40 Gm at puberty. It then gradually regresses and is replaced by fat, connective tissue, or both.

Adrenal Glands

The *adrenal glands* are composed of the centrally located medulla and the surrounding cortex. The medulla arises from cells of neural crest origin. The cells migrate ventrally and enter the sympathetic ganglions. Eventually they detach from the ganglions and form gland cells. These cells are smaller than neuroblasts and stain a brownish yellow with dichromate salts. Due to this staining reaction, they have been termed *chromaffin cells.* Many clusters of chromaffin cells are located near each chain of ganglions and may be found at birth near the aorta, the abdominal sympathetic plexus, and the root of the inferior mesenteric artery. The largest and most constant masses of chromaffin cells appear on either side and cephalic to primordial kidneys and are destined to become the *adrenal medulla.*

About the sixth week, the primordial cortex makes its appearance as a fissure in the splanchnic mesoderm near the primordial kidneys. Mesodermal cells rapidly proliferate into underlying mesenchyme and have formed considerable cell masses by the eighth week. These cortical masses are now free of the parent tissue and are surrounded by a capsule of developing connective tissue. Chromaffin cells penetrate each cortical mass. Thus, the primordial adrenal medulla is encapsulated by the developing cortex.

During the third month, the inner portion of the cortex develops the provisional cortex composed of cell cords which have vacuoles, indicating the possibility of secretory activity. The less-differentiated cells outside the provisional cortex become known as the permanent cortex. Toward the end of gestation and into the neonatal period, the provisional cortex involutes and has disappeared by the end of the first year. At the same time, the permanent cortex begins to differentiate into a more highly specialized structure.

Islets of Langerhans

The islets of Langerhans arise from the primordial epithelial cords of the developing pancreas as buds which separate early from the parent tissue. They differentiate into a tangled knot of cellular cords with dilated capillaries. Insulin is discharged directly into the bloodstream. Within the pancreas are a million such islets which secrete insulin by the beginning of the third trimester. The presence of fetal insulin is indicated in pregnant diabetic women whose insulin requirements decrease in the third trimester.

GROWTH PATTERNS OF THE CHILD
Normal Patterns

Growth from conception is on a continuum, but the rate is not constant. In general, growth as measured by body weight follows a pattern similar to that of stature; that is, as a child's height increases, his weight increases. At adolescence, there is a rapid increase in body size and changes in the body contour and the composition and development of the gonads, reproductive organs, and the secondary sex characteristics as a result of the hormones secreted for the first time or secreted in increasing amounts. Each hormone acts on certain receptors; however, several types of tissue can be affected. For example, testosterone acts on receptor cells in the penis, facial skin, and certain cerebral areas. Knowledge is limited about the morphologic changes occurring in the development of normal children, and so it is not possible to identify the hormonal cause of each change at this time. (See Figs. 39-1 to 39-4.)

Girls generally experience an adolescent growth spurt 2 years earlier than boys. Growth spurts or the peak of them usually occur at age 12 for girls and age 14 for boys. The adolescent growth spurt is more an increase in the length of the trunk than in the length of the leg; thus the relation of the length of the leg to the length of the trunk changes at this stage of development. Changes in body composition at adolescence are characterized by an increase in bone and muscle diameters accompanied by a loss of fat, especially in boys. An increase in strength accompanies the increase in muscle size as does an increase in total body potassium, total body water, and intracellular water. In males, there is an increase in red blood cells and hemoglobin, thought to be due to the secretion of testosterone which increases the production of the erythropoiesis-stimulating factor in the kidney. Other changes influencing increased physical stamina at adolescence include an increased lung size and ability to sustain oxygen debt, and increased creatinine excretion.

The first sign of puberty in boys is usually an increase in the growth of the testes and scrotum followed by a slight growth of pubic hair. The increase in the size of the testes is due to an increase in the size of the seminiferous tubules. Genital development requires about four years and is usually completed by the age of 15 for boys. Axillary hair usually appears about two years after the beginning of pubic hair. Facial hair, in boys, begins at about the same time that axillary hair appears. Cracking of the voice, which occurs in adolescence, is probably due to the multiplication of thyroid and cricoid cartilages influenced by testosterone. The seminal vesicles, prostate, and bulbourethral glands enlarge and develop under the same stimulus as the growth of the penis. The first ejaculation normally occurs about a year after penis growth becomes accelerated.

In girls, the development of the breast bud heralds puberty. The menarche occurs after the peak of the growth spurt has passed. The first menstrual period does not indicate full reproductive function, for the first cycles are frequently irregular and anovulatory. Other differences between the sexes which are produced by puberty include, in girls, an increase in the width of the hips and pelvic outlet presumably due to the stimulation of estrogen; similarly, boys experience an increase in the growth of the shoulders and chest due to the effect of testosterone upon the cartilage in the shoulder and chest regions.

Abnormal Patterns

The short stature of a child may be due to various causes. Thus, when a child's height is three or more standard deviations below normal, a thorough history and physical examination are in order. Although endocrine disorders are infrequently the cause of organic impairments of growth, hypothyroidism, hypopituitarism, and endogenous cortisol excess may occur. Systemic disorders and maternal deprivation are more frequently associated with short stature.

REGULATORY FUNCTIONS OF THE ENDOCRINE SYSTEM

The two major control systems which regulate the functions of the body are the nervous and the endocrine systems. They are closely related; directly or indirectly, hormonal secretion is under the control of the nervous system, and the level of most hormones directly or indirectly affects the activities of the central nervous system. *Hormones* are chemical substances concerned primarily with metabolic functions of the body, control of the rate of chemical reactions within cells, transport of substances through cell membranes, or cellular metabolism such as growth and secretion. Thus, the endocrine system is primarily responsible for growth, maturation, metabolic processes, and reproduction as well as the integration of body responses to stress.

The endocrine glands synthesize hormones which are continually lost from the body by excretion or metabolic inactivation. Some hormones have a rhythmic pattern to their secretion, whereas others are secreted in response to a blood level of a specific substance such as sodium, water, another hormone, or sugar. The blood level of each specific hormone is maintained within definite limits in health. Dysfunction of an endocrine gland may be the result of

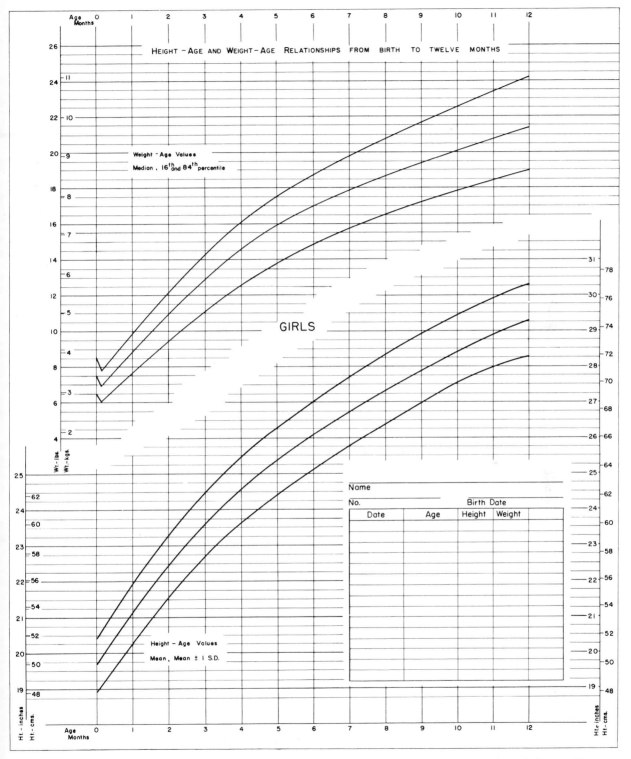

Figure 39-1   Female infant growth chart, prepared from data compiled by the Iowa Child Welfare Research Station. *(Source: Department of Pediatrics, State University of Iowa. Copyrighted 1943 by State University of Iowa. Courtesy of Mead Johnson Laboratories, Evansville, Ind.)*

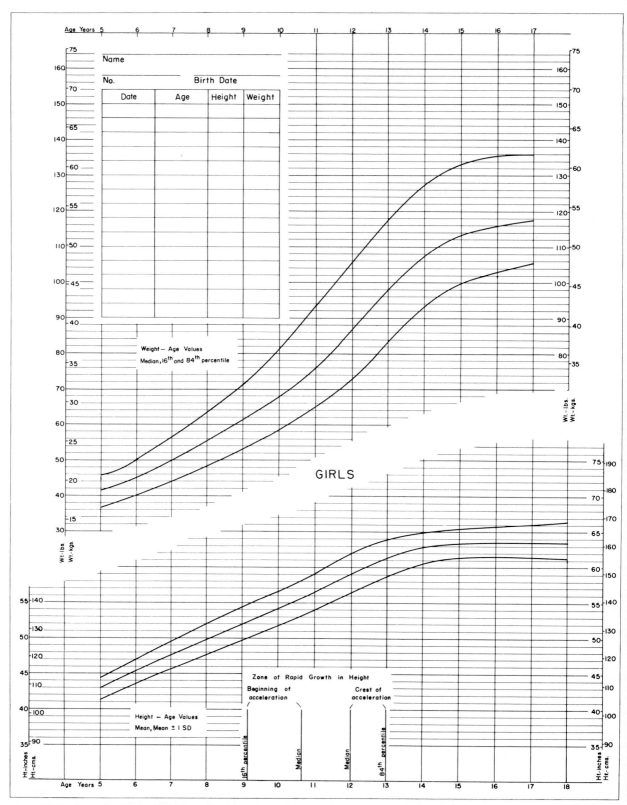

Figure 39-2 Female growth chart (5 to 17 years), prepared from data compiled by the Iowa Child Welfare Research Station. *(Source: Department of Pediatrics, State University of Iowa. Copyrighted 1943 by State University of Iowa. Courtesy of Mead Johnson Laboratories, Evansville, Ind.)*

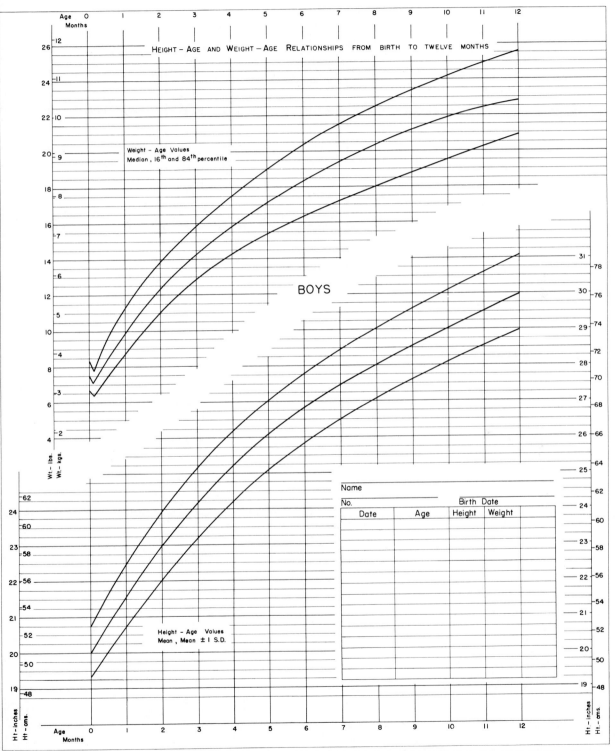

Figure 39-3 Male infant growth chart, prepared from data compiled by the Iowa Child Welfare Research Station. *(Source: Department of Pediatrics, State University of Iowa. Copyrighted 1943 by State University of Iowa. Courtesy of Mead Johnson Laboratories, Evansville, Ind.)*

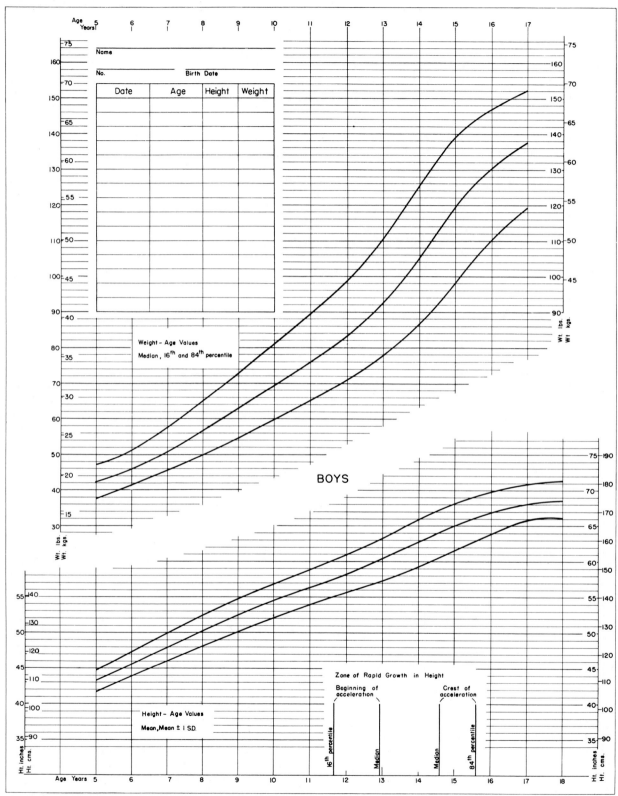

Figure 39-4 Male growth chart (5 to 17 years), prepared from data compiled by the Iowa Child Welfare Research Station. *(Source: Department of Pediatrics, State University of Iowa. Copyrighted 1943 by State University of Iowa. Courtesy of Mead Johnson Laboratories, Evansville, Ind.)*

malfunction of the regulatory mechanism or failure of the body processes to respond to regulation. A disorder of one of the glands is apt to affect the function of others. Structural alteration of the gland resulting in dysfunction may be caused by abnormal embryonic development of the tissue, *ischemia*, or a deficient blood supply to the gland, infection of the gland, malignant or benign tumors, overstimulation or atrophy of the gland, and hypertrophy with or without hyperplasia of the gland.

Disease of an endocrine gland usually causes a decrease or an increase in the secretion of hormones. Symptoms of the dysfunction are those of increased or decreased regulation of the bodily processes normally controlled by the gland and/or specific hormone. Symptoms of endocrine dysfunction are reflected in many parts of the body because of the diverse physiologic functions under the control of the endocrine system. Likewise, owing to the vital nature of the functions controlled, endocrine disorders can be extremely serious.

Medical treatment of endocrine disease is directed toward decreasing the production of the hormones when hypersecretion of the glands occurs and replacing hormones when hypofunction of an endocrine gland occurs. Hypersecretion is usually corrected by partial or total resection of the gland or by surgical removal of the tumor. Irradiation of the specific endocrine gland or the pituitary may be used to destroy sufficient tissue to control the secretion. Essential hormones are supplied as replacement or to supplement endogenous hormones when there has been complete destruction of an endocrine gland or when there is hypofunction.

PITUITARY GLAND
Physiology

The hypophysis, about one centimeter in diameter, is located within the sella turcica at the base of the brain and is connected with the hypothalamus by the hypophyseal stalk. The adenohypophysis secretes six hormones important in the control of metabolic functions of the body. *Growth hormone,* also known as *somatotropin,* causes growth of all tissues with the potential to grow by increasing the size and the number of cells. Growth hormone increases the synthesis of protein, conserves carbohydrate utilization, and increases the mobilization and use of fats for energy. This hormone is ineffective if insulin and carbohydrate are not available, and it has a diabetogenic effect because it causes a decrease in the utilization of carbohydrate for energy and causes glycogen to be stored until cells become saturated, resulting in a rise in the blood sugar level. Although growth hormone is secreted throughout life, the amount of hormone present is about one and one-half times greater in children than in adults. Adults stop growing because of the union of the epiphyses of the long bones with shafts.

Corticotropin (adrenocorticotropic hormone, or ACTH) controls the secretion of the adrenocortical hormones which affect the metabolism of glucose, protein, and fat. *Thyrotropin* (thyroid-stimulating hormone, or TSH) controls the secretion of thyroxine by the thyroid gland which affects the rates of most reactions of the body. *Follicle-stimulating hormone* (FSH), *luteinizing hormone* (interstitial-cell stimulating hormone, or ICSH), and *luteotropic hormone* (LH) control the growth of the gonads as well as reproductive activities.

Disorders and Deviations

Idiopathic Hypopituitarism Children who have idiopathic hypopituitarism do not usually show evidence of the disease other than short stature. The development of secondary sex characteristics is delayed or does not occur without treatment (see Chap. 37). Tests to indicate growth hormone deficiency include assays of this hormone by using antibody response and the induction of hypoglycemia, and intravenous *l*-arginine to produce an increase in the concentration of growth hormone if pituitary function is normal.

Tests to establish the presence of other anterior pituitary hormones are also used on the premise that if there is an absence of ACTH or TSH, growth hormone is probably deficient. Urine specimens for 24-hour periods may be examined to determine gonadotropin function and the ability of the pituitary to produce ACTH in response to metyrapone (Metopirone), a drug that inhibits the synthesis of cortisol by the adrenal cortex. Laboratory tests to determine thyrotropin activity include measurement of protein-bound iodine (PBI) and butanol-extractable iron (BEI), and radioactive iodine (I^{131}) uptake. ACTH activity can be measured in the plasma, but it is usually measured by the excretion of 17-hydroxycorticosteroids (17-OHCS) or 17-ketogenic steroids (17-KS). (See Tables 39-1 and 39-2.)

Radiographic examinations are used to determine skeletal age. X-ray films of the distal parts of the radius and the ulna, the metacarpals, and all the phalanges are assessed on the ossification of the epiphyseal centers. The size of the pituitary fossa is also assessed radiologically. The pituitary fossa has

Table 39-1 URINARY CORTICOSTEROID RESPONSES TO DIAGNOSTIC MANEUVERS DESIGNED TO DEMONSTRATE NONAUTONOMY* OR AUTONOMY† OF ADRENAL FUNCTION

Condition	Urinary 17-hydroxycorticosteroids					Urinary 17-ketosteroids
	Basal	Suppression with dexamethasone		ACTH stimulation	Metyrapone	Basal
		2mg	8 mg			
Normal	3–10 mg/24 hr	<3 mg/24 hr	<50% initial value	2–3-fold increase over base line	2-fold increase over base line (or >5 mg increment/24 hr)	Female: 5–15 mg/24 hr Male: 8–20 mg/24 hr
Adrenal hyperplasia	Increased	Not suppressed	<50% initial value	Hyperresponsive	Hyperresponsive	Normal or increased
Adrenal adenoma	Increased	Not suppressed	Not suppressed	No or normal response	No or decreased response	Decreased or normal
Adrenal carcinoma	Markedly increased	Not suppressed	Not suppressed	No response	No response	Markedly increased
Pituitary tumor	Increased to markedly increased	Not suppressed	Not suppressed	No to slight response	No response	Increased
Ectopic ACTH	Markedly increased	Not suppressed	Usually not suppressed	Usually no response	No response	Increased

* Nonautonomy of adrenal function, as would be seen in adrenal hyperplasia.
† Autonomy of adrenal function, as would be seen in adrenal, pituitary, or "ectopic" tumors.
Source: Reprinted from Dorothy T. Krieger, "Cushing's Syndrome," *Hospital Medicine*, September 1972, pp. 29 and 35.

Table 39-2 PLASMA CORTICOSTEROID RESPONSES TO DIAGNOSTIC MANEUVERS DESIGNED TO DEMONSTRATE NONAUTONOMY* OR AUTONOMY† OF ADRENAL FUNCTION

Condition	Plasma 11-hydroxycorticosteroids					Plasma ACTH
	Basal (8 A.M.)	Circadian variation	Response to dexamethasone (1 mg at midnight)	Response to aqueous pitressin (10 U., I.M.)	Response to ACTH	
Normal	10 to 25 µg/100 ml	A.M. greater than P.M.	<6 µg/100 ml	Increased 15 µg/100 ml above base line	Doubling of baseline value	20 to 100 pg/ml 8 A.M.
Adrenal hyperplasia	Normal or increased	Absent	>6 µg/100 ml	Increased	Increased	Normal or increased
Adrenal adenoma	Normal or increased	Absent	>6 µg/100 ml	Absent	No or normal response	Decreased
Adrenal carcinoma	Increased	Absent	>6 µg/100 ml	Absent	No response	Decreased
Pituitary tumor	Increased	Absent	>6 µg/100 ml	Absent	No to slight response	Markedly increased
Ectopic ACTH	Increased	Absent	>6 µg/100 ml	Absent	Usually no response	Markedly increased

* Nonautonomy of adrenal function, as would be seen in adrenal hyperplasia.
† Autonomy of adrenal function, as would be seen in adrenal, pituitary, or "ectopic" tumors.
Source: Reprinted from Dorothy T. Krieger, "Cushing's Syndrome," *Hospital Medicine,* September 1972, pp. 29 and 35.

been found to be abnormally small in hypopituitarism.

Growth hormone is available in limited quantities, and it is used in selected patients who will go into a period of sustained growth. It is given in intramuscular injections two or three times weekly. The development of antibodies to growth hormone has been a problem because the antibodies terminate growth. Thyroid hormone is useful if there is a deficiency of thyroid function. It is administered in tablet form in a dose sufficient to eliminate symptoms of hypothyroidism and restore the protein-bound iodine level to normal. However, thyroid hormone is of no value if there is not a deficiency of thyroid function.

Panhypopituitarism In the presence of panhypopituitarism, rather than isolated growth hormone deficiency, gonadal function is restored by the administration of testosterone or methyltestosterone to males. Estrogens are administered to girls to stimulate the growth of the breasts and the uterus. Menstrual cycles are induced by the addition of progestin to the estrogen regimen.

There is disagreement as to the value of administering anabolic steroids in the absence of growth hormone. Some studies have indicated that the use of testosterone could produce stunting of growth, while other studies have shown that the induction of pubertal growth by using small doses of methyltestosterone could be accomplished without stunting growth. Chorionic gonadotropins have been used to treat hypogonadism; however, prolonged intramuscular therapy is unpleasant, and the development of antibodies has occurred.

Organic Hypopituitarism In children organic hypopituitarism follows the destruction of the anterior pituitary as a result of tumor, trauma, infections, irradiation, or histiocytosis. Congenital absence of the pituitary does not appear to be incompatible with life. Rarely, hypopituitarism follows acute infections such as tuberculosis, syphilis, and other granulomas.

The most common tumors to occur in the pituitary area are *craniopharyngiomas* and *gliomas*. Carcinomas of the pharyngeal epithelium may infiltrate the pituitary. These tumors usually occur in the hypothalamus. Many of the functions of the pituitary are controlled by the hypothalamus, and so dysfunctions are not readily identified as being pituitary or hypothalamic in origin.

Histiocytosis is the invasion of the skeletal system by histiocytes loaded with cholesterol. Symptoms of this syndrome, also known as Hand-Schüller-Christian syndrome or eosinophilic granuloma,

include increased intracranial pressure, proptosis, diabetes insipidus, dwarfism, and hypopituitarism.

Irradiation used to treat diseases of the pituitary-hypothalamic area may cause hypopituitarism. Symptoms of hypopituitarism include hypofunction of the target organs regulated by the anterior pituitary hormones, namely, the thyroid, gonads, and adrenal cortex. Failure to develop secondary sex characteristics may occur. Signs of hypothyroidism, including dry skin, loss of eyebrows, weakness, asthenia, sluggishness, intolerance of cold, bradycardia, subnormal temperature, and hypotension may be present. Headache and vomiting may be the first symptoms to appear in children with tumors. *Froehlich's syndrome* with obesity and hypogonadism may appear when tumors of the hypothalamic area are present.

Gigantism and Acromegaly An excessive secretion of growth hormone by the anterior pituitary is the cause of gigantism and acromegaly. Both diseases are rare in children. The disorders are characterized by excessive height and rate of growth, acral enlargement and soft-tissue growth, headache, excessive perspiration, enlarged sella turcica, and visual impairment. These symptoms are caused by the excessive secretion of growth hormone and the expansion of the pituitary tumor. The cause of cardiovascular problems frequently associated with the conditions is not clearly understood.

The measurement of serum growth hormone levels by immunoassay during fasting and after glucose administration is useful to confirm the diagnosis upon inspection. Hypophysectomy and conventional radiation are the usual forms of therapy. Yttrium[90] and gold[198] implanted within the pituitary, cryohypophysectomy, irradiation using heavy particles, and Bragg-Peak proton beam are newer forms of therapy.

The main functions of the posterior lobe of the pituitary, or neurohypophysis, are to store and release antidiuretic hormone (ADH, or vasopressin) and oxytocin which are believed to be secreted by the nerve endings of the hypophyseal stalk. Antidiuretic-hormone secretion is regulated in response to the concentration of body fluids. When body fluids become concentrated, antidiuretic hormone is secreted and the permeability of the collecting tubules to water is increased. The extracellular fluids are thereby diluted and returned to normal osmotic composition. Antidiuretic-hormone secretion is inhibited in the presence of dilute extracellular fluid; large quantities of water are lost in the urine, and body fluids become more concentrated. Antidiuretic-hormone secretion is increased in the presence of bodily trauma, pain, anxiety, and drugs such as morphine, nicotine, tranquilizers, and some anesthetics. Alcohol inhibits antidiuretic-hormone secretion. In the absence of antidiuretic hormone, the reabsorption of water is prevented and extreme amounts of water are lost in the urine.

Diabetes Insipidus This condition is the principal disorder associated with the posterior pituitary. It results from inadequate formation and release of vasopressin or from failure of the kidney to respond to the hormone. Polyuria, polydipsia, and dehydration result. The major cause of diabetes insipidus is a tumor; however, the cause in many cases is undetermined. Diabetes insipidus may occur following encephalitis, meningitis, communicable diseases, and vaccination.

Loss of approximately nine-tenths of the normal vasopressin secretion may occur without the symptoms of polydipsia and polyuria. Children, unlike adults, are known to cope with painless symptoms without complaint. Unusual thirst and enuresis in a previously toilet-trained youngster should cause concern. Similarly, impairment of peripheral vision due to an expanding lesion, headaches, and vomiting symptomatic of increased intracranial pressure

and symptoms of anterior pituitary dysfunction may herald the onset of tumor growth. Diagnosis of diabetes insipidus is dependent upon water-deprivation tests and an antidiuretic response to an infusion of hypertonic saline.

Diabetes insipidus is treated by the intramuscular administration of vasopressin tannate (Pitressin Tannate) in oil. It is important to resuspend the active vasopressin within the peanut oil vehicle by warming the ampule (by holding it under the hot water faucet) and shaking it vigorously to disperse the active drug. Injections should be made deep into the muscle and should be followed by vigorous massage of the area. This route of administration has the disadvantage of a brief duration of effectiveness (2 hours) and the unpleasant side effects of vasospasm and contraction of the smooth muscle of the gastrointestinal tract. Lypressin (Diapid) nasal spray works satisfactorily for long-term usage. One or two sprays in each nostril four times daily usually control frequent urination and excessive thirst. Nocturia can be controlled by a bedtime dose. The absorption of vasopressin by the nasal mucosa is hindered by local chronic inflammatory changes and during bouts of upper respiratory tract infections. Figure 39-5 is an example of patient instructions for cortisol replacement and the use of lypressin nasal spray.

Figure 39-5 SAMPLE INSTRUCTIONS FOR PATIENTS WITH HYPOPITURITARISM.

Identification
I have hypopituitarism; I am to wear an identification bracelet or necklace with this inscription at all times.
Medicine
Prednisone
I am to take one 5-mg tablet of prednisone in the morning and one-half tablet of prednisone or 2.5 mg in the evening every day.
Fever
If I have a fever, I need to take more prednisone. If my temperature is:
98.6° to 100°F (37.0 to 37.78°C), I am to take my usual daily dose;
100.2° to 101°F (37.88 to 38.33°C), I am to take two tablets in the morning and one tablet in the evening;
101.2° to 102°F (38.44 to 38.89°C), I am to take four tablets in the morning and two tablets in the evening.
If my temperature ever goes above 102°F, I must see the doctor.
Nausea and Vomiting
If I am nauseated and vomit, I should insert a 25-mg promethazine (Phenergan) suppository into my rectum. One-half hour later, I should take double the usual dose of prednisone. If I vomit the double dose of prednisone, I am to take another promethazine suppository, and one-half hour later I am to take another double dose of prednisone. If I vomit again, I need to take a 4-mg dexamethasone (Decadron) injection and call the doctor.

Dexamethasone
I have a syringe with 4 mg dexamethasone in it. An injection of dexamethasone is to be given if:
I have been involved in an automobile accident,
I have severe nausea and vomiting and cannot keep the prednisone on my stomach after taking two promethazine suppositories,
I have fainted.
Thyroid
I am to take one thyroid tablet each day (3 grains desiccated thyroid).
Lypressin (Diapid)
Lypressin is a medication that prevents me from passing too much urine and having continuous thirst. I should take it in the following way:
two sprays in each nostril when I get up,
two sprays in each nostril at lunch,
one spray in each nostril at the evening meal,
three sprays in each nostril at bedtime.
In addition, I need to take one spray in each nostril if:
I have to get up to urinate during the night,
I have to urinate in usual amounts more than every 1½ to 2 hours,
if the amount of urine I pass is a very large amount.
Notifying my doctor
I can reach Dr. _____ at the following numbers:
Home:
Office:
C.R.C:

Nursing Management

The observant nurse may be the first to detect symptoms of abnormal pituitary function. Symptoms due to an expanding intracranial lesion and characteristic of hypersecretion or hyposecretion of the anterior pituitary may be noted upon physical examination or called to his attention by the parents or the schoolteacher. Delayed puberty is frequently the chief complaint when a physician is finally consulted, although the child's mother may have been aware that he usually *wore out* his clothes while his normal siblings *outgrew* theirs. In reality, the child has probably been called a "shrimp" by his peers and suffered psychologically for a number of years.

Once the dwarfed child is accepted for growth hormone therapy, the parents and the child are filled with hope. The parents or the child are taught injection technique, the necessity for following the prescribed program, and the advisability of follow-up examinations. It is indeed a rewarding experience to observe the delight of both the youngster and parents when the child can report he has grown or has had to shave.

Initially, when the child is evaluated for his acceptability to receive growth hormone, the nurse is responsible for being cognizant of the effects upon the child of new situations, unfamiliar equipment, painful injections, and the thought that one may not be accepted for the program. The child needs close observation when hypoglycemia is induced: he may experience severe hypoglycemia due to an exaggerated response to insulin. Constant attendance will also assist in preventing the dislodgement of the needle requiring additional venipunctures and involving additional pain.

In gigantism, the nurse is cognizant of an altered body image by the child. Children with gigantism may be uncoordinated and have difficulty bending forward. Fractures may occur, analgesics may be required, and assistance in performing activities such as tying shoes may be needed. The skin usually becomes tough and thick, and so sharp needles will facilitate venipunctures and injections. Frequent bathing is helpful for comfort because of the hyperactivity of sweat and sebaceous glands.

In the presence of pituitary tumor, nursing care is determined by the medical therapy selected. The patient having a craniotomy is observed for cerebral edema and signs of increased intracranial pressure by checking the vital signs and neurologic status. Fluid intake is controlled to prevent overhydration. When hypophysectomy is performed via the transsphenoidal approach, the patient is observed for nasal congestion, leakage of cerebrospinal fluid, especially from the nose, and symptoms of infection, because meningitis is a constant threat. To avoid dislodging the muscle graft used to close the opening made for exposure of the pituitary, the patient is cautioned not to blow his nose. The presence of rhinorrhea after the third day postoperatively must be reported to the physician.

Temporary or permanent diabetes insipidus may occur after hypophysectomy. Urine volume greater than 100 ml hourly and with a specific gravity of less than 1.010 is indicative of dilute urine. The physician is to be notified when either occurs. Vasopressin may be ordered as the need for it is indicated.

Following hypophysectomy, replacement drugs are prescribed. Parenteral cortisone is given for the immediate surgical stress. Drugs to make up deficiencies in cortisone, thyroid, androgen or estrogen, mineralocorticoids, and vasopressin are administered for life. The nurse is responsible for teaching the child the need to take the replacement drugs for life and must collaborate with the physician, dietitian, and social worker to meet the physiologic and rehabilitation needs of the child. The management of cortisol requirements and emergency use of parenteral cortisol are discussed in the section on adrenocortical insufficiency. The family should be advised to secure an identification (MedicAlert) bracelet or necklace for the child.

THYROID GLAND
Physiology

The thyroid gland is located below the larynx on both sides of and anterior to the trachea. Although it probably does not greatly influence fetal development, it is essential for normal growth at the end of intrauterine life and during the neonatal period. Thyroid activity is dependent upon thyrotropin (thyroid-stimulating hormone, or TSH) secreted by the interior pituitary. Thyroid hormones are believed to exert a feedback inhibition on the secretion of thyrotropin.

Thyroid hormones are formed by transference of iodides ingested in food from extracellular fluids and concentration of them in the thyroid gland. Thyroglobulin reacts with iodine to form the two most important thyroid hormones, thyroxine and triiodothyronine. Thyroxine increases the metabolic activity of most body tissues. It raises the rate of glucose absorption from the gastrointestinal tract and glucose utilization by the cells. It accelerates the rate of fat metabolism and decreases the quantity of circulating fats in the blood and liver. Thyroid hormones increase both the anabolic and catabolic rates of protein. With thyroxine the need for vitamins becomes greater, especially for the B complex and vitamin C.

Osteoclastic activity to a greater degree than osteoblastic activity is increased by thyroxine. Consequently, calcium and phosphorus are excreted, resulting in porous bones. It also may increase parathyroid hormone secretion, resulting in even greater bone absorption. Thyrocalcitonin, a relatively newly discovered hormone, is secreted by the thyroid in response to increased serum calcium, thereby increasing calcium deposition in the bones.

Disorders and Deviations

Hypothyroidism This condition may occur in the presence or absence of goiter. In *nongoitrous hypothyroidism* (also called *cretinism* and *myxedema*), the thyroid is absent or too small to maintain a euthyroid state. Hypothyroidism can be congenital or acquired. The clinical manifestations of nongoitrous hypothyroidism are dependent upon the extent of thyroid deficiency, the time of onset and duration, and the particular individual. At birth, most athyrotic infants appear to be normal. However, a thick tongue; the product of a prolonged pregnancy; an above-normal birth weight and length; large, puffy, and cyanotic facies; retarded prenatal osseous development; and prolonged neonatal jaundice may be viewed as suspicious of hypothyroidism.

As the hypothyroid child develops, the "unusually good baby" is recognized as lethargic. Crying is husky and gruntlike; reactions are slow. There is a loss of appetite and a lack of energy to suck. Respiratory infections with profuse mucus are common. Constipation due to decreased peristalsis and hypotonia of the abdominal muscles and diminished food intake is an early and frequent sign. Linear growth is decreased. Puffiness of the face and supraclavicular regions and protruding abdomen may disguise the poor nourishment. Thick, scaly skin with the exception of the greasy forehead and a yellowish tinge with mottling are characteristic. The hair is usually sparse and coarse. Cardiac enlargement and bradycardia may be present. Abnormal ECGs and EEGs are not infrequent.

The diagnosis of hypothyroidism is dependent upon clinical manifestations and thyroid function tests. Laboratory tests include serum protein–bound iodine, serum-free thyroxine (column T4), T3 test, and radioactive iodine (I^{131}) uptake. Radioactive

scanning is useful to determine the type of thyroid dysplasia and to detect small goiters. The absence of the distal bone of the femur demonstrated on x-ray has been found to occur only in the presence of hypothyroidism and in babies of diabetic mothers.

Hypothyroidism is treated by the administration of desiccated thyroid or a synthetic preparation such as sodium levothyroxine (Synthroid). The child receiving thyroid replacement is observed for symptoms of hyperthyroidism (described below), growth, bone age estimations, and serum protein–bound iodine levels. Treated children may develop an interest in life misinterpreted as thyrotoxicosis since the contrast between their interest and energy level prior to therapy and after therapy may be quite dramatic. Good rapport to avoid misunderstanding by parents is essential.

Hypothyroidism occurring prior to the age of 3 months is present at a vulnerable stage of cerebral development. The brain cell count continues to increase for the first 5 months of life, so the mental prognosis of hypothyroid babies and young infants is particularly guarded. Iatrogenic hypothyroidism and goiter may result from dietary manipulation and drug therapy. Certain formulas, especially soybean, diets deficient in iodine, and drugs such as the thiouracils, iodides, thyroxine, para-aminosalicylic acid, resorcinol, and phenylbutazone have antithyroid actions. Thyroidectomy results in hypothyroidism.

Hyperthyroidism This condition, also known as Graves' disease, Basedow's disease, and thyrotoxicosis, is thought to develop as a result of excessive production of thyrotropin by the adenohypophysis or the ingestion of exogenous thyroid. Increased oxygen consumption and heat production with intolerance to heat, increased perspiration, weight loss, diarrhea, muscular weakness, and nervousness occur. The pulse rate and systolic blood pressure increase in response to the increased demands for oxygen. *Exophthalmos*, protrusion of the eyeball and lid retraction, may be present because of an overgrowth of the tissue behind the eyeball.

Hyperthyroidism is more common in girls. It may be inherited or the result of an immunologic disturbance. The onset of hyperthyroidism may be insidious. Mild hyperthyroidism may terminate in remission or become severe suddenly. Children with severe hyperthyroidism have poor academic performance. Although they are highly motivated, their attention span is brief. The younger child tends to be hyperactive; the adolescent is restless. Insomnia and failure to concentrate are characteristic of the condition. The apical pulse can be seen in the thin-chested child, and a tachycardia as high as 160 to 200 may result from the increased metabolic needs. A voracious appetite accompanied by a loss of weight is common.

The diagnosis of hyperthyroidism is dependent upon the clinical manifestations and pertinent laboratory determinations including serum protein–bound iodine, radioactive iodine uptake by the thyroid gland, and butanol-extractable iodine. The patient may complain of a fullness or tightness of the neck as a result of an enlarged and frequently visible thyroid gland.

Therapy for the mildly hyperthyroid child includes mild sedation and a well-balanced high-caloric diet with frequent snacks. Reserpine and guanethidine may be administered for their antihypertensive and sedative effects. Both drugs deplete the body stores of catecholamines. Other drugs given to restore the euthyroid state include iodine, thiocyanate, perchlorate, and the thiourea derivatives (propylthiouracil, methimazole). These drugs have the potential to cause side effects of agranulocytosis, leukopenia, urticaria, edema of the legs, lymphadenopathy, loss of hair and taste, and abnormal pigmentation. The use of x-ray radiation has been practically abandoned because of its association with the development of thyroid cancer.

Radioactive iodine is concentrated in the thyroid and is used to destroy thyroid tissue. One of the thiourea derivatives is given for a week or so and terminated several days prior to administration of radioactive iodine to avoid a thyroid crisis. Radiation illness is infrequent. Thyroidectomy or surgical resection can be done. A small portion of the gland is usually left to decrease the risk of injuring the recurrent laryngeal nerves and inadvertently removing the parathyroid glands.

The most frequent complications following thyroidectomy are hypoparathyroidism, injury to the laryngeal nerves, hemorrhage, and thyroid storm. Transient hypoparathyroidism may occur as a result of edema of the tissues in the parathyroid area. Tetany appears within 48 hours postoperatively. Signs of impending tetany include sensory disturbances, nausea, and vomiting. The Chvostek and Trousseau signs may be positive. A mild hypoparathyroid state is treated by the administration of calcium lactate and a high-calcium, low-phosphorus diet and vitamin D. An acute episode of tetany is treated by the administration of calcium gluconate given slowly by the intravenous route. The pulse should be monitored and the injection terminated if bradycardia occurs. Parathyroid extract may be given subcutaneously, intramuscularly, or intravenously.

Bilateral paralysis of the recurrent laryngeal nerves and complete paralysis of the vocal cords can occur during thyroidectomy or in the early postoperative period. The airway must be maintained by tracheotomy for several months to facilitate recovery of one or both laryngeal nerves. Surgery on the larynx may be required, and the prognosis of restorative surgery is less favorable for children than for adults. Voice changes may result from damage to one of the recurrent laryngeal nerves or injury to the larynx or superior laryngeal nerve.

Postoperatively, the vital signs and neck are checked frequently to avert serious hemorrhage. Severe hemorrhage may compress the trachea and require immediate surgery to alleviate the resulting pressure.

Thyroid storm caused by the sudden release of thyroid hormone is best prevented by proper preoperative preparation. Thyroid storm is characterized by fever, restlessness, irritability, delirium, and finally shock. It can occur when a poorly nourished patient has an acute infection or emergency surgery or after radioactive iodine therapy in the absence of antithyroid drugs used prior to therapy. Treatment includes the intravenous administration of iodine, heavy sedation, reversal of cardiac failure, and reduction of temperature.

Thyroiditis When it occurs during childhood, thyroiditis may be acute, subacute, or chronic. Acute bacterial thyroiditis commonly due to beta-hemolytic streptococci is treated with antibiotics. Subacute thyroiditis, most frequently seen in adolescents, is manifested by fever, tender enlarged thyroid, increased sedimentation rate, and decreased or absent uptake of radioactive iodine. Chronic thyroiditis, also known as Hashimoto's thyroiditis, occurs in children of 6 to 16 years of age and is more common in girls. The resulting hypothyroidism is due to the presence of antibodies to thyroid hormone. The disease is treated by replacement therapy using desiccated thyroid.

Nursing Management

The observant nurse may be the first to notice symptoms of hyperthyroidism or hypothyroidism. This observation may be made in a presumably well-child clinic, in school, or in the public arena. Parents or the schoolteacher may report symptoms to the nurse first. Children with symptoms suggestive of thyroid dysfunction should be evaluated and treated, if necessary, as early as possible for effective therapy.

Hyperthyroidism is treated prior to surgery with drugs to decrease the size of the thyroid gland and avert thyroid crisis. Iodides are absorbed by the gastrointestinal tract and decrease the size of the thyroid gland effectively. The nurse observes the patient receiving iodides preoperatively for side effects of fever, rhinitis, edema of the eyelids, adenopathy, and skin rashes. The iodides are administered after being diluted with water or fruit juice to make them more palatable. Drinking the liquid through a straw further prevents tasting it. Thiouracil derivatives interfere with the formation of thyroxine and depress thyroid activity. Patients receiving a thiouracil derivative are observed for untoward effects of the drug; they are instructed to report the development of a sore throat, head cold, or malaise immediately. Other side effects include leukopenia, skin rash, drug fever, enlargement of the salivary glands and lymph nodes in the neck, hepatitis, loss of the sense of taste, edema of the lower extremities, and granulocytopenia.

The increased metabolism caused by excess thyroxine raises the tissues' demands for nutrients. To provide adequate nutrition for all the body's cells, diets rich in calories, carbohydrates, and vitamins are served to satisfy the appetite and protect the liver from damage. Food preferences are observed. The child and his parents should be helped to understand that food requirements are increased by the illness. Remarks about a ravenous appetite may make the child self-conscious and cause him to eat less than he needs. Rate, character, and rhythm of the pulse, respirations, and blood pressure are observed and recorded. The patient is further observed for signs and symptoms of cardiac failure.

Excessive amounts of thyroxine can cause diarrhea. The child is encouraged to eat slowly and to drink only a minimum of fluid during meals; between meals, fluids are encouraged. The stools are observed for frequency, color, consistency, and character.

Thyroxine affects the nervous system and may result in nervousness and psychoneurotic tendencies such as anxiety, extreme worry, and paranoia. Environmental stimuli for the hypersensitive patient should be reduced to a minimum. The patient's requests need to be answered promptly. The nurse informs and helps the family understand that behavior problems, such as a limited attention span and excessive activity, are a part of the illness. An increase of thyroxine causes vigorous muscle reaction; muscle exhaustion results when the amount of thyroxine is extreme. The nurse planning care for the patient assesses his limitations and abilities in an unhurried and relaxed manner and provides him with simple diversional activities.

Hyperthyroidism may be manifest by an enlargement of the thyroid located below the larynx on either side of the trachea and anterior to it. Dysphagia may result. The consistency of food most easily swallowed is identified by the nurse and provided in a form palatable to the patient. Means to facilitate heat loss, such as light bedclothing, pajamas to eliminate the need for covers, and adequate ventilation, are provided. Frequent bathing, sponging of the hands and face at intervals, limitation of muscular movement, and the encouragement of fluids provide comfort and adequate hydration in the presence of diaphoresis.

Constant fatigue in the presence of insomnia is a characteristic of hyperthyroidism. Sleep and rest are encouraged by providing a nonstimulating environment and psychologic, physiologic, and muscular relaxation. Diversional activities and a sedative may be employed to promote rest. The patient with exophthalmos may have a loss of vision. He is taught to close his eyes at intervals to moisten the cornea. Tape may be required at night to keep the eyes closed if the palpebral fissure is severe.

Prior to thyroidectomy, the patient and his family are informed regarding the usual preoperative and postoperative practices to facilitate their understanding and cooperation. Nursing care following thyroidectomy includes supporting the head to prevent strain on the incision and to maintain the desirable anatomic position. Observations for bleeding into the tissues surrounding the operative site are made; signs of hypoparathyroidism, thyroid crisis, and obstruction of breathing, if noted, are treated appropriately. Calcium lactate and a tracheotomy tray are readily available.

Adequate explanation of the use of radioactive iodine to destroy thyroid tissue is essential to alleviate fears of radioactivity that the parents and child may have. The patient receiving radioactive iodine must be closely observed for symptoms of hyperthyroidism on the fourth or fifth day of therapy, for at this time large amounts of thyroxine may be released from the necrotic thyroid cells.

A deficiency of thyroxine results in extreme somnolence and mental sluggishness. Hypothyroid patients cannot be hurried or stimulated to move rapidly; they must be permitted to proceed at their own pace. They may not have normal functioning of the cerebral cortex. They must be closely observed and assisted to meet their basic physiologic needs.

Soap is used sparingly; lanolin or lotion may provide some relief of the scaly skin present in myxedema.

The level of endogenous organic iodine in the blood is a measure of the amount of circulating thyroxine. The previous ingestion of iodine may alter the PBI, BEI, and I^{131} uptake values. The patient and/or his parents are questioned about previous medications that may interfere with the diagnostic laboratory tests, i.e., any iodide preparation such as intravenous pyelograms and similar x-ray, iodine, and antithyroid preparations.

Vitamins are an essential part of some of the enzymes required to synthesize and release thyroid hormones. The use of iodized salt is a simple form of primary prevention of goiter. Goiter is more likely to occur during puberty, pregnancy, and gastrointestinal infections when the iodine requirement is increased or the absorption of iodine is impaired. The general public needs to be trained to observe the principles of adequate nutrition and the use of iodized salt. Fad diets are to be avoided.

Thyroid deficiency is treated by giving replacement therapy with oral tablets. The effect of this therapy is cumulative, and the full effect of a maintenance dosage is not seen for 7 to 10 days. Similarly, the effects of thyroid are long-lasting, and so toxic effects can develop and persist. The nurse is observant for, and instructs the patient to observe for, toxic effects resembling hyperthyroidism.

PARATHYROID GLANDS
Physiology

There are usually four parathyroid glands, but the number varies from two to six in human beings. Although the parathyroid glands are usually located on the underside of the thyroid gland, parathyroid tissue has been found in such sites as the connective tissue and fat of the neck, in the mediastinum, behind the esophagus, and within the thyroid capsule. Parathyroid hormone secretion is regulated by a negative feedback system on the level of plasma ionized calcium. Parathyroid hormone appears to increase serum calcium and decrease serum phosphate by affecting absorption from the bone, by the kidney, and from the gastrointestinal tract.

Disorders and Deviations

Hypocalcemia   In the newborn, hypocalcemia has been related to the low calcium–high phosphorus ratio of cow's milk, immaturity of the renal system, inadequate parathyroid hormone, and complicated pregnancies and labors. Tetany occurring within the

first 2 days after birth and associated with an abnormal pregnancy and/or labor may be due to the increased destruction of the neonate's tissues, causing an increase in the circulating phosphate or an increase of adrenocorticosteroids which may cause a hypocalcemic effect.

Hypocalcemia in the infant usually occurs within the first 2 weeks after birth. Characteristic symptoms include hyperactivity, muscle twitching, and a heightened startle response. Laryngospasm, carpopedal spasm, and Chvostek's sign may occur. Seizures, vomiting, and intestinal spasms similar to those of intestinal obstruction, edema possibly related to the ingestion of cow's milk and its heavy solute component, and cardiopulmonary symptoms of apnea, tachycardia, and tachypnea due to the decreased concentration of serum calcium may occur. Neonatal tetany is usually associated with serum calcium levels of less than 8.0 mg/100 ml. The serum inorganic phosphorus values are variable but tend to be increased.

The symptoms of neonatal tetany are similar to those of other central nervous system disorders. Carpopedal spasms may be present in the presence of central nervous system diseases, and Chvostek's sign may be positive in normal children. An examination of cerebrospinal fluid may be done to determine the presence of central nervous system disease; however, central nervous system disease and tetany may both be present after a complicated labor and delivery. The infants are usually responsive with good Moro and sucking reflexes and normal crying.

Neonatal tetany is treated initially by administering calcium salts, preferably calcium gluconate intravenously. Calcium solutions must be administered slowly to avoid the toxic reaction of circulatory collapse, nausea, and vomiting. Care must be taken to avoid extravasation of calcium, for calcium is very irritating to the tissues and may cause extensive sloughing if allowed to infiltrate the surrounding tissues.

Calcium mixed with the formula is administered for a week or longer after the acute symptoms have been controlled. Calcium chloride is more irritating to the gastrointestinal tract than calcium gluconate or lactate and should be given in concentrations of 2 percent or less and for a period less than 48 hours. Breast milk or a formula resembling the calcium-phosphorus ratio of breast milk is recommended. The prognosis of neonatal tetany is largely dependent upon the presence or absence of other complications. Thus, the prognosis of infants associated with complicated pregnancies and deliveries is poorer than of those infants who develop tetany later.

Nursing Management

Prior to adequate treatment of hypocalcemia, the nurse is confronted with the actual or potential symptoms associated with tetany. He must observe the child for signs of calcium deficit. These signs and their manifestations include carpopedal spasm (muscle spasms of the feet and hands), muscle twitching, and seizures. Tests of hypocalcemia include *Chvostek's sign* demonstrated by twitching of the facial muscles when the child's facial nerve (below the temple) is tapped. A positive *Trousseau's sign* is demonstrated by palmar flexion when the circulation at the wrist is constricted for a few minutes. The absence or presence of the signs and symptoms of hypocalcemia must be identified and recorded; appropriate actions are to be taken when the signs and symptoms change from negative to positive or vice versa.

Seizures may also occur. The child having a hypocalcemic seizure is an emergency situation. Calcium is required immediately, and measures to provide it must be taken at once (see Chap. 32).

THYMUS GLAND

The thymus gland is a two-lobed structure lying just behind the upper part of the sternum in front of the beginning of the aorta and the pulmonary artery. The thymic cells become reticulum cells capable of conversion to plasma cells under the stimulus of antigens. Consequently, the absence of the thymus in the fetus or newborn influences the ability of the child to produce antibodies. The reader should consult specific references for additional information regarding theories of the role of the thymus in autoimmune diseases (see the "Bibliography" at the end of this chapter).

ADRENAL GLANDS
Physiology

The adrenal gland consists of the adrenal medulla and the adrenal cortex. The adrenal medulla secretes the hormones norepinephrine and epinephrine in response to sympathetic nervous system stimulation. Both hormones are vasoconstrictors. Epinephrine also increases heart rate, cardiac conduction rate, and ventricular contractility and relaxes bronchiolar musculature. The hormones secreted by the adrenal cortex are of three major types—miner-

alocorticoid, glucocorticoid, and normal small amounts of sex hormones, namely androgenic, estrogenic, and progesterone compounds. The mineralocorticoids principally affect the electrolytes of the extracellular fluids, especially sodium, potassium, and chloride. The major mineralocorticoid is aldosterone. The glucocorticoids affect the metabolism of carbohydrates, proteins, and fats. The most important glucocorticoids are cortisol and corticosterone; the latter exerts both glucocorticoid effect and a small amount of mineralocorticoid effect.

The major effect of the glucocorticoids is to stimulate gluconeogenesis by the liver. They also decrease the utilization of glucose by the cells. Consequently, they cause the blood sugar to increase. The glucocorticoids cause decreased protein anabolism and reduce the protein stores in the body except in the liver. Amino acids are mobilized from the tissues. Fat metabolism is affected by mobilizing fatty acids, yet the storage of adipose tissue is increased. Cortisol is secreted in response to corticotropin and corticotropin production is influenced by the level of blood cortisol—a negative feedback system. Cortisol secretion is increased in response to the stress of trauma, intense temperature, sympathomimetic drugs, surgery, fright, and debilitating disease; cortisol has an anti-inflammatory effect. It decreases the number of eosinophils and lymphocytes and increases the number of red blood cells.

Disorders and Deviations

Cushing's Disease and Syndrome *Cushing's syndrome* results from adrenal cortical hypersecretion and may be caused by adrenocortical tumors or adrenocortical hyperplasia as a result of pituitary or nonendocrine tumors (Fig. 39-6). *Cushing's disease* is a combination of adrenocorticotropin excess and adrenal hyperplasia. Adrenocortical carcinoma and adenoma are twice as frequent in females and may be detected as early as 3 months of age (Fig. 39-7). Symptoms include plethora, truncal and facial obesity, mild diabetes, muscle weakness, hypertension, easy bruisability, purplish striae, mental changes, mild hirsutism, acne, and menstrual irregularities. Virilization is common in both conditions.

Laboratory findings include glycosuria, hyperglycemia, and elevated cortisol levels. The absence of a diurnal variation of cortisol levels is usually noted. Hypokalemia and hypochloremia occur less frequently in children than in adults. X-ray films demonstrate osteoporosis of the bone and delayed epiphyseal maturation.

Diagnosis is dependent upon the physical exam-

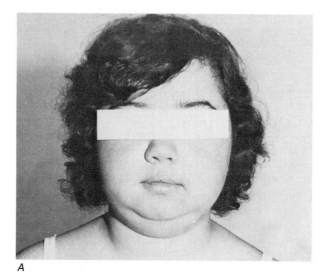

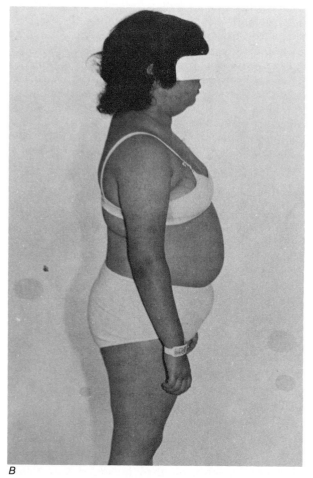

Figure 39-6 Pituitary Cushing's disease in a 13-year-old female. (*A*) Note facial rounding and hairline. (*B*) Note central obesity and "buffalo hump."

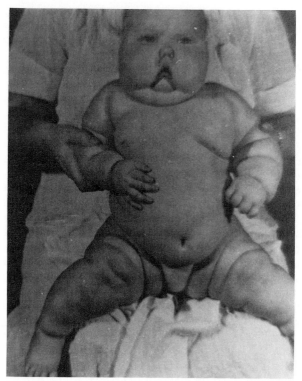

Figure 39-7 A 9-month-old baby with an adrenal adenoma.

ination, plasma cortisol levels, and the excretion of 17-ketogenic steroids. Diagnostic tests include the ACTH infusion stimulation test and dexamethasone and metapyrone suppression tests. Radiologic examinations include intravenous pyelogram, pneumoencephalogram, and abdominal flat plates. Radioactive isotopic scanning may be done.

Iatrogenic Cushing's syndrome may occur after ACTH and cortisone therapy used for autoimmune diseases, leukemia, nephrotic syndrome, and arthritis. Symptoms of prolonged dosage resemble those of Cushing's disease caused by excessive endogenous cortisol secretion. The greatest danger of iatrogenic Cushing's disease is suppression of the inflammatory response resulting in overwhelming infections and suppression of the hypophysis-hypothalamus and adrenal response.

Surgery is the choice of treatment in adrenal tumor. Adrenal tumors suppress the hypothalamic-pituitary axis (see Fig. 39-8) and the uninvolved adrenal. Thus, cortisone is administered prior to and during surgery and during convalescence. Cortisol in replacement doses is given during severe stress.

Total adrenalectomy may be the selected therapy when there is adrenal hyperplasia. Irradiation of

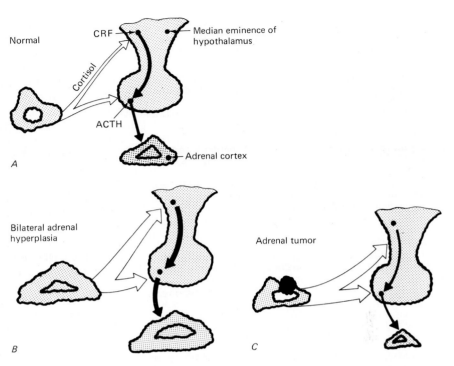

Figure 39-8 The adrenal-pituitary axis. (*A*) Normal relation of plasma cortisol levels, hypothalamic CRF release, and ACTH release. (*B*) Excessive ACTH release results in bilateral adrenal hyperplasia with hypersecretion of cortisol. (*C*) Excessive cortisol production by adrenal tumors leads to suppression of hypothalamic-pituitary ACTH release and consequent atrophy of the contralateral adrenal gland. (*Source: Reprinted from T. Frawley, "Cushing's Syndrome," in G. W. Thorn et al. (eds.), Clinician-1: The Adrenal Gland, MEDCOM Press, New York, 1971, p. 40.*)

the pituitary or hypophysectomy may be used when there is evidence of an enlarging pituitary tumor or to prevent Nelson's syndrome after adrenalectomy. *Nelson's syndrome* includes excessive pigmentation due to increased ACTH secretion and the formation of tumors of the pituitary after adrenalectomy. Cortisol is administered parenterally initially after adrenalectomy. The replacement doses of hydrocortisone or cortisol, supplementary salt, and the potent mineralocorticoid, 9α-fluorohydrocortisone (Florinef), if needed, are taken by mouth when the patient is able to tolerate them. Within a year following total adrenalectomy, the overt signs of Cushing's disease disappear. However, the demineralization of the vertebral bodies, diabetes mellitus, hypertension, and renal calculi may persist.

Adrenal Insufficiency In infancy adrenal insufficiency is characterized by a salt-losing syndrome including weight loss, fever, vomiting, hyponatremia, hyperkalemia, metabolic acidosis, and hyperpigmentation. This condition is most commonly associated with congenital adrenal hypoplasia, but it can be due to enzymatic defects, tubular insensitivity to mineralocorticoids, adrenal cysts, and hemorrhage or calcification in the adrenal.

The clinical manifestation of adrenal cortical insufficiency varies with the age of the patient and the rapidity with which the insufficiency occurs. The young child experiences dehydration, vomiting, intermittent fever, hyponatremia, hypochloremia, and hyperkalemia. The older child experiences general weakness, anorexia, weight loss with dehydration, nausea, vomiting, and diarrhea. Hyperpigmentation of mucous membranes and skin, especially of the genitalia, scars, areolas, and buccal mucosa, is usually present. Acute infection usually is the precipitating cause of adrenal cortical insufficiency. Circulatory failure, delirium, coma, severe abdominal pain, metabolic acidosis, hypoglycemia due to the loss of sodium and chloride, and hemoconcentration are usual symptoms.

Adrenal function is tested by examining the level of the adrenocortical hormones in the blood and urine, serum glucose, tolerance to glucose, and electrolytes, especially the ratio of sodium to potassium in the urine, sweat, and saliva.

Congenital Adrenal Hyperplasia This condition, also known as adrenogenital syndrome, can contribute to errors of steroid metabolism with overproduction of one or more of the steroid categories. The possibility for a variety of defects occurs because the adrenals are capable of synthesizing all categories of steroids from cholesterol. Therefore, the adrenals have pathways to form aldosterone from mineralocorticoids, cortisol from glucocorticoids, and testosterone and estrogen from androgens. The most common defects are:

1 21-Hydroxylase deficiency resulting in cortisol deficiency leading to excessive ACTH secretion and ending with excessive androgen production
2 21-Hydroxylase deficiency with sodium loss where both cortisol and aldosterone production are affected
3 11-Hydroxylase deficiency resulting in cortisol deficiency and excessive amounts of mineralocorticoid leading to androgenic manifestations and vascular hypertension
4 3β-Hydroxydehydrogenase and isomerase deficiency resulting in a disturbance of glucocorticoid and mineralocorticoid synthesis, severe salt-losing syndrome, disturbed differentiation of external genital organs in the male, male pseudohermaphroditism, and possibly slight virilization of the female
5 17-Hydroxylase deficiency resulting in cortisol deficiency, primary aldosteronism leading to benign hypertension, hypovolemia, low plasma renin activity unresponsive to low sodium intake, hyperaldosteronism, and mild hypokalemic alkalosis

Congenital adrenal hyperplasia is a familial, autosomal, recessive hereditary disease. Both sexes are affected with the same frequency. Diagnosis is dependent upon the family history. Unexplained infant deaths, excessively tall children with sexual precocity, and dwarfed adult stature provide helpful clues. Laboratory measurements of 17-ketosteroids, 11-deoxyketosteroids, pregnanetriolone and pregnanetetrol, aldosterone, and 17-hydroxycorticosteroids in the urine are diagnostic. Deficient mineralocorticoid synthesis causes hyponatremia, hyperkalemia, and metabolic acidosis. The response of abnormal steroid values to corticosteroid substitutional therapy is tested by giving cortisol hemisuccinate and measuring 17-ketosteroids in the urine. The bone age of the baby with congenital adrenal hyperplasia is normal at birth. Thereafter, there is abnormal acceleration of osseous maturation and testicular development.

The anatomy of the female with viralizing signs of adrenal hyperplasia is visualized by urethroscopy, colposcopy, and roentgenography to determine her condition prior to plastic surgery. Exposure of the external genitalia to androgenic hormones during the process of differentiation of the urogenital sinus into the urethra and vagina around the ninth to the twelfth fetal week results in masculinization. Normally, testosterone is thought to be the responsible hormone; however, in female hermaphroditism, the fetal adrenals secrete sufficient androgen to result in various degrees of masculinization of the external genitalia. Clitoral hypertrophy may

occur any time in fetal life or postpartum in response to excessive androgen (see Figs. 39-9 and 39-10).

Clinical manifestations of increased androgen production are advanced skeletal and sexual development. Growth ceases at an early chronologic age because of premature epiphyseal fusion resulting in a dwarfed adult. Muscle development is enhanced. Axillary, facial, and body hair may appear at an early age.

Severe dehydration and circulatory insufficiency in those with salt-losing syndrome are treated with hydrocortisone intravenously. Deoxycorticosterone is administered intramuscularly or intravenously. The blood pressure and serum electrolytes are monitored closely to determine hydration and the cardiovascular state. Hyperkalemia is treated with sodium bicarbonate in 5 percent dextrose in normal saline or 10 percent dextrose in water. Calcium may be given intravenously if cardiac problems are identified. Cation exchange resin retention enemas with, for example, sodium polystyrene sulfonate (Kayexalate) may be administered.

Oral hydrocortisone is the drug of choice for long-term therapy. The circadian cycle of endogenous corticosteroid is imitated by giving hydrocortisone in three or four divided doses daily with an equal time interval between doses. Fluid hydrocortisone (Cortef) is a palatable form of hydrocortisone available for infants. Fluorocortisone acetate (Florinef Acetate) is given to those with salt-losing forms of congenital adrenal hyperplasia. Deoxycorticosterone acetate (DCA) pellets implanted every 3 to 4 months, and deoxycorticosterone trimethylacetate (Percorten M) intramuscularly monthly may be used if there is unreliable administration of the drug. The blood pressure is measured carefully. Salt intake is increased in those with salt-losing syndrome; however, the requirement for additional salt decreases with age.

Surgical correction is performed to make the genitals appear normal before the infant becomes aware of his abnormal genitalia. In the female, the procedures may be done in steps, for example, separation of the fused labia, widening of the external orifice of the urogenital sinus to treat or avoid the urinary tract infections which commonly occur, and reconstruction of the clitoris. Clitoral enlargement seems to diminish when hormonal treatment is instituted early. Hypospadias and bilateral cryptorchidism may be surgically repaired. If the external genitalia are phenotypically female, the testes may be removed, estrogens administered, and a female gender role assigned.

The follow-up evaluations include studies to

indicate androgen suppression, the development of cushingoid features, and optimum growth. The prognosis for the child with adrenal hyperplasia is excellent if the disorder is recognized early and replacement therapy is instituted early. The gonadotropins induce their appropriate effects, and an uncomplicated and isosexual puberty is likely to occur in both sexes.

Nursing Management

The patient and the parents need much understanding and explanation. As with pituitary disorders, the body image is altered with Cushing's disease. The child may be considered fat and "dumpy" because of the distribution of adipose tissue, the retention of fluids, and the effect of cortisol upon bone growth. In addition, acne may be very unattractive and bothersome owing to the effect of cortisol upon the sebaceous glands. The child may be considered a weakling on account of his weakened muscles and bones, or he may be considered just fat and lazy.

The child with hypercortisolism is especially prone to infections due to the immunosuppressive action of cortisol. Chest x-rays to determine the presence of tuberculosis or other mycotic infection are in order. The child should be protected from undue exposure to infection. Susceptibility to injury is increased also. The muscles have lost strength; the bones may be fragile, and the child is uncoordinated. In addition, the skin has become thin, and there is a tendency to bruise readily. Care should be taken to avoid unnecessary overinflation of the blood pressure cuff to avoid bruising. Venipunctures and injections need to be accomplished with the least trauma possible. The diet should be rich in potassium and protein and relatively low in carbohydrates and sodium because of the loss of potassium and protein and the presence of hyperglycemia and fluid retention. Plasma cortisol levels must be obtained at the times specified to determine diurnal variations and levels. The environment should be as calm as possible to prevent the effect of excitement on cortisol level.

Medications for diagnostic tests such as dexamethasone (Decadron) suppression and metyrapone (Metopirone) must be administered as designated by the physician to provide valid blood and urine levels for differential diagnoses. It is helpful to give both metyrapone and dexamethasone with food to avoid gastric distress. Urine collections must be obtained accurately, i.e., beginning and ending the collection at the designated time and obtaining complete col-

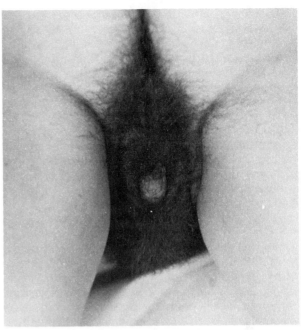

Figure 39-9   Congenital adrenal hyperplasia in a 7-year-old female. Note pubic hair and enlarged clitoris.

lections. Instruction, understanding, and cooperation of the patients regarding specimen collection is essential for accurate collections. X-ray procedures are explained as to the expected behavior of the patient and the rationale for performing the procedure.

Medications given to treat metastatic disease of the adrenals are toxic. Much support and understanding is necessary to attain the patient's cooperation to take dichlorodiphenyldichlorolthane (Lysodren) and aminoglutethimide (Elipten) because nausea, vomiting, anorexia, and diarrhea are

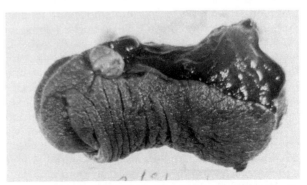

Figure 39-10   Clitoris of a 7-year-old female with congenital adrenal hyperplasia.

the usual side effects when the drugs are taken in therapeutic doses.

Adrenalectomy, when selected as the therapy of choice for treating hyperadrenocorticism, involves preoperative and postoperative nursing care. Preoperatively, the patient is informed of the usual routine practiced at the particular hospital and by the individual surgeon. Preoperative instruction and the practice of deep breathing, coughing, and using blow bottles are helpful to prevent pulmonary complications. This preparation is particularly beneficial if a flank approach is planned because the incision will be close to the diaphragm, and the pulmonary toilet is more painful.

Following adrenalectomy, the patient is likely to have a nasogastric tube and infusion therapy. The blood pressure is monitored closely, for hypertension can occur as a result of the manipulation of the glands and excessive hormones in the circulation. Shock is more of a threat than hypertension as pronounced hypotension occurs as cortisol levels become deficient. Cortisol is administered parenterally to sustain the patient throughout the immediate postoperative period. Pressor amines may be administered to maintain the blood pressure within normal limits. Physiologic shock may occur if the patient's blood pressure is considerably lower postoperatively. Urine output is observed closely. Volumes of less than 30 ml/hour are indicative of hypotension and/or hypovolemia and are reported immediately.

Recovery from anesthesia may be delayed because of the amount of anesthetic used and the fact that it is retained within the fat cells. The prolonged effect of the anesthetic predisposes the patient to problems of shock, and the maintenance of vital processes is made more difficult.

Postoperative care includes the maintenance of the pulmonary toilet by using blow bottles, intermittent positive pressure breathing, coughing, and deep breathing to promote lung expansion and prevent infection. Position changes are important to promote circulation and prevent thrombosis. The usual care for the patient with nasogastric drainage is employed. The anterior approach results in discomfort due to the manipulation of the bowel and the inhibition of peristalsis causing nausea and vomiting. Analgesics are administered as needed to facilitate convalescence. Normal activities and a diet rich in protein and potassium are resumed as soon as possible. The previously diabetic patient will continue to have serum glucose levels measured. Sugar and acetone levels of the urine will be determined.

The postoperative adrenal insufficiency resulting from adrenalectomy is treated as is the adrenal insufficiency of Addison's disease. Cortisol is essential for life. The dosage is usually divided as described earlier. It is essential that the patient and his family understand the cortisol requirement. In addition to the regular cortisol supplement, the nurse instructs the patient and his family regarding the use of parenteral cortisol or dexamethasone in emergency situations. It is useful for the patient and parents to observe injection technique and practice the technique using the usual equipment and an orange. After a sufficient learning period, the patient injects himself using sterile water. Sometimes it is helpful for the nurse to demonstrate self-injection using her leg and sterile water. The anterior portion of the upper leg is utilized for the injection site because it is convenient and a safe location. Prefilled Decadron syringes are available and facilitate the technique in an emergency setting. The patient is instructed to administer the dexamethasone or hydrocortisone whenever he is unable to retain (due to nausea and vomiting) the oral replacement drug for longer than 4 hours, whenever he faints, or if he is involved in an automobile accident. Each time it is necessary to administer the parenteral medication, a physician should be consulted to determine if further action is indicated.

Patients are taught and learn by their own experience the management of their replacement drugs. Minor adjustments in dosages to meet increased stresses are necessary. See Fig. 39-5 for common stresses and dosage modifications. An identification (Medic-Alert) necklace or bracelet with the inscription Adrenal Insufficiency should be worn at all times.

The patient with aldosteronism is observed especially for digitalis intoxication and hypokalemia. Constipation is a frequent problem due to potassium deficiency causing atony of the intestinal muscles. Bulky foods and adequate fluids are encouraged. Aldosteronism is frequently treated with adrenalectomy. Postoperative care is similar to that previously described except that the most common problems are associated with fluid and electrolytes and cardiac problems rather than complications from glucocorticoid excess.

ISLETS OF LANGERHANS
Physiology

The islets of Langerhans are composed of alpha cells which secrete glucagon and beta cells which secrete insulin. Insulin is composed of two amino acids and affects carbohydrate metabolism by increasing the rate of glucose metabolism, decreasing the blood glucose concentration, and increasing the glycogen stores in the tissues. Thus, as can be readily ascertained, insulin affects total body metabolism. Metabolism is affected by increasing the glucose utilized by most of the body tissues by facilitating the movement of glucose into cell bodies. Skeletal and adipose tissue make up approximately 65 percent of the weight of the body, and the enhanced transport of glucose into these tissues is particularly profound. However, insulin fails to enhance the transport of glucose into the brain cells, the interstitial mucosa, and the tubular epithelium of the kidney, making up less than 5 percent of the total body mass.

Insulin enhances the storage of glycogen in the skeletal cells throughout the body and moderately enhances the glycogen storage in cells such as the skin and glandular tissues. The liver has an important role in the regulation of blood glucose concentration and the control of insulin secretion. The liver stores glucose and prevents an excessive increase in blood glucose concentration by storing glucose as glycogen. When the blood glucose concentration falls below normal, the liver releases glucose stored as glycogen to maintain a normal blood glucose level. The regulation of blood glucose concentration is vital because glucose is the only nutrient that can be utilized to provide the energy required by the brain, retina, and germinal epithelial cells.

Insulin is not known to affect fat metabolism directly. However, insulin affects carbohydrate metabolism profoundly, and fat and carbohydrate metabolism supply the majority of energy for the body and thus affect fat metabolism indirectly. Glucose is preferred to fat to supply energy when both glucose and insulin supplies are adequate. However, when either glucose or insulin is insufficient, fat is mobilized to provide energy. In the absence of insulin, lipid components in the plasma are elevated. Increased fat metabolism is also associated with ketosis. Two theories advanced for the explanation of ketosis are the following. (1) Excessive production of acetoacetic acid occurs when large quantities of fat are mobilized and utilized for energy resulting in an increased concentration of acetoacetic acid in the extracellular fluid. (It is recalled that the adrenocortical secretion of glucocorticoids is increased in the absence of insulin, and the mobilization of fats from fat storage areas is further enhanced.) (2) Acetoacetic acid is not utilized as efficiently in the peripheral tissues in the absence of insulin.

Protein in addition to fat is mobilized and used for energy when carbohydrates are not available. Insulin is essential for growth due to its protein-sparing effect on increased carbohydrate metabolism and the direct effect of insulin on protein anabolism by increasing the transport of amino acids through the cell membranes. Growth hormone has very little effect in promoting growth in the absence of insulin.

Disorders and Deviations

Diabetes Mellitus   When part of or all the ability to utilize carbohydrate is lost due to a deficiency of insulin, diabetes mellitus results. It is a genetically determined, chronic, metabolic disorder characterized by hyperglycemia. Most children with diabetes mellitus have the juvenile form characterized by ketosis and acidosis as well as hyperglycemia. Children with juvenile diabetes are dependent upon the administration of exogenous insulin to control symptoms and maintain life. Overweight children may develop diabetes mellitus resembling maturity-onset diabetes. These children have hyperglycemia without ketosis; weight reduction sometimes results in the disappearance of chemical abnormalities. Secondary diabetes may occur with hyperadrenalism, hyperthyroidism, excessive secretion of growth hormone, and pheochromocytomas.

Chemical onset of diabetes may occur at any time during childhood; the incidence in males and females is equal. Between 4 and 5 percent of all diabetics have juvenile diabetes. Heredity is apparently a predisposing factor to the development of diabetes mellitus; however, the exact mode of inheritance is complicated because clinical manifestation are varied and may appear at any age. Expression of the clinical manifestation probably requires the genetic abnormality to be present in both parents. Factors other than genetic ones are also involved in provoking the clinical expression of the disease.

The importance of insulin in metabolic functions is demonstrated by the catabolic state that ensues when insulin supply is deficient or absent. Insulin insufficiency decreases the utilization of glucose by muscle and adipose tissue and at the same time results in an increased glucose output by the liver. Thus, the decreased glucose utilization by the peripheral tissues and increased gluconeogenesis by the liver result in hyperglycemia. The blood glucose level is further increased when there is increased secretion of growth hormone, glucagon, corticotropin, luteotropic hormone, and thyrotropic hormone. These other hormones act to increase blood glucose concentration by promoting gluconeogenesis and opposing the transport of glucose through the membranes. Growth hormone, also, is able to stimulate the islets of Langerhans directly. The increased concentration of glucose in the blood reaches the kidneys and increases the amount of glucose that must be excreted by the kidney. The ability of the kidney to concentrate glucose is limited, resulting in an osmotic diuresis. Thus, these actions explain the polyuria observed in most poorly controlled diabetics and during the development of ketoacidosis.

Insulin insufficiency also leads to an accelerated lipolysis of fats, resulting in an increase of fatty acids sent to the liver and the accelerated formation of ketone bodies (acetoacetic acid and β-hydroxybutyric acid). The ketone bodies are released into the bloodstream and metabolized to some extent, but are excreted into the urine when overproduced where they can be detected by a positive Acetest reaction. The excretion of the anion portion of the ketone bodies requires cations (sodium, potassium, magnesium, and calcium). Thus the hydrogen ion is increased and compensated for by the conversion and excretion of monobasic salts as dibasic salts and increased ammonia production. These compensatory mechanisms readily become inadequate as the diabetic state progresses, resulting in the accumulation of carbonic acid which dissociates into water and carbon dioxide. Increased carbon dioxide levels lead to hyperpnea and a lowered P_{CO_2}. An uncompensated acidosis results from the progressive accumulation of hydrogen ion.

Nausea, vomiting, and decreased fluid intake result in dehydration, a primary factor in ketoacidosis. Dehydration results from increased urine output combined with decreased fluid intake. Dehydration interferes with normal kidney function, and ketone bodies accumulate in the blood more rapidly. Ketoacidosis can lead to altered consciousness, coma, and, if untreated, death. The prevention and treatment of acidosis are discussed later.

The length of time insulin deficiency has been present is directly related to the clinical symptoms. Transient glucosuria may occur in the presence of stress, illness, or overeating. Spontaneous hypoglycemia may precede the onset of diabetic symptoms by several years. The more typical symptoms of weight loss, polydipsia, polyphagia, and polyuria may be present. Bed-wetting in a previously trained child is a frequent occurrence. Continuous diuresis produces progressive dehydration, resulting in dry skin and mucous membranes, flushed cheeks, and sunken eyeballs. Progressive ketoacidosis results in hyperpnea, drowsiness, and ultimately coma. Nausea, vomiting, abdominal pain, and occasionally abdominal rigidity may be present.

The chemical abnormalities of hyperglycemia, glucosuria, and ketosis are considered sufficient for the diagnosis of diabetes mellitus. The serum lipids increase to the extent that the serum is opalescent and may result in a falsely low interpretation of electrolyte values as ketoacidosis increases. Blood potassium levels may initially be abnormally high; however, the total body potassium is almost invariably low. Urine, in addition to glucose and ketone bodies, may occasionally contain albumin and casts.

Glucosuria and hyperglycemia may occur with exogenous or endogenous increases of cortisone and in children with hyperthyroidism, pheochromocytoma, head injuries, and hypothalamic lesions. Minimal glucosuria is associated with thiazide diuretics. Renal tubular disease results in glucosuria without hyperglycemia.

Most authorities now believe the indications for an oral glucose tolerance test are few; however, if the test is indicated, it needs to be performed in the following manner.

1   The subject must ingest at least 300 Gm of carbohydrate daily for 3 days prior to the test.
2   After an overnight fast, the subject is kept at rest. A palatable glucose solution containing 1.75 Gm of glucose/kg body weight is administered orally over a 5-minute period. (In children under 18 months of age, the glucose is increased to 3.0 Gm of glucose/kg body weight.)
3   Blood samples are obtained for fasting and 30, 90, 120, and 180 minutes postingestion of the glucose to follow the glucose values in the blood.

The nurse assists in obtaining valid results and the cooperation of the patient and his family by explanation of the diet preceding the test, the administration of the glucose solution, and the collection of blood specimens. The commercially prepared glucose solutions are more palatable if given with ice and drunk through a straw. A heparin-lock (venipuncture maintained patent for blood drawing by the instillation of a small amount of heparin to prevent the occlusion of the needle or catheter) may simplify and avoid the repeated trauma of multiple blood sampling, especially if the venipunctures are difficult.

The insulin requirement for children gradually decreases after acute acidosis, but then gradually increases to a usual level of 0.5 to 1.0 unit/kg body weight daily. Exercise decreases the insulin requirement. Acceptable control is demonstrated by a child who feels well, grows normally, and has normal energy; who is free of hypoglycemic reactions and ketones in the urine; and whose glycosuria is not often in excess of ½ to ¾ percent reaction in premeal and bedtime urine testing. Most physicians who care for juvenile diabetics agree that the psychotic and physical hazards of strict control are not warranted by studies indicating that aglycosuria reduces cardiovascular complications. Evidence that cardiovascular problems are an integral part of the disease of diabetes and not just a complication has also been cited.

Nursing Management

The nurse and the physician must attain a collaborative relationship with each other and with the child, with his parents individually and together to educate, answer questions, and facilitate the development of a healthy acceptance of diabetes. On the average the child can be taught to do his own urine testing at 6 or 7 years of age and to give himself injections when he is 7 or 8. While encouraged to assume increasing responsibility, the child cannot be expected to perform the task of caring for his diabetes independently until he is 13 or 14 years old.

The child and his parents are taught insulin administration, urine testing, prevention of ketoacidosis, foot care, and hygiene. They are also taught to make minor adjustments in insulin dosage on the basis of urine glucose and acetone. When acetone appears in the morning specimen accompanied with increased glucosuria, additional crystalline insulin is administered with the daily dose of insulin (one-fifth of the morning dose for moderate or large amounts of acetone and one-tenth for small amounts). In the presence of fever, vomiting, or persistent acetonuria, a visit to the physician and/or emergency room is indicated.

Insulin is a protein and therefore must be given by a parenteral route. It is available in short, long, and intermediate forms and in concentrations normally of 40, 80, and 100 units/ml. The vials of insulin in use are kept out of direct sunlight at room temperature. (Insulin kept at room temperature is thought to cause less damage to the subcutaneous tissues.) All vials of insulin not being used daily need to be refrigerated. Vials of insulin taken with one when traveling need to be kept on one's person because baggage may be subjected to extreme temperatures and pressures incompatible with the stability of insulin.

Injection technique is taught to the child by discussion, demonstration, and practice. Injection sites are rotated so that a particular site is not used more frequently than once every 90 days. (See Fig. 39-11.) All general areas of injection sites are demonstrated; the abdomen is not often utilized. (The abdomen, with the exception of 1 inch around the umbilicus, is readily accessible, and its use should be encouraged.) The "pinching up" of the subcutaneous tissue to be injected is preferable to the more traumatic technique of "stretching" the skin.

Children and their parents are taught only one method of determining the presence of sugar and acetone in the urine. A chart to record the urine-testing results is provided. The child and his family must have specific instruction regarding what results are desirable for him and the appropriate action to take when the test results are other than those desired.

The nurse must work closely with the child and his family, pointing out the necessity of following the directions accompanying the brand of reagent used. For example, observing the time interval for reading; observing the Clinitest reaction for "pass-through" phenomenon; using the correct color chart for the brand of reagent and the method used (two-drop versus five-drop); and the correct handling and use of the reagent by keeping it dry and employing unexpired reagent only. (See Table 39-3.)

Foot care is taught in an attempt to prevent problems caused by the tendency to impaired circulation in the lower extremities. The elements of foot hygiene and care include properly fitted shoes of materials other than vinyl or plastic to permit ventilation and avoid calluses and blisters, regular bathing, application of lotion or lanolin to keep the skin soft and clean, and correct cutting and trimming of the nails.

The *diet* of the diabetic child is designed to meet his caloric needs based upon his physical activity, insulin requirement, and metabolic demands. It is desirable to have the dietitian explain the prescribed diet to the parents and the child; however, when a dietitian is not available, the nurse is responsible for diet instruction. The diabetic diet is distributed throughout the day to correlate with activity patterns. Caloric patterns are frequently divided into thirds or eighteenths based upon the usual meals and two between-meal snacks and one bedtime snack (5/18, 1/18, 5/18, 1/18, 5/18, 1/18). The diabetic child's diet pattern is thus similar to that of any active child. Dietetic foods are not recommended unless caloric restrictions are made to reduce weight.

The treatment of diabetic acidosis is directed toward restoring carbohydrate metabolism by removing the ketone bodies, restoring life-compatible acid-base balance, replacing fluid and electrolyte losses, and providing glucose and insulin. The severity of the acidosis is assessed by the state of con-

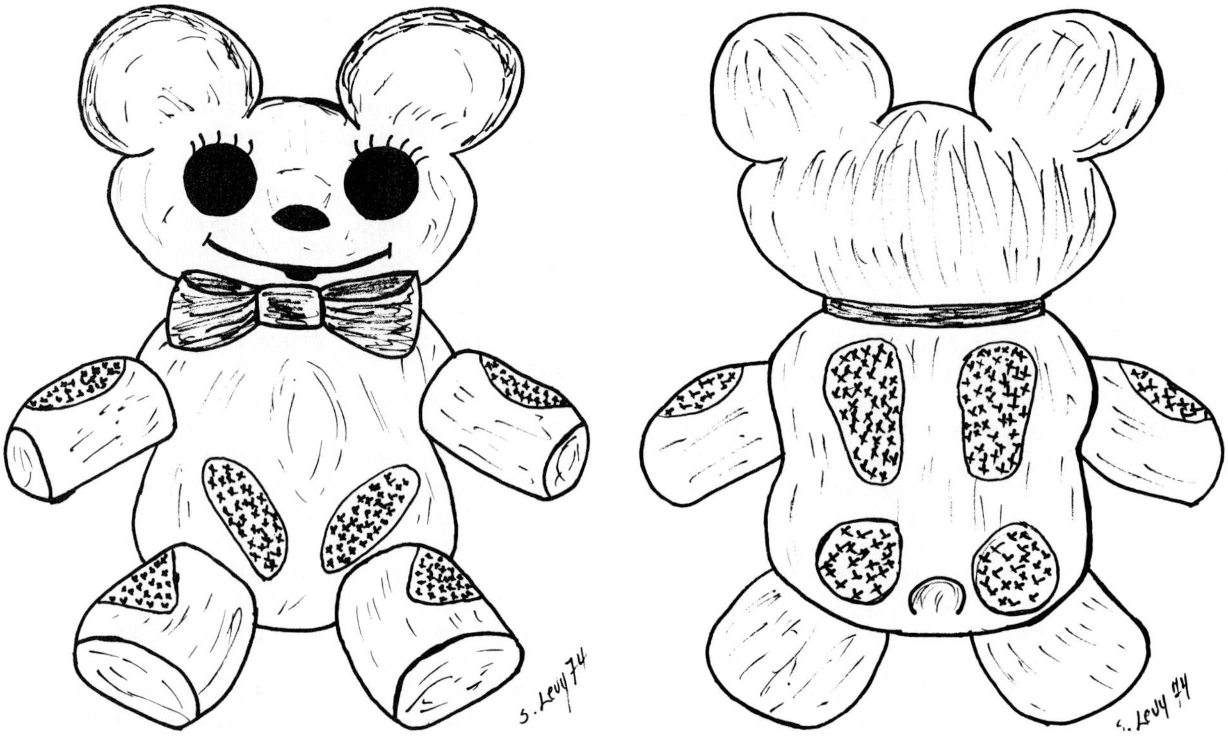

Figure 39-11 A toy animal illustration may add interest to the young child's awareness of the rotation of sites for insulin injection. Stars of a specific color can be pasted on each area to indicate the sequence of usage. *(Used with permission of Susan Levy.)*

sciousness, for oxygen to the brain is affected as metabolic disturbances progress. Kussmaul's breathing occurs as an initial response to acidosis. However, as acidosis progresses, the respiratory rate decreases; therefore, a decreased respiratory rate is indicative of profound acidosis.

The administration of parenteral fluids to restore hydration and prevent acute tubular necrosis is initiated as soon as blood specimens to determine glucose, electrolytes, blood urea nitrogen, and total and differential white blood cell counts are obtained. The amount of fluid infused is based upon the administration of 8 ml/min/sq m body surface until 500 ml/sq m body surface has been infused.

Crystalline insulin is administered intravenously to severely acidotic patients who are hypotensive and therefore would perfuse subcutaneous sites poorly. An alternate method is to administer half the insulin subcutaneously and half intravenously. The dose of insulin is calculated on the basis of 1.0 unit/kg body weight. In the second hour of treatment, fluid replacement is at the rate of 2 to 3

ml/min/sq m body surface, depending upon the degree of dehydration. The initial dose of insulin is repeated each hour until the urine acetone decreases and the patient's condition improves; then the dose of insulin is reduced to half that administered the previous hour.

The serum potassium is expected to be normal or slightly elevated initially because the potassium leaks out of the cells in response to dehydration. Thus, the cells develop a potassium deficit. Potassium levels may be monitored by the presence of electrocardiographic changes, and potassium infusion is usually begun 3 to 4 hours after parenteral therapy has been initiated. (See Chapter 34 for determining the effects of hyperkalemia and hypokalemia upon the myocardium.) Mild potassium deficiency may be recognized by muscular weakness, gastric dilation, and illness when the patient is admitted.

Electrolytes may be replaced by use of sodium chloride, sodium bicarbonate, and sodium lactate solution to replace the 40 Gm of sodium chloride lost and to increase the pH to 7.2 for the patient in

Table 39-3   FALSE POSITIVE AND FALSE NEGATIVE REACTIONS WITH VARIOUS TESTS FOR GLYCOSURIA

Urine constituents causing false positive or negative reactions with tests for glycosuria	Enzyme strip tests: The glucose test area on Labstix and other Ames reagent strip tests	Copper reduction tests	
		Benedict's solution	Clinitest
Sugars other than glucose			
Galactose	No effect	Reacts positively	Reacts positively
Lactose	No effect	Reacts positively	Reacts positively
Levulose (fructose)	No effect	Reacts positively	Reacts positively
Maltose	No effect	Reacts positively	Reacts positively
Pentose	No effect	Reacts positively	Reacts positively
Urine constituents			
Creatinine	No effect	May cause false +	No effect
Uric acid	No effect	May cause false +	No effect
Drug metabolites or contaminants in urine			
Salicylates (aspirin)	No effect	May cause false +	No effect
Penicillin (massive doses)	No effect	May cause false +	No effect
Chloral hydrate	No effect	May cause false +	No effect
Menthol	No effect	May cause false +	No effect
Phenol	No effect	May cause false +	No effect
Turpentine	No effect	May cause false +	No effect
Glucosamine	No effect	May cause false +	No effect
Streptomycin	No effect	May cause false +	No effect
Isoniazid	No effect	May cause false +	No effect
Para-aminosalicylic acid*	No effect	May cause false +	No effect
Ascorbic acid	Interferes with enzyme reactions for glucose impeding color development	May cause false + with large quantities	May cause false + with large quantities
Nalidixic acid (NegGram)	No effect	May cause false +	May cause false +
Metaxalone (Skelaxin)	No effect	May cause false +	May cause false +
Cephalothin (Keflin)	No effect	May cause false +	May cause false +
Probenecid (Benemid)	No effect	May cause false +	May cause false +
Hypochlorite or chlorine	May cause false +	No effect	No effect
Peroxide	May cause false +	No effect	No effect

* Now designated aminosalicylic acid U.S.P.
Source: The Ames Company, Elkhart, Ind. 46514.

diabetic coma. Glucose is given because the patient has no liver glycogen, and glucose must be available to prevent hypoglycemia.

After diabetic acidosis, crystalline insulin is administered before each meal in doses dependent upon the presence of glucose and acetone in the urine until reasonable control is achieved for 1 or 2 days. Then, two-thirds of the day's requirement of insulin is administered in the form of an intermediate-acting insulin, and crystalline insulin is given at meals if acetone appears in the urine. To determine glucose loss and ascertain appropriate combinations and doses of insulin, fractional urines for a 24-hour period are obtained. A specimen collected in this manner enables the determination of glucose lost between meals and at night. The objective of control is to have glucose concentration between 5 and 10 percent of the carbohydrate intake. In achiev-

ing control of ketoacidosis and the recovery from ketoacidosis, it is imperative that the nurse be instrumental in accurate urine testing and collection and accurate administration of replacement fluids, electrolytes, and insulin.

Labile control of juvenile diabetics is frequent. Factors affecting control may include emotional stresses at home and at school, variable exercise, and the process of maturation. Modifications of insulin dosage should not be made unless acetone appears in the urine or symptoms of hypoglycemia occur. Somogyi reaction due to overdosage of insulin and resulting in hyperglycemia, polyuria, and glycosuria is quite common in teen-agers. Somogyi reaction is distinguished from acidosis by the presence of a normal level of carbon dioxide in the plasma.

Hypoglycemic episodes are frightening, embarrassing, and unpleasant experiences. In addition, if hypoglycemia occurs frequently, cerebral damage may result. The child and his parents are taught the harbingers of severe hypoglycemia, i.e., hunger, irritability, nervousness, and headaches. Hard candy or sugar lumps carried on one's person are to be utilized when such early symptoms appear. Glucagon as prescribed can be injected in the unconscious child. Attempts to maintain blood glucose within the normal range result in intracellular hypoglycemia and may cause the discomfort associated with normal blood sugar levels in some diabetic children.

The growth and development of children is affected in some respects by the presence of diabetes. The adult height of diabetics is somewhat less than normal if the disease is diagnosed prior to the growth spurt. Diabetic girls have a tendency to be overweight while diabetic boys are underweight. Although diabetic children respond to viral and bacterial infections similarly to other children, infection needs to be treated vigorously to prevent acidosis.

Sexual maturation occurs normally. Impotence and male infertility may occur because of a thickening of the basement membrane of testicular tubules and abnormal spermatogenesis. The incidence of spontaneous abortion and neonatal death is increased for diabetic mothers. Diabetes mellitus is accompanied by degenerative processes in the small blood vessels of the kidneys, eyes, muscles, and skin.

In summary, the role of the nurse in the care of the juvenile diabetic is to do the following:

1 Teach insulin administration
2 Teach urine testing
3 Teach foot care
4 Ensure understanding of the diet
5 Teach prevention of and treatment of diabetic acidosis and hypoglycemia
6 Monitor and observe the child in diabetic coma for acetonuria, urine volume, and glucosuria, the state of consciousness, and hyperkalemia and hypokalemia
7 Administer and accurately record insulin, fluids, and electrolytes prescribed
8 Assist the parents and the child to accept diabetes

INBORN METABOLIC ERRORS
Glucose 6-Phosphatase Defect

In this disorder of carbohydrate metabolism, both sexes may be affected even when both parents are normal. The heterozygote is detected by a lowered glucose 6-phosphatase level in the intestinal mucosa.

Glucose 6-phosphatase is an enzyme that regu-

lates blood glucose, especially in infants. In the absence of glucose 6-phosphatase, there is a fasting hypoglycemia because the enzyme prevents the formation of free glucose from glycogen. Mobilization of fatty acids results in ketone formation and increased triglyceride and cholesterol levels. High uric acid levels also result; however, urinary uric acid excretion is not elevated comparably.

Clinically, the child may initially have symptoms varying from steatorrhea and intermittent pyrexia to hepatomegaly, dyspnea, hypoglycemic convulsions, and ketonuria. Linear growth is retarded; the skin is thin with prominent venules, and the liver becomes progressively more enlarged with very high triglyceride levels. The child is treated by serving high-carbohydrate feedings between regular meals through the first 2 years. The prognosis of the disease is variable and dependent upon the development of ketoacidosis associated with infection, enlargement of the liver associated with cardiac hypertrophy, and cardiac failure. Gouty nephritis may also occur. Certain viral and bacterial infections have resulted in the precipitation of hemolysis in these children. Some drugs may also initiate the hemolytic process.

Nursing Management The nurse is responsible for explaining the necessary preparation for diagnostic studies using (1) blood specimens to determine fasting hypoglycemia, ketosis, triglyceride, and cholesterol levels as well as the glucose tolerance curve; (2) administration of glucagon and galactose to determine blood lactate and glucose levels; and (3) liver biopsy to demonstrate the absence of glucose 6-phosphatase in the liver.

The nurse must explain the importance of the diet to correct the blood sugar and ensure adequate intake. Bleeding can be a problem. The child must be observed for persistent oozing if surgery is performed, and the vital signs are carefully monitored after the liver biopsy. Nosebleeds are treated by employing the usual measures to promote hemostasis.

BIBLIOGRAPHY

Allison, Sarah E.: "A Framework for Nursing Action in a Nurse Conducted Diabetic Management Clinic," *Journal of Nursing Administration*, 3(4):53–103, 1973.

Balinsky, B. I.: *An Introduction to Embryology*, W. B. Saunders Company, Philadelphia, 1970.

Beeson, P. B. and McDermott, W. (eds.): *Textbook of Medicine*, 13th ed., W. B. Saunders Company, Philadelphia, 1971, pp. 1718–1855.

Beland, Irene L.: *Clinical Nursing*, 2d ed., The Macmillan Company, New York, 1970, pp. 840–879.

Brunner, Lillian Sholtis, et al.: *Textbook of Medical-Surgical Nursing*, J. B. Lippincott Company, Philadelphia, 1970, pp. 683–715.

————: *Fourth Allied Health Postgraduate Course in Diabetes*, American Diabetes Association in cooperation with Vanderbilt University, Nashville, Tenn., April 17–19, 1972.

Carozza, V.: "Diabetic Out of Control," *Nursing '73*, 3(5): 11–15, 1973.

Conn, J. W., et al.: "Primary Aldosteronism," *Archives of Internal Medicine*, 129(3):417–425, 1972.

Driscoll, Ann E.: "A Teaching Aid for Endocrine Disorders," *American Journal of Nursing*, 73(11):1944–45, 1973.

Fishman, L. M., et al.: "'Effects of Amino-glutethimide on Adrenal Function in Man," *Journal of Clinical Endocrinology and Metabolism*, 27(4):481–490, 1967.

Gardner, L. I. (ed.): *Endocrine and Genetic Diseases of Childhood*, W. B. Saunders Company, Philadelphia, 1969, pp. 1–466, 808–821, 856–861.

Goodman, L. S., and Gilman, A.: *The Pharmacological Basis of Therapeutics*, 4th ed., The Macmillan Company, New York, 1970.

Guthrie, Diana W. and Guthrie, R. A.: "Coping with Diabetic Ketoacidosis," *Nursing '73*, 3(11):16–23, 1973.

————: "Diabetic Children: Special Needs, Diet, Drugs and Difficulties," *Nursing '73*, 3(3):10–15, 1973.

Guyton, A. C.: *Textbook of Medical Physiology*, 3d ed., W. B. Saunders Company, Philadelphia, 1970, pp. 1035–1182.

Hamdi, Mary Evans: "Nursing Intervention for Patients Receiving Corticosteroid Therapy," in Kay Corman Kintzel (ed.), *Advanced Concepts in Clinical Nursing*, J. B. Lippincott Company, Philadelphia, 1971, pp. 236–245.

Howell, R. R.: "The Glycogen Storage Diseases," in J. B. Stanbury, J. B. Wyngaarden, and D. S. Fredrickson (eds.), *The Metabolic Basis of Inherited Disease*, McGraw-Hill Book Company, New York, 1972, pp. 155–159.

Hutter, A. M., and Kayhoe, D. E.: "Adrenal Cortical Carcinoma: Results of Treatment with o,p-DDD in 138 Patients," *American Journal of Medicine*, 41(10):581–591, 1966.

————: "Injecting Insulin: Atrophy and Hypertrophy not Inevitable," in *Innovations in Nursing, Nursing '73*, 3(2):14–15, 1973.

Kjellberg, R. N.: "The Bragg-Peak Proton Beam Noninvasive Hypophysectomy," *Hospital Practice*, 7(10):95–102, 1972.

Lawrence, Patricia A.: "Diabetes Mellitus," in Kay Corman Kintzel (ed.), *Advanced Concepts in Clinical Nursing*, J. B. Lippincott Company, Philadelphia, 1971, pp. 105–129.

Liddle, G. W.: "Tests of Pituitary-Adrenal Suppressibility in the Diagnosis of Cushing's Syndrome," *Journal of Clinical Endocrinology*, 20:539, 1960.

Lieberman, L. M., et al.: "Diagnosis of Adrenal Disease by Visualization of Human Adrenal Glands with ^{131}I-19-Iodocholesterol," *New England Journal of Medicine*, 285(25):1387–1393, 1971.

McFarlane, Judith, and Homes, Carolyn C.: "Children with Diabetes Learning Self-Care in Camp," *American Journal of Nursing*, 73(8):1362–1365, 1973.

Marble, A., et al. (eds.): *Joslin's Diabetes Mellitus*, Lea & Febiger, Philadelphia, 1971.

Nelson, W. E. (ed.): *Textbook of Pediatrics*, W. B. Saunders Company, Philadelphia, 1966, pp. 1254–1320.

Porter, Anne Lynn, McDonald, Avis, and Levine, Myra R.: "Giving Diabetics Control of Their Own Lives," *Nursing '73*, 3(9):44–49, 1973.

Scteigart, D. E., et al.: "Persistent or Recurrent Cushing's Syndrome after 'Total' Adrenalectomy," *Archives of Internal Medicine*, 130(9):384–387, 1972.

Spencer, Roberta T.: *Patient Care in Endocrine Problems*, W. B. Saunders Company, Philadelphia, 1973.

Stowe, Sharon M.: "Hypophysectomy for Diabetic Retinopathy," *American Journal of Nursing*, 73(4):632–637, 1973.

Sussman, K. E. (ed.): *Juvenile-Type Diabetes and Its Complications*, Charles C Thomas, Publisher, Springfield, Ill., 1971.

Thorn, G. W., et al. (eds.): *Clinician-1: The Adrenal Gland*, MEDCOM Press, New York, 1971.

Trayser, Lisa M.: "A Teaching Program for Diabetics," *American Journal of Nursing*, 73(1):92–93, 1973.

Watson, Jeanette E.: *Medical-Surgical Nursing and Related Physiology*, W. B. Saunders Company, Philadelphia, 1972, pp. 532–580.

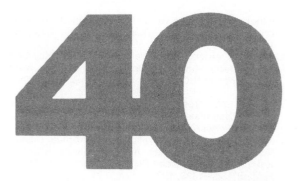

THE MUSCULO-SKELETAL SYSTEM

SHERRILYN PASSO*

EMBRYOLOGY OF THE MUSCULOSKELETAL SYSTEM

Mesenchymal tissue, which is derived from the mesoderm, differentiates into the connective tissues, including cartilage, bone, muscle, ligaments, and tendons.

Bone

Bone forms by two processes, endochondral and intramembranous ossification. In *endochondral ossification*, mesenchymal tissue differentiates into a cartilage model of the bone, which, in turn, is invaded by blood vessels and replaced by bone. Almost all bones of the body are formed by this process. *Intramembranous ossification* takes place without the cartilage model; instead, mesenchymal tissue is replaced directly by bone. This method of ossification is seen primarily in the skull.

Endochondral Ossification   The formation of a tubular bone such as the femur best illustrates endochondral ossification. During the fifth week of embryonic development, the limb buds appear. Mesenchymal cells condense in the form of a short cylinder in the central axis of each limb bud. The cylinder is segmented at sites of future joints by sparse cellular areas. Each segment of the cylinder becomes the mesenchymal model of the future long bone that will develop from it. By the sixth week, mesenchymal cells of each model begin to differentiate. They manufacture a cartilage matrix, forming the *cartilage model* of the future bone. The covering of the model is the perichondrium, as illustrated in Fig. 40-1*A*. The cartilage model resembles the general form of the future bone, with a *diaphysis*, or central shaft, and an *epiphysis* at each end. The model grows in two ways, by *interstitial growth* from within and by *appositional growth* in which new cells are formed on the surface from deeper layers of the perichondrium.

About the eighth week of embryonic life the first step in formation of bone occurs. Cartilage cells which surround the center of the model like a collar hypertrophy and die because of calcification of the intercellular matrix. (See Fig. 40-1*B*.)

The *primary center of ossification* is formed by ingrowth of vascular connective tissue into the central area of the model. *Osteoblasts*, or bone-forming cells, then appear. These cells secrete collagen to

* The author gratefully acknowledges Dr. Richard Lindseth, Chief of Pediatric Orthopedics, Indiana University Medical Center, for his help in reviewing this chapter.

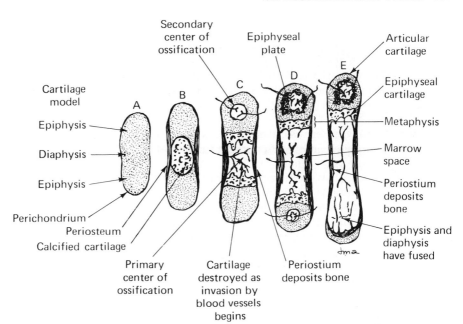

Figure 40-1 Development of a long bone. *(Adapted from L. L. Langley, The Physiology of Man, McGraw-Hill Book Company, New York, 1958, p. 33.)*

form a mucopolysaccharide matrix, which is impregnated with calcium salts. This process of endochondral ossification advances toward each end of the cartilage model. The model continues to grow in length at its cartilage ends by interstitial growth. Growth in width is accomplished by the process of intramembranous ossification in the periosteum. A combination of endochondral and intramembranous ossification takes place simultaneously.

By the sixth month the process of tabulation occurs. Resorption of the central part of the long bone results in formation of a medullary cavity. At birth, the largest epiphysis in the body, the distal femoral epiphysis, has developed a *secondary center of ossification*, as shown in Fig. 40-1C, by the process of endochondral ossification. At varying ages after birth, secondary centers of ossification appear in the other cartilaginous epiphyses. An ossification center appears in the proximal epiphysis of the tibia soon after birth and distally in the second year. Each new center of ossification is separated from the diaphysis by a special plate of growing cartilage, the *epiphyseal*, or growth, *plate*. This plate lies at the region of bone known as the *metaphysis* (Fig. 40-1D).

Continuous growth in length of a long bone takes place in the articular cartilage and the epiphyseal plate. Articular cartilage is found on the outer edge of the epiphysis (Fig. 40-1E). This cartilage is the only site for growth of the epiphysis itself, by

the processes of interstitial growth and endochondral ossification. The epiphyseal plate cartilage allows for growth in the length of the metaphysis and diaphysis by a balance between the two successive processes of interstitial growth and endochondral ossification. Interstitial growth of cartilage cells on the epiphyseal plate makes the plate thicker and moves the epiphysis farther away from the metaphysis. Through endochondral ossification the processes of calcification, death, and replacement of cartilage by bone take place on the metaphyseal surface. As bone grows longer, the flared metaphyseal areas are continually remodeled. When the epiphysis and diaphysis have fused after puberty, growth ceases.[1]

Intramembranous Ossification   The flat bones of the face and some bones of the skull develop directly in mesenchymal tissue by the process of intramembranous ossification from the periosteum. Cancellous, or spongy, bone is developed in the ossification center of the flat bone. The periosteum forms parallel plates of bone on the inner and outer surfaces of the cancellous bone. Bone at the surface is transformed from the cancellous to compact type. Some reconstruction also takes place at the inner ossification center. The final form of the bone consists of inner and outer layers of compact bone between which is spongy cancellous bone.

Joints

The primitive joint plate, an articular disk of mesenchyme, appears at the site of a future synovial joint in the mesenchyme of the limb bud. Dense tissue similar to the perichondrium of the cartilage model surrounds the primitive joint plate and later becomes the joint capsule.

By the tenth week spaces filled with tissue fluid appear in the primitive joint plate and gradually join into a single joint cavity filled with fluid. The outer layer of the joint capsule differentiates into fibrous tissue, while the inner layer forms the *synovial membrane*. At birth the synovial joint appears as two opposing bone surfaces covered by articular cartilage and joined by an encircling band of fibrous tissue. The joint cavity is held in place by ligaments and muscles. The synovial membrane lines the joint cavity except over surfaces of articular cartilage. *Synovial fluid* lubricates and nourishes the articulation. Full development of a synovial joint such as the hip joint does not occur until adulthood.

Muscle

During the fourth week of embryonic life, mesoderm around the notocord condenses into segments called somites, which are further differentiated into sclerotome, dermatome, and myotome. Sclerotome is destined to become the vertebrae and ribs; dermatome, the skin; and myotome, the skeletal muscles.

The myotome plate thickens by the fifth week, and cells differentiate into myoblasts, or muscle-forming cells, which arrange themselves parallel with the long axis of the body and become skeletal muscle fibers. From the sixth to eighth weeks of embryonic life, muscles of the fetus become well fashioned, as muscle fibers aggregate in groups which comprise the individual muscles. At this time, muscles are capable of movements. Proliferation of new muscle fibers occurs until about the middle of fetal life. After this time, enlargement of a muscle occurs as a result of an increase in the size of individual fibers rather than the number of fibers.

The spinal nerve corresponding to each somite makes contact with the myotome and dermatome at an early stage. By the fourth month, a flattened terminal network differentiates from the spinal nerves. This network enters the muscle fiber and rests on a special area of muscle called a *motor end plate*. The relationship of segmental spinal nerve to myotome is retained throughout life. This is illustrated when myotomes fuse to form a muscle; that muscle remains innervated by several spinal nerves. If myotomes split into several muscles, all these muscles are innervated by the original spinal nerve. Connective tissue is differentiated from local mesenchyme and binds individual muscle fibers together or encloses an entire muscle.

NORMAL FUNCTION AND REACTION TO DISEASE OR TRAUMA
Bone

Bone functions both as a structure and as an organ. As a structure, it provides a framework for the body, acts as a lever for skeletal muscles, and protects vital organs such as the brain, spinal cord, heart, and lungs. As an organ it contains tissue for production of erythrocytes and stores calcium, phosphorus, and other minerals.

There are two types of bone: immature and mature. The *immature* type of bone is formed by endochondral ossification during embryonic development. It is very cellular and contains less cement substance and mineral than mature bone. By 1 year of age, immature bone has been replaced by mature bone.

Bone reacts to injury or disease in three basic ways: (1) local death, (2) alterations in bone deposition, and (3) alterations in bone resorption. When the blood supply to an area of bone is completely stopped, local death, or *avascular necrosis,* occurs. The resultant dead bone acts as an abnormal condition and encourages further destruction in the area. Alterations in bone deposition and bone resorption take place in bone which is alive. Bone is deposited in sites subjected to stress and resorbed from sites with little stress, and normally a balance of these two processes exists. Reactions to abnormal conditions may occur in an entire bone, part of a bone, or in all bones of the body.

After a fracture, there is a localized increase in bone deposition in order to form callus. The healing and remodeling process is divided into three stages: (1) Callus forms around the bone edges and becomes progressively firmer and less mobile. (2) When callus is firm enough so that no movement occurs at the fracture site, clinical union has taken place. (3) Consolidation of the fracture is present when all temporary callus is replaced by mature bone. Sharp edges are smoothed off by bone resorption and deposition. The remodeling process is illustrated in Fig. 40-2.

Healing of a fracture varies a great deal with age. More time is required for healing as age increases until the child reaches adulthood. For example, a fracture of the femoral shaft at birth is united in 3 weeks. At 8 years, the same fracture requires 8 weeks

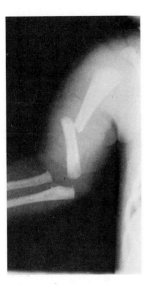 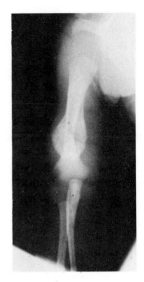 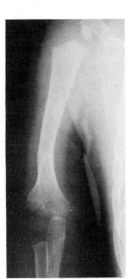

Figure 40-2 Healing and remodeling of a fractured humerus in a newborn: At birth, 3½ weeks, and 5½ months. *(Photography by the Department of Medical Illustration, Indiana University–Purdue University at Indianapolis.)*

for union; at 12 years, 12 weeks are required; at 20 years through adulthood, 20 weeks are needed for healing.

Epiphyseal Plate

Normal growth in an epiphyseal plate requires an intact structure, normal blood supply, and intermittent pressure from normal activity. Like bone, each epiphyseal plate reacts in limited ways to a large number of abnormal conditions. Reactions include (1) increased growth, (2) decreased growth, and (3) torsional or twisted growth. Prolonged hyperemia stimulates growth; hypoxia retards it. Complete lack of blood supply results in necrosis of the epiphyseal plate and completely stops growth. Torsional growth occurs when growth is abnormal in one part of an epiphyseal plate and normal in the remainder of the plate.

Joints

A joint is a junction between two or more bones and has several functions: it segments the skeleton, permits motion between segments, and allows for varying amounts of segmental growth. The construction of a joint varies according to the function required of it. Joints are classified as fibrous, cartilaginous, and synovial types. Motion is very limited in *fibrous joints,* which are found between bones of the skull and at the borders of the radius and ulna. Slightly movable *cartilaginous joints* include the epiphyseal plates and the symphysis pubis. *Synovial*

joints appear at such structures as the elbow, shoulder, and fingers.

Synovial joints may be uniaxial, biaxial, or polyaxial, according to the type of movement their structure permits. Movement is possible around only one axis in a uniaxial joint, two axes in a biaxial joint, and innumerable axes in a polyaxial joint. Movements and the terms used to describe them are illustrated in Fig. 40-3.

Skeletal Muscle

Skeletal muscles provide active movement and maintain posture of the skeleton. They are called *voluntary muscles* because they are controlled at will. Microscopic cross striations account for the name *striated* muscles. Each muscle fiber is innervated by an axon. The axon attaches to the muscle fiber at the motor end plate and originates from the anterior horn cell of the spinal cord. The anterior horn cell, its axon, and the motor end plates and individual muscle fibers supplied by the anterior horn cell constitute a *single motor unit.*

The membrane of the skeletal muscle fiber has a resting potential maintained by the permeability of the cell membrane to potassium and sodium. When a nerve action potential arrives at the motor end plate, biochemical processes are set off in the muscle fiber which generate local action potentials. The local action potential travels toward both ends of the muscle fiber, resulting in contraction of the fiber. The energy for muscle action is thought to be derived from the breakdown of adenosine triphosphate

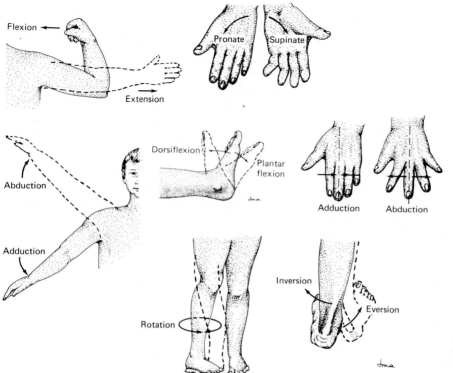

Figure 40-3 Clinical terms used to describe movement. *(Adapted from L. L. Langley, et al., Dynamic Anatomy and Physiology, McGraw-Hill Book Company, 1974, p. 124.)*

(ATP). Actual contraction seems to result from movement of special myofilaments in the myofibril, a subunit of the muscle fiber. These myofilaments, actin and myosin proteins, are packed in a regular arrangement in the myofibril. Muscle contraction is thought to take place as a result of the sliding of myosin myofilaments over actin. As these myofilaments move closer together, the entire fiber shortens or contracts.

Each muscle fiber obeys the *all-or-none law:* it either contracts maximally or not at all. Therefore, the number of individual fibers that contract determines whether a contraction is weak or powerful. The total number of muscle cells is established at birth; however, dead muscle cells do not regenerate but are replaced by fibrous tissue. Enlargement of a muscle after sustained physical exercise is a result of hypertrophy of existing cells, not an increase in number.

Dysfunction or injury of any part of the single motor unit can cause a reaction in skeletal muscle. *Disuse atrophy,* which is manifested by weakness and decrease in size of a muscle, results from lack of normal use. A persistent shortening of a muscle which is resistant to stretching is a muscle *contracture* and occurs when the muscle remains shortened over a prolonged period. While a muscle becomes stronger and larger when it is repeatedly exercised against resistance, the resulting *hypertrophy* of muscle fibers is dependent upon persistent exercising. *Ischemic necrosis* of a muscle occurs within 6 hours after arterial occlusion, which can be caused by spasm, thrombosis, or embolism.

Musculoskeletal Reactions

When an entire limb or the trunk reacts to disease or injury, a musculoskeletal deformity is produced. Bones, joints, soft tissues, or a combination of these three may be involved. Special terms are used to describe deformities in limbs. Abnormal angulation within a limb is a varus or a valgus deformity. In the *varus* type, the angle of deformity points away from the midline of the body. Distal segments of the limb or long bone are displaced toward the midline. In *coxa vara,* there is a decrease in the angle of the femoral neck; in genu varum, or bowleggedness, the feet are held together but the knees remain apart. In the *valgus* type, the segments of the deformity are pointed outward. For example, in *coxa valga,* there is an increase in the femoral neck-shaft angle, while in *genu valgum,* or knock-knee, the knees are held together but the feet are apart. Calcaneus and equinus are deformities which occur at the ankle only. In *calcaneus* the foot is maintained in dorsiflexion. On weight bearing, only the heel touches the floor. *Equinus* of the foot is a sustained position of plantar flexion. On weight bearing, only the forefoot touches the floor. Anteversion and retroversion refer to the direction the neck of the femur takes in relationship to the femoral shaft. In *femoral anteversion* the femoral neck is directed anteriorly to some degree, with the knee directed posteriorly. In *femoral retroversion* the femoral neck is directed posteriorly to some degree, with the knee directed anteriorly.

COMMON NURSING MANAGEMENT
Multiple Trauma

Motorcycle and automobile accidents, lawnmower injuries, and falls are just a few of the causes of multiple trauma in children. Injuries to the musculoskeletal system often include fractures, dislocations, and associated soft-tissue injuries. Although other body systems may take priority in immediate treatment, disabilities from musculoskeletal injuries are longer lasting and are often of more concern to the child and his family.

Assessment of the *skeletal* system after trauma begins with observation for obvious deformity, swelling, and pain. Fractures and dislocations should be splinted before moving the extremity to prevent further injury and to minimize pain. The splint is applied a joint above and a joint below the fracture with the limb in a position of maximum comfort and relaxation. For upper-extremity fractures, a padded arm board or right-angle splint can be used for immobilization; for fractures of the leg, a Thomas splint is preferred. When the patient has arrived wearing a plastic air splint, the physician should be present during removal since improper removal can cause further injury to the limb. Splinting should not be done when an extremity is so deformed that it does not conform to the splint; instead, the extremity should be left in its position and immobilized with sandbags.

A cervical neck injury should always be considered in trauma. The patient should not be moved until an x-ray has confirmed that the cervical vertebrae are intact. If a cervical fracture is found, traction to the head may be necessary. Crutchfield or similar tongs should be readily available. When an injury to any part of the spine is suspected, the child should be moved only as an immobilized unit with a board or flat object as a splint. When turning is necessary, it should be done by *logrolling,* a method of turning the body as one rigid unit. A drawsheet often facilitates logrolling, and an adequate number of staff members should help with this procedure. When x-rays are needed, radiologic equipment should be brought to the emergency room so that movement of the patient is minimized.

Whenever possible, the nurse seeks information from a witness to the accident concerning the time and events leading to the injury. The type of accident often indicates the type of injury to be suspected; that is, a diving accident makes one suspect trauma to the cervical spine. If parents or relatives are available, they should be questioned about the time of the child's last meal, allergies, and his past medical history. Some type of progress report at intervals can help to relieve the anxiety of family members waiting outside the emergency area.

Preoperative and Postoperative Care

The aims of musculoskeletal surgical procedures are to improve function and ability, to prevent or correct deformity, or to relieve pain. Surgical manipulations are usually done to reduce fractures or dislocations by passive movements of the parts. Surgical operations involve incisions and repair or reconstruction of tissues; soft tissues (muscles, tendons, and ligaments), nerves, joints, or bones may be involved. Terms used to describe common surgical procedures are defined in Table 40-1.

Table 40-1 TERMS USED TO DESCRIBE COMMON SURGICAL PROCEDURES

Term	Definition
Arthrodesis	Stabilization or fusion of a joint
Arthroplasty	Reconstruction of a joint
Arthrotomy	Surgical opening and exploration of a joint
Epiphyseodesis	Binding of an epiphysis to its diaphysis
Laminectomy	Removal of the vertebral lamina for decompression of spinal nerves
Myotomy	Cutting into a muscle
Osteotomy	Division of a bone
Tendon lengthening	Division of a tendon followed by resuturing in an elongated position
Tendon or muscle transfer	Transference of the origin or insertion of a tendon or muscle into the place of a paralyzed or damaged one
Tenotomy	Division of a tendon

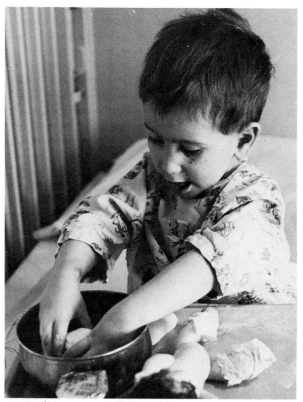

Figure 40-4 Child casting doll as preoperative preparation. *(Courtesy James Whitcomb Riley Hospital for Children, Indianapolis, Ind.; photograph by G. Dreyer, Indiana University School of Nursing, Instructional Communications and Educational Resources.)*

Preoperative preparation centers around the child's and family's understanding of the surgery and the child's readiness to cooperate with postoperative care. The nurse reinforces information given by the physician concerning anesthesia, the time of surgery, the surgery itself, and the child's postoperative appearance. The child may enjoy manipulating rolls of plaster and applying a cast on a doll similar to the cast he will wear after surgery, as illustrated in Fig. 40-4. This play activity can also help the child understand what is to be done to him during surgery. Special functions which will be required postoperatively may be practiced before the child goes to surgery. If he is to be immobilized, he should try voiding into a bedpan in bed. Other routines which can be rehearsed are turning or logrolling, coughing, and deep breathing.

Postoperatively, assessments should be made of circulation and function in peripheral parts of the extremity. At 1- to 2-hour intervals, observations are made of color, warmth, swelling, pulses, sensation, and movement in the limb. The fingers or toes are pressed to see if they blanch and show rapid return of color. Drainage on the cast or bandage should be recorded. Stains from drainage on the cast are outlined with a pen and labeled as to the time observed. The nurse must be aware of early warning signs that the cast is too tight or circulation is insufficient. These signs are (1) severe pain and pain unrelieved by analgesics, (2) persistent swelling which does not respond to elevation of the limb, (3) pulselessness, (4) whiteness or cyanosis, (5) cold, (6) numbness, tingling, or burning, and (7) inability to move a previously functioning part. If any of these signs are observed, they should be reported to the physician at once! Their presence usually means that the cast must be *bivalved* (split apart) to restore circulation and function to the extremity.

Positioning during the immediate postoperative period aims to maintain the original shape of the cast and to support the child in anatomic postures. Pillows and blanket rolls are used for padding and support. The cast may be elevated to prevent swelling. A footboard, special shoes, or splints prevent foot drop in the paralyzed patient. The child should be turned every 2 hours to promote circulation and to facilitate drying of the cast, which should also be left uncovered. In the supine position, the child's head should be slightly elevated during drinking and eating in order to prevent choking.

Cast Care

Casts are used for immobilization of body parts, maintenance of position, or correction of deformity. The most common cast material is plaster of Paris. The plaster comes impregnated in rolled gauze bandages, and the cast is formed by wrapping the body part with sheet wadding and then applying wet layers of plaster bandage around the part. After application, the plaster "sets" in a few minutes by changing into crystalline gypsum. Approximately 24 to 48 hours are required for the cast to dry completely. The cast dries from the outside to the inside; therefore, it may feel dry on the outside but still be wet on the inside. It should remain uncovered during drying, and the patient should be turned frequently (every 2 hours) so that moisture can evaporate from its surface. Heat lamps or heated fan dryers should never be used for drying since they can cause skin burns under the plaster.

The child can best be prepared for cast application by actually putting a cast on a doll. The nurse may assist with preparation of materials used in cast-

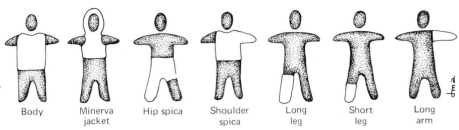

Figure 40-5 Types of casts. *(From H. Moidel et al., Nursing Care of the Patient with Medical-Surgical Disorders, McGraw-Hill Book Company, New York, 1971, p. 881.)*

Body Minerva jacket Hip spica Shoulder spica Long leg Short leg Long arm

ing such as plaster bandages, sheet wadding, and stockinet. During cast application, the child is positioned as directed by the physician. To minimize movement at a fracture site, manual traction on the extremity or a strong steady pull on each side of the fracture site is exerted while the cast is being applied. A special orthopedic cast table is usually required when body or hip spica casts are applied.

Various types of casts are shown in Fig. 40-5. A *body cast* covers the entire trunk region, and a *minerva jacket* encases the head and trunk. *Hip spica* and *shoulder spica casts* immobilize their respective limbs to the trunk. Lower-extremity casts include *short leg* and *long leg casts* and are designed for walking by the addition of a bar or a heel on the sole. For the upper extremity, casts may be the *short arm* or *long arm* types.

Casts which are made of fiber glass are useful in special circumstances. The advantages of this material are that it is stronger and lighter than plaster and can be immersed in water, if the physician permits. Soaking should not be prolonged, and soap should be used sparingly around the cast. Drying is accomplished by blotting with towels or blowing with a hair dryer set at a low temperature. Rough edges can be finished off with an emery board or a nail file.

After cast application, circulation and function in the limb should be assessed for all patients every 1 or 2 hours and then less frequently. Parents of children who are sent home from the hospital immediately after cast application must be informed about the signs of a tight cast. They are instructed to return to the physician without delay should any of these signs appear. To prevent unnatural molding of the cast, the wet cast is supported on pillows on a firm base or mattress, and the child is turned at 1- or 2-hour intervals. The nurse handles the cast with the palms of the hands instead of the fingers to prevent indentations in the soft plaster. Abduction bars built into the cast to keep the legs apart should never be used as handles to move the cast.

When the cast is dry, rough edges are finished off by petaling. Strips of adhesive tape are cut and secured over rough or unfinished edges as illus-

trated in Fig. 40-6. Each petal overlaps the previous one until the entire edge is covered. The skin at cast edges is checked for signs of soreness, and tight edges causing irritation are stretched or cut away. Complaints of pain or burning or an offensive odor from the inside of the cast should be investigated since these may indicate that a sore is forming or has become infected. Powders and lotions should not be used inside the cast; skin underneath cast edges can be massaged with alcohol. Itching under the cast is eliminated by blowing cool air through the cast with an asepto syringe or hair dryer. Some physicians insert a strip of gauze through the cast which can be used to gently massage the skin and eliminate itching. Sharp objects such as knitting needles may injure the skin and are not suitable as scratchers. Skin care is particularly important for the neurologically damaged child who lacks sensation under the cast.

Cast care begins immediately after the cast is applied. Keeping it clean and dry is a challenge with infants or children who are incontinent. The child may be placed on a frame which allows urine and feces to drain into a bedpan below, or he may be returned to his crib with plastic-covered pillows used for support. With the head of the frame or bed elevated, urine and feces drain away from the cast by gravity. Plastic wrap is tucked around cast edges, although it cannot be taped onto the cast until it dries. When the cast is dry, inner edges around the diaper areas may need to be cut away to allow for care after defecation and voiding. Edges of the dry cast are covered with adhesive tape petals, after which plastic wrap is tucked under the inside edge and secured to the outside of the cast with tape. The child who is in bed can be kept dry by the use of a folded diaper or sanitary pad which is tucked under the cast edges and changed frequently. This is held in place by another diaper which is fastened around the cast. Plastic 24-hour urine collecting bags may also be used, but they often cause skin irritation. When a cast becomes soiled, it can be cleaned by removing soiled tape petals and wiping with a damp cloth which has been rubbed over a cake of Bon Ami.

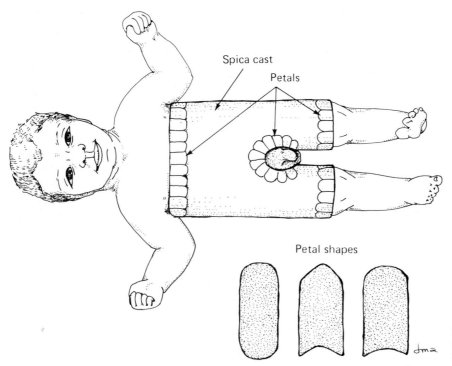

Spica cast

Petals

Petal shapes

Figure 40-6 Spica cast finished off with adhesive tape petals and samples of petals.

For all children in casts, bowel and bladder function should be regularly assessed. Constipation and poor urinary drainage may result from immobilization. A fracture bedpan can be used to facilitate toileting. The child's head and shoulders should be elevated, and a folded pad placed over the back edge of the bedpan. Administration of suppositories or mild laxatives may be necessary for the child who is constipated. The urine should be checked for signs of infection, especially in the child who has a neurogenic bladder. An adequate fluid intake should be maintained. A low-calcium diet may be prescribed in an effort to prevent urinary calculi.

To prepare the parents for home care of their child, the nurse should demonstrate turning, positioning, and handling of the child in the cast and also clarify the child's mobility limits with parents. Bathing, skin care, diaper care, bowel evacuation, and treatment of problems in these areas are discussed and activities of care are practiced. Parents should be aware of warning signs that the cast is too tight or the child is outgrowing the cast, and they should know what to do if this happens. Other safety measures should be discussed, such as elevating the child's head during eating and drinking to prevent choking, preventing the small child from dropping crumbs, coins, or other small objects down into the cast which could cause skin breakdown, using body

mechanics when lifting the child and transporting the child.

Casts

Normal daily activities at home may need to be altered for the child in a cast although the child should be treated as normally as possible within activity limits. Clothing has to be purchased in larger sizes or constructed differently. A wagon, wheelchair, or stretcher is needed to transport the child in a heavy cast, while crutches may be required for the older child in a long leg cast. A creeper or padded board on wheels provides mobility for the young child in a body or spica cast. Simple tasks such as washing hair or bathing may need to be modified. A sponge bath may have to be substituted for a tub bath. Spray hoses aid hair washing over the sink, but the older child in a body cast may have to wash his hair by leaning over the edge of the bed with a pan placed on a low stool below. Flexible drinking straws made from plastic tubing used in aquariums facilitate drinking for the child who cannot sit. Teachers for the home-bound may be required to continue schoolwork.

When the cast is to be altered or removed, the cast cutter, an electric saw with an oscillating circular blade, is especially frightening to children. The child may well believe that the saw will cut off his limb. The cast-cutting noise is also upsetting. Children can be helped to deal with anxiety by wearing a special set of earmuffs or cotton plugs, playing with make-believe saws, or observing the saw lightly touched to the operator's palm. The child should be held very still and the procedure carried out as quickly and as safely as it can be done. Short casts, such as clubfoot casts, can be soaked off with the physician's permission in order to avoid use of the saw. Parents can be instructed to immerse the cast in a vinegar-water solution (about 1 part vinegar to 4 parts water) and unwind the softened bandages. When a cast is removed, support is provided for all joints which were immobilized. Dead skin and sebaceous material are gently removed by repeated washing or by application of oil for a few hours, followed by washing.

Traction

Aims of traction may be to correct displacement of fragments in a fracture, to immobilize the fracture, to reduce muscle spasm causing deformity, to decrease spinal curvature, or to reduce dislocation. The type of traction is selected according to the age of the patient and the goals of treatment. Skin traction is used for younger children when the condition of the skin is good and mild forces of traction are sufficient. Skeletal traction is used in children when greater traction force is required or the skin is damaged. Traction may be continuous or intermittent. When used for reduction and immobilization of a fracture, it is continuous and should not be interrupted for dressing or any other activity. Intermittent traction may be temporarily disconnected as specified by the physician. Traction may be fixed with the traction device fastened to the end of the bed (fixed traction), or the traction device may be balanced by cords with pulleys and weights (balanced traction.)

In *skin traction,* moleskin, adhesive, or foam rubber extensions are fastened firmly to the skin. An encircling wrap such as an elastic bandage holds them in place. Weights then are attached to the extensions by cords which pass over one or more pulleys. The foot of the bed may have to be raised so that the child's own weight provides countertraction. *Bryant's traction* for fractured femurs or dislocated hips of very young children suspends the child's legs from an overhead rod with the hips at right angles. The nurse should be able to pass one hand under the child's buttocks, which are clear of the bed. A *Posey restraint* maintains the child's position in bed. The position of the bandages is checked daily to ensure that they do not slip and cause pressure on the dorsum of the feet. They are rewrapped as necessary. In *Buck's extension traction,* one or both legs rest on the bed, pulled by weights at the end of the bed. This type of traction is used in immobilizing a fractured hip or an injured knee or proximal tibia. *Russell's skin traction* reduces fractures of the femoral shaft. A sling under the distal thigh applies force to the back of the thigh. Skin tapes are applied to the leg with weights attached which exert force on the long axis of the leg. Some flexion of the knee and hip results. *Overhead arm traction* is used to treat supracondylar fractures. The affected arm is placed in abduction off the side of the bed. Skin tapes are applied to the forearm and attached to weights and pulleys. A sling is attached over the upper arm to permit a traction force toward the floor.

In *skeletal traction* a direct hold on the bone is obtained by means of metallic devices. Traction forces are stronger and maintained for longer periods of time than in skin traction. Certain children's fractures are best reduced and immobilized by skeletal traction. The Thomas splint is part of the traction setup for management of femoral fractures. It consists of two rods on each side of the leg joined proximally by a padded ring around the leg and distally by a crossbar. Metallic devices most often used are Kirschner's wires and Steinmann pins. Both pins are usually inserted completely through the bone, and traction forces are applied to them. Crutchfield tongs and halo pins are utilized to apply traction to the head. All sites of entry for pins, wires, or tongs should be treated as surgical wounds. These areas may be kept very clean by wiping with Betadine solution or applying Neosporin or Bacitracin ointment daily. Some physicians prefer to let these areas crust over or to cover them with plaster.

When caring for a patient in traction, the nurse checks for disturbance of circulation in the extremities. Skin color, joint motion, complaints of numbness, coldness, or swelling of the extremity are observed. The most serious complication of displaced fractures is Volkmann's ischemia, in which persistent occlusion of deep arteries results in damage to nerves and muscles. Signs of Volkmann's ischemia are severe pain, absence of peripheral pulses, pallor and coolness of the skin, puffy swelling, paresthesia, and paralysis. The nurse must avoid giving analgesics for severe and persistent pain. Instead, when Volkmann's ischemia is suspected, constricting bandages should be removed from the limb, traction should be decreased, and the physician should be notified immediately.

Skin care for the child in traction is an important

nursing responsibility. The child should lie on smooth, clean, and dry bedsheets. When the bed of the larger child is changed, two folded sheets are often more convenient than a single sheet. One sheet reaches from the head of the bed to the level of the splint, while the other covers the lower half of the bed under the splint. A trapeze bar assists the older child in lifting his shoulders off the bed for his bath and back care. The sacral area is another body part which is prone to become sore and irritated. Both the back and sacral area should be lifted off the bed and massaged two or three times a day. Skin over the heels and ankles is inspected daily for signs of pressure from bandages. A fracture bedpan assists in toileting.

The child's body alignment is closely supervised by the nurse. He must be positioned so that the purpose of traction is accomplished. The footplate does not rest against the foot of the bed and weights hang free. Measures are taken to prevent foot drop. Flexion contractures of the hip are prevented by lowering the backrest of the bed several times a day. The angle at which the child's head and shoulders can be elevated and whether the child can sit up are clarified with the physician. *Traction is not interrupted for any nursing activity* without specific orders. Clothing and diversional activities must be adapted to the traction apparatus. The child's bed can be pulled into the hall or playroom for group activities. Mobiles and toys can be suspended from the overhead bar.

Bed Rest

Bed rest provides total body rest for acute conditions such as osteomyelitis. The patient in traction or in a spica or body cast is also forced to maintain bed rest to some degree. Remaining in bed for prolonged periods has several potential hazards however, including contractures, osteoporosis, muscle atrophy, calculi development, constipation, and decubitus ulcers. Activities which can help to prevent these complications are active or passive exercises, proper positioning and turning, adequate fluid intake and diet, and good skin care.

Bed rest and immobilization are particularly difficult for the frightened or active child. Long-term hospitalizations often lead to boredom. Such problems are minimized by providing regular activities in a structured daily schedule. Schoolwork can be continued in the hospital. The child often enjoys having a television, radio, record player, tape recorder, or telephone available. When the child's bed is pulled into the hall or playroom, he can participate in group ac-

tivities. For the child who cannot sit up, special glasses with prismatic lenses allow him to see people and activities in front of him. The prone position may be facilitated by the child lying on a stretcher or Stryker frame with his arms free. Continuous relationships with nurses are important so that care is consistent. Nurses encourage independence by having the child give part of his bath, brush his teeth, comb his own hair, help dress himself (where possible), and participate in other daily care activities as he is able.

Exercise

Therapeutic exercise aims to increase muscle strength or to maintain or regain joint movement. Exercises are classified as active, passive, and resistive. Only *active exercises* strengthen muscles, and they are executed by the child himself as a natural part of his daily activities. Active exercise is dynamic when it produces motion and is static when no motion is produced (*isometric exercise*). *Passive exercise* is performed by external forces and is most valuable for the patient with paralyzed or contracted muscles. Range of motion exercises prevent deformity by maintaining movements in joints. Contractures may be treated by passive stretching of muscles. *Resistive exercise* is active exercise performed by the patient against an external resistive force, such as iron weights, sandbags, or elastic bands. This type of exercise allows the patient to improve muscle strength and coordination and to build muscle hypertrophy.

Rehabilitation

As long as physical and social barriers exist, the ability of the physically handicapped child to develop to his potential remains limited. Nurses can participate in eliminating barriers through community action and individual assistance to children and families. Local community resources can be made available to the handicapped child, in conjunction with an overall treatment program which helps the child maximize his individual resources.

The most simple and concrete suggestions are the most helpful to a child and family. For example, the little girl on crutches who would like to carry her doll with her can do so when a sling-type carrier is devised. Aprons or clothes with big pockets are useful for both boys and girls. Lightweight bicycle baskets can be attached to walking frames and pushers for use as carryalls. During play outdoors in cold weather, children who are paralyzed should be checked every 15 to 20 minutes to assure that their legs and feet are warm. Electric blankets and heating pads should not be placed on the paralyzed child's bed since they can cause burns. For the child who is incontinent, absorbent garments can be cut from colorfully designed flannel material and constructed to look more like underpants than diapers. Plastic wastebaskets can be cut out and converted into bathing chairs to help the child with poor trunk control sit in the bathtub. Parents are often exceptionally creative in adapting equipment and devising activities for their child. The nurse works closely with other interdisciplinary team members and with parents to provide a wide range of experiences which lead to maximum independence and self-esteem in the child.

MUSCULOSKELETAL DISORDERS AND INJURIES IN THE NEWBORN
Fractured Clavicle

The clavicles are the bones most often fractured during delivery, and it is interesting to note they are also the bones most commonly fractured during childhood. A clavicular fracture may be incomplete or complete. If the fracture is incomplete at birth, no pain or disability may be noticed at first, but in the second or third week of life a large callus will be discovered at the fracture site. The complete fracture is disclosed immediately after birth by the infant's refusal to move the affected arm, crying with pain when his arm is moved, and tenderness at the fracture site. Visible angulation, hematoma over the fracture site, or hypermobility of the bone may be present. The Moro reflex is reduced on the affected side. Diagnosis is confirmed by x-ray. A fracture of the clavicle increases the likelihood of brachial plexus injury; therefore, observation for this injury should be made.

The usual treatment for fracture in the newborn consists of a triangular sling and/or a figure-of-eight bandage worn underneath the clothes for 2 weeks. If there is pressure on the subclavian vessels, the bones should first be manipulated into position and then held with a figure-of-eight bandage.

The tumbling preschooler is also especially prone to a fracture of the clavicle during childhood. Treatment in the toddler is immobilization in a figure-of-eight bandage. In a child over 10 years of age, the figure-of-eight bandage is applied to reduce the fracture and if the child is very active, a plaster cast is added over the bandage. Remodeling of the bone, which corrects a residual deformity, is completed in 6 months in the younger child and within a year in the child over 10 years of age.

Nursing Management In the nursery, the nursing staff must know how to apply appropriate slings. The figure-of-eight bandage is made from strips of soft flannel, stockinet filled with cotton wool, or an elastic cotton bandage. The bandage passes around the anterior side of the shoulder and then crosses and ties posteriorly between the shoulder blades. Cotton or gauze pads should be placed in each axilla to protect the infant's skin from rubbing by the bandage. The bandage needs to be tightened daily so that it fits snugly around the shoulders; however, it should not be applied so tightly as to apply pressure on vessels or nerves. Maximum pressure should be exerted over the distal part of the shoulders, and lifting of the affected arm should be avoided. A triangular sling may be used to support the elbow, thereby holding the arm up against the chest so that the shoulder does not sag.

The nurse's teaching prepares parents to care for the child in the bandage or sling. Parents should be asked to demonstrate positioning and handling of the infant in the sling during activities such as bathing, dressing, and feeding. Parents need to know how to tighten the bandage each day as it stretches and how to reapply it if it comes off.

Brachial Plexus Injuries

Paralysis of the upper limb may be caused by traction to one or more components of the brachial plexus. These injuries occur in large babies when delivery is difficult. In modern obstetrics, the only time traction is likely to be exerted upon the plexus is when one shoulder is trapped behind the symphysis pubis during delivery and attempts to free it by traction on the head result in injury.

Signs of the injury vary according to the parts of the brachial plexus which is injured. The *upper arm* type of injury (Erb-Duchenne) involves damage to the fifth and sixth cervical nerve roots in the upper trunk of the plexus. The upper arm lies by the side of the body, with the forearm pronated and the elbow slightly flexed. Swelling and tenderness may appear in the supraclavicular region in the first few days of life. The *whole arm* type involves all cords of the plexus, resulting in complete paralysis of the limb. There is complete anesthesia on the lateral side of the arm, forearm, and hand. This injury is less common than the upper arm type. The *lower arm* type is rarest, involving injury to the lower part of the plexus and the eighth cervical and first thoracic nerve roots. Paralysis of the intrinsic muscles of the hand results. If the lesion involves the first thoracic root near the spinal cord, *Horner's syndrome* may be positive, as demonstrated by sinking in of the eyeball, ptosis of the upper eyelid, and constriction of the pupil. Spinal cord damage may also be present.

All three types of injury have some physical signs in common. Abnormal posture of the limb is immediately evident. The elbow is held in extension. Movement is absent at the shoulder on the involved side. Posterior dislocation of the shoulder may develop immediately after birth or at a later time due to muscle imbalance. A fracture of the clavicle is sometimes an associated injury.

The course of paralysis depends on the degree of damage to the nerves, which may range from slight stretching to complete rupture. If the injury, due to hemorrhage and edema in the nerve sheath, is mild, recovery is spontaneous in the first month. In moderate injuries, recovery is slow and incomplete. In severe injuries with complete rupture of the nerves, no recovery is to be expected, and with increasing age there may be severe wasting of the paralyzed muscles.

Without treatment, fixed adduction and medial rotation of the shoulder usually develop in a few days. Treatment should be instituted in the first few days after birth. The treatment of choice is early motion, in which passive range of motion exercises are instituted as soon as the diagnosis is made. Occasionally, because of the severity of injury, the extremity is splinted to allow edema to subside. The "Statue of Liberty" splint holds the arm in abduction and external rotation. Care must be used in handling the infant in the splint because the shoulder can become dislocated in this position. As recovery takes place, range of motion exercises are instituted.

Spontaneous recovery occurs to some degree in more than half the infants with the upper-arm type of injury and is complete in about 10 percent of the cases. For an infant with any type of injury in whom no recovery has taken place by the end of 2 years, reconstructive surgery has to be considered. In severe cases which cannot benefit from such surgery, amputation above the elbow may be desired during adolescence, followed by fitting with a prosthetic limb.

Nursing Management Nurses play a major role in detecting brachial plexus injuries as they care for the infant in the nursery, and it is their responsibility to teach parents how to care for their baby after discharge. When passive range of motion exercises are prescribed, the nurse carries out the exercises and demonstrates them to parents. Parents should practice doing exercises before their child is discharged so they can continue to perform them correctly at home. The purpose of these exercises should also be explained to parents. Use of the "Statue of Liberty" splint requires much care by the nursing staff to prevent posterior dislocation of the shoulder; therefore, the child's arm and shoulder should be carefully supported and cautiously moved.

Parents of a child with a brachial plexus injury should be given an estimate of the severity of damage and expectations for future growth by the physician. When the child is older, he should be helped to understand his disability and the reasons for reconstructive surgery. If amputation is considered, the adolescent should make this decision, utilizing information and support from his family and medical personnel.

Congenital Foot Deformities

Clubfoot (Talipes Equinovarus) Involved in talipes equinovarus are equinus, adduction, and inversion of the hindfoot and adduction and inversion of the forefoot (Fig. 40-7A). The incidence of this common congenital abnormality of the foot varies from 1 per 1,000 births to 4.4 per 1,000 births and is twice as common in males as in females. An equinovarus deformity may be present at birth in association with other defects, such as myelomeningocele; however, management of clubfoot due to paralysis differs from treatment of talipes equinovarus as an isolated deformity.

The cause is not known, but evidence suggests a mixed genetic and environmental causation. The most widely accepted theory is that of arrested development during the ninth and tenth weeks when the embryonic foot goes through a stage of equinus and inversion. Because the insult occurs early, it more often leads to the *rigid* type of clubfoot. Later in development, mechanisms such as malposition and abnormal intrauterine pressures are thought to be at fault. The type of deformity caused later in development is more *flexible* and involves joint tissues instead of bone.

In the rigid type of clubfoot, the only bony deformity at birth is in the talus, a major bone of the foot; there are no primary abnormalities of muscles, tendons, nerves, or vessels. The foot can be only partially corrected by manual pressure. In the flexible type of clubfoot, abnormal bony relationships are present but they are not severe. Soft tissues do not show severe shortening initially, and it is possible to correct the foot by manual pressure. Without treatment, however, all deformities progress as they did in utero. Contractures worsen and the clubfoot becomes more rigid.

Treatment for both rigid and flexible deformities should begin within the first week of life if possible. Gentle manipulation is followed by immobilization with plaster casts, elastic splints, or adhesive strapping. Weekly manipulations and cast changes are needed owing to rapid growth. By the sixth to eighth weeks, correction should be obtained. For an additional 3 months correction is held at night by bivalved casts and during the day with corrective shoes and passive exercises. If the foot is not corrected after 3 to 4 months, surgery will probably be needed to correct bony deformity, release tight ligaments, or to elongate or transplant tendons. In some cases of clubfoot, treatment is prolonged and the deformity tends to recur. Additional casting and surgery may be required throughout childhood.

Metatarsus Adductus   Also called metatarsus varus, metatarsus adductus is an adduction or varus deformity of the forefoot. The anterior portion of the foot, including all metatarsals, is adducted as well as supinated (Fig. 40-7B). There is usually an associated internal tibial torsion deformity. The incidence is 2 per 1,000 live births, and it is often bilateral. Metatarsus adductus is one of the causes of pigeon-toe.

If the deformity is minimal, treatment consists of stretching exercises five or six times daily by parents and attention to sleeping posture. Habitually sleeping with the feet turned in aggravates the deformity. Treatment must be received early, at least in the first few weeks of life, if the deformity is more angulated and rigid. Initially, treatment involves plaster casting to achieve a gradual reduction of the deformity. After 6 to 12 weeks (depending on resistance to correction), a Denis Browne boot splint is worn nightly. This splint is worn for a few months to maintain the correction and to treat the accompanying internal tibial torsion. Corrective shoes are worn during the daytime for the first year.

The deformity becomes more rigid with each month it is undetected. If it remains untreated after walking begins, the child may toe in, walk clumsily, and trip over his feet. In untreated severe metatarsus adductus, a soft-tissue releasing operation or osteotomy may be required.

Nursing Management   Nurses play a role in early detection and referral of an affected child to an appropriate physician or clinic. Parents need an overall view of the treatment program to understand the importance of regular cast or splint changes. They can be taught to soak off old casts before a clinic appointment by immersing the cast in a vinegar-water solution of about 1 part vinegar to 4 parts

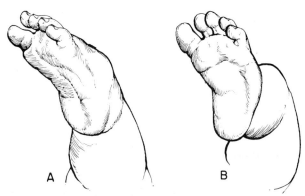

Figure 40-7   Congenital foot deformities: (A) Clubfoot. (B) Metatarsus adductus. *(Illustration by C. Gosling, Department of Medical Illustration, Indiana University–Purdue University at Indianapolis.)*

water, and then unwrapping the plaster. When a new cast is applied, parents should be instructed about how to support the cast until it dries and observe for signs of circulatory impairment.

If the child is fitted with a Denis Browne splint, the nurse should discuss its care with parents. The child's feet may be slipped into special boots or shoes attached to the splint, or the feet may be strapped to the splint by adhesive tape. The nurse can demonstrate these care measures: application of the removable splint, use of socks to protect the feet, checking the skin for reddened areas, and use of the splint key to tighten shoes against the bar if they become loose. The nurse should clarify for parents the times the splint is to be worn. The child who requires surgery receives preoperative and postoperative care as described earlier in this chapter.

Congenital Amputation

A congenital amputation is the absence of a distal part of a limb at birth. The arms are more often involved in this deformity, and severity ranges from absence of a toe to amputations involving all four limbs.

Constricting bands are seen in the affected limb, and they are probably caused by insufficient growth of skin and soft tissues around the limb's circumference. If constrictions are shallow, a normal limb may exist distal to the constriction. Deep circular constrictions cause an enlargement of the distal portion of the limb due to edema. With very deep constrictions, the distal part of the limb is absent.

Fitting the child with appropriate artificial limbs (*prostheses*) should begin in early infancy. With growth, limbs will need frequent modifications in size. Upper-limb prostheses are a greater functional problem because of the highly specialized movements of a normal hand. When the infant starts to use his hands and develop hand-eye coordination, a prosthesis of a simple mitten design is fitted to help him become bimanual. A prosthesis with full adult controls should be worn by the time a child reaches school age. Lower limbs are fitted before the child begins to walk.

Nursing Management As parents work through their grief after birth of the child, they need to be presented with realistic information about their child's future abilities. Both the child and his parents should be encouraged to use the prescribed prostheses as directed. Parents often have a difficult time getting the child to use his prosthesis because of their own guilt feelings; therefore, early intervention is essential.

Much recent progress in care can be credited to the establishment of juvenile amputee centers, which employ an interdisciplinary approach. One outgrowth of these centers has been major improvements in prostheses. External power for upper-limb prostheses has been developed from compressed gases and electronic devices. Cosmetic hands with the coloring and form of a normal hand are especially favored by girls.

Dysmelia

The term *dysmelia* refers to congenital malformations in which the long bones of the extremities are hypoplastic or aplastic. Both dysmelia and congenital amputation present degrees of loss of a limb. In congenital amputation, the lost part is distal. In dysmelia, the part may be lost proximally or axially.

Deformity in dysmelia ranges from peripheral hypoplasia of one bone, as in *proximal focal femoral deficiency* (PFFD), to total absence of the extremity (*amelia*). *Phocomelia* describes a degree of dysmelia in which remnants of the long bones are present between the limb girdle and the hand or foot. There may be a family history of the deformity, or it may be caused by an environmental factor, such as the drug thalidomide.[2]

For some children, function is improved by a built-up boot or a prosthesis fitted over the entire limb. Upper-extremity deformities may require no prosthesis. Surgery is sometimes indicated for correction or stabilization of limb deformity. Amputation is performed in severe cases to allow fitting of a prosthesis.

Torticollis (Wryneck)

Torticollis is an abnormality in which the head is flexed and rotated by a shortening of the sternocleidomastoid muscle on one side of the neck. At birth the deformity is small; after a few weeks a large, firm tumor appears in the sternocleidomastoid muscle. This swelling probably results from a hypertrophy of fibrous tissue in the muscle. The cause of swelling is unknown; however, the defect is seen more frequently following difficult deliveries with abnormal presentations and in primiparas.

The tumor slowly subsides in 3 to 6 months, but without treatment a contracture (shortening) of the muscle usually remains, and it fails to grow normally in length. Shortness of the muscle causes even greater flexion or tilting toward the affected side, and rotation or twisting toward the opposite side. During the growing years, a facial asymmetry develops.

If daily stretching exercises are begun in the first month of life, complete correction of the torticollis can be achieved in 90 percent of children. Before treatment begins, parents should understand that the deformity can recur.

In severe cases or those diagnosed after the first few months of life, surgical intervention is necessary, and it involves a division of the sternocleidomastoid muscle and the contracted soft tissues. When the child is admitted to the hospital, the parents (and the child if he is old enough to understand) need preparation about what will be done in surgery and how the child will appear afterward. Postoperative nursing measures depend on the type of immobilization used. When a cast has been applied, the nurse is careful to position the child on pillows which support the cast. It is also important to turn the child frequently to allow the entire cast to dry. If a bulky dressing has been applied, stretching exercises must be started on the day after surgery and continued two or three times a day for several weeks. The nurse who does these passive exercises must ensure that they are carried out fully despite the child's complaints of tenderness along the incision line. Parents should be taught to do these exercises at home. Simple treatment measures include (1) moving a child's bed so that he must turn away from the affected side, and (2) feeding the child in a position which requires him to turn his head away from the affected side in order to see his caretaker. If exercises cannot be done, the physician should be informed. When surgery involves the left side, any sign of respiratory distress which appears postoperatively should be reported to the physician immediately. These symptoms may indicate damage to the thoracic duct during surgery, which allowed lymph to effuse into the chest.

Congenital Hip Dysplasia

Congenital hip dysplasia denotes an abnormality of the hip joint at birth. Hip dysplasia involves three stages of increasing severity: unstable, subluxed, and dislocated. It may be unilateral or bilateral (see Fig. 40-8). Although hip dysplasia may occur secondary to joint, muscular, or neuromuscular abnormalities, the cause of the typical condition is unknown.

Several theories of the cause of hip dysplasia have been suggested. Laxity of the ligaments around the capsule of the hip joint is the most widely accepted cause, and it is thought to result from action of maternal sex hormones which relax maternal ligaments in preparation for labor. Other important causative factors include malposition in utero and environmental factors after birth. The former is often associated with a breech presentation, dislocation being 10 times more common after a breech delivery than after a vertex presentation. Factors in the environment include the position in which an infant is carried during its early months. In areas of the world where a mother carries her child balanced on her hip with legs in abduction, the incidence is very low. The incidence is high among cultures which swaddle infants' legs together in adduction and extension.

Physical findings depend on the age of the child and the type of dysplasia (unstable, subluxed, or dislocated). Barlow's test is the most reliable test in the newborn and is used to detect an unstable hip which is dislocatable. Ortolani's test is used to detect a dislocated hip. Both Ortolani's and Barlow's tests are useful in the infant under 3 months of age. After 3 months, limited abduction of the hip becomes a significant sign. The femur appears shortened when the infant lies on a table with his knees and hips flexed at right angles. Asymmetry of skin folds of the thigh and popliteal and gluteal creases result in deeper creases on the affected side. These creases may be present at any age, but they are unreliable for diagnosis in the newborn. After 1 year of age when the infant has begun to walk, he has a typical limp to his gait—a ducklike waddle or "sailor's gait." The child shifts the weight of his trunk over the dislocated hip when he stands on it. Another sign is a positive Trendelenburg's test: when the child stands on the side of the dislocated hip, the pelvis drops on the opposite normal side; when he stands on the normal side, the pelvis on that side stays up in the horizontal position. Dropping of the pelvis on the normal side is due to

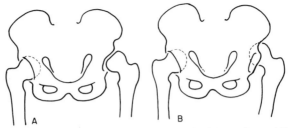

Figure 40-8   Unilateral hip dysplasia in the newborn. (A) Left subluxed hip and (B) left dislocated hip, with normal hips on both right sides. *(Illustration by C. Gosling, Department of Medical Illustration, Indiana University–Purdue University at Indianapolis.)*

weakness in the abductor muscles of the affected hip.

Treatment which begins under 2 months of age is most successful. The hip is reduced by gentle manipulation and maintained by splinting the hips in abduction with a Frejka pillow or other abduction splint. The splint is used continuously for approximately two to three months, followed by night splinting for another month. Normal development of the hip can then be expected.

By the second to the eighteenth months, a contracture of the hip adductors has developed. The child who is diagnosed at this time is first placed in bilateral skin traction to pull the femoral head down to the acetabulum. The older child who has been standing or walking may need to be placed in skeletal traction on the affected side, with skin traction on the normal side. The hips are gradually moved into wide abduction after the femoral head has been brought into the socket. After a period of approximately two weeks, gentle closed reduction is done. If a reduction is evident on x-ray, the hips are immobilized in a hip spica cast or metal splint for 4 to 6 months. Open reduction may be needed if closed methods are unsuccessful. X-ray follow-up is done on subsequent clinic visits while the cast is still in place.

The older the child when treatment is begun, the less potential for normal hip development. With increasing age and progressive weight bearing, soft-tissue contractures become more rigid, and the contour of the acetabular socket and femoral neck become more abnormal. Skeletal traction followed by closed or open reduction and a hip spica cast are accepted treatments between the ages of 1½ and 3 years. In the child of 4 to 7 years, skeletal traction and open reduction are usually necessary. Osteotomy may also be necessary. By 8 years and older it is best to postpone treatment for bilateral dislocation, although when dislocation in unilateral, attempts may be made to improve stability of the hip by surgery. Subluxed hips may also be helped by surgery.

Nursing Management Every nurse concerned with the care of newborn infants should be aware of the clinical signs and tests used to diagnose congenital dislocation of the hip. Although the nurse does not generally perform Ortolani's and Barlow's tests, he can be aware of suspicious signs such as asymmetric creases and limitation of abduction. In the infant, these signs are much more significant. Additional observations should be made of the child who is walking, including watching for the ducklike waddle and positive Trendelenburg's sign.

When dysplasia is found early, the newborn or infant is fitted with a Frejka pillow splint or another abduction device such as the Illfeld splint. The nurse should explain the splint's purpose and demonstrate its application to parents. As the nurse observes parents applying the splint, instructions should be given about handling the child in such a way as to keep hips abducted. Clothing worn under the splint should protect the child's skin from any irritation caused by the appliance. Two pillow covers are provided with the Frejka pillow splint so that one can be worn while the other is being laundered. It is important that the nurse clarify, with parents, the times the splint is to be worn and how long it can be removed for bathing, dressing, and diaper changes.

The child who is hospitalized for treatment faces several months of immobilization in traction and spica casts. Parents need information and anticipatory guidance about the care of their child. If they feel comfortable with equipment used in treatment and are adequately informed, they are better able to enjoy and play with the child during the course of his immobility.

Myelomeningocele

A congenital abnormality, myelomeningocele involves herniation of the spinal cord and its meninges through a defect in the vertebral canal (see Chap. 32). Resulting nerve damage usually causes muscle paralysis or weakness in the lower limbs and requires long-term orthopedic care (see Table 40-2).

The aims of orthopedic treatment are to correct deformity, maintain the correction, and obtain maximum function in the lower limbs. Growth can be a troublesome factor, for with growth an increasing deformity may develop in response to unbalanced muscle action. Because of normal upper limbs and trunk musculature, most children, even if severely paralyzed, can stand or walk with appropriate bracing. In the treatment to minimize deformities, timing of procedures is critical. The orthopedic surgeon aims to complete all procedures before the eighteenth month because most children appear ready to stand and walk by that time. On the average, two to three but as many as seven or eight orthopedic procedures are likely to be needed. As the child matures, he grows taller and heavier, he cannot balance and handle himself as well, and deformities such as scoliosis increase. Often he can no longer use his braces and must depend upon a wheelchair for mobility.

Nursing Management Prevention and correction of hip deformity begins at birth. The infant is positioned with the hips in abduction (Fig. 40-9). The Frejka pillow splint maintains such a position when the infant goes home, and it is worn for 6 to 8 months. Nursing care in the Frejka pillow is described in the section on congenital hip dysplasia above. The abduction position has been responsible for reducing the necessity for surgery in many children. If abduction contractures develop and do not correct after removal of the splint, the deformity can easily be surgically corrected after the child develops deep acetabular coverage for the femoral head.

When dislocation of the hips is present at birth or occurs after birth, other measures may be necessary. Conservative measures such as traction or casting are done initially. Because these children have some lack of sensation in the lower extremities, special care must be taken to prevent skin breakdown. The skin should be checked thoroughly every day when traction is rewrapped. If the child is in a cast, areas around cast edges should be checked every day.

If conservative measures fail to correct dislocation, some type of surgery may be required. Muscle and tendon transfers may be done to maintain the femur in the hip socket. In the older child, an osteotomy is often the treatment of choice. Special needs of these children after surgery include prevention of urinary tract infection, observation for pressure areas under the cast, and measures to keep the cast clean and dry despite incontinence. Many older children have urinary diversions and regular bowel evacuation routines which, when modified to care in the cast, make nursing care easier.

Deformities of the knees and feet require early manipulation. Knee deformities are less common and can usually be corrected by gentle passive manipulation in the early neonatal period. A fixed

Table 40-2 LEVEL OF PARALYSIS AND CORRESPONDING ABILITIES AND
DEFORMITIES IN MYELOMENINGOCELE

Level of paralysis (vertebra)	Functional ability	Orthopedic deformity	Probable ambulation ability
T 12	Pelvic flexion	Flaccid paralysis of legs	Wheelchair
L 1–2	Hip flexion	Flexion contracture and dislocation of hips	Wheelchair
L 3	Extension of knee	Flexion contracture and dislocation of hips, hyperextension of knees	Ambulation with long leg braces and crutches
L 4	Flexion of knee	Dislocation of hips, clubfeet	Ambulation in short leg braces and crutches
L 5	Dorsiflexion and eversion of the feet	Calcaneous deformity of feet with heel ulcerations	Ambulation in short leg braces
S 1	Plantar flexion of feet, extension of hips	None	Ambulatory

Source: R. Lindseth, M.D., Chief of Pediatric Orthopedics and Professor, Indiana University Medical Center.

hyperextension deformity or increasing flexion contractures in the older child requires operative treatment. Foot deformities may be present at birth or may develop in infancy and childhood from unequal muscle pulling. Treatment is aimed at correcting all fixed deformities before the child starts to bear weight on the feet. In the newborn, positioning should allow feet to rest in an anatomic position, and plaster casts and/or passive stretching exercises are used to correct clubfeet. Nurses, physical therapists, and parents must realize the importance of these early measures, since they may prevent the need for surgery.

Any type of manipulation or range-of-motion exercises should be prescribed by the orthopedist. Hips should not be exercised in the newborn because of the tendency for dislocation. Knee and ankle exercises are done for correction of specific deformities. Exercises should be gentle because of the danger of pathologic fractures. Before the infant is discharged, the physical therapist should teach parents the exercise program for their child.

Spinal deformities which may be present at birth or develop with growth include kyphosis, lordosis, and scoliosis. Pressure sores over the bony defect are common in kyphosis. To facilitate the supine position, which is important in the infant's development, a foam rubber pad can be used with a hole cut out under the back defect. The skin over the kyphosis should be checked for reddened areas daily, and measures taken to remove pressure over these areas by modifying clothing or the child's position. Any clothing or equipment which irritates the child's

back should be removed. He should be placed on his abdomen for sleep, with any sore areas exposed to air. Wet-to-dry soaks may be needed to debride decubitus ulcers over the kyphosis. When a child actively rubs skin areas raw, these areas should be covered for protection and every effort made to keep the child off his back. Kyphosis may be corrected by excision of one or more vertebrae in a vertebral resection operation. After this surgery, the child is immobilized in a spica body cast for approximately six months. Lordosis and scoliosis may require spinal osteotomy and spinal fusion later in childhood.

Braces are introduced at a selected time in the child's development. Metal, leather, and polypropylene plastic are materials used in brace construction. The purpose of bracing is to give support to weak or unstable body parts. Short leg braces stabilize the ankle and foot, while long leg braces give stability to the entire leg. A pelvic band is added for support at the hip so that the young child with almost total paralysis can stand. Special standing devices, such as modified tables, can be constructed to support the child wearing these standing braces. Various walking aids such as crutches or walkers provide support for any child who needs it for ambulation.

Due to loss of sensation in parts of the lower extremities and the perineal area, decubitus ulcers are common (see Chap. 32). Attention should be given to teaching both parents and child about skin care, methods of bowel and bladder control or drainage, hygiene, and other activities of daily living which

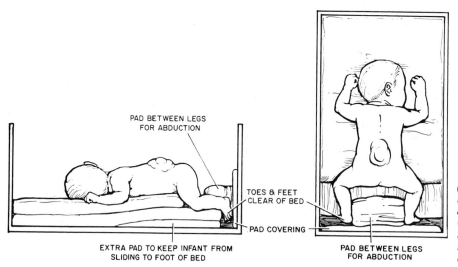

PAD BETWEEN LEGS
FOR ABDUCTION

TOES & FEET
CLEAR OF BED

PAD COVERING

EXTRA PAD TO KEEP INFANT FROM
SLIDING TO FOOT OF BED

PAD BETWEEN LEGS
FOR ABDUCTION

Figure 40-9 Positioning of infants with myelomeningocele. *(Courtesy James Whitcomb Riley Hospital for Children, Indianapolis, Ind.; illustration by C. Gosling, Department of Medical Illustration, Indiana University–Purdue University at Indianapolis.)*

contribute to health. School-age children and adolescents should be taught to inspect the soles of their feet and the perineal area daily, using a hand mirror. Rubbing from splints, braces, or shoes must be watched carefully, and if signs of prolonged redness or soreness occur, the cause of pressure should be removed. This may mean that weight bearing or sitting must be stopped. Obesity and limited mobility also contribute to formation of decubiti. Teaching about nutrition begins in infancy, with modification of diet any time a child appears to be gaining too much weight.

Spontaneous fractures due to osteoporosis are also all too common in these children. No pain occurs because of sensory loss; therefore, the fracture may not be recognized at first. Spontaneous swelling may result 1 or 2 days after mild trauma causes a fracture. Redness and warmth may also be present and resemble a cellulitis. A suspected fracture should be splinted and the child taken to a physician as soon as these signs are noticed.

As in the care of any child who has a chronic, incurable illness, nurses need to examine their attitudes and behaviors toward the child and his parents if they are to intervene successfully. Parents' feelings of guilt, hostility, and frustration are especially prominent at the time of the infant's birth, but if they are helped to gradually learn to care for their child and develop a relationship with him, this period has much positive potential. Parents are particularly receptive at this time to teaching about medical problems and treatment, special nursing measures, and normal baby care. Associations of parents of children who have spina bifida, which have been formed in many states and large cities, offer parents educational and supportive experiences.

MUSCULOSKELETAL DISORDERS AND INJURIES IN THE INFANT AND TODDLER
Cerebral Palsy

The wide variety of nonprogressive brain disorders referred to as *cerebral palsy* require carefully planned, individualized training programs (see Chap. 32). It should be remembered that the severity of a child's physical handicap is not an accurate prediction of the severity of the mental handicap or the ability to benefit from a training program. The child is helped to develop speech, locomotion, self-help skills in daily activities, such as eating and dressing, and success in regular or special education. Problems often occur in social adjustment, especially during adolescence. Treatment of problems associated with cerebral palsy, such as seizures and visual or auditory disorders, continues throughout life and must be considered in any overall treatment program. The aim of treatment is to help the child become as physically independent, socially adjusted, mentally able, and emotionally competent as possible. For the older child with these abilities, vocational training is considered a step toward economic independence.

Therapy for the development of motor skills begins in infancy and continues throughout childhood. Although the infant may be slow, he should follow a pattern of normal development as closely as possible. Regular assessments are made to measure the level and progress of his motor development. Suggestions are then given to the child's family on specific ways in which to help their child progress. The *spastic* child has problems of exaggerated stretch reflexes and muscle imbalance in involved limbs. He often acquires flexion, adduction, and internal rotation contractures. To prevent such occurrences, passive stretching of spastic muscles should begin in infancy. The older child exercises actively to prevent contractures and strengthen the weak antagonistic muscles. Braces may be worn at night to preserve functional positions, and they are used during daytime hours for standing, gaining balance and strength, and allowing activities in the upright position. The child with *athetosis* has constant involuntary movements which disappear during sleep. He is trained in voluntary and conscious relaxation to allow purposeful movements. These children usually do not develop contractures unless they are positioned improperly by their caretakers. Braces may help correct contractures and control some involuntary movements. With *ataxia,* balance and coordination are impaired. Training includes improvement of muscle tone, sitting and standing balance, walking, and eye-to-hand skills. The child with *rigidity* type of cerebral palsy is trained much like the spastic child, although training is less effective owing to more extensive brain damage. Medication is the primary treatment for the *tremor* type of handicap.

The role of orthopedic surgery in treatment is to correct local physical defects. Surgery is most often indicated in spastic paralysis although it is becoming more useful in athetosis. Parents need to understand that surgery can only improve function; it will not make the limbs normal. Much of the success of surgery depends on the quality of follow-up care and training afterwards. In spasticity, operations are performed to release resistant contractures, to correct other deformities, and to improve muscle balance. Common procedures include tendon lengthening, tendon transfers, and arthrodesis. In athetosis, surgery may be useful for correcting distorted positions, but it is more commonly done to release postural contractures, such as equinus deformity in the ankle. Release of such contractures often makes bracing and walking possible for the child.

Nursing Management When a child with cerebral palsy is admitted to the hospital for orthopedic surgery, the nurse should collect information from parents about his home routines in feeding, taking medications, dressing, and other daily activities so that these routines can be incorporated into the nursing care plan. Much of the success of nursing care depends on the attitude of acceptance of the handicapped child by the nurse. Only with this attitude can the nurse help the child adjust to hospitalization and treatment and help parents care for their child. Teaching about cast care, positioning and handling, mobility limits, and stimulation begins during hospitalization so that parents are ready to continue care at home.

Nurses may also be involved in the child's long-term program of therapy. Assistance is given to parents as they attempt to carry out recommended activities in feeding and positioning measures, in addition to assisting the child in the development of motor skills and in intellectual accomplishment. Modifications may be needed to help the child with bowel and bladder training and toileting. The nurse should instruct parents on skin care and skin checks in order to detect irritation from braces and other sources of pressure. When administering anticonvulsant drugs, the nurse constantly assesses these children for evidence of the effects of these medications, in addition to increased seizure activity.

Parents can be encouraged by the nurse to participate in parent organizations. Much support is shared among group members, and opportunities are provided for socialization, parent education, and public education. Nurses sometimes serve as sponsors for these organizations, utilizing their knowledge about interpersonal relationships and group dynamics.

Osteomyelitis

Osteomyelitis is primarily a disease of children, with boys being more frequently affected than girls. Long bones that are rapidly growing, such as the femur, tibia, humerus, and radius, are most often involved. In 80 to 90 percent of the cases, *Staphylococcus aureus* is the responsible organism. *Streptococcus, Proteus,* and *Pseudomonas* are other causative agents. Bacteria enter through infections on the skin, such as scratches, pimples, boils, or through the mucous membranes after nose or throat infections. An open fracture or other wound may also serve as a portal of entry. When bacteria have been introduced, a traumatized area in a bone seems to attract bacteria and provide a locus for osteomyelitis. This area is found most often in the metaphysis of the long bone, and it is due to the sluggish blood flow and blood pools of that region.

Because a bone is a rigid closed space, the edema and hyperemia at the beginning of infection cause a sharp rise in pressure within the bone. Severe and constant pain is felt in the area. With formation of pus, pressure on local blood vessels may be so great that necrosis of bone results. Pus also strips the periosteum from bone, interfering with its blood supply. When infection spreads through the cortex to the periosteum, pain becomes even more severe.

Without treatment the area of infection continues to enlarge, and septicemia may develop. The infection penetrates the periosteum into the soft tissues, where it produces cellulitis and then an abscess. If the joint capsule is penetrated, septic arthritis results. When the initial area of bone necrosis separates from living bone, a *sequestrum,* or isolated piece of dead bone, is formed. Metastatic focuses of infection are carried to other bones by the septicemia. Without treatment, the child who survives the septicemia acquires a chronic form of osteomyelitis.

The first symptom experienced with this disease is pain in the involved area. The child is unwilling to move the limb. Septicemia results in just 24 hours, as evidenced by weakness, lack of appetite, and fever. It takes a few days for soft-tissue swelling, redness, and heat to be produced as the infection spreads beyond bone. In infants, signs of osteomyelitis are more diffuse. Little or no fever may be present, but irritability, loss of function in the involved limb, tenderness, and swelling may be noted. Early diagnosis is based on clinical signs alone, although these may be masked by inadequate antibiotic therapy. X-ray is valuable only after several days when destruction of bone has taken place.

Treatment begins immediately after diagnosis, in the hospital. After blood cultures have been taken, intravenous antibacterial therapy is instituted. Bed rest and analgesics make the child more comfortable. The affected extremity is rested by removable splints or traction to reduce pain, prevent movement which spreads infection, and prevent contractures in soft tissues. If clinical signs have not improved within 24 hours, decompression of the infected bony area must be done in surgery. At that time, pus is removed for culture, and pressure in the bone relieved. Postoperatively, drainage is continued.

Inadequate treatment usually leads to chronic osteomyelitis. The presence of infected dead bone prevents healing. Because this bone separates from live bone in the form of a sequestrum, resorption and deposition of new bone does not take place, and antibiotics cannot reach it. The child is no longer acutely ill, but local signs of inflammation are present. Treatment is more radical in the chronic form of disease. Removal of the dead bone must usually be accomplished by surgery, and it is followed by drainage of the area.

Septic Arthritis

Acute septic or suppurative arthritis is an inflammation of the joint caused by pus-forming organisms. Infants and children of 1 or 2 years of age are most often affected, although this disease appears in all age groups, and males are involved more often than females. The hip joint is the site of highest frequency, with the knee and elbow second in order of occurrence. More than one joint may be involved.

Infection is most commonly caused by a staphylococcus or a streptococcus organism. Infection is spread to the joint through the bloodstream from a distant focus of infection such as otitis media or an acute infectious disease. Direct extension of infection may travel from a neighboring bone focus, especially at the hip. At the knee, penetrating wounds are a primary cause. Inflammation begins in the synovial membrane. Synovial fluid is thin and cloudy at first but thickens as pus is formed. The pus rapidly destroys articular cartilage. Disintegration of cartilage may be followed by osteomyelitis in the underlying bone.

There are clear signs and symptoms in the toddler with this disease. The child may be able to point out the painful joint, and he guards it from movement. Other signs include spasms of the muscles around the joint, swelling of tissues, fever, and an elevated white blood cell count.

In the infant, septic arthritis is found most frequently in the hip. Pathologic dislocation and necrosis of the femoral head can complicate the disease. Because the entire femoral head, including the epiphyseal plate, is composed of cartilage, it may be completely destroyed.

Treatment must be immediate in all age groups. Fluid for culture is obtained by needle aspiration. Antibiotic treatment is started locally by joint instillation. Surgical exploration of the joint (*arthrotomy*) is more effective to remove pus and irrigate the joint. Postoperatively, closed infusion and drainage are commonly used and are continued until drainage is sterile. Immobilization of the joint by casting is necessary to prevent dislocation. If damage to the joint is permanent, reconstructive procedures may be needed. Although treatment is similar in osteomyelitis and septic arthritis, failure of treatment to be effective in septic arthritis can lead to more permanent disability.

Nursing Management The nurse's role in early detection and in support during hospitalization is similar in osteomyelitis and septic arthritis. When a child is seen with chief complaints of fever and a swollen, tender extremity, the nurse should think primarily of acute osteomyelitis. A history of boils, puncture wounds, tonsillitis, or upper respiratory infection increases the likelihood of this diagnosis. Signs of septic arthritis which can be recognized early by the nurse include a painful and swollen joint, guarding of the joint against movement, fever, and irritability. Assessment of the site of inflammation is more difficult in the infant or toddler who cannot describe where he hurts. A child who is suspected of having either of these disorders should be referred to a physician for immediate diagnosis and treatment.

When the child is admitted to the hospital, he should be placed in bed and helped to rest as much as possible. The nurse assists the physician in securing blood and wound cultures and instituting intravenous therapy. Bactericidal drugs which are often given intravenously include penicillin and methicillin. Analgesics are administered to make the child more comfortable. Skin traction, splints, or casts are applied to immobilize the involved limb or joint. The nurse should check the peripheral circulation of the limb for signs of circulation impairment in a cast or traction. Vital signs are monitored every 4 hours or more frequently in the presence of fever or postoperatively. If closed infusion and drainage are used, the nurse is responsible for monitoring the fluids and keeping accurate intake and output records.

When early treatment has been effective and the child does not feel particularly ill, appropriate stimulation becomes a part of nursing care. Play activities can be brought to the child, or he can be taken to them in bed or in a wheelchair. As in any long-term hospitalization, the child's parents need to be involved in his care. They should be helped to understand his mobility limitations as well as his needs for socialization.

Osteogenesis Imperfecta

Also known as "brittle bones," osteogenesis imperfecta is a connective tissue disorder that primarily affects bone. It is manifested by a fragile skeleton, thin skin and sclera, poor teeth, macular bleeding, and hypermobility of the joints. The tendency of the fragile bones to fracture on slight trauma is an outstanding characteristic of the disease. The underlying pathology is in bone formation. Collagen fails to maturate throughout the body and remains in an immature form. Therefore, instead of normal compact bone, a coarse, immature type of bone is produced.

A *congenital* type of osteogenesis imperfecta in which multiple fractures are caused by minimal trauma during delivery or in utero is rare. Osteogenesis imperfecta *tarda* is less severe and becomes evident at some time in childhood. The condition occurs as a spontaneous mutation, but once established, it persists as an autosomal dominant trait.

In the tarda type, delayed walking may be the chief presenting complaint. The child is often seen by a physician for the first time following a fracture. The number of fractures which continue to occur during childhood varies greatly. Lower limbs are more frequently affected since they are more prone to trauma. Refracturing is common because of limb deformity and disuse atrophy resulting from immobilization.

The pain, deformity, and swelling which result from a complete fracture are the same as those in a normal child. With an incomplete fracture, however, pain may not be a complaint because soft-tissue injury is minimal. A deformity often develops in the injured limb with continued activity. Fractures heal at a normal rate. Callus formation may be minimal or occasionally so excessive that it may be misdiagnosed as osteogenic sarcoma. Bone formed following a fracture is of the same poor quality as that which it replaces.

Growth may be retarded from curvature of the limbs and spine and by multiple injuries at the epiphyseal ends. Extremities tend to be thin and long. Kyphosis and scoliosis are common as a result of compression fractures of the vertebral bodies. The skull is often misshapen with protrusion of the frontal and parietal regions.

Other connective tissue besides bone is affected. Skeletal muscles are poorly developed, and the child is generally weak. Hypermobility of joints results from excessive laxity of the ligaments and capsule. The skin is thin, and subcutaneous hemorrhages may occur. Teeth, often discolored, are affected because of deficiency of dentin. They break easily, are prone to caries, and after dental care, fillings are not retained. The sclerae may appear blue, although vision is unaffected. Deafness, due to osteosclerosis or pressure on the auditory nerve as it emerges from the skull, may be a problem in adult life.

Prognosis varies in the tarda type. If the condition is severe in early childhood, disabling deformities are likely to develop unless constant care is taken to minimize them. The severity is likely to decrease at puberty because of the action of sex hormones. With maturity, the patient also learns how to prevent falls and fractures.

There is no specific treatment for this condition. The child should be taught to avoid unnecessary risks. Active sports and gymnastic activities should be prohibited. Some fractures are inevitable, but during treatment, immobilization should be reduced to a minimum since disuse atrophy increases the likelihood of more fractures. Bowing or torsional deformities may require multiple osteotomies of long bones and insertion of intramedullary metal rods. These rods serve the dual purpose of correcting deformity and providing support to prevent further fractures and deformity. Braces, crutches, or wheelchairs are sometimes prescribed as added protection against fractures.

Nursing Management Early recognition of fractures is important in treatment; therefore, both parents and the child need to be taught the signs of fractures. Treatment of fractures and correction of deformities often involve traction and/or immobilization in casts. In the hospital, nurses should handle the child gently to avoid further fractures.

Limitation of activity and frequent hospitalizations place much stress on both the child and his family. As the child assumes independence, close monitoring of his activities by parents is impossible. It is essential that the child be helped to understand his disability so that he can gradually assume responsibility for precautions required. Interest in activities other than the gross motor type should be encouraged by parents and nurses. School should be continued during the older child's admissions to the hospital. Parents need information concerning recurrence risks and may desire to be referred to a genetic counseling service.

Rickets

Rickets is a generalized disease of growing bone caused by inadequate calcification of bone matrix and evidenced by bone deformities. Uncalcified areas of bone are soft, allowing deformities to result from physiologic and gravitational stresses. The epiphyseal plate can also be affected, resulting in growth disorders in limbs.

Normal calcification of matrix is dependent upon adequate levels of calcium and phosphorus in the blood. Three factors regulate calcium and phosphorus levels: (1) absorption from the intestines, (2) excretion by kidneys and intestine, and (3) rates of movement into and out of bone. Vitamin D and parathyroid hormone are important in maintaining a normal balance of minerals between bone and bloodstream. Classification of rickets is based on the cause of mineral imbalance: vitamin D deficiency, chronic renal insufficiency, or renal tubular insufficiency.

Rickets caused by *vitamin D deficiency* is much less common since the importance of sunlight and vitamin D have been recognized. This type is usually seen in children about one year of age. Growth retardation and weakness are present, and if severe hypocalcemia has occurred, convulsions or tetany may result. Treatment by normal doses of vitamin D and improvement in diet corrects the underlying disease. In infants, most structural deformities are corrected by growth alone.

Chronic renal insufficiency may cause rickets, which has been referred to as *renal rickets*. Chronic renal disease produces not only the rickets but also a hyperparathyroidism which creates bone lesions. The disease is vitamin D–refractory in that it does not respond to normal doses of the vitamin. Primary treatment must be for the renal disease; surgical correction of deformities must be correlated with treatment for renal disease.

Rickets due to *renal tubular insufficiency* is also vitamin D–refractory. The name *hypophosphatemic rickets* is derived from the basic pathology. Tubular reabsorption of phosphorus is inadequate, causing hypophosphatemia. Without sufficient phosphorus, calcium is not deposited in adequate amounts in the bones. Otherwise the child is healthy, and the renal problem does not affect life expectancy. An inborn error of metabolism is responsible for the disease and can be inherited by either a sex-linked or a dominant gene. Treatment includes administration of oral phosphorus solutions and massive doses of vitamin D with close monitoring of calcium balance for hypercalcemia.

Orthopedic management of deformities is secondary to treatment of the basic disorder causing rickets. When treatment is successful, bony deformities tend to improve. If torsional deformities are present in the limbs, appropriate night splints may be prescribed. Surgical correction by osteotomy may be necessary for persistent deformities. Several weeks before surgery, vitamin D therapy should be stopped so that postoperative immobilization and resulting decalcification of bone do not cause severely elevated levels of calcium in the blood.

Nursing Management Diet is the primary consideration in the treatment of rickets caused by vitamin D deficiency. The child should be provided with an improved diet which includes normal amounts of vitamin D. Milk fortified with vitamin D and other fortified products such as cereals provide adequate amounts of the vitamin. Rickets due to chronic renal insufficiency has a much poorer prognosis because of the effects of the renal disease. Adequate amounts of calcium and vitamin D are included in the diet, but primary attention is given to treatment of the renal disorder.

Because the child with hypophosphatemic rickets has no other harmful manifestations of his disease, the prevention and correction of musculoskeletal deformities assumes high priority during the entire growth period. Large doses of vitamin D promote calcium absorption in the intestine so that adequate calcium is available for bone growth and calcification of teeth. Drisdol, a form of vitamin D, is available in capsules or solution. Enough of the vitamin is given to maintain a normal blood calcium level. Because large doses of vitamin D can impair kidney function, 24-hour urine specimens are taken to ensure that waste products, including creatinine, are being excreted normally. Phosphorus solutions such as Neutra-Phos are also given to maintain adequate levels of blood phosphorus. A common side effect of administering phosphorus solutions in the younger child is diarrhea, which may need to be controlled with medication. Regular dental examinations are particularly important for children with this disease because dental caries are likely to develop. The child should be supervised in a daily program of dental hygiene. The nurse is a member of the interdisciplinary team which institutes and reinforces this treatment program.[3]

Orthopedic deformities are assessed regularly in children with hypophosphatemic rickets. Bowing of the legs is a common deformity for which osteotomies may be required. Before the child is admitted to the hospital for surgery, administration of vitamin D is stopped. After surgery blood calcium tends to rise, and vitamin D is temporarily discontinued. Special postoperative nursing measures include maintaining hydration and resuming phosphorus solutions when the child can take them orally. Screening for hypercalcemia is done through regular serum calcium measurements during the first and second postoperative weeks. *Nephrocalcinosis,* a condition of renal insufficiency caused by precipitation of calcium phosphate in the kidney tubules, is manifested by decreased urine output. To screen for this complication, the nurse should keep accurate accounts of intake and output during hospitalization. Care of the child in a cast is discussed earlier in this chapter.

Torsional Deformities

Tibial Torsion Both external and internal tibial torsion are rotational deformities of the tibia. When the knee is facing forward, the foot is rotated inward (internal torsion) or outward (external torsion). External tibial torsion is rare. When it develops, it is usually secondary to paralytic muscle imbalance as in myelomeningocele or cerebral palsy.

Internal tibial torsion is a common cause of intoeing in young children. Some degree of torsion is common in all infants from the intrauterine position they assumed. Normally the torsion corrects itself with growth. If the child continually assumes postures which aggravate the torsion, it not only fails to correct, but it may increase. Two positions which have this effect are sleeping on the knees with the feet turned inward and sitting on top of inturned feet.

Treatment of internal tibial torsion consists of training the child to avoid harmful postures during sleeping and sitting. The deformity usually starts to correct when the infant spends more time on his back. If the deformity is so severe that the child over 2 years of age trips over his feet when walking, a night splint may be utilized to hold the feet in external rotation. The external torsional force influences growth of the epiphyseal plate to achieve correction. The Denis Browne splint is commonly used as a night splint for this purpose. If conservative measures are unsuccessful, surgical correction of deformities may be necessary.

Internal Femoral Torsion This deformity involves rotation of the entire lower limb. When the child stands, the knees are rotated inwardly, and when he walks, both feet and knees are turned inward. Internal femoral torsion is a variant of normal within certain limits and usually disappears with growth. It is the most common cause of intoeing (*pigeon-toe*) gait. Persistent internal femoral torsion is often seen with dislocation of the hip.

Early treatment is to correct the sitting position by training the child to sit in a cross-legged position. In this position corrective external torsional forces act on the femora. The disorder usually disappears spontaneously. If it is severe enough to cause limb deformity, difficulty with walking, or hip dysplasia, it should be corrected by surgery.

Nursing Management The nurse's attention is initially directed toward detection of torsional deformities. Children with suspected deformities should be referred for diagnosis and treatment. As part of treatment, the nurse clarifies for parents the postures which the child is directed to assume. Instructions are given concerning use of the Denis Browne splint.

Battered-Child Syndrome

The child who has received physical injury which is nonaccidental but is the result of acts of negligence by his parents or guardians has become known as the *battered child*. The true incidence of cases is not known because of the failure to report all suspected acts of abuse. Abusive acts tend to be repeated, often resulting in multiple musculoskeletal injuries. The child may not be brought in for medical care at the time of injury, but when seen by a doctor, the history of injury given by parents is often vague or may be intentionally misleading.

Most skeletal lesions are caused by jerking, twisting, or whiplash stresses, as when a child is grabbed and held by the extremities during shaking. The high incidence of subdural hematoma is caused by these stresses on the head. In the extremities, forces are aggravated by the child's own squirming.

Study of the bones on x-ray reveals the site, number, nature, and approximate age of bone lesions. Multiple fractures in different stages of healing are characteristic of this syndrome, as well as dislocations, injuries to the epiphyseal plate, external cortical thickenings, and cupping of the metaphyses. Bruises or other evidence of injury to the overlying skin may or may not be present on physical examination.[4]

The child should be admitted to the hospital for investigation and treatment. Most medical center hospitals have a team which deals with suspected cases of child abuse, and the child should be brought to the team's attention. Additional information about the battered-child syndrome is provided in Chapter 17.

Fracture of the Femoral Shaft

Displaced fractures of the femur are common in childhood and usually involve the middle third of the femoral shaft. The strong periosteum of the femur remains intact even with much displacement of fragments, but because the fracture is very unstable, it should be splinted as soon as discovered.

Closed reduction is carried out for a simple closed fracture. This is done by continuous traction, the type of traction varying with the age of the child. Under 2 years of age, overhead or Bryant's skin traction is applied to the lower limbs (Fig. 40-10). Over 2 years of age, overhead traction may be dangerous owing to the risk of arterial spasm and ischemia. Instead, a fixed type of continuous traction in the Thomas splint is used. When the femur is relatively stable and painless, traction is discontinued, and a hip spica cast is used for immobilization until clinical union of the fracture.

Healing after a displaced fracture of the femoral shaft always takes place by temporary overgrowth of bone. Therefore, the ideal position for uniting of bone fragments is one of intentional shortening; fragments are placed side-to-side with overriding of about one centimeter. The shortening is compensated by overgrowth within 1 year.

Nursing Management   A displaced fracture of the femoral shaft appears to the nurse as an angulation, external rotation, and shortening deformity of the thigh which is swollen and very painful. Splinting of the fracture should be done immediately. The child should be moved as little as possible for x-rays and other examinations to prevent further displacement of the fracture and pain.

A serious complication which can occur after reduction of the fracture is Volkmann's ischemia. Ischemic damage to muscles and nerves is due to femoral arterial spasm, which is aggravated by excessive traction.

MUSCULOSKELETAL DISORDERS AND INJURIES IN THE PRESCHOOLER
Juvenile Rheumatoid Arthritis

The cause of juvenile rheumatoid arthritis, or Still's disease, is unknown, but the evidence suggests that the primary problem is a hypersensitive response in which normal immune mechanisms are exaggerated. Although the age of onset varies, the peak age is during the preschool years, and more girls are affected than boys. The number of joints involved determines the type of arthritis. *Monoarthritis* means that only one joint is diseased (usually the knee); *polyarthritis* indicates that many joints are affected. More than half the children with this disease have the polyarthritic type.

The underlying joint pathology begins in the synovial membrane with an inflammation of the membrane leading to edema and proliferation of cells. Granulation tissue infiltrates the synovial membrane and causes the swelling. As the disease progresses, scar tissue replaces granulation tissue, and the joint may become contracted, particularly without proper physical therapy. The muscles are affected by inflammation in muscle tissue as well as

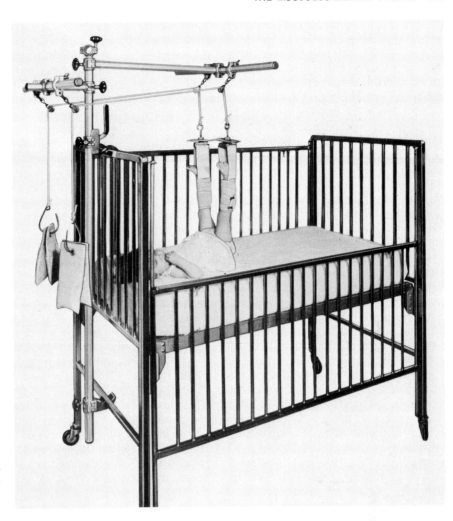

Figure 40-10 Bryant's traction.
(Courtesy Zimmer USA, Warsaw, Ind., A Traction Handbook, 1971, p. 25.)

by joint immobility, thereby aggravating contractures.

Symptoms at the onset of juvenile rheumatoid arthritis vary. Some children become ill suddenly, while in others symptoms appear very gradually. The clinical manifestations may be limited to the peripheral joints, or they may appear as a generalized systemic illness. When the onset involves *peripheral* joints, swelling of the joints is usually the first sign noticed by the parent. There is some limitation of motion, manifested by a limp, and mild warmth over the joint which accompanies the swelling. Tenderness and pain are present when swelling has occurred suddenly. The onset of *systemic* involvement is usually more sudden and includes fever, rash, malaise, pallor, subcutaneous nodules, lymphadenopathy, liver and spleen enlargement, and pericarditis.

These symptoms are often accompanied by arthritis in one or more joints.

The clinical course of juvenile rheumatoid arthritis is variable, involving many exacerbations and remissions. Pain on motion is the major complaint of a child, but instead of voicing his discomfort, he may walk with a limp or refuse to move the extremity. Morning stiffness is often manifested by the child's inability to get out of bed in the morning or difficulty arising from a nap. A *rheumatoid rash* is a salmon-pink, macular rash which appears intermittently on the chest, thighs, axilla, and upper arms. Subcutaneous nodules are found in about 10 percent of affected children, usually on the fingers, toes, wrist, or elbows. For about three-fourths of children, fever occurs intermittently, and it is often accompanied by other systemic symptoms. *Iridocyclitis,* or inflammation of the iris and ciliary body, is a sign which usually originates several years after the onset of the disease. Joint deformities, including subluxation, dislocation, and contracture, are seen in more severe cases. Growth disturbances sometimes result from abnormal influences on the epiphyseal plate.

Diagnosis of juvenile rheumatoid arthritis depends mainly on the history and demonstration of clinical symptomology. No single diagnostic test has been found to be effective. The rheumatoid factor is positive in only about 15 percent of patients.

Nursing Management   In juvenile rheumatoid arthritis, the child and his parents face a disease with many unknowns. Parents may feel guilty, and the child often attributes the illness to his "bad" behavior, despite reassurance that the cause is unknown. A nurse can help clarify this fact for the family as well as help them to understand that the course of the disease is unpredictable and may continue for several years. Long-term encouragement becomes necessary as the parents and child experience the inertia of a daily therapy program as well as recurring episodes of acute illness.

The child is hospitalized during acute episodes of joint inflammation and systemic illness. The nurse checks to see that the child's bed has a firm mattress which resists sagging. Although positions of flexion are often preferred by the child because they are more comfortable, pillows should be kept from under painful joints to prevent stiffness and contractions. The child may be allowed up if he can tolerate the activity, but if the inflamed joints are too painful to move actively, they should be moved passively through their range of motion at least twice a day by the physical therapist or nurse. Both of these disciplines should work together to reinforce the treatment program. The child is encouraged to do his exercises actively as soon as he is able. Warm compresses to joints, hydrotherapy, and paraffin oil baths often facilitate joint movement. Warm baths or showers in the morning help the child overcome morning stiffness. Diversional activities also encourage movement. When splints are used to rest warm, swollen joints, the child may have difficulty adjusting to them at first, especially during sleep. Nurses must know how to apply splints properly in addition to helping the child adjust to the splint.

Drug therapy is an important part of the treatment program. Because gastric irritation often accompanies administration of salicylates, these drugs are frequently given with meals or with antacids. Gold is given intramuscularly, and steroids are usually given orally or *intraarticularly* (into the joint).

The nurse should be aware of the side effects and toxicity of all drugs. Special screening tests may be appropriate during drug administration, such as checking the urine for protein during the administration of gold or checking for glycosuria when steroids are being given. Drugs used in treatment of juvenile rheumatoid arthritis are described in Table 40-3.

The community nurse, who may have played a role in the detection of the disease, is also responsible for follow-up care. This nurse may administer gold intramuscularly, and it is essential that the patient be monitored closely for side effects. Encouragement and supervision are given for the prescribed exercise or play program and for warm baths to overcome morning stiffness. For a child who attends school, provisions may need to be made to allow him to move around every hour. The nurse should ensure that every child with this disease receives a slit-lamp ophthalmologic exam by an experienced physician every 6 to 12 months for detection of iridocyclitis. Regular follow-up should be made for symptoms such as visual disturbance, chest pain, and skin rashes, and any new or unusual symptoms should be reported to the physician promptly.

The prognosis is improving for this disease as medical care progresses. Over one-half of the children recover completely in 1 or 2 years. If only one joint is involved for longer than a year, the disease is unlikely to spread further. In polyarthritis the disorder usually remains active for many years and may continue into adulthood. Approximately 15 percent of affected children are left with severe and permanent disability.

Legg-Perthes Disease

Legg-Perthes disease is one of a group of diseases called the *osteochondroses* which share the common pathology of idiopathic avascular necrosis of the epiphyses. In Legg-Perthes disease, vascular disruption to the femoral head causes necrosis and variable deformity of the upper femoral epiphysis. The age of onset is usually between 3 and 11 years, and the disease may be present for 2 to 8 years, after which time it spontaneously resolves itself. The condition is unilateral in about 85 percent of cases, and it tends to recur in families. Boys are affected four times more frequently than girls, probably because they are more physically active.

The pathophysiology of the disease can be divided into four phases. The first phase, *avascularity,* begins with spontaneous interruption of the blood supply to the upper femoral epiphysis. Bone-forming cells in the epiphysis die and bone ceases to grow,

Table 40-3 DRUGS USED IN TREATMENT OF JUVENILE RHEUMATOID ARTHRITIS

Drug	Specific action	Route of administration	Side effects or toxicity
Salicylates	Antipyretic, analgesic, anti-inflammatory	Per os, I.V.	Abdominal pain, gastric bleeding (occult blood in stool), hyperventilation in the small child, tinnitus in the older child
Gold	Unknown	I.M.	Skin rashes, nephritis with hematuria or albuminuria, thrombocytopenia, neurotoxicity
Steroids	Anti-inflammatory	Per os, I.V., I.M., intraarticular	Masking of infection, peptic ulcer, vascular disorders, hypertension, increased intraocular pressure (blurry or dim vision), osteoporosis with pathologic fractures, euphoria or other mental disturbance, glycosuria, weight gain secondary to water retention, appetite stimulation

although its density does not change. The second phase is the period of *revascularization*. New blood vessels are sent into the area of dead bone, and both bone resorption and deposition take place. However, the new bone is not strong, and pathologic fractures occur. Pain and limited motion develop in the hip joint. Abnormal forces on the weakened epiphysis may produce progressive deformity. The third phase involves *healing*. Dead bone is removed and replaced by new bone. The fourth phase of *residual* deformity takes place when healing is complete and the contour of the hip joint is fixed. Subluxation of the hip, flattening of the epiphysis resulting in incongruity of joint surfaces, and limitation of motion may lead to degenerative joint disease in later life.

Clinical symptoms begin in phase 2. While pain may be felt in the hip or referred to the knee or inner thigh, such pain is present only during the initial period. The child walks with a protective limp, and he has limited movement in the hip joint. Disuse atrophy develops in muscles of the upper thigh. Although these symptoms are intermittent, any child who has them should be referred to a physician.

In general, the earlier the age of onset, the better the results of treatment. Effective intervention should begin as soon as the diagnosis is made. Success is diminished by the fact that symptoms do not occur until phase 2 when damage has already been done to the femoral head. Treatment aims to prevent abnormal forces on the femoral head during the second and third phases of revascularization and healing. Although some physicians advocate no treatment, most begin treatment with bed rest and traction to the limb during the painful initial period. An attempt is made to locate the femoral head deep in the acetabulum, thereby protecting it while revascularization and growth occur. This process is accomplished by weight bearing in abduction plaster casts or abduction braces to allow deeper seating of the femoral head and prevent subluxation, or by use of a hip sling to rest the affected leg. A surgical osteotomy of the femur may also be desired to prevent or correct subluxation. Treatment is considered to be successful if the contour of the hip joint allows normal function after resolution of the disease.

Nursing Management When the child is first admitted to the hospital with a diagnosis of Legg-Perthes disease, he is uncomfortable and may need analgesics for relief of pain. If bed rest and traction are instituted and abduction casts are applied, appropriate nursing functions should be carried out.

Immobilization is often difficult for the child to accept. After the initial period of discomfort, he feels well and wants to be up and out of bed. The preschool child has difficulty understanding why he must stay in bed or wear special appliances. All children can benefit from explanations and visual aids about their disease and its treatment. During immobilization, the child should participate in activities which keep him occupied and stimulate his development. Play should include exercise for uninvolved extremities. A teacher for the home-bound may be required for the school-age child, and special activities with peers should be arranged. During hospitalization, the nursing staff can demonstrate such management to parents and help them plan for care at home.

Duchenne's Muscular Dystrophy

Duchenne's muscular dystrophy is a progressive muscle disorder which is genetically determined. The more common form is found only in boys because it is transferred as a sex-linked recessive trait, while the less common form is inherited as an autosomal recessive trait and therefore appears in both girls and boys. Muscular dystrophy usually starts in the preschool years but may occur in older children and young adults. Pathogenesis is unknown, although particular enzyme levels are elevated in the blood, and a biochemical defect in muscle tissue is suspected.

In the more common form, progression is faster than in the less common form, but clinical features are similar in both. The child appears normal during infancy and no abnormality appears until he begins to walk. At age 3 or 4 years, the child typically has flat feet, develops weakness in his legs, and begins to stumble and fall. Weakness in the pelvic muscles causes difficulty in climbing stairs and getting up off the floor to a standing position. The child must "climb up his legs" with his hands to get up from the floor, a characteristic sign of the disease known as *Gowers' sign*. Although wasting of the muscles is progressive, muscles appear to grow larger or hypertrophy, especially in the calves of the legs. The increase, or *pseudohypertrophy,* is due to excessive fibrous tissue and fat rather than hypertrophy of muscle fibers. Histologic changes show a variation in size of muscle fibers, degeneration of the fibers, and fatty infiltration between muscle bundles.

The course of this disease is relentless, without remissions. Lordosis develops as the pelvis rotates forward because of muscle weakness. To compensate for the abnormal posture, the child assumes a waddling gait and begins to walk on his toes. As walking becomes more precarious, the child fears falling and spends more time in a wheelchair. Confinement to the wheelchair usually begins between 7 and 10 years of age. Scoliosis develops after several months in the wheelchair and progresses to the extent that vital organs are displaced. Contractures of the elbows, feet, knees, and hips may develop during immobilization. In the more common type of this disease, few boys survive beyond 20 years of age, the most frequent causes of death being respiratory infection, respiratory acidosis, and cardiac complications.

Diagnosis is made from the history and various tests. Laboratory measurement is made of cellular enzymes which probably arise from affected muscles. The enzyme creatine phosphokinase (CPK) is elevated early in the course of the disease. An *electromyogram* (EMG) may be done to establish whether muscle weakness is caused by abnormal nerves or muscles. A muscle biopsy is surgically performed to confirm the diagnosis.

Without a cure for this disease, children face progressive disability and death. Normal amounts of exercise, dietary supervision, light braces, special aids and equipment, and supportive relationships with staff are all part of the treatment program to help make the disease more bearable for children and their families. Much research is being done in an effort to identify the specific cause and alleviate symptoms of the disease. The effects of experimental drugs are being evaluated. Use of a lightweight body brace early in the disease is a hopeful development in order to delay abnormal postures and subsequent muscle deterioration.[5]

Nursing Management The diagnostic period in muscular dystrophy involves frightening and uncomfortable tests for the child. One of these tests is the electromyogram, in which thin, wirelike needles are stuck into the child's muscles while a recording of muscle contractions is made on a screen. After explaining the test to parents, the nurse can plan with them for preparation of the child. Reassurance that the test is not a punishment is important for the preschooler. A simple explanation of the test may be accompanied by supervised needle play before and after the test. Whenever possible, the nurse who is working with the child should accompany him.

Preparation for muscle biopsy is also required. The child and his parents need to understand that the child will be asleep during the procedure, that only a tiny part of the muscle will be removed, and that there will be a small incision after surgery. Postoperatively, the child's vital signs are monitored frequently until stable and then every 4 hours. Drainage from the incision is recorded, as well as observations about pain and the effect of analgesics. Before discharge parents need instructions on keeping the incision clean and dry and allowing return to normal activity. When a positive diagnosis is made on biopsy, parents need additional explanations about the disease from the physician, followed by clarification and emotional support by the nurse.

During the course of the disease the goal is to keep the child as independent as possible and provide supportive interaction for the family and child. An interdisciplinary team supervises continued care. The child is encouraged to continue normal activities to prevent atrophy of uninvolved muscles. Attention is given to diet in an effort to prevent or reduce obesity which often accompanies inactivity and makes walking more difficult. Light braces may be fitted to delay progression of abnormal postures or to support weakened muscles. In order for the child to use and benefit from bracing, his parents must reinforce the treatment program and supervise proper wearing of the brace. Ramps may need to be installed in the home, and architectural barriers reduced which hinder independent mobility, particularly when the child must use a wheelchair. An electric wheelchair allows mobility for the older child with upper-extremity weakness. Correct positioning of the feet and adjustment of footrests on the wheelchair is important to prevent foot drop and other ankle deformities. Portable lifts are useful when a child is unable to transfer himself or he is too heavy to lift. Treatment for contractures may involve minor surgical procedures such as subcutaneous tenotomy, although these procedures are controversial. Prolonged bed rest and inactivity should be avoided because of their weakening effects.

Other measures for independence in daily activities are planned to compensate for the child's weakness. Clothing may need to be modified so that the child can dress himself. Large rings on zipper tabs in the front of clothing allow easier manipulation. Toileting is often difficult, requiring special planning or the use of a bedside commode or bedpan. Bathing, washing hair, and self-feeding may also need to be modified, considering the child's abilities and the home situation. Operation of special equipment should be demonstrated by staff to parents and by parents to staff. Parents also need information about the genetic transmission of Duchenne's muscular dystrophy, for which genetic counseling can be helpful.

Fractures of the Forearm

When a child falls and catches himself with his hands, forces are transmitted to the wrist and forearm, sometimes causing fractures in those parts. Fractures of the forearm usually involve injury to both the radius and ulna, occurring in the distal, middle, or proximal third of the bones. They may be incomplete (greenstick) or complete.

A *buckle* fracture in the distal third of the forearm is common in young children. This is a compression fracture resulting in "buckling" of the thin cortex which surrounds the cancellous bone of the metaphysis, and it heals completely after several weeks in a cast. A *greenstick* fracture in the distal or middle third of the forearm must first be reduced by closed manipulation. In this procedure, the bones are corrected to the point that the intact part of the cortex cracks through. *Complete* fractures are reduced by closed manipulation and immobilized in plaster casts. In the proximal third of the forearm the injury is often a *Monteggia* fracture-dislocation. This

serious injury involves a fracture of the shaft of the ulna as well as a dislocation of the radiohumeral joint. Treatment is by closed reduction; the angle of ulnar fracture is corrected, and the radial head relocated.

Nursing Management The nurse may assist with the reduction and immobilization of fractures as well as supervision of the child in a cast. Closed reductions of fractures are usually done by applying manual traction to the forearm with the elbow flexed, while wrapping the arm in a circular plaster cast from the axilla to the midpalm. After casting, the arm should be elevated for 24 to 48 hours with ice bags applied to the forearm, and frequent checks of circulation are made. A triangular sling, which ties at the back of the neck, can be used to support the hand, forearm, and elbow. If the child is cared for at home during this time, instructions should be given to parents about care of the cast, circulation checks, and use of the sling. X-rays are taken at intervals to visualize alignment of bone fragments. If the cast becomes loose after swelling subsides, a new cast should be applied. After several weeks the cast is removed and the child is allowed free use of his arm.

When manipulation fails to achieve reduction or normal alignment of bone fragments, fixed traction is used. A wire loop is incorporated into the cast to exert traction on the fingers. Skin traction is applied to the fingers by rubber bands connected to the loop. Fixed traction is removed after a few weeks, and a regular plaster cast is applied.

Open fractures must first be converted to closed injuries by surgery. Severely comminuted fractures of both bones of the forearm are then reduced by skeletal traction. Pins pass through the radius and ulna above the wrist joint and through the distal end of the humerus. When the fracture is sufficiently reduced, the arm is immobilized in a plaster cast. Care of the child in skeletal traction is discussed earlier in this chapter.

Supracondylar Fracture of the Humerus

The most common and most serious type of fracture around the elbow is a supracondylar fracture of the humerus. The incidence of complications is high. The usual injury is one of hyperextension or falling on the hand with the elbow flexed. The forces of injury are transmitted through the elbow joint to the humerus, and jagged fragment ends may be driven through the region of the brachial artery and nerve or even through the skin. Severe soft tissue damage may result, causing swelling and internal hemorrhage.

Treatment varies according to the extent of damage. The undisplaced fracture requires only immobilization of the arm with the elbow flexed for 3 weeks. Most displaced fractures are treated by closed reduction. Manual traction on the forearm reduces the deformity, with the elbow held in slight flexion to prevent damage to the brachial artery. If reduction is confirmed by x-ray, the arm is immobilized in a plaster cast held by a sling around the neck. After reduction, the child is admitted to the hospital for observation. The peripheral circulation should be checked for signs of Volkmann's ischemia. Although the cast is worn for only 3 weeks, elbow stiffness is always present after removal. Stiffness should be alleviated by the child's own active movements; passive exercises should be avoided. In a few dislocated fractures, reduction is very unstable, and excessive swelling or circulatory impairment is present. These fractures are treated by skeletal traction through a pin in the olecranon.

Complications which may occur in addition to Volkmann's ischemia are peripheral nerve injury and malunion. The prognosis for recovery is good in peripheral nerve injury because injured nerves are not divided. If residual deformity caused by malunion is severe, a supracondylar osteotomy is required to restore appearance and function of the elbow.

Nursing Management   Observations are made in the hospital to ensure that the fracture is held in a reduced position and to check for signs of complications. The position of the cast or alignment of traction is observed at regular intervals. Peripheral circulation (including the radial pulse) and neurologic function in the forearm and hand are checked every hour for the first 24 to 48 hours, and then less frequently, to detect signs of Volkmann's ischemia and peripheral nerve injury. Persistent pain may be a sign of Volkmann's ischemia and should not be masked by careless use of analgesics; instead, the physician should be called immediately. Before discharge, the nurse demonstrates to parents the application of the collar and cuff neck sling or triangular sling and its proper fit to hold the arm in alignment. If the child is wearing a long arm or shoulder spica cast, this care is also discussed with parents.

Wringer Crush Injury

With modernization of machinery, wringer washing machine injuries are being replaced by similar crushing injuries from other sources, although crushing injuries caused by washing machine wringers account for thousands of accidents every year in children. A variety of forces produce injury: compression, contusion (bruising), heat from friction, and avulsion. The extent of damage is determined by the force of the wringers, the amount of the extremity which entered the wringer, the duration of exposure, and the forces used to extricate the extremity.

Significant injury occurs at sites where wringers are likely to stop. These sites include the back of the hand or wrist, the inside of the elbow, and the axilla. The web space between the thumb and fingers is frequently torn. Deep burning of the skin and subcutaneous tissue as well as severe bruising of underlying muscles are caused by prolonged exposure to the force of the wringers. Avulsion of skin and an increased incidence of peripheral nerve damage result when strong countertraction is used to extricate the extremity. After the injury, edema and hemorrhage develop in damaged tissues. Extensive hematomas may accumulate in space created by separation of the skin and subcutaneous tissue from the underlying fascia. Subfascial hematoma and severe muscle damage are manifested by pain on passive extension of the fingers. Fractures do not commonly occur, but when they are present, they usually involve bones of the thumb.

In the emergency room, the extremity is cleaned, hematomas are drained, and wounds are dressed. A bulky pressure dressing is applied, and the extremity is elevated. Tetanus antitoxin and antibiotics are given. Damage is difficult to assess initially, and progressive damage can result from edema and the swelling caused by hematomas; therefore, most children are hospitalized for observation. All children with injuries above the midarm are hospitalized. When dressings are changed 24 hours after injury, the extremity is reevaluated. Areas of skin with full-thickness loss are prepared for grafting. Hematomas are drained. If significant swelling, skin loss, or paralysis is present, the child remains in the hospital for further observation and treatment. The child who is able to be discharged at that time is instructed to elevate the extremity for 48 hours and to continue wearing the pressure dressing. Return appointments are made for periodic dressing changes.

Nursing Management   When the child with a wringer injury arrives in the emergency room, the nurse or physician should collect information from relatives about the injury. Important facts to know are the age of the machine and the condition of the wringers, the area of the extremity crushed by the wringer, the time of exposure, and the actions required to extricate the extremity.

Aseptic technique is used for treatment of wounds. The extremity is first cleansed with a mild detergent solution, after which hematomas are drained and wounds are dressed. A bulky pressure dressing is applied to immobilize the extremity from the fingertips to above the proximal area of injury. Antibiotic therapy is instituted after administration of tetanus toxoid.

On the pediatric unit, the extremity is elevated by suspension from an I.V. (intravenous drip) pole or similar apparatus. These patients are allowed out of bed pushing their I.V. poles. Circulation in the fingertips is assessed every 1 to 2 hours. If skin involvement is present, analgesics can be given before dressings are changed to make the child more comfortable.

When the child is discharged, parents should receive instructions from the nurse on how to elevate the extremity, apply a triangular splint, and rewrap dressings which come off. If medications are prescribed, parents should be told the hours at which they are to be administered. Keeping subsequent outpatient visits which require dressing changes should be stressed. The amount of activity allowed also needs to be elaborated at this time.

MUSCULOSKELETAL DISORDERS AND INJURIES IN THE SCHOOL-AGE CHILD AND ADOLESCENT
Traumatic Paraplegia and Quadriplegia

Paraplegia describes paralysis of the lower extremities; quadriplegia is paralysis involving all four extremities (see Chap. 32). With growth, the paraplegic or quadriplegic child is likely to develop deformities in his paralyzed limbs. Surgical operations may be needed to correct muscle imbalance and diminish the effects of spasticity. Scoliosis may also be a problem, and often it requires the support of a body brace. If the curvature is progressive, spinal fusion will be necessary.

Nursing Management To prevent deformity, nursing measures must begin immediately after injury. Turning the patient every 2 hours maintains integrity of the skin and prevents the formation of decubitus ulcers. When red or sore areas are discovered, the child is repositioned immediately. Paralyzed limbs must be supported in functional positions to prevent contractures. Passive exercises help preserve mobility in affected joints, and active-resistance exercises begin strengthening of functional muscles. Bowel and bladder training are instituted early to begin rehabilitation and reestablish independence. Establishing a bowel and bladder training program

presents a real challenge to the nurse because school-age children and adolescents are usually very modest. The basic principal in a bowel reeducation plan is regular, consistent evacuation of the bowel. Time should be planned each day for the bowel movement. Suppositories and, if necessary, an enema are used to promote evacuation. Digital stimulation and manual pressure on the abdomen may be necessary in high-cord lesions to produce effective emptying of the bowel.

Before bladder training can begin, the ability of the bladder to expel urine and to hold up to 500 ml of urine must be determined. Children with a flaccid bladder must use a catheter because the bladder cannot empty, but a spastic bladder may be trained to fill to a specific capacity before it releases urine. Some bladders are conditioned to respond to time and degree of pressure; others are conditioned to respond to a reflex action when a muscle group is stimulated and a specific spastic response is elicited. Obviously the latter is far more acceptable but not always attainable.

The child who must use a Foley catheter must be taught to care for it. Someone in the family may learn to change the catheter, or an older child may learn to insert his own.

During the initial hospitalization, nurses plan the teaching program for the patient and his family. The older child is an active participant in planning as well as learning. Both the child and his family need support as they work through the grieving process. Information about future abilities should be given to the child and his family honestly, and although false ideas need correction, hope should never be destroyed. Anticipatory guidance is especially meaningful when it includes visits from other children or adults who have sustained similar spinal cord injuries. Information from local chapters of the National Paraplegia Foundation may be helpful and informative.

With this type of injury, the child may actually reject his body. Early refusal to be concerned with the paralyzed body parts is later manifested by lack of care to the involved areas, resulting in decubitus ulcers, contractures, and infections. Nurses must help the child assume responsibility for paralyzed parts of his body, being careful to consider the *whole* child—his feelings, concerns, and needs as a person.

Ambulation is possible for the child who is highly motivated and whose cord lesion is not at too high a level. Essential abilities for ambulation are pelvic control and full range of motion at the hips, especially full extension. The physical therapist trains the child to ambulate with braces and crutches designed for his needs. However, braces are of little value to the paraplegic who lacks strength in the upper arms or trunk to support himself. For this patient as well as for those who ambulate only short distances, a wheelchair allows functional mobility.

The wheelchair should be selected to meet the highly individual needs of each child. Padded upholstery or wooden inserts can be added which reduce the width of the chair temporarily, and these devices can be removed as the child grows. Special cushions are available to help prevent decubitus formation. Electric wheelchairs should be reserved for the quadriplegic child who is unable to propel a chair with his arms. All children should spend some time during the day out of the chair to help preserve skin integrity.

A variety of assistive devices are available to the paraplegic or quadriplegic patient. Standing tables or tilt tables help the paralyzed child assume an upright position. Parallel bars provide support for ambulation in braces. Special splints may be prescribed to improve function in the upper extremities of quadriplegic patients. Eating utensils, toothbrushes, paint brushes, and writing tools may need to be modified so that the child can grasp them. Parents, who often have excellent suggestions and ideas about modifying equipment, should be vitally involved in the rehabilitation program.

All patients need long-term care and follow-up by an interdisciplinary team. Special attention should be given to helping family members achieve satisfactory relationships as well as realistic expectations for the child. The child should be guided toward independence in activities of daily living such as bathing, toileting, and dressing. Patterns of weight gain or weight loss should be noted before they create problems. The parents and child must be taught how to check for skin irritation daily and how to prevent skin breakdown.

A home visit by the nurse and physical therapist should be done prior to discharge to evaluate the need for change within the home. The height of the bed may need to be altered to foster transfer to the wheelchair. Ramps may be installed, and doors may need to be widened. Railings are helpful at the bathtub to allow for transfer. Clothes racks and storage space may need to be lowered. Although the child's ability to perform activities of daily living is critical for the development of a positive self-image, high priority should also be placed on the access to the outside world. The educational and socialization needs of these children may be met by tutoring during hospitalization and the support of friends. Return to his school upon discharge from the hospital is desirable. The nurse may visit the school to help evaluate the facilities for use by a student in a wheelchair. Many schools, because of their architectural structure, cannot accept the wheelchair-bound student, and transfer to a school that can accommodate him may be necessary. Socialization with peers is also encouraged in summer camps and special programs for handicapped children where recreational activities are adapted to the child's abilities (Fig. 40-11).

Adolescents with spinal cord injuries need to develop positive relationships with members of the opposite sex even though the ability to participate in and enjoy sexual activity is altered. Sexual ability in males is fostered if they have spastic paralysis because erection and ejaculation may be possible. Female paraplegics are able to participate in intercourse, but the degree of active involvement is limited. While neither male nor female is able to enjoy the physical sensations of intercourse, both are able to provide satisfaction for their partners.

Athletic Injuries

There are two types of athletic injuries, intrinsic and extrinsic. Intrinsic injuries involve the athlete's own physical activities, in which he hurts himself. These activities involve contraction of his own muscles owing to awkward movements or to strong repetitive movements. Extrinsic injuries arise from external forces, such as blows from other players, causing the athlete injury. Because the epiphyseal plates have not closed in the young growing athlete, he is prone to types of injuries different from those of his adult counterpart. The epiphyseal cartilage usually tears before major ligaments are injured. Since these injuries occur first in growing athletes, damage to major ligaments is not common.

Injuries are largely preventable by adequate conditioning and training of athletes. The individual who is in excellent physical condition and highly skilled in his sport is less likely to be injured. Use of appropriate protective equipment such as padding and helmets also helps to prevent injuries, as does the enforcement of safety rules and regulations in sports activities. The injured athlete should not enter into competitive sports until adequate healing has taken place. The specialty of sports medicine is evolving to focus on the care of athletes with as much emphasis on prevention of injuries as on diagnosis and treatment once they have occurred.

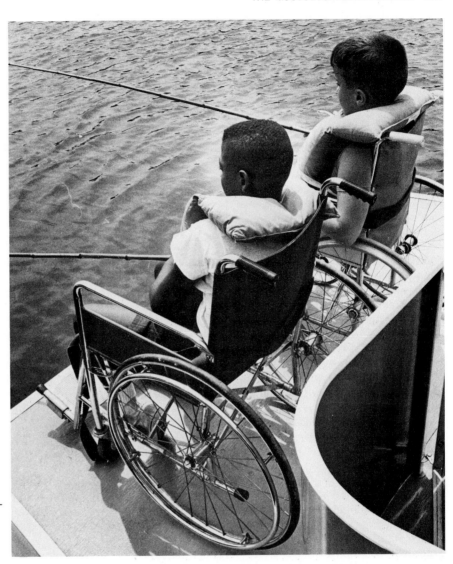

Figure 40-11 Fishing is an activity easily adapted for children in wheelchairs. *(Courtesy Camp Riley for Physically Handicapped Children, Bradford Woods, James Whitcomb Riley Memorial Association, Indianapolis, Ind.)*

Epiphyseal Plate Fractures

Fracture injuries of the epiphyseal plate make up 15 percent of all fractures in children. Trauma causes separation through the weakest area of the plate, the area of calcifying cartilage, although the plate itself remains attached to the epiphysis. Since the plate gets its blood supply from the epiphysis, disruption of the vessels to the epiphysis causes both the epiphysis and the plate to become necrotic, and growth ceases. One would expect more injuries in this region than actually occur because the plate is weaker than the bone, associated ligaments, and the joint capsule; therefore, with trauma, separation of the plate is more likely than tearing of the ligaments or dislocation of the joint. The union of perichondrium and periosteum attaching the epiphysis and metaphysis is very firm, however, preventing some injuries which would otherwise take place.

Treatment for these injuries is different from that for typical fractures. Some types of epiphyseal fractures require open reduction and internal fixation. Immobilization may be shorter than for a fracture of the metaphysis in the same bone; however, longer follow-up is essential to detect any disturbance in growth. Although only 15 percent of these injuries are complicated by growth disturbances, such disabilities are progressive with retardation of growth occurring for several months, followed by an arrest in further development. If the entire epiphyseal plate stops growing, the affected limb will be shorter than the other, normal limb. If the damaged bone is one of a pair, as with the radius and ulna, an angulatory deformity becomes evident and progresses with growth.

In the leg-length discrepancy, surgical procedures are sometimes done to correct the differences in length. In *epiphyseal plate arrest,* the epiphyseal plate in the longer leg is prevented from further growth by bone grafts or by metal staples. *Epiphyseal plate stimulation* increases the circulation to the epiphyseal plate of the shorter leg so that it is stimulated to grow faster.

Nursing Management It is imperative that parents keep follow-up appointments for their child after epiphyseal plate fractures and that they are aware of the risk of growth disturbances. The community or outpatient nurse encourages parents to keep regular appointments and checks the length of the affected limb himself. True length of the leg is assessed by measuring from the anterior superior iliac spine to the medial malleolus of the ankle. This measurement should be compared with the length of the normal leg, and any discrepancies reported to the physician. The length of time necessary for follow-up is at least 1 year and may be longer in some cases.

Fractures of the Ankle

Almost all fractures of the ankle in children involve an epiphyseal plate. Therefore, the prognosis depends on the extent of damage to the plate. *Less severe* injuries include separation or fracture-separation of the epiphysis. After a closed reduction, the ankle is immobilized in a below-knee walking cast for 3 weeks. These types of injuries have a good prognosis for further growth. Injuries which are *severe* include fractures of the epiphysis and fractures of the epiphyseal plate. Open reduction is required to restore alignment of the fracture fragments or joint surfaces. Weight bearing may need to be postponed for several weeks to prevent further injury to the epiphyseal plate. Because of the type of injury, severe growth disturbances frequently result.

Nursing Management Patients with less severe types of ankle fracture often see only the staff in the emergency room, where their fracture is reduced, the leg is casted, and they are sent home. Following open reduction of severe fractures, however, the patient is hospitalized. Nurses on the unit provide post-

operative care and observe for complications. The child is usually returned to the unit in a below-knee cast, which should be elevated on pillows to prevent swelling. Frequent checks are made of circulation and neurologic function, as described in the section on common nursing measures. Active exercises begin while the ankle is still immobilized in plaster. When the fracture is soundly united, movement of the joint begins under the direction of the physical therapist. After discharge, the community or outpatient nurse should check for growth disturbance by measuring the leg's true length, a technique discussed in the previous section.

Slipped Upper Femoral Epiphysis

In slipped upper femoral epiphysis, the head of the femur becomes displaced both downward and backward off the neck of the femur. Weakness of the epiphyseal plate allows the epiphysis to slip off the femoral neck in reaction to force. Gradual slipping of the epiphysis is most common and leads to a progressive coxa vara deformity of the femoral neck. However, after trauma a sudden further slip may occur. If separation of the epiphysis and the femoral neck is complete, the blood supply is likely to be interrupted, resulting in avascular necrosis of the femoral head. Slipping can no longer take place after the epiphyseal plate closes by bony union, but a residual deformity may lead to degenerative hip disease in adult life.

Early symptoms include fatigue after walking or standing, mild pain in the hip which may be referred to the knee, and a slight limp. A progressive external rotation deformity develops in the lower limb. Movements of internal rotation, flexion, and abduction become restricted, and x-ray confirms the diagnosis.

This problem is found most frequently in children between 10 and 16 years of age and more often in boys. Both hips are affected in 30 to 40 percent of cases. The disorder is most common in very tall, thin, rapidly growing children and in obese, inactive children with underdeveloped sexual characteristics. The cause is unknown.

The slip or separation is reduced as much as possible by gentle manipulation, and threaded pins are inserted surgically across the epiphyseal plate for stabilization. At that point, the aim of treatment is to prevent further slipping. Weight bearing is not allowed until the epiphysis is joined to the femoral neck.

The chronic slip of more than 1 cm, which is discovered late, is most difficult to treat. Surgery in the region of the epiphyseal plate is contraindicated by the risk of producing avascular necrosis. Instead, a subtrochanteric osteotomy of the femur may reduce bony deformity and improve hip function.

Nursing Management   When slipped upper femoral epiphysis is suspected, the young person should be referred to a physician as soon as possible and instructed to avoid unnecessary weight bearing. After admission to the hospital, bed rest is instituted with the affected leg in an internally rotated position. The rationale for traction (further immobilization) and surgical procedures (reduction of separation and stabilization of the plate) must be clarified for the child and his family. In consultation with the dietitian, a weight-reduction diet for the obese child should begin in the hospital. Both the child and his parents should be involved in planning for the diet in the hospital and at home. Rest and prevention of abnormal forces on the affected hip are prescribed when the child is at home. Normal daily activities and school activities will need to be revised if weight bearing is not allowed. Mobility limits must be clearly understood by the child as well as his parents.

Follow-up care emphasizes monitoring of the opposite hip for bilateral involvement. The nurse's teaching can help both child and family understand the disease process and the importance of early recognition of symptoms in the opposite leg.

Simple Bone Cyst

A simple bone cyst is a benign lesion which may stimulate a neoplasm. The cyst is a collection of fluid in a capsule, usually affecting the humerus, femur, and other long bones. Most bone cysts occur in children and adolescents, and the cause of these lesions is unknown.

The cyst begins in the metaphysis next to the epiphyseal plate and gradually expands through the shaft toward the middiaphysis. Because the bone's cortex around the cyst becomes very thin, pathologic fractures are common. Medical care is often sought only after a fracture has occurred because there is pain with a fracture; the cyst itself is not painful.

If the cyst is small, it may heal spontaneously. Spontaneous healing may also take place after a fracture; however, surgery is usually required when the fracture is impending or has already occurred. During the operative procedure, the cystic cavity undergoes curettage, and is then filled with bone chips (grafts). It is important to remember that these cysts may recur despite treatment. When surgery is required, postoperative nursing measures include assessment of vital signs and circulation in the ex-

tremity, care of the cast, and instructions for the family concerning mobility limits and cast care at home.

Neoplasms

Osteogenic Sarcoma   Children, adolescents, and young adults are victims in three-fourths of all cases of osteogenic sarcoma (osteosarcoma). This malignancy of bone affects males twice as frequently as females. The tumor arises from osteoblasts, or bone-forming cells, the most common site being in the metaphysis of a long bone. More than half of these lesions are found at the lower end of the femur or the upper end of the tibia, while many others are found at the upper end of the humerus. These skeletal areas are sites of active epiphyseal growth.

Pain is the only consistent symptom; it begins intermittently at the tumor site but becomes more intense and continuous. Joint function is limited as the tumor grows. Because this neoplasm is very vascular, swelling over the tumor site feels warm, and overlying veins are dilated. Pathologic fractures may take place after an erosion of the bony cortex. X-ray shows a characteristic formation, but proof of a positive diagnosis comes only from surgical biopsy.

Other diagnostic tests are carried out when the patient is first admitted to the hospital. Blood tests include a complete blood count, platelet count, and liver function studies such as alkaline phosphatase, transaminase, and protein electrophoresis. Urinalysis is routinely done, as well as studies of the bone, including x-rays of the lesion, bone survey, bone scan, and sometimes a bone marrow test. Chest x-rays with planigrams are also taken. These tests are done for evaluation of the lesion as well as screening for other lesions.

Because matastases often travel to the lungs early in the disease, osteogenic sarcoma is a tumor with a very poor prognosis. Between 75 percent and 90 percent of patients die within 5 years. No consistent response has been shown to any one treatment. The tumor is not particularly radiosensitive; therefore, amputation is the treatment of choice if no evidence of metastases is shown on x-ray. Amputation is usually followed by 2 years of chemotherapy, including such drugs as cyclophosphamide, dactinomycin, vincristine sulfate, or adriamycin. When metastases are present or the tumor is nonresectable, treatment is by radiation therapy combined with chemotherapy. Drugs are administered for pain. In cases of severe pain or deformity, amputation may be done for palliative instead of curative reasons.

Ewing's Sarcoma This neoplasm develops from primitive bone marrow cells (myeloblasts). It usually occurs between the ages of 10 and 20 years and sometimes in younger children. The incidence for males is twice that for females. Shafts of the long bones, including the femur, tibia, and humerus, are common sites, as are the metatarsals and the ileum.

The lesion tends to extend longitudinally in the involved bone and develop early metastases to the lungs, other bones, and lymph nodes. Tumor cells grow so rapidly that they soon perforate the cortex of the bone to form a large soft-tissue mass. This mass is usually palpable and tender. Pain at the site of the bony lesion becomes increasingly severe. As the central areas of the lesion outgrow their blood supply and degenerate, toxic products enter the bloodstream and cause fever and leukocytosis.

Hematology tests which are taken before diagnosis include hemoglobin, hematocrit, white blood cell count, and platelet count; blood chemistry includes determinations of serum glutamic oxaloacetic transaminase (SGOT), alkaline phosphatase, and uric acid. A 24-hour urine test for vanillylmandelic acid (VMA) or total urinary catecholamines is often done to rule out neuroblastoma, a tumor in which these substances are elevated. Other diagnostic measures include urinalysis, bone marrow, chest x-ray and tomograms, bone survey, bone scan, and x-ray of the involved area. Distinctive radiographic features are present with this lesion, and results of surgical biopsy confirm the diagnosis.

The mortality rate is extremely high; despite treatment, 95 percent of children die within the first few years. Radiation therapy can be helpful, and it is sometimes followed by amputation of the affected limb. Chemotherapy is used for treating the major lesion and preventing metastases. Vincristine, cyclophosphamide, and dactinomycin are the drugs of choice.

Nursing Management Diagnosis of a neoplasm has a tremendous impact on the child and his family. If the diagnosis is given too early and then reversed, the family may be so frightened that they cannot believe the more favorable diagnosis. If the diagnosis of a neoplasm is given too late, the family may have such false hope that they postpone the decision for life-saving amputation. The nursing staff must be honest with the child and family from the beginning. The child will not accept amputation or long-term chemotherapy without a good understanding of the problem. The physician usually talks with parents first and gives parents the choice of whether they or the doctors or both together will talk with the child. Terms such as tumor or growth may be used in talking with the child; however, it is important to use a term which the child can understand. Older children need specific information, and they resent not being told about the diagnosis or treatment.

Nurses need to find out from the physician and the parents what the child has been told and what terms were used. It is important that nurses do not avoid the child or his family, for they can offer support and should be available to listen. Often a child or family members will confide in the nurse instead of the physician, thereby partially relieving themselves of fears and misconceptions.

Chemotherapy Uses of chemotherapy are to inhibit growth of tumor cells in major lesions as well as prevent or inhibit microscopic metastases. The three drugs which are commonly used in combination for treatment of osteogenic sarcoma and Ewing's sarcoma are listed in Table 40-4. If these drugs prove ineffective, experimental drugs may be tried. All side effects of chemotherapeutic drugs should be reported to the physician so that measures can be taken to counteract them or the drugs can be discontinued. Nurses are in the best position to observe side effects and help relieve them if the drug must be continued. Base line studies are taken which can serve as comparisons to later symptoms.

In response to either radiation or chemotherapy, mouth ulcers may appear. Good oral hygiene should include regular cleansing of gums and teeth and use of mouthwashes. Nausea and vomiting should not be ignored; instead, every effort should be made to find a schedule of administration and an antiemetic drug which will give relief. Constipation may require use of a stool softener. Before the child loses his hair (*alopecia*), he should be prepared for this possibility and encouraged to purchase a wig, if he desires. Hemorrhagic cystitis caused by Cytoxan can be detected by routine testing for blood in urine. High fluid intake or hydration with intravenous fluids is necessary at the time this drug is administered. Oral doses of the drug should be given in the morning so that the child has all day to drink extra fluids.

Amputation

Amputation is *therapeutic* in the case of a neoplasm and is therefore done to prolong life, decrease pain, or increase function. Amputation is *traumatic* when

Table 40-4 DRUGS OF CHOICE FOR TREATMENT OF OSTEOGENIC SARCOMA
AND EWING'S SARCOMA

Drug	Specific action	Route of administration	Toxic and side effects
Vincristine sulfate (Oncovin)	Arrests cells in metaphase	I.V.	Neurotoxicity (foot drop, leg pain, paresthesia, constipation), alopecia, injection site extravasation causes induration
Cyclophosphamide (Cytoxan)	Prevents cell division	I.V. or per os	Leukopenia, hemorrhagic cystitis, alopecia, nausea and vomiting
Dactinomycin (actinomycin D, Cosmegen)	Inhibits protein synthesis	I.V.	Bone marrow depression, nausea and vomiting, alopecia, injection site extravasation causes induration

it is caused by injury. Both kinds of amputation are physically and psychologically distressing for the child and his family. On admission to the hospital, an assessment should be made of the child's behavior and his relationships with parents. When amputation is therapeutic, the nurse has time to help the patient and his family prepare for surgery through explanations and interviews. Feelings need to be expressed. Preoperatively the child may act out his overwhelming fears of disfigurement and death by hostile reactions and refusal to cooperate with hospital staff. When amputation is traumatic, the child should not be left without an explanation of what has happened. Postoperatively all children should be provided with some means for expressive play or expression of their feelings. Since loss of a body part can be compared with death of a loved one, the child feels extreme sadness and grief. Parents often have guilt feelings about the disease or accident. Both child and parents need support in working through the grief process.

During surgery every attempt is made to cover the stump with a flap of healthy skin so that scars or nerve endings are not over the weight-bearing portion of the bone. Nursing care postoperatively aims to prevent bleeding, minimize swelling, maintain body alignment, and decrease pain. A plaster cast or compression bandage is usually applied. The stump may be elevated on pillows, although elevation must be done judiciously to avoid contractures which would interfere with the use of a prosthesis. If an immediate postoperative lower-limb prosthesis is used, a plaster cast is applied around the stump after surgery. When the cast is dry, a temporary prosthesis is secured to the plaster and the patient begins walking or using the prosthesis.

Phantom limb sensations may be very disturbing and confusing to the child. The phantom sensation has been described as a hallucination in which the patient reorganizes his perception of his body as

established by kinesthetic and tactile sensations. Feelings, such as burning, itching, throbbing, or sharp pain, may be perceived in the phantom limb. Over a period of 1½ years, the phantom sensations decrease, until the distal portion merges with the stump. The child needs to be supported in understanding that these sensations are normal and will gradually decrease.[6]

Adjustment to the loss of a limb is a difficult, long-term process. Nursing staff can help the child accept the stump by treating it in a matter-of-fact way, without negative projections or undue concern. When the child looks at the stump or touches it, he can begin to accept its reality; therefore, these activities should be encouraged when the child is ready for them. He should also be encouraged to discuss future activities and relationships such as modifications in clothing, use of the prosthesis, returning to school, and meeting old friends.

The child and family should begin caring for the stump in the hospital. Daily washing with soap and water should be accompanied by checks for skin irritation or breakdown. Exercises for muscle strengthening are taught by the physical therapist. The permanent prosthesis is usually fitted a few months after the stump is healed, and regular follow-up is carried out in an amputee clinic. The prosthesis will need frequent replacement as the child grows. Follow-up is important to ensure that the child wears and benefits from his prosthesis.

Curvature of the Spine

Types of Curvature Spinal deformities include kyphosis (humpback), lordosis (swayback), and scoliosis (lateral curvature). These deformities may occur alone or in association with other conditions.

Kyphosis is a fixed flexion deformity of the spine which most often appears in the thoracic spine. The vertebral deformities in the infant with myelomeningocele may assume the form of a kyphosis. It is also produced by a decrease in weight-bearing and muscular control, as seen in muscular dystrophy and poliomyelitis. *Adolescent kyphosis* (juvenile kyphosis, Scheuermann's disease, osteochondrosis of the spine) is a disorder affecting both girls and boys, which begins at puberty and progresses until vertebral growth has stopped in the late teens. The child with adolescent kyphosis is noted at first to have "poor posture" or "rounded shoulders," but as the curvature progresses, moderate back pain may be a complaint. Treatment is conservative, including spinal exercises, sleeping without a pillow and with boards under the mattress, body casts, and the Milwaukee brace modified to treat kyphosis.

Lordosis is a fixed extension deformity which rarely occurs in isolation but most often forms to compensate for other abnormalities. Whenever a kyphosis is present in the spine, lordosis may form above or below it. In addition, congenital hip dislocation and progressive muscular dystrophy are frequently associated with a compensatory lordosis. Treatment is primarily for the underlying disease.

Scoliosis involves a lateral curvature of the spine. *Nonstructural* scoliosis is caused by changes outside the spine, such as poor posture, pain, or leg length discrepancy. Because the curve is flexible, it corrects by bending to the opposite side. *Structural* scoliosis is a curvature in which the vertebral bodies are rotated in the area of the greatest or major curve. The curve fails to straighten out with side bending. This type of scoliosis is *compensated* when curves above and below the major curve allow shoulders to be level and directly above the pelvis. The curvature is *decompensated* when the major curve dominates; shoulders are not level, and the trunk shifts to one side. Structural scoliosis may be idiopathic (cause unknown) or due to another abnormality such as neurofibromatosis or paralysis. Treatment is by a combination of bracing, casting, and often spinal fusion. Untreated scoliosis leads to degenerative joint disease of the spine in an adult. Respiration may be affected and pain may be progressive.

Idiopathic Scoliosis In 80 percent of the cases of scoliosis, the cause is idiopathic. A familial incidence seems to be a factor. Types of idiopathic scoliosis are differentiated by age group: infantile (birth to 3 years), juvenile (4 to 9 years), and adolescent (age 10 until growth ceases). The adolescent type usually is found in girls, with a right thoracic scoliosis most common.

The lateral curvature progresses with growth, making secondary changes in the vertebrae and ribs.

Vertebrae are wedge-shaped in the middle of the curve from pressure on one side of the epiphyseal plate of the vertebral bodies. Typically, the curve begins slowly and is concealed by clothing. An uneven hemline may be the first clue that a problem exists. When it is noticed that one shoulder blade is higher than the other or one hip more prominent, a significant curve exists.

Prognosis is better when curvature begins at an older age and less growth remains. The outcome is also usually better when the curve is mild at the time of initial diagnosis and treatment. Treatment is instituted to prevent progression of mild scoliosis and stabilization as well as correction of more severe scoliosis. Treatment may be conservative, operative, or a combination of the two.

Many types of conservative treatments have been tried. Such measures as exercises alone and plastic body jackets have been unsuccessful. The Milwaukee brace is the most successful type of spinal brace, and it is widely used in the treatment of scoliosis (Fig. 40-12). Prior to bracing, correction in plaster casts may be helpful. In the older child the brace may prevent the need for surgery; in the younger child it may keep the curvature from becoming worse.

The Milwaukee brace is individually fitted to combine forces of longitudinal traction and lateral pressure. Exercise programs should be prescribed in conjunction with its use. Supervised by the physical therapist, exercises are designed for two purposes: (1) to increase muscle strength of the torso to counteract the effects of splinting and (2) to actively assist in correcting the abnormal curves and rib deformities. The increased strength he has gained from exercises helps the patient maintain an improved position after he has begun to remove the brace part-time. In school a full program of physical education can usually be maintained with the exception of contact sports, trampoline, and violent gymnastics. Adapting to the brace includes an educational program for the child and his parents concerning scoliosis, the brace, and the exercises.

Operative treatment is required only for obvious deformity, and it is usually done after 10 years of age. In surgery, the curvature is corrected, and the involved area of the spine is stabilized. Moderate curvatures may be passively corrected by plaster casts or traction before surgery, followed by surgical spinal fusion and immobilization in a body cast. In severe curvature, mechanical correction of the curve is accomplished by use of a Harrington rod or other instrumentation, followed by spinal fusion and wearing of a body cast for several months. Postoperatively when the patient is out of the cast, activities should be limited, and strenuous exercise or sports which are likely to end in falls (i.e., horseback riding) should be avoided.

Nursing Management The nursing role in idiopathic scoliosis begins with detection. School nurses have conducted successful screening programs which refer schoolchildren to physicians for early diagnosis and treatment.[7] With early case-finding, conservative treatment is more likely to be effective.

When surgery is required, various casts may be used preoperatively for correction of the curvature. The *localizer cast* developed by Risser is a body cast which utilizes cephalopelvic traction as well as pressure directly over the major curves to give correction. Cotrel's *E-D-F cast* (elongation, derotation, and flexion) is most effective in correcting the rib hump of severe thoracic curves. The *surcingle* cast, which extends up over the occiput, also provides correction of the rib hump. Patients are sometimes hospitalized overnight after cast application so that necessary adjustments can be made in the cast before discharge. The nurse should check the cast for uncomfortable or tight points and help the patient adjust to wearing it. Movements in the cast are restricted; ambulation is often difficult at first; and sleep is uncomfortable until the child adjusts to the cast.

Normal activities such as bathing, dressing, eating, or washing hair must often be modified to accommodate the cast or Milwaukee brace. Skin care in the cast or brace includes keeping the skin clean and dry, preventing sore areas at pressure points, having adjustments made in the appliance at pressure areas, and avoiding use of strong deodorants or perfumes which may cause rashes. A smooth-fitting undershirt or stockinet should be worn under the brace to protect the skin. Clothing must be loose or purchased in larger sizes to be worn outside of the appliance. Washing the hair can be made easier by the use of spray hoses on faucets or by lying with the head extended over the side of the bed above a washpan. For the patient who cannot ambulate, stretchers or reclining wheelchairs may be necessary for transportation. Trips to and from the hospital require the use of an ambulance, stationwagon, or van. The nurse can help the child and parents plan for these activities during hospitalizations and outpatient visits.

Traction may be used prior to surgery to stretch out soft tissue structures or correct spinal curvature. *Cotrel traction,* used for soft-tissue stretching around moderate curves, consists of a leather head halter and padded pelvic straps which are controlled

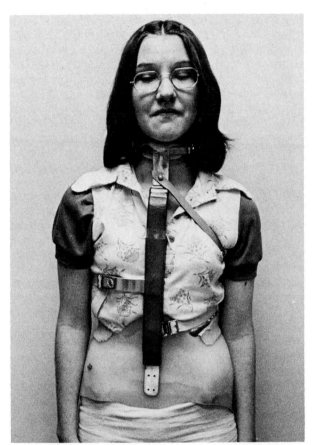

Figure 40-12 Milwaukee brace (blouse is worn under brace for purpose of photograph only). *(Courtesy James Whitcomb Riley Hospital for Children, Indianapolis, Ind.; photograph by Gerald Dreyer, Indiana University School of Nursing Instructional Communications and Educational Resources.)*

by the patient. *Halo-femoral traction* corrects severe and resistant curves. Pins which attach the halo to the skull and insert into the distal femur for femoral traction should be kept clean by daily nursing care. Dramatic correction is achieved by gradually adding heavier weights. Surgery is performed after adequate correction, and the patient may be returned to traction postoperatively.

Preoperative preparation includes explanations and practice for postoperative activities. Explanations about care immediately before surgery, about anesthesia, postoperative care, and appearance should be given to the child and his parents. The child can practice deep breathing or other respiratory routines, logrolling, and use of the fracture bedpan while lying flat in bed.

Postoperative nursing care must be gentle but at

the same time aggressive enough to prevent complications. The patient is usually returned without a cast but with a dressing over his back incision. Nursing functions include logrolling or turning the entire body as one piece at 2-hr intervals, caring for the urethral catheter, monitoring of intravenous and central venous pressure lines, monitoring blood transfusions, administering analgesics, and supervising coughing and deep breathing. Nursing observations include vital signs, neurologic function in the lower extremities, drainage from the incision, and signs of paralytic ileus. The patient's bed should have a firm mattress and be placed so that it is not easily joggled.

Adolescents treated for scoliosis have many concerns about their bodies and body images. In the cast, the adolescent may feel unreal or unlike his real self. Girls often have concerns about breast development and the effect of treatment on other bodily functions. They may be concerned that the cast will prevent growth or change the shape of their breasts, or that menstruation will temporarily cease in the cast.[8] Feelings of vulnerability are common, aggravated by disrobing during cast application or the restrictions imposed by casts or traction. Most teenage girls adjust well, however, because of their desire to look better and to please their parents and medical staff. The acceptance of the treatment program by parents is a crucial factor in the child's acceptance.

REFERENCES

1 R. B. Salter, *Textbook of Disorders and Injuries of the Musculoskeletal System,* The Williams & Wilkins Company, Baltimore, 1970, pp. 3–5.
2 L. Henkel and Hans-Georg Willert, "Dysmelia: A Classification and a Pattern of Malformation in a Group of Congenital Defects of the Limb," *Journal of Bone and Joint Surgery,* 51 B(3): 399–414, 1969.
3 Mabel Brunk, "Hypophosphatemic Rickets: Information for Parents," James Whitcomb Riley Hospital for Children, Indianapolis, Ind., unpublished work, 1973.
4 J. Caffey, *Pediatric X-Ray Diagnosis,* vol. 2, 6th ed., Year Book Medical Publishers, Inc., Chicago, 1972, pp. 1132–1146.
5 C. A. Bonsett, *Studies of Pseudohypertrophic Muscular Dystrophy,* Charles C Thomas, Publisher, Springfield, Ill., 1969, pp. 151–152.
6 Judith Ritchie, "Body Image Changes Following Amputation in an Adolescent Girl," *Maternal-Child Nursing Journal,* 1(1):39–46, 1972.
7 C. Sells and Eleanor May, "Scoliosis Screening in Public Schools," *American Journal of Nursing,* 74(1):60–62, 1974.
8 Jo Ann Neff, "Feminine Identity Concerns of Girls Undergoing Correction for Scoliosis," *Maternal-Child Nursing Journal,* 1(1):9–18, 1972.

BIBLIOGRAPHY

Ansell, Barbara: "Rheumatoid Arthritis—Medical Management," *Nursing Mirror,* 133(11):20–23, 1971.
Arey, Leslie B.: *Developmental Anatomy,* W. B. Saunders Company, Philadelphia, 1954.
A Traction Handbook, Zimmer USA, Warsaw, Ind., 1971.
Ballinger, W., Rutherford, R., and Zuidema, G.: *The Management of Trauma,* W. B. Saunders Company, Philadelphia, 1968.
Beare, Joan: "Osteogenesis Imperfecta," *Nursing Times,* 66(15):453–455, 1970.
Blount, W., and Moe, J.: *The Milwaukee Brace,* The Williams & Wilkins Company, Baltimore, 1973.
Brewer, E.: *Juvenile Rheumatoid Arthritis,* vol. 6 in A. Schaffer (ed.), *Major Problems in Clinical Pediatrics,* W. B. Saunders Company, Philadelphia, 1970.
Crenshaw, A. H. (ed.): *Campbell's Operative Orthopedics,* 5th ed., The C. V. Mosby Company, St. Louis, 1971.
Dadich, Karen: "An Eleven Year Old Girl's Use of Control While Immobilized in Halo-Femoral Traction," *Maternal-Child Nursing Journal,* 1(1):67–74, 1972.
De Palma, A.: *The Management of Fractures and Dislocations,* W. B. Saunders Company, Philadelphia, 1970.
Keim, H.: "Scoliosis," *Clinical Symposia,* 24(1), 1972.
Larson, Carroll, and Gould, Marjorie: *Orthopedic Nursing,* 7th ed., The C. V. Mosby Company, St. Louis, 1970.
Lloyd-Roberts, G. C.: *Orthopaedics in Infancy and Childhood,* Appleton-Century-Crofts, London, 1971.
Robinault, Isabel P.: *Functional Aids for the Multiply Handicapped,* Harper & Row, Publishers, Incorporated, New York, 1973.
Rosse, C., and Clawson, D. Kay: *Introduction to the Musculoskeletal System,* Harper & Row, Publishers, Incorporated, New York, 1970.
Rubin, P.: *Dynamic Classification of Bone Dysplasias,* Year Book Medical Publishers, Inc., Chicago, 1964.
Scharrard, W. J. W.: *Paediatric Orthopaedics and Fractures,* Blackwell Scientific Publications, Ltd., Oxford, England, 1971.
Schneider, R. R.: *Handbook for the Orthopaedic Assistant,* The C. V. Mosby Company, St. Louis, 1972.
Shands, A., and Raney, B. Beverly: *Handbook of Orthopedic Surgery,* The C. V. Mosby Company, St. Louis, 1967.
Tachdjian, M. O.: *Pediatric Orthopedics,* W. B. Saunders Company, Philadelphia, 1972.
"The Trouble's in the Bones": *Emergency Medicine,* 3(1):111–113, 1971.
Wagner, Mary: "Assessment of Patients with Multiple Injuries," *American Journal of Nursing,* 72(10):1822–1827, 1972.

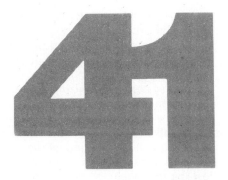

41

THE INTEGUMENTARY SYSTEM

JANET A. MARVIN, INEZ L. KING TEEFY,
and JUDITH M. JOHNSON

EMBRYOLOGY

The skin is composed of two layers, the epidermis derived from the ectoderm and the dermis developed from the mesenchyme. The ectoderm covering the surface of the embryo is at first a single layer of cuboid cells which multiply and become arranged in two layers: the epitrichium and the epidermis. The outer layer, the epitrichium, is shed around 6 months and becomes mixed with secretions from the sebaceous glands to form the vernix caseosa. This white, cheesy material (vernix caseosa) covers the fetus until birth and protects it from maceration as it floats in the amniotic fluid.

The epidermis proliferates and differentiates into the *stratum germinativum*, the *stratum spinosum*, the *stratum granulosum*, the *stratum lucidum*, and the *stratum corneum*. The epidermis sends down blunt ridges in the underlying mesenchyme, forming the epidermal ridges and the dermal papillae.

At about the 13th week of gestation, the epidermis is invaded by cells from the neural crest which form the *melanocytes*. In the epidermis these cells take their place in the stratum germinativum, and as tyrosinase appears in the cytoplasm, they form the pigment melanin. The melanocytes donate their melanin to adjacent keratinocytes by a process called *cytocrine* activity. The amount and color of the melanin present in the epidermis are responsible for the differences in skin color among races.

The dermis is formed from a condensation in the underlying mesenchyme, which is derived from two sources: (1) the cells of the somatopleuric mesoderm of the body wall and limbs and (2) the cells of the dermatome, which migrate from each somite. Fibroblasts are soon formed, and a network of collagen and elastic fibers is laid down. Capillaries and lymphatic vessels are also formed. Adipose tissue which appears in the deeper parts of the dermis and the subcutaneous tissues during the later months of gestation accounts for the rounded contours of the newborn.

Although hair first appears on the eyebrows, upper lip, and chin as early as 9 weeks of gestation, for the most part it begins to develop as cylindrical downgrowths of epidermis into the underlying mesenchyme between the third and fourth month of fetal life. At the same time the mesenchymal cells and fibroblasts increase in number and form the rudiments of the hair papillae beneath the hair germ. As the germ develops, it grows obliquely downward, and the advancing extremity becomes bulbous, gradually enveloping the dermal papillae. Two epithelial swellings appear on the posterior wall of the follicle; the lower one is the bulb to which the arrector muscle becomes attached, and the upper is the rudiment of the sebaceous gland.

The hair follicles form patterns, usually in groups of three with the hair arranged on a straight short line, transverse to the grain or slant of the hair. During postnatal development, a decrease in actual density of the follicle occurs as the body surface increases.

The sebaceous glands develop as solid outgrowths in the ectodermal cells near the neck of the hair follicle and extend into the mesenchyme. Degeneration of the central cells results in a fatty secretion that passes out into the hair follicle as *sebum*. The glands are functional from their earliest differentiation in fetal life; the sebum forms part of the vernix caseosa. At the end of fetal life the sebaceous glands are large and well developed over the entire surface of the skin. After birth, their size rapidly diminishes and the glands do not enlarge until after puberty.

The sweat glands (*eccrine glands*) appear about the fifth month as a solid downgrowth of the ectodermal cell into the mesenchyme. The terminal part of the downgrowth becomes convoluted and forms the body of the gland. Later the central cells degenerate to form the lumen of the gland. Peripheral cells differentiate into secretory cells and outer contractile myoepithelial cells.

The nails begin as thickened fields of ectoderm at the top of each digit and later migrate onto the dorsal aspect of each digit but retain their innervation from the ventral surface. The nail proliferates from the ectodermal cells which form the proximal nail fold. These cells become flattened and keratinized to form the nail plate, which continues to grow until it reaches the tip of the digit 1 month prior to birth. The development of the fingernails is slightly ahead of the toenails.

PHYSIOLOGY OF THE SKIN

The skin consists of a superficial layer of stratified epithelium (epidermis) laid on a foundation of firm connective tissue of dermis (Fig. 41-1). Its major function is protection against the external environment. The skin forms a barrier to protect the body from trauma, radiation, penetration of foreign bodies, moisture and humidity, microorganisms, and macroorganisms. To perform these functions it has a highly integrated, efficient, and complex mechanism of keratinization, pigment production, sensory nerves, and circulatory regulation. The skin also

maintains itself and efficiently and quickly repairs itself. The production of secretions from its surface glands maintains a buffered protective surface film which is said to be somewhat bacteriostatic. The skin functions as an important part of the body's defense system, recognizing foreign protein and setting in motion the immunologic response of the body. The internal fluid environment of the body is preserved by the skin, which prevents dissipation of the body fluids as long as the surface membrane is intact. When the surface membrane is injured or lost, as in extensive burns or severe skin diseases, large amounts of fluids, electrolytes, and proteins are lost from the body. The intact skin also serves in a minor way as an organ of elimination, excreting small amounts of sodium chloride and urea.

One of the most important functions of the skin is the regulation of body temperature. The body must adjust to fluctuations in environmental temperatures as well as in the heat produced by its own metabolism. Adjustments in body temperature are made by adjusting the loss of heat from the body to the environment. Dilatation of the arterioles increases blood flow to the extensive capillary plexuses of the dermis when heat loss is needed. When heat must be conserved, large units of the capillary bed are shut off by direct arteriovenous anastomoses which shunt blood away from the surface. The adipose tissue of the tela subcutanea functions as an insulating sheet against external temperature changes. Further cooling of the body can be provided when needed by an increase in sweat production. Perspiration on the skin surface provides cooling by evaporation.

CLASSIFICATION OF SKIN LESIONS

According to the nature of the pathologic process, cutaneous lesions assume more or less distinct characteristics. Primary or secondary lesions are of the following forms: macules, papules, nodules, tubercles, tumors, wheals, vesicles, bullas, and pustules (see color plate at the back of the book). Maturation of lesions presents numerous and varied secondary lesions which may be modified by many extraneous factors.[1]

Macules (color plate A) are of various sizes and are usually circumscribed alterations in the color of the skin, without elevation or depression. They may constitute the whole of the eruption or a part or may be merely an early phase or an associated symptom. Occasionally the spots become slightly raised and are designated as maculopapules.

Papules (color plate C) are circumscribed, solid elevations with no visible fluid, varying in size from

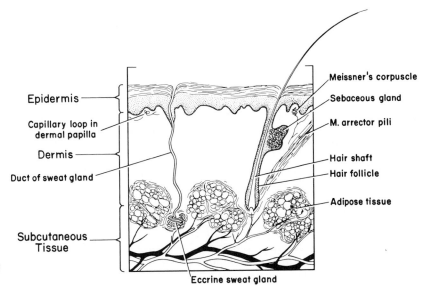

Figure 41-1 Anatomic diagram of the skin. *(Courtesy of University of Texas Southwestern Medical School at Dallas, Department of Medical Art.)*

Epidermis

Capillary loop in dermal papilla

Dermis

Duct of sweat gland

Subcutaneous Tissue

Meissner's corpuscle

Sebaceous gland

M. arrector pili

Hair shaft

Hair follicle

Adipose tissue

Eccrine sweat gland

a pinhead to a pea. They may be acuminate, rounded, conical, flat, or umbilicated and may appear white, red, yellowish, yellowish brown, or blackish. Papules may be seated in the corium around sebaceous glands, at the orfices of the sweat glands, or at the hair follicles. Some papules persist as papules, whereas those of the inflammatory type may progress to vesicles, pustules, or eventually ulcers.

Nodules (color plate *E*) are larger, solid forms of papules with a persistent character, perhaps midway between a papule and a small tumor. They differ from papules in being in close association with the corium or subcutaneous tissue and project both upward and downward.

Tumors (color plate *G*) may be soft or firm, freely movable or fixed, and are of various sizes and shapes. Consistency depends on the constituents of the lesion, which may be either inflammatory or neoplastic.

Wheals (*urticaria*) (color plate *I*) are evanescent, edematous, flat elevations of various sizes. They are usually oval, whitish or pinkish, and surrounded by pink aerolae. These lesions characteristically develop in a few seconds but disappear slowly; itching and tingling are almost always present.

Vesicles (*blisters*) (color plate *K*) are circumscribed, epidermal elevations of pinhead to pea size and contain a clear fluid. They may be pale or yellowish from seropurulent material or reddish from serum mixed with blood, and occasionally have deep reddish areolae. Vesicles may arise directly from macules or papules and generally break spontaneously or develop into blebs or pustules within a short time.

Bullae (*blebs*) (color plate *M*) are rounded or irregularly shaped blisters containing serous or seropurulent fluid. They differ from vesicles only in size, being larger than a pea. They are usually single-chambered and located superficially in the epidermis so that their walls are thin and subject to rupture. There is sometimes a lack of cohesion between the epidermis and the cutis so that the epidermis can be easily rubbed off, leaving a raw, moist abrasion (Nikolsky's sign).

Pustules (color plate *O*) are small elevations of the skin and contain pus. They are similar to vesicles in shape, have an inflammatory areola, and may be unilobular or multilobular. They are usually whitish or yellowish but may be reddish if they contain blood with the pus. They may originate as pustules or may develop as papules or vesicles, passing through transitory early stages during which they are known as papulopustules or vesicopustules.

INTEGUMENTARY DISEASES IN THE INFANT
Diaper Dermatitis

The diaper area of the neonate is constantly exposed to a wide variety of irritants, such as moisture, heat, and chemical substances. The contact dermatitis, or *diaper rash*, that develops from these irritants is a troublesome, distressing problem. Erythema in the genital or perianal area usually signals the beginning of the rash. Left unattended it quickly spreads throughout the diaper area as it progresses from macules and papules to eroded, moist, or crusted lesions.

Ammonia dermatitis, caused by the breakdown

of urea in the urine to ammonia by bacteria in the feces, presents a similar clinical picture. The areas of greatest involvement are the perianal and gluteal regions where it appears as a diffuse erythema. As it spreads throughout the diaper area, the skin appears shiny, red, and excoriated. Any infant with a diaper rash may be expected to voice pain and generalized discomfort, particularly when his diapers are wet or soiled. Ulceration of the urinary meatus in circumcised males sometimes develops in conjunction with the diaper rash.

The epidermis of the infant is highly permeable because of the immaturity of the stratum corneum. Chemical and physical insults such as ammonia and friction decrease the ability of the epidermis to maintain the integrity of the stratum corneum, resulting in the development of cutaneous lesions. The stratum corneum is thinnest in the intertriginous areas of the body. Gluteal, inguinal, and neck folds are particularly sensitive and therefore more prone to dermatitis. Maceration of any two skin surfaces in close opposition is termed *intertrigo*. Obese infants frequently develop intertrigo in the gluteal and neck folds. Poor ventilation, inadequate cleaning, and high humidity produce the irritating accumulation of sweat and sebum in the skin folds of the thin stratum corneum. Erythema, maceration, chafing, and fissuring develop as the intertrigo progresses.

Nursing Management Although it is difficult to pinpoint a single factor responsible for a particular diaper dermatitis and impossible to predict that any one treatment will both cure and prevent all diaper rashes, most of the principles for clearing a diaper dermatitis are also used for prevention. The general principles of keeping the area dry, well ventilated, and free of irritating substances sound simple enough. The astute nurse, however, will realize that diaper rash is an annoying and embarrassing problem to all mothers and that it deserves a careful exploration of present care and a thorough explanation of these general principles.

Skin irritants include urine and fecal material, either alone or in combination; the increased amounts of organic substances in diarrheal stools; excessive perspiration, particularly in the intertriginous areas; and friction from the rubbing of rough diapers against the skin. Changing diapers as quickly as possible after soiling is of the utmost importance. In a young infant, then, diapers are changed or at least checked for dampness every hour during the day and evening. Once the diapers are removed, the area is washed thoroughly with

water or with a bland soap and water if needed. Commercially available premoistened disposable towelettes may also be used. Careful attention should be given to cleansing the intertriginous, genital, and anal areas, separating the skin folds with one hand while washing with the other. All areas should be patted dry with a soft cloth or towel. Allowing the infant to go without diapers for short periods of time is healthful. Direct exposure to sunlight or artificial light is also beneficial. A gooseneck lamp with a 25-watt bulb placed approximately *1 foot from the infant's body* two to four times a day for 30 minutes promotes drying and healing. Intense heat to the raw areas, caused by the light being too close or too strong, may damage the epidermis. Ointments may increase the skin's sensitivity to the light; therefore, the areas should be clean and free of all ointments during lamp treatments. The lamp must also be securely located where bedclothing and moving legs will not touch the bulb.

A variety of ointments and creams are used to prevent and treat diaper rashes. The choice of ointment depends on the condition of the skin. Protective ointments are generally used for clear skin; commercially available diaper rash compounds are used for soothing and protecting minor rashes. Drying ointments or compresses of Burow's solution are indicated for acute weeping rashes. Steroid creams may be prescribed for their anti-inflammatory properties in stubborn or severe rashes but can be used safely for only short periods of time. Nurses should assume the responsibility for determining if parents are using steroid creams as directed by the physician. Powders are sometimes used; however, they tend to cake and are never used on open lesions.

Rubber pants, occlusive plastic coverings, tightly pinned or double diapers, and heavy snug-fitting clothing increase the production and retention of body heat and moisture in the diaper area. Loose diapers and clothing provide better ventilation. Plastic pants are completely avoided. Disposable diapers may be substituted by loosely pinned, single cloth diapers, without occlusive coverings, until the rash improves. The legs of all pants should be checked and discarded if there is constriction of the thighs or legs. Overheating by room temperature, clothing, or blankets should be avoided.

Infants may vary somewhat in their susceptibility to cutaneous irritants; however, substances left in improperly washed diapers are one of the main causes of diaper rashes. Diapers should be soft and free of soap, bacteria, and ammonia. Mothers are instructed to presoak soiled cloth diapers, wash them with a bland soap, and then thoroughly rinse them.

The amount of residue left in water after swishing a clean, dry diaper in cool water determines the adequacy of rinsing technique. A terminal antiseptic rinse with vinegar, Borax, or Diaperene may neutralize the ammonia produced by the urea-splitting bacteria; however, these diapers may be irritating to sensitive children. Generally, diapers are soaked for 20 minutes in the terminal rinse solution and then dried, preferably in the sun. Commercial diaper services function under strict regulations, and families using coin-operated laundries may find it more economical, efficient, and convenient to use such services.

Nurses and parents should see a noticeable improvement in the diaper dermatitis within a week if the previous general principles are followed. If the condition is not improving, an extensive area is involved, or weeping and oozing occur, a referral to the physician should be made. Secondary infections with bacteria and yeast frequently occur in the affected areas.

Diaper rashes are not without complications. A serious complication is stenosis of the urinary meatus as a result of ulceration and scarring. The possibility of permanent scarring and depigmentation in the diaper area are of concern to many mothers. They may be reassured that there is no permanent damage to the epidermis in most cases and that the skin will return to normal as the child gains bowel and bladder control.

A less common form of diaper dermatitis is *candidiasis* (moniliasis). These lesions appear as red, scalding, sharply circumscribed moist patches. Flaccid, pustular, satellite lesions surround the larger lesions. Cultures taken from these lesions reveal colonies of the yeast *Candida albicans*. Because yeasts require high humidity for growth, they are found frequently in the diaper area, mouth, and as a part of the normal intestinal flora. An oral *Candida* infection (thrush) is often found in conjunction with *Candida* infection in the diaper area. Antibiotics may upset the normal balance and may produce an overgrowth of *Candida*. Newborns are exposed to *Candida* from their mothers during birth. In both instances moniliasis is the cause. If a diaper dermatitis has been present for some time prior to the development of the demarcated lesions, the moniliasis is most probably a secondary infection.

Nystatin (Mycostatin) cream or ointment applied to the affected areas is the treatment of choice. It may be used alone or in combination with compresses of Burow's solution three times a day. An oral preparation of nystatin is used if thrush is present. The general principles of preventing diaper dermatitis should be reviewed with the mother and fol-

lowed. Careful handwashing by all caretakers is most important in preventing spread of the infection.

Bacterial dermatitis caused by other organisms, like the staphylococci, is unusual but may be found in conjunction with other low-grade infections. The distinctive lesions are papular, erosive, discrete, deep lesions with rolled edges. Antibiotics and steroids may be used in the treatment along with the general principles for care of the diaper area. Of particular importance is keeping the area dry. The nurse should observe for, or instruct the parents to observe for, signs of further infection and response to the therapy. If the infant does not appear to be responding to therapy within a couple of days, he should be reevaluated by the physician. During the acute stage of the bacterial dermatitis the bacteria may be recovered from the lesions. Therefore, in addition to the general principles referred to earlier, careful handling of linens and thorough handwashing are indicated.

Roseola Infantum

Roseola infantum (exanthem subitum) is a benign self-limiting infection seen in children 6 months to 3 years in age. Transplacental passive immunity apparently protects infants under 6 months of age. Little is known about the mode of transmission, causative agent, or communicability. It is believed to be caused by a virus but does not have the contagious characteristics of the measles. Generally no known actual exposure to a child with roseola occurs; therefore the incubation period has been difficult to determine, but it is presumed to be between 10 and 15 days. Spring and fall are the seasons of greatest incidence; however, it is seen throughout the year. No specific diagnostic tests are available. Diagnosis is based mainly on symptoms and differential diagnoses.

Assessment A febrile convulsion in a seemingly well child may be the first sign of the impending illness. The temperature rises abruptly to 103 to 105°F (39.5 to 40.5°C) and remains at that level for 3 to 4 days. Temperature-controlling methods only decrease the fever for short periods before it returns to the same high levels. This prodromal period causes great anxiety in parents and medical people alike, as there are only very mild nonspecific symptoms other than the fever on which to base a diagnosis. A mild pharyngitis, tonsillitis, otitis media, or lymphadenopathy may be present, but there are generally no signs of coryza, cough, or conjunctivitis. Leukopenia is present.

One of the striking features of the illness is the contrast between the febrile course and a child who looks alert and relatively well. On the third or fourth day a rash appears and the temperature returns to normal. The rosy pink, discrete macules or maculopapules appear first on the trunk and then spread to the neck, upper extremities, face, and eventually the lower extremities. The lesions fade with pressure, rarely coalesce, and disappear without desquamation in about 2 days. It is most important, but sometimes very difficult, to distinguish the symptoms of roseola from those of rubella, rubeola, meningitis, or a drug rash.

Nursing Management During the prodromal period, control of the temperature with tepid sponge baths and antipyretics may be necessary around the clock. Acetaminophen every 4 hours by mouth is the safest antipyretic, since there is little danger of overdosing the child. However, acetylsalicylic acid alternated with acetaminophen every 2 hours may be more effective than if either one is used alone. The nurse should carefully outline the appropriate dosage (1 grain per year of age) and the schedule of antipyretics with the parents. It is also wise to give them a written copy of all treatments discussed. Sponge baths for 15 to 20 minutes several times a day may also be used because tepid water and friction increase the amount of heat lost, thereby lowering the body temperature. Dressing the child in light colors, decreasing bedclothing, and keeping the room temperature normal will all assist in controlling the child's temperature. It must be remembered that these measures are in direct contrast to some of the older beliefs about treatment for chills and fever. Therefore, the nurse must make her explanations clear to parents in order to overcome their fears of making the child worse.

Phenobarbital may be given for several days by mouth to the child who has had a febrile convulsion, thereby decreasing the possibility of another seizure. However, care of the child before and after a convulsion should be reviewed with the parents. Antibiotics are sometimes prescribed during the early phase of the illness for prophylactic reasons, although they do not affect its course. The child may be happier and more comfortable with quiet activities outside the bed. There are no indications for strict bed rest nor for isolating the child from other children. A diet high in fluids is preferable during the febrile period but may otherwise vary according to desire and tolerance. No immunization against roseola is available at this time, and one episode is believed to confer permanent immunity.

Roseola may be the illness that indicates that a particular child is prone to having febrile convulsions. These children may be given phenobarbital daily until around 5 years of age to prevent convulsions in other febrile illnesses. Some physicians prefer to give the mother a prescription for phenobarbital with instructions to administer it to the child at the first sign of a temperature elevation. A diagnostic workup to rule out other possible causes of the convulsions may also be indicated. Parents often mistakenly associate convulsions with fever and brain damage. Therefore, nurses should explain the relationship of convulsions to an abrupt rise in temperature, stressing that a short febrile convulsion does not cause permanent brain damage.

Seborrheic Dermatitis

Seborrheic dermatitis is a common recurrent cutaneous disease of unknown cause and remarkable variation. In the neonate it appears as cradle cap; in infancy, as a dermatitis of the scalp and diaper area; and in older children, as dandruff or dermatitis of the midsternum, upper midback, and head. All these areas have a high level of sweat and sebum production from the sebaceous glands. The accumulation of sweat, sebum, and dirt is thought to be partially responsible for the scaly dermatitis. Seborrheic dermatitis often becomes a chronic inflammatory reaction that involves several areas of the body at one time. Complications include secondary infections of the involved areas with bacteria and yeasts.

Assessment Cradle cap in the infant and dandruff in the older child appear as mild inflammations of flat, adherent, greasy scales. Cradle cap is commonly seen in babies whose mothers are afraid to wash the infant's head. The scales continue to build and spread without adequate treatment and care. Eventually they may cover the entire scalp and most of the skin surface as well. Another common site for the dermatitis is in the diaper area. At times these erythematous scales may be oozing. The abdomen and back may become involved as the process spreads. The affected areas may be pruritic. Scratching the lesions frequently leads to secondary bacterial infections. By the end of the first year the condition usually improves spontaneously, only to reappear at a later age as dandruff. Dandruff appears more often in the winter when occlusive hats are worn. It may spread downward to the eyebrows, eyelids, neck, and external ear canal. In addition to the redness and scaling, there may be weeping and crusting of the affected areas. Crusting usually indicates a secondary infection. After puberty the site of predilection continues to be the hairbearing areas plus the midsternum and upper midback. The pale erythematous lesions differ from those in the young child by having sharply demarcated borders and a yellowish color of the greasy scales. Blepharitis is also a common finding of this age group.

Nursing Management The areas involved by seborrheic dermatitis must be kept clean, dry, cool, and free of rubbing by clothes or scratching by fingers. The scalp may be cleansed in several ways. Mild cases may need only a thorough shampoo followed by an application of a selenium sulfide suspension. This treatment shampoo is left on the scalp for approximately 10 minutes and is rinsed off thoroughly; the hair is then brushed well. In more severe cases, an oil, ointment, or lotion may be needed to soften the scales so that shampooing will be effective in removing them. Following the selenium sulfide suspension a fluocinolone or betamethasone lotion or cream may be applied. These medications are also used for eye and ear lesions. Tar bath solutions may be beneficial for seborrhea elsewhere on the body, particularly in the diaper area. Ointments containing sulfur and salicylic acid may then be applied. The first step in treating weeping or oozing lesions is to dry them by soaking with Burow's solution three or four times a day. Adrenocorticosteroid creams, which are particularly effective in the intertriginous areas, may then be used. Topical or oral antibiotics may be ordered for secondary bacterial infections. In severe, uncontrollable, spreading seborrhea, oral steroids may be administered. The nurse should carefully review the prescribed treatments with the parents. Treatments other than steroids, Burow's solution, and antibiotics are used as a rule for several days after clearing and then gradually tapered off. At the first sign of a recurrence they should be started again. Burow's solution is used only for oozing lesions and should not be started or stopped indiscriminately by parents. Medications with steroids and antibiotic components may be prescribed for a given period of time; the schedule should be closely followed and usually includes a slow withdrawal of medications. The temperature of the environment and the weight of the clothes should be controlled to decrease the amount of perspiration. Clothes should be soft, loose, and porous to prevent irritation from rubbing and to allow for adequate ventilation. Attempts should be made to prevent scratching of the affected areas and introducing bacteria in the lesions. The nurse may need to review general principles of well-child care with the mother of a young child, particularly those involving general hygiene, care of diapers, and care of the diaper area.

Infantile Eczema

Infantile eczema (atopic dermatitis) is often the earliest manifestation of an allergic tendency. Usually a hereditary predisposition for the development of sensitization to common allergens is present. At various ages children often develop the triad of eczema, asthma, and hay fever. Eczema usually appears by the fourth month and clears spontaneously by the fourth year. It appears most often in the well-nourished, well-cared-for healthy infant and is not influenced by race or sex. The winter months show a worsening of the condition followed by a general improvement during the summer. The introduction of new foods during infancy is thought to provide allergens responsible for the cutaneous response. However, skin-testing infants for sensitization to these substances has not always shown a positive correlation. Other causes appear to be related to a hyperactive skin and normal sensitivity to external irritants. A disturbed mother-child relationship may also influence the disease process, as psychologic factors appear to affect the course. The prognosis of eczema is good, although the course is prolonged and characterized by many exacerbations and remissions. Secondary bacterial infections of the lesions commonly occur and are the complication most often associated with eczema. Eczema should be differentiated from contact dermatitis and seborrheic dermatitis.

The cheeks are generally the area where the infantile eczema is first evident. Initially, pruritus, erythema, and edema appears, caused by dilatation of the blood vessels, followed quickly by the formation of papules and vesicles as fluid from the capillaries escapes into the tissues. The reaction often spreads to the forehead, scalp, and flexor surfaces of the extremities, particularly of the antecubital and popliteal fossae. Eventually it may cover most of the body surface. Because the pruritus is intense, the child scratches the lesions, thus rupturing vesicles and causing excoriation of the area. Weeping, oozing areas of thick yellow sticky exudate cover the raw surfaces. As these areas dry, crusts form. Generalized lymphadenopathy, low-grade fever, and splenomegaly may also be found in this uncomfortable, fretful, and irritable child. Eventually the acute process subsides, and the crusts desquamate, leaving healthy new epithelium. Scarring may occur with secondary infections but is not a part of the eczematous process. In older children exacerbations usually occur in the flexural creases, volar surfaces of the wrists, and extensor surfaces of the knees and elbows. Over the years the affected skin becomes thickened and darker in color. This condition is called lichenification and is the hallmark of chronic eczema.

Nursing Management Successful management of the child with eczema requires a comprehensive approach on the part of both the family and the medical team. Parents must understand that infantile eczema is a chronic condition for which there is no cure. There are, however, therapeutic regimens which control the symptoms and attempt to define and alleviate the causative factors. The medical team must be particularly aware of the mother's emotional state. Care of the child in the home is always preferable to the hospital where exposure to a variety of bacteria would be inevitable. The parents' feelings toward the child must be determined and discussed. Commonly a parent disgusted at the sight of weeping, oozing lesions; overwhelmed by the time-consuming treatments; and confronted by an impossible-to-satisfy, fussy, irritable, scratching child is overcome by guilt of producing the illness and has strong feelings of rejecting the child. Nurses must be aware that these feelings are normal and should be expressed along with constructive suggestions and explanations to decrease the burden and the anxiety. Maternal responses of anxiety, rejection, and overprotection are quickly detected by the child and may aggravate the condition. Continual reassurance, support, understanding, and praise will be needed by the mother over the years. A sympathetic nurse who is readily available to the distressed parent is invaluable in the care of the child.

Determination and elimination of the possible allergens are primary goals of the regimen. A careful, thorough past and present history may be the most helpful tool in identifying allergens. In the child under 18 months of age dietary allergens are extremely common. Cow's milk, egg whites, wheat cereals, and fruits such as oranges and apples are food proteins which cause sensitivity. A diet eliminating possible allergens is usually suggested, and substitute foods are recommended. Diets low in carbohydrates and fats also seem to provide benefits. In older children foods seem to cause fewer reactions than external irritants.

Inhalants that produce reactions may be controlled by the elimination of dust-collecting items, especially in the child's bedroom. Rugs, drapes, stuffed fuzzy toys, and upholstered furniture all hold dust. The rooms should be cool, well ventilated, and dusted with a wet cloth daily. Wool clothes often cause eczema as a result of overheating and sweating; therefore, clothes should be soft and lightweight. Soaps are another irritant either as a residual in clothes and linens or when used in bathing. Laundry soaps should have a neutral pH and be thoroughly rinsed from the clothes. Bathing with soap and water may be restricted and plain water, oil, or starch baths substituted.

During the acute phase of eczema, treatment consists of prevention of scratching, alleviation of pruritus, promotion of healing, and prevention of secondary infections of the lesions. Eczema is sometimes referred to as a pruritus that causes an eruption rather than an eruption that is pruritic. In addition to controlling the environmental irritation and topical therapy, specific antipruritic agents such as elixir of trimeprazine or cyproheptadine may be administered orally several times a day. Adequate rest is essential to the child and may be aided by antihistamines, tranquilizers, or barbiturates. Restraining a child may be necessary in order to prevent scratching and rubbing of the affected areas. Elbow, wrist, and ankle restraints and socks covering hands as well as affected parts are used as needed. Restraints should be applied loosely and carefully and only when absolutely necessary. They should be removed frequently to allow free movement and expressive play. Plastic sheets and bibs may be used to prevent the absorption of ointments by the bedding and clothing. The child's nails should be clipped and washed frequently to prevent scratching and introducing bacteria into the lesions.

Wet compresses of Burow's solution are used for their bacteriostatic, drying, and antipruritic effect on weeping areas. They should be thoroughly soaked with the solution and loosely applied for 30- to 60-minute periods four times a day. The compresses should be resoaked and reapplied every 10 to 15 minutes to prevent drying and sticking. Saline solutions (2 teaspoonfuls of salt to 1 quart of water) are sometimes used. Both solutions should be kept at room temperature and applied with soft cloths rather than gauze squares. Antibiotics and steroids may also be ordered, topically or orally, depending on the condition and severity of the involved areas. The schedule of all treatments and medications should be clearly outlined with the parents and closely adhered to.

The child with eczema has the same needs for growth and development that any other child has. Without a doubt his needs for love, attention, and expression of frustration are greater than those of the normal child. Mothers and other attending persons should be encouraged to use a gown or apron to cover their clothes and to handle and cuddle the child as much as possible. Visual and auditory stimulation should be provided while the child is restrained. Play should be provided with smooth, washable toys, stimulating the child's developmental level and his need for expression of frustrations.

Erythema Infectiosum, Fifth Disease

Erythema infectiosum is a mild, self-limiting disease thought to be caused by a virus. It appears to be mildly contagious and is seen in small outbreaks in the spring at intervals of several years. Because it has been confined to families and other groups of people, it is thought to spread by droplet infection. Children between the ages of 2 and 10 years are most commonly affected. The estimated incubation period is from 5 to 14 days. Erythema infectiosum is a benign disease with an excellent prognosis and no complications.

Assessment The exanthema of erythema infectiosum erupts in three stages. A prodromal period is usually absent but may include fever and malaise. In the first stage a coalescent erythematous maculopapular rash appears on the cheeks. The affected areas are slightly raised, warm, and have defined edges, giving the child a "slapped cheek" or sunburned appearance. The circumoral area is not involved and appears as pallor next to the red, efflorescent cheeks. The eruption fades in 1 to 4 days. The second stage begins 24 hours after the first stage with a maculopapular rash on the proximal parts of the extremities, extending to the hands and feet. Within a day or two the rash spreads distally to the hands, feet, buttocks, and trunk; and in 6 to 10 days it begins to fade centrally on the extremities, leaving a diagnostic lacelike pattern. Also diagnostic is the evanescent nature as the exanthema changes in intensity from hour to hour. The third stage is said to begin after the rash has cleared. For a variable length of time the rash may reappear when precipitating factors such as trauma, heat, cold, or sunlight irritate the skin. Throughout the illness the child remains afebrile, without lymphadenopathy or enanthem, and with only mild complaints of pruritus. Erythema infectiosum should be differentiated from enterovirus infections and drug reactions.

Nursing Management The child with erythema infectiosum may be kept home from school, but isolation is not considered necessary. The child generally feels well, and no treatments are indicated. Parents should be given anticipatory guidance concerning the stages of the rash. They may be reassured particularly that the third stage is normal and that the problem will disappear in time.

Scarlet Fever

Scarlet fever is an infection caused by the group A beta-hemolytic streptococci. The primary site of the infection is usually the pharynx: however, the disease has been known to occur following infections of wounds, burns, and other skin lesions. The toxic and septic manifestations of the illness appear as the erythrogenic toxins of the streptococci are produced. Scarlet fever is seen most often in children between the ages of 2 and 8 years, in the winter and spring, and in the temperate and cold climates. The mode of transmission is usually direct contact, but it may be indirect or by contaminated foods. The incubation period ranges from 1 to 7 days. The most severe complications of scarlet fever are acute glomerulonephritis and rheumatic fever. Cervical adenitis, otitis media, sinusitis, and bronchopneumonia are some other complications.

Assessment Scarlet fever generally begins abruptly with fever, vomiting, a sore throat, headache, chills, and general malaise. The fever reaches a peak by the second day and returns to normal within 5 to 6 days. If penicillin is administered, it returns to normal within 24 hours. The pulse rate increases. The tonsils are edematous, enlarged, and covered with patches of exudate, while the pharynx is edematous and beefy red in appearance. During the first day or two the tongue looks like a white strawberry. The reddened papillae project through the white furry dorsum. By the fourth or fifth day "strawberry tongue" is noted as the white coat peals off and leaves the dorsum bright red. The enanthema consists of erythematous punctiform lesions and petechiae which cover the soft palate and uvula. The skin rash (exanthema) appears 12 to 72 hours after the onset of the illness as a diffuse erythematous papular rash first on the base of the neck, axillae, groin, and trunk. Within 24 hours it covers the body. There is circumoral pallor because the cheeks are red and flushed in contrast to the uninvolved area surrounding the mouth. The lesions blanch with pressure and feel like goose pimples, and form transverse lines (Pastia's sign). One area that does not blanch on pressure is the flexor surface of the elbow, which is hyperpigmented and contains petechiae. At the end of the first week the rash begins to desquamate. Desquamation is first apparent on the face, becomes generalized by the third week, and is characteristic of scarlet fever and is directly proportional to the intensity of the rash. Cultures from the throat or portal of entry reveal group A beta-hemolytic streptococci. A significant rise in the antistreptolysin O titer is evident during convalescence, leukocytosis is present, and the Dick test reverts from positive to negative a few weeks later.

Nursing Management Penicillin is the drug of choice and may be administered intramuscularly, orally, or both. Erythromycin may be used in patients who are allergic to penicillin. Adequate early treatment prevents complications of rheumatic fever and glomerulonephritis and eradicates the carrier state. The child will probably be most comfortable in bed during the febrile period. After the temperature has returned to normal, quiet play activities should be provided in the home. During the acute phase, the upper respiratory tract symptoms probably cause the most discomfort. Aspirin, codeine, analgesic gargles, lozenges, and inhalation of cool mist may make the child feel better. A fluid diet is tolerated best during the febrile period. Parents should be informed about the natural course of the illness and should be instructed to observe for complications. Continuation or recurrence of fever may be the most obvious sign of a complication. Parents should not hesitate to return to their physician if they do not feel their child is progressing. Isolation of the child and his return to school depend on local regulations. Close contacts of the child should be watched for symptoms of a streptococcal infection; if symptoms occur, a throat culture should be done. A positive culture necessitates treatment with penicillin. Measures which prevent the spread of the bacteria at home include careful handling and thorough washing of the child's clothes, linens, and dishes; scrubbing dust-collecting surfaces; and cleaning and airing the child's room thoroughly following the illness.

INTEGUMENTARY DISEASES IN THE PRESCHOOL AND SCHOOL-AGE CHILD
Varicella

Varicella (chickenpox) is a benign, self-limiting disease caused by the varicella-zoster virus. It is highly contagious and seen often in the winter months in preschool and school-age children. Since there does not appear to be transplacental immunity, varicella may be seen in the young infant. Direct contact is the most common method of exposure, but indirect contact through a third person or contact with airborne droplets are also possible. A child with varicella may transmit the disease to susceptible children from 1 day prior to the eruption of his rash until all his lesions have become dry and crusted. The incubation period is from 10 to 21 days. Complications are not common, although secondary bacterial infection of the lesions, encephalitis, and pneumonia may occur. It is potentially fatal in a newborn and in children who are on corticosteroid therapy.

Herpes zoster (shingles) and varicella are two different clinical manifestations of the same virus. The primary response to contact with the virus is chickenpox. A later exposure to the same virus in a partially immune individual produces symptoms of herpes zoster. Therefore, a susceptible child exposed to an adult with herpes zoster may develop chickenpox. Likewise, an older child or an adult with only partial immunity may develop herpes zoster when exposed to a child with chickenpox.

Assessment The prodromal period of anorexia, fever, and general malaise may precede the rash by a few hours or may be absent altogether. In young children all symptoms occur the same day, whereas the exanthema in adolescents is more often preceded by a prodromal period of 24 to 48 hours. The exanthema which appears in crops first on the trunk and then on the scalp, face, and extremities continues to erupt for a period of 3 days with the heaviest concentration on the trunk and the lightest concentration on the forearms and lower legs. A most striking characteristic of the exanthema is the rapid transition from its beginning as a macule through stages of a papule, a vesicle, a ruptured vesicle, and finally to a crust. This progression is accomplished approximately every 8 hours; therefore, any anatomic area will have lesions in all the stages of transition, and recognition of chickenpox is relatively easy. The typical vesicle has the appearance of a thin fragile dewdrop on an erythematous base. It begins drying and forming crusts first in the center of the lesion, resulting in an umbilicated appearance. Scabs normally fall off in 5 to 20 days, leaving a shallow pink depression. Gradually, normal skin color returns without scar formation.

Lesions may also be noted on the palate as white ulcers and around the genitalia and in the vagina. The lesions are intensely pruritic until crusts form and cause extreme discomfort, particularly when located on the genitalia and in the vagina. Fever, anorexia, headache, and general malaise are common throughout the eruptive phase. The highest temperature is reached during the period of greatest eruption and is in proportion to the severity of the rash.

Nursing Management The child with chickenpox is most concerned about the intense itching. Pruritus in the vesicular stage is the beginning of a cycle which may lead to scarring and septicemia unless there is adequate treatment. Scratching causes rupture of the vesicles and the introduction of bacteria into the lesions. Normally they heal without residual effects, but those that are secondarily infected may leave permanent scars. A variety of treatments and preventive measures can decrease the possibility of infections. Calamine lotions, antipruritic ointments, antiseptic or starch baths, oral antihistamines, and sedatives are all used in the treatment, depending on the extent of the lesions and the response of the child. The hands, a source of infection, should be washed frequently, and the nails should be clipped short. In a young child or infant, mittens are used to decrease scratching. Clothing should be loose-fitting, cool, and lightweight and should be changed at least daily. Care should be taken never to deliberately break a vesicle. Gentle patting is preferable to rubbing when bathing the child or applying medication. Bed rest and antipyretics are indicated during the febrile period. Quiet play activities involving use of the hands should be provided. In addition to meeting his emotional needs, such activities serve as a substitute for scratching. Scabs may be expected to fall off spontaneously in 1 to 2 weeks. Local regulations determine when the child may return to school. Generally, he is kept at home until all the vesicles have dried and the scabs are well formed. Parents should notify the physician if new symptoms develop after the third day of the rash. Neurologic or respiratory symptoms are especially indicative of a complication. Lifelong immunity is provided by having the disease. No vaccine is yet available. Although varicella is usually a benign disease in childhood, it may be a severe and potentially fatal disease in adulthood. Consequently, attempts to prevent the normal child from exposure to varicella are not recommended.

Rubella

The rubella virus produces a mild self-limiting illness of major significance only because of the danger it presents to the fetuses of susceptible women in the first trimester of pregnancy, when a variety of serious congenital abnormalities may occur. Rubella (also known as the German measles, or 3-day measles) may occur at any age, but is most often seen in children between the ages of 3 and 12. Immune childbearing women provide their infants with transplacental immunity for about the first 6 months of life. It is therefore rarely seen in children under 6 months of age. The virus is easily transmitted by airborne droplets, by direct contact, or by articles contaminated with secretions from infected individuals. An infected child frequently exposes others before his disease is suspected. The virus is found in nasopharyngeal secretions, urine, and feces 7 days before the appearance of the rash until 5 days later. First signs of the disease may appear from 14 to 21 days following the initial exposure.

Assessment About 1 to 3 days prior to the development of the rubella rash, the child complains that the back of his neck is sore and stiff. Lymphadenopathy of the postauricular, posterior cervical, or suboccipital nodes is the reason for the complaints and is characteristic of the disease. A careful examination at this time usually reveals another sign—reddish spots, the size of a pinpoint, located on the soft palate. One to five days prior to the eruptions, malaise, anorexia, low-grade fever, sore throat, headache, cough, mild conjunctivitis, and coryza are seen in older children but are only occasionally apparent in the young child. The exanthema appears first on the face as a pinkish red discrete maculopapular eruption. During the next 12 to 24 hours it spreads rapidly down the neck, arms, trunk, and extremities until the entire body is covered. On the second day the temperature returns to normal and the majority of the symptoms subside. The rash begins fading from the face but remains on the extremities. The trunk becomes completely covered as the lesions coalesce and form a diffuse erythematous blush. In most cases the rash disappears by the third day without desquamation. Duration of the exanthema varies from 1 to 5 days; rarely is the rash absent.

Lymph node tenderness usually subsides after the first day, but the nodes may be palpable for several weeks. Adolescents are prone to developing arthritis in one or more joints at about the same time the rash is fading. Fever may accompany the joint swelling and tenderness. Although the development of arthritis causes some anxiety in both the parents and the children, it usually clears spontaneously in 5 to 10 days.

Rubella may be confused with roseola or scarlet fever. The colors of the rashes are most significant. The nurse should know that a rubella rash is pinkish red, scarlet fever rash is yellowish red, and roseola has a purplish red rash. Another important difference is that the lesions of rubeola tend to coalesce around the head and trunk, while the lesions of rubella are generally discrete. With scarlet fever there is usually a circumoral pallor, while in rubella this area contains pinkish red lesions.

Nursing Management It is not unusual for a school nurse to find an older child attending classes with a rubella rash hidden under long sleeves. The child insists he is not ill enough to curtail his normal activities. It is generally accepted, however, that it is more beneficial for the child, and others, to remain at home until the rash has disappeared. He need not stay in bed unless he has arthritis of the weight-bearing joints or other symptoms which make him feel quite ill. Aspirin or acetaminophen controls the symptoms of fever and arthritis. Pruritus is not a problem. A persistent fever, continued malaise, abnormal neurologic signs, purpura, or excessive joint involvement should alert the nurse to the probability of complications and the need for a physician to see the child. Generally, photophobia or nausea is not associated with rubella. One attack of rubella provides permanent immunity.

Parents are sometimes confused about the differences between roseola, rubeola, and rubella and may report that their child is immune to measles. Careful questioning about the symptoms may reveal that a so-called rubella rash may in fact have been roseola, scarlet fever, or even a viral rash. Nurses should explain to parents that as a rule one attack of a particular disease, such as rubella, confers immunity for life.

In addition to having the disease, a second form of active immunity is available through a single subcutaneous injection of rubella live attenuated virus vaccine. The vaccine is recommended for children from 1 year of age to puberty. Children in elementary school are the major disseminators of the virus and are therefore the target population for the vaccine. It may be given safely to children with a questionable history of rubella. If the vaccine is given to children under 1 year of age, maternal rubella antibodies may interfere with the active immune response when the neutralizing antibodies of transplacental immunity are still present. A child vaccinated before 1 year of age may eventually be as susceptible to rubella as if he had not received the vaccine. Pregnant women should never be given the rubella vaccine because of the danger of causing congenital defects in the unborn child. Postpubertal females are not vaccinated routinely because of the potential risk to the fetus if the girl is pregnant but unaware of it. Those asking to have the vaccine should be counseled to have a hemagglutination inhibition test to determine the presence or absence of rubella-neutralizing antibodies. If test results indicate susceptibility, vaccination is done only with the understanding that pregnancy is contraindicated for the next 3 months. A contraceptive method should be carefully used during this period. There are no contraindications to vaccinating postpubertal males; however, it is not done routinely.

Contraindications to giving the vaccine include active febrile infections; sensitivity to chicken or duck meat, eggs, or feathers; sensitivity to neomycin; presence of blood dyscrasias; current therapy affecting the bone marrow or lymphatic system; and a gamma globulin deficiency. The live rubella virus may be given in preparations which contain other live vaccines but must not be given less than 1 month before or after single immunizations with other live virus vaccines.

Mothers are instructed that the child may develop any of the symptoms of rubella, usually within 2 weeks but even within 2 months, after the vaccination. Symptoms are generally mild and will not inhibit activity. Antipyretics may be given to ease the fever or discomfort. Warm soaks to the injection site may relieve the tenderness or induration. Older children appear to have a stronger reaction than younger children.

Rubeola

Rubeola (measles, morbilli, red measles) is a highly contagious, self-limiting infection caused by the rubeola virus. It is a more severe disease in childhood than rubella or roseola because of the intensity of the symptoms and the frequency of complications. Outbreaks occur in the winter and spring and reach epidemic proportions every 2 to 3 years. Incidence is greatest in children of school age, but rubeola may be seen at any age. Infants under 6 months of age may be protected by passively acquired maternal antibodies from the immune mother. The virus is transmitted directly by a cough or sneeze, indirectly by contaminated articles, or in the air by dust particles. The incubation period is from 10 to 21 days. Children are considered infective for a period of up to 2 weeks, from as early as the fifth day of the incubation period and up to a week following the onset of symptoms. The age of the child and the severity of the symptoms affect the prognosis. The infant with a severe case of measles has a greater probability of developing complications and therefore a poorer prognosis. Complications most often involve the respiratory tract, nervous system, eyes and ears, and occasionally the skin. Effective antibiotic therapy has decreased the mortality rate from secondary complications. The administration of gamma globulin following exposure to measles has improved the prognosis by causing the child to have only a mild or modified case of measles. The incidence of rubeola has decreased sharply in the United States with the use of live attenuated measles vaccine.

Assessment   In the typical case of rubeola, a fever around 101°F (38.3°C) and general malaise are common on the first day. Within 24 hours the temperature increases and the child appears to have a severe cold. Sneezing, nasal congestion, brassy cough, and conjunctivitis are present. Generalized lymphadenopathy may occur. On the second or third day Koplik's spots appear on the buccal mucosa opposite the molars. These small, irregular, reddish spots with minute bluish white centers are diagnostic. On the third day an increase in the severity of all symptoms occurs. Usually by the third or fourth day the rash becomes apparent. The erythematous maculopapules appear first around the hairline of the neck and forehead and spread downward to the feet over the next 2 days. By the time the rash reaches the feet as discrete maculopapules, those of the face and trunk may have become confluent. The child appears most ill when all symptoms reach a height on the fourth or fifth day of the illness, or the second to third day of the rash. The fever may be as high as 105°F (40.5°C), coryza is profuse, cough is harsh, eyes are swollen, watery, and sensitive to light, the buccal mucosa is covered with Koplik's spots that are beginning to slough, and the rash is pruritic and almost covers the body. Within 24 hours, or around the fifth to sixth day, the temperature returns to normal and there is a noticeable improvement in the coryza, conjunctivitis, and cough. The rash begins fading in the same order in which it appeared and leaves a brownish staining of the skin and a fine, branny desquamation. The child coughs for a week or so, but there should be a steady improvement in his general condition during this time. If immune serum globulin has been given following exposure to rubeola, the course of the illness is milder and shorter. It is appropriately called modified measles and rarely causes complications. In this abbreviated version, symptoms are milder and disappear more quickly or are absent altogether. The prodromal period lasts about a day, the fever is low grade or normal, and the rash is sparse and fades more quickly.

Nursing Management   The child with rubeola generally feels miserable and needs a good deal of sup-portive care. Bed rest is indicated, and easy to enforce, until the fever subsides. A variety of quiet play activities should be available to the child, but during the acute phase he will probably prefer to sleep. If photophobia is present he will be most comfortable in a dimly lighted room. Watching television and reading may have to be postponed until the sensitivity to light decreases. The eyes should be kept clean and free of crusts. They may be bathed with warm water to remove the matting associated with the conjunctivitis. Antipyretics are beneficial for fever and generalized discomfort. Medications for cough and coryza may be prescribed but are never too effective in rubeola. The nares may become excoriated by the continual nasal drainage and should be protected. Dressing the child in soft, lightweight cotton clothing provides maximum heat loss during the febrile periods and decreases the irritability or sensitivity of the rash. Calamine lotions may be used to control the pruritus if needed. Some parents become concerned with the brown staining of the skin as the rash fades (bathing in warm water makes this staining more apparent) but should be reassured that the staining will fade.

Antibiotics are not routinely given or recommended to prevent the bacterial complications of roseola. Nurses must consider specific facts which influence complications when teaching parents about the disease. The more severe the illness, the greater the possibility of complications. The younger the child, the more prone he is to developing complications. Parents should be instructed to seek medical attention if there is not a noticeable improvement in the child after the third day of the exanthema, if there is prolonged fever or increased lethargy, or if the child has respiratory distress. Permanent immunity follows the disease, whether it runs a full course or is a modified case. Following exposure to rubeola, immune serum globulin is administered in a dosage that does not prevent the disease entirely but allows the child to build up a permanent active immunity and greatly decreases the severity of the disease. Parents of susceptible children should be instructed to notify their physician immediately if exposure to rubeola occurs so that the illness may be modified. If a child has a chronic disease, is ill, or is very young at the time of exposure, the physician may feel that it is imperative for the child not to have rubeola. In this child, larger doses of immune serum are given to prevent the disease entirely. This passive immunity is, of course, temporary. Active immunity is also provided by a single subcutaneous injection of live attenuated measles vaccine. It is not recommended for children under 1 year of age, since maternal antibodies may still be present in the child. It is recommended for some children with chronic diseases, since rubeola and its complications could be fatal for them. The vaccine will not affect the outcome of the disease if given after exposure. Contraindications include active untreated tuberculosis; sensitivity to eggs, chicken, feathers, or neomycin; an acute febrile infection; blood dyscrasias; malignancies; gamma globulin deficiencies; and pregnancy. Care must be taken when administering to children with histories of febrile convulsions. The vaccine should not be given less than 1 month before or after another live virus vaccine but may be given in a preparation that contains rubella and mumps vaccine. The rubeola vaccine may temporarily depress tuberculin skin sensitivity. Therefore, skin testing should be administered prior to the immunization. Parents may expect a mild fever during the month following the vaccine. Generally fever or a minimal rash occurs in 5 to 12 days. Local reactions may appear at the injection site and are treated with warm moist compresses. With the preventive methods available today, there is no reason for a child to have a natural case of measles and its complications. Nurses should assume responsibility for educating parents in immunizing their children against rubeola or at least in having it modified following exposure.

Impetigo

As a primary lesion, impetigo is an infectious disease of the superficial layers of the skin which have been invaded by coagulase-positive streptococci, staphylococci, or pneumococci. Lesions may develop on any part of the body but are most commonly found on the face about the mouth and nose. Impetigo is rampant in the South, particularly during the summer months. However, it can be readily seen any time or any place where children are victims of poor hygiene, malnutrition, or crowded living conditions.

Assessment At the onset skin blisters develop from small reddish macules that fill with serum and rapidly become cloudy. Pustules form and then rupture, discharging serous and purulent fluid which forms straw-colored or brown, thick crusts on an erythematous base. Multiple lesions are common and may be present in all stages, sizes, and shapes. During this acute phase, chickenpox may be erroneously diagnosed. There is a tendency toward peripheral spreading, with the development of circles and arcs healing over in one portion while continuing to advance in another. Without prompt treatment, lesions

rapidly extend beneath the stratum corneum. With proper intervention, healing usually occurs within a week or two, leaving a slightly reddened annular area that may be mistaken for ringworm.

Impetigo may be a primary lesion or a complication of any skin condition in which there is a breakdown or irritation of the integumentary system, such as in chickenpox, mosquito bites, pediculosis, or eczema.

Nursing Management Impetigo responds well to meticulous hygienic conditions and various therapeutic regimens described in the literature. A recent study by Ruby and Nelson[2] revealed that a daily cleansing bath with castile soap, which involves removing the scab, is just as effective as vigorous hexachlorophene scrubbing of the lesions. Local antibiotic ointment was hardly better than a placebo. However, parenteral or oral antibiotics are recommended if the child has lesions in the nose and/or ears and widespread lesions on extremities. Lubricating ointments will facilitate removal of crusty scabs on the face. Fingernails should be clipped short and scratching prevented.

There is a 3 percent chance of acute glomerulonephritis being a complication when group A beta-hemolytic streptococci are cultured from the impetigo lesions.

Prevention is best effected by daily soap baths and protecting the child from insect bites by means of window screens and insect repellents. Personal items such as towels and washcloths should not be interchanged with family members; hands and face should always be washed before eating. Proper nutrition is also of utmost importance.

Insect Bites

Insects and their allies produce disease in three ways:

1 The venenating arthropods—centipedes, scorpions, spiders, ticks, mites, bees, wasps, ants, and blister beetles project poisonous venoms into the human body.
2 The tissue invaders—the itch mite produces scabies; maggots (larval stage) of many flies cause myiasis.
3 Mechanical transmitting agents of disease—common housefly is often responsible for the transmission of typhoid and cholera; lice, fleas, red mites, ticks, sand flies, black gnats, and assassin bugs are all responsible for transmitting other diseases.

Assessment The skin reaction to the bite of an insect results from hypersensitivity. A nonsensitized person will have little or no reaction, but a sensitized person may have an immediate, delayed, or combined reaction, evidenced by headache, fever, weakness, involuntary muscle spasms, and sometimes even convulsions.

Scorpion stings and black widow spider bites are the most serious insect bites. Death from scorpion stings usually occurs in young children (under 4 years of age). Symptoms of scorpion sting are convulsions with an ascending motor paralysis, rapid weak pulse, extreme thirst, and anuria. If shock ensues, emergency treatment with steroids and parenteral solutions including blood plasma is indicated.

Nursing Management Ticks or the honeybee's stinger must be removed from the body for rapid, complete recovery. When the hypersensitive person goes into shock from an insect bite, epinephrine must be used immediately. Ammonia will partly neutralize the fluid from a blister beetle, and a corticosteroid ointment should be used to reduce pain from insect bites. In the case of the black widow spider bite, an intramuscular injection of antiserum is given. Pain can be reduced by an intravenous injection of a 10 percent solution of calcium gluconate. Since no method of treatment is satisfactory for the person allergic to bites from mosquitoes, lice, assassin bugs, and fleas, the hypersensitive person must learn to protect himself from these insects.

A child who has a history of hypersensitivity to insect bites should undertake a program of desensitization, usually initiated with a very dilute solution of allergens normally consisting of bee, wasp, hornet, and yellow jacket extracts. A survival kit containing epinephrine, a tourniquet, ephedrine, and an antihistamine should also be immediately available to the extremely hypersensitive person. As a preventive measure to eliminate the disease carriers, dusting a person's clothing with DDT, using insect repellents, and destroying the hosts at their breeding site are most helpful.

Poison Ivy

Poison ivy is an allergic cutaneous contact dermatitis. It occurs as a delayed or cell-mediated response to direct contact with a substance to which the skin has become sensitized. In poison ivy the substance is pentadecacatechol, a simple compound found in plant sap. Children usually come in direct contact with the plant while playing, but highly sensitized persons may react to indirect contact with a pet carrying the allergen on its coat or to airborne ash from burning vegetation. Poison ivy is most common in school-age children in the spring and summer months. The eruption is self-limiting and clears in 2 to 4 weeks, although secondary bacterial infection of the lesions is a common complication.

Assessment Depending on the child's level of sensitivity, the vesicular lesions may appear at any time, from a few hours to a few days following exposure. The lesions are seen most often on exposed parts of the body in linear tracks which coincide with scratch marks of the plant stem or brush marks of the leaves. It may also appear in areas in which the allergen has been spread by contaminated fingers, such as the face and genitalia. It does not spread by means of contaminated vesicle fluid. The skin response varies as to the extent of lesions and appears to depend on the individual's level of sensitivity. The vesicles rupture, crust, and normally heal without scarring.

Nursing Management Pruritus is the common and constant complaint of children with poison ivy. Lotions containing calamine provide not only an antipruritic action but also lubrication, cooling, and drying, which are extremely beneficial. In more extensive cases in which control of infection is also important, wet dressing of potassium permangnate, topical steroids, and antihistamines may be used. Oral steroids are reserved for very severe reactions with extensive involvement. The areas of involvement should be kept clean, dry, and well aerated, and the vesicles should be allowed to rupture spontaneously. Clothes should be lightweight and soft to decrease the irritation. Dressings are generally not needed, but if used, they should be loose and lightweight. Applications of lotion should be done with a patting motion rather than a rubbing motion. The child's hands should be washed frequently to prevent infecting the lesions, and he should be warned against scratching.

Parents should know that the more exposure to poison ivy the child has had, the more rapid and violent the reaction will be. Therefore, they should attempt to find and destroy plants in the immediate area and teach the child to recognize and avoid the plant. When exposure occurs, the child should learn to wash immediately with soap and water those areas touched and possibly prevent the reaction if the antigen is washed off rapidly enough. Partial desensitization to pentadecacatechol is available, but it is not generally recommended except for highly sensitized children. The procedure takes at least 6 months and produces only a milder reaction to the plant.

Drug Eruptions

Adverse reactions to drugs are most often seen in the skin. They resemble other cutaneous diseases and are present in varying degrees of severity. The exact mechanism of drug reactions is not known, but a variety of factors may influence or precipitate the development of a reaction to a drug. Normally children show fewer drug eruptions than do adults. Age may be a factor in that adults have had greater exposure to drugs and an increased chance of developing allergies to them. Children with serious diseases are more likely to have reactions. There is a high correlation between the number of drugs a person receives and the development of a reaction. In some cases the adverse interaction of the drugs may be responsible. Toxic effects sometimes develop from an abnormal accumulation of the drug in the body. Some children metabolize drugs more slowly than normal because of inherited biochemical deviations. Illnesses affecting the renal filtration rate may also decrease the normal urinary excretion time. Sunlight combined with certain orally administered drugs may produce an inflammatory reaction on exposed skin surfaces. These drugs are said to produce photosensitivity in the child. Almost any drug, prescribed or proprietary, may produce a reaction when the circumstances in the child are conducive. The reaction itself depends on the particular drug and the child's individualized response. Some drugs are known to produce certain recognizable reactions, but a wide variability in the severity exhibited by the child remains. One child may respond to a specific drug with a single lesion, while another child may develop a life-threatening generalized epidermal necrosis. Drug reactions frequently involve other systems and organs in the body in addition to the skin. The prognosis depends on the identification and eradication of the causative agent, the extent of involvement, and the adequacy of treatment.

Assessment Among the most commonly seen drug eruptions is urticaria, which is thought to be produced by the release of histamine in an allergic reaction. Urticaria, or wheals, begin with pruritus or numbness of a particular area which becomes erythematous and edematous and develops lesions with sharply demarcated elevated edges. If the lesions involve the lips, mucosa, or eyelids, there may be diffuse swelling rather than a recognizable lesion. The distribution of wheals varies. Some disappear in minutes, and others last for hours. Urticarial reactions are produced by antibiotics; salicylates; barbiturates; iodine-containing radiopaque media;

vaccines like poliomyelitis, rabies, and tetanus-diphtheria toxoids; and drugs such as chloral hydrate, insulin, atabrine, and antepar.

Another common reaction is a maculopapular eruption, which again exhibits wide variation in distribution. Among the medications that produce the maculopapular rash are barbiturates, salicylates, measles vaccine, chloral hydrate, insulin, and para-aminosalicylic acid (PAS). A fixed drug eruption is a third type of reaction. It is thought to be a delayed reaction and appears in the same location each time the causative agent is introduced. The single lesion appears as a purplish red, round, or oval plaque with sharp borders and is pruritic. It is most often located on an extremity but may be seen anywhere on the cutaneous surface. Barbiturates, salicylates, tetracyclines, sulfonamides, and phenacetin are all known to cause fixed eruptions. Drugs that cause photosensitivity include povan, griseofulvin, methotrexate, and tetracycline.

Nursing Management The most satisfactory treatment for a cutaneous drug response is administration of antihistamines. In mild reactions antihistamines are given by mouth until the lesions have disappeared and for several weeks thereafter. Urticaria, one of the symptoms of anaphylactic shock, will respond to subcutaneous injections of epinephrine, as will the other symptoms. Epinephrine and antihistamines are effective because they are antagonists of the histamine which is released in allergic responses. Since histamine is also thought to be associated with the pruritus, antihistamines are also beneficial in relieving the burning and itching. Steroids are sometimes used with severe or widespread lesions or to speed the clearing process in less severe cases. Identifying the cause of the eruption is extremely important. The offending drug should be discontinued as soon as possible, and in some cases, another drug may be substituted for it. Withdrawal of the offending drug usually results in noticeable improvement in a short time. Following a drug reaction, even a small dose of the same medication will cause a recurrence. Parents should be informed of the drug or group of drugs responsible for the reaction and of the potential risk of giving the drug again.

INTEGUMENTARY DISEASES IN THE ADOLESCENT
Acne Vulgaris

Acne vulgaris, a chronic inflammatory disease of the sebaceous glands and hair follicles of the skin, afflicts 80 to 90 percent of all adolescents in varying degrees of severity. It often develops during puberty and frequently lasts throughout adolescence. Comedones, papules, and pustules are the characteristic lesions. Cysts and nodules may develop, and scarring is common. Regardless of the extent of the condition, it produces disfigurement, if only temporary, and anxiety. Even mild or inconspicuous lesions may be perceived by the adolescent as highly noticeable, causing him great worry and embarrassment. The type of lesions and their distribution, extent, and site of involvement vary. The basic cause of acne is still unknown; however, considerable knowledge of its pathogenesis does exist.

Acne begins with hormonal changes at puberty. The sebaceous follicles enlarge, secrete increased amounts of sebum, and become plugged, producing the characteristic lesion of acne, the *comedo*. In an open comedo, which appears as a blackhead, the orifice is dilated. The dark color probably comes from oxidation of the sebum as it reaches the skin surface. In a closed comedo, which appears as a whitehead, there is no visible opening on the skin. Closed comedones are responsible for the inflammatory changes and lesions of acne. Sebum and perhaps other substances continue to accumulate within the closed follicle until the walls finally rupture. With the rupture, fatty acids, irritating components of sebum, are released into the surrounding dermis, producing an inflammatory reaction. When the rupture is near the surface, a superficial pustule appears. These eruptions generally last only a short time and heal without permanent damage or scarring. If the rupture occurs deep in the dermis, a papule forms which heals more slowly and is more likely to develop into cystic or abscess-like lesions. Destruction of the follicle and scar formation may be the end result.

Some adolescents with acne have pustules and little or no scarring. Others have papules, cysts, and a particular scar formation. Scars may be depressed or elevated. Diet, emotions, cosmetics, drugs, bacteria, cleansing practices, skin type, and trauma from manipulation may affect a person's particular response. Acne usually subsides by 20 years of age but may continue longer. Even though the inflammatory process ceases, the person may be left with permanent emotional and physical scars.

Assessment   During the course of acne, assessment of the adolescent's emotional state is as important as assessment of the lesions. His feelings about himself as a person, his peer relationships, his appearance, and his attitude toward the treatment regimen should all be established. Distribution and extent of the lesions and the depth of tissue involvement should be assessed. The face, neck, chest, back, and arms should all be examined for possible involvement. Scarring should also be noted. If treatment has been in progress for some time, the effects of various medications should be evaluated.

Nursing Management   The long-range objective of therapy is to prevent permanent scarring and promote a healthy self-image in the patient. The adolescent must understand that although acne is a long-term condition, he does have some control over it. Periods of remission and exacerbation occur. A good understanding of the progression of the lesions and of the rationale of the various treatments recommended is essential. Since improvement sometimes takes up to 6 weeks, he should not be discouraged if improvement is not immediate. The adolescent should help plan his own skin care and should be encouraged to evaluate the results and assist in planning a new regimen if needed. Development of the total plan may require several visits with the doctor. Topics such as cleansing procedures and medications may be discussed in the initial visit, with diet and care of hair and scalp the subjects of subsequent visits. Instructions should be written down so that the patient may refer to them.

Preventing formation of comedones is one of the first objectives of therapy. Various soaps and topical lotions or ointments are recommended for their drying and peeling effects. As the skin dries and peels, the follicular orifices are opened and the sebum is allowed to flow freely. Topical preparations containing sulfur, resorcin, salicylic acid, and benzoyl peroxide are often used.

Adolescents should be cautioned that scrubbing or rubbing the skin too hard may damage it. An oil-base lotion may be prescribed if severe chapping occurs. Generally, however, adolescents are instructed not to use other creams or lotions on the face because the oil, grease, or wax contained in these applications plugs the follicles. Dry face powder, rouge, and eye makeup may be substituted. Oily or greasy suntan preparations should not be used on affected areas while sunbathing. Greasy hair preparations should be avoided. Seborrhea is often present as a result of marked oiliness of the scalp. To remove the excess oil, the scalp may need to be washed two to three times per week. Soapless shampoos are preferred over oily or superfatted ones. Many commercially available shampoos contain antiseborrheic agents. In severe cases, topical lotions or steroids may be used in addition to special shampoos.

Vitamin A acid is applied once daily for its drying and peeling effects. It not only prevents comedo formation but also seems to eliminate existing comedones. Tetracycline is the antibiotic most frequently used in the treatment of acne. It decreases the population of *Corynebacterium* on the skin and reduces the concentration of free fatty acids in the sebum. The dosage is regulated according to need. Monilial vaginitis is an occasional complication. Adolescents must be cautioned that the use of both tetracycline and vitamin A produce temporary sensitivity to sunlight.

In females over 16 years of age, anovulatory drugs may be used to decrease the amount of sebum production. The dosage required to suppress sebum production would cause feminizing effects if used in males and could inhibit bone growth in patients under 16 years of age.

Acne surgery or mechanical expression of comedones, pustules, and cysts is used by some dermatologists. The surface of the lesions is cut with a sharp needle and the contents are expressed with a comedo extractor. Any squeezing of the lesions by the patient should be discouraged because it often causes rupture of the follicle and inflammation and scarring. Elimination of certain foods from the diet, particularly chocolate, nuts, milk products, sweets, fats, and spicy foods, is sometimes recommended, but most of the diet restrictions have now been refuted. However, individual adverse responses may still occur. A more realistic approach is to encourage the adolescent to eat a balanced diet and to try to identify and eliminate from the diet specific foods that lead to the development of new lesions.

In patients not using tetracycline or vitamin A, sunshine is beneficial. Acne frequently clears during the summer months and flares up in the fall. Therapy with ultraviolet light produces a peeling effect and may be prescribed two to three times a week.

Adolescents need support to cope with acne. They must be encouraged to find activities in which they can excel and those which will increase their self-confidence and self-esteem. Expressing frustrations and feelings to an understanding person, such as a nurse, is also beneficial, particularly when contact can be maintained over a period of years. The scars left on the face and other areas generally show some improvement in a few years. If they are severe or create psychologic problems, several types of cosmetic treatments are available. Although they help to some extent, they cannot always provide the degree of attractiveness desired by the patient.

Additional disorders of the integumentary system seen in children are presented in Table 41-5 at the end of this chapter (p. 859).

THERMAL INJURIES IN CHILDREN

Burn injuries, the most severe form of trauma to the integumentary system, affect children of all ages. Burn injuries rank second only to automobile accidents as a chief cause of death due to accidents among children from birth to age 15.

The causes and incidence of burn injuries in the pediatric population are as follows:

1. Scald burns account for 40 to 50 percent of burns.
2. Flame burns account for 20 to 30 percent of burns.
3. Chemical and electrical burns account for the remaining injuries.

Burns and the Abused Child

In a recent study, Stone et al.[3] show that almost 10 percent of the children admitted to the Children's Division of Cook County Hospital for verified child abuse had been abused by burning. Yet child abuse by burning often goes unrecognized because physicians and nurses are not aware or do not observe for clues which would lead to such a diagnosis (see Chap. 16).

Pathophysiology of the Burn Injury

The magnitude of the burn injury on the integumentary system of the body can be appraised by measuring the extent and depth of the injury. The extent of the burn injury is usually expressed as a percentage of *total body surface area* (TBSA) burned. A rapid method for estimating the percentage of body surface area burns devised by Pulaski and Tennison is known as the "rule of nine."[4] Although widely used, it is not an adequate clinical method for calculating the percentage of burn in children. For example, the area of the head and neck makes up a relatively larger portion of the total skin area of infants (21 percent) as compared with adults (9 percent). The Lund and Browder method (Fig. 41-2) allows for the changes in percentage of body surface of various parts that occur during different stages of development from infancy through childhood.[5] It is a much more accurate clinical tool, especially in children, and should be used to calculate extent of injury, since most fluid resuscitation formulas are based on this accurate estimation.

The depth of a burn injury is traditionally classified as first, second, or third degree. Other classifica-

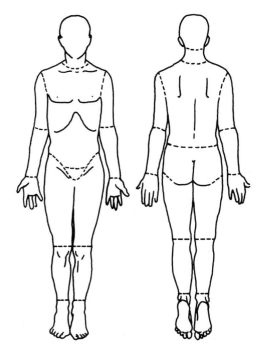

AREA	1 Yr.	1-4 Yrs.	5-9 Yrs.	10-14 Yrs.	15 Yrs.	Adult	2°	3°
Head	19	17	13	11	9	7		
Neck	2	2	2	2	2	2		
Ant. Trunk	13	13	13	13	13	13		
Post. Trunk	13	13	13	13	13	13		
R. Buttock	2½	2½	2½	2½	2½	2½		
L. Buttock	2½	2½	2½	2½	2½	2½		
Genitalia	1	1	1	1	1	1		
R.U. Arm	4	4	4	4	4	4		
L.U. Arm	4	4	4	4	4	4		
R.L. Arm	3	3	3	3	3	3		
L.L. Arm	3	3	3	3	3	3		
R. Hand	2½	2½	2½	2½	2½	2½		
L. Hand	2½	2½	2½	2½	2½	2½		
R. Thigh	5½	6½	8	8½	9	9½		
L. Thigh	5½	6½	8	8½	9	9½		
R. Leg	5	5	5½	6	6½	7		
L. Leg	5	5	5½	6	6½	7		
R. Foot	3½	3½	3½	3½	3½	3½		
L. Foot	3½	3½	3½	3½	3½	3½		
TOTAL								

Figure 41-2 Lund and Browder method of calculating burn size. *(Reproduced with permission from C. P. Artz and J. A. Moncrief, The Treatment of Burns, 2d ed., W. B. Saunders Company, Philadelphia, 1969.)*

tion systems are presented in Table 41-1. The actual depth of a burn injury is very difficult to assess, but the appearance of the wound, how the injury occurred, the skin thickness over different parts of the body, and the variation in skin thickness in various age groups must be taken into account. Table 41-2 describes the different depths of injury and the characteristics of each.

The burn wound is actually three-dimensional.[6] The first two dimensions, extent and depth of injury, have been discussed. The third dimension, volume, is very difficult to measure. Volume refers to the amount of fluids sequestered in the interstitial space and is related to the depth and extent of injury.

Edema fluid is a result of the initial cellular response to the burn injury because the development of an abnormal capillary permeability allows protein-rich fluid to escape into the tissue spaces. Water and electrolyte shifts are affected by both the increased capillary hydrostatic pressure and indirectly through the protein shift. The depth of injury affects the volume as well as the composition of fluid lost from circulation. In a first-degree burn, which only damages the avascular epidermis, vasodilatation is the only major change and results in insignificant protein losses with little or no edema formation. Second- and third-degree burns are characterized by variable amounts of damage to the capillaries and thus account for the variability in the large amounts of fluid sequestered in and around the burn wound. Correlating the amount of fluid lost with the visible formation of edema is extremely difficult since large

Table 41-1 CLASSIFICATION OF BURN DEPTH

Traditional terminology	Anatomic terminology	Depth of involvement	Depth of anatomic involvement
1st degree	Epidermal	Partial thickness	Stratum corneum of the epidermis
2d degree	Intradermal Superficial Deep dermal	Partial thickness	Dermis to a variable extent
3d degree	Subdermal	Full thickness	Subcutaneous adipose tissue, fascia, muscles, and bones

Table 41-2 CHARACTERISTICS OF DEPTH OF INJURY

Depth of injury	Appearance	Pain sensitivity	Edema formation	Healing time	Scarring	Cause
1st degree	Pink to red	Painful	Very slight	3–5 days	None	Sunburn, flash, explosives
2d degree	Red to pale ivory and moist; may have vesicles and bullae	Extremely painful	Very edematous	21–28 days	Variable	Flash, scalds, flame, brief contact with hot objects
3d degree	White, cherry red, or black; may contain bullae and thrombosed veins; dry and leathery	Painless to touch	Marked edema may require escharotomies	Requires grafting	Yes	Flame, high intensity flash, electrical, chemical, hot object, scalds in infants and elderly

quantities of fluid may accumulate in deeply located tissues and give no visible evidence of swelling. The rate and quantity of fluid loss in the burn patient occurs much more rapidly than has been previously described.[7]

Damage to the integumentary system caused by the burn injury destroys the evaporative water barrier, thus increasing the insensible water loss from 4 to 15 times normal. Evaporative water losses are especially high in children since the ratio of body surface area to body weight is greatly increased. Very strict attention must be paid to fluid losses in the infant and young child. Physiologic immaturity of renal-cardiovascular systems, prevents adequate response to hypervolemia or hypovolemia.

The burn injury also decreases the efficiency of the temperature control mechanism of the body. Recent studies seem to implicate the tremendous caloric requirement associated in part with increased evaporative water losses. For each milliliter of water vaporized, 0.576 kcal of heat must be produced by the body in order to maintain thermal equilibrium. Since evaporative losses in major burns vary between 2.5 and 4.0 liters per day, 1444 to 2300 kcal should be required to prevent a fall in body temperature.[8] In the infant and young child hypothermia frequently occurs as a result of the increased caloric requirements, the labile heat regulatory system, and the increased ratio of body surface area to body weight.

The destruction of skin by burning causes loss of the first line of defense against infection and produces an excellent culture medium for bacteria. Since the skin is so thin and has such shallow dermal appendages in children, conversion of deep dermal burns to full-thickness burns may rapidly result from bacterial, fungal, or viral invasions.

Local Treatment of Burn Wounds

Burn wound sepsis has long been a major problem of the burn patient. Teplitz[9] originally described *burn wound sepsis* as a rapid proliferation of bacteria in the burn wound and an active invasion of the adjacent unburned tissue. Streptococcal and staphylococcal sepsis have been brought under control with antibiotics only to have a new problem emerge, that of gram-negative bacteria (*Pseudomonas, Aerobacter, Klebsiella, Escherichia coli*, etc.). More recently, burn infections have been traced to such so-called nonpathogens as *Serratia, Providencia stuartii*, fungi such as *Candida* and *Mucor*, and even viruses. Numerous attempts have been made to control burn wound sepsis with multiple broad-spectrum systemic antibiotics, but they have usually failed. The morphologic studies of Order demonstrate the avascular destructive nature of the burn wound with immediate occlusion of arterial blood supply to the burned area in all but the most superficial types of burn injury. In full-thickness skin destruction, vascular occlusion is permanent until replaced by the neurovasculature of granulation tissue in about 21 days. In partial-thickness wounds the patency of the vascular tree is reestablished after several hours, but supervening infection may also cause these wounds to convert to full-thickness wounds with the resultant destruction of the vasculature. Lack of an effective blood supply to the burned area explains the failure of systemic antibiotics to control burn wound infection.

Of the many topical agents investigated today, the following have gained the most widespread use: silver nitrate 0.5 percent, Sulfamylon, gentamicin cream, and silver sulfadiazine. Silver nitrate therapy is used in a 0.5 percent solution as a continuous wet soak in combination with large bulky dressings.[10] The dressings are changed at least once a day and the wounds are debrided with each dressing change. The mode of action of silver nitrate is not specifically known, but it is probably dependent upon free silver ions, and is effective in relatively low concentrations. The major advantages and disadvantages are outlined in Table 41-3.

Sulfamylon, the "burn butter," is another topical agent for controlling the population of microbial opportunists in thermally injured tissues.[11] It is applied as an even coating approximately ⅛ inch in thickness to all partial and full-thickness burn wounds following initial debridement, provided that hemodynamics stabilization has been achieved and the patient is not acidotic. The advantages and disadvantages of Sulfamylon are presented in Table 41-4.

Recent studies of the acid-base effects of Sulfamylon have confirmed the reduction of buffering capacities of the blood in association with increased bicarbonate excretion by the kidney and conversion of bicarbonate to carbon dioxide excreted during hyperventilation. These acid-base changes result from the carbonic anhydrase inhibition caused by the absorption of mafenide acetate (Sulfamylon) and its breakdown products. Carbonic anhydrase inhibitors, among other effects, decrease reabsorption of bicarbonate by the kidney, lowering the serum bicarbonate and producing a mild metabolic acido-

sis. If present in sufficient quantities, these agents may inhibit red blood cell carbonic anhydrase, leading to impaired carbon dioxide transport at the tissue and lung level. Thus, the buffering capacity of the blood is reduced so that the addition of even a small acid load may result in a profound acidosis. The most frequent cause of acidosis in these patients is either pulmonary complication, preventing the excretion of carbon dioxide through the lungs, or renal failure, preventing the excretion of Sulfamylon and its metabolites as well as the retention of other acid metabolites. Thus Sulfamylon reduces the buffering capacity of blood and predisposes the patient to acid-base derangements.

Another topical agent, gentamicin cream, has gained early recognition because of its specific effect against *Pseudomonas*.[12] This agent is easy to apply and has few known side effects. The major disadvantage has been the rapid development of resistant strains of *Pseudomonas*. Gentamicin may be used in selected cases in which other topical agents have failed to prevent the colonization of the wound with *Pseudomonas* strains which are not resistant to gentamicin.

The newest topical agent is 1% silver sulfadiazine, which is spread over the wound in much the same manner as Sulfamylon. The treatment may be open as with Sulfamylon or semiclosed or closed as with silver nitrate. Some physicians prefer the semiclosed method, employing one or two layers of fine mesh and light dressings to hold the mesh in place. These dressings may be changed once or twice a day. The advantages of silver sulfadiazine are that it (1) is applied easily, (2) is soothing when applied, (3) softens the eschar, allowing less painful debride-

Table 41-3 ADVANTAGES AND DISADVANTAGES OF SILVER NITRATE (0.5%) THERAPY

Advantages	Disadvantages
1 Effective against most organisms which colonize the burn wound	1 Limited penetration of deeper tissues; eschar must be removed if this drug is to affect deep tissue colonization
2 Does not appear to delay or retard epithelialization	2 Hypotonicity of solution results in marked loss of electrolytes
3 Absorbed in small amounts; excreted by the kidneys and liver	3 Restricts joint mobility because of the requirement of large bulky dressings
4 Essentially nonallergenic	4 May produce methemoglobinemia in patients with *Aerobacter* infections (organism's ability to change nitrate to nitrites causes this complication)
5 Relatively inexpensive	
6 Reduces insensible water losses through the use of constant wet dressings	5 Stains normal skin so that perspective donor sites require additional preparation prior to grafting
7 Useful during the grafting phase, since treatment of undebrided areas may be combined with grafting of adjacent granulating areas	6 Produces multiple housekeeping problems related to the removal of the black stains created by $AgNO_3$

Table 41-4 ADVANTAGES AND DISADVANTAGES OF SULFAMYLON (MAFENIDE ACETATE) THERAPY

Advantages	Disadvantages
1 Effective against a wide range of gram-negative and gram-positive organisms	1 Painful on application, especially to partial-thickness burns; duration of pain, 20–30 minutes
2 Freely disfusable into the eschar, providing effective drug levels at the viable-nonviable interface	2 Associated with hypersensitivity in 5–7% of all patients (resulting in a maculopapular rash reaction which in most cases responds to the administration of antihistamines)

3 Permits open treatment of wounds
  a Allows for frequent careful examination of the burn wound
  b Facilitates treatment of associated injuries
  c Allows intensive physical therapy, thus improving joint mobility
	3 May be responsible for delayed eschar separation due to control of bacterial proliferation

4 Easy to use, does not present housekeeping problems, well accepted by patients and staff	4 Associated with acid-base derangements
5 Does not produce nephrotoxicity associated with other sulfa preparations	5 May be associated with the emergence of newer opportunistic infections

ment and increased joint mobility, and (4) is absorbed more slowly, decreasing the chance of renal toxicity. This drug has proved effective against a wide spectrum of gram-negative and gram-positive organisms as well as *Candida*. Although studies have failed to demonstrate the development of resistant strains, the selection of nonsensitive strains of *Pseudomonas* as well as other organisms has been observed. As with other sulfa drugs, a hypersensitive reaction occurs in approximately 5 percent of patients treated with silver sulfadiazine. This drug appears to have more of the characteristics sought in the ideal topical agent than others which have been developed to date. Because of the limitations of the bacterial spectrum of each of the topical agents and the possibility of the developing resistant organisms, the extensive use of any one agent should be avoided and careful attention should be paid to rotation of topical therapy among patients.

Another method of controlling bacterial invasion of adjacent tissue is the administration of subeschar antibiotics, employed when topical agents are contraindicated or have failed to prevent colonization of the wound with organisms at 10^5 organisms per gram of tissue or greater. This technique is based on the use of burn wound biopsy cultures and selection of antibiotics specific for the organisms colonizing the deep tissue of the burn wound. The daily dose of the specific antibiotic is prepared in an isotonic saline solution or half-strength saline solution in sufficient quantities to cover each area of 37.5 sq cm with 25 ml of solution. This technique has been most successful in controlling burn wound sepsis, since by a needle clysis a specific antibiotic is delivered to the viable-nonviable tissue interface. This therapy is used routinely as an adjunct to topical therapy to treat those infections which escape the control of topical agents.[13]

Definitive Closure of the Wound

A discussion of wound care would not be complete without a discussion of debridement and closure of the wound—which is the overall long-term objective of burn therapy. Cleansing and debridement of the wound may be accomplished after initial fluid resuscitation and airway maintenance has been initiated. Debridement begins with the initial cleansing of the wound with a dilute iodine base solution and removal of all loose epidermis. It is carried out daily until all eschar is removed and the wound is healed by primary wound healing (as with first- and second-degree wounds) or secondary closure (as in grafting of third-degree or full-thickness wounds). Dead or dying tissue must either be removed or slough spontaneously before open wounds can heal. Early excision of small (less than 15 percent) full-thickness burns is ideal in that it shortens the course of the illness by early grafting, preventing wound infection and reducing the complications resulting from scarring in areas of full-thickness injuries. Contraindication to excisional procedures are (1) inadequate resuscitation, (2) burn wound to the face and neck, (3) presence of infection, (4) unavailability of autografts or heterografts for wound closure, (5) extremes of age, (6) debilitating diseases, (7) unavailability of blood, and (8) unavailability of supporting facilities and competent personnel. With the advent of improved infection control, the increased availability of homograft and heterograft, improved tissue typing techniques, and breakthroughs in transplant immunology, early staged excision is being attempted in the massive burns (greater than 80 percent) with some success.

Tangential excision is a surgical technique of removing the burned eschar of deep dermal and subdermal burns with a small free hand knife or dermatome without anesthesia, since it is a relatively painless procedure. Thus, thin layers of eschar are repeatedly shaved away until a viable plane is reached and bleeding begins. Ideally these wounds are then covered with homograft or heterograft and are protected from infection until autografting can be accomplished. This procedure must be performed early in the burn course, preferably in the first 5 days before significant wound colonization occurs. Its advantages include early removal of the eschar without the large quantity of blood loss and the postanesthetic complications of excisional therapy. With obvious partial thickness wounds or heavily colonized wounds tangential excision should not be performed.[14]

The use of topically applied proteolytic enzymes has become popular in the past decade. Theoretically these enzymes destroy the devitalized tissue but do not affect the viable tissue. The agents are in the early developmental stages and have yet to prove the panacea of debridement. Moderate depth wounds may be converted to deeper wounds when these agents are used, because vascular planes of the underlying tissue are open and exposed to bacterial contamination.

Advances in grafting techniques have also improved the overall mortality and morbidity of the burn patient. The *postage stamp* graft consists of small postage stamp–sized pieces of split thickness skin placed on granulation tissue, allowing small intervening areas of granulation tissue to heal in from the sides between grafts. With the *Tanner mesh graft* a strip of split thickness skin is run through a special cutting machine. Multiple parallel rows of staggered small slits are cut in the skin, allowing it to expand and thus cover as much as nine times the area of the original donor skin. This technique and other advances have made it possible to cover burn areas of more than 50 percent in a relatively small amount of time, thus decreasing the morbidity and mortality.

Heterografts (animal skin) and homografts (human skin) have also decreased the overall morbidity and mortality of burns during the past two decades.[15] The use of heterografts as a biologic dressing to protect the burn wound has increased as commercial production of both fresh and lyophilized

heterograft (porcine skin) has become available. Homografts are generally preferred over heterografts, but the supply cannot meet the demand. Newer techniques of tissue typing have made the use of matched homografts for long-term "take" a possibility, but until techniques for freezing and thawing skin to retain its viability are better understood, the supply of matched homografts will be virtually nonexistent. Both homografts and heterografts are used in many ways to aid the recovery of the burn patient:

1 Immediate coverage of superficial second-degree wounds (hastens healing)
2 Debridement of "untidy" wounds as eschar separation nears completion
3 Promotion of healing of deep second-degree burns
4 Temporary, immediate coverage following excision
5 Coverage of granulation tissue between "crops" of autografts in the larger burn
6 "Test" material prior to autografting (adherence of homograft predicts success of autograft)
7 Coverage of other surgical wounds prior to secondary closure

Homografts and heterografts have several advantages. The primary one is the restoration of the water vapor barrier function of the epidermis and the virtual elimination of protein loss from the burn wound. This restoration of the water vapor barrier decreases the energy demands on the body, thus decreasing the massive caloric expenditures associated with large open wounds. Other major advantages include relief of pain, thus increasing joint mobility; reduction in the bacterial count of the burn wound as the grafts become adherent to the wound; and protection of exposed burns, tendons, vessels, and nerves from desiccation until a more definitive coverage can be obtained.

Response of the Cardiovascular System

In the immediate postburn period violent and dramatic changes in the dynamics of the whole circulation result in what is known clinically as burn shock. Initially a precipitous drop in the cardiac output (about 50 percent of resting normal values) precedes any measurable change in blood or plasma volume.[16] As plasma and blood volume begin to decrease rapidly, cardiac output drops even further. The striking decrease in cardiac output unexplained by any change in blood volume suggests a direct myocardial effect of thermal trauma. Although slower in onset than the decrease in cardiac output, the blood volume deficit after thermal injury can be profound and is roughly proportional to the extent and depth of the burn. In burns of greater than 30 percent total body surface area, increased vascular permeability exists throughout the vascular tree, although it is more pronounced in the burned area. Free loss of plasma protein, including fibrinogen, into the extravascular, extracellular space results in a concentration of protein in this area as high as 3 Gm/100 ml and probably acts later to perpetuate the holding of large volumes of fluid in the extravascular space. The destruction of the capillary as a semipermeable membrane negates the maintenance of plasma volume during this period by colloid oncotic pressure since there is free permeability of the membrane.

The immediate red blood cell hemolysis does not exceed 10 percent; thus, the decrease in blood volume is primarily due to the loss of plasma volume. Measurements of the total functional extracellular fluid (ECF) volume indicates that the ECF volume deficit is considerably greater than even the plasma volume deficit. The greatest loss in both plasma and ECF volume takes place within the first 12 hours after burn and continues at a much slower rate for only an additional 6 to 12 hours. This sequestering of fluids in the extracellular space may be accounted for in part by the avid uptake of water and sodium by injured tissue.

Replacement of fluids sequestered in the burn wound is the most important goal of the initial therapy of thermal injury. An optimal physiologic response is dependent upon the rate of fluid losses, the total quantity of fluid sequestered, the composition of edema fluid, and the ability of various solutions to restore fluid volume or to effect a complete and rapid cardiovascular response. Most resuscitation formulas have attempted to correct the plasma volume deficit, and their success was based on one criterion, survival of the immediate postburn period. This assumption has led to erroneous conclusions since it can be readily demonstrated that burn individuals can survive the immediate postburn period with a cardiac output of less than 25 percent normal basal values and an associated plasma or blood volume deficit of 30 to 50 percent.[17] The ideal solution for resuscitation is a balanced salt solution.[18] Lactate Ringer's solution is the solution of choice (the ratio of lactate as bicarbonate to chloride is 27 to 103) because it most closely approximates the composition of extracellular fluid; has a physiologic pH of 7.4 (in vitro pH is 5.5); and the lactic acid acidosis of untreated burn shock disappears rapidly (12 to 18 hours after burn) despite the large quantities of exogenous lactate administered. No free water is required with the use of lactated Ringer's solution since the sodium concentration is 130 mEq/liter and as such furnishes 80 to 100 ml free water per

liter. The total quantity of lactated Ringer's solution to be administered is based on the following formula: 4 ml Ringer's lactate per kilogram body weight per percentage of burned area (Fig. 41-3). This formula differs from the more conventional formulas in the rate of administration, the time interval that colloid is administered, and the calculation of volume on the total percentage of body surface burn, not on a maximum of 50 percent of the body surface area as other formulas recommend. The total quantity of fluid is given during the first 24 hours, with one-half the amount given in the first 8 hours to coincide with the time of the losses of fluids from both the plasma and extracellular fluid spaces. Approximately 20 to 30 hours after burn the capillary integrity seems to be reestablished. The administration of colloid at this time in the form of plasma produces a substantial increase in cardiac output and plasma volume and maintains them at these levels without further administration of additional colloid. In the second 24 hours after burn, a decreasing volume of administered fluids is required to maintain volume. Further administration of electrolyte solutions at this time results in edema far in excess of any improvement in circulatory dynamics. Thus, during the second 24 hours, only plasma (amount necessary to return the hematocrit to normal) and water (5 percent dextrose and water) should be administered. Beginning at approximately 24 hours after burn, the increased evaporative water loss through burned skin is clinically apparent. Water must be supplied in an amount sufficient to maintain the serum sodium within a normal range (138 to 142 mEq/liter). A marked variability of insensible water loss from patient to patient ranges from 4 to 15 times normal (normal insensible water loss equals 10 ml/kg body weight/day). The increased daily water requirements vary according to depth and extent of burn as well as age. Second-degree burns have a greater insensible water loss than third-degree burns. Younger children (below the age of 2) require more proportionately since their normal insensible water losses may exceed 100 ml/lb/day. Occlusive dressings or burned surfaces in contact with the bed and not exposed to air and the air velocity are other factors which may influence the amount of insensible water loss. Thus, replacement of daily water requirements must be based on frequent evaluations of serum sodium levels.

Beginning in the second 24 hours, potassium is excreted in large amounts and must be replaced. In children 40 to 100 mEq potassium per day may be required to maintain a normal serum potassium concentration. Although it is important to prevent extracellular potassium depletion, intracellular potassium deficits also exist which are not correctable by extracellular potassium replacement. Therefore, the use of digitalizing drugs is potentially hazardous and should be utilized only under careful electrocardiographic controls.

After 48 hours, mobilization of burn wound edema begins. The body weight begins to decrease and should reach preburn weight in about 10 days, at which time the majority of the burn wound edema should be mobilized. During this period there seems to be an expanded blood volume as evidenced by increased cardiac output, slight tachycardia, declining hemogloblin concentrations, and a notable diuresis; in reality a progressive profound anemia exists. The continued loss of red blood cells results from microangiopathic anemia which generally parallels the severity and extent of the burn.[19] Thus, fluid therapy after 48 hours should include water and electrolytes to maintain serum sodium and potassium within normal limits and packed red blood cells to maintain a normal hemogloblin concentration.

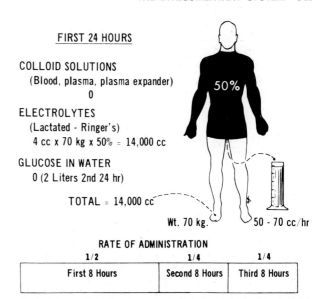

Figure 41-3 Parkland resuscitation formula for the first 24 hours after injury. *(Reproduced with permission from Charles R. Baxter, "Response to Initial Fluid and Electrolyte Therapy of Burn Shock," in J. B. Lynch and S. R. Lewis (eds.), Symposium on the Treatment of Burns, vol. 5, p. 43, The C. V. Mosby Company, St. Louis, 1973.)*

Pulmonary Response to Burn Injury

Pulmonary complications persist as a major cause of morbidity and mortality in the burn patient.[20] The early (first week) complications include carbon monoxide poisoning, inhalation injury resulting in pulmonary edema, and extrinsic obstruction due to edema of the face, neck, and upper airway as well as atelectasis resulting from restriction of the chest wall by the burn eschar, and pneumonia. Late pulmonary complications include pneumonia, pulmonary edema, and atelectasis. During the early postburn period upper airway problems often present as edema and obstruction of the upper airway or bronchospasms due to chemical irritation of the upper airways from toxic products of combustion. Direct heat injury to the respiratory tract rarely occurs because of the remarkable ability of the moist air in the respiratory tract to cool entering hot air. Only in unusual accidents, such as in 100 percent oxygen chambers, have there been any cases of actual heat damage to the respiratory tract, and even then, this damage only extends a few centimeters below the glottis. Only live steam, with a heat-carrying capacity 4,000 times that of hot air, can produce direct heat damage to the lower respiratory tract. Early recognition of potential respiratory complications is essential to successful treatment. Careful attention to history (preburn history as well as details of the burn injury), physical findings, and early base-line labora-

tory studies will focus suspicion on the patient predisposed to pulmonary complications. The history of the patient should include any previous respiratory condition such as asthma, bronchitis, chronic lung disease, or cardiac problems. Also of utmost importance in diagnosing pulmonary difficulties is a complete history of the accident, including the burning agent, whether the accident occurred in a closed space, whether the patient had been unconscious or overcome by smoke, or as in cases of chemical burns if the patient aspirated any of the chemical. Any of the following physical findings should alert one to the possibility of respiratory burn: deep facial burns; singed nasal vibrissae; blistering of the mouth; oropharyngeal inflammation; soot in the oropharynx; progressive hoarseness; labored or rapid breathing or hacking cough. Rales and bronchi are not usually present for a number of hours but may occur at any time. Sudden high fever, extreme restlessness, and disorientation are often early signs of hypoxia from respiratory complications. Circumferential eschar of the chest wall or neck; soft tissue injuries; obstructing edema of the lip, tongue, pharynx, or larynx; and fractures of the jaw or maxilla, larynx, or ribs are physical findings with important respiratory complications. Roentgenographic findings are often unchanged initially, but base-line films are important to the later diagnosis of progressive respiratory complications. Laboratory studies initially should include blood gases as well as carboxyhemoglobin level to evaluate pulmonary functions. (Normal values: P_{O_2} = 90 to 100 mm Hg; P_{CO_2} = 40 mm Hg; pH = 7.44; and carboxyhemoglobin below 10 percent.) Evaluating the patient's pulmonary status and noting his physical and laboratory findings can prevent, diagnose, and treat disastrous pulmonary difficulties.[21]

Renal Response to Burn Injury

Burn-induced renal insufficiency during the early postburn period represents a reversible functional response to *hypovolemic shock*, a reduction in kidney performance based on reduced renal perfusion, which is renal ischemia.[22] With the diminished cardiac output, renal blood flow is drastically reduced, resulting in impaired renal function and thus decreasing the effectiveness of the kidney in varying urine volume and concentration in response to homeostatic needs. Because of immature renal function in young children (less than 2 years of age), they are more susceptible to impaired kidney function.

In burns greater than 15 to 20 percent of body surface, reduced urinary output is immediately evident, and the essence of therapy is to establish adequate urine flow promptly. Large amounts of sodium containing intravenous fluids must be administered early to prevent acute renal failure with its resultant high morbidity and mortality. Urine volumes in excess of 10 ml per hour in the infant, 20 ml per hour in the preschool child, 30 ml per hour in older children up to puberty, and 50 ml per hour in adults are essential for the support of renal function. Some authorities recommend the administration of mannitol or ethacrynic acid in an effort to preclude renal failure; but documentation of success with this technique is difficult to assess.[23] Mannitol may be necessary in the very deep burns involving muscle tissue or in electrical burns to assist the kidney in excreting myoglobin, thus preventing additional renal damage by this hemochromogen.

Besides the initial consideration of reduced renal blood flow and resultant renal damage, other renal complications beset the burn patient. Urinary tract infections, whether catheter-induced or systemic, occur frequently. Renal impairment may occur from the toxic products of systemic sepsis, low-flow states associated with sepsis, or drug toxicity. The nurse must always be aware of changes in kidney function and in renal function tests for the early detection of renal complications.

Gastrointestinal Complications

One of the most common gastrointestinal complications associated with burns is acute gastric dilatation and paralytic ileus. These complications occur in the early postburn period and are associated with burn shock. For this reason any child with a burn greater than 30 percent of the total body surface area (TBSA) should have a Levine tube inserted initially and gastric contents removed to prevent vomiting and aspiration. Usually, the Levine tube may be removed in 18 to 24 hours when adequate resuscitation has been accomplished and bowel sounds have returned. In burns greater than 60 to 70 percent TBSA, bowel sounds may not return for 48 to 72 hours. Continued gastric decompression may be required to prevent vomiting and aspiration, which often have disastrous consequences. Acute gastric dilatation and paralytic ileus may occur at any time during the burn course for a number of reasons. Some of the more common causes are sepsis, hypokalemia, and Curling's ulcer. Acute gastric dilatation which appears after the first 3 to 5 days may often be the first sign of invasive sepsis. When gastric dilatation develops, one is obligated to look for other signs of sepsis as well as the focal point of sepsis so that proper therapy can be initiated. Oral or intravenous potassium salts will quickly cure an ileus due to hypokalemia. Gastric dilatation may cause little or no change in the contour of the abdominal wall because of the tight eschar over the abdomen. A change in the character of respiration may be the only sign, and the index of suspicion should be high during the early postburn period. Often escharotomies of the chest wall must be extended to allow expansion of the abdominal wall.

Another common gastrointestinal complication of the early postburn period may be *hemorrhagic gastritis* resulting in coffee-grounds gastric aspirant. It is frequently present during the first 24 to 48 hours after burn injury and represents bleeding from congested capillaries in the gastric mucosa. It may be confused with the coffee-grounds aspirant associated with Curling's ulcer. Hemorrhagic gastritis is characterized by small volumes of coffee-grounds fluid accompanied by large volumes of air in the stomach and may be relieved by decompression of the stomach with intermittent gastric suction via a Levine tube. Since acute hemorrhage from a *Curling's ulcer* can often follow such findings, the patient must be watched carefully.

Acute ulceration of the stomach or duodenum is the most frequent life-threatening gastrointestinal complication in the burn patient,[24] occurring in approximately 11 percent of the total burn population. Duodenal ulcers appear twice as frequently in children as in adults. Gastric ulcers are seen with equal frequency throughout the first month after burn injury in all age groups, whereas incidence of duodenal lesions reaches a peak during the first week in adults and during the third and fourth weeks in children. Although ulcerogenic factors may be present in some burn patients, the etiology cannot be attributed to any one factor. Hemorrhagic gastritis during the early postburn period has been implicated as a possible precursor lesion of Curling's ulcer. This has not yet been proved, but hemorrhagic gastritis does damage the mucosa and renders it more susceptible to ulceration. Sepsis may have an additive effect on predisposing the burn patient to Curling's ulcer.[25] Sepsis appears to function only as an added stress, but in small burns the addition of sepsis results in a much higher incidence of Curling's ulcer. The precise cause of Curling's ulcer remains obscure.

The initial treatment for Curling's ulcer should include decompression and evacuation of the stomach, gastric lavage with iced saline, blood transfusions as necessary, and general supportive care. At least one-third of all patients treated in such a manner initially rebleed and require operative intervention. Although much controversy exists about the proper operative procedure in such cases, most authorities recommend vagotomy and at least partial gastric resection.

Another less common but severely debilitating gastrointestinal complication in the burn patient is superior mesenteric artery syndrome (SMAS).[26] *SMAS* is the compression of the distal duodenum at the level of the superior mesenteric artery, resulting in partial or complete duodenal obstruction. This complication, characterized clinically by painless upper abdominal distention, recurrent emesis, excessive gastric drainage, and more than anticipated weight loss, is confirmed by x-ray studies. Nonoperative therapy includes gastric decompression, fluoroscopic studies to determine the position which allows the maximal drainage of barium past the "point of obstruction," and gradual reinstitution of oral feedings using this predetermined position afterward. Frequently the patient must be supported nutritionally with intravenous hyperalimentation until oral feedings can be resumed. Operative intervention is required in those patients with persistent obstruction despite positioning, those unable to be properly positioned because of the location of their burn, or those who develop supervening complications of a progressive nature. Duodenojejunostomy

is usually the operative choice. SMAS is a formidable threat to the burn patient, who has a spectacular increase in metabolic demands, not only because of the direct effect of the disease process itself but also because of the secondary debilitating effect of interference with alimentation and uptake of the major source of energy supply which are necessary to satisfy the patient's much augmented metabolic requirements.

Metabolic Response to Burn Injury

Weight loss accompanied by negative nitrogen balance characterizes the metabolic response in patients with extensive burns. This catabolic phase is followed by a prolonged period of anabolism with gradual restoration of body weight and lean tissue mass. The basal metabolic rate during the catabolic phase is increased markedly, and predicted energy requirements for a 70-kg male with a 40 percent TBSA burn is 3000 to 4000 kcal/day. Similar caloric intakes are predicted for children depending on age and percentage of burned area.

When exposed, extensively burned patients have a greatly increased heat loss by evaporation and an increased metabolic rate, which correlates to some extent with evaporation losses. A widely accepted hypothesis is that the two phenomena are causally related; that is, the heat loss by evaporation from extensive burns is so great that the patient is forced to compensate by increasing his metabolic demand. Zawacki[27] and his associates have demonstrated that the elevated metabolic rate of the thermally injured could not be decreased by marked reduction of evaporation from the burn surface when a plastic film was applied to the burn wound for a 12-hour period. By treating burn patients in a warm, dry environment (temperature 28 to 30°C and a relative humidity of between 15 and 30 percent) the basal metabolic rate may be lowered somewhat.[28] Since the reasons for the hypermetabolic response of the burn patient have not been adequately defined, and since the control of this response by environmental manipulation has not been completely successful, improved methods for providing the needed caloric requirements of the burn patient are being investigated.[28]

Up to 5000 kcal/day can be provided exclusively by vein with a resultant weight gain, positive nitrogen balance, wound healing, and, in the pediatric patient, normal growth and development. These findings led to studies by Wilmore and Curreri in which they were able to give as much as 8000 kcal/day by a combined intravenous and enteric feeding program to severely burned and septic patients, thus establishing an anabolic state with weight stabilization and wound healing.[29]

Immunologic Response to Burn Injury

Although the number and types of bacteria in the burn wound are of obvious importance in the development of sepsis, equally important are the immunologic defenses of the individual against those microorganisms. Abnormalities can occur in almost every component of host defense following a burn injury, but the relative importance of each varies with age of patient, extent of burn, and interval following injury. The generalized vascular response in an acute burn injury is associated with an inability of the host to localize inflammatory cells in the burn tissue or other areas subjected to bacterial contamination.[30] The presence of this transient but severe susceptibility underscores the necessity of meticulous attention to aseptic technique during this early period.

After the first few days, a layer of granulation tissue gradually develops beneath the burn eschar and affords the host a progressively increasing resistance to invasion of bacteria in eschar. Healthy granulation tissue can readily resist invasion of bacterial concentrations of 10^6 to 10^7 organisms per gram of tissue, but a comparatively lower resistance of bacterial invasion is found in less well developed granulation tissue, since the resistance is related directly to the ability of the reactive capillary network to sequester large numbers of phagocytic cells. This capability diminishes as granulation tissue is replaced by scar, partially explaining the late susceptibility of burn patients to local invasion of bacteria.

With exudation and loss of plasma protein into the burn wound and interstitial tissues, nearly all the plasma proteins fall in concentration immediately after the burn injury. Total complement levels and individual complement components have been found to be decreased following burn injury, but there is no apparent relationship to the susceptibility of these patients to infection.[31] The circulating levels of IgG, the most important of the immunoglobulins, continue to fall for 2 to 4 days but usually return to normal by the second week and characteristically remain elevated thereafter. Both synthesis and catabolic destruction of IgG are increased after burn injury. Failure to recover normal levels usually reflects an accentuated catabolic state rather than an increased loss into the burn wound; since this is often associated with sepsis, these patients often die. Adequate IgG therapy cannot be administered because commercially available globulin cannot be given intravenously and the amount of globulin necessary to adequately replace that destroyed cannot be given intramuscularly. Recently, therapy with type-specific antibody hyperimmune globulin has been investigated with some promising results.[32] Also, the use of specific vaccines, such as *Pseudomonas* polyvalent vaccine, adds a new dimension to protecting the burn patient from specific bacterial infections.[33]

Abnormalities of phagocytosis by the reticuloendothelial system have also been demonstrated following burn injury, but their relationship to the development of sepsis remains obscure. In contrast, abnormalities of the antibacterial function of neutrophils have recently been shown to be a major determinant in the development of sepsis in the burn patient. Neutrophils from healthy persons normally have a cyclic variation in their ability to kill ingested bacteria. After a burn injury the cyclic variation of neutrophilic function becomes markedly accentuated, and the overall antibacterial function of the neutrophil is adversely affected. Life-threatening sepsis occurs only when neutrophilic function is relatively poor. The number of bacteria in the eschar increases as neutrophilic function decreases, and conversely.[34] Thus, not only does normal neutrophilic function inhibit systemic invasion from the burn wound, but the number of bacteria in the eschar are influenced greatly by variations in the basic neutrophilic function. Unfortunately, the variables which regulate neutrophil function are still poorly understood.

Neuromusculoskeletal Changes Secondary to Burn Injury

The physical impairments which accompany burns are the results of immobilization, infection, or metabolic changes and include contractures, dislocation of tendons, dislocation or fusion of joints, heterotopic bone, limb amputations, and weakness secondary to neuropathy. Since fibrosis is an unavoidable response to deep thermal injury, it would be unrealistic to expect to avoid all deformities, but simple preventive measures will lessen the incidence and severity of these complications.[35] Proper splinting and positioning can help to prevent deformities. Active and passive exercise as well as early ambulation are prophylactic measures which may be employed. Adequate nutrition to prevent unnecessary wasting of lean muscle masses and other musculoskeletal changes are important to eventual recovery and rehabilitation. During all phases of burn care, concern is given to the prevention and treatment of deformities so that the patient can return to society as a functional member.

Psychologic Sequelae of Burn Injuries

A burn injury in a child is extremely stressful for him and his parents. The injury itself is frightening, and during his prolonged hospitalization he and his family must face both physical and emotional pain, helplessness, dependency, and the possibilities of disfigurement, disability, and death. Medical personnel caring for these patients must deal not only with shock, electrolyte imbalance, sepsis, nutrition, and wound healing but also with fear, depression, grief, and guilt in both the child and his family. About 60 to 80 percent of all burned children have significant emotional problems during the acute phase of care and later in the reconstructive and rehabilitative phase. In a study of 198 burned children, after a minimum of 2 years after burn injury 81 percent demonstrated signs of emotional disturbances, showing a marked contrast to only 7 percent in 608 siblings studied and 14 percent in a random control group of 50 children.[36] A high incidence of psychopathology in the family unit antedating the burn incident has been reported, suggesting that chronic relationship problems may become overtly manifest at the time of the child's injury.

Holter and Friedman suggest a method of identifying the emotionally high-risk patient and his family which can be used effectively in dealing with burn children.[37] One must first seek to understand the patient's emotional and social adjustment before the injury occurred and his physiologic and psychologic response to the burn injury, hospitalization, and treatment procedures. These factors and the precise circumstances under which the child was burned have been found to be the most helpful in planning for the management of the child and his family. Most burn injuries in children may be classified in three main groups: (1) true accident, (2) situational crisis, or (3) child abuse. *True accidents* have been defined as injuries which appear to have happened under circumstances beyond parental control. As a rule, these families are emotionally healthy families and the child and his family can be dealt with easily and require little in the way of psychiatric follow-up. *Situational crisis* is defined as an incident which appears to be associated with markedly disturbed family situations. This group may actually be divided into two subgroups. In one group the incidents seem to occur because the parent is unable to cope with the child's preburn emotional problem; in the sec-

ond group, an emotional disturbance of the mother results in the child's receiving little or no parental supervision. These distressed families are often found to need intensive psychiatric counseling for prolonged periods of time to help the child and his parent adjust to the illness and associated disfigurement and disability. The third classification, *child abuse*, involves extremely disturbed family situations which necessitate protective measures to prevent recurrence of abuse until adequate psychotherapy can be obtained for the family. Approximately 75 percent of the patients studied fell within the two latter categories of situational crisis and child abuse (child abuse accounting for approximately one-third of these cases). An in-depth history of the psychosocial aspect of family life and the circumstances surrounding the burn accident should be a clue to the best approach to treat the potential psychologic sequelae of the burn injury. The precise treatment of any individual case must be based on the interactions of the patient, his family, and the medical and paramedical personnel involved.

Nursing Management

The nursing care of the burned child requires continued diagnosis, intervention, and evaluation of the numerous parameters of various phases of burn care. To simplify somewhat the multiplicity of nursing needs of these patients they will be discussed according to phases of care: resuscitation (first 72 hours), acute phase (72 hours until healing or grafting occurs), and reconstructive phase (postgraft).

Resuscitative Phase Nursing care during the resuscitative phase is concerned with five major areas; that is, fluid resuscitation, pulmonary care, prevention of infection, preservation of function, and psychologic support.

A detailed history including past medical history as well as a complete account of the burn injury should assist the nurse in planning nursing care and anticipating complications. For example, a history of asthma or the occurrence of the burn injury in a closed space indicate possible respiratory problems. A history of sickle-cell disease suggests potential hematologic crisis with the hypercoagulability of burns added to the clotting difficulties associated with sickle-cell disease. Also of extreme importance is a history of any drug or food allergies, since an unnecessary allergic reaction may complicate the diagnosis and treatment of other supervening complications.

Early in the resuscitation period diagnosis and

treatment for pulmonary complications is of utmost importance. Upon initial examination, ascertaining that the patient has an adequate airway is paramount to his ultimate survival and continues to be a major concern throughout the resuscitative and acute phases. The usual signs of acute respiratory distress (rales, dyspnea, increased respiratory rate, and bronchospasms) may be extremely rapid in onset in the burned child and are considered late signs of distress. Although radiologic studies are important during the early postburn period, as a base line for therapy, they do not often show changes in the lung until after acute respiratory distress is readily apparent. The primary objective for treatment of any respiratory complication is adequate oxygenation of the blood. Aggressive therapy should be initiated at the first sign of respiratory insufficiency. Treatment of all respiratory complications includes (1) adequate ventilation, which may require a tracheostomy and assisted ventilation; (2) aspiration of tracheal bronchial secretions; (3) administration of humidified oxygen to maintain oxygenation; and (4) medication as indicated to liquefy secretions, relieve bronchospasms, and decrease the inflammatory response. The nursing management of the child with respiratory problems should include (1) observation of changes in rate and in character of respirations; (2) encouragement of coughing, deep breathing, and frequent changes of position to prevent atelectasis; (3) expertise in the management of patients on respirators; and (4) application of sterile technique and proper methods of suctioning when caring for patients with tracheostomies or endotracheal tubes.

Next in order of importance during the resuscitative phase is resuscitation for burn shock. Successful nursing management is dependent on the nurse's understanding of fluid therapy and the expected response to adequate or inadequate resuscitation. Some signs and symptoms of inadequate resuscitation are thirst, vomiting, increased pulse rate, decreased blood pressure, changes in sensorium, and decreased urinary output. The first four signs can be misleading. Many patients who have dry mucous membranes as a result of smoke inhalation or from not drinking will complain of thirst. Vomiting may be a sign of circulatory collapse, acute gastric dilatation, paralytic ileus, or a nonspecific effect of the injury. Increased pulse rate is difficult to evaluate, since a high normal pulse rate should be expected during this phase of burn injury. Decreased blood pressure is rarely seen in the burn patient unless he is in profound shock. Central venous pressure, a reliable guide to the rate of fluid volume

needed, becomes extremely important in evaluating whether or not respiratory complications are a result of intrinsic pulmonary edema from inhalation injury or whether the cardiovascular system is unable to handle the large quantities of fluid, thus causing pulmonary edema.

Sensorium is a very useful guide. If the patient is being resuscitated properly he will be alert, complain of pain appropriately, and exhibit a sense of well-being. This sign, too, may be altered if a patient becomes hypoxic from pulmonary complications; if he has suffered a stroke, seizure, or closed head injury at the time of the accident; or if he has been oversedated. Urine output is perhaps the single most reliable sign of adequate resuscitation. Urine output should be maintained at 20 to 50 ml per hour in children. Glycosuria may give a falsely high urine output. Thus, sugar and acetone determinations and urine osmolarity should be checked at least every 4 hours, and urine electrolytes should be measured daily. The expected signs of adequate resuscitation are a combination of the following: clear sensorium, urine output of 20 to 50 ml per hour, a high normal pulse rate of 100 to 140 beats per minute, the central venous pressure below 12, and the absence of acute gastric dilatation. An understanding of these signs of adequate resuscitation enables the nurse to evaluate the patient's response to fluid therapy and anticipate complications arising from inadequate fluid therapy.

Infection control also begins with initial care and spans the course of the illness until spontaneous healing or grafting takes place. Extreme caution and superb aseptic technique must attend all procedures to protect the patient from infection. During the early postburn period (3 to 4 weeks) until granulation tissue is well established, patients with major burns (greater than 15 to 20 percent) should be afforded some type of isolation from the routine hospital environment. Isolation may range from a private room with reverse isolation precautions to specialized burn unit care.

Infection control of the burn wound begins with initial cleansing and debriding. Sterile technique should be used when cleaning all burned as well as nonburned areas with an iodine-containing solution to remove surface contaminants. All blisters should be broken at this time, and all loose tissue should be removed. Immediately after debridement, definitive care with the selected mode of therapy should be initiated to prevent unnecessary contamination. Other early measures ordered by the physician to prevent burn wound infection are tetanus prophylaxis and the institution of preventive drug therapy, such as the use of a short course of prophylactic penicillin or other drugs to control an early streptococcal infection, which often may occur during the first week.

Routine serial biopsy culture of the burn wound is the most accurate tool for evaluating the adequacy of therapy and isolation technique. Cultures of the burn wound should be taken at least every 3 days from the day of admission until healing or grafting takes place. The practice of routine cultures of the burn wound, blood, urine, and tracheal aspirants enables early diagnosis and treatment of infectious complications. Of equal importance is the culture of the tip of all intravenous catheters when they are discontinued. Infection control is a prime responsibility of nursing care.

Maintenance of function is also of utmost importance beginning in the resuscitation phase and continuing through the rehabilitation phase. During the resuscitation phase maximum joint function is maintained by proper positioning and elevation of burn extremities. The arms should be abducted from the body at 90° angles. The legs should be kept straight with hips slightly flexed and feet at 90° angles. Patients with burns of the neck should be positioned with the head slightly hyperextended. If the ears are also involved, precautions should be taken so that pillows and other objects do not exert pressure on the ears, producing pressure necrosis. The patient should be turned frequently and all joints exercised either actively or passively. Elevating burned extremities prevents further loss of tissue from increased edema and impaired circulation, resulting in progressive tissue necrosis. Frequently, elevation is not enough with circumferential, full-thickness burns of extremities, and escharotomies are necessary to prevent vascular occlusion and progressive necrosis. When escharotomies are performed and deep tissue planes are exposed, the patient's burn wounds become even more susceptible to infection and added precautions should be taken to protect these incisions from contamination. Proper positioning and elevation during this early postburn period will prevent some of the later functional complications.

Psychologic support for the burned child and his family also must begin with this initial phase. Pain, fear of the unknown, and the fear of abandonment are all paramount in the child's thinking at this time. As soon as resuscitation is begun and the patient is stable, analgesic medication should be administered so that debridement and other painful procedures can be accomplished without pain to the patient. Because parental support is extremely important for most children at this time, parents should be allowed to stay with the child as much as possible.

Parents also need support during this initial phase. They fear death, disfigurement, or deformity of their child and feel guilty for "letting" the accident occur or "causing" the accident. They need reassurance and simple explanations so that they can help the child cope with the situation.

Acute Phase During the acute phase infection control, maintenance of function, preservation of tissue, and psychologic support continue as primary nursing concerns. Careful observation for impending complications and adequate nutritional support become paramount.

Infection control during the acute phase continues to be a major concern. The fine balance between what to do and what not to do to protect the child becomes a problem. Absolute isolation severely limits many functions which seem to be important for the child's maximum physical and psychologic rehabilitation. Some authorities believe that total isolation is imperative to infection control; others believe that with modern topical therapy, total isolation is not necessary. Resident skin flora and gastrointestinal tract flora have been implicated as the most frequent colonizers of the burn wound. Therefore, total isolation systems may not provide the patient with the safeguard initially apparent. Careful reverse isolation technique in a "super" clean environment appears to offer the patient the environmental protection he needs without interfering with other medical and nursing procedures as well as play activity which afford the patient both physical and emotional therapy.

Infection control of the burn wound centers around removal of eschar and necrotic tissue and the protection of the developing granulation tissue. Painful debridement becomes an everyday encounter for the child and his nurse. Whirlpool therapy, debridement, application of topical agents, and application of heterograft or homograft all evoke physical and emotional pain for the child and a challenge for the nurse who must cope with his own feelings as well as the behavior of the child. As newer, safer, less painful methods of debridement are developed, perhaps the "horror" of this phase can be lessened. The ultimate goal of the acute phase is rapid debridement of dead tissue and preservation of viable tissue and definitive closure of the wound.

Exercise, splinting, and positioning to maintain function becomes a goal of physical therapy. Active and passive exercise to maintain joint function must be encouraged constantly if deformities are to be avoided. The temporal relationship of splinting and mobility of affected parts should balance each other. As long as the child is awake, cooperative, and can be encouraged to move affected parts, splinting is not necessary. Splinting in a position of function is necessary during periods of inactivity, such as sleep, or when the patient is unwilling or unable to cooperate. Continuous splinting is recommended for any joint with an open capsule.

The child and his parents need continued reassurance and simple explanations. Procedures may have to be explained time and time again. This stage is extremely frustrating for health care personnel. Coping with demanding behavior of the child, the often antagonistic behavior of parents, and the anxious behavior of himself and other nursing and medical personnel is very stressful. In burn units across the country where nurses are continually caring for these difficult patients, psychologic consultation for the nursing staff has proved helpful. Many of the acute emotional problems of the burned child and his parents can best be managed through psychologic support for the nursing staff so that they may assist the patient and his family to understand their coping behaviors.[38]

A new concern in the acute phase is nutrition. The metabolic demands of the burned child are greatly accentuated, and adequate nutrition becomes a major challenge. Frequently providing an adequate number of calories through conventional oral routes is unsatisfactory for several reasons. The child may be unaccustomed to eating hospital food. His refusal to eat may be part of his reaction to the situation. He may be unable to tolerate oral alimentation because of gastric dilatation, paralytic ileus, or sepsis. His oral intake may be restricted because of surgical procedures. Ingenuity may be required to encourage oral intake. Careful planning between the nurse, the dietitian, and the mother can often lead to a diet high in protein and calories which is acceptable to the child. Encouraging the family to bring favorite foods from home helps to increase the child's appetite. If the child refuses to eat as part of his coping behavior, thus controlling at least one part of his new environment, hospital personnel are forced to abandon conventional means of oral alimentation and use nasogastric feeding tubes or feeding jejunostomies to provide the necessary caloric support. These procedures should never be approached as punishment for the child's refusal to eat but as simple medical procedures to supplement care.

The use of intravenous hyperalimentation has added a new dimension to providing the additional calories required by the burned child. However, this innovation should be approached with extreme caution in the case of a burned child because infectious complications attending it are fierce even in a patient not already predisposed to infection. These complications can be kept at a minimum if strict aseptic technique is followed.

The constant evaluation of the nutritional status of the burned child requires accurate records of all intake and output, daily calorie counts, and accurate daily weights. Without all three it is impossible to evaluate nutrition properly and plan measures to correct nutritional deficits. Careful consideration of nutritional status of the patient should precede the planning of any surgical procedures, since an optimal level of nutrition improves wound healing postoperatively.

In the acute phase, which might also be named the "phase of complications," continued nursing assessment is vital. Anticipation of likely complications and observation of early impending signs of complications are the essentials of nursing assessment. Major complications include burn wound sepsis, pneumonia, Curling's ulcer, suppurative thrombophlebitis, acute renal failure, and electrolyte imbalances. Others which may supervene and cause concern in differential diagnosis are throat and ear infections, urinary tract infections, the usual childhood diseases (measles, mumps), and complications of preexisting conditions such as asthma, allergies, and cardiac disease. The complications of this period are often disastrous; and if definitive therapy is to be instituted in time to salvage the patient, it will be the diagnostic and assessment skills of the nurse that will intervene and alter the eventual outcome.

Rehabilitative Phase Preservation of new tissue and prevention of infection continue to be part of the rehabilitation phase. New tissue, whether the result of spontaneous healing or grafting, must be protected from breakdown and possible infection. Protective clothing, orthopedic equipment, and special skin care procedures may be required to prevent such occurrences. As scars mature and hypertrophic scarring and scar contracture takes place, continued physical therapy is required to maintain joint function and minimize deformities. In time, further surgical procedures may be necessary. Cosmetic surgery to eliminate or improve disfigurement caused by the burn injury must usually wait until 18 months to several years after injury. Continued psychologic support during this period becomes all-important. Parents and children alike become depressed, discouraged, and emotionally distraught as the ugly, disfiguring scars build and function becomes more impaired. Realistic explanations and continued encouragement are necessary. Care should be taken to support the parent and child realistically so that they do not become too hopeful about the end result of reconstructive and cosmetic surgery and then suffer frustration and disappointment if the results are not spectacular. Psychologic support for the child and his family during this period has a paramount effect on the eventual outcome of the illness and whether or not the child will become a functional member of society or an emotional and physical cripple.

REFERENCES

1 A. N. Domonkos, *Andrew's Diseases of the Skin*, W. B. Saunders Company, Philadelphia, 1971, pp. 18–19.
2 R. J. Ruby and J. D. Nelson, "Effects of Hexachlorophene Scrubs on the Response to Placebo or Penicillin Therapy in Impetigo," *Pediatrics*, 52(6):854, 1973.
3 N. H. Stone et al., "Child Abuse by Burning," *The Surgical Clinics of North America*, 50(6):1419–1424, 1970.
4 C. P. Artz and J. A. Moncrief, *Treatment of Burns*, W. B. Saunders Company, Philadelphia, 1969, p. 92.
5 C. C. Lund and N. C. Browder, "The Estimation of Areas of Burns," *Surgery, Gynecology and Obstetrics*, 79,352, 1944.
6 C. P. Artz and J. A. Moncrief, *The Treatment of Burns*, W. B. Saunders Company, Philadelphia, 1969, p. 119.
7 G. T. Shires et al., "Treatment of Severely Injured Patients," in C. E. Welch (ed.), *Advances in Surgery*, vol. 4, Year Book Medical Publishers, Inc., Chicago, 1970, pp. 308–324.
8 F. E. Gump and J. M. Kinney, "Caloric and Fluid Losses through the Burn Wound," *The Surgical Clinics of North America*, 50(6):1235–1248, 1970.
9 C. Teplitz et al., "Pseudomonas Burn Wound Sepsis in Pathogenesis of Experimental Burn Wound Sepsis," *Journal of Surgical Research*, 4:200, 1964.
10 W. W. Monafo and C. A. Moyer, "The Treatment of Extensive Thermal Burns with 0.5% Silver Nitrate Solution," *Annals of New York Academy of Science*, 150:937–945, 1968.
11 J. A. Moncrief, "The Status of Topical Antibacterial Therapy in the Treatment of Burns," *Surgery*, 63(5):862–867, 1968.
12 R. P. Hummel et al., "Topical and Systemic Antibacterial Agents in the Treatment of Burns," *Annals of Surgery*, 172:370–384, 1970.
13 C. R. Baxter, "The Control of Burn Wound Sepsis by the Use of Quantitative Bacteriologic Studies and Subeschar Clysis with Antibiotics," *Surgical Clinics of North America*, 53(6):1509–1518, 1973.
14 W. W. Monafo et al., "Early Tangential Excision of the Eschar of Major Burns," *Archives of Surgery*, 104:503–508, 1972.
15 B. A. Pruitt and P. W. Curreri, "The Use of Homografts and Heterograft Skin," in H. Polk and H. Stone (eds), *Contemporary Burn Management*, Little, Brown and Company, Boston, 1971, pp. 397–417.
16 C. R. Baxter et al., "Fluid and Electrolyte Therapy of Burn Shock," *Heart and Lung*, 2(5):707–713, 1973.
17 J. A. Moncrief, "Burns," *The New England Journal of Medicine*, 288(9):444–456, 1973.
18 C. Baxter et al., "Fluid and Electrolyte Therapy of Burn Shock," op. cit.
19 E. C. Loebl et al., "The Mechanism of Erythrocyte Destruction in the Early Post Burn Period," *Annals of Surgery*, 178(6):681–686, 1973.
20 H. H. Stone, "Management of Respiratory Injury According to Clinical Phase," in H. Polk and H. Stone (eds.), *Contemporary Burn Management*, Little, Brown and Company, Boston, 1971, pp. 111–123.
21 B. A. Pruitt et al., "Pulmonary Complications in Burn Patients," *The Journal of Thoracic and Cardiovascular Surgery*, 59(1):7–20, 1970.
22 Moncrief, "Burns," op. cit.
23 Moncrief, "Burns," op. cit.
24 H. M. Bruck et al., "A 10 Year Experience with 412 Patients," *Journal of Trauma*, 10(8):658–662, 1970.
25 B. A. Pruitt et al., "Curling's Ulcer: A Clinical Pathology Study of 323 Cases," *Annals of Surgery*, 172:523–539, 1970.
26 J. M. Reckler et al., "Superior Mesenteric Artery Syndrome As a Consequence of Burn Injury," *The Journal of Trauma*, 12(11):979–985, 1972.
27 B. Zawacki et al., "Does Increased Evaporative Water Loss Cause Hypermetabolism in Burned Patients?" *Annals of Surgery*, 171(2):236–240, 1969.
28 P. O. Barr et al., "Studies on Burns X. Changes in BMR and Evaporative Water Loss in the Treatment of Severe Burns with Warm Dry Air," *Scandinavian Journal of Plastic and Reconstructive Surgery*, 3:30–38, 1969.
29 D. W. Wilmore et al., "Supranormal Dietary Intake in Thermally Injured Hypermetabolic Patients," *Surgery, Gynecology and Obstetrics*, 132:881–886, 1971.
30 M. S. Rittenbury, "The Response of the Reticuloendothelial System to Thermal Injury," *Surgical Clinics of North America*, 50(6):1227–1234, 1970.
31 Rittenbury, op. cit.
32 J. W. Alexander, "Control of Infection Following Burn Injury," *Archives of Surgery*, 103:435–441, 1971.
33 J. W. Alexander, "Prevention of Invasive Pseudomonas Infection in Burns with a New Vaccine," *Archives of Surgery*, 94:249–256, 1969.
34 J. W. Alexander, "Periodic Variation in the Antibacterial Function of Human Neutrophils and Its Relationship to Sepsis," *Annals of Surgery*, 173:206–213, 1971.
35 E. B. Evans, "Prevention and Correction of Deforming after Severe Burns," *Surgical Clinics of North America*, 50(6):1361–1375, 1970.
36 Joan M. Woodward, "Emotional Disturbance of Burned Children," *British Medical Journal*, 5128:1009–1013, 1959.
37 J. C. Holter and S. B. Friedman, "Etiology and Management of Severely Burned Children," *American Journal of Diseases of Children*, 118:680–686, 1969.
38 Susan Quinby and N. R. Bernstein, "Identity Problems and the Adaptation of Nurses to Severely Burned Chil-

dren," *American Journal of Psychiatry*, 128(1):90–95, 1971.

BIBLIOGRAPHY

Alexander, Mary, and Brown, Marie: *Pediatric Physical Diagnosis for Nurses*, McGraw-Hill Book Company, New York, 1974.

American Academy of Pediatrics: *Report of the Committee on Infectious Diseases 1970*, 16th ed., Evanston, Ill., 1971.

————: *Standards of Child Health Care*, 2d ed., Evanston, Ill., 1972.

Behrman, H., and Labow, T. A.: *The Practitioner's Illustrated Dermatology*, Grune & Stratton, Inc., New York, 1965.

Champion, R. H., et al.: *An Introduction to the Biology of the Skin*, F. A. Davis Company, Philadelphia, 1970, pp. 23–24.

Clark, W. E. Le Gros: *The Tissues of the Body*, 6th ed., Clarendon Press, Oxford, England, 1971, pp. 293–334.

Di Dio, Liberato S. A.: *Synopsis of Anatomy*, The C. V. Mosby Company, St. Louis, 1970, pp. 489–493.

Falconer, Mary W., et al.: *The Drug, The Nurse, The Patient*, 4th ed., W. B. Saunders Company, Philadelphia, 1970.

Gardner, W. D., et al.: *Structure of the Human Body*, W. B. Saunders Company, Philadelphia, 1967, pp. 390–391.

Gellis, S. S., and Kagan, B. M.: *Current Pediatric Therapy*, W. B. Saunders Company, Philadelphia, 1973.

Hughes, J. G.: *Synopsis of Pediatrics*, 3d ed., The C. V. Mosby Company, St. Louis, 1971.

Karelitz, S.: *When Your Child Is Ill*, Warner Paperback Library, New York, 1972.

Kempe, H. C., et al.: *Current Pediatric Diagnosis and Treatment*, Lange Medical Publishers, Los Altos, Calif., 1972.

Krugman, S., and Ward, R.: *Infectious Diseases of Children and Adults*, 5th ed., The C. V. Mosby Company, St. Louis, 1973.

Nelson, W. E., et al.: *Textbook of Pediatrics*, 9th ed., W. B. Saunders Company, Philadelphia, 1969.

Pillsbury, D. M.: *A Manual of Dermatology*, W. B. Saunders Company, Philadelphia, 1971.

Saver, G.: *Manual of Skin Diseases*, 3d ed., J. B. Lippincott Company, Philadelphia, 1973.

Shelley, W. B.: *Consultations in Dermatology II*, W. B. Saunders Company, Philadelphia, 1974.

Slobody, L., and Wasserman, E.: *Survey of Clinical Pediatrics*, 5th ed., McGraw-Hill Book Company, New York, 1968.

Snell, R. S.: *Clinical Embroylogy for Medical Students*, Little, Brown and Company, Boston, 1972, pp. 283–291.

Stave, Uwe: *Physiology of the Perinatal Period*, vol. 2, Appleton-Century-Crofts, Inc., New York, 1970, pp. 889–906.

Stewart, W. D., et al.: *Synopsis of Dermatology*, 2d ed., The C. V. Mosby Company, St. Louis, 1970, pp. 3–20.

Disorder	Cause	Pathophysiology	Assessment	Intervention

I Congenital diseases of the skin
A Pigmented nevi
  1 Moles (true pigmented nevi)
    a Nevus spilus
		Smooth, flat, no hair, pigmented nevus	Pigmentation ranges from pale yellow to black or brown	If subject to trauma or repeated irritation, excise for cosmetic reasons; electrodesiccation and cryotherapy contraindicated since they do not permit tissue diagnosis

b Nevus pilosus		Growth of downy or stiff hair		Remove surgically for cosmetic reasons
c Nevus verrucosus		Hyperkeratotic, raised, sometimes wartlike areas		Psychologic support when lesions are large and disfiguring
B Vascular nevi (hemangiomas) 1 Nevus flammeus (port-wine mark)		Flat and red to purplish in color; commonly seen on face or neck; size varies from few mm to covering most of face or neck; commonly seen and present at birth	Watch for intracranial vascular malformation when nevus presents asymmetrically (one side of face); intracranial lesion may be associated with seizures but cannot be seen due to damage to underlying tissue in later childhood (encephalofacial angiomatosis or Sturge-Weber syndrome)	Surgery, irradiation (often with unsatisfactory results), or cosmetic creams; usually less intensely colored types fade in intensity as the child grows but rarely disappear completely
II Miliaria rubra (prickly heat, heat rash)	Environmental, physical, and chemical agents	Due to warm weather condition or overdressing, which causes excessive perspiration; fine erythematous papular rash; shoulders, neck, and skin folds most common sites; usually face is exempt; results from occlusion of pores of sweat glands with retention of sweat within epidermis	No visible sweating	Avoid use of soap; bathe frequently with cool plain water; keep environment cool; dress lightly; light application of bland dusting powder and calamine lotion
III Carotenosis (hypervitaminosis A)	Inability of liver to convert carotene to vitamin A	Orange-yellow hue to the skin of the palms, soles, and fatty tissue of nose; carotene not converted to vitamin A and large amounts may be found in the circulating blood; if carotene provided plentifully in the diet (yellow vegetables), it may exceed the capacity of the immature neonatal liver to transform it to vitamin A; enough may then accumulate in the plasma to alter skin color	Differs from jaundice in that the sclera is not preferentially involved; serum bilirubin always normal in true carotenosis though the icterus index may be falsely elevated; consider hyperlipidemia, diseases of the liver, hypothyroidism and diabetes in differential diagnosis	Provide diet low in carotene

(Continued)

859

Table 41-5 DISORDERS OF THE INTEGUMENTARY SYSTEM (*Continued*)

Disorder	Cause	Pathophysiology	Assessment	Intervention
IV Dermatophytoses (most common fungus infections of skin) A Tinea (ringworm infections) 1 Tinea capitis (scalp ringworm)	*Microsporum canis* (animal-borne fungus)	*Microsporum* and *Trichophyton* are only two genera that produce tinea capitis; common in children; rare in adults whose relative resistance has been credited to fatty acids on the skin; contracted from infected domestic animals or from soil; usually sporadic; moderately common	Loss of hair and/or weeping exudative inflammation; most common in occipital area, but any area may be affected; history of animal contact; not infectious from child to child; spores not easily seen microscopically; differentiate culturally from *Microsporum audouini* which is transmitted from a human source, is highly infectious from child to child, and occurs in epidemics; Wood's black light an invaluable diagnostic tool in *M. lanosum* and *M. audouini* infections; shows bright blue-green fluorescence on infected hairs early in the course of the disease	Both the child and animal source require treatment with orally administered griseofulvin for infections involving hair or nail; high-fat meal significantly aids intestinal absorption of griseofulvin; surface creams which work well for tinea elsewhere simply cannot penetrate hair or nail and should be used only as adjunctive therapy Cure may sometimes occur spontaneously in 2–4 months if patient develops sufficient inflammation or enters puberty; secondary bacterial infection rarely demonstrable by culture, although the lesion may appear infected because of host resistance to fungus; x-ray epilation is never employed but was mainstay of therapy before griseofulvin became available
	M. audouini (human-borne fungus)	Transmitted by direct contact with infected hairs; incubation period brief, but evidence of the disease may not manifest itself until 3 weeks after exposure; signs of infection may not be picked up until 6 weeks or more after inoculation	Patches of broken-off hair and partial alopecia are cardinal signs; 2 or 3 patches of 6–8 cm in diameter are often present; single patch very uncommon	As above. If the lesion is weeping and exudate present, the child does not return to school; should all be dry before reentry; psychologic trauma from loss of hair, especially in young girls, can be prevented by use of scarves and wigs
	Trichophyton tonsurans (human-borne fungus)	Now shares with *M. canis* most important role in producing scalp ringworms in childhood; pathophysiology similar to that for *M. audouini*	Although inflammatory oozing and scaling may occur, this pathogen regularly produces so-called black dot ringworm; it invades and weakens hair shaft producing very short, stubby, broken-off hairs; unlike the two pathogens noted above, parasitized hairs do not fluoresce under Wood's (black light)	As above

	Causative Agent	Characteristics	Clinical Signs	Treatment
2 Tinea cruris ("jock strap itch")	*Trichophyton rubrum* and *T. mentagrophytes*	Common fungal infection in males; exceedingly rare in females; involves intertriginous areas, starting in crural or perineal folds and extending to surrounding regions	Scales contain filaments of fungi; annular, scaling, inflamed itching lesions of upper thighs and scrotum; if area moist, scaling may not be present; tends to be recurrent	Keep intertriginous areas clean and dry; frequent bathing in warm weather, being sure to rinse well and thoroughly removing all soap; loose-fitting, nonbinding, absorbent undergarments allowing aeration; light applications of bland dusting powders; in severe cases topical hydrocortisone therapy or griseofulvin therapy may be indicated. Prevent secondary bacterial infection
V Deep folliculitis (bacterial infections of hair follicles) A Furuncles (boils) and carbuncles	*Staphlococcus aureus*	Not seen in areas where there are no hair follicles (palms, etc.); most common sites are posterior neck, face, axilla, and buttocks; pustules or papules which originated within and in proximity to the hair follicle and progress to hard, tender, hot nodules which form a necrotic core and a pus "point"	Furuncles may be recurrent and chronic; rule out underlying diabetes; culture in resistant cases	Use a penicillinase-resistant penicillin or broad-spectrum antibiotic; topical neomycin cream for external nares may reduce recurrences; diet high in protein, low in fat and carbohydrates; avoid contact with very young children, especially the neonate and newborn. Personal hygiene and cleanliness is paramount; *do not squeeze*, especially in area of the nose for fear of involving cavernous sinus. Unless treatment cannot be carried out in the home it is very unwise to hospitalize for danger of spreading antibiotic-resistant (now less of a problem) strain of *Staphylococcus*; if hospitalization necessary, strict isolation precautions must be carried out
VI Variola (smallpox)	Poxvirus	Transmitted by direct contact with individuals, with smallpox from crusts and mucous membrane secretions or from contaminated articles such as bed linens; two types are variola major and variola minor, which is also called alastrim; both highly contagious; incubation period 10–21 days; communicable 2–3 days prior to the appearance of the rash and until all crusts are shed; mortality greatest under 5 years of age and	Variola major most severe, with frequent complications systemically as well as from exanthema; prodromal period, 2–4 days; abrupt onset with extreme prostration, sudden fever (104–106°F), convulsions, headache, backache, and transient morbilliform rash most prominent in the "swimming trunk" area; characteristically, exanthema begins by 3–5 days with macules on the face, wrists, and ankles and spreads to the extrem-	Child should be isolated and hospitalized; no specific therapy; treatment is symptomatic and supportive; attentive careful nursing care is most important; observe closely for hemorrhage, shock, respiratory tract involvement, secondary infections, adequate nutrition, oral and parenteral; attention to lesion of eye if present; general care to other lesions; an effective antiviral agent (methisazone) has been shown to *(Continued)*

Table 41-5 DISORDERS OF THE INTEGUMENTARY SYSTEM (Continued)

Disorder	Cause	Pathophysiology	Assessment	Intervention
		over 45 years of age; fatality rate variable with severity of disease; 1% with variola minor (discrete or minimal rash) and up to 80% with variola major with a confluent rash; complications include secondary bacterial infections of the lesions, bacteremia, bronchopneumonia, respiratory tract obstruction, osteomyelitis, joint deformities, encephalitis, keratitis, blindness, and abscess formation	ities, chest, and abdomen; rash more profuse on face and extremities than trunk; in contrast to chickenpox, variola lesions also appear on lips, palms, and soles; lesions appear in single crops and progress at the same rate with macules becoming papules, followed by unbilicated vesicles; pustular stage begins 5–6 days with a rise in temperature and all constitutional symptoms; on 10th day, pustules rupture and begin drying and forming crusts; pruritic lesions; crusts drop off by 3–4 weeks leaving scars most prominent on the face; hemorrhagic smallpox may appear during the prodrome period causing death even before characteristic rash develops Variola minor less severe, with minimal rash; may be misdiagnosed as chickenpox; lesions progress more rapidly through same stages and there is a milder prodromal period and general course of the illness Leukopenia is evident early from the blood picture and leukocytosis by the time the rash appears; other hematologic abnormalities apparent with hemorrhagic smallpox, secondary infections, and electrolyte imbalances; virus can be isolated from both the blood and the papules	produce a reduction in smallpox if given orally to an unvaccinated person exposed to smallpox; vaccinia immune globulin may also be given before fever and rash appear; vaccinia immune globulin may also be used in combination with the vaccination to modify smallpox if given shortly after exposure
VII Pediculosis (lice infestation of skin) A Pediculosis capitis (lice infestation of head)	*Pediculus humanus* *P. humanus capitis*	Blood suckers which characteristically localize in the scalp, rarely in beard, pubis, or other regions; occiput and temporal areas are favored sites; common in young females; uncommon in the Negro; itching is most common symp-	Nits represent egg cases which are tenaciously cemented to the hair and cannot be removed by flicking with the finger as can particles of dandruff Occipital and cervical adenopathy is common; differentiate from a	Early diagnosis to control or prevent spread and secondary bacterial infection; benzyl benxoate emulsion or benzene hexachloride (Kwell) shampoo; one application usually sufficient; second shampoo may be given in 24

	tom; secondary bacterial infection with impetiginization is common; variable macular or papular erythematous rash appearing principally on the trunk and resembling German measles may be present, believed caused by sensitization to the parasite	chronic nasopharyngeal infection or impetigo of scalp; length of infestation may be determined by the position of the nits on the hair shaft; nits are laid on hair shaft close to the head; as the hair grows, nits are carried to the top	hours, but should not be repeated more than twice in 1 week
B Pediculosis corporis (lice infestation of body)	*P. humanus corporis*	Manifests by erythematous macules most commonly seen on the upper back and areas where clothes are tight	Differentiate from scabies infestation by examination of hands and feet, which are not involved in pediculosis corpus; pubic louse infestation rare in children, confirmation of diagnosis by identification of lice and nits in the seams of clothing	Early diagnosis to control or prevent spread to other persons and to control or prevent secondary bacterial infection; benzyl benzoate emulsion or benzene hexachloride (Kwell) lotion or cream; DDT dusting of personal articles and clothing after boiling; particular attention should be given to seams; all family members should be treated at one time to prevent reinfestation
VIII Neurofibromatosis (von Recklinghausen's disease); café au lait lesions	Hereditary disorder	Onset of symptoms generally around puberty but may be present at birth; congenital skin lesions—café au lait spots in numbers exceeding six alert the physician that the disease is present and that the child should be observed closely for the development of signs of neurologic problems or subcutaneous tumors	Café-au-lait spots appear as irregularly shaped, sharply demarcated tan to brown, flat asymptomatic deposits of melanin which measure 1 cm or more; not uncommon to see 1–2 spots in normal child; 6 or more spots are diagnostic with or without other symptoms; in the infant, glaucoma or skeletal abnormalities may be associated findings; in children from infancy through puberty other associated symptoms include intracranial symptoms, mental retardation, deafness, gastrointestinal involvement, abnormalities of sexual development, pituitary and thyroid function, and subcutaneous neurofibromas; the subcutaneous neurofibromas may appear as minute lesions or large tumors, are flesh colored, flaccid to palpation, and occur at varying depths beneath the skin	Careful follow-up by a pediatrician and dermatologist suggested; treatment limited to the surgical excision of tumors causing symptoms, particularly of those located on nerve roots along the brain stem or cord; genetic counseling indicated

(Continued)

Table 41-5 DISORDERS OF THE INTEGUMENTARY SYSTEM *(Continued)*

Disorder	Cause	Pathophysiology	Assessment	Intervention
IX Systemic lupus erythematosus (disseminated lupus erythematosus)	Unknown	Disease of connective tissue which affects many organ systems; severe disease in childhood with a fatality rate reported to be above 50%; most often seen in girls between 9 and 15 years of age; onset abrupt or insidious over several years; course may be fulminating or with periods of exacerbation and remission over several years; renal disease is the most common and serious complicating lesion and is also the most important factor in the prognosis	In addition to cutaneous manifestations there may be fever, arthritis, malaise, anorexia, loss of weight, myocarditis, central nervous system involvement, inguinal, cervical and axillary lymphadenopathy, hematuria, proteinuria, splenomegaly, hepatomegaly; almost all children show some form of cutaneous manifestations, such as erythematous blush or scaly erythematous papules called the "butterfly rash" over the bridge of the nose and malar area, which may spread to the face, scalp, neck, chest, and arms; erythematous macules on the palms, soles and fingertips; punctuate lesions on the palate and oral mucous membranes; purpura of pressure areas, and alopecia	Topical steroids may or may not be used for the rash; secondary infection of the lesions should be prevented; rash may be photosensitive and need protection from strong sunlight, especially during the summer months

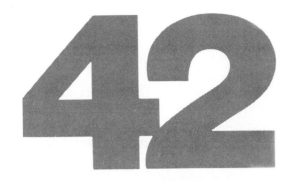

THE SPECIAL SENSES

GLADYS M. SCIPIEN, MARILYN A. CHARD, and MARY C. SCAHILL*

EMBRYOLOGY OF THE SPECIAL SENSES
Embryology of the Eye

During the first 4 weeks, the eye begins to develop in the embryo as an evagination of the lateral aspect of the forebrain. The diverticulum grows out laterally toward the side of the head, and the end becomes enlarged to form the *primary optic vesicle,* while the proximal portion becomes narrower, forms the *optic stalk,* and, on fusion of its inner and outer walls, gives rise to the optic nerve.

The larger, distal portion then becomes evaginated, undergoing further transformation into the two-layered *optic cup.* These two highly specialized layers will become the *retina* of the eye. The outer layer, the pigment layer, forms as a result of the development of pigment granules in the cells, while the inner layer consists of nervous tissue. By the sixth month of fetal growth rod and cone cells, bipolar cells, ganglionic cells, and supportive elements have developed from the inner layer.

Simultaneously, the surface ectoderm of the head, opposite the optic vesicle, thickens to form the lens placodes. Each of the placodes becomes depressed and sinks below the ectoderm to become the lens vesicle. It will come to rest in the cavity of the optic cup to become the *lens* of the eye (see Fig. 42-1). As it moves beneath the level of the ectoderm, the cells of the posterior wall undergo many changes, rapidly becoming elongated, losing their nuclei, and forming transparent lens fibers. The cavity of the lens gradually becomes obliterated as a result of the increase in the length of these cells. The cells forming the anterior wall of the lens remain the low, columnar type, forming the lens epithelium.

As cell differentiation of the optic and lens vesicles occurs, the loose mesenchyme which surrounds both condenses about them, forming a two-layered, fibrous capsule. Its inner layer becomes the highly vascular, delicate choroid of the eye, with its anterior section thickening and undergoing development to form the connective tissue of the ciliary body and the ciliary muscle, as well as the suspensory ligaments of the lens. The choroid encircles the eye structure and becomes continuous with the pia arachnoid of the brain, which forms a sheath around the optic nerve. The mesenchyme on the anterior surface of the lens forms the *pupillary membrane*, while the ectoderm forming the edge of the optic cup covers the ciliary muscle and extends posteriorly to fuse and form the *iris.*

* The authors wish to thank James L. Guillette, M.D., Senior Ophthalmologist, St. Vincent Hospital, Worcester, Mass., and Assistant Professor of Ophthalmology, University of Massachusetts Medical School, for his help in preparing this chapter.

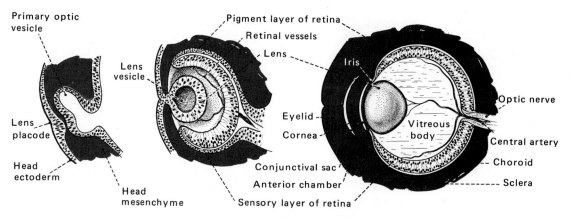

Figure 42-1 Embryonic development of the eye. *(From L. L. Langley, Ira R. Telford, and John B. Christensen, Dynamic Anatomy and Physiology, 4/e, McGraw-Hill Book Company, New York, 1974, p. 305. By permission of the publishers.)*

The outer layer of the fibrous two-layered capsule, which surrounds the optic and lens vesicles, continues to encircle these structures, developing into a thick, fibrous membrane which will become the *cornea* and the *sclera*. At the point of attachment of the optic nerve, the sclera becomes continuous with the dura mater of the brain, which also forms a fibrous sheath around the optic nerve.

The aqueous chamber of the eye arises as a cavity in the mesenchyme between the surface ectoderm and the developing iris, and it is called the anterior chamber. The posterior chamber develops as a split in the mesenchyme behind the developing iris and in front of the developing lens. Communication between the anterior and posterior chambers occurs when the pupil is formed. The mesenchyme which occupies the space between the developing retina and the lens becomes a delicate network of fibers embedded in a jellylike substance called the *vitreous body.*

The extraocular muscles, consisting of the four rectus muscles and the superior and inferior ocular muscles, form from mesenchyme in the area of the developing eyeball. It is important to note that they are innervated by the third, fourth, and sixth cranial nerves.

Eyelids develop as ectodermal folds below and above the cornea. As they grow, fusion occurs at about the third month of embryonic life, and they remain in this position until the seventh month. While the lids are fused, a closed space, called the *conjunctival sac,* exists in front of the cornea. Another accessory eye structure—the lacrimal gland—is formed as a result of a series of ectodermal buds growing upward. These cells experience changes

which result in canal formulation for these secretory units as well as the multiple ducts of this gland. The lacrimal sac and nasolacrimal ducts develop from ectoderm between the lateral nasal process and the maxillary process of the developing face. A series of cellular changes result in canal formation which gives rise to the nasolacrimal duct. A dilated upper end of this duct forms the lacrimal sac. With continued cellular proliferation and specialization, lacrimal ducts, which enter each eyelid, develop.

The eyes of the infant achieve their greatest growth during the first year and continue to grow rapidly until age 3. However, growth continues at a slower pace until puberty. Not all parts of the eye grow at the same rate. At birth the eye is three-fourths of its adult size. The lacrimal gland, which is small, is capable of producing tears at birth. The eyes, which are blue or gray at birth, attain their permanent color by 6 months of age.

Embryology of the Ear

The three regions of the ear consist of the internal ear, middle ear, and external ear. Most structures are well developed by the third month of fetal life.

The Internal Ear This structure is composed of the membranes and bony labyrinths and the perilymphatic spaces. During the third week of embryonic life the auditory placode appears and, in several days, is well circumscribed. It invaginates and forms the auditory pit during the fourth week. As the pit deepens and the surface opening closes, a closed sac called the auditory vesicle forms. This vesicle differentiates to constitute the membraneous labyrinth. The dorsal portion is the primordium of the vestibular complex, while the ventral extension is the primordium of the cochlea. Flanges which appear on the vestibular portion at the end of the sixth week eventually form three semicircular ducts: the superior, the posterior, and the lateral. At the same time, changes are occurring in the vestibular portion of the auditory vesicle. A progressively deepening constriction subdivides it dorsally into the utriculus and ventrally into the sacculus. The semicircular ducts now open off the utriculus. An ampulla (local enlargement) is formed by each semicircular canal. Within the ampulla, in an area known as the *crista,* specialized hairlike receptors develop and are innervated by the vestibular branches of the VIIIth cranial nerve. Similar specialized areas, called *maculae,* which arise in the sacculus and the utriculus, are also supplied by the vestibular branches of the VIIIth cranial nerve. The cochlea becomes evident during the sixth week. Rapid elongation occurs during the sixth, seventh, and eighth weeks. The distal portion of the cochlea spirals 2½ turns. The cochlea is also innervated by the VIIIth cranial nerve. The cells of the spiral ganglion of the cochlea make connections with the organ of Corti for tonoreception.

As the membranous labyrinth has been forming, mesenchyme has been surrounding it and later is transformed into cartilage—the beginning of the bony labyrinth. Between the cartilage and the membranous labyrinth is a space containing some mesenchymal cells. Those cells toward the cartilage become a perichondrial connective tissue layer; those adjacent to the membranous labyrinth organize a fibrous outer layer. Connective tissue strands develop between the reinforced walls of the membranous labyrinth and the encircling cartilage. The membranous labyrinth is thus suspended in the cartilagenous labyrinth. The connective tissue strands cross what is known as the *perilymphatic space.* Each space contains a clear, watery fluid. The cartilagenous tissue surrounding the membranous labyrinth eventually becomes bone and is known as the *bony labyrinth.*

Within the cochlear duct is the organ of Corti, or the spiral organ. At the third month of intrauterine life it first becomes apparent as an epithelial thickening on the floor of the cochlear duct. A structure known as the *tectorial membrane* forms over this thickening. As the cochlear duct expands from the third to fifth month, this membrane extends. The organ of Corti becomes more specialized as outer hair cells develop in its outer portion and inner hair cells form near the center of the spiral. In the sixth month the groove on its inner border deepens to form the inner spiral sulcus. Through resorption within the organ of Corti an inner tunnel forms between the inner and outer hair cells, and an outer tunnel develops peripheral to the outer hair cells. Fibrils form next to the inner tunnel and eventually become pillar (supporting) cells.

The Middle Ear While the inner ear is developing, the middle ear is also forming. In the young embryo, during cephalic differentiation, the first pharyngeal pouch, or tympanic recess, arises. It is destined to become the middle ear chamber (tympanic cavity) at its distal end and the eustachian tube at its proximal portion. As the primordium of the middle ear chamber separates from the surface, a concentration of mesenchymal cells appears next to it. These cells then organize into the cartilagenous primordia of the auditory ossicles (incus, stapes, malleus). The primordium of the external meatus arises from the branchial groove. During the latter part of fetal life through resorption of connective tissue and resultant expansion of the tympanic cavity, the ossicles eventually are suspended in the middle ear chamber.

The connective tissue which is destined to become the tympanic membrane is buried on both sides of the primordial mass which evolves into the middle ear chamber. As the tympanic cavity (middle ear chamber) is enlarged and the ossicles are freed, the entodermal lining of the chamber comes in contact with the inner surface of the connective tissue which is forming the tympanic membrane, and the meatal plug disappears. The eardrum then is composed of a tensely stretched membrane covered externally by a thin layer of ectodermal epithelium and internally by entodermal epithelium.

The External Ear The pinna arises from mesenchymal tissue flanking the hyomandibular groove. It begins as nodular enlargements from the mandibular and hyoid arches, which coalesce. Its supporting cartilage arises from underlying mesenchyme. By the seventh week of intrauterine life, the pinna is well demarcated. Its primitive position is at the hyomandibular cleft. As the jaw develops, each pinna is forced around to the side of the head.

Embryology of the Gustatory and Olfactory Organs

Taste Buds Taste, or gustation, is a function of the taste buds. Most taste buds are formed in two types of lingual papillae: fungiform and circumvallate. In the fetus, the forerunners of taste buds are seen in the lingual epithelium as small clusters in the eighth week of gestation. During the third month, the lingual epithelium begins to grow into the underlying mesenchyme, forming a solid circular lamina which opens into a slitlike groove and surrounds the papilla. Flat-topped *circumvallate papillae* arise along the V-shaped ridge between the body and root of the tongue. *Fungiform papillae* develop in a similar manner but are rounded and elevated. By the fourth gestational month nerve fibers can be seen entering the clearly defined cell clusters, or primordial taste buds, and by the sixth month of fetal life a pore opening is formed at the apex of each cluster. In mature taste buds, a bristlelike process (*taste hair*) extends through each pore to the surface, and nerve fibers enter at the base of each bud and terminate in the neuroepithelial cells in a basketwork pattern. As physiologic changes occur in the taste bud neuroepithelium (*neuromasts*), impulses are relayed along the taste nerve fibers to the central nervous system.

Olfactory Cells   Olfaction, or smell, is a function of the *olfactory cells,* which are found in the mucosal epithelium of the superior portions of the nasal cavity. During the fourth week of fetal life a pair of *olfactory placodes* (thickened areas of ectoderm) appear on the frontal portion of the head and begin to form the floor of the nasal pits. The pits are deepened by the rapid proliferation and forward growth of surrounding mesenchymal tissue. The resultant elevated borders assume a horseshoe shape. One elevation is known as the *nasomedial process* and the other as the *nasolateral process.* The nasal pits and their processes move medially, and the nasomedial processes merge beneath the ectoderm. This tissue gives rise to several facial structures as well as the bridge of the nose and the nasal system. The alae nasi arise from the nasolateral processes. Other developmental processes occur in the seventh week involving the formation of the palate.

Elevations in the lateral walls of the nares evolve into nasal conchae which are supported early in fetal life by turbinate cartilages. These cartilages eventually ossify and form the turbinate bones. Fetal conchae include the maxilloturbinal and five ethmoturbinals. The second and third ethmoturbinals are important to olfaction in that they form the superior concha in the olfactory area.

The epithelial lining of the nares begins as cuboidal/columnar and evolves into pseudostratified to stratified columnar epithelium. The *olfactory area* encompasses the middle superior portion of each nasal chamber and extends 8 to 10 mm medially onto the septum and laterally onto the superior concha. Cells which transform into olfactory receptors develop bristlelike processes (*olfactory hairs*) from the distal portion of the cell through the epithelium. Nonmedullated axonic processes central to each cell synapse with mitral cells in the olfactory bulb. Impulses are relayed from the mitral cells along the olfactory impulses to the central nervous system.

Irregularly shaped chambers lined with extensions of the nasal mucosa connect with the nasal cavity and are known as *paranasal sinuses.* The frontal and maxillary sinuses appear during the fourth or fifth month of gestation. Sphenoid sinuses are formed postnatally. None attains full size for several years.

PHYSIOLOGY OF THE SPECIAL SENSES
Physiology of the Eye

The cornea is the transparent structure of the eye composed mainly of stroma and with regularly arranged epithelium on the outer surface and a single layer of endothelial cells lining the inner surface. The anterior portion of the cornea is bathed in tears, and the posterior part is bathed with aqueous humor. The lens maintains a high intracellular potassium content and is bathed in a solution of relatively high sodium content. Interference with its metabolism results in sodium and water accumulations and loss of potassium. The aqueous humor contributes to the maintenance of intraocular pressure, supports lens metabolism, and is partly responsible for nutrition of the cornea. Tears are formed by the accessory lacrimal glands along the lid margin and conjunctival fornices. They are distributed over the eyeball by periodic involuntary blinking, which also causes a pumping action in the lacrimal drainage system. Tears are secreted in response to psychic stimuli and reflex stimuli.

The metabolism of the retina may be divided into a general metabolism required for cell integrity and a specialized metabolism related to photoreception and nerve impulse transmission. The general metabolism of the retina is dependent upon a continuous supply of glucose from the bloodstream. Interruption in blood supply for 6 minutes results in irreversible retinal degeneration. Attention has been directed to glutamic acid and glutamine in the retina because of their connecting link between carbohydrate and protein metabolism.

Some of the structures of the eye form an optical system which focuses the light rays from outside objects to form sharp images within the eye. Other structures react to the light rays that compose the images and give rise to nerve impulses which result in various sensations of form, contrast, and color.[1]

Photochemistry Electromagnetic energy must be absorbed to exert an effect. To initiate a chemical change, that portion of the electromagnetic field known as light must be absorbed by the pigment molecule of the disks in the intersegment of the rods and cones. The chemical change gives rise to a nervous impulse that is amplified in the retina and relayed to the brain where perception occurs.

The electromagnetic spectrum (EMS) contains many wavelengths that are either reflected, absorbed, or transmitted. The portion of the EMS with wavelengths between 400 and 700 nM is visible light and passes through the cornea and lens. It is absorbed by the photosensitive pigment in the rods and cones and initiates the chemical change that sets off the nervous impulse which, in turn, is transmitted to the brain and causes subjective sensation.[2]

The radiant energy of visible light is not colored. Color sensation is caused by the absorption of energy by the photosensitive visual pigments of the retina, of which there are three types responding to red, green, and blue. The color perceived depends upon the wavelength absorbed. Color blindness is believed to occur as a result of a deficiency or abnormality in the photosensitive pigments.

Neural Activity The formation of minute images by the rods and cones of the retina is not conveyed to the brain by the optic nerve as a neat colored picture. Each ganglion cell receives its imput from many receptors, but not all connections to the retina cause excitement. If this were so, vision would be blurred. By means of a complex code the rate of firing of the ganglion cell is increased or decreased. Although the nature of the integration of neural activity of the human retina is unknown, experiments on lower animals suggest that the retina carries on a complex filtering of information before passing it on to the brain. There appear to be inhibiting and excitatory cells present so that not all impulses are relayed, but there is little reorganization of incoming messages.

Refraction When a ray of light passes through one transparent medium to another, its velocity increases if the medium through which it is passed is less dense; the velocity decreases in a more dense medium. If the medium is not perpendicular to the ray of light, the emerging ray has a different direction from the entering ray. This change in direction is called *refraction* and is measured in focal length or diopters. The refractive surfaces of the eye are the cornea, the aqueous humor, and the lens. The anterior cornea is the chief refracting surface because it separates media of such different optical density as air and corneal substances. The lens at its anterior and posterior surfaces is convex, but because it is immersed in liquid on both sides, it has less refractive power than the cornea. Optically the lens behaves as though it were composed of a series of concentric lenses so that its total refractory index is greater than the individual portion of the lens.

Errors in refraction occur when there is a failure of refractory power of the anterior segment to correlate with the length of the segment. Two factors are involved: (1) refractory power of cornea and lens, and (2) the length of the eye. Most persons have good correlations so that parallel rays of light fall on the retina.

Accommodation The process by which the refractory power of the anterior segments increases in order that distant and near objects may be distinctively focused on the retina is termed *accommodation.* It is stimulated by a blurred image on the retina which gives rise to active contraction of the ciliary muscle resulting in relaxation of the zonule, in turn freeing the lens from compression force. The elasticity of the lens capsule allows the lens to assume the shape of a sphere. The lens which is soft and pliable in youth becomes harder and less compressible with age; the capsule becomes less elastic. The result is less of a change in shape and therefore a gradual loss of accommodation. The lens itself continues to grow throughout life and does not shed any of its cells; therefore its central portion becomes more compact and closed. There is a tendency toward myopia and eventual opacity. With age there is also an increased weakness of the ciliary muscle. All these factors result in decreased accommodation.

Physiology of the Ear

The eustachian tube in the middle ear has two major functions. It serves to equalize the air pressure in the middle ear with that of the outside, and it also provides a means of ventilating the middle ear. It protects the eardrum from being forced inward or outward when outside pressures increase or decrease, as happens with changes in altitude when flying.

The two muscles of the middle ear, the stapedius and tensor tympani, have two opposing functions: (1) to increase the sensitivity of the eardrum and the ossicular chain to signals of weak intensity and (2) to mediate the action of the ossicular chain when the eardrum receives an unusually intense stimulation. This latter aspect is important because of the protection it affords the inner ear.

The *round window,* another connection between

the middle and inner ears, is just below the *oval window.* It is covered with an elastic membrane and serves as a termination of the acoustic pathway of the inner ear. Both these windows communicate with different parts of the inner ear. The inner ear is both the end organ for hearing and the sensory organ for balance.

Physiology of Hearing

Air Conduction   The majority of the sounds heard are airborne because air conduction is much more sensitive than the mechanism of bone conduction. Sound waves in the environment are picked up by the pinna of the external ear, then directed into the external acoustic meatus where the sound waves exert a force on the eardrum. It in turn is set into vibration by the movements of the air particles. The handle of the malleus embedded in the eardrum sets the ossicular chain into vibration. The in-and-out vibration of the eardrum results in a rocking motion of the stapes in the oval window which produces a pressure wave in the perilymph. The ossicular chain transforms the energy collected by the eardrum into a greater force but with less movement, thus matching the impedance of the sound waves in the ear to that in the fluid in the vestibule. The inward movement of the footplate of the stapes produces pressure on the fluid of the inner ear, which is incompressible and which necessitates some provision for relief of the pressure. This is accomplished by the round window whose membrane reacts to the movements of the footplate in the stapes of the oval window. As the footplate pushes inward on the oval window toward the inner ear, the membrane of the round window is pushed outward toward the middle ear cavity.

The fluid motion from the oval to the round window is transmitted through the cochlear duct causing movement of the endolymph within it and also movement of the basilar membrane where the hair cells of the organ of Corti are located. The movement of the membrane results in its displacement, which in turn causes a shearing effect on the hair cells by the tectorial membrane above. The nerve impulse is thus initiated, then carried by the nerve fibers to the main trunk of the acoustic portion of the VIIIth cranial nerve, and finally received by the brain.

Bone Conduction   The inner ear is encased in bone so that vibrations of the bone are transmitted directly to the inner ear causing movement of the fluid. It is not necessary to produce vibration of the drum or ossicles. Bone conduction requires vibrations intense enough to set the bones of the skull in vibration. The sound waves must go through skin, soft tissue, and bones so that the wave is often distorted. However, the mechanism of bone conduction provides an alternative pathway for sound in those people who have impairment of air conduction.

Physiology of the Gustatory and Olfactory Organs

Taste and smell have some effect on the appetite, the beginning of digestion, and the avoidance of harmful substances. Gustation is present at birth, and salivation begins at about three months of age. Four primary sensations which are generally agreed on are sour, salty, sweet, and bitter. Acids cause a sour taste. Ionized salts elicit a salty taste. Many chemicals, such as sugars, glycols, alcohols, and ketones, are responsible for a sweet taste. A bitter taste is caused by alkaloids and long-chain organic substances. Many drugs, such as quinine, caffeine, strychnine, and nicotine, and many deadly toxins found in poisonous plants are alkaloids. The highly acute bitter taste sensation provides an important protective function in that, if it is intense, a person rejects the substance offered.

Most taste buds are located on the anterior and lateral surfaces of the tongue, but a few are found around the nasopharynx. Taste hairs (microvilli) in the taste buds, thought to provide the receptor surface for gustation, are found in three cranial nerves: facial (VII), glossopharyngeal (IX), and vagus (X).

Taste activation, adaptation, discrimination, and preference are not clearly understood. Since taste buds are chemoreceptors, a substance must be in solution to cause activation, but the actual mechanism is not known. Taste buds exhibit some adaptation. Although they react quickly to a substance, within a few seconds impulse rates become slow and steady. Prolonged exposure to most substances results in almost complete loss of taste. Further adaptation is thought to occur in the central nervous system. The classical version of taste discrimination holds that taste buds are specific to the four primary sensations of taste. In reality, any one bud will respond to all four, but perhaps more vigorously to a specific taste. Temperature, texture, and odor activate extragustatory receptors and may play a role in discrimination. The food preference mechanism to bodily needs is not understood. Taste reflexes are called forth by a little-understood mechanism whereby the secretion and consistency of saliva (dilute and watery versus thick and mucous) are controlled.

Olfaction is slight in the newborn and develops slowly, although the neonate does smell milk. The primary sensations of smell have not been classified with total success, but seven primary odors may be the following: camphorous, musky, floral, pepperminty, ethereal, pungent, and putrid. Only a minute quantity of the stimulus is required. Impulses proceed along the olfactory pathway to the central nervous system.

Olfactory cells are chemoreceptors. The exact mechanism of chemical stimulation is unknown, but the substance causing stimulation must have three qualities: volatility, slight water solubility, and lipid solubility. Thus it can be sniffed, pass through olfactory mucosa, and penetrate the olfactory hairs and outer tips of the olfactory cells. Olfactory responses may also vary with attentiveness, state of the olfactory membrane, hunger, status of neural mechanisms, and sex. Olfactory adaptation is more rapid than gustatory. As with taste, part of the olfactory adaptation is thought to occur in the central nervous system.

ASSESSMENT OF THE SENSES AND NURSING MANAGEMENT
Sensorimotor Stimulation

Touch is perhaps one of the most important avenues of learning. With it one can explore the environment, reach out, and become part of the world in all its dimensions. Without it one is physically isolated from the world. Touch, together with the rest of the senses, provides a complex system of communication and interaction, enabling a person to express to others his inner feelings and reactions and to perceive theirs. A handshake, a hug, a kiss—all have meaning to the giver and the receiver. All human beings have a desire to reach out and touch and to be touched.

The baby's perception of the world is built upon and shaped by his initial tactile experiences. Tabori postulates that tactuality is initiated in the uterus by friction during gestation and continues in the neonate in the general infant care activities of feeding, bathing, dressing, and handling.[3] As the baby is cared for and handled, the special senses become organized neurologically into a pattern of behavior which will greatly determine the child's subsequent development. A deviation in one sense, such as hearing, will affect the development of the other senses. For example, the deaf may reflect this handicap in defective speech. The blind infant relies upon his other senses to help him learn what the outside world looks like.

The alert nurse has within his repertoire of skills the ability to detect and assess potential or already present evidence of deviations in the special senses. Early detection of seemingly insignificant variations may greatly influence subsequent development. Prompt treatment instituted properly is often the major difference between elimination or modification of difficulties and the development of serious complications.

Assessment of Vision

The full-term infant has eyebrows and lids. Eyebrows which are bushy, overly heavy, or joined over the bridge of the nose may indicate an abnormality. The lids should close completely over the orbit when the baby is asleep, and there should be no epicanthal fold unless the infant is of Oriental parentage. Both eyes should open simultaneously and should be symmetrical and equidistant from the nose.

The infant has limited vision at birth. In the early postnatal days the eyes are very sensitive to light and are closed most of the time. By the end of 2 weeks the infant is able to look at large objects but does not follow them to any great extent. By 4 to 5 weeks he can look at relatively small objects, and can follow them by 8 to 10 weeks. Visual acuity gradually increases to include binocular vision, ocular mobility, convergence, and conjugate movements. Bright toys that dangle promote visual interest and encourage eye coordination. Infants respond to changes in their immediate environment and are more interested in looking at new objects with bright and unusual patterns.

Eye contact is an essential component of vision and the infant's relationship to people. An infant is able to momentarily fix his gaze on a human face within the first 6 weeks of life. Lack of eye contact between mother and infant may be predictive of a potential problem in the mother-infant relationship.

Examination of the Eye   This consists of observing the various structures of the eye and testing with special instruments. Testing for acuity of vision is done by use of various charts. Screening may be done by a person trained in the use of some tools, but definitive testing is possible only by an ophthalmologist. The optimal schedule for examinations is (1) in the neonatal period, (2) before entering school, and (3) at intervals of 2 years beginning at puberty. In addition the child should be examined whenever an abnormality is noted, vision appears to be defective, or an injury has been sustained. Strabismus should be brought to the attention of an ophthalmologist as soon as possible because it will not correct itself and cannot easily be treated after the age of 6. Myopia in a child under 5 or 6 years of age is usually associated with prematurity. Myopia is more common during puberty, while young children are more prone to hyperopia, with or without astigmatism.

Vision Screening   Visual testing should be done before the child is 4 years old. The critical period for developing acute vision is between 1 and 6 years of age because the learning ability of the eye decreases sharply after that period. However, according to the National Society for the Prevention of Blindness, organized preschool vision screening programs are most inadequate. Of the 16 million children in the United States between the ages of 3 and 6 years, only about 500,000 are tested annually.[4] About 1 in 20 children have visual problems of one kind or another, and early diagnosis is imperative if sight is to be preserved.

Vision screening is not intended to replace an ophthalmologic examination; it merely identifies the presence of a sight deficit. For example, amblyopia ("lazy eye") is a condition in which one eye is unable to focus on an object as well as the other eye. Since the brain automatically blocks out the poor vision of the weak eye, using only the clear image, the poorer eye is not used and vision deteriorates. If the presence of amblyopia is not detected before 6 years of age, a permanent visual deficit may result.

Home eye test kits are available to parents, especially those who reside in rural areas, which allow them to do vision screening tests at home. Once a problem has been identified, a further examination and diagnosis should be made by a physician. These kits may be obtained from the National Association for the Prevention of Blindness.

Testing Distance Vision   This testing is usually done by showing the child a series of symbols at a fixed distance. Several devices are available, and they include the Snellen standard tests, the Lebensohn chart for testing near vision, and the Schering children's eye chart.

By the age of 4 years nonliterate symbols can be used easily, and two of the most common tests are the use of E cards and pictures. When a picture of an E is presented to a child, he can cooperate in the testing if he has been instructed to point his fingers in the direction toward which the E is pointed. It is best to instruct these young children immediately before the procedure, for this brief training period may facilitate a better understanding of what is desired by the tester.

In the course of testing with the E cards, the nonliterate symbol is presented to the child in four directions with the "fingers" pointing to the left, right, up, or down. Initially it is done within reasonable proximity of the child; then the symbol is held a few feet away. When it has been determined that the child does understand what is devised, the E card is placed 20 feet away from him for the actual test. Typically, young children are interested in close objects, showing little interest in what is across the room. If such is the case, vision can be tested at 10 feet and then the findings can be transposed to obtain an accurate acuity reading.

Using individualized E cards appears to be less confusing to a young child and holds his attention for longer periods. One disadvantage may be the child's inability to indicate whether the legs of the symbol point to the left or to the right. If a set of E pictures is given to the child, he may choose a symbol that matches one being held by the tester, thereby eradicating the problem.

Picture charts are occasionally used in testing children. A major problem which may arise in utilizing this device is a child's inability to recall the word which identifies the picture, or he may be unfamiliar with the picture material. The Koehler picture test cards are preferred by some testers for use with young children, deaf mutes, and the retarded. The house, apple, and umbrella were chosen from the five pictures used in the Schering children's eye chart primarily for their interest and familiarity to children.

Increasing numbers of nurses are becoming involved in day care centers and preschool nurseries. In improving the health services provided, many have initiated eye testing as an integral part of assessment, or they have done vision screenings after teachers have brought the problem to them. Such actions are essential if the impaired vision of thousands of children is to be detected and rectified at a critical time in eye and intellectual development.

Common Signs of Eye Problems   Certain actions are characteristically performed by children who are having difficulty seeing: frequent rubbing of the eyes; shutting or covering an eye when reading or looking at or playing with a toy; tilting the head or thrusting it forward; and holding objects to be examined close to the eyes. School-age children may have difficulty reading, looking at the blackboard, or doing close work. They also blink more frequently, squint the eyelids together, or frown constantly.

Assessing the eyes is an important nursing responsibility. One should note strabismus or eyes which are red-rimmed, edematous, or encrusted. Watery, inflamed eyes are commonly seen in children with eye problems. Recurrent styes should prompt an ophthalmologic examination.

Young children may complain that their eyes itch, burn, or feel scratchy. All these symptoms should be investigated. Repeated complaints of a child's inability to see, especially in the classroom, should be followed up by the school nurse. After doing close work, some children with visual deficits state they feel dizzy, have headaches, or are nauseated. Verbalizations regarding blurred vision or the presence of diplopia are serious clinical manifestations which should be thoroughly investigated immediately.

Allergic responses of the eye   These responses of the eye may occur at any age, depending upon the specific allergy, and include edema of the lids, chemosis, hyperemia (redness), conjunctivitis, Dennie's sign, and allergic shiners.

Chemosis is defined as edema of the bulbar conjunctiva. In *allergic conjunctivitis,* the palpebral conjunctiva is milky, pale, and edematous, occurring only on the lower conjunctiva. *Vernal conjunctivitis* involves both upper and lower palpebral conjunctivae, the upper containing hard, flattened papillae. The patient complains of lacrimation, itching, and photophobia. Exudate is stringy and mucoid and contains eosinophils. It is treated with steroids. *Edema of the eyelids* is due to local irritants such as hair spray, powder, and nail polish. This edema is treated with steroids and local applications of cold for 5 minutes several times a day. Both Dennie's sign and allergic shiners involve the lower orbitopalpebral grooves. In *Dennie's sign,* lines radiate from the inner corner of the eye, slant downward, and end in a slight upward swing. *Allergic shiners* ("black eyes") are noted because of edema and discoloration of these grooves.

Assessment of Hearing

The infant in the newborn nursery is very responsive to loud noises within the first 2 to 3 days after birth. Unusual ear configuration may be indicative of congenital abnormalities, as is abnormal placement.

There are approximately 39,000 deaf children of school age in the United States who either were born deaf or lost their hearing before speech and language patterns were established.[5] If a hearing deficit is suspected, the infant should be referred to an audiologist whose specialty is the identification and measurement of hearing loss and the rehabilitation of those with hearing impairments.

Audiology is the offspring of two parents: speech pathology and otology. Speech pathology deals with the diagnosis and treatment of individuals who have problems in oral language, and otology is concerned with the diagnosis and treatment of individuals with ear disease or disorders of the peripheral mechanism of hearing. An otologist is a medical physician, whereas an audiologist has not had the medical education and training of the otologist.

There is no common agreement as to when a child's hearing should be tested, but some specialists recommend that infants who belong to the high-risk category be followed very carefully from the point of view of normal auditory behavior: response to sound, the human voice, and making verbal sounds. It is recommended that they be seen frequently during the first 2 years for a general follow-up which would include a hearing assessment.

All children attending well-baby clinics or coming to private pediatricians might be screened for hearing problems during the latter part of their first year. The ideal time to detect impairment is before 6 months of age in order to institute appropriate special care and treatment. Practical reasons may necessitate delaying testing until the last 6 months of the first year.

In recent years the public school systems have been assuming increased responsibility for hearing assessment programs. These programs vary from state to state, but an appropriate practice would include testing in the primary grades (Fig. 42-2). Children of this age have a higher incidence of upper respiratory infections and of tonsil and adenoid problems which usually respond to proper medical treatment. The purposes of a school hearing-conservation program are to reduce to an absolute minimum the number of children with permanently impaired hearing and to provide educational programs for those children whose hearing problems will not respond to medical or surgical treatment.

Testing Hearing in the Neonate   Hearing loss in the neonate can be detected by an instrument known as a Crib-O-Gram, an automated sensor which records on tape a newborn's movements before, during, and after a test sound is sent forth from a microphone near the bassinet. These recordings are scored at regular intervals to ascertain any changes in activity both with and without the test sound. Thus, spontaneous movements can be differentiated from activity in relation to sound. Thirty-two normal newborns can be tested at the same time. The sensor is also

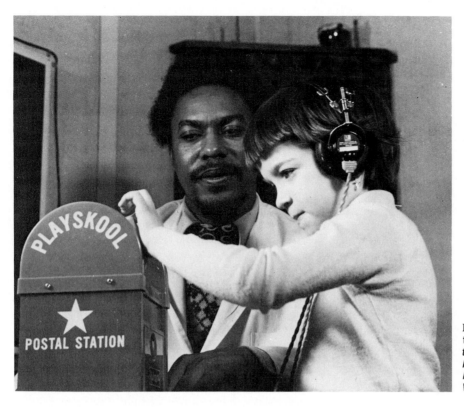

Figure 42-2   An audiologist tests a child's hearing. *(Courtesy of Media Center, Eunice Kennedy Shriver Center for Mental Retardation, Inc., Waltham, Mass.)*

capable of detecting heartbeats, respirations, and hiccoughs and scores them along with other motion. A portable unit is available for use in premature and intensive-care nurseries. More longitudinal study of the Crib-O-Gram is needed to determine its effectiveness as a mass screening technique.[6]

Testing Hearing in the Toddler or Older Child   The acoustic nerve is divided into two parts, the cochlear and the vestibular nerves. The latter is not tested routinely; however, the cochlear nerve can be tested quickly without the need for additional tools. Moving a ticking watch away from the ear until the child cannot hear it is a quick method of evaluating his hearing. The child is instructed to state when he no longer hears the sound. In order to determine bone and air conduction, a tuning fork is placed on the mastoid bone until the patient can no longer hear sound. The vibrating portion of the tuning fork is then placed next to the ear to check air conduction. Normally air conduction is about twice as long as bone conduction. It is important to understand that such testing does not give quantitative data. These results indicate hearing deficits or bone or ear conduction problems which require audiometric testing.

Auditory Training   Before a child is placed in a training program, it is important that his hearing loss be carefully analyzed by a professional trained in testing and evaluation. The way in which he responds to testing will determine whether he will benefit from a hearing aid and what type would be best for him. The child with a profound hearing loss will need a training program which begins with learning to recognize gross sounds, in contrast to the child with a specific type of hearing problem who has difficulty in hearing speech at higher frequencies but has good hearing for low frequencies. Either child may or may not benefit from a hearing aid.

If the child needs a hearing aid, training him in its use is almost always necessary. If he has never experienced sound amplification, learning to use a hearing aid may be very difficult. The overall objectives of an auditory training program are to teach the child how to operate his hearing aid and to persuade him to wear it. He must learn how to control the tone and volume of the aid, how to change the battery, how to connect the receiver to the earpiece, how to insert and remove the earpiece, and how to wear the instrument comfortably. Some experimentation is usually necessary to determine volume control. The audiologist, not the child, has this responsibility because the child may set the volume too high and suffer additional hearing loss.

The parents of the child must be involved in every phase of the auditory training program. Frequently counseling the parents precedes training the child since their attitude toward the hearing problem and the auditory training program will affect his adjustment and attitude. Whoever will influence the child's daily activities should understand his special needs in order to help him feel comfortable with his handicap and not set apart by it.

NURSING MEASURES IN CARE OF THE SPECIAL SENSES
Postoperative Care of Eye and Ear Patients

The child who is undergoing treatment for a condition involving the eyes or ears often faces the prospect of surgical correction. Depending upon his age, the child may or may not understand the reason or be prepared for what will happen to him.

Surgical intervention usually results in a change in either vision or hearing which may be permanent or temporary. Following surgery there may be a temporary diminution of function due to edema and/or a dressing. It is important therefore that the nurse know what the physician plans to do in order to interpret both to parents and child what to expect postoperatively.

Following surgery it is often necessary to restrain the child's arms to prevent trauma induced by touching the operative site or dislodging the dressing. The pediatric nurse realizes that the lesser the amount of restriction imposed on a child, the less is the anxiety and the more cooperative the child will be. Elbow restraints are less inhibiting to movement than wrist restraints but at the same time prevent his being able to touch his head. It may be necessary to prevent him from lying on the operative site so that sandbags on either side of his head, a jacket-type restraint, or both may be used until the child has recovered from anesthesia sufficiently and is able to participate in maintaining the prescribed position.

Whether a dressing will be used may vary with the physician as well as with the procedure. If one or both eyes will be bandaged, the effect on the child's emotional status must be anticipated. Not to be able to see what is going on around him may produce a variety of fantasies and fears. It is important that the child be acquainted with his surroundings and those who will be caring for him prior to surgery. Following surgery, sounds which he was unaware of previously may take on a variety of unusual and anxiety-provoking meanings. The sensitive nurse will indicate his approach in a calm reassuring voice and will tell the child what is planned before touching him. The nurse must explain once more the reasons for the restraints and side rails. The older child may consider side rails an affront to his maturity, but the empathetic nurse can explain their purpose and reassure the child that their usage is temporary.

The child who has had ear surgery will usually wear some type of dressing. Otoplasty may require a large pressure dressing wrapped around the entire head with only the face exposed. The youngster who is having plastic repair may indeed be frightened to find himself encased in such a manner. Comparing the dressing with a football helmet may ease his fear.

The instillation of medications may begin soon after eye surgery. The eyelids may become crusted and edematous. Gentle washing with a warm saline solution will alleviate some of the discomfort. It is important to prevent vomiting, which causes increased pressure within the eye. Fluids and solids are given as soon as possible to promote regular kidney and bowel function. Bed exercises are instituted to maintain good muscle tone. Ambulation in some instances may be allowed the day after surgery since it will exert both physical and psychologic advantages to the child regardless of age.

Eye and Ear Medications and Treatments   In instilling eye drops in an infant, care must be taken not to cause pressure on the eyeball. To instill eye drops in an infant's eyes, his head is held steady with his nose toward the ceiling. The medication is dropped on the inner canthus of the eye. Eventually the infant will blink, and the drops will enter the eye socket. Ointments are applied along the inner margin of the lower lid. Excess is then gently removed with a sterile cotton ball.

Ear drops are instilled by holding the pinna down and back to straighten the external ear canal in a child under 3 years of age. The child should be lying down and instructed to lie on the unaffected side for a few minutes following the treatment.

Parents should participate in the child's care pre- and postoperatively and may require guidance in learning how to communicate with their child when his sight and hearing are limited.

Contact Lenses   Although eye glasses are preferred in correcting refractive errors in children, in certain situations ophthalmologists may recommend plastic contact lenses. There are advantages to contact lenses. Common problems associated with the wearing of eye glasses, such as dirty glasses, loosened frames, and broken lenses, are eliminated. Contact lenses permit children and adolescents to participate in sports and active play without the danger of loss or breakage.

Several disadvantages of lenses also need to be stated. The wearer must be taught how to insert and remove them, and such teaching may be time-consuming. The cost of contact lenses is high initially but not greater than the cost of frequently replacing or repairing eye glasses. Initial minor eye discomfort in adjusting to contact lenses is another disadvantage, especially for children with low corneal tolerance.

Various methods of cleaning and storing contact lenses are commonly used. It is important for the nurse to know what instructions were given to the patient by his ophthalmologist. Secondary corneal infections may occur as a result of improper care and storage. Once the contact lenses have been removed, they should be placed in dry, well-ventilated, and properly marked (left, right) containers. Solutions or moist containers are excellent media for pathogens and should therefore never be used. Generally, storage containers for contact lenses should be boiled once a week.

A nurse should know how to remove contact lenses from the eyes of a patient who is unable to perform the task himself. Such a situation may occur when a child in unconscious. Lenses do not affect pupillary responses, but they need to be removed often to prevent corneal irritation. Apparatus specifically designed for removing contact lenses may be available for use; however, a tiddlywink maneuver or a suction cup will facilitate their removal. The rubber bulb of a glass eyedropper may also be used. After the bulb is wet and compressed, it may be lowered on to the lens and the lens lifted off the cornea with manual suction.

Care of the Nose Whenever the nasal mucosa is inflamed, exudate forms. Before a child learns how to blow his nose, drainage is facilitated when the infant or young child is placed in a prone position and the foot of the bed is raised. Nasal bulb syringes may also be used to withdraw exudate in the anterior nares, but they are relatively ineffective. The anterior nares may also be cleansed with a twisted cotton cone slightly moistened with water: with gentle circular motion, the exudate is collected. Excoriation is prevented by applying cold cream or petrolatum to irritated areas about the nostrils and upper lip.

Nose drops are instilled into the nares every 3 to 4 hours if obstruction due to exudate is present.

Nose drops shrink the nasal mucosa and relieve congestion by decreasing nasal discharge. They should be instilled 15 to 20 minutes before feedings to facilitate breathing through the nose while sucking. They are repeated at bedtime. To ensure that drops come in contact with the nasal mucosa, the infant's or child's neck should be extended. This position is maintained for approximately one minute following instillation.

The preschooler can be taught to blow his own nose. Some people maintain that he should learn to blow from both nostrils at the same time while his mouth is open—others advocate blowing from one nostril while the other is occluded with pressure from the finger.

Both dental caries and infected teeth may exacerbate rhinitis, nasopharyngitis, and sinusitis. Therefore, nurses should stress the importance of dental hygiene, regular dental checks, and diet in their health teaching to parents and children.

SENSORY DISEASES AND DEVIATIONS IN THE NEWBORN
Retrolental Fibroplasia

Retrolental fibroplasia is seen most commonly in premature infants who have received oxygen at concentrations above 40 percent for a prolonged period during the early days of life. High concentrations of oxygen are toxic to the retina. Since this complication is rare in infants who have received concentrations of less than 40 percent, retrolental fibroplasia is believed to be secondary to partial pressures of oxygen in the blood which are above the 100 mm Hg seen under normal conditions while breathing air. Raising the oxygen concentration to 40 percent results in partial pressures of 140 to 150 mm Hg in the pink infant. Since the cyanotic infant's partial pressure is well below 100 mm Hg, he can usually withstand an oxygen concentration of less than 40 percent, and thus retinal toxicity can be prevented. The need for a higher concentration is determined by the physician. Excessive oxygen therapy results in constriction of the arterioles followed by dilation and tortuosity of the retinal vessels, hemorrhage and edema, and, ultimately, retinal detachment resulting in blindness.

The nurse should ensure that oxygen concentration does not exceed 40 percent unless ordered by the physician. Oxygen concentrations are analyzed and recorded every 4 hours. If a newborn, of necessity, has received higher oxygen concentrations for a period of time, the nurse should impress upon the parents the need for frequent eye examinations for at least 3 months to determine the status of the infant's retina.

Congenital Cataracts

In fetal life, congenital cataracts develop anytime during the formation of the lens (sixth or seventh week). By the twelfth week of gestation three very important events are occurring: the lens is still developing, the heart is forming its chambers, and the brain is undergoing development of a critical nature. Trauma, anoxia, or maternal systemic disease during the first trimester of pregnancy may have a very profound effect.

Congenital cataracts may be bilateral or unilateral and range from minimal involvement to complete opacification. Cataracts may be congenital or acquired. They are among the most common defects as a result of congenital rubella syndrome; are often genetically determined; may be caused by toxoplasmosis, hypocalcemia, and galactosemia; or may follow uveitis, retinitis, retrolental fibroplasia, retinal detachment, or retinitis pigmentosa. Other abnormalities, both ocular and otherwise, often are associated with congenital cataracts.

While an intracapsular extraction is performed in adults, an extracapsular operation is used for infants and children. The eye is not completely developed, and the lens is usually attached to the vitreous. Therefore, if the lens is removed via an intracapsular extraction, the vitreous is also extracted, resulting in an empty shell. Although the nucleus is easily removed extracapsularly, the tenacious, gummy cortical material is removed piecemeal and requires repeated washings through a good opening created during surgery. The newest treatment for the removal of cataracts is phacoemulsion. A special machine emulsifies the lens, and the lens contents are aspirated. Care is taken not to break the posterior capsule of the lens as vitreous would be lost.

Postoperative prognosis is guarded because of the high percentage of associated defects. Surgery is postponed until 2 years of age in children whose cataracts are a result of maternal rubella, because the virus may be activated if the operation is done earlier. If a child has a corrected vision of 20/50 or better, surgery is usually not done. When one eye is normal and the other eye has a complete cataract, surgery is deferred until the child is older, usually until adolescence for cosmetic reasons. The teenager then has monocular fixation in the uninvolved eye and possibly 20/50 vision in the affected eye through either a contact lens or placement of a prosthetic lens within the anterior chamber of the eye. If both eyes are moderately involved, the ophthalmologist's and pediatrician's decisions for management are guided by the child's school progress and social functioning.

When the child returns from surgery, he has a loose eye patch in place. With modern suture techniques early ambulation is encouraged, and the child may be out of bed on the operative day. On the fourth postoperative day, the dressing is removed, and topical eye drops are instilled three to four times a day in diminishing doses over a 6-week period. Atropine-like eye drops keep the pupil enlarged and thereby keep the eye at rest, in effect "splinting" the eye. Steroids and antibiotics may be supplied in one mixture. A bandage or shield is applied at night for additional protection, for example, to prevent rubbing. The average hospital stay is 6 days. Discharge instructions include avoidance of all activities which increase intraocular pressure. A relatively high late complication occurring 20 or more years postoperatively is retinal detachment.

Nursing Management Once an infant has been diagnosed as having cataracts and the physician has discussed the cause, prognosis, and treatment with the parents, the nurse may need to help the parents digest all the information which has been given. Anticipatory guidance regarding developmental problems and hospitalization should also be provided.

Postoperatively, the nurse carries out treatments. By involving the parents in the child's care, the nurse can teach them how to instill eye drops and instruct them regarding diminishing doses over the 6-week period. Parents may also have questions about home care.

Ophthalmia Neonatorum

The term *ophthalmia neonatorum* refers to any acute conjunctivitis in the newborn, regardless of cause. The origin may be chemical, bacterial, or rickettsial. In acute conjunctivitis, the conjunctiva is red and edematous. A mucopurulent discharge is present. Prophylactic instillation of silver nitrate into the newborn's eyes may result in these clinical manifestations for 24 to 48 hours, especially when the silver nitrate has not been freshly prepared. This condition must be differentiated from gonorrheal conjunctivitis. If the symptoms are chemical in cause, smear and culture are sterile. Treatment consists of keeping the eyes clean via sterile water irrigations. Some physicians may treat chemical conjunctivitis with Gantrisin to prevent secondary infection.

Gonorrheal conjunctivitis is usually contracted from an infected mother during the birth process. Clinical manifestations begin 2 to 5 days following birth and include a profuse purulent discharge, redness and chemosis (edema) of the conjunctiva, and edematous eyelids. If contracted in utero from premature rupture of the membranes, corneal ulcers may result. Diagnosis is confirmed with a positive smear and culture. Treatment consists of systemic penicillin and local chemotherapeutic agents.

Inclusion blennorrhea occurs 5 to 10 days after birth presenting with a purulent discharge and a cobblestone appearance of the conjunctiva. The condition is caused by *Chlamydia oculogenitalis* of the family Chlamydiaceae, order Rickettsiales. This rickettsia is an intraepitheleal invader. Therefore, the organism and inclusion bodies are found in conjunctival scrapings rather than in the discharge. The newborn contracts inclusion blennorrhea during labor from the infected mother's birth canal. The same organism causes "swimming pool" conjunctivitis (from contaminated urine) and nonspecific urethritis and cervicitis in adults. There is some speculation that *Chlamydia* organisms are attenuated forms of trachoma. Inclusion blennorrhea responds to sulfonamides and tetracyclines. Treatment lasts for 10 days.

Nursing Management The nurse should observe newborns for edema of the conjunctiva and purulent discharge from the eyes and report such occurrences promptly to the physician. If the conjunctivitis is gonorrheal in origin, the infant is isolated. When caring for the infant, the nurse should wear protective goggles to prevent contamination of his own eyes. Pus in the infant's conjunctival sac may spurt into the air or into the nurse's eyes on eversion of the infant's lids. Parents should be reassured that prompt and adequate treatment results in a complete cure.

Congenital Lesions of the Ear

Although minor congenital anomalies of the ear occur frequently, serious malformations and congenital tumors (i.e., hemangiomas, lymphangiomas, and dermoid tumors) are rare. Malformed *low-set ears* may be indicative of other congenital anomalies, such as renal abnormalities, mental retardation, and mandibulofacial dysostosis. Sometimes auricular malformations are found. An absent auricle is termed *anotia*. *Microtia* denotes an extremely small auricle, while *macrotia* is the medical term for an extremely large auricle. "*Lop ear*," which is the result of ab-

sence of both the antihelix and superior crus, may be corrected with plastic surgery. Unless cartilage or a broad base is present, *accessory auricular skin tags* are ligated; otherwise, surgical intervention is necessary. Hereditary *sinus tracts* or *cutaneous* dimples situated anterior to and above the tragus do not require surgery unless recurrent infection occurs. Since *extoses* and *chondromas* of the auditory canal are usually small, they seldom necessitate removal. If *atresia* of the external auditory canal is present, the infant must be assessed for abnormalities of the external or middle ear. Through x-ray, the status of the bony canal, ossicles, and middle ear cavity can be determined. Reconstructive surgery may be attempted if the elements necessary for conductive hearing are present. In or near the lobule *sebaceous cysts* frequently occur. Although they enlarge periodically causing slight tenderness, they subside spontaneously.

Nursing Management Nurses in newborn nurseries and ambulatory settings should be cognizant of the relationship between abnormalities of the ear and other congenital anomalies. Any such observations should be brought to the physician's attention.

SENSORY DISEASES AND DEVIATIONS IN THE INFANT
Trachoma

Trachoma is one of the most common blinding diseases in the world. In the United States it is endemic in parts of the South and Southwest and on various Indian reservations. The cause is viral, and it is a member of the psittacosis-lymphogranuloma group of agents. Trachoma usually begins with a redness of the conjunctiva, most frequently involving the upper lid, very similar to a mild, purulent conjunctivitis. There is a gradual subconjunctival infiltration, with the formation of follicles. As the disease advances, there is follicular erosion and rupture, with the development of scar tissue.

The disease progresses slowly, and inflammation may persist for years. There is always corneal involvement with an infiltration of tiny, white, opaque specks noted on the periphery of the cornea and extending to the pupil. Corneal ulcerations may appear, and pain and photophobia are also present. A superimposed bacterial infection intensifies the dangers to the cornea as well as the entire eye. Without treatment damage to the eyes is severe.

Antibiotics and sulfonamides are used in treating trachoma, being administered locally and systemically. Cycloplegic drops relieve the photophobia, and most of the symptoms subside by the eighth or ninth day of therapy. The amount of residual damage depends on the time of diagnosis. Scarring of the conjunctiva or cornea may require surgical reconstruction later.

Nursing Management A nursing assessment of the eye is imperative. Its size, whether redness is apparent, and whether drainage is present are important considerations, particularly since this eye problem is similar to the mild, purulent conjunctivitis seen frequently in infants.

It is important to teach parents how to instill the medications properly and to adhere to the schedule devised. In view of the presence of photophobia, explanations should focus on methods whereby light may be decreased, thus alleviating the condition. These measures should include keeping the infant out of direct sunlight by lowering the shades in his room and using indirect lighting in his bedroom. As the condition improves, photophobia disappears. At the same time parents may need reassurance that the baby's fussiness is the result of pain he is experiencing and that this problem will diminish as the antibiotics take effect and the eye improves. Long-term follow-up care with subsequent eye testing is important in order to identify and resolve any visual impairment.

Congenital Glaucoma (Infantile, Developmental)

Primary developmental glaucoma, an autosomal recessive characteristic, is a disease which is generally diagnosed before the end of the first year of life. About fifty percent are identified soon after birth. An anomaly in the angle of the anterior chamber interferes with drainage of the aqueous humor and results in an increase in intraocular pressure. The globe enlarges as a result of the continued increase in intraocular pressure, giving the eye a characteristic appearance of buphthalmos ("cow eye").

Clinical manifestations include tearing, photophobia, a dilated pupil, and an increase in corneal diameter. A corneal haziness which is evident is due to the edema present.

The threat to normal vision is serious, and the prognosis is poor if the condition is not treated. While ocular tension can be temporarily controlled with the use of carbonic anhydrase inhibitors, such as acetazolamide (Diamox) which suppresses the secretory function of aqueous humor, the treatment of choice is surgical intervention. It is important to understand that the antiglaucoma drops used by adults do not influence the elevated intraocular ten-

sion in these children. A procedure known as a *goniotomy* is performed, in which an incision is made through the obstructing mesodermal tissue in the angle of the anterior chamber to facilitate drainage.

When diagnosed early, there is a high rate of success, although the procedure may be repeated two or three times. Best results are obtained in children under the age of 1 year. If the cornea was hazy and enlarged before the procedure, the operation may not be as successful as in those cases where the disease had not progressed to that extent.

Nursing Management Patients admitted for a goniotomy are usually accustomed to eye drops and tonometric readings; however, this knowledge does not negate additional preparation where possible. In the postoperative phase eye patches are in place, and the patient is kept as quiet as possible. Eye medications are administered according to the physician's orders, usually every 2 hours. Tonometric readings the morning after surgery usually evaluate the effectiveness of the procedure. Restraints are required if the patient is too young to comprehend. An important nursing observation immediately postoperative is the overall status of the patient. Occasionally increasing restlessness may identify increasing intraocular pressure. Patients are discharged a day or two after the procedure, and parents are advised of the eye medications and to return to the clinic or office for follow-up examinations of the infant and subsequent tonometric readings.

Infections of the Ear

The most common ear infection in childhood is *acute otitis media*, which usually occurs secondary to a respiratory tract infection with the causative agents being transported to the middle ear by the lymphatics. Pneumococci, streptococci, and *Hemophilus influenzae* are the most common organisms involved. The infant with otitis media tugs at or rubs his ears and is more irritable than usual. The older child frequently complains of deafness as well as popping noises in his ears. In the presence of a mild inflammation a dull, throbbing earache, nausea, and vomiting also occur.

The inflammatory process usually subsides once the patient receives systemic antibiotics such as ampicillin and penicillin; however, there may be a spontaneous perforation of the tympanic membrane with immediate relief. If symptoms persist and the child has a painful, bulging drum and acute pain and is febrile, a myringotomy may be done. This procedure involves incising the tympanic membrane to relieve the pain and allow the drum to heal.

The otitis media resolves itself in about a week. If the fluid is not drained, it may become thick and viscous, resulting in a "glue ear." If the condition is not detected, hearing loss may occur and language retardation may become evident at a later date.

Chronic otitis media occurs when acute otitis media remains untreated or is treated inadequately. A discharge may or may not be present; however, the tympanic membrane is usually perforated. Systemic antibiotics are sufficient in treating a chronic case. On rare occasions a *tympanoplasty* may be necessary. This procedure restores the conductive hearing loss which resulted from the perforation. It may range from as simple a procedure as a myringoplasty, which closes the drum, to a procedure in which fascia grafts and prosthetics are used to reconstruct the sound-conduction mechanism.

An effusion of a serous or mucoid exudate in the middle ear is *serous otitis media* and is a cause of deafness in older children. Usually it is treated by a paracentesis of the tympanic membrane followed by a regimen of systemic antibiotics. When drainage is insufficient, polyethylene tubes are inserted through the membrane to facilitate drainage and enhance healing. These tubes remain in place for several weeks (draining the material off), and then they are removed.

Nursing Management Frequently ear infections are treated in a physician's office or clinic. When antibiotics are prescribed, the nurse should emphasize the regular time interval to be followed in order to maintain adequate blood levels.

When a child is hospitalized for a tympanoplasty, routine preoperative care and teaching should be done. Postoperatively the patient has a dressing in place, which the nurse observes for bleeding or drainage. The outer dressing can be replaced as necessary; however, the inner dressing should be changed by the physician only. The child is hospitalized for 3 or 4 days before resuming his normal activities.

Congenital Obstruction of the Nasolacrimal Duct (Dacryostenosis)

A congenital obstruction of the nasolacrimal duct occurs in about 1 percent of all newborns. The most common cause is a plugging of the lower portion of the duct by epithelial debris. Failure of the duct to open (in 10 percent of patients seen) after conserva-

tive measures is usually attributed to the presence of a thin membrane over the nasal end of the duct.

Constant tearing, or *epiphora*, is noted in the first few weeks of life. Inflammatory signs are absent initially. Should the condition persist without medical intervention, the sac may well become infected and pus will be present.

The nasolacrimal passage may open spontaneously; however, the obstruction may persist. In those cases stricture and permanent obstruction may develop, further complicating the problem. Early treatment includes massaging the area over the sac to clear the duct. Irrigations may also be done to facilitate removal of the debris. If irrigations are done two or three times without success, the lacrimal duct may be probed.

In young infants irrigations are the only successful means of determining patency of the canal. In older children a drop of 2 percent merbromin (Mercurochrome) or fluorescein may be instilled into the conjunctival sac to determine the presence of dacryostenosis. After 2 minutes the child is asked to blow his nose. If the canal is patent, there is a discoloration on the tissue. The dye does not appear if an obstruction is present.

Nursing Management The conservative method of treating dacryostenosis is teaching parents how to correctly massage the area over the region of the sac. Impressing them with the importance of conscientiously performing this task many times a day is imperative.

Probing the duct, once that decision is made, means that the parents should be prepared for the procedure. Should the probing be done in the operating room with a general anesthetic administered to the young patient, all essential principles relevant to postoperative care should be implemented. If a general anesthetic is not used and the physician elects to perform this procedure in a treatment room or his office, the nurse will need to choose an effective method of restraining the infant.

Nasopharyngitis

Acute nasopharyngitis (the common cold) involves the nasopharynx, the accessory paranasal sinuses, and frequently the middle ear. Although the causative agent includes a large number of viruses, the principal ones are most likely rhinoviruses. The incubation period is 12 to 72 hours, and the infectious period lasts from a few hours before to 24 to 48 hours after symptoms have appeared. It is transmitted by droplet infection. Predisposing factors are suspected, but not proved, to be teething, poor nutrition, chilling, exposure to dampness and cold, degree of susceptibility and resistance, and allergy.

Clinical manifestations in infants and young children differ from those in older children. Before 3 months of age, infants are usually afebrile. Children beyond 3 years of age usually have low-grade fevers and are more prone to persistent sinusitis. Infants over 3 months of age are febrile, often as high as 102 to 104°F (38.9 to 40°C). Sneezing, irritability, and restlessness are common. Within a few hours, nasal discharge appears. Nasal obstruction interferes with sucking during feedings. The eardrums may be congested for 2 or 3 days. Since infants react systemically to infection, vomiting and diarrhea may be present.

Treatment consists of antipyretics for fever, malaise, and irritability; tepid-water sponge baths for fever over 103°F (39.4°C), fluids at frequent intervals, and nose drops. The drops most commonly used are Neo-Synephrine 0.25 percent and ephedrine 0.5 to 1.0 percent, one to two drops 15 to 20 minutes before feeding and at bedtime. For young infants, normal saline drops may be ordered. Oil-base drops are never given, since they may be aspirated and cause lipid pneumonia. Nose drops are never given for more than 4 or 5 days. Overuse of nose drops can irritate the nasal mucosa.

Nursing Management Unless complications such as febrile convulsions and superimposed infection ensue, infants are treated on an ambulatory basis. Therefore, the nurse's role is mainly one of teaching and counseling the parents. Parents must understand how to give the exact amount of antipyretic and nose drops and at what times. They need to know how and when to give a tepid-water sponge bath. The nurse should discuss the importance of fluids, prevention of excoriation of the skin due to exudate, and prevention of secondary infection. Parents should also be alerted to the signs and symptoms of complications and urged to call if any appear.

SENSORY DISEASES AND DEVIATIONS IN THE TODDLER
Strabismus (Squint, "Crossed-eyes")

Eye movement is controlled by the muscles of the eye, and any imbalance in intraocular muscles results in one or both eyes deviating, rather than functioning as a unit; this condition is known as *strabismus*. In early infancy movements of the eye bear little relationship to one another; however, by the sixth month convergence should be established.

There are several types of strabismus. *Internal strabismus* (convergent, also called *esotropia*) results in the eye turning inward. It may be congenital or acquired. In order for the child to see more clearly, he must accommodate (the muscle of accommodation shifts the focus from near to far or vice versa), and in doing so convergence results. Most children are farsighted (hyperopic), requiring greater accommodation; hence the frequency of this type of strabismus. *External strabismus* (divergent, also called *exotropia*) occurs when the eye turns "out." It has a later onset than the internal type and is associated with little or no refractive error. *Vertical strabismus* may be hypertropic, when the eye is above the visual axis, or hypotropic with the eye below the visual axis. These children have ocular deviations as a result of overactive or underactive oblique and vertical rectus bulbi muscles.

A persistent strabismus without treatment may result in a loss of vision in the deviating eye (amblyopia). If not corrected, the visual deficit may be permanent.

Refractive errors are a major cause of strabismus. The high degree of hyperopia in children gives rise to the overconvergence which results in convergent strabismus. Conversely, myopia is responsible for an underconvergence and divergent strabismus. Corneal scarring, cataracts, or optic atrophy all interfere with vision, interrupt fusion, and result in strabismus. Congenital deformities of the orbit of the eye, or the extraocular muscles as well as diseases or injuries to these structures or to the nerves which supply them, make binocular cooperation difficult and strabismus almost inevitable.

Treatment may entail any one or all four of the following. After an eye examination glasses may be prescribed to correct the refractive error and control the excessive accommodation. The eye will then be in a better position to develop binocular vision. The second step in treatment may include an occlusion of the straight eye with elastic tape, thereby forcing the squinting eye into activity. The third step may involve orthoptic training, with exercises especially devised for these children to perform. This ocular physiotherapy is concerned with restoring binocular function or assisting in its development. The last option is surgery. One of two types of procedures may be employed. When a *resection* is done, the intraocular muscles are shortened, while a *recession* refers to a lengthening of these muscles.

Nursing Management Successful treatment of the child with strabismus is related to the teaching of parents and children. The care is long term, and necessitates office or clinic visits every 6 to 12 months.

If glasses are prescribed, children should be taught how to care for them and how to clean them. Should they be broken, replacement is imperative. Some of the children may need encouragement to wear these prescription lenses.

Patients with occlusive patches should wear them constantly during the 6- or 8-week period in which they will be utilized. If they become loose or are removed, they, too, should be replaced immediately. Since the parents and children may not understand the rationale, a nurse should spend time explaining why the "straight," good eye is patched, and her comments should focus on improving the amblyopia. The teacher should be contacted so that he knows why the child's schoolwork may be substandard initially.

When all conservative efforts to correct the strabismus have not been as successful as desired by the ophthalmologist, surgery may be performed. Preoperative teaching includes preparing the child for eye patches (if they are used by the surgeon) and restraints. The child may be confined to bed the first 24 to 48 hours, and appropriate diversional activities will need to be selected. When the patient is being fed, a running commentary of what he is being given is appreciated. Eye drops or ointments are administered as ordered, following sterile normal saline eye irrigations. The entire hospitalization may be 3 or 4 days.

Orbital Neoplasms

Hemangioma A *hemangioma* is a benign growth of primitive, endothelial cells. While it may involve the skin of the upper or lower eyelids, the hemangioma may also be demonstrated within the orbit of the eye with the appearance of an exophthalmos. A biopsy is generally performed to rule out the presence of a sarcoma. About 20 percent are identified at birth, and the remainder diagnosed weeks after delivery.

A hemangioma may progress at an alarming rate for 6 to 9 months and then gradually regress. Hemangiomas in children are diffuse, making treatment difficult. With regression possible at a later date, surgery, irradiation, or sclerosing agents are not employed immediately. Conservative treatment entails a waiting period which may last several months or even years. The treatment of choice for cosmetic

reasons or for a rapidly progressive exophthalmos is radiation therapy. This treatment is used only after careful consideration because radiation therapy may harm the growth centers of bones, resulting in facial deformities later in life.

Glioma A *glioma* (astrocytoma) of the optic nerve is usually diagnosed after the child demonstrates an exophthalmos, complains of a loss of vision, and on examination there is no pupillary response to light. It is seen in a large number of patients with neurofibromatosis or von Recklinghausen's disease.

This type of primary tumor grows slowly and does not metastasize. It may involve the optic chiasm as well as optic tracts extending into the cranium through the optic canal. Surgery is the treatment of choice, although it results in loss of sight in the affected eye.

Rhabdomyosarcoma The most common primary maligancy of the orbit seen in children is rhabdomyosarcoma. The most common symptoms are diplopia and proptosis and their onset is rapid. Since the tumor grows rapidly, it may extend into the brain, with subsequent metastasis. Treatment consists of exenteration, radiation, and chemotherapy. With early diagnosis and treatment, 30 to 40 percent of affected children survive.

Neuroblastoma A *neuroblastoma* frequently metastasizes to the orbit from a primary site in the adrenal gland. Clinical manifestations include exophthalmos with an associated ecchymosis. These symptoms may be the first indication of a retroperitoneal neuroblastoma. An exenteration of the orbit may be necessary because of the tremendous exophthalmos, which develops rapidly.

Nursing management These tumors, benign or malignant, reiterate the essential task of examining the eyes and eyelids closely, in addition to pursuing complaints of a visual problem—diplopia or loss of vision. No redness or ecchymosis should be discussed without an examination.

If radiation is used, parents and patients must be prepared by the nurse for the treatment and the possible sequel. The radiologic markings on the head should be explained and the patient warned not to wash them off. A trip to radiology to look at the equipment may make the patient more cooperative and aware of what to expect.

Nursing responsibilities include preoperative teaching and postoperative monitoring of vital signs, dressing inspection, and observation of the patient's overall behavior and his response to the resumption of fluid and food intake and normal activities.

Patients who must have an exenteration of the orbit for the removal of a rapidly growing rhabdomycosarcoma or neuroblastoma demand skillful nursing care from a professional who knows the radical nature of this procedure. The contents of the orbit are completely evacuated, extending to the bone. Everything which lies within the boundary of the orbital rims is excised—including the lids. It is a mutilating type of surgery reserved for extreme situations. The child and his family will require extensive preparation. Since the principles of pre- and postoperative nursing care are similar to those described in caring for patients with retinoblastoma, the reader is referred to the following section.

Retinoblastoma   The highly malignant tumor known as a *retinoblastoma* almost always occurs in the first year of life, and is seldom diagnosed beyond the fifth year. It is hereditary, and the mode of transmission is thought to be autosomal recessive. Although it is seen more commonly in one eye, this tumor is present bilaterally in about twenty-five percent of affected infants.

A common sign is the white appearance of the pupil identified by parents. Convergence of an eye may also be a clinical manifestation of the tumor, and whenever strabismus is noted, an extensive ophthalmic examination should be done to rule out its presence. Redness, which is sometimes seen, indicates an advanced tumor. Pain in the eye, present because of the glaucoma which has developed, occurs in the final phase of the tumor. There are four commonly seen stages of development: (1) intraocular growth, (2) secondary glaucoma, (3) extraocular involvement, and (4) metastasis.

A careful examination by an ophthalmologist, in addition to x-rays of the affected eye which reveal calcium particles in the retinoblastoma, confirms the diagnosis. The highly malignant nature of this tumor makes immediate surgical intervention imperative. Enucleation is the treatment of choice; however, the mortality rate is about 50 percent within 3 years after removal of the eye.[7]

A thorough, complete examination of the other eye is essential to detect involvement and should be performed under ideal conditions. The presence of a lesion in that eye must be identified as soon as possible for it, too, can be treated and arrested, salvaging a degree of normal vision for the child. Monthly examinations are done routinely on these children. Two methods of treatment for the remaining eye

include photocoagulation and the administration of triethylenemelamine (TEM).

Nursing management   A nurse should watch for signs of hemorrhage, edema, and acute infections. Pressure dressings are applied after surgery to decrease the possibility of hemorrhage or the formation of a hematoma. Restraints may be used on the infant or toddler who attempts to remove his dressings; however, resistance may increase with their application. Then, the most effective means of quieting such an infant is to have his parents present; providing facilities which may accommodate them are encouraged. If the parents cannot be present, a nurse familiar to the patient may also assist in comforting and quieting the young child. On occasion, sedating the patient after surgery may be necessary. Resuming normal activities is important, and they are generally instituted the day after surgery.

Dressing changes are usually done by the ophthalmologist. Fittings for a prosthesis do not occur until the edema has subsided. The time interval varies and depends on the preference of the physician.

Granting permission for an enucleation is difficult for parents; however, when a bilateral enucleation is necessary, the parents' emotional stress increases greatly, for blindness will be the result of their action. Refusing to grant permission decreases the infant's life expectancy, and yet the decision must be made quickly without resolution of the emotions experienced or answers to questions raised. Nurses must comprehend the tragic aspect of that decision and take the time to provide opportunities in which parents may verbalize fears of their infant's disfigurement, the pain which he will experience, in addition to questioning whether they are making the "right" decision. They may also verbalize anxiety about what may occur in the future—especially the child's resentment of their decision which resulted in blindness for him. It is a difficult task to make oneself available for a discussion such as this; however, taking the time to facilitate an exploration of parental fears and anxieties will do much to assist these parents in recovering from the diagnosis, enabling them to resume normal parent-child relationships.

Young children who face an enucleation need to be informed of the procedure in advance. Spending time with the patient is important, for there may be questions he would like to ask his nurse. Typically, he wants to know if his new eye is going to move, if he will be able to see with his new eye, and if it will fall out. Each question should be answered honestly and in a language the child can comprehend.

Postoperatively, the full impact of the procedure may result in hostility, resentment, regression, or depression by the child. The professional nurse must understand why these responses are being displayed. If they persist, it may be helpful to consult with a nurse in child psychiatry who may offer additional guidance and direction. On rare occasions an extension of these symptoms may require professional psychologic support.

Ambulation should occur early in a newly blinded child—if he has achieved this developmental milestone. A nurse assigned to this patient should plan on spending a considerable amount of time talking and playing with him. He needs to be able to explore his environment, locating and touching various large items in his room. It is important to protect him as he begins his explorations. Frustrated by his dark world, he may throw temper tantrums to demonstrate his anger. These feelings of inadequacy will be overcome as he resumes more and more of his usual activities.

It is important to keep the door to an ambulatory blind child's room either open or closed, but never ajar, to avoid accidents. If the child is very young, the nurse may hold his hand when they take walks. If the child is older, he may need only to touch the nurse's elbow to have a sense of direction.

The patient should be allowed to dress himself as soon as possible. Feeding may also be done soon after resuming his preoperative diet. If the patient still uses a spoon to feed himself, a guard may need to be attached to the most distant part of the plate to enable him to scoop up the food. If use of a fork has been mastered, although feeding may be awkward and uneasy initially, he will regain table etiquette with practice.

Parents will need support in allowing the child to do things for himself, for there is a tendency for parents (and nurses) to perform for him such tasks as dressing and feeding. It is important for adults to respect the child's quest for independence. Clumsiness is to be expected at first, but the acquisition of skills comes with practice.

At the time of discharge it is important to stress the need for furniture to remain in the same place in the home if the patient's spatial orientation is to be successful. Should the position of a couch in the living room be changed, the child should be allowed to explore the change cautiously and make the necessary adjustment.

Additional education and further assistance should be sought from those persons especially skilled in rehabilitating the blind. A list of the various community resources should be made available to parents. Several national associations which might be helpful include the American Foundation for the Blind, The National Society for the Prevention of Blindness, and Howe Press of the Perkins School for the Blind.

Artificial Eyes

When the eye is removed, muscles are cut as close to the globe as possible. These muscles are then approximated with sutures to a plastic prosthesis, thereby providing coordinated movement of the prosthesis with the real eye. The plastic conformer remains in place until the edema has subsided and there is no evidence of infection in the socket.

The permanent prosthesis may be made of glass or plastic. Both look the same and allow the same amount of movement. A major disadvantage of glass appears to be the expansion of gases within it which might cause the prosthesis to crack in hot weather. A plastic artificial eye has a more natural-looking iris and is unbreakable.

Once inserted, instructions regarding care are given to the patient and his family. They are highly individualized and dependent on the preferences of the physician. Such guidance includes whether the prosthesis should be removed or worn through the night.

When not in use, a plastic prosthesis should be cleansed with soap and warm water and stored in a container with plain tap water. The glass prosthesis should also be cleansed with soap and water; however, it is dried and stored in its own case. Extremely hot or cold water or alcohol is never used in cleansing an artificial eye.

Nursing Management Teaching a child and his parents how to care for the prosthesis and its eye socket is essential. Normal saline irrigations are done routinely before insertion, and parents should become skillful and comfortable in performing the procedure before the child is discharged. Since the eye socket can easily become infected, nurses must stress the need for handwashing before irrigating or handling the eye.

Clear, definitive instructions should be given to the child and his family regarding the watery discharge which is present when a prosthesis is worn. It may be necessary to wipe the eye socket four or five times a day. Children tend to use their fingers or sleeves to brush away tears. They should be supplied with small packages of sterile, disposable tissues and taught how to use them correctly. Parents should be advised that any increase in the amount of tearing as well as the duration should be reported to the ophthalmologist at once.

Since children are so active and prone to injury, oftentimes safety glasses are prescribed, despite the fact that vision in the remaining eye is normal. Some anxiety may be precipitated, and it is important for the nurse to explain the rationale for such a prescription. Where enucleations have been done as a result of a penetrating wound of the globe, protecting the remaining eye ensures a degree of vision, and adjustment to the wearing of a prosthesis should ensure successful adaptation to a minimal handicap.

Mastoiditis

In many cases of suppurative otitis media, the infection may extend to and produce an inflammation of the mastoid process. The causative organisms are usually streptococci, pneumococci, staphylococci, and pseudomonas. Symptoms present themselves about one week after an untreated or inadequately treated otitis media, and they may be acute or chronic in nature.

A child with *acute mastoiditis* is usually under 3 years of age and has a history of draining ear, redness, pain, fever, and a retroauricular swelling. *Chronic mastoiditis* generally develops after repeated episodes of otitis media. These children have chronic draining ears with perforated eardrums and infections of the mastoid. In these children conductive hearing losses are common; therefore, mastoidectomies are usually necessary, in addition to tympanoplasty with reconstruction of the tympanic membrane and hearing apparatus of the middle ear. Systemic antibiotics are also prescribed to combat the infection as well as to enhance healing.

Nursing Management Children with mastoiditis should have their hair washed the night before surgery, with care being taken to prevent the water from entering the involved ear. The area immediately surrounding the involved ear may require shaving.

On return from the recovery room, the child may be restless, and sedatives may be ordered during the immediate postoperative period. Vital signs are monitored, and the bulkly dressing is checked frequently for bleeding. Considering the age, restraints may need to be applied in order to keep the dressing intact. These head dressings are changed every day or two, depending on the physician's wishes.

Since a complication of this type of surgery may be facial paralysis, the nurse should carefully observe for a drooping mouth, an eye which does not close, or difficulty in drinking once oral fluids have been started. Corticosteroids are usually ordered to decrease facial nerve inflammation.

Mastoiditis is common in children, and it is an infection which can be prevented. Early recognition of tympanic perforation, adequate treatment, and diligent follow-up by the clinic nurse or the public health nurse can decrease the number of children with mastoid complication.

Foreign Bodies in the Ear

Young children may place a variety of objects within the external auditory canal, including beads, erasers, pebbles, and food. A playmate may also be the culprit. Whether it is accidental or purposeful is irrelevant, for it is a foreign body and may result in certain clinical manifestations.

The object may be identified readily, or weeks may go by before its presence is known. Insects within the ear cause a great deal of noise and discomfort, and as a result they are easily and frequently found. While a rough-edged plastic object may damage the ear, substances of a vegetal source (pea, bean) tend to swell and set up a local inflammatory response which results in deafness. An obstruction may also be caused by an overaccumulation of cerumen.

A complaint of deafness may be the first indication of the presence of a foreign body. Pain and cellulitis are other clinical manifestations, especially if the object is vegetal in nature.

Foreign bodies should not be removed by anyone other than a physician. If the person is not skilled in performing this procedure, additional damage to the ear may occur. Unless it is clearly visible and within easy reach, and the patient is cooperative, the object is removed under anesthesia with forceps.

It is essential that the object be identified before treatment is begun. Cerumen is most easily removed after instilling a solution of hydrogen peroxide or sodium bicarbonate to soften the wax and then irrigating the auditory canal with warm water. Instilling oil or water drowns the insect, and irrigations remove it from the canal. Other objects such as rubber or beads may be removed by instilling oil or soap and then irrigating the auditory canal. Irrigating vegetal objects such as a bean or pea should be avoided because the irrigating solution may be absorbed, increasing the object's size.

Nursing Management A nurse may become involved in irrigating the auditory canal, and it is important that the patient's cooperation be obtained through a simple explanation. Restraints may be necessary for the child's safety. Syringing is done with a 20-ml syringe. A soft no. 5 or no. 8 rubber catheter is an effective device to use, for it decreases the possibility of injury. Ear drops are usually prescribed and should be instilled properly. An important aspect of caring for these children is teaching the patient to refrain from placing objects in his ears. He, in turn, may be responsible for teaching his playmate to refrain from performing the identical act.

Foreign Bodies in the Nose

Through exploration, toddlers discover that small objects can be placed in the nostrils. Such *foreign bodies* include erasers, pebbles, cherry stones, beads, nuts, and paper wads. Rarely is any small object pushed deeply into the nostril by the child. Initially it is anterior and not forced farther unless parents, child, or other unskilled people push it deeper in their efforts to remove it.

If the mother is unaware that her toddler has placed a foreign body in his nose, her first clue may be his complaint of soreness when his nose is touched. He may also have local obstruction and sneezing due to irritation. *Hygroscopic bodies,* such as peas and peanuts, increase in size as they absorb fluid. These objects cause discomfort soon after placement in a nostril. Smooth, hard objects which are not hygroscopic may not produce symptoms for weeks or months or may cause swelling and obstruction through mucosal irritation. If infection ensues, a purulent, malodorous, or even bloody discharge is noted. Whenever a child complains of or presents with unilateral nasal obstruction and discharge, a foreign body should be suspected as the causative agent. Examination with a nasal speculum or nasoscope confirms the diagnosis.

Removal is accomplished promptly to prevent aspiration and local tissue necrosis. Following the instillation of a local anesthetic, the object is removed with either forceps or a nasal suction apparatus. Infection disappears shortly, and usually no other treatment is needed. Some pediatricians have found that a foreign object may be moved into the anterior nasal chamber for easy removal by occluding the unobstructed nostril with the finger and blowing on the mouth as in mouth-to-mouth resuscitation.

Nursing Management Nurses providing routine well-child care should alert mothers to the toddler's bent for placing small objects in his nose as he explores his body in relation to his environment and discuss methods of prevention. Mothers should be aware of the signs and symptoms produced by these foreign bodies and realize the importance of having a physician remove them before necrosis occurs or the object is aspirated into the lower respiratory tract. Nurses themselves should be aware of signs and symptoms so that appropriate and immediate referral is made for removal of the foreign object.

SENSORY DISEASES AND DEVIATIONS IN THE PRESCHOOLER
Refractive Errors

The extent of visual impairment can be diagnosed by an ophthalmologist, regardless of the infant or young child's age or cooperation, with a retinoscopic examination, in which the refractive state of an eye can be determined. (See Fig. 42-3.) The examination is facilitated with the use of cycloplegic drugs (atropine, scopolamine, homatropine, or cyclopentolate) which eliminate the ability of the eye to accommodate.

Hyperopia (Farsightedness) Hyperopia is a refractive error in which parallel rays of light focus behind the retina (Fig. 42-4). In those situations distance vision is usually better than close vision. Hyperopia is common in all infants, and normal for most children. As a child grows, the eye also grows slightly, and the hyperopia diminishes; however, in some instances, farsightedness persists into adulthood.

The child may be symptom-free, or complain of frontal headaches with pain which localizes over one eye. Frequently there is squinting to "see better," or a toy or book is held up close to the eyes while being examined.

Glasses are usually prescribed to correct the refractive error. If distance vision is impaired, glasses should be worn at all times. In some instances the child's symptoms are those of insufficient accommodation for close work, and glasses may be prescribed for reading only.

Myopia (Nearsightedness) Myopia is a refractive error in which parallel rays of light focus in front of the retina (Fig. 42-4). Myopic children usually see well when doing close work and have difficulty viewing objects in the distance. The cause is an increased anterioposterior diameter of the eye. It is frequently diagnosed with the start of school when the teacher notices that the child cannot see the blackboard from the back of the room.

Prescription eyeglasses are corrective, and children should be encouraged to use them to learn what good vision is. Since there is some resistance

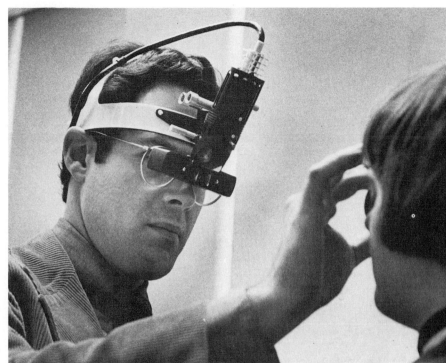

Figure 42-3 An ophthalmologist examines a preschooler's eyes. *(Courtesy of Media Center, Eunice Kennedy Shriver Center for Mental Retardation, Inc., Waltham, Mass.)*

to wearing glasses, they should be used in the classroom; however, whether they are worn during play activities is a decision the child should make.

Astigmatism When there is an irregular curvature of the anterior surface of the cornea which results in an aspheric surface, the entering rays of light are not regularly refracted and astigmatism is present. When an astigmatic child looks at the symbol +, and he focuses on the vertical bar, the horizontal bar will not be in focus. Conversely, when he focuses on the horizontal bar, the vertical bar will not be clear. Uncorrected astigmatism causes squinting, burning, and fatigue. These children have an intense dislike for prolonged close work.

Eyeglasses are usually prescribed. In some instances visual improvement is not obtained with the use of glasses, and contact lenses, which act by neutralizing the irregularity of the corneal surface, may be indicated.

Nursing management Many children with refractive errors are diagnosed early, but the nurse who observes children may identify a heretofore unknown visual problem. In the course of meeting other health needs, parents may ask about the use of medications, exercises, or vitamins which may improve the visual acuity of their children. None of these measures is effective in hyperopia, myopia, and astigmatism, and parents should be advised accordingly. These conditions necessitate prescription lenses, and parents as well as children must understand that they are to be worn appropriately. Since these problems are long-term, regular clinic or office visits—every 6 to 12 months—should be encouraged.

Foreign Bodies in and Trauma to the Eye

Accidental injury to the eye occurs often and is usually one of three types: a foreign body in the eye, a nonperforating injury of the globe, or actual perforation of the eyeball. The consequences depend upon the seriousness of the injury.

Extraocular Foreign Bodies Such foreign bodies as particles of wood, plastic, dirt, metal, or paper may become lodged in the conjunctival sac, causing excessive lacrimation and redness. They are removed without subsequent damage to vision.

Foreign bodies which are imbedded in the cornea cannot usually be easily removed. A physician should be seen as soon as possible, for normal blinking may force the object deeper into the cornea, making removal more difficult. The object can

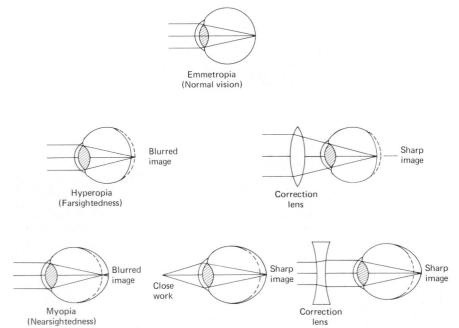

Emmetropia
(Normal vision)

Hyperopia
(Farsightedness)

Blurred image

Correction lens

Sharp image

Myopia
(Nearsightedness)

Blurred image

Close work

Sharp image

Correction lens

Sharp image

Figure 42-4 Hyperopia and myopia.

usually be lifted out of the corneal membrane without perforation. Antibiotic instillation and an eye patch complete the treatment for a foreign body in the eye.

Nonperforating Injuries of the Globe Blows to the eyeball by blunt objects such as stones, baseballs, or fists may cause damage which ranges from pain to severe intraocular destruction. Corneal abrasions may occur from paper, tree branches, or fingernails.

A common result of such a blow is hemorrhage into the anterior chamber, a condition known as *hyphema.* It is a serious clinical finding, for if the globe is filled with blood, secondary glaucoma may develop. While hyphema may clear without any complication, repeated or delayed hemorrhaging 2 or 3 days after the event necessitates treating the patients cautiously.

If the injury is untreated, vision may be impaired or lost. A cataract may develop as a result of poor nutrition of the lens from damage to the ciliary body. Permanent mydriasis by a tear of the iris sphincter precipitates the appearance of a permanently dilated pupil.

The serious complications of secondary glaucoma or cataract do not necessarily appear immediately; they may be delayed in formation, causing visual defects at a later date. These patients are usually hospitalized, sedated, have both eyes bandaged, and remain on bed rest for several days.

Penetrating Injuries of the Globe Injuries which penetrate the eyeball are serious and may necessitate removal of the affected eye. Causative agents include pointed objects such as forks, sharp sticks, arrows, and knife blades. Children's games which include flying objects are also offenders. With a corneal break, the eye becomes red and soft, and the iris may prolapse with the outward rush of aqueous. In patients with severe injuries, the whole eye may be filled with blood, and damage to the lens, retina, and choroid may be difficult to determine. Examining the eye may require much effort. In fact, it may be an impossible task for the ophthalmologist because of photophobia and interference with the clarity of the intraocular structures.

Some children give a history of pain and admit having stuck something in the eye. Toddlers who have not mastered language may be unable to identify the act which resulted in the injury. Other children, frightened by their parents' response, may not reveal the injury until the eye is red, swollen, and painful, several days later.

Such painful, penetrating injuries must be treated as soon as possible if vision and the eye are to be saved. These children are hospitalized, their eyes are bandaged, and they are confined to bed. Infection is the dreaded complication, and local as well as systemic antibiotics are instituted.

Treatment is lengthy and extends for 2 to 3 weeks as care is directed toward saving the eye. If there is little or no response to treatment in 3 weeks, and if the ophthalmologist has no hope for useful vision, the red, irritated, perforated eye is removed. In such injuries, concern focuses on the child developing *sympathetic ophthalmia,* a rare type of bilateral uveitis which follows perforation of the globe, especially when there has been extensive damage to the ciliary body. It occurs as a result of a sensitivity reaction which develops in the uveal tract of the uninjured eye. Once uveitis appears in the other eye, bilateral blindness may result. Hence the enucleation is done before sight is totally lost.

Nursing management A nurse who assists the ophthalmologist in removing a foreign body from the conjunctiva or cornea should mummify the child, restraining his hands and feet securely. He must also hold the child's head absolutely still as the object is removed. If the child is 1 or 2 years old and struggling vigorously, the physician may elect to take the patient to the operating room, where a general anesthetic may be administered.

Children who are hospitalized for hyphema are confined to bed and sedated, and both eyes are bandaged. Like other sightless patients, they should be spoken to before being touched. Appropriate diversional activities are important. These patients like to be read to, and they should be assigned to nurses who will spend time with them. Radios also help. Occasionally, the child is hostile or angry as a result of this injury, and an opportunity should be provided for him to verbalize these feelings.

In working with children who have penetrating injuries of the globe, administering eye drops as ordered is important. The child's cooperation is essential to treatment, although at times it is difficult to secure. The frequent extensive ophthalmologic examinations are important in determining the progress being made, and a nurse who is known and trusted by the patient may be helpful in soliciting his collaboration in these procedures.

The decision to enucleate is never an easy one for the physician to make, but preserving sight in the unaffected eye is paramount in the treatment of a penetrating injury. Once the decision is made, the child and his parents will need to be adequately prepared, and all questions should be answered honestly. Postoperatively, the nursing care given is similar to that of caring for a patient with a retinoblastoma where enucleation was also necessary (see above).

Penetrating injuries of the globe are preventable, and nurses should teach children, their parents, and the public to be more conscious of eye safety. Children should be cautioned about throwing snowballs and stones and aiming arrows at others, all of which may result in sight-destroying injuries. Young children who begin to feed themselves must be cautioned about the use of knives and forks as eating utensils—not as weapons. Only toys which are "child safe" should be purchased. At times, it may be necessary to remove potentially dangerous games from a play area.

Herpes Simplex of the Cornea (Dendritic Keratitis)

An inflammation of the superficial layers of the cornea can accompany any type of conjunctivitis. Viral infections may also elicit such responses, and, if not treated, they may be responsible for extensive erosions of the cornea, scarring, and subsequent loss of vision. A common offending virus is herpes simplex, which may cause ulcerations and dendritic keratitis.

The presence of this viral infection anywhere on the body, or as a result of some mild febrile upset, may lead to the initial inflammation. It usually begins as an invasion of the corneal epithelium by the herpesvirus. Vesicles are formed, break down, and erode the superficial layers of the cornea until an ulcer develops. Photophobia, pain, and excessive lacrimation are common complaints. If untreated scar tissue forms and loss of vision occurs.

When the infection is confined to the epithelium, treatment may involve a curettage with or without chemical cauterization. Idoxuridine (IDU), an antiviral agent, is used topically to inhibit viral synthesis of DNA. Corticosteroids are not used because they reduce tissue immunity and may possibly accelerate spread of the viral infection.

Nursing Management These patients need constant nursing care when hospitalized. The IDU drops are administered every hour during the day, and every other hour during the night. Since an eye patch is in place at all times, restraints are necessary to retain the occlusive dressing and decrease irritation from rubbing or touching the eye. Photophobia also needs to be considered, and, where possible, light should be kept to a minimum. Pain is commonly caused by this viral infection. Thought should be given to requests for soothing eye ointments which may decrease the irritation. Mild sedatives may be ordered initially and discontinued as the eye shows improvement. The nurse should spend time with the child in order to allay his fears and help him redirect his energies toward more constructive, diversional activities.

Loss of Hearing

The development of speech is dependent on the infant's ability to hear; therefore, impaired hearing has grave implications for speech as well as future intellectual function. In about 1 in 1,000 live births, a baby is profoundly deaf, and about 25 out of 1,000 newborns have a moderate to severe hearing loss.[8] Hearing disorders in these infants must be diagnosed early, and rehabilitation instituted immediately if the children are to be helped.

Hearing loss is a progressive phenomenon. Total deafness rarely occurs, and therefore deafness usually refers to a partial hearing loss. The intensity of sound is measured in decibels, and a mild loss refers to a reduction of 20 to 40 decibels. A severe loss is beyond 50 decibels.

There are two types of hearing loss. In *conductive hearing loss* there is interference with the transmission of sound from the external ear to the inner ear. Repeated ear infections, such as otitis media, are the commonest causes. Temporary hearing loss in upper respiratory tract infections may also cause a hearing impairment, for the eustachian tubes are obstructed. The second type of hearing loss is called *perceptive hearing loss,* in which there is an impairment of the inner ear and the eighth cranial nerves of the auditory cortex including the afferent pathways. Causes of this type of deafness are not as clearly understood as conductive hearing loss. Infections of the central nervous system, such as meningitis, and antenatal infections can cause perceptive hearing loss. A number of drugs currently in clinical use are ototoxic and also may contribute to this type of impairment.

Recently, some studies have indicated that perceptive hearing loss may result from incubator utilization soon after birth. The humming sound of the motor which heats the incubator, as well as the fan which circulates the air, may be contributing factors in the cause of hearing loss among sick prematures and neonates.[9, 10] High noise levels have been recorded within the plastic hoods, and apparently these levels have been elevated further by additional sound sources within intensive care units or nurseries.

What are some clinical manifestations which would identify a hearing problem? In an infant, speech development is abnormal, for he does not appear to respond to the sounds of others. In the older child, there may be distorted speech or the failure to respond to adequate auditory stimuli. Some children are considered behavior problems or difficult to handle, when, in fact, they may be deaf. Deaf schoolchildren do poorly academically, and they also test poorly in verbal intelligence testing. Playing the radio, phonograph, or television at abnormally high volumes may suggest the presence of a hearing problem. If this hearing impairment goes unnoticed, at a time of great intellectual development, a child's potential may be seriously curtailed.

Once the child with a hearing problem is identified, a complete history and physical should be done. The definitive work-up should include a careful assessment of the child through observation. Behavioral testing and impedance testing should be done by an audiologist.

A frequently used audiometric screening test involves the use of a pure-tone audiometer which tests the hearing in each ear separately. Pure-tone sounds are presented in a stepwise manner, and hearing ability is recorded in decibels (intensity) for each sound frequency (cycle/second).

Once the degree of deficit is determined, children are started on auditory training programs, after receiving hearing aids. They will then be able to profit from exposure to language at a critical stage of development.

Rehabilitation requires an interdisciplinary approach utilizing the expertise of skilled professionals in medicine, otology, speech education, speech therapy, and nursing.

Nursing Management Identification of hearing problems by nurses is enhanced by a thorough knowledge of growth and development as well as the ototoxic side effect of certain medications. Observing a child during hospitalization or a home visit may focus attention on a heretofore undiagnosed problem.

It is very difficult to differentiate between hearing loss and speech impairment, for they go hand in hand. Observing the young infant and noting his response to jingling keys, noise-making toys, or the voice may help the nurse identify impaired hearing. Asking the toddler to identify parts of the body or follow directions without giving visual clues enables the nurse to better evaluate his performance. In the playroom a toddler or preschooler who constantly spends time alone, even when there are other children nearby, deserves additional observation. His play activities, language development, and peer interaction should all be assessed. Impaired or slow language development is an important clue to a hearing deficit, so it is imperative that the nurse constantly evaluate the infant's ability to vocalize and the young child's ability to express himself.

Trauma to the Nose

Trauma to the nose may occur as a result of a fall, an auto accident, being hit by a baseball, or colliding with another person. While the fractures are severe, they are easily reduced. The cosmetic damage done tends to become more apparent in adolescence, if not reduced at the time of the accident.

Almost all external fractures of the nose have an associated subluxation, a fracture of the nasal septum, or both. Since fractures may occlude one side of the nares, breathing is difficult; rhinitis and a chronic sinusitis may develop. If the bone is displaced, a physician reduces the fracture by applying pressure to the convex surface of the nose with one or both thumbs.

A common symptom of trauma to the nose is epistaxis. While bleeding is associated with hemophilia, rheumatic fever, or purpura, it is also present when an injury has been severe enough to fracture the nose. Should a nosebleed occur, the child is placed in an upright position and instructed to stop talking and to breathe through his mouth. The nose is compressed between the nurse's fingers for 15 to 20 minutes. It is important that the pressure applied be adequate and constant in order to be effective. After the blood flow has stopped, ice packs can be applied over the bridge of the nose. Cotton plugs with petrolatum may be inserted into the nares to remain there for about four hours if a small amount of bleeding persists.

In the case of continued bleeding, a physician may insert cotton pledgets saturated with vasoconstrictors such as phenylephrine or epinephrine (1:1000) into the nares in an effort to control the bleeding. In severe cases nasal packing may be necessary. It is important for a nurse to remember that children may swallow blood which produces nausea and precipitates the vomiting of "coffeeground" material.

In addition to trauma causing nosebleeds, young children may initiate hemorrhage by picking their noses and rupturing distended vessels in the anterior, inferior section of the nasal septum. Applying liberal amounts of petrolatum to the encrusted areas and teaching the child to refrain from picking his nose should be initiated to decrease the likelihood of such occurrences.

Allergic Rhinitis

Both seasonal and perennial allergic rhinitis are seen in children, usually not before 4 or 5 years of age.

Foods are often the allergens in the first year or two of life. Later, inhalants are more important.

Seasonal allergic rhinitis (hay fever, rose fever) is caused by sensitivity to molds, pollens, and house dust. Allergy to molds may depend upon the weather. Reactions to pollens (rose fever) coincide with the pollinating season of several grasses and also occurs in the early spring with tree pollens. Sensitivity to ragweed pollen is manifest from mid-August to early October. House dust is the most common allergen during the winter months, particularly with central heating. Clinical manifestations include sneezing, itching of the nasal mucosa, profuse lacrimation and rhinorrhea, and often allergic conjunctivitis. Olfaction and gustation are decreased. The nasal mucosa is edematous, pale, and wet.

Perennial allergic rhinitis has no seasonal pattern and is caused by sensitivity to house dust, wool, feathers, and molds. It is manifest by mild congestion and sniffling, mouth breathing, postnasal drip, and complaints of an itchy nose. Several facial mannerisms may be indicative of perennial allergic rhinitis: the allergic salute, nose wrinkling, and mouth wrinkling. All are utilized to relieve nasal itching. In the *allergic salute*, the child uses one hand to push the nose upward and backward not only to relieve itching but also to move the swollen turbinates away from the septum, thereby allowing freer air passage. After 2 years of pronounced saluting, a transverse nasal crease occurs just above the bulbous portion of the nose. Nasal mucosa may be pale, edematous, and wet, or, with purulent discharge, may be inflamed as in acute nasopharyngitis. Differential diagnosis may then be made via nasal smear. Eosinophilia is present in allergic conditions, whereas polymorphonuclear cells are seen with infection. Recurrent epistaxis due to persistent nose picking and mouth breathing is common in perennial allergic rhinitis, and allergic shiners may be present.

Diagnosis is made through a detailed present, past, and family history, eosinophilia on nasal smears, and scratch test. By x-ray, the mucosa of the maxillary sinuses may appear thickened, and polyps may be seen.

Treatment includes a comprehensive program aimed toward removal of causative allergens, desensitization to incitants which cannot be avoided, and control of infection. Immediate treatment for symptomatic relief is provided by antihistamines, oral decongestants, and nasal sprays.

Nursing Management Nurses providing routine well-child care who observe that a child has allergic shiners, conjunctivitis, allergic facial mannerisms, and/or a transverse nasal crease should refer that child for an allergic evaluation. Other clues include reddened nasal mucosa, sneezing, an itchy nasal lining, and rhinorrhea. A thorough history will add to the data base. Once an allergic basis has been determined, the parents will need to know how to allergy-proof their house. The nurse should also provide health teaching in relation to medications and prevention of infection.

SENSORY DISEASES AND DEVIATIONS IN THE SCHOOL-AGE CHILD
Impaired Color Vision

Color vision is dependent on intact macular cone cells in the retina, as well as effectively functioning pathways which transmit color from the macula to the cerebral cortex. An impairment may result in a *color deficiency* or *color blindness,* which is the inability to differentiate some colors of the spectrum.

Impaired color vision may be congenital or acquired. Causes of acquired impairment are cataracts and diseases of the optic nerve, macula, and occipital cortex. These entities are usually associated with abnormal retinal functioning, that is, impaired vision. It may or may not be bilateral and involves blue-green as well as red-green discrimination. Congenital color blindness is bilateral and involves red-green color differentiation. The visual acuity of the congenitally afflicted is good. The red-green deficiency is transmitted as a male, sex-linked recessive trait, affecting 8 percent of the male population. Blue-yellow deficiency is an extremely rare condition. *Total color blindness* (*achromatopsia*), or the absence of cone function, is a simple recessive trait.

Color blindness cannot be corrected but can be diagnosed easily and should be identified as early as possible in a child. The Ishihara charts offer a quick and accurate test for color vision. These plates contain geometric symbols in red, green, blue, and yellow (the commonly involved colors) on a gray background, and a child deficient in color vision cannot identify the symbols.

Nursing Management Although color blindness cannot be corrected, identification is important. Nurses working with young children in a hospital or day care center may test a knowledge of colors and conclude the presence of this deficiency. Teachers, especially in kindergarten, may notice a child having a problem with colors and convey this information to the nurse, who follows through. Since traffic signals are red and green, the most often affected colors, young children who have this problem may have some difficulty in determining when to cross a street. The safety factor must be emphasized to the young child.

In counseling adolescents about their future plans, the nurse needs to discuss the presence of this deficiency. Many industrial plants use a red-green color combination in their light signals, for example, and high school graduates should not be placed in jobs in which color blindness could jeopardize their safety or effectiveness as employees.

Otitis Externa

An infection of the skin of the external auditory canal, otitis externa is frequently seen in children from about five years of age through young adulthood. It is especially common in the summertime, affecting many children who spend a great deal of time swimming. Generally the ear canal is swollen and discharges a purulent exudate. Common offending organisms include *Staphylococcus, Pseudomonas,* and other gram-negative bacteria.

Treatment consists of instillation of an acidic solution containing polymyxin or neomycin. In severe cases corticosteroids are used to reduce the inflammatory process. When the child is swimming, ear plugs are recommended after an initial episode. A simple prophylactic measure is the instillation of 2 or 3 drops of white vinegar (5 percent acetic acid) before and after swimming.

Nasal Polyps

Nasal polyps arise from the turbinates or paranasal sinuses and are described as chronic, inflammatory, pedunculated masses. The usual symptoms of chronic nasal discharge and obstruction are generally unilateral. The child may complain of a headache. These edematous masses may be single or multiple, are white to pale pink in color, and are relatively avascular. Surgical removal is advocated. Unless the underlying cause (i.e., allergy) is treated, they are prone to reappear. Occasionally polyps disappear with the use of topical steroids.

Nursing Management The nurse should explain to the child and parents that not only is the airway obstructed, but also the senses of taste and smell may be impaired by the chronic rhinitis. Postoperatively the child is observed for bleeding and occlusion of the airway. Health teaching and preparation for discharge should include explaining the need for treating the underlying cause.

Sinusitis

Sinusitis is an inflammatory process involving frontal (ethmoid) or sphenoid sinuses. Bacterial infections of the sinuses can occur in infancy as well as throughout childhood, but they are most common in the school-age period. Sinusitis may be acute or chronic, involving the maxillary, ethmoid, and/or frontal sinuses. The most frequently involved microorganisms include the filtrable viruses of acute rhinitis, pneumococci, staphlococci, and streptococci. While sinusitis itself may be symptomatically severe, the real danger lies in the infectious process invading adjacent structures.

The signs of acute sinusitis, accompanying an upper respiratory infection, include a fever, purulent nasal discharge with nasal congestion, headache, and periorbital or facial swelling which is tender to touch. The periorbital edema and redness of the skin involved indicates a bone and periosteal infiltration. When the purulent material is trapped within a sinus, there may be a subsequent necrosis of the bone, venous thrombosis, and finally bone sequestra. The extravasation of pus from the sinus into the orbit of the eye, especially in ethmoid sinusitis, may cause permanent blindness as a result of a thrombosed orbital vein. Other complications of sinus infections include otitis media, meningitis, orbital cellulitis, and optic neuritis. A severe frontal sinus infection which has ocular involvement may produce an epidural abscess secondary to an erosion of the frontal sinus.

Treatment of acute sinusitis involves nasal and nasopharyngeal cultures and smears, which are examined immediately for an identification of the microorganisms involved. Systemic antibiotics and vasoconstrictors are employed. Drainage of the frontal sinus followed by antibiotic irrigations of this cavity may also be necessary.

Chronic sinusitis may be caused by hypertrophied adenoids. Allergic irritants may also be responsible for a chronic condition. In warm climates, diving into swimming pools may be an irritation factor to be considered. Dental caries and subsequent abscesses may cause maxillary sinusitis. Oftentimes the chronic presence of this condition is overlooked.

Clinical manifestations include a chronic cough from a persistent postnasal drip, a constant, purulent discharge, a recurrent headache, frequent sneezing, and mouth-breathing. The presence of this chronic problem tends to aggravate the respiratory problems of asthmatic children.

Treatment is dependent on the cause, which may be difficult for the physician to identify. If systemic antibiotics and nasal decongestants do not relieve the symptoms, adenoidectomy and sinus irrigation may be necessary.

Nursing Management   The aim of therapy is to provide a tract whereby the purulent material is drained from the affected sinus. Should hospitalization be necessary, these patients are frequently febrile, so their temperatures should be monitored often, and antipyretics as well as cool sponges utilized as frequently as ordered or necessary. Fluids should be encouraged, and humidifiers which are effective in liquefying secretions may facilitate the draining process. Nose drops, especially Neo-Synephrine, are frequently ordered, and they should be administered after a thorough, gentle cleansing of the nasal passages. In assessing a patient's response to therapy, the nurse should focus on the temperature returning to normal and the type of drainage being produced. It is especially important to note the color and the tenaciousness of the material, for, as there is a response to treatment, the drainage becomes clear and more liquid.

Warm compresses applied to the present periorbital edema may be soothing for the young patient. Accompanying eye drainage may be purulent, and therefore its presence should be noted. It is also important to frequently assess the extent of the tissue involved, its color, and the patient's ability to open his eye. Identifying a change in the child's behavior or his neurologic status may determine the existence of a complication. For example, if he covers his ear with his hand or complains of an ear hurting, it may indicate otitis media, while other changes in his neurologic status may demonstrate the presence of an epidural abscess. A physician should be notified immediately.

Sinusitis may partially obstruct the airway, impairing the senses of smell and of taste. The nurse should explain this fact to the child and his parents. Health teaching about proper diet, care of the teeth, and/or allergies should be provided, as well as instruction in carrying out prescribed treatments.

SENSORY DISEASES AND DEVIATIONS IN THE ADOLESCENT
Hordeolum (Stye) and Chalazion

The glands of Zeis and Moll are located in the margins of the eyelids. When they are infected, a localized pyogenic inflammation with abscess formation occurs at the lid margin and is known as a *hordeolum* (stye). The causative organism is usually *Staphy-*

lococcus aureus. Treatment is aimed at localizing the abscess and promoting drainage. Therefore, hot wet packs are applied every 4 hours and are followed by topical antibiotics. If the stye is not responding to treatment, a culture and sensitivity test will determine the drug of choice.

A *chalazion* is a chronic granulation tissue tumor of the Meibomian glands within the tarsal cartilage of the lid. It does not drain. Treatment is aimed toward shrinking this hard nodule and letting it absorb naturally. Hot, moist packs are applied every 4 hours and are followed by topical antibiotics. Drops are used during the day, and ointment is instilled before bedtime and cleaned off in the morning. Topical antibiotics keep the nodule soft and moist and prevent secondary infection. *S. aureus* coagulase causes secondary infection. Treatment lasts for 4 to 6 weeks. Ninety percent of lower-lid chalazions respond, while 90 percent of upper-lid ones do not since the cartilage is thicker. If a chalazion does not respond to treatment within the allotted time period, a complete excision or incision and curettage is performed.

Nursing Management Although styes and chalazions can occur at any age, they are slightly more common in adolescents because of the hormonal influences at puberty. They are also more common in adolescent girls who use eye makeup and do not completely wash it off before going to bed at night. The nurse should stress good eye hygiene with adolescent patients. Since patients who have styes and chalazions will not be hospitalized, the nurse in ambulatory care centers is the one who will teach them how to apply hot packs and instill eye drops and ointment.

Trauma to the Eye

Blunt and chemical eye injuries are more common in adolescence, while penetrating eye injuries are more common at preschool age. Results of *blunt injuries* range from slight to severe and include slight, transient pain, mild iritis, corneal abrasion, intraocular hemorrhage, permanent muscle palsies, detached retina, dislocated lens, ruptured sclera, and proptosis of the globe following retrobulbar hemorrhage. Such injuries may be caused from sticks, stones, golf clubs, golf balls, air guns, slingshots, firecrackers (concussive effect), and homemade bombs (container becomes a projectile). When the eye is hit, it dimples in, raising intraocular pressure. Tears may occur in the iris causing hemorrhage. Tears in the retina can result in retinal detachment.

If the lens is torn, a cataract may result. Sudden increase in intraorbital pressure may also cause a fracture of the orbital floor.

Symptoms of blunt injuries include lid abrasion, ecchymosis, and edema. Some adolescents may complain of diplopia, and the affected eye may not be in the normal position. When the injured eye is examined, the patient may be unable to move it completely in all directions. The anterior chamber may be flat and full of blood. The iris may be tremulous and the eye soft. Less obvious signs which may be discovered by the ophthalmologist include a sluggish or inactive pupil, an abnormally shaped or dilated pupil, variations in the anterior chamber depth, and sudden visual loss. Even though hemorrhage into the anterior chamber absorbs easily, a delayed cataract or glaucoma can occur. Any medication which affects the pupil is never given until the extent of the injury is known.

Treatment for blunt injuries includes bed rest, dilatation (splinting) of the pupil, topical steroids to prevent iritis, and frequent assessment for secondary glaucoma and repeated hemorrhage. If glaucoma becomes unmanageable, surgical decompression and local treatment with Diamox are advocated. If a blowout fracture of the orbit has occurred, surgical repair is deferred until 1 week following the injury. With anterior chamber hemorrhage, the patient is sedated and on bed rest. Both eyes are bandaged. If corneal abrasion has occurred, it is treated with a bacteriostatic eye ointment, a mild cycloplegic (i.e., homatropine), and a firm eye patch. Prompt treatment in the first 24 hours may mean the difference between saving or losing eyesight following blunt injuries.

Chemical trauma may be due to alkalis or acids and is caused by such agents as household cleaning materials, plumbing supplies, and aerosol sprays. Corneal burns result. Immediate emergency treatment consists of irrigating the eye for 20 to 30 minutes with clean tap water, after which the injured person is immediately brought to an emergency room for prompt evaluation. The affected cornea is stained with a fluorescein litmus strip to demonstrate any loss of corneal epitheleum. The depth of loss is determined with a slit lamp microscope. *Acid burns* are usually self-limiting, barring infection. Acid forms a coagulum with the tissue which further limits burning. *Alkalis* continue to dissolve tissue by forming toxic alkaline products which continue to penetrate deeper and deeper into the tissues.

Treatment consists of debridement of dead and devitalized tissue and ensuring that all the noxious agent has been removed. Topical antibiotics and steroids are given until there is evidence of complete healing via slit lamp microscopy. If burns are severe, the patient is hospitalized. Otherwise, treatment is on an ambulatory basis in the office or clinic. With strong caustics, treatment lasts 5 to 6 weeks.

Nursing Management Nursing intervention should begin with preventive measures. As the nurse discovers the interests of teen-agers through history-taking, accident prevention should be stressed. The nurse should ensure that any youngster brought to the emergency room because of blunt eye injury or chemical burns is *promptly* assessed by an ophthalmologist. A determination or prior emergency treatment is ascertained. If treatment is on an ambulatory basis, the nurse teaches the adolescent home care and stresses the importance of keeping appointments for assessment of the healing process.

When the teen-ager is hospitalized, he will need much reassurance and honesty from the nurse. He needs to understand the need for bed rest, eye patches, and eye drops and ointments. He will also need to learn home treatment. In dealing with the adolescent, the nurse should always bear in mind his stage of development.

Blow-Out Fractures (Complication of Blunt Trauma to the Eye)

When the eye is struck by a fist or some other blunt object, increased intraorbital pressure is transmitted to the orbital walls. The orbital floor fractures or blows outwardly because its structure is the weakest.

There is palpable crepitus in the lids indicative of a fracture into the nasal sinuses. Ecchymosis and edema are generally present, and if the child can see, he may complain of diploplia. X-rays confirm the diagnosis, and surgery is performed a week or 10 days later, after the edema and hemorrhage have subsided.

Zygomatic fractures are sometimes found with blow-out fractures; therefore, the nurse should heed a patient's complaints of limited jaw movement. Surgery involving either an open or closed reduction, and a wiring of the jaw, enhance the healing of this type of fracture.

Nursing Management If the child or adolescent sustains a blow-out fracture, he is uncomfortable. Analgesics relieve the pain, and ice packs or cold compresses should relieve the edema. Eye drainage may be present, and it should be noted and reported. Preparation for surgery and postoperative treatment are important aspects of caring for a patient with such an injury.

The presence of a zygomatic fracture complicates the nursing care because a form of fixation is necessary to repair the jaw. If teeth are present, wires are placed around the teeth, and the lower jaw is held against the upper jaw by cross-wires or rubber bands. When the patient returns from the operating room, he should be kept on his side with the head of the bed elevated.

Since the wired jaw cannot be disturbed, the patient receives a fluid diet until the wires or bands are removed after the jaw has healed. The fluids offered should be varied, blenderized, and given frequently. They may be administered by plastic straw or asepto syringe (rubber-tipped), and water should be given after all oral feedings. Mouth care needs to be given about every two hours and after each oral intake. All feedings should be given with the patient on his side or in a sitting position, to prevent aspiration.

When oral feedings are initiated after the jaw has been wired, it is extremely important that fluids be introduced slowly and cautiously. The nurse should observe the patient for any signs of aspiration (choking, cyanosis, and dyspnea). Every effort is made to prevent vomiting, and antiemetic drugs may be essential initially. Suction apparatus should be at the bedside of the patient, and wire cutters are always taped in a conspicuous place at the head of the bed, ready for emergency use. Should the patient vomit or demonstrate respiratory distress from an obstructed airway, the wires or rubber bands *are cut* to maintain a patent airway.

Detached Retina

Detached retina can occur at any age, but it is most common in older people. In adolescents, it is seen more often in myopic teen-agers after trauma. A blow with a fist to the back of the head can cause detachment, or it may occur after blunt trauma to the eye. Sometimes detachment does not occur for months or years after an injury.

Following an injury, when fluid separates the retina from the choroid, a *detached retina* results. Retinal sensitivity decreases. If early reattachment is not accomplished, irreversible changes can result. Symptoms which are indicative of imminent detachment include complaints of light flashes, smoky vision, veillike or curtainlike opacities, and distortion of the visual field. Once separation has occurred, the patient may or may not complain of blurred vision corresponding to the area which has detached. When the macula has detached, central vision is reduced and blurring is noted. The affected eye becomes amblyopic, and esotropia may develop. A poor red reflex is present in the detached area.

Reattachment may be accomplished through cryotherapy or diathermy. The ophthalmologist finds the retinal tears and seals them off with ultra cold or heat. Fluid is aspirated. The eyeball sometimes is invaginated via scleral buckling to bring the choroid in better contact with the detached retina. Thus, the affected eye appears smaller than the unaffected eye. Postoperatively the patient is on bed rest for 2 days and then allowed limited ambulation for 3 or 4 days. The pupil is dilated (splinted), and local antibiotics and steroids are instilled in the eye. The total hospital stay is 5 to 8 days. Once home, the patient must rest; he is permitted no strenuous exercise nor heavy lifting and must avoid sudden jarring motions of head and eyes for several months. Contact sports may be restricted for life. With first-time retinal detachments, there is an 80 percent success rate. With repeated detachments, the success percentage drops off quite rapidly.

Nursing Management The nurse should be aware of early signs of detachment and promptly report them to the ophthalmologist. The same holds true for late signs. The nurse should help the teen-ager to understand what is happening to him and what the aim of treatment is. Before discharging him, the nurse must teach the patient home care and the importance of following instructions.

Trauma to the Ear

Middle Ear There are two primary sources of trauma to the middle ear. The first is *iatrogenic* and is usually induced by removing a foreign body like an eraser or paper from the external ear. If the object is not carefully withdrawn, the tympanic membrane and ossicles can be damaged with permanent hearing loss. The second cause, *barotrauma,* is a consequence of an interference in the middle ear pressure-regulating mechanism. Airplane ascents and descents and springboard and scuba diving cause pressure changes which are greater than environmental changes, especially in people with large adenoids or poorly functioning eustachian tubes. Eardrums may perforate, and although they usually heal without complications, at the time of the perforation the pain is intense.

Temporal Bone Fractures Affecting Middle and Inner Ear Most temporal bone fractures are characterized by a hearing loss and the presence of blood behind the eardrum. In extensive fractures there may be blood draining into the nasopharynx through the eustachian tubes.

Several clinical manifestations occur, and they depend on the area of involvement. If the fracture involves a lower portion of the bone, there may be a paralysis of the facial nerve. A longitudinal fracture through the inner ear can result in permanent hearing loss, while a transverse fracture causes a conductive hearing loss and a partial or total facial nerve paralysis.

Another important point to remember is that these fractures do not heal as others do, for the union is fibrous. There is a potential tract for the organisms of upper respiratory infections to migrate to the meninges, precipitating a meningitis years after a temporal bone fracture.

Nursing management When the eardrum has been perforated in middle ear trauma, the nurse should direct his efforts toward patient teaching. The adolescent needs to know that showers are avoided and swimming is not resumed until the perforation has healed. Younger children need to be taught why objects are not placed into the middle ear, and inexperienced adults should be cautioned about removing such objects from the ear.

Patients who have received temporal bone fractures are carefully observed, especially for signs of neurologic involvement. Complaints of an earache, evidence of facial paralysis, and the presence of impaired hearing are serious clinical manifestations which should be reported to a physician immediately. The identification and confirmation of symptoms and patient teaching are integral components of nursing care given to a patient with ear trauma.

Sound Pollution

Although attention has been focused on such sound contributors to pollution as bulldozers, airplanes, industrial operations, and road traffic, recently recreational noise has been emphasized as an offender. Acute exposure to the sounds of toy guns, rock-and-roll music, model airplanes, motorboats, and snowmobiles has been responsible for producing temporary elevations of the hearing threshold.[11] Sound levels in homes, on the street, and at recreational sites are above those at which sensorineural hearing loss occurs.

The extent of hearing loss appears to be related to the magnitude of the sounds, their frequency, their type (constant or intermittent), their duration, and the complexity of tones. Certain combinations of these factors, such as magnitude, frequency, and long duration, appear to be more damaging than others.

Music—loud music—is synonymous with adolescence. Since the introduction of rock-and-roll music, there has been a substantial increase in hearing deficits among adolescents and young adults. Phonographs, radios, and television sets are often played at full volume, and often for a long period, especially when earphones are used. Music is considered a semiconstant sound pollutant. It consists of a complexity of tones rather than pure tones because of the variety of sounds elicited from different instruments. Therefore, when the delicate hearing apparatus is exposed to these complex sounds for long periods of time, cumulative, subtle sensorineural damage may occur over a period of years. Hearing tests on members of rock music groups have demonstrated temporary loss after exposure at concerts.[12] Some of these performers have had hearing loss only after continuous exposure.

Nursing Management It is imperative that nurses become more knowledgeable about prevention of sensorineural hearing loss in the adolescent. This problem emerges slowly, progressing over a period of years, and may be identified at a critical period in the teen-ager's life.

The nurse should teach adolescents the principles of maintaining good hearing. Teen-agers interested in playing in rock groups should be encouraged to use ear plugs, to minimize the likelihood of hearing loss. Whether an adolescent is experimenting with a model airplane, playing an electric guitar, listening to records, or driving a snowmobile, moderation is very important. Lower sound levels are more acceptable to the ear and allow the sensitive hearing apparatus to recover from the impact of noise and music.

REFERENCES

1 F. Newell, *Ophthalmology: Principles and Concepts,* The C. V. Mosby Company, St. Louis, 1969, p. 78.
2 Ibid., pp. 81–82.
3 R. H. Barsch, *Achieving Perceptual Motor Efficiency,* Special Child Publications, Seattle, vol. 1, 1968, p. 209.
4 "Nebraska Society for the Prevention of Blindness," *Nebraska Medical Journal,* vol. 58, no. 1, April 1973, p. 123.
5 H. Davis and R. S. Silverman, *Hearing and Deafness,* Holt, Rinehart and Winston, Inc., New York, 1970, p. 386.
6 "Newborn's Hearing Loss Detected in Nursery by Automated Sensor," *Pediatric Herald,* 14(6):8, 1973.
7 S. D. Liebman and S. S. Gellis, *The Pediatrician's Ophthalmology,* The C. V. Mosby Company, St. Louis, 1966, p. 206.
8 H. L. Barnett, *Pediatrics,* 15th ed., Appleton Century Crofts, New York, 1972, p. 1891.
9 F. L. Seleny and M. Streczyn, "Noise Characteristics in the Baby Compartment of Incubators," *American Journal of Diseases of Children,* vol. 117, April 1969, pp. 445–450.
10 J. A. Falk and J. C. Farmer, Jr., "Incubator Noise and Possible Deafness," *Archives of Otolaryngology,* vol. 97, no. 5, May 1973, pp. 385–387.
11 S. A. Falk, "Combined Effects of Noise and Ototoxic Drugs," *Environmental Health Perspectives,* October 1972, pp. 5–20.
12 J. M. Flugrath, "Modern Day Rock and Roll Music and Damage Risk Criteria," *Journal of the Acoustic Society of America,* vol. 45, no. 3, March 1969, pp. 705–711.

BIBLIOGRAPHY

Boies, L. R., et al. : *Fundamentals of Otolaryngology,* W. B. Saunders Company, Philadelphia, 1964.
Cooke, R. E. (ed.): *The Biologic Basis of Pediatric Practice,* McGraw-Hill Book Company, New York, 1968.
Guyton, A. C.: *Basic Human Physiology: Normal Function and Mechanisms of Disease,* W. B. Saunders Company, Philadelphia, 1971.
Jackson, C. S. R.: *The Eye in General Practice,* E. and S. Livingstone, Ltd., London, 1969.
Jones, L., Reeh, M., and Wirtschafter, J.: *Ophthalmic Anatomy,* American Academy of Ophthalmology and Otolaryngology, Rochester, Minn., 1970.
Katzin, H., and Wilson, Geraldine: *Rehabilitation of a Child's Eyes,* The C. V. Mosby Company, St. Louis, 1961.
Langley, L. L., Telford, I. R., and Christensen, J. B.: *Dynamic Anatomy and Physiology,* 4th ed., McGraw-Hill Book Company, New York, 1974.
Paparella, M., and Shumrick, D. A.: *Otolaryngology,* vol. I, W. B. Saunders Company, Philadelphia, 1973.
Patten, B. M.: *Human Embryology,* 3d ed., McGraw-Hill Book Company, New York, 1968.
Slobody, L. B., and Wasserman, E.: *Survey of Clinical Pediatrics,* 6th ed., McGraw-Hill Book Company, New York, 1974.
Vander, A. J., Sherman, J. H., and Luciano, Dorothy S.: *Human Physiology: The Mechanisms of Body Function,* McGraw-Hill Book Company, New York, 1970.
Whetnall, Edith, and Fry, D. B.: *The Deaf Child,* William Heinemann, Ltd., London, 1964.
Ziai, M.: *Pediatrics,* Little, Brown and Company, Boston, 1969.

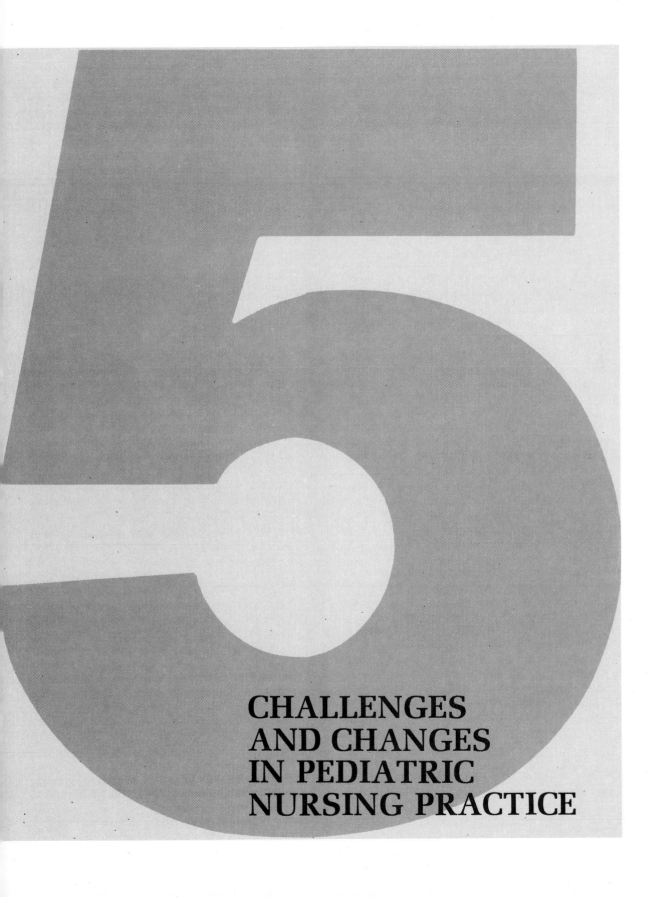

CHALLENGES AND CHANGES IN PEDIATRIC NURSING PRACTICE

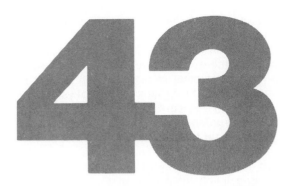

PEDIATRIC NURSING IN THE HOSPITAL

JOYCE M. OLSON
and JO-EILEEN GYULAY

Nursing practice in pediatric episodic care cannot be discussed without examining the factors which influence the delivery of health care and confronting the many issues that are yet to be resolved by the nursing profession.

Health care delivery is being critically examined by some members of the health professions, by third-party payment groups, and especially by the consumer. Change is occurring in the delivery of episodic care, but some changes must occur more rapidly and effectively if the needs of the client are to be met. Changes must also be considered in view of the desired outcome—change for the sake of change is invalid.

CURRENT STATUS OF EPISODIC CARE

Episodic care is defined in *An Abstract for Action* as "that area of concentration in nursing practice which emphasizes the curative and restorative aspect of nursing and which usually involves patients with diagnosed disease, either acute or chronic."[1] In caring for the child and his family, distributive and episodic care cannot be totally separated; one must complement the other.

In the area of episodic care, there are two major dissatisfactions. One involves dissatisfaction on the part of the client—the child and his family. Episodic pediatric care today is still largely fragmented, with the major emphasis placed on the specific disease process or acute health crisis. Often little attention is given in any comprehensive manner to the impact of the illness on the child and on the functioning of the family unit. Neither the pediatrician nor the nurse has assumed leadership roles to promote comprehensive child and family care. The trend in most modern hospitals is toward increased specialization and further discontinuity in care. The individuality and uniqueness of the child and his family become lost in the routines and regimens imposed by many different health care disciplines. Pediatric facilities need to increase utilization of known principles relevant to the needs of the sick child and his family. Anticipatory guidance to promote positive family health and growth, both physical and psychosocial, should be incorporated into the acute care setting to provide comprehensive child and family services.

The second problem area involves the satisfaction of the nurse providing care in the acute setting. Lack of satisfaction is evidenced by the high rate of personnel turnover. Nurses leave the acute care setting for other areas of practice, hoping to attain better hours, improved working conditions, more personal freedom, and professional autonomy. Staff-

901

ing patterns and assignment methods often prevent rather than encourage the continuity of care and involvement with a group of patients. Innovations in methods of providing nursing care need to be more widely researched and utilized. However, institutional patterns and bureaucratic structure cannot be blamed for all the dissatisfaction. Satisfaction is derived from the caring and helping; involvement and knowledge on the part of the nurse are essential. The nurse must look within himself and examine his commitment. Is this commitment to the patient and to the nursing profession? The professional nurse of today must have a comprehensive knowledge of the physical and behavioral sciences, a keen sensitivity to patient needs and wants, and the necessary skills related to the technological advances; then, he must utilize them fully in the nursing process to promote satisfaction within his own role.

INFLUENCING FACTORS IN FUTURE DELIVERY OF CARE

In pediatric nursing, as in all areas of nursing practice, the demands for change, improvement, and role expansion are influenced by several factors. Today's health care consumer is generally rather well informed. He no longer views the physician and nurse as the somewhat omnipotent, all-knowing, and caring team. He is more aware of what is or should be available to him and is demanding more accountability on the part of health team members. The parent consumer looks to the hospital and physician to have the latest in knowledge and technical capabilities to care for his child but demands a personalization of this care. Rooming-in facilities and care by parent units decrease trauma to the child and permit family involvement in the child's care. Episodic-care institutions need to examine the needs of the client in planning for and optimally utilizing facilities.

Medical science continues to change at a phenomenal rate, and these advances, coupled with the technical possibilities of the computer age, are going to greatly affect the skills and knowledge needed by the nurse, the tools available for use in giving care, and the numbers of other people involved in the total picture of patient care. The innovations in computers, monitoring equipment, surgical intervention, transplants, respiratory care, chemotherapy, nuclear medicine, and genetics all affect care given by the nurse. He must consider not only the scientific and technical aspects, but the many moral and ethical issues involved. Only by knowledgeable application of techniques and interpretation of data as they affect the individual child

and family can the nurse provide care along with cure and treatment.

Medical practice in the acute-care setting is becoming more and more a practice of specialists. It is rather typical to find that the patient may not know his doctor; in fact, several physicians may be involved in his care. The rotation of house staff, medical students, and attending staff, while perhaps necessary for the educational process, does not lend itself to coordinated, comprehensive, and continuous care. With many other paramedical people becoming involved in care of the patient, the nurse must provide the continuity and coordination in the sense that he may be the only one who can assess the total impact of all involved on the individual child and family.

The growth of prepaid medical and surgical insurance plans and the arrival of Medicare and Medicaid have already increased the need for and utilization of health care facilities. It appears likely that some form of national health insurance will become a reality in the near future, perhaps before this book is in print. With nearly 100 percent of the population covered, the demands for health care at all levels will be greatly increased.

Predictions are that episodic care in the future will encompass one-third or less of total health care. It seems reasonable to assume that those clients receiving care in the hospital or other acute setting will represent the more difficult diagnostic problems and the more complicated illnesses requiring the most advanced technology and equipment. This has implications for the location of facilities, specialization of units, utilization of various kinds of personnel, and especially the preparation of the nurse for practice in the acute-care setting.

ISSUES TO BE RESOLVED

Definition and Control of Nursing Practice

The critical issue of who defines nursing practice and who controls nursing practice within the episodic-care setting must be decided if professional nursing is to remain a part of the setting. Decision-making by physicians and administrators has long been the practice in the hospital. When able nursing leaders have tried to promote positive changes in nursing practice and patient care, an authority conflict has developed. The idea of self-governance for nursing practice by nurses must be promoted from within the profession. This idea implies not only freedom and authority to determine nursing practice and provide nursing care but also a commitment by the nurse to accountability for his nursing actions.

This accountability must be to himself, the patient, and nursing colleagues.

Expansion or Extension of Roles

The literature abounds with articles related to expanded roles and extended scope of practice for the nurse. Murphy conceptualizes role extension as a unilateral lengthening process and role expansion as a spreading out or a process of diffusion.[2] In relating these concepts to the care-cure model, those functions directed toward cure are seen as extenders and those functions undertaken in care as expanders. Viewed in the framework of cues used in decision-making, the expander of care utilizes a broader range than does the extender of cure.

In the episodic pediatric setting, cure is seen as the primary function of the health care team. Cure without care reduces the patient to a disease process rather than a unique individual.

Therefore, both functions are a part of nursing practice in the acute-care setting. Nurses are now being taught and "allowed to perform" many tasks which were once performed only by the physician. This occurrence is an extension of the physician and not an expansion of nursing. Performance of these tasks is acceptable as long as the *nurse* decides which tasks are best used and in what manner in the provision of *nursing* care.

Emerging Roles

A multiplicity of new roles and titles have emerged over the past few years, and programs continue to develop. Confusion, controversy, and competition have resulted. Many of these new roles for the nurse are being defined by other disciplines, particularly medicine. New classifications of health personnel are being prepared, and these newly prepared people are requesting recognition and licensure.

The terms *nurse clinician* and *clinical specialist* are used interchangeably in many institutions without a defined level of practice, education, or function. The concept of the primary nurse is being developed in several institutions. The professional nurse in this role assumes responsibility for the nursing care of a small group of patients and their families throughout the hospital stay and for the provision of continuity of care upon discharge.

The *pediatric nurse practitioner* and *pediatric nurse associate* roles are being developed primarily in the area of distributive care. These nurses are prepared to function in well-child care and health-screening programs in community clinics, pediatricians' offices, and hospital outpatient departments. Preparatory programs vary in length and content and focus primarily on physical examination, history-taking, and developmental assessment of the well child. These nurses will enter the acute setting as their clients experience episodes of illness requiring hospitalization. Continued effort will be needed to work out interrelations allowing for the utilization of their knowledge of the child and family and to provide continuity in care.

Physician's assistant programs are multiplying rapidly. Programs vary in entry requirements and may be from a few weeks to 2 or more years in length. A certificate, diploma, or degree may be awarded. The scope of practice for the physician's assistant is a narrowly defined set of activities delegated by the employing physician. The entry of this category of personnel into the acute-care setting will further fragment medical care and create issues of legality and interpersonal relationships. Nursing's role will remain much more comprehensive than that of the physician's assistant.

Unless the nurse uses professional judgment and assumes responsibility for his own actions within the scope of nursing, the independent functions of nursing will be further jeopardized. Nurses must decide who will provide nursing care and what are the appropriate levels of practice.

Professional or Technical Practice?

The delineation of practice at professional and technical levels is advocated by some, deplored by others. Acceptance or rejection depends on the individual interpretation of the terms and the vested interest of the nurse involved. Attempts to define *technical* and *professional* based on functions have not been successful. Definition based on educational level has been similarly futile and has created further divisiveness among nurses. However, it is imperative that nursing make some distinctions in levels of practice. Within the acute-care setting, the practice of nursing has been largely technical. Much of it will remain so as long as the decision-making power resides with the physician and administrator and accountability of the nurse is limited to carrying out the physician's orders and institutional policy. Professional nursing practice exists when the nurse has decision-making power with respect to patient care which falls within the realm of his competency. A system which allows for independent nursing practice—in which nursing orders are written and carried out as effectively as physicians' orders, and in which patient care management is the responsibility of nursing or medicine depending on the patient's need—is necessary for professional nursing practice. Professional or technical levels may in part be determined by the knowledge base and educational credentials of the nurse. The application of the knowledge, its utilization in decision-making, the ability of the nurse to function in a colleague relationship with other health professionals, and his commitment to the independent practice of nursing are more definitive components.

Independent Nursing Practice

Is independent nursing practice viable in the episodic pediatric setting? This question has not been answered yet. It must be dealt with if professional nursing is to survive in the acute-care setting. As has been stated, many nursing functions will be dependent and technical as they relate to the medical plan of treatment. We have also said that cure is only one part of the patient's need in health care. If the nurse uses only cues from a medical model aspect, independent practice is not involved.

There are many independent functions of nursing which can be practiced in the episodic setting. Assessment and decision-making in the areas of comfort, prevention, coping, and adaptation to illness or disease process, teaching and counseling related to illness, normal growth and development, family planning, family interactions, and utilization of hospital and community resources all involve independent practice. Independent activities of the nurse are not always understood or accepted by members of other disciplines. More importantly, they are not given proper priority by the nurse himself. A philosophy of professional nursing practice must be developed, and the concepts of accountability and independence accepted by members of the nursing profession. Resistance will be encountered from the physician, the institution, and from within the nursing profession. Change will come only through demonstration of knowledge and ability to provide meaningful contributions to patient care and documentation and evaluation of these contributions.

Independent practice of the nurse within the episodic setting may have differing modes of implementation. Some nurses will practice in the community—in group nursing practice or in collaboration with physicians. As their clients require episodic care, they will admit patients and be directly responsible for the planning of nursing care during the course of illness. If the client requires nursing assessments outside the particular nurse's practice area, the nurse will directly consult another nurse or refer the client to another nurse or physician.

Other nurses may remain in the direct employ of the institution. These nurses will have staff appointments and a case load much the same as the physician. Patients will be referred to them by other independent nursing practitioners and physicians. The need of the client will determine who manages the care.

Independent functioning must also be a part of nursing practice for those nurses who choose to remain a part of the more formalized nursing service structure. The clinical specialist or nursing practitioner operating at a unit or subunit level within the hospital facility must increase his contribution to patient care and assume accountability for the quality of nursing care given to the child and family. Utilization of other nursing personnel on a consultative basis should greatly enhance the quality of care.

ROLES OF THE PROFESSIONAL NURSE IN EPISODIC CARE

Examination of the independent and congruent roles of the nurse, physician, and other health-team members was a major recommendation of The National Commission for the Study of Nursing and Nursing Education. Within acute-care settings, the dependent functions of nursing have always received greater emphasis, especially those involved in carrying out the medical plan of care. Even within this area, nurses have not utilized the knowledge and skills they do have to function independently. Many doctors' orders are actually nursing assessments and judgments well within the realm of the professional nurse. With improved *communication* and *actual demonstration*, it is hoped that those facets of acute care which the professional nurse can manage independently will be recognized by both nursing and medicine.

Physicians have demonstrated their recognition of patient needs and nursing function by saying, "There are things my patients need which I cannot give them or with which I have neither the time, interest, nor talent to get involved." Many of these "things" are related to family stresses, teaching needs, and psychosocial problems.

Professional roles, both present and projected, must be defined within some guidelines and yet not become so rigid that flexibility, creativity, and sharing in the team approach are totally subjugated to role definition. There are different approaches, tools to use, and methods of delivery of care. Nursing practitioners within particular institutions must decide what will work best for them in providing excellence in episodic care for their patients. Change and expansion of roles are valuable only when they improve patient care and increase the satisfaction of the person providing the care.

If the literature discussing clinical specialists is reviewed, one can devise a composite picture of professional nursing activities in the episodic setting. The clinical specialist functions on a colleague basis with the physician and other health team professionals. He is able to systematically assess nursing needs and plan, implement, and evaluate nursing care. He gives direct care, teaches others who provide care, and ensures that the child and family have necessary health teaching and counseling. He provides for continuity in physical care and psychologic support of the child and family and coordinates aspects of care requiring services of other departments. He may also carry a case load of his own, undertake clinical research to increase his competence and advance nursing knowledge, and serve as a role model of expert clinical practice to students, physicians, peers, and members of allied health disciplines.

Some specific role functions of the professional nurse practicing in a pediatric episodic-care setting are discussed next.

Patient Advocate

The primary role of the professional nurse is that of advocate of the child and family. By virtue of his longer, more continuous contact with the child and family, his basic knowledge of development, family dynamics, and disease process, the nurse is in the best position to assess the total impact of the illness and hospitalization on the child and family. If the professional nurse is to be a patient advocate, he must be adept in assessing, planning, implementing, and evaluating direct patient care. He must also act as liaison, teacher, and consultant.

Assessment The components of assessment have been discussed in depth in Part 1. The degree of overlap between the physician and nurse will vary with the particular acute setting. The goals of the individual assessment and the tools the nurse may use will vary from area to area within the acute setting. For example, a nurse in the pediatric screening area of the emergency room, the nurse in the neonatal intensive-care area, the nurse involved with pediatric cardiology patients, or the nurse working in a birth defects specialty clinic will have the common goal of comprehensive child and family care but will use the components of assessment with differing specific goals. In some instances, the nurse will do a complete physical examination. At other times, particularly when the medical student and intern have already done this examination, the nurse will use data already obtained. The nursing goals may be concerned with the ongoing assessment of particular needs such as respiratory status, cardiovascular status, or child and family adjustment to illness. The goals of the nurse in observation, interviewing, and testing may in part overlap with those of the physician. It is hoped that these goals will serve as complementary parts of the total assessment. The physician has and probably will continue to concern himself with disease manifestations and treatment in his problem-oriented approach. The nurse must include many other developmental and psychosocial factors in his assessment of the child and family, with all being combined if individualized patient care is to be delivered. The physician may diagnose diabetes in a child, determine management of the acute episode of ketoacidosis, and initiate a maintenance program of control with insulin and diet. However, the nurse must also assess patient and family knowledge of the disease, understanding and thinking related to knowledge and past contact with the disease, readiness and ability of the child and parents to accept and manage the disease, parent-child relationships, and many other factors if optimum long-term planning for living with the disease is to be accomplished.

Direct Patient Care The professional nurse at any level in acute care must be involved in direct patient care. Direct care may be total nursing care for a small group of patients, or it may involve specific facets of care for a larger group of patients. As the roles of *technical and professional nursing* become more clearly defined—and they must—the structure for the delivery of nursing care will change. The professional nurse may be a staff nurse who, with guidance from the team leader, provides total nursing care. He may be a *primary nurse* who alone or with the assistance of the technical nurse or patient aide plans for and provides total nursing care, doing those parts which require his knowledge and expertise or which he elects to do for purposes of further assessment and evaluation of the patient or teaching of team members. These parts might include complicated procedures, patient and family teaching, admission interviews to begin the care plan and write nursing orders, or dressing changes to assess wound healing. He may also be the *clinical specialist* or *nurse clinician* who assesses, evaluates, and is involved in those areas of direct patient care which are necessary for providing optimal nursing care, continuity, staff growth, student teaching, and coordination of the care. The *clinical specialist* or *clinician* may function as a primary nurse.

A statement from the Secretary's Committee to Study Extended Roles for Nurses appears in The National Commission for the Study of Nursing and Nursing Education (NCSNNE) pamphlet and suggests that acute-care practitioners in the future will:

> Secure and record a health and developmental history and make a critical evaluation of such records.
> Perform basic physical and psychologic assessments and translate the findings into appropriate nursing action.
> Discriminate between normal and abnormal findings on physical and psychosocial assessments.
> Make prospective decisions about treatment in collaboration with the physician.
> Initiate actions and treatments within the protocols developed jointly by medical and nursing personnel, such as adjusting medications, ordering and interpreting laboratory tests, and prescribing certain rehabilitative and restorative measures.[3]

Professional nurses have already been performing several of these functions, though in many instances they occur in the form of suggestions to the physician. Again, these functions are tools and means which the nurse can utilize in meeting nursing goals and will not, it is hoped, be viewed as the sum total of nursing practice in the episodic setting.

Evaluation The professional nurse is concerned with the evaluation of nursing care given, and with the evaluation of the impact on and response of the child and family to the total treatment plan. Without the ongoing evaluation of individual child and family, nursing care becomes routinized and mechanistic.

Liaison The professional nurse functions as a liaison between many disciplines involved in patient care and between child and family when they are separated within the acute-care setting. Potential liaison needs are between (1) patient, family, and physician; (2) patient and nursing staff; (3) patient and other members of the health-care team; (4) patient and individual, group, or agency who will provide follow-up care; (5) patient and other family members; and (6) patient and patient.

As a liaison between the patient, family, and doctor, the professional nurse can interpret the termi-

nology of diagnosis, prognosis, treatments, medications, and procedures in terms that both child and family can understand. To do this, it is vital that he maintain good communications with the physician and with the child and family. The nurse may be the buffer and interpreter when problems arise because of misunderstandings, misinterpretations, and personality conflicts. This situation may be more frequent in the medical center setting where child and family can be very confused by a multitude of contacts with members of the medical profession. The nurse may need to be the doctor-to-doctor liaison and insist that physicians coordinate what is being said to and done for the child and family.

The professional nurse functions as a liaison and communication agent between the child, family, and other members of the health team. Through assessment of the total needs, strengths, and weaknesses of the child and family during the illness crisis, he can best interpret to, and coordinate efforts of, other team members.

Other nursing personnel within the acute setting can be used in providing care. Referrals can also be instituted on a nurse-to-nurse level. For example, a child with an eye prosthesis was admitted to a general pediatric unit. The nurse had limited knowledge of the care required, and the family was not present. A nurse on the eye, ear, nose, and throat unit was contacted; care was explained and demonstrated. A team conference and written care plan provided for continuity. As another example, a patient with a diagnosis of postpartum depression needed instruction in baby care. A nursing consultation to the pediatric clinician was written. An assessment of need and cooperative plan of action resulted which utilized expertise of both pediatric and psychiatric nurses.

The need to plan for follow-up care on discharge has been discussed and written about hundreds of times, but in reality it is often poorly done. The planning must be started early in the hospitalization and implemented as soon as appropriate. This planning may involve the following:

1. Community health nursing referral—ideally an opportunity would be made for the community health nurse to meet with the patient, family, and nurse in the hospital.
2. Referral to parent groups such as the myelomeningocele club, sudden infant death groups, cystic fibrosis groups, or the local diabetes association.
3. Referral to physician or independent nurse practitioner.
4. Communication with the school nurse, schoolteacher, school counselor, and perhaps even the babysitter if the mother works. Arrangements for home-bound teaching may be needed.
5. Communication with the nurse in the specialty clinic or coordination of clinic visits, as many children are followed in two or more clinics.

6 Instruction in the use of equipment and arrangements for the family to obtain necessary equipment and supplies. Special formulas and equipment may not be available through small rural drugstores unless specific arrangements are made.

7 Referral to or arrangements made for special services such as physical therapy, speech therapy, or counseling.

The child is an individual, a member of a family, and a member of the community. The illness of a child concerns parents, siblings, grandparents, aunts, uncles, peers, teachers, and neighbors. The liaison function may be that of interpreting the child's illness not only to parents but to other family members. It may be in helping parents cope with other family members and their feelings and concerns. It is difficult for a young mother to care for her child in the way she thinks best if three other family members are all giving her conflicting advice. It is difficult for parents to be open and honest with their leukemic child if grandparents think that he should not be told the diagnosis. Parents frequently need assistance in knowing how to explain the child's illness to other children in the family or the child's peer group. Often direct contact and intervention by the nurse with these significant persons are needed.

In the hospital, there are frequently times when the child and parent must be separated, sometimes for many hours. The professional nurse caring for the child should serve as a liaison between the child and family at these times. It takes only a few minutes to check on a child in the recovery room, the cardiac catheterization laboratory, or the radiology department. These checks, combined with brief parent contact, do much to relieve parental anxiety. With adequate planning, it is even possible for the nurse to accompany the child to the operating room, remain until he is asleep, and then see him as he is waking in the recovery room. The same is true for the child having a cardiac catheterization, bone marrow aspiration, brain scan, or other special procedures.

Frequently, another patient or family with the same illness can be of assistance. Nurses often overlook this available and worthwhile source of support. Certainly careful assessment of the situation must be made before involving another child and family. However, one child and family's successful everyday living and coping with a problem can provide another family with assurance and hope that is difficult for the professional person to give. For example, parents, ages 18 and 19 years, have a newborn baby with a cleft lip and palate. They have had no previous exposure to such a defect, and it is indeed horrifying.

Why not have them talk with a family whose child is now in the hospital for some stage of palate repair? The same would be possible for the child with a myelomeningocele or a colostomy, or one who is facing eventual open-heart surgery.

Teacher The professional nurse working with the child and family is involved in many kinds of teaching. Anticipatory guidance requires a thorough initial and ongoing assessment of the child's physical condition, developmental level, behavioral reactions, readiness for particular teaching, and of the family dynamics, parental responses, behaviors, and expectations related to the child, illness, and hospitalization. It requires alertness to both verbal and nonverbal cues as to what the needs, fears, and concerns are and then intervening with the appropriate teaching. For example, a mother was rooming in with her 11-month-old daughter. This was the fourth admission to determine the cause of febrile episodes. She said to the nurse, "I'm not that worried about Susie, as I'm here and she is being cared for. But I don't know what I'm going to do about the two boys at home. I'm having all kinds of problems with them." Do nurses explore the kinds of problems, help her look at possible causes, and suggest some concrete methods of coping with these problems? Frequently not, because it is not viewed as a part of the child's acute illness. If nurses are truly providing comprehensive family care, they will look at how one child's illness affects the functioning of the total family.

Aspects of assessment, exploration, and evaluation that result in determined needs for teaching may relate to:

1 Orientation to the acute-care setting
2 Interpretation and explanation of the disease process
3 Knowledge of illness, reasons for hospitalization
4 Normal growth and development
5 Well-child care
6 Behavioral problems and management
7 Special procedures and tests
8 Preoperative teaching
9 Postoperative activities—what procedures are necessary and why
10 Long-range expectations
11 Family relationships
12 Introduction of a new baby into the family
13 Family planning
14 Effect of illness on the family unit—acute, chronic, or terminal
15 Anticipated behaviors of the child postdischarge
16 Clarification of ideas or misinformation
17 Special care needed at home—temporary or long term
18 Ways in which the parent can assist the child in coping and in promoting faster recovery

Teaching may be done with the individual child and family most of the time. However, group teaching may be more effective and efficient in some instances. With many mothers who are rooming in or spending most of the day with their child, daily sessions relevant to health needs, normal growth and development, and management of usual childhood and family problems are appropriate.

Role Model, Educator, and Researcher

Every professional nurse should be a role model for students and other members of the nursing team. The positiveness of the role model is dependent upon the nurse's ability to demonstrate his depth of knowledge, skills, and competence in providing nursing care. If professional nursing is to survive in the acute care setting, the nurse must assume responsibility and accountability within the health team.

Education of all members of the health team is a responsibility of the professional nurse. Teaching is done in both formal and informal ways.

With members of the nursing staff, much teaching is done informally as the nurse provides direct care to children and families and assists the staff in giving care. Formal teaching can be provided through patient care conferences, nursing rounds, and staff development classes.

With nursing students, some teaching is done informally as students are caring for patients. Capable members of the nursing staff can also be utilized by nursing education in the formal classroom setting. If professional clinical practice is the major focus of nursing, the teacher must also be an active practitioner.

There are many ways in which the professional nurse can teach medical students as they rotate through the pediatric service. As has been pointed out, medical care is highly disease process–oriented, and while other aspects of care are mentioned, the student often has inadequate role models when it comes to "putting it all together." The students are aware of the need for involvement of other disciplines in providing care but have little knowledge of how to obtain it or what others can be expected to contribute. The nurse can enhance the medical student's education and at the same time make him more aware of the nurses' contributions to patient care, above and beyond carrying out medical orders. As the trend to include students of many health care disciplines in clinical process classes increases, teamwork and learning will be more effective.

Physicians are beginning to recognize that they,

too, can learn from the nurse and that he has information vital to the provision of care. As episodic care becomes even more specialized, it is reasonable to assume that the nurse coordinator of the neonatal intensive-care nursery or the nurse involved with pediatric cardiology patients on a continuous basis will have expertise that the physician rotating through the area does not possess. This knowledge and expertise will involve the technical aspects of care and also an in-depth knowledge of and ability in intervention with the child and family experiencing the particular illness or disease crisis. Interpretation to the physician of the developmental levels and strengths of a particular child and capabilities of a particular family is a vital educational role of the professional nurse. Active participation in patient rounds and communication through progress notes are tools also used by the nurse in the educational process.

The professional nurse at all levels should be involved in, and/or supportive of, research related to the care of children and families. The level of involvement and responsibility will vary with particular interests and capabilities. The staff nurse who is most directly involved in patient care should be questioning practice and the delivery of care. While he may not have the capabilities to conduct a major research project, he should be suggesting ideas to those who can and participating in data collection. Primary nurses and team leaders should be assisting in projects and perhaps conducting their own related to questions and problems encountered in the delivery of care to their patients. The clinician who is involved in trying different kinds of intervention with children and families must collect data and promote research in the clinical practice of nursing. He may be the project director but may also utilize the skills of others in the research planning, design, data collection, and analysis of results. Much of what nurses do is based on intuition or assumed need or benefit; scientific validation is needed.

MODELS FOR THE DELIVERY OF EPISODIC PEDIATRIC CARE

Nursing positions are no longer being defined by functional position titles such as Head Nurse, Supervisor, or Assistant Director. As more administrative duties are assumed by unit managers and clerical personnel, the emphasis has shifted to clinical practice and expertise in service and education.

Pediatric episodic care is delivered for the most part within the structure of the hospital and specialty clinics. Innovative approaches must be tried and validated if nursing care needs are to be met and satisfaction derived by the nurse. A commitment to the patient and his nursing care needs becomes the priority over meeting the needs of the institution and the physician.

Within the acute-care setting, medical technology will be a large factor in determining nursing care. Hospital facilities will be used for diagnosis, intensive care, and specialty clinic follow-up. Much of the nursing care will involve technical skills. However, there will be a need for different levels of nursing if comprehensive child and family care is to be provided.

To provide a theoretical base, the authors will use some designations proposed by Cleland.[4] She believes that the *clinical specialist* is a nurse who has mastered particular diagnostic or therapeutic techniques in a specific area. Examples would be renal dialysis, kidney transplant monitoring, intensive-care specialties, juvenile diabetic care, and similar subspecialties within the area of episodic pediatric care. This nurse provides care utilizing a defined, restricted range of cues in an extended role.

The *nurse clinician* is seen as a generalist who uses a broad range of cues obtained from several parameters. He then prescribes nursing care independently, using an approach which extends beyond the immediate response to disease pathology or medical treatment.

A distinction is also made between a *general nurse* and a *nurse practitioner*. The *general nurse* is accountable for a daily assignment which is usually functional in nature. The *practitioner* is accountable for a number of patients during the entire hospital stay. The difference is that of scope of practice and the range of cues utilized in decision-making within the nursing process. Cleland basically sees two levels of nursing. The first level includes *general nurses* and *nurse practitioners*, and the second level includes *nurse specialists* and *nurse clinicians*. The general nurse and nurse specialist work in the defined setting and with the time dimension extending over an 8-hour period or the current acute episode. The nurse practitioner and nurse clinician use multiple sources of data to plan a broad patient care program which involves the family and includes the entire course of the illness.

The National Commission for the Study of Nursing and Nursing Education proposes three levels of nursing in the episodic setting. These levels are:

Staff nurse   A beginning-practice designation for graduates of all preparatory programs that encompass levels or steps attained by demonstration of increasing proficiency in the provision of nursing care.

Clinical nurse   Middle levels or steps of nursing practice attained by demonstrating increasing competence in providing leadership for the nursing team and contributing significant clinical nursing skills to the patient care team.

Master clinician   An advanced level of practice attained through clinical experience, additional study, and designation by an academy of nursing (or other group empowered to do so) which involves the demonstrated ability to make a significant contribution to patient care through independent nursing judgments and scientifically based participation in the patients' therapeutic regimens.[5]

Career development in episodic practice may then be shown as depicted in Fig. 43-1. Not all nurses will agree that either of these attempts at delineation of levels of practice is meaningful and sufficient. However, the multiplicity of educational programs and position titles has resulted in confusion and dissatisfaction among nurses and other health care disciplines. Reality and practicality require some concrete operational framework. The authors suggest that the three levels of staff nurse, clinical nurse, and master clinician provide this basis and that other definitions and job descriptions fit within this framework.

The staff nurse is the general nurse. He functions within a specific setting and is accountable for a daily assignment, utilizing a limited range of cues to carry out this assignment. This level would include beginning practitioners from associate degree, diploma, and baccalaureate programs. It also would include nurses with more experience and/or education who, because of home, family, or other priorities, choose to function on a part-time basis and assume responsibility for only an 8-hour shift assignment in a circumscribed area.

The clinical nurse may be the nurse practitioner, team leader, or primary nurse who assumes responsibility and accountability for the nursing care of a group of patients throughout the hospitalization period. He also plans for continuity of care following discharge. The clinical nurse may also be the clinical specialist who assumes responsibility and accountability for the quality of nursing care for a group of patients with a particular disease process or nursing-care problem. He provides for continuity by seeing and caring for these patients in the hospital and specialty clinic and by making home visits. The clinical nurse is the baccalaureate graduate who, with additional experience, demonstrates ability in management of care for a group of patients. He may also be an associate degree or diploma graduate who, with continuing education and additional experience, is able to demonstrate the skills and capabilities required to function at the clinical nurse level.

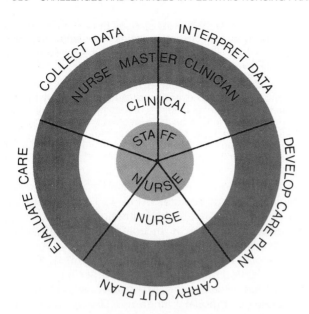

Figure 43-1 Career development in episodic practice. *(From National Commission for the Study of Nursing and Nursing Education, From Abstract into Action, McGraw-Hill Book Company, New York, 1973, p. 120.)*

The master clinician level includes the nurse clinicians who function either as generalists or specialists, utilizing a broad range of cues and assuming responsibility and accountability for the quality of nursing care of a larger group of patients and/or carrying their own case load. The master clinician has a graduate degree and the expertise to care for patients in a variety of pediatric settings, although he may elect to focus on a particular group in the specialist sense.

The preceding description could be shown as follows:

NCSNNE levels	Other titles in current use	Requirements for entry
Staff nurse	General nurse	Associate degree Diploma Baccalaureate in nursing
Clinical nurse	Team leader Primary nurse Nurse practitioner Clinical specialist May be generalist or specialist	Above plus additional experience, continuing education, or both Demonstrated expertise
Master clinician	Nurse clinician Generalist or specialist	Graduate degree Designation by an academy of nursing

Although the entry of the independent practitioner into the acute-care setting will be a new role, the change and challenge for the pediatric nurse in episodic care will be to define and improve on some of the current trends, with emphasis placed on expert clinical practice and full utilization of the skills possessed by the nurse to provide nursing care. The following case history is typical of what we shall see in the future.

The nurse clinician in independent practice sees Peter, age 6 months, in his office for a well-baby visit. He finds that Peter is well below normal in height and weight and is behind in motor and social development. He arranges for hospital admission to secure further diagnostic information. He consults with the resident physician who orders appropriate diagnostic tests to rule out physical causes. The clinician writes orders and communicates pertinent history and assessment information to the clinical nurse on the pediatric unit. Throughout the hospitalization the clinician sees the child and mother daily. The clinical nurse plans, coordinates, and evaluates care at the unit level. The staff nurse provides parts of the care involved in carrying out diagnostic procedures and implementing the nursing care plan. The child and family return to the care of the clinician.

Increased mobility of the nurse within the episodic setting and into the home will occur, as in the following case history:

Mary Lynn, age 7 years, is seen in hematology clinic with acute leukemia. Blood tests and bone marrow aspiration indicate an exacerbation of the disease. The physician decides to hospitalize the child for further chemotherapy. The pediatric hematology nurse specialist, who has been following Mary Lynn in clinic and through home visits, calls and arranges for admission to the unit where Mary Lynn has been cared for previously. Utilizing his information about Mary Lynn, the course of her disease, her family, their knowledge of the disease, and the coping mechanisms of the child and family, the nurse specialist obtains an admission history, updates the assessment, writes nursing care orders, and formulates the written care plan for Mary Lynn. Since the clinical specialist also follows all pediatric hematology patients in the hospital, communication is easily maintained and continuity in care provided. The specialist sees the child at least daily and consults with the clinical nurse who is planning, coordinating, and giving care on the unit level. The staff nurse is involved in the shift-to-shift provision of nursing care and in carrying out the medical regimen. Upon discharge, Mary Lynn will continue to be followed by the clinical specialist in clinic and at home. This kind of mobility between hospital, clinic, and home should be possible for many groups of patients, especially those with chronic illness.

There will be an increased use of nurses on a consultation and referral basis by nurses and physicians. The professional nurse cannot have in-depth knowledge of nursing care and techniques in all specialities; nor will all nurses be specialists. The nurse caring for a 12-year-old with a cervical fracture and who is on a general pediatric unit must recognize and utilize the expertise of the clinical nurse or specialist on the neurosurgery and rehabilitation units in planning care to meet immediate and long-term nursing goals for the patient.

A 4-year-old boy is admitted with second- and third-degree burns. A social and family history reveals that there are two younger children and that the mother is approximately 2½ months pregnant. Her husband is unemployed, she does not want another child, and she has seriously considered an abortion but does not know how to proceed. The pediatric nurse clinician consults with the mother and refers her to the clinician in family-planning clinic. The family-planning clinician carries out an assessment, counsels the mother, and helps make arrangements for having the abortion.

In another instance, the psychiatrist, in treating a patient with a diagnosis of postpartum depression, determines that feelings of inadequacy in caring for her baby are a major problem. Since babies have not routinely been admitted with the mothers, the pediatric clinician is consulted to assist in planning for the admission and to assess capabilities and work with the patient in care of the baby.

There will be an increased involvement of the nurse in management of and decision-making in the total care of the child and family. As knowledge and skill are demonstrated, the primary management of care for many patients will reside with the nurse, with the physician serving as a consultant. Such patients might include infants and children who fail to thrive, children with diabetes requiring teaching, insulin, and diet regulation, children for whom abuse or neglect is suspected and observation and evaluation are necessary, or infants with congenital anom-

alies when parent teaching is required. The technical skills and expertise of the nurse in neonatal intensive care, pediatric cardiology, and other specialties will also increase the involvement of the nurse in management of patient care.

These last statements have been made in a positive frame of reference. They should occur, but this will happen only if the professional nurse has the commitment to this kind of nursing practice and the issues presented are resolved by the nursing profession.

REFERENCES

1 The National Commission for the Study of Nursing and Nursing Education, *An Abstract for Action*, McGraw-Hill Book Company, New York, 1970, p. 166.
2 Juanita F. Murphy, "Role Expansion or Role Extension," *Nursing Forum*, 9(4):380–389, 1970.
3 The National Commission for the Study of Nursing and Nursing Education, *Episodic Nursing Practice: Refinement and Expansion of Roles*, Rochester, New York, 1972.
4 Virginia Cleland, "Nurse Clinicians and Nurse Specialists: An Overview," *Three Challenges to the Nursing Profession*, American Nurses Association, 1972, pp. 13–25.
5 The National Commission for the Study of Nursing and Nursing Education, *An Abstract for Action*, op. cit., pp. 165–167.

BIBLIOGRAPHY

Brown, Esther Lucille: *Nursing Reconsidered: A Study of Change*, pt. 1, J. B. Lippincott Company, Philadelphia, 1970.
Chioni, Rose Marie, and Panicucci, Carol: "Tomorrow's Nurse Practitioners," *Nursing Outlook*, 18(2):32–35, 1970.
Clausen, Joy Princeton, et al.: *Maternity Nursing Today*, McGraw-Hill Book Company, New York, New York, 1973, pp. 24–42.
Conant, Lucy H.: "The Nature of Nursing Tomorrow," *Image*, vol. 4, no. 2, 1970–71.
"Extending the Scope of Nursing Practice," *Nursing Outlook*, 20(1):46–52, 1972.
Kramer, Marlene: "The Consumer's Influence on Health Care," *Nursing Outlook*, 20(9):574–578, 1972.
Lewis, Edith P.: *The Clinical Nurse Specialist*, The American Journal of Nursing Company, New York, 1970.
———: *Changing Patterns of Nursing Practice*, The American Journal of Nursing Company, New York, 1971.
Manthey, Marie: "Primary Nursing is Alive and Well in the Hospital," *American Journal of Nursing*, 73(1):83–87 1973.
Rothberg, June S.: "Nurse and Physician Assistant: Issues and Relationships," *Nursing Outlook*, 21(3):154–158, 1973.

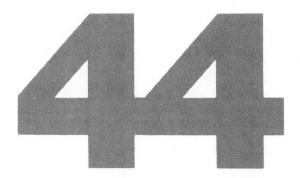

44

PEDIATRIC NURSING IN THE COMMUNITY

MAUD ADAMS

SEPARATISM AND SYNERGISM IN DELIVERY OF HEALTH CARE

The nature of health care appears to be moving away from a period of separatism toward an age of synergism in the process of delivery. One factor is the movement from medical care predominately to health care. Health care is synergistic—medical care is not. Medical care connotes specific disease conditions and the clinical procedures related to their biochemical, physiologic, and related processes. Health care is broader in scope, including not only the physical aspects but also cultural, social, and behavioral aspects of harmonious functioning in work, play, family, and community life. There is a renewed awareness that, although health and dysfunction show up in the individual, many interrelated influences—genetic endowment, family life, education, economics, work, fortuitous factors of physical environment, and the entire structure of the community, including cultural, political, and historical development—exist. The growing child is not divisible within himself nor from his family and the many factors within his community. He is involved in an interlocking phenomena. Health care of the child today involves a comprehensive approach with real problems of coordination and integration in its implementation. To bring this age of synergism into reality, adaptations that are attitudinal, communicative, educational, and structural in nature are required to meet the challenge of the changing clinical practice.

Cooperative Partnership

The new age brings into focus some aspects which are familiar and some new complexities. There are still children who have families as there have always been. Physicians, nurses, allied health welfare professionals, and neighborhoods with their unique collective personhood, and health-related agencies continue to exist. Community problems, some old and some new, are still present. Some of the old include those of communicable disease and environmental sanitation control, ignorance in health affairs, poverty, and categorical federal funding. Added to these now, among others, are pollution, increased population with large proportions of the young and aged, mechanization of the farming industry, mobilization into urban areas and spread to the suburbs, social stress, drug and alcohol dependency, changes in family life-style, early pregnancies, child abuse, chronic illness, transportation problems, consumer activism by individuals and citizen groups, specialization and maldistribution of the health professional, spectacular advances in medical technology with rising medical costs, and a new federalism in health care. There is cognizance of the interrelatedness of such problems, social, physical, emotional, and professional; they are indeed complex and cannot be resolved by any one discipline or institution.

Cooperative partnership is becoming more a pattern of approach to health care. Linkage components of the problem are being assessed. Personnel whose unique talents would contribute most effectively toward the solution of the problem are being employed in a collaborative and coordinated manner. Optimal utilization of physician and nursing talents are being translated into more effective child-family care through cooperative integrated functioning. The pediatric nurse with her knowledge and skill in the health care of the child and his family complements the medical talents of the physician. With the evolving change, comprehensive health care for the child and his family in the community is being brought into greater balance.

Environment and Health

Man's natural environments are an integral part of his state of health and sense of well-being. How well this writer recalls an early experience as an elementary school nurse when an 8-year-old girl came to the office in the early fall with a flushed face and complaints of a sudden bout of nausea and vomiting. This writer plunged headlong into a disease-centered analysis, feeling almost certain that the pathology was physical. When her little friend arrived subsequently, a communicable disease was suspected. When, in a short period of time, her third friend arrived with similar symptoms, an epidemic seemed to be brewing. The answer was forthcoming after an inquiry as to what was happening in their classroom. In chorus, they replied that they were having a math test from a stern teacher. In unison they voiced, "And we never did like arithmetic!" They readily taught this writer something she had heard but had not really learned: assessment includes a concentration on how and what factors in the environment may be contributing to a "dis-ease" within one. How often is a child presented by a parent as the "identified sick patient," yet an exploration of the complaint, or presenting problem, is found to be negative in the best clinical judgment? A single question, "What is going on at home?" will unravel a whole tangled strand of family stress and disharmony to which the child is reacting. The "real patient" becomes the parent and the dysfunctioning family. The child's symptoms may be viewed as a re-flection of the emotional behavior of the entire family.

Family and Health

Dr. Nathan Ackerman saw the family as the unit of health and illness and the unit of treatment—not the single patient in isolation, but in the wider context of reciprocal family role adaptation.[1] In the universal tasks of living and growing, the child and each individual family member, as well as the family functional unit, are simultaneously attempting to cope with critical personal developmental shifts and experiences along with complex interfacing environmental forces outside the social framework of the family unit. Take the young child with a reading lag. Is his problem one of a vision or hearing deficit, a cognitive problem, or distraught parenting in an overwhelming impoverished home? More parental concern may be placed upon the sheer struggle to provide a roof over the heads and to make food available in the poverty-stricken family than upon stimulation of word curiosity and learning. The reasons for this parenting behavior are multiple and may be completely unknown to the parent. Factors that need exploration include the following: the situation of the family at any given point in time; the family's own particular history; the physical condition and age of family members; the family dynamics; the physical factors of the home; and the economic, cultural, and the societal nature of the neighborhood and its community services.[2]

FAMILY- AND COMMUNITY-CENTERED CARE OF CHILDREN

The nurse who has a professional interest in children becomes at once family- and community-centered. Family- and community-centered nursing of children is the particular focus of the nurse in the community.

Such a nurse has concern for a five-dimensional level of development: that of the child, the family, the community and its health welfare supportive services, her own development, and nursing in general. Such a nurse has the privilege of experiencing the dynamic processes of growth and development with children and their parenting figure(s) in the intimacy of their homes and in the larger community environment. From the time the child is in the cradle, this relationship continues throughout his springboard periods toward maturity. The nurse has an opportunity to be a part of the dynamic interplay of family members working through their mutually interdependent roles. This involvement offers an opportunity to renew the very essence of life in her own being, as well as to enrich her own philosophic outlook; to think, rethink, and grow continuously in the acquisition of knowledge, understanding, and competency in procedural and interpersonal skills. Family and community nursing reveals a unique factorial mosaic around each child in the situation occurring along the way in the developmental life-span. They become her best teachers of experiential professional insight and wisdom.

During a critical epoch of history, with privilege come both opportunity and responsibility. In spite of an increasing percentage of the gross national product being expended for health care, the United States with an infant mortality rate of 19.2 in 1971[3] remains at the level of a developing nation in maternal child health. Communities are groping with the task of providing citizens an adequate transportation system, schools, mass protective police and fire programs, as well as those for air, noise, water, and sewage environmental management, and personal health welfare services. Consumers have become more verbal and are expressing loudly their concerns about what they perceive as inadequacies. They are becoming more assertive in the decision-making process of the community's activities. Traditional health care services are being challenged. The foundations of family life are being shaken. There are those who are asking if we need the family unit. Eulch Laucks records that only 35 percent of the families in this country are now nuclear in structure, the traditional concept of family.[4] How many families maintain a borderline accommodation until the children are grown or disintegrate to become dysfunctional? Family life-styles are changing with a number of the universal functions of family being provided by community supportive programs. More living occurs outside the home with mothers being a large part of the labor market. Increased use of child care centers and baby-sitters are made. Recreation is more a part of organized group efforts such as those offered by Blue Birds, Scouts, dancing and sewing classes, little league baseball, and organized playground programs. Individual family members have increasingly wider and scattered interest. Divorce is made quickly, more easily, and with less stigma. The women's liberation movement seems to be pointing up changes in the degree of dependence of women in numerous ways. Contraception methods have given mothers alternative choices in planning a family. Teaching of health is being assumed by extra-family programs. Health services and sickness care are provided by professional experts outside the home. Life-styles are changing at such a rapid pace

that, in the biological linkage, generational gaps widen to the extent that grandparents feel too out of phase to support either the current generation of youth or the parents, their own progeny. Sharing what seemed to work for them experientially does not seem relevant to the problems of today.

To add another dimension in this critical epoch, nursing is in a state of flux in its evolutional development. As time and needs change, so must the profession and its practitioners. In the transitional 1970s communities, parents, children, and nurses are caught up in a web of problems of a similar nature, but perhaps with different parameters of concern. Each is trying to develop responses to the uncertainties of inevitable and rapid change as they attempt to remain relevant. Attempts are made to modify attitudes and beliefs and to reason out a road map into the future for improved realignments of societal, organizational, educational, and service models which are more responsive and satisfactory to the interrelated needs and concerns for the well-being of people.

Episodic or Distributive

What relevance does all this information have for the nurse? Where is nursing, and, more specifically, how is nursing care of children beyond the hospital walls going to be delivered? The National Commission for the Study of Nursing and Nursing Education explored such questions. In that study two essentially related, but differing, career patterns for nursing practice are discussed: episodic care and distributive care. Episodic care would emphasize nursing practice that is essentially curative and restorative, generally acute and chronic in nature, and most frequently provided in the setting of the hospital or in-patient facility. The other is referred to as a distributive career pattern emphasizing nursing practice which is essentially designed for health maintenance and disease prevention. This care is generally continuous in nature, is seldom acute, and will increasingly take place in the community or emergent institutional setting.[5]

The nurse encounters children and parents in two major settings, that is, in the hospital and in the community that encompasses many settings including the home, physician's office, traditionally organized units as school, departments of health and visiting nurse services, and, now, emergent units such as neighborhood health centers, health maintenance organizations (HMOs), and satellite clinics. In the hospital setting, the child is usually admitted for a thorough medical definition of his difficulty and/or acute medical intervention. In other community settings he tends to be in a more normal life situation attempting to function maximally within the parameters of his genetic endowment and life environments. The predominant tasks of nurses vary in degree, but are not mutually exclusive in the two major settings. The facts of life do not permit a decisive either/or differentiation into episodic and distributive. If total needs of children and parents are to be met, care must be available from various care resources.

The nurse in the hospital must have a positive attitude toward the reciprocal impact of the child's condition upon the family and the child and give appropriate attention to family concerns here and now. The family health nurse in the community must have an appreciation of childhood disease and sufficient working knowledge to be competent in recognizing prodromal symptoms of acute episodes of disease and take appropriate action. He also monitors, supports, and cares for children with chronic latent illnesses in settings other than in-patient services. The human being simply does not maintain a consistent plateau in his health-disease-illness continuum. Human development and human illness do not come in neatly labeled boxes. Admittedly, degrees of competence, skill, and interest differ in each setting, but there is an inevitable overlap in the two classifications; strict functional boundaries are impractical. A study done in New York City in a teen-age contraception clinic explored a concept of adolescence as the healthiest time of life.[6] Findings reveal how intermixed the health-disease continuum becomes. A chart review of 255 single "healthy" teenagers (ages 11 to 17 years), who voluntarily registered over a period of 1 year, found that 61 percent had notable medical problems during childhood; 31 percent were currently being treated for one or more illnesses; 63 percent had undiagnosed conditions that required medical therapy, and 53 percent had problems relating to home-school-family situations or psychologic difficulties ranging from neurosis to alcoholism.

In nursing today a name game is occurring. One hears such attempts in further differentiation in titles as pediatric nurse practitioner, pediatric nurse clinician, family health practitioner, health nurse clinician, nurse associate, the nursing clinician of children with certain diseases such as leukemia, maternal-child nurse clinician, and community health nurse. In an integrated curriculum, making a home visit to a patient known in the hospital is interpreted as community health nursing. Is it not extended episodic nursing or is it extended distributive nursing when the patient enters the hospital? The instantaneous development of the "expert" is occurring in nursing like instant tea or potatoes. The trend is fashionable, but confusing, and, without a clarification of services rendered, the name is unintelligible.

Generalist or Specialist

The trend reflects the crunch going on in nursing between specialization and generalization in both education and service. Medical care has been challenged for overspecialization; nursing in its overzealousness could fall into the same trap. Specialty is a fragmented service. Some nurses specialize by exclusion, developing only knowledge and skills within their area of special interests and competence. Others specialize by inclusion, i.e., of knowledge, skill, and perspective for the comprehensive care of the patient and the family. In practice, recognizing those aspects is considered a part of the nurse's responsibility. One particularizes care; one synthesizes care with a broad concern, widened skill, and responsibility. Health services have been built upon categorization of clinical areas, organs and bodily systems, age groups, disease entities, degree and length of illness, operational procedures, treatment modalities, and fields of knowledge such as "interpersonal nursing." Health care calls for a synthesizing effort to adapt knowledge and skill for the treatment of persons, as well as care and treatment of disease. Specialization by inclusion of the social-psychologic-biologic units of the human being is the generalist whose training must be as extensive, lengthy, and rigorous as the other specialties. In order to be competent in handling the whole person or family unit on a comprehensive, continuous, and coordinated basis, the generalist must be knowledgeable in human development, family dynamics, emotional elements of health and illness, group dynamics, and family, social, and community determinants of health and illness. In addition, he must possess an understanding of and appreciation for promotional, preventive, and maintenance care.

The generalist's function as described by Pelligrino[7] can be adapted and enlarged to the nurse generalist roles as follows:

1 Primary nursing assessment of health care needs of selected and unselected children—their functional, personal, social, and family needs.
2 Judicious decision as to which can be met by the nurse generalist and which must be referred to the nurse specialist, physician, allied health professional, or social agency.
3 Design and coordination of a nursing plan of management.

4 Continuing care and support of children and parents for whom definitive care is not available, but who need comfort and understanding.

5 Nursing care of common and stable long-term illnesses.

6 Sensitive consideration and personal involvement in psychosocial determinants of health and illness.

7 Child and parent education.

8 Health promotion.

9 Health maintenance.

10 Disease and disability prevention.

11 Use of the health team in both the employment setting and the community.

12 Nursing care coordination and management.

The preceding is not new but does reflect a new awareness: an attitude of mind—with power for viewing things as a whole, understanding respective values of the components determining mutual relatedness of the parts, and placing the parts in a sequence for a logical nursing plan which meets their needs.

The nurse in the community uses many cues, those related to the child, his family, other professionals, and forces within the community and their interrelated impacts upon the child's development. How realistic is it to work with the child as an isolate? The nurse has to be ready to cope with the needs of all age groups in various stages of health and illness in the family, be it the family of one's childhood, the family of marriage and parenthood, or the family of grandparenthood. Although the child may be the pivotal patient, the nurse is drawn into the family care constellation. This nurse is a generalist by function. If one wishes to think in terms of specialization, the nurse could be called a generalized specialist or a specialist by inclusion rather than exclusion; one with generalized nursing knowledge, but with a specialized background and skill in family and community health. It is a little like putting new wine in old bottles because the well-prepared public health nurse has long had such a background for his area of practice. The public health nurse developed skill in disease prevention, health promotion, health teaching and counseling, and restorative care while monitoring health and disease, family needs, and program effects in the community.

What appears to be new for the public health nurse, community health nurse, health nurse clinician, or "new" generalized specialist would appear to be more in degree than kind. These changes include increasing background knowledge in the physical as well as the psychologic and behavioral sciences, universalizing skill in general assessment, including use of medical instruments in a systematic physical assessment of the patient, and a greater degree of responsible accountability for his judgment and actions.

In *An Abstract for Action,*[5] distributive nursing practice emphasizes health maintenance and disease prevention. For the generalized family- and community-centered nurse, the emphasis would be strengthened if it included health promotion as well as health maintenance, and disability prevention as well as disease prevention. Nurses have a responsibility to prevent developmental lags and disability that interfere with the child's and family's maximum development within the parameters of genetic endowment and environment. Prevention has a three-level element to it as described by Doctors Leavell and Clark.[8] The primary level occurs during any prepathogenic stage with health promotion and specific protection as the primary focus to prevent the disorder from happening; the second level occurs at a time of the earliest discernible symptoms when early diagnosis and prompt intervention reduce the length or severity of the disorder, and the tertiary level occurs after there is a diagnosed condition, but continuing preventive measures may minimize the handicap or chronicity of the disorder and further limit the individual's functioning.

Illiteracy was spotlighted as a crippling national problem in 1969 when the first commission of education launched the Right to Read Program. The U.S. Office of Education estimates that 7 million elementary and secondary school children have severe reading problems. Each year 700,000 children drop out of public schools with reading levels generally 2 or more years behind those who stay. The United States has close to 19 million adults who are functionally illiterate. Theirs is a story of poverty, unemployment, crime, and lost opportunity.[9] The nurse has responsibility to do vision and hearing screening on all infants, toddlers, and preschoolers to identify any deficit early for correction. In elementary school, the teacher, nurse, and parent should monitor closely the child's developing ability to read. If there is a problem, they should marshal resources for a remedial program as soon as it is diagnosed to prevent further lag. If the child continues to experience frustration without remediation, he may drop out of school with an inability to continue his developmental tasks. At this stage of limitation, tertiary prevention which may arrest or reverse the process of social pathology becomes more difficult. Community programs to help the young adult may be projected to be a Sesame Street kind of television-teaching program for adults; Right to Read academies for adults, operating out of libraries, community centers, churches, and prisons; on-the-job literacy programs in business and industry. Nurses who are sensitive to the problem can be catalysts to inspire civic-minded persons to acknowledge the problem, plan, and implement programs within the resources of the community.

Perhaps it would be well to ask what "positive health" or "successful development" with forward movement from one developmental level to the next is. There is no great clarity, but some of the concepts in definition which have considerable agreement are:

1 Capacity to maximize one's own physical, intellectual, emotional, and social potential within a social framework.
2 Capacity to simultaneously satisfy one's self, maintain rewarding personal relationships, and stay within the behavior boundaries set up by society.[10]

Where does "successful development" or "positive health" begin for the child? This writer firmly believes it is with the family. If one believes that "the family is the unit of growth and experience and therefore, the unit of health and illness,"[11] then the nurse's major focus should be on the primary preventive level to maximize the fully functioning family.

Process

What is the process? The components of the nursing process for the family as a dynamic family organism are the same as for an individual child with a diagnosed disease. The steps include a family assessment, definition of discernible strengths and deficits, development of a plan for action collaborately with family members, support of implementation of action plan, and evaluation of effectiveness of action with a constant reappraisal of each step as insights are gained and with appropriate replanning where it is indicated.

FUNCTIONS OF THE NURSE

Numerous suggestions are beginning to appear in the nursing literature describing assessment tools for individuals with specific disease entities and for specific age groups. According to Broderick,[12] Harold Christensan designated 1950 as the beginning of the era of systematic theory building of the family. In spite of numerous research articles, especially by sociologists over the last few years, Ruben Hill indicates that findings are modest indeed.[13]

Assessment of the Family

Nursing family assessment tools are embryonic, yet no one profession probably has as rich an access to

the family as nursing. At the same time nurses historically have been heard to describe a family using such words as "the greatest," "neat," "uncooperative," and other adjectives which reflect a judgment. What elements of observation and exploration are used to arrive at such conclusions? How helpful are such conclusions as a basis for family intervention? Questions such as these motivated some nurses to develop a tool for use in taking a family history, one that would help the nurse identify systematically those factors which facilitate an integrated functioning of the family and those strains which contribute to family dysfunction. From such analysis the nurse would have a more meaningful basis for defining areas in which appropriate plans may be developed for family-oriented health promotion and preventive programs.

Analysis of unique findings in a family would assist the nurse in determining the level of intervention as promotional or preventive for those in which he finds a high-risk determination. The history needs to be updated as a member of the family passes into a new age cycle and takes on its developmental tasks. Milestone events such as the birth of a new baby, entrance to school, or going away to college or military service are added to the family history as these events bring about a realignment of family members and an introduction to a new stage of the family life cycle.

A type of embryonic family history guide is shown in Fig. 44-1.

Nursing Care in Emergent Community Settings

Activities for generalized nurses who are family- and community-centered in their care of children include, in addition to family and child assessment, personal nursing care in selected situations, teaching, counseling and support, referral, coordination and collaboration, family advocacy, and community planning. The degree to which the nurse will be directly responsible will depend upon the setting in which he finds himself working, its support personnel, and organization. If he is the lone district nurse, he will have to be all things to all people with consultation of the specialized nurses from regional or state offices. However, this writer envisions a trend toward the development of large multipurpose neighborhood ambulatory health centers—more like the supermarket—wherein many services will be provided under a single roof with numerous levels of health workers on staff. The center would provide a wide range of screening services: early and acute diagnostic services both for those screened but who

Figure 44-1 FAMILY ASSESSMENT TOOL

Family name _____ Other names used _____

Woman (mother/wife/parent substitute)

_____ Marital status _____

Mate (husband/father)

_____ Marital status _____

Children:

Name	Sex	Birth year	Ordinal position
1. _____	_____	_____	_____
2. _____	_____	_____	_____
3. _____	_____	_____	_____
4. _____	_____	_____	_____
5. _____	_____	_____	_____
6. _____	_____	_____	_____

Others living in the home:

Name _____ Age ____ Relationship _____

Name _____ Age ____ Relationship _____

Significant others who may not live in home:

Name _____ Age ____ Relationship _____

1. _____

2. _____

3. _____

General health status of all family members:

Name	Current status	Disease and/or disability limitation
1. _____	_____	_____
2. _____	_____	_____
3. _____	_____	_____
4. _____	_____	_____

Current status of immunizations _____

Family history of diabetes, TB, cancer, heart disease, allergies, nervousness: _____

Residence (via a home visit and/or history)

Address

Degree of ownership

Provisions for human comfort:

Space
Heating
Lighting
Ventilation
Refrigeration
Waste disposal
Cooking facilities
Laundry facilities
Bathing and personal hygiene facilities

Sleeping arrangements
Play and recreational areas
Safety and architectural privacy
Provision for individual privacy

Neighborhood, in general, in which family resides (from interview, windshield view, chamber of commerce, community planning data):

Section of area
General population: number, age, and ethnic distribution
General evidence of its stability, economic level, public maintenance, etc.
Housing: type, upkeep
Availability and accessibility to transportation
Schools
Shopping facilities
Job opportunities
Recreational facilities
Medical care resources (outpatient departments, neighborhood clinics, physicians offices)
Health-welfare services
Family likes or dislikes about where they live
Aspiration for residence in the future

The family, a macroscopic view:

Cultural background and languages spoken in nuclear and extended families
Religious orientation: general significance, traditional practices at milestone events of family members
Level of educational attainments, general feeling about significance of school, and aspirations for the children and/or parents
Economic functioning, sources of income, job, hours, special skills needed, satisfactions and/or problems related to work; adequacy of funds to meet needs; available health insurance or medical-care coverage

Interactions of family as a unit:

a Within the unit between family members (content, tone, method of expressing feelings, i.e. joy, anger, love, anxiety, between parents and children and parents)
b With extended family members and/or significant others
c Within the community, as church, P.T.A., union, social clubs

Basic patterns of daily living:

a Daily schedule of activities (how they spend their time)
b Rest and sleep patterns
c Patterns of daily hygiene including dental care
d Food and meal patterns, schedule and food for a typical day, special diets, likes and dislikes, problems in marketing and preparation; alcohol, tobacco, and drug intake
e Recreational activities; creative talents and interests of individuals; family activities and those with community groups
f Sexuality patterns
g Decision-making process
h Child-rearing practices
i Discipline patterns
j Use of health/welfare resources
k Use of medical/dental resources
l Sick-care practices in the family (Who offers care when one is ill? What is done for "minor" illnesses? What nonprescription drugs are kept in home?)

Individual members of the family, a microscopic view:

a Primary role of each
b Description of age/task development of each member

Identify the *family strengths* for self-maintenance

Identify *family functioning lags or deficits*

need further medical examination and for those with early disease symptomatology; primary medical treatment; monitoring of patients with stable chronic conditions; preventive services; a wide range of health education programs; and home care services. Family-child centered nurses in such a setting will have a wide range of technicians, nursing aides, and nurses with other talents working with them. Medical and dental staff will be available as will multidisciplinary supportive health care personnel including the nutritionist, social service worker, health educator, pharmacist, recreationalist, psychologist, and other personnel appropriate to meet specific needs of the population served. Since a great thrust will continue to be toward the containment of the health dollar, everyone's specific talents and skills for which he is trained will be used maximally for his unique contributions to the total care of the child and family. In large centers specialized maternal child health nurses will be working with the family and community nurses.

Quality care mechanisms will be built into the unit to promote ongoing learning and evaluation such as one-to-one conferences; consultations between and among nurse, physician, and allied health experts; informal group discussions and planned team conferences centered on care—physical, emotional, social, preventive, or therapeutic. Procedures for quality assurance, peer review, and cost accounting will facilitate specific definition of function and promote maintenance of quality performance.

This writer does not see the family- and community-centered nurse making all home visits. The nurse is seen doing one-to-one nursing with ambulatory patients as they come into the center, considerably more small-group work with children and parents, and selected home visits. The nurse will have with him a team of nursing assistants consisting of the district nurse, who is particularly well prepared in physical care, and nursing aides from the neighborhood itself. The nurse leader of the team will make an early visit for overall family assessment; will determine the most appropriate level of team member to continue visits, if necessary; will have daily discussion with those assigned on the progress of the child/family and problems encountered; and will make selected home visits for the more complicated situations. Children and families will be supported toward self-management as much as possible. In some situations direct nursing care may be given; in others, care will be taught to family members, and supportive supervision given. Considerable counseling and support will be indicated for those problems which interface with the illness and adequate family functioning.

For example, consider the situation of Jim and Jane Earl, a blind couple, their 4-year-old son, Timmy, and 3-month-old daughter, Susie, in their quest for a normal happy life. Jim, blind since birth, is a highly trained masseur at a YMCA. He goes to work every day on the bus and has no problem getting around town. The nurse learned during her antepartum visits that Jane had aniridia, a hereditary disease which caused several other members of her family to lose their sight. Hanging over this family is the threat of blindness to both children. Timmy had not been examined when the nurse began her visits. Although he is the "eyes of the family," he has since been diagnosed as having the same condition as his mother. Progression of the disease differs with individuals and may be abated by modern methods of treatment. Timmy now wears dark glasses to protect his eyes from damaging light and will later be fitted with corrective glasses. He has been enrolled at a Children's Rehabilitation Unit of a Family Guidance Center where he is being prepared for entrance into public school. Susie has not yet been examined by a specialist to determine her fate. Joan said, "Of course it would be wonderful if Susie could be one of the lucky ones, but we do not regard blindness as the tragedy most people do. It is much less a handicap than other things that can afflict children. We feel sure our youngsters will have good lives regardless of their vision."

Jim and Jane manage their family and home in an incredible manner, fully competent to make the formula and bathe and diaper Susie who doubled her weight at 3 months. The couple do their own grocery shopping, laundry, and cleaning. The household has the same hectic experiences as any other family. About two months after Susie was born, Jane was called home to another state because her mother was quite ill. She arranged for a friend with two children to care for her family during her absence. Upon returning she found that the friend was not feeling well and Susie was under a doctor's care. Within 2 days both were admitted to the hospital—Susie with a congested lung and ear infection and the baby-sitter with pneumonia. Jane then took over the care of her friend's two children along with making daily trips to the hospital. Susie progressed nicely. Although Jane gives all other medication, she shied away from giving the baby ear and nose drops. A visiting nurse assisted her.

Jane related an adjustment of Timmy who is proud of his little sister and is learning to share the attention of his parents with her. "The first time I took Timmy and the baby out together was a new experience for us all," she said. "Timmy was accustomed to taking my hand when we went walking. But I could not carry the baby and my cane and hold his hand too, so I explained to him that he was older now and that

I could expect him to walk closely beside us, on his own. So far he has responded well to the responsibility.''

The nurse becomes an impartial sounding board against which to bounce off ideas, to think them through for a satisfactory family fit, and a resource from whom to learn of possible community services which may prove helpful to their needs. The nurse provides supportive care in a personal manner, knowing the emotional and social problems in this family which are interacting with the physical disease process. The goal for the nurse is to offer care, guidance, and support in times of family stress and to promote healthy family adaptation and self-reliance within the circumstances of the situation.

The traditional nurse makes many home visits to motivate family members to utilize sick/health care services, to maintain appointments, to comply with specific medical instruction or orders, and to do case finding. This writer sees the well-counseled neighborhood health aides doing much of these activities, perhaps better than the nurse. The aide brings to the situation some built-in qualities such as an experiential knowledge of the neighborhood, the characteristics of the population, and their values, health attitudes, and social-health needs.

Coordination and Collaboration

The family- community-centered nurse must have considerable skill in collaboration and coordination of care within the nursing team, with related staff in the center, and with health personnel in other community programs in order to ensure continuity and to prevent the family's getting lost in the shuffle. With Jane and Jim the nurse was an epidemiologist, teacher, facilitator, and coordinator of a number of helping professionals to get an active plan of care implemented for Timmy. The process continues through monitoring Timmy's progress, Susie's development, and the parents of the family unit.

Health Teaching

With the current thoughtful appraisal of the health care delivery system and cost containment, this writer predicts that the family- and community-centered nurse will experience a revitalization of his potential in primary prevention and in teaching the family greater mastery in self-maintenance. The difference from what is now current is that, in the future, members of the family will have opportunities more readily to attain health information upon which to make alternative decisions about themselves

rather than making judgments necessarily upon ignorance, hearsay, and folklore or waiting until a crisis when only costly acute care is indicated. With their right to health comes also responsibility. Accountability will be reflected in the outcomes of their health practices. For example, one hears too often the remark, ''He will grow out of it'' when the child's symptom is a lisp or leg pains. As another example, families need to know the potential risk of a second or third child after they have had one who has cystic fibrosis so that they may make choices based upon the best medical knowledge available at the time.

Not so obvious in the Smith family constellation are a number of problems that reflect a need for a blending of episodic and distributive nursing in teaching health promotion and developing effective self-maintenance. They are a ''well'' child-centered family. Both parents look upon their children as individuals and relate with love for each child. Discipline is permissive and communicative rather than corporal. The parents take advantage of medical resources and practice preventive care to a degree. The children have all been adequately immunized and have regular dental examinations. Mrs. Smith believes that ''more than two colds a winter is serious and worth worrying about.'' Both Mr. and Mrs. Smith ask about the value of vitamins, yet food and meal patterns leave something to be desired.

Ava, a 3-year-old, is active and well. The Denver Developmental Screening Test revealed that she had mastered all tasks for her age; in fact, she completed tasks not completed by her older sister, Doreen. As the youngest in the family she gets much attention and protests by yelling and sometimes crying if she gets left behind by the faster, older children.

Doreen, a 4-year-old, seemed to have lags in fine motor-adaptive skills. She wears corrective shoes, has an abundance of energy, and loves to ride her bike with Ava. Her mother refers to her as the ''devil of the moment.''

Burt, a 7-year-old, is an active second-grader who wore corrective shoes when younger. He has a very loud manner and does things which are dangerous to him. As the only ''man'' around the house much of the day, Burt tries to impress demands on his sisters and even his mother, usually to no avail. He has a hard time accepting any kind of corrective discipline and usually stomps off yelling and groaning. Mischievous activity gets him into trouble at school. Mr. and Mrs. Smith are quite worried about Burt's hyperactivity. They have gone to the extent of using coffee drinks to slow him down. The parents believe this medication is safer than any other for their self-diagnosis.

Amy, an 8-year-old, is quite mature for her age, is inquisitive, and enjoys school. As the oldest child she voluntarily passes on authoritative discipline and watches after her younger brother and sisters. These actions lead to great regard from her sisters and parents and mumbling from Burt. Amy is at the stage where she is losing about a tooth a month. Dental care is required since several "new" teeth are crooked. She wears glasses all the time and is excited about the new frames she received for Christmas.

Mrs. Mary Smith, 39 years old, reported that she had a "head aneurysm" about two years ago, causing headaches and blurred vision when she is tense and tired. She is on a "take-it-easy" prescription. Mary is 15 lb overweight but is not concerned about it. She skimps on breakfast and smokes.

David Smith, 45 years old, is a steel rule dye cutter by vocation and a wood-carver by avocation. Mary reported that he had a "bout of alcoholism" a few years ago and has a diagnosed hypertension. This fall he had elective surgery for a hernia, removal of a facial nonmalignant cyst, and tests which revealed hyperlipoproteinemia. He finds it hard to accept a special diet and the restriction of two beers a day. Both Mr. and Mrs. Smith drink 10 cups of coffee a day, and he smokes heavily.

The child-family nurse has a role in supporting the parenting of this couple who are doing well, on a strained budget and no means of private transportation, with physical aspects of care, i.e., providing glasses, corrective shoes, and dental care. However, they may be setting by their personal health practices questionable models for developing children, for example, inadequate nutritional habits, excessive drinking of coffee, and smoking.

Small-group teaching can be about as varied as the nurse's knowledge, special interests, and schedule permit to meet the needs of the population. How long have health professionals failed parents waiting in child health clinics and other settings? Such blocks of time offer an opportunity for educational exchange, a mutual sharing of problems and feelings about rearing children, and approaches which have proved successful. Hopefully, waiting lines will be reduced or eliminated, but with health care services more readily accessible and in evening hours as well, small-group sessions will become a pattern. To name a few possible topics, the sessions could be addressed to growth and development of the newborn and the task of weaving him into the new family; living with a toddler and still loving him; preparing for a day care or nursery school experience; parents and the 8-to-10-year-old; raising a son or daughter as a single parent; understanding the adolescent; family coping regarding aggressive child behavior or poor school adjustment; care of the physically handicapped child or mentally retarded; sex education; family planning; premarital education; food planning; and ways in which a family can have fun and not leave town. No nurse should feel bored from lack of challenge or opportunity to be creative. The educational programs would assist family members to widen the boundaries of their information and deepen their understandings against which they may make choices in health behavior in their life situations.

Family Advocacy

Another area which will call, as it does now, for both skill and commitment is that of family advocacy. It is not a new term, but a concept deeply rooted in the best tradition of the public health nurse. The emphasis is renewed in a professional commitment of purpose to enrich and strengthen family life and to the current thrust of being more responsive to social conditions. Just as nurses assess strengths and needs of a child and his family, so they assess those factors in a care-giving service which enhance and constrain effectiveness. They have a role in bringing responsible attention to those barriers in an institution which seem to block the child and family from receiving appropriate care. The linkage calls for diplomacy. One may feel at risk in negotiation, but the nurse's skill and the family strength can bring about effective change.

A young woman, Mrs. C., was found to have leukemia at the time of delivery of her first child. She remained in the hospital while her baby was taken to its maternal grandparents. After further diagnostic procedures, Mrs. C. was placed on a strict protocol of treatment, a part of which was to minimize any chance of infection. Her prognosis was guarded with some doubt expressed as to whether she would ever leave the hospital alive. Mrs. C. said a couple of times, "Oh, if I could just see and hold my baby." The student knew it would mean altering institutional policies and practices, but, through negotiations with the obstetrician, the hematologist, and appropriate nursing staff, the family was invited to bring the infant into the hospital. Mrs. C. cried with joy and held her baby. Advocacy is a commitment to the person and not the system.[14] Another example is pertinent. The nurse in the community was visiting a mother and her family who were on Aid to Families of Dependent Children (AFDC). Mrs. A. was rightfully proud of her family and of her parenting abilities. However, she was concerned for her 16-year-old daughter, who had been elected queen of her class; Mrs. A. wanted desperately to be able to provide her daughter with a stylish new dress like the other girls at the special ceremony. The AFDC allotment did not cover such clothing costs, and the agency worker only recited the rigidities, rules, and regulations to Mrs. A. The nurse, with verification of the facts she could collect and with a sensitivity for Mrs. A.'s concern and the family situation, jumped channels and went to the director of the local welfare office. The nurse left with a check for Mrs. A. and her daughter. The nurse never asked what policies the director might have had to circumvent, but thanked him for cooperating toward a teenager's mental and social well-being as well as that of the parent.

Community Planning

Another area of functioning this writer sees increasing is that of community-wide planning for the improvement of health services for families and children. This activity is largely a collaborative one with consumers, elected officials, community planners, and other health providers. The process for nurses is similar to that used with the individual and family. The steps are identification of a problem area, assessment of the problem, planning for an appropriate approach, promotion of program development, evaluation, and reassessment. Decision-making for recommending a certificate of need, promotion of a resolution, or establishing standards for a service must be based upon as specific and valid an assessment as one can get and must promote the general welfare rather than enhance the interest of any one profession or institution. Areas for planning will vary as widely as local health/welfare needs and problems present themselves.

In a large Midwestern eight-county area recent exploration and/or action have been directed toward the establishment of an area-wide emergency care program; task force activities on ambulatory and family planning services; an area-wide immunization program; a proposal to administer the Denver Development Screening Test in 90 counties in a state; a program to update a county's teachers in their understanding of behavioral problems of school-age children; and a formal lead-poisoning program. The lead-poisoning program calls for identification of high-risk areas with structures built prior to 1950; massive screening especially in "lead belts" for all children between the ages of 1 to 6 years; immediate referral of children with elevated levels of lead in the blood; mechanisms for repair of houses; and extensive education programs for the general public, medical community, public health, and other health-related professions.

SUMMARY

Concern for growing children in distributive care, a generalized specialty, becomes at once family- and community-centered. It involves a synergistic process as the nurse relates to many cues in the child which are linked with his situational environments. Since the family is the child's unit of health, disease, and dysfunction, the goal in primary prevention is a fully functioning family as well as a maximally functioning child. The nurse's activities in distributive care include, among others, family assessment, analysis of child-family-community linkages, implementation in traditional and emergent community health settings with particular actions in coordination and collaboration, preventive teaching toward family self-maintenance, family advocacy, and community planning for the improvement of health services for families and children.

REFERENCES

1 N. W. Ackerman (ed.), *Family Process,* Basic Books, Inc., Publishers, New York, 1970, p. 8.
2 C. S. Chilman, "Families in Development at Midstage of the Family Life Cycle," *The Family Coordinator,* October 1968, p. 298.
3 ———, *Demographic Yearbook,* Statistical Office of United Nations, Department of Economics and Social Affairs, New York, 1972.
4 E. Laucks, "Do We Need Families?," *Center Report,* October 1973, p. 22.
5 J. P. Lysaught, *An Abstract for Action,* The National Commission for the Study of Nursing and Nursing Education, McGraw-Hill Book Company, New York, 1970, pp. 91–92.
6 D. E. Fiedler et al., "Pathology in the 'Healthy' Female Teenager," *American Journal of Public Health,* vol. 63, no. 11, November 1973, pp. 962–965.
7 E. D. Pelligrino, "The Generalist Function in Medicine," *Journal of the American Medical Association,* vol. 198, no. 8, October 31, 1956, p. 128.
8 H. R. Leavell and E. G. Clark, *Preventive Medicine for the Doctor in his Community,* 3rd ed., McGraw-Hill Book Company, New York, 1965, pp. 19–37.
9 C. T. Rowan, "Poor Readers Breed on a Poor Society," *Kansas City Times,* January 23, 1974, p. 35.
10 C. S. Chilman, "Families in Development at Midstage of the Family Life Cycle," *The Family Coordinator,* October 1968, p. 309.
11 N. W. Ackerman, "Psychological Dynamics of the Family Organism," in I. Gladstone (ed.), *The Family as a Focal Point in Health Education,* International Universities Press, Inc., New York, 1961, p. 34.

12 C. B. Broderick, "Beyond the Five Conceptual Frameworks: A Decade of Development in Family Theory," *Journal of Marriage and the Family,* February 1971, p. 139.

13 R. Hill and D. A. Hansen, "The Identification of Conceptual Frameworks Utilized in Family Study," *Marriage and Family Living,* November 1960, p. 299.

14 E. Manser (ed.), *Family Advocacy, Manual for Action,* Family Service Association of America, New York, 1973, p. 24.

BIBLIOGRAPHY

Carrieri, V., and Sitzman, J.: "Components of the Nursing Process," *Nursing Clinics of North America,* 6:115–124, 1971.

Chinn, P.: "New Dimensions for Pediatric Nursing," in A. M. Reinhardt, and M. D. Quinn (eds.), *Family Centered Community Nursing,* The C. V. Mosby Company, St. Louis, 1973.

Chioni, R. M., and Panicucci, C.: "Tomorrow's Nurse Practitioners," *Nursing Outlook,* 18(2):32–35, 1970.

Cleland, Virginia: "Nurse Clinicians and Nurse Specialists: An Overview," *Three Challenges to the Nursing Profession,* American Nurses Association, 1972, pp. 13–25.

Conant, L. H.: "The Nature of Nursing Tomorrow," *Image,* 4(2):4–6, 1970–71.

Lambertson, E.: "Let's Get the Nurse's Role into Focus," *Prism Magazine,* 1(6):27–30, 1973.

Mereness, D.: "Recent Trends in the Expanding Roles of the Nurse," *Nursing Outlook,* 18(5):30–33, 1970.

Reverly, S.: A Perspective on Root Causes of Illness," *American Journal of Public Health,* 62(8):1140–1142, 1972.

Silver, G.: "Family Health Maintenance," in I. Gladston (ed.), *The Family as the Focal Point in Health Education,* International Universities Press, Inc., New York, 1961.

Tapia, J.: "The Nursing Process in Family Health," *Nursing Outlook,* 20(4):267–270, 1972.

45

THE FUTURE OF NURSING EDUCATION AND PRACTICE

LUTHER CHRISTMAN

THE PROFESSION

Every profession is, to a great extent, a captive of the times. No profession, furthermore, exists in a vacuum and decides its future unilaterally. The destiny of all professions is tied irrevocably to the tide of change in society as a whole, but modifications can occur as a result of forces within each profession. Professions evolve because the society for which they are invented to serve perceives the need of that particular complex of services. In turn, certain rights, privileges, and obligations are set up by society for that specific group so that mutual expectations can be met. Professions that respond most completely to the expectations of society and which demonstrate an ability to improve their particularized service continuously are accorded increased status. Those professions that establish a clear image of their social worth by being constructive participants in the work necessary to achieve the goals set by society are viewed as being the most successful and are rewarded in kind. Nurses should view the major stresses and strains within the profession as responses that are necessary to enable nurses to articulate with the considerable flux of the society in which the profession is embedded. Professions that wait until other professions pioneer the way to new methodologies and are relatively non-innovative usually are considered as secondary or dependent professions. Front-running professions are constantly building up the competence of their members and always have portions of their membership in endeavors of considerable risk which have the potential of improving service to the public.

It is mainly by the guidelines briefly stroked above that professions are measured. It is not sufficient to measure growth and competence vis à vis members within one's own profession but by the more searching comparison of the general competence of the members of all other professions, especially those professions that are highly related. At the nub of this analysis is the role core of all professions. This core consists of elements generally labeled as service, education, consultation, and research. The competent professional person is aware of the interplay of all four segments of the role and the challenge of remaining reasonably proficient in all categories. Many nurses have tended to concentrate on only one of the four subroles and have thus inhibited their full professional growth. One of the challenges that nurses now face is to develop a new professional life-style—one that encompasses the full role. How effectively this feat is accomplished will be indicative of how well nurses can march in step with the major professions.

SOCIETAL CHANGES

The future cannot be assessed without some base line from which to draw conclusions. The most volatile changes in our society have occurred since World War II. An examination of some of the social indicators will be useful for this discussion. In the late thirties and early forties of this century the national economy was borderline. Most of the population had very modest incomes. Although there were persons of great wealth, the largest portion of all incomes was clustered at the lower end of the economic scale without much invidious comparison between socioeconomic groups. Economic aspirations were relatively low-keyed. The gross national product inched upward. The general life-style was essentially rural. Urban populations were increasing gradually. Rural life provided a way for personal intimacy and intense interest in, and understanding of, the general welfare of others. The tempo of life was placid and predictable. Marriage generally was postponed until the age of 25 or over. Family size tended to remain small, thus keeping the population growth to modest dimensions. The creeping increase in population did not place unusual demands on natural and scarce resources. The education of most persons stopped at graduation from high school or sooner. The turnover of knowledge was about once every 15 or 20 years. New additions in knowledge could be absorbed without discomfort because of the incipient way in which they crept into use. The increments in the expansion of science and technology were at a leisurely pace, manageable, and welcomed. The mass media were unobtrusive, and television was unavailable. Tranquility ruled the waves.

Compare that relatively stable state and pedestrian pace with what has happened since the fifties. The national economy has become very affluent and almost overheated. The average income level has moved into the middle-class range. There is a huge gap between the very rich and those portions of the population who are struggling at poverty levels. The maldistribution of wealth and resources is the cause of much frustration and irritation. This very unequal dispersion of wealth continues to be the cause of much explosive debate and action. The age at which marriage occurs has dropped significantly, and until very recently the average family size has increased to such an extent that we went through a population explosion. The strain on natural and scarce resources went up algebraically. The extremely rapid expansion of science and technology triggered off whole new changes in the national patterns. One of these marked changes was the sudden shift from rural to urban living. This shift was brought about as manufacturing and other industries grouped to utilize technology profitably. Since the means of utilizing science and technology was concentrated, it became imperative for workers to move close to the production centers which were creating jobs. The population became very mobile and unsettled as families migrated frequently in attempts to improve their economic status. The movement of people was so continuous that persons living near each other never had the opportunity of knowing and understanding each other. Neighborliness just about disappeared as a characteristic of urban living.

The aspiration for education settled out at college level or its equivalent. We became a highly educated citizenry. All these rapid changes produced a highly diversified mixture of many subcultures and socioeconomic groups. Impersonalization of interaction with others became the norm. A whole series of political polarizations occurred. It became impossible to get a stable majority opinion—even a silent one. Onto this set of turbulent events an intrusive and omnipresent mass media was superimposed, especially with the easy availability of television. Instant news dissemination and its commentary gave us essentially a state of "information overload." With all these major changes occurring at a barely absorbable pace, the management of society (and of the profession) was out of control to a very great extent. It will take a considerable period of time before we design adequate organizational devices which will enable us to steer our political, economic, and educational destinies with much precision. It is in this broad context that we must examine the challenge to the nursing profession and particularly to one of its specialties—pediatric nursing.

CHALLENGES

The most important challenge is to make dramatic, and, it is hoped, startling changes in the kind and quality of education. Professional education, no matter of what sort, tends to occur in universities. Professional education, moreover, tends to take place in complete schools, which are defined as including undergraduate and graduate education through the doctoral level, continuing education, and research to increase the proficiency of all the members under one roof. Nursing education is grossly underrepresented in these types of educational settings and highly overrepresented in incomplete schools. The only way for nursing education to compare favorably with that of the other major professions is to move to maintaining only complete schools. If such action were taken, we might ultimately have only about 125 schools of nursing in this country. A major advantage of this move would be greater government support of nursing education. Adequate government funding could more easily be obtained for 125 complete schools than for 1,400 schools of all types, and quality education could be underwritten in all schools of nursing. These complete schools would have to be of sufficient size to prepare all the nurses needed to serve our health care system. Some examples of this type are in existence already; hence we are not without models.

Specialization in nursing occurs at the graduate level, and so complete schools will provide the base for the rapid extension of all nursing specialties. Nursing students enrolled in complete schools will more readily understand the advantages of graduate education and seek advanced degrees.

How strongly will pediatric nurses support a change of this magnitude? Since it will take large numbers of pediatric nurses to substantially improve the quality of pediatric care, it is up to pediatric nurses to develop their education, practice, and clinical research in a fashion that will capture the imagination of good students and encourage them to enter the specialty in the numbers desired.

Education

Not only should the preparation of nurses take place in complete schools of nursing, but their education should happen in conjunction with the complete schools of the other health professions. If the preparation of all the health professions occurred only in health universities, it would enable the various types of health students to develop a common language and a better appreciation of each other as they shared courses. It might be possible to offer the students of each one of the health professions a minor in one of the others, much as liberal arts students take majors and minors. While a minor in another profession would not qualify a candidate to practice in that profession, it would generate a greater understanding among professions. There are numerous ways in which patterns of education could be blended so that future generations of practitioners could cooperate more harmoniously in providing health care.

The role socialization process for nurses is quite different when it happens in a health university where a form of complete education is present for all or most of the health professions. Under this set of conditions nurses can learn the many alternatives to actions that are possible, witness much innova-

tion, experience the participation in excellent clinical practice, and be exposed to cooperative relationships during the entire role induction process. As compared with the incomplete models of nursing education, the type being advocated is much less likely to lock nurses into a frozen mold—with all its implications for lifelong resistance to change—than any of the other present models we are using. It is particularly important to consider the value of making this choice when the process of specialization is not fully decided. It will take courage to move against the entrenched establishment and the long tradition of neighborhood schools. Will the voices and energies of pediatric nurses be used to advocate forms of education that have the best chances of keeping nursing among the front-running professions?

Practice

There is a very great need to develop centers of excellence in nursing. These centers probably can be brought about more easily, at least initially, in health university settings than anywhere else. Centers of excellence should be bellwethers by which progress in nursing is marked. The chief characteristics of these centers should be high levels of nursing care, innovative demonstrations of more efficient means of organizing nursing-care delivery, insightful and effective clinical research, and experimental attempts to improve nursing education. When strong centers of excellence are developed, they will provide springboards for the rapid dissemination of new knowledge throughout the profession. Nurses who have the opportunity of experiencing excellence, both in their formative years as students and in their initial work experience, will be splendidly equipped to become proficient practitioners in their own right. It will take a substantial amount of commitment and a high-energy effort to develop the first few centers. Nurses from all the specialty areas will have to participate wholeheartedly to bring this venture to a successful conclusion.

Multidisciplinary Care

Multidisciplinary care is being heralded as the wave of the future. So far this theme appears to be more of an exercise in rhetoric than a reality. The plethora of articles on professionalism and on health care often have the form of rhetorical harangues instead of being useful contributions to the advancement of patient care. Many of the writers seem to believe that they must act as spokesmen for their particular profession. Thus a central role is ascribed to the work of the profession under discussion and written with an assertion that this central role should be accepted as written by the members of other professions. The accumulation of so much professional flag-waving appears to have increased the isolation of professions from each other. There appears to be as much suspicious surveillance of each other as there are efforts at interdisciplinary collaboration. Professional persons who are trained in isolation from each other seem to find it quite difficult to assume the role of team members on the much-talked-about health team. Out of all the past disharmonies and current unsettling change some means must be found to orchestrate the various themes. Care is not very effective when it is a series of solo parts that are not in tune with each other. We need to design models of interdisciplinary collaboration that help everyone to play in concert.

All the issues that are of major importance in bringing about harmony between the professions fortunately are responsive to planned change. The members of the different professions in general can be viewed as applied scientists. Health care essentially is a clinical process. By and large, the different types of practitioners are pulling the knowledge they use from the same common base of sciences. Some specialties, or some subspecialties of professions, may tend to use some science or sciences more than they do others, but the commonality of science is there. As the understanding of the clinical process broadens and deepens, the amount of common knowledge should become clear to all. The presence of this broad base gives the opportunity to emphasize the similarities of knowledge systems rather than the differences in training.

If clinical practice is the transformation of science into health care processes, and if a common knowledge base exists, then there is a considerable possibility of the presence of role overlap and shared competence. The argument for being more alike than different is strengthened. There may be less major variations in the knowledge systems each discipline claims as its own as the training of each profession grows in depth and intensity. The role expression of knowledge in caring for patients and clients, however, is expressed somewhat differently, mainly because of the variation in the vertical range of knowledge, the role ascriptions of the different professions and their specialties, external constraints such as licensing boards and governmental regulations, and the organization of the delivery system.

Nurses and Physicians

One way to explore the points in the above paragraph further is to examine the state of affairs between nurses and physicians. The current confrontation between these two professions over "delegation" versus "expansion" is an example of how the basic issue of high degree of overlap in knowledge has been ignored. Physicians state that they wish to delegate many of their conventional activities to nurses. Nurses, in the meanwhile, are asserting that they are expanding their role. A semantic barrier thus has been established. An objective analysis, however, of the content of what the members of each profession are discussing reveals a high level of knowledge congruency and a great deal of role overlap. An isomorphic area of common competency is a reality. The discord is more imagined than real. It will be much easier to resolve this issue when both groups adopt this conclusion. It is more important to harness all this expertness for patient care than to continue the debate.

Adding to the confusion of the relationships between nurses and physicians are the differences in the means of delivering care. These differences are disparate enough to make it nigh impossible for a relationship between the two groups to exist at all. A physician usually cares for the same patient, or at least monitors the care, throughout the period of the patient's illness. But rarely does the same nurse care for the same patient in the hospital from the time of his admission to the time of his discharge. The managerial type of nursing practice has released, to a considerable extent, accountability for any specific patient's welfare from individual nurses and made the welfare of patients a vaguely defined group responsibility. Anonymous groups of nursing personnel seem to be trying to give care to anonymous mobs of patients. The hierarchical care of patients through others, the atomizing of care by functional assignment, the rotating of shifts so constantly that the nursing personnel assigned to a unit are in a state of constant flux, and the daily rotation of assignments make it practically impossible for physicians to communicate with nurse staff members about the particular designs of care for each patient. Communication, in many cases, is reduced to written "orders"—one of the poorest forms of communication. This state of affairs will continue to exist until the departments of nursing are reorganized into a form permitting the clinical practice of nursing. This change in itself, however, is not sufficient. Physicians will have to give thoughtful consideration to the way they randomly operate within the hospital system, they will have to reflect on whether their requests are personal whim or are useful in patient care, and they will have to take time to participate in the staff meetings on the units where they have patients in order to help establish the best means of improving the quality of care. Registered nurses will have to take on the responsibility of giving direct care to patients and using practical nurses and aides to do support work. They will have to be answerable for the 24-hour management of the nursing care of patients. The so-called primary nursing being introduced in some settings is an example of this way of organizing. Nurses should be the prime advocate for patients and should be tied tightly to the patients they care for. They will have to develop perfect accountability models similar to those of physicians. This accountability will be most in evidence with nurse specialists. Pediatric nurses will have to take the major responsibility for developing this kind of nursing practice in pediatric settings. The concept of perfect accountability works equally well whether pediatric nurses are working within a hospital setting or in the community. The recent changes in the legislation regulating practice in the states of Washington and Idaho increase the right of nurses to make diagnoses and to prescribe care, but it carries with this right an equally strong obligation for accountability. One cannot have rights and privileges without an equally balanced set of obligations. If one wishes to reap the benefits of professional excitement by being one of the primary agents in the welfare of others, one must be willing to be held accountable for the quality of interventions in the fate of others.

Among the many recommendations of the White House Conference on Children are the ones which recommend that nurses work in new ways in the community.[1] Nurses, for instance, could work in small groups in natural communities. As an extension of this notion, they could set up offices in the neighborhood school, their own homes, or similar types of locations so as to serve the community in which they were placed. Services designed to promote health maintenance would be the chief objective of such arrangements.

Interdigitation

New ways of viewing the interdigitation of roles around the patient are needed. One of the most useful ways is to start the reconstruction of the role set around the patient with the patient as the center of focus rather than with any one of the health professions receiving the major amount of attention. Organizational devices should be employed that are designed to permit all the disciplines to contribute effectively to the problems of clients. Even though there is as much difference in individual competency within a given profession as there is between professions, there nevertheless has been a traditional pecking order based solely on a presumed hierarchical array of ability. Ritualism in behavior, as well as an informal deference system, sprang from this traditional power structure. Frequently the client or patient is scapegoated by lower-ranking health professionals as a symbolic expression of objection to this form of care structure.

One way, theoretically, that has great possibilities of generating professional excitement and gaining commitment to care is to utilize the social device of shared responsibilities.[2-4] In this type of organizational pattern, the participants share power according to the competencies and skills they have, instead of being assigned power according to the profession from which they come. Each participant would contribute to the decision-making process according to his or her clinical acumen. The patient demand system could be responded to more promptly and with more certainty if each participant were free to intervene, provided he had the needed competence. In this type of model whoever was geographically closest to the patient, and had the required skill, could serve the patient when the demand arose rather than going through a circuitous route which forced a delay in meeting situations presented by patients. Ground rules for devising an acceptable arrangement which permits whoever is in the clinical situation to use the full range of his skills freely and openly is a prerequisite to making this proposed model work efficiently. These ground rules would be developed by a joint practice committee in each respective setting. The sobering effect of being solely accountable for one's own action will tend to keep each participant honest in the use of discretionary power. The model suggested here contains many of the characteristics of an interdependent approach to the management of health care. Pediatric nurses and pediatricians have skated on the edges of this model. It remains to be seen whether they are able to exploit its full potential and to bring members of other professions into a design most useful to the care of children.

The age of specialization may be full of more uneasiness in the future than it has been up to the present. Nurses had to overcome considerable inertia to accept the proposition that specialization required preparation at the master's level. That proposition, in all likelihood, will not hold for the future. Specialization occurs at the doctoral level in most disciplines. It is apparent that pediatric nurses will have to do likewise if they are to keep pace with board pediatricians, speech therapists, reading specialists, child psychologists, and similar professional persons who work closely with children. If pediatric nurses do not respond to this challenge, they will be a dependent profession as compared with their better-prepared colleagues.

The internal problems within the nursing profession may seem monumental, but they are of much less significance than the mounting external controls. The health industry appears fated to become the most controlled industry in the nation. We seem to have a form of government-controlled health program by indirection. By the time that national entitlement is enacted, all the health professions may have very rigid controls. Part of this desire for societal control comes from the failure of the health professions to respond appropriately. Emphasis has been overwhelmingly on crisis care and its resulting high cost. Very little work has been done to make health maintenance feasible. Nurses and physicians have not been attracted to what many label as "mundane" and "unexciting." One of the ways to ward off even more stringent regulation is to move imaginatively in this field of endeavor. While much ground has been lost, it is not too late to demonstrate that there is a willingness to make dramatic and measurable switches in professional life-styles.

We must stand up and be counted. We still have time to take positive positions. It is important to be highly informed and to have something to say that will push health care into a form most useful to consumers. It is urgent that nurses be very active even if this activity becomes an intrusion into "private time."

THE FUTURE

The future does not have to be fraught with uneasiness. It is a matter of being objective about what is happening, correctly reading the signals put up by society, making relevant responses to new expectations as they emerge, working to ensure the quality of care, being a continuous student throughout life, conducting the kind of research needed to improve care, constantly raising the standards of professional proficiency, developing competency in interdisciplinary efforts, improving the quality of generic and graduate education, and keeping abreast of science and technology. The challenge is the outcome of living in a dynamic society. Each subset of the profession must contribute its effectiveness to help the nursing profession compete successfully in this unending strain to move forward. How successful pediatric nurses are, to a great extent, will depend on how much they desire to be a major contributor to the health care of children in the future.

REFERENCES

1 *Report to the President*, White House Conference on Children, U.S. Government Printing Office, 1971, pp. 170–171.
2 L. Christman, "Community Resources—The Role of Other Professionals," *Medical College of Virginia Quarterly*, vol. 5, no. 3, 1969, pp. 143–146.
3 ———, "Education of the Health Team," *Journal of the American Medical Association*, vol. 213, no. 2, July 13, 1970, pp. 284–285; reprinted in *Selected Papers from the 66th Annual Congress on Medical Education*, Chicago, Feb. 8–9, 1970, January 1971.
4 ———, "Community Context," in Harry Gottesfeld (ed.), *Controversies in Community Mental Health*, Behavioral Publications, Inc., New York, 1972.

APPENDIXES

1

SITES FOR INTRAMUSCULAR INJECTIONS

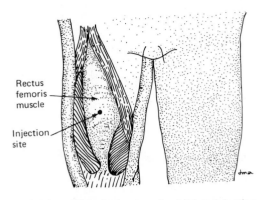

Figure A1-1 Midanterior muscle of thigh. Injection should be into the middle third of the anterior thigh.

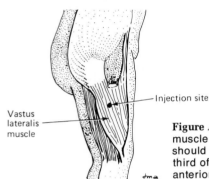

Figure A1-2 Midlateral muscle of thigh. Injection should be into the middle third of the lateral thigh, anterior to the femur.

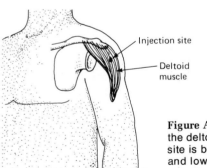

Figure A1-3 Two views of the deltoid muscle. Injection site is between the upper and lower portions of the muscle.

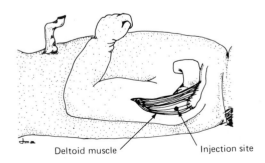

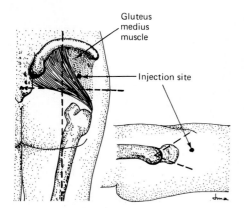

Figure A1-4   Injection site is the upper outer quadrant of the gluteal area.

2
TYPES OF RESTRAINTS

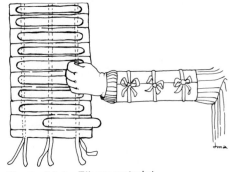

Figure A2-1 Elbow restraint.

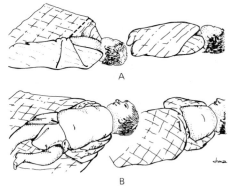

A

B

Figure A2-2 Two types of mummy restraints.

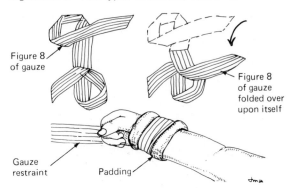

Figure 8 of gauze

Figure 8 of gauze folded over upon itself

Gauze restraint

Padding

Figure A2-3 Clove-hitch restraint.

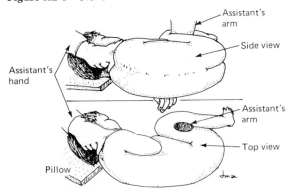

Assistant's arm

Side view

Assistant's hand

Assistant's arm

Top view

Pillow

Figure A2-4 Restraint for lumbar puncture procedure.

935

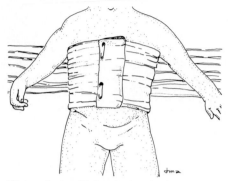

Figure A2-5 Abdominal restraint.

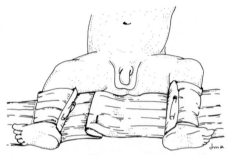

Figure A2-6 Ankle and extremity restraint.

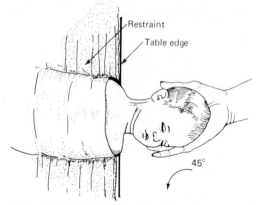

Figure A2-7 Restraint for jugular venipuncture procedure.

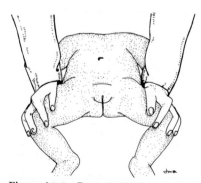

Figure A2-8 Restraint for femoral venipuncture procedure.

SUGGESTED
SCHEDULE FOR
PREVENTIVE
CHILD
HEALTH CARE

Age	History*	Measurements†	Physical examination	Developmental landmarks*‡	Discussion and guidance*	Procedures†	Attending
1 mo	Initial Eating Sleeping Elimination Crying At every visit mother should be asked for questions	Height Weight Head circumference Temperature Evaluation of hearing	Complete‖	Eyes follow to midline Baby regards face While prone, lifts head off table	Vitamins Sneezing Hiccoughs Straining with bowel movements Irregular respiration Startle reflex Ease and force of urination Night bottle Colic "Spoiling" Accidents	PKU Urinalysis	M.D. and assistant

Note: Underlined items indicate report of parent may be accepted as proof of accomplishment. May be obtained by assistant.

*May be accomplished in part by assistant if physician desires. Much of this may be accomplished in part by appropriate pamphlets or leaflets where deemed desirable.

†Usually accomplished by assistant.

‡Age given for landmarks indicates approximate age at which 90% of children have accomplished test. Adapted from "Denver Developmental Screening Test."

‖By physician.

¶Observation of child, completely undressed, by assistant trained to observe respiration, skin, musculature, motor activities, and so forth. Obvious deviations from normal must be checked by physician.

Source: Reprinted with permission from Committee on Standards of Child Health Care, Council on Pediatric Practice, American Academy of Pediatrics, 1972.

SUGGESTED SCHEDULE FOR PREVENTIVE CHILD HEALTH CARE (*Continued*)

Age	History*	Measurements†	Physical examination	Developmental landmarks*‡	Discussion and guidance*	Procedures†	Attending
2 mo	Health Sensory-motor development Eating Sleeping Elimination Happiness	Height Weight Head circumference Temperature	Complete or observation¶	<u>Vocalizes</u> <u>Smiles responsively</u>	Solid foods Immunizations Thumbsucking	DTP TOPV Urine screening	M.D. and/or assistant
3 mo	Health Eating Sleeping Elimination Crying Other behavior	Height Weight Head circumference Temperature	Complete or observation¶	Holds head and chest up to make 90° angle with table Laughs	Feeding Accidents Sleeping without rocking, holding, etc. Coping with frustrations		M.D. and/or assistant
4 mo	Health Eating Sleeping Elimination Other behavior Sensory-motor development Current living situation Parent-child interaction	Height Weight Head circumference Temperature	Complete‖	Holds head erect and steady when held in sitting position <u>Squeals</u> Grasps rattle Eyes follow object for 180°	Feeding Schedule to fit in with family Attitude of father Respiratory infections	DTP TOPV	M.D. and assistant
5 mo	Health Eating Sleeping Elimination Sensory-motor development	Height Weight Temperature	Complete or observation¶	<u>Smiles spontaneously</u> <u>Rolls from back to stomach or vice versa</u> Reaches for object on table	Feeding Vitamins (if not previously mentioned)		M.D. and/or assistant
6 mo	Health Eating Sleeping Elimination Other behavior Sensory-motor development	Height Weight Head circumference Temperature Evaluation of hearing	Complete or observation¶	No head lag if baby is pulled to sitting position by hands	Feeding Accidents Night crying Fear of strangers Separation anxiety Description of normal micturition	DTP TOPV	M.D. and/or assistant
8–9 mo	Health Eating Sleeping Elimination Sensory-	Height Weight Temperature	Complete or screening‖	Sits alone for 5 seconds after support is released Bears weight	Use of cup Eating with fingers Fear of strangers		M.D. and/or assistant

SUGGESTED SCHEDULE FOR PREVENTIVE CHILD HEALTH CARE (*Continued*)

Age	History*	Measure-ments†	Physical examination	Develop-mental landmarks*‡	Discussion and guidance*	Procedures†	Attending
8–9 mo (*Cont.*)	motor de-velopment Behavior			momentarily if held with feet on table Looks after fallen object Transfers block from one hand to the other Feeds self cracker	Accidents Need for affection Normal un-pleasant behavior Discipline		
10 mo (if last exam at 8 mo)	Health Eating Sleeping Elimination Behavior Sensory-motor de-velopment Speech de-velopment Current living situation Parent-child interaction	Height Weight Temperature	Complete or obser-vation¶	Pulls self to standing position Stands hold-ing on to solid object (not human) Pincer grasp: picks up small object using any part of thumb and fingers in opposition Says Da-da or Ma-ma Resists toy being pulled away from him Plays peek-a-boo Makes at-tempt to get toy just out of reach Initial anxiety toward strangers	Toilet training: when to start Normal drop in appetite Independence vs. depen-dency Discipline Instructions for use of syrup of ipecac	Hemoglobin or hematocrit	M.D. and/or assistant
12 mo	As for 10 mo	Height Weight Head cir-cumference Temperature	Complete‖	Cruises: walks around hold-ing on to furniture Stands alone 2–3 sec-onds if outside support is removed Bangs to-gether two blocks held one in each hand Imitates vocal-	Negativism Likelihood of respira-tory infec-tions "Getting into things" Weaning from bottle Proper dose of vitamins Control of drugs and poisons	Tuberculin test (intra-dermal pre-ferred) Measles Rubella and mumps may be given at this or sub-sequent visit Urinalysis	M.D. and assistant

SUGGESTED SCHEDULE FOR PREVENTIVE CHILD HEALTH CARE (*Continued*)

Age	History*	Measure-ments†	Physical examination	Develop-mental landmarks*‡	Discussion and guidance*	Procedures†	Attending
12 mo (*Cont.*)				ization heard within pre-ceding minute Plays pat-a-cake			
15 mo	As for 10 mo	Height Weight Temperature	Complete or obser-vation¶	Walks well Stoops to recover toys on floor Uses Da-da and Ma-ma specifically for correct parent Rolls or tosses ball back to examiner Indicates wants by pulling, pointing, or appropriate verbalization (not crying) Drinks from cup with-out spilling much	Temper tantrums Obedience		M.D. and/or assistant
18 mo	As for 10 mo	Height Weight Temperature	Complete‖	Puts one block on another without its falling off Mimics house-hold chores like dusting or sweeping	Reaction toward and of siblings Toilet train-ing Speech de-velopment	DTP TOPV	M.D. and assistant
21 mo	As for 10 mo Peer reaction	Height Weight Temperature	Complete or obser-vation¶	Walks back-wards and upstairs Feeds self with spoon Removes arti-cle of cloth-ing other than hat Says 3 spe-cific words besides Da-da and Ma-ma	Manners "Poor ap-petite"		M.D. and/or assistant
2 yr	Health Eating Sleeping Elimination	Height Weight Temperature Hearing	Complete‖	Kicks a ball in front of him with foot without sup-	Need for peer companion-ship Immaturity:	Hemoglobin and/or hematocrit Urinalysis	M.D. and assistant

SUGGESTED SCHEDULE FOR PREVENTIVE CHILD HEALTH CARE (*Continued*)

Age	History*	Measure-ments†	Physical examination	Develop-mental landmarks*‡	Discussion and guidance*	Procedures†	Attending
2 yr (*Cont.*)	Toilet training Sensory-motor development Speech Current living situation Peer and social adjustment			port Scribbles spontane-ously—pur-poseful marking of more than one stroke on paper Balances 4 blocks on top of one another Points cor-rectly to one body part Dumps small objects out of bottle after demon-stration Does simple tasks in house	inability to share or take turns Care of teeth From this point on, guidance may be in-cated by the moth-er's an-swers to a question-naire about behavior and emo-tional prob-lems		
2½ yr	As for 2 yr	Height Weight Temperature	Complete‖	Throws over-hand after demon-stration Names cor-rectly one picture in book, e.g., cat or apple Combines 2 words mean-ingfully	Guidance from ques-tionnaire answers Dental referral Perversity and deci-siveness		M.D. and/or assistant
3 yr	As for 2 yr	As for 2 yr Blood pres-sure	Complete‖	Jumps in place Pedals tri-cycle Dumps small article out of bottle without dem-onstration Uses plurals Washes and dries hands	Guidance from ques-tionnaire answers Sex edu-cation Nursery schools: qualifica-tions of a good one Obedience and disci-pline	As for 2 yr	M.D. and assistant
4 yr	As for 2 yr	As for 2 yr Vision ("E" chart) Blood pres-sure	Complete‖ Fundus exami-nation	Builds bridge of 3 blocks after demon-stration Copies circle and cross	Guidance from ques-tionnaire answers Kindergarten Use of	As for 2 yr	M.D. and assistant

SUGGESTED SCHEDULE FOR PREVENTIVE CHILD HEALTH CARE (*Continued*)

Age	History*	Measurements†	Physical examination	Developmental landmarks*‡	Discussion and guidance*	Procedures†	Attending
4 yr (*Cont.*)				<u>Identifies longer of two lines</u> Knows first and last names Understands what to do when "tired" <u>Plays with other children so they interact—tag</u> <u>Dresses with supervision</u>	money Dental care		
5 yr	As for 2 yr (omit toilet training) Kindergarten	As for 2 yr Vision ("E" chart) Color blindness Audiometer Blood pressure	Complete‖	Hops 2 or more times Catches ball thrown 3 ft Dresses without supervision <u>Can tolerate separation from mother for a few minutes without anxiety</u>	Guidance from questionnaire answers Readiness for school Span of attention: how to increase it	As for 2 yr TOPV DTP	M.D. and assistant
6 yr	As for 2 yr Peer and adjustment	As for 5 yr (omit color blindness)	Complete‖	Bicycle riding Copy a square Draw a man with 6 parts Define 6 simple words, e.g., ball, lake, house Name materials of which things are made, e.g., spoon, door	Guidance from questionnaire answers School readiness or performance Allowance	As for 2 yr	M.D. and assistant

From 6 years on, annual examinations follow approximately the same pattern. Developmental landmarks are judged by school performance, assumption of responsibilities, and physical maturation. Guidance is more complicated and is summarized below. Immunization includes maintenance of immunity to diphtheria and tetanus. If community situations preclude examination by a physician yearly, it should be accomplished at least every 2 years.

Items to be considered for guidance and discussion after 6 years are:

Posture and prediction of future height, where of concern.
Safety.
Responsibility for household tasks—giving choice and changing often.
Responsibility for money—how to teach.
Independence versus close supervision in out-of-school activities.
Obedience.
Discipline.

SUGGESTED SCHEDULE FOR PREVENTIVE CHILD HEALTH CARE (*Continued*)

Need for praise.
Summer activities—age for going to camp. Home town programs.
Swimming—learn to do it capably.
Responsibility for homework without prodding.
Responsibility for getting to school on time.
Hours of sleep.
TV versus activities requiring child participation.
Sex education—elementary knowledge. Dating and supervision.
Increasing independence during youth.
Competitive athletics—when? Desirability during youth.
Planning for future careers.

INDEX

COLOR PLATE ILLUSTRATIONS

Schematic diagrams of the primary skin lesions with examples of lesions. [*Source: Figures (A), (C), (E), (G), (I), (K), (M), (O) reproduced with permission from CIBA Pharmaceutical Company, The Basic Skin Lesions. Figures (B), (D), (F), (H), (J), (L), (N), (P), courtesy of Dr. James Herndon, Department of Dermatology, University of Texas Southwestern Medical School at Dallas.*]

(A)   Macule

(B)   Macule, or Mongolian spot

(C)   Papule

(D)   Papule seen in molluscum

(E)   Nodule

(F)   Nodule seen in granuloma annulare

(G)   Tumor

(H)   Tumor seen in insect bite granuloma

(I)   Wheal

(J)   Wheal seen in urticaria pigmentosa

(K)   Vesicle

(L)   Vesicle seen in neonatal herpes simplex

(M)   Bulla

(N)   Bulla seen in creeping eruption

(O)   Pustule

(P)   Pustule seen in bullous impetigo

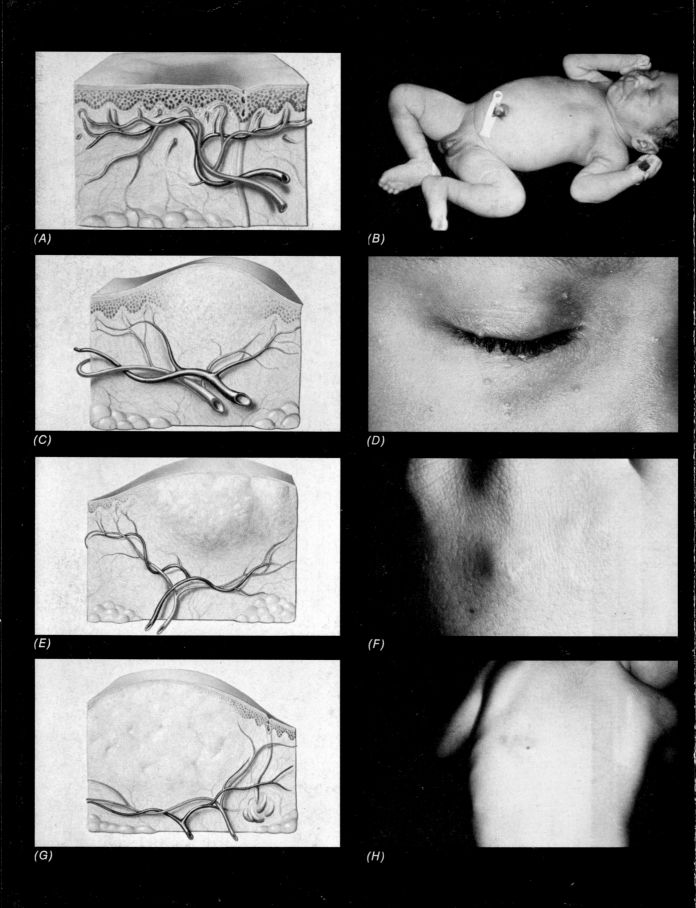

(A)

(B)

(C)

(D)

(E)

(F)

(G)

(H)